T0140575

Lecture Notes in Computer Science 11070

Commenced Publication in 1973
Founding and Former Series Editors:
Gerhard Goos, Juris Hartmanis, and Jan van Leeuwen

Editorial Board

More information about this series at http://www.springer.com/series/7412

Alejandro F. Frangi · Julia A. Schnabel
Christos Davatzikos · Carlos Alberola-López
Gabor Fichtinger (Eds.)

Medical Image Computing and Computer Assisted Intervention – MICCAI 2018

21st International Conference
Granada, Spain, September 16–20, 2018
Proceedings, Part I

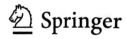 Springer

Editors
Alejandro F. Frangi (iD)
University of Leeds
Leeds
UK

Julia A. Schnabel
King's College London
London
UK

Christos Davatzikos (iD)
University of Pennsylvania
Philadelphia, PA
USA

Carlos Alberola-López (iD)
Universidad de Valladolid
Valladolid
Spain

Gabor Fichtinger
Queen's University
Kingston, ON
Canada

ISSN 0302-9743   ISSN 1611-3349   (electronic)
Lecture Notes in Computer Science
ISBN 978-3-030-00927-4   ISBN 978-3-030-00928-1   (eBook)
https://doi.org/10.1007/978-3-030-00928-1

Library of Congress Control Number: 2018909526

LNCS Sublibrary: SL6 – Image Processing, Computer Vision, Pattern Recognition, and Graphics

This Springer imprint is published by the registered company Springer Nature Switzerland AG
The registered company address is: Gewerbestrasse 11, 6330 Cham, Switzerland

Preface

We are very pleased to present the conference proceedings for the 21st International Conference on Medical Image Computing and Computer Assisted Intervention (MICCAI), which was successfully held at the Granada Conference Center, September 16–20, 2018 in Granada, Spain.

The conference also featured 40 workshops, 14 tutorials, and ten challenges held on September 16 or 20. For the first time, we had events co-located or endorsed by other societies. The two-day Visual Computing in Biology and Medicine (VCBM) Workshop partnered with EUROGRAPHICS[1], the one-day Biomedical Workshop Biomedical Information Processing and Analysis: A Latin American perspective partnered with SIPAIM[2], and the one-day MICCAI Workshop on Computational Diffusion on MRI was endorsed by ISMRM[3]. This year, at the time of writing this preface, the MICCAI 2018 conference had over 1,400 firm registrations for the main conference featuring the most recent work in the fields of:

- Reconstruction and Image Quality
- Machine Learning and Statistical Analysis
- Registration and Image Guidance
- Optical and Histology Applications
- Cardiac, Chest and Abdominal Applications
- fMRI and Diffusion Imaging
- Neuroimaging
- Computer-Assisted Intervention
- Segmentation

This was the largest MICCAI conference to date, with, for the first time, four volumes of *Lecture Notes in Computer Science* (LNCS) proceedings for the main conference, selected after a thorough double-blind peer-review process organized in several phases as further described below. Following the example set by the previous program chairs of MICCAI 2017, we employed the Conference Managing Toolkit (CMT)[4] for paper submissions and double-blind peer-reviews, the Toronto Paper Matching System (TPMS)[5] for automatic paper assignment to area chairs and reviewers, and Researcher.CC[6] to handle conflicts between authors, area chairs, and reviewers.

---

[1] https://www.eg.org.

[2] http://www.sipaim.org/.

[3] https://www.ismrm.org/.

[4] https://cmt.research.microsoft.com.

[5] http://torontopapermatching.org.

[6] http://researcher.cc.

In total, a record 1,068 full submissions (ca. 33% more than the previous year) were received and sent out to peer-review, from 1,335 original intentions to submit. Of those submissions, 80% were considered as pure Medical Image Computing (MIC), 14% as pure Computer-Assisted Intervention (CAI), and 6% as MICCAI papers that fitted into both MIC and CAI areas. The MICCAI 2018 Program Committee (PC) had a total of 58 area chairs, with 45% from Europe, 43% from the Americas, 9% from Australasia, and 3% from the Middle East. We maintained an excellent gender balance with 43% women scientists on the PC.

Using TPMS scoring and CMT, each area chair was assigned between 18 and 20 manuscripts using TPMS, for each of which they suggested 9–15 potential reviewers. Subsequently, 600 invited reviewers were asked to bid for the manuscripts they had been suggested for. Final reviewer allocations via CMT took PC suggestions, reviewer bidding, and TPMS scores into account, allocating 5–6 papers per reviewer. Based on the double-blind reviews, 173 papers (16%) were directly accepted and 314 papers (30%) were directly rejected – these decisions were confirmed by the handling area chair. The remaining 579 papers (54%) were invited for rebuttal. Two further area chairs were added using CMT and TPMS scores to each of these remaining manuscripts, who then independently scored these to accept or reject, based on the reviews, rebuttal, and manuscript, resulting in clear paper decisions using majority voting: 199 further manuscripts were accepted, and 380 rejected.

The overall manuscript acceptance rate was 34.9%. Two PC teleconferences were held on May 14, 2018, in two different time zones to confirm the final results and collect PC feedback on the peer-review process (with over 74% PC attendance rate). For the MICCAI 2018 proceedings, the 372 accepted papers[7] have been organized in four volumes as follows:

– Volume LNCS 11070 includes: Image Quality and Artefacts (15 manuscripts), Image Reconstruction Methods (31), Machine Learning in Medical Imaging (22), Statistical Analysis for Medical Imaging (10), and Image Registration Methods (21)
– Volume LNCS 11071 includes: Optical and Histology Applications (46); and Cardiac, Chest, and Abdominal Applications (59)
– Volume LNCS 11072 includes: fMRI and Diffusion Imaging (45); Neuroimaging and Brain Segmentation (37)
– Volume LNCS 11073 includes: Computer-Assisted Intervention (39) grouped into image-guided interventions and surgery; surgical planning, simulation and work flow analysis; and visualization and augmented reality; and Image Segmentation Methods (47) grouped into general segmentation methods; multi-organ segmentation; abdominal, cardiac, chest, and other segmentation applications.

We would like to thank everyone who contributed greatly to the success of MICCAI 2018 and the quality of its proceedings. These include the MICCAI Society, for support and insightful comments; and our sponsors for financial support and their presence on site. We are especially grateful to all members of the Program Committee for their diligent work in the reviewer assignments and final paper selection, as well as the 600

---

[7] One paper was withdrawn.

reviewers for their support during the entire process. Finally, and most importantly, we thank all authors, co-authors, students, and supervisors, for submitting and presenting their high-quality work which made MICCAI 2018 a greatly enjoyable, informative, and successful event. We are especially indebted to those reviewers and PC members who helped us resolve last-minute missing reviews at a very short notice.

We are looking forward to seeing you in Shenzhen, China, at MICCAI 2019!

August 2018

Julia A. Schnabel
Christos Davatzikos
Gabor Fichtinger
Alejandro F. Frangi
Carlos Alberola-López
Alberto Gomez Herrero
Spyridon Bakas
Antonio R. Porras

Organization

Organizing Committee

General Chair and Program Co-chair

Alejandro F. Frangi — University of Leeds, UK

General Co-chair

Carlos Alberola-López — Universidad de Valladolid, Spain

Associate to General Chairs

Antonio R. Porras — Children's National Medical Center, Washington D.C., USA

Program Chair

Julia A. Schnabel — King's College London, UK

Program Co-chairs

Christos Davatzikos — University of Pennsylvania, USA
Gabor Fichtinger — Queen's University, Canada

Associates to Program Chairs

Spyridon Bakas — University of Pennsylvania, USA
Alberto Gomez Herrero — King's College London, UK

Tutorial and Educational Chair

Anne Martel — University of Toronto, Canada

Tutorial and Educational Co-chairs

Miguel González-Ballester — Universitat Pompeu Fabra, Spain
Marius Linguraru — Children's National Medical Center, Washington D.C., USA
Kensaku Mori — Nagoya University, Japan
Carl-Fredrik Westin — Harvard Medical School, USA

Workshop and Challenge Chair

Danail Stoyanov — University College London, UK

Workshop and Challenge Co-chairs

Hervé Delingette   Inria, France
Lena Maier-Hein   German Cancer Research Center, Germany
Zeike A. Taylor   University of Leeds, UK

Keynote Lecture Chair

Josien Pluim   TU Eindhoven, The Netherlands

Keynote Lecture Co-chairs

Matthias Harders   ETH Zurich, Switzerland
Septimiu Salcudean   The University of British Columbia, Canada

Corporate Affairs Chair

Terry Peters   Western University, Canada

Corporate Affairs Co-chairs

Hayit Greenspan   Tel Aviv University, Israel
Despina Kontos   University of Pennsylvania, USA
Guy Shechter   Philips, USA

Student Activities Facilitator

Demian Wasserman   Inria, France

Student Activities Co-facilitator

Karim Lekadir   Universitat Pompeu-Fabra, Spain

Communications Officer

Pedro Lopes   University of Leeds, UK

Conference Management

DEKON Group

Program Committee

Ali Gooya   University of Sheffield, UK
Amber Simpson   Memorial Sloan Kettering Cancer Center, USA
Andrew King   King's College London, UK
Bennett Landman   Vanderbilt University, USA
Bernhard Kainz   Imperial College London, UK
Burak Acar   Bogazici University, Turkey

Carola Schoenlieb	Cambridge University, UK
Caroline Essert	University of Strasbourg/ICUBE, France
Christian Wachinger	Ludwig Maximilian University of Munich, Germany
Christos Bergeles	King's College London, UK
Daphne Yu	Siemens Healthineers, USA
Duygu Tosun	University of California at San Francisco, USA
Emanuele Trucco	University of Dundee, UK
Ender Konukoglu	ETH Zurich, Switzerland
Enzo Ferrante	CONICET/Universidad Nacional del Litoral, Argentina
Erik Meijering	Erasmus University Medical Center, The Netherlands
Gozde Unal	Istanbul Technical University, Turkey
Guido Gerig	New York University, USA
Gustavo Carneiro	University of Adelaide, Australia
Hassan Rivaz	Concordia University, Canada
Herve Lombaert	ETS Montreal, Canada
Hongliang Ren	National University of Singapore, Singapore
Ingerid Reinertsen	SINTEF, Norway
Ipek Oguz	University of Pennsylvania/Vanderbilt University, USA
Ivana Isgum	University Medical Center Utrecht, The Netherlands
Juan Eugenio Iglesias	University College London, UK
Kayhan Batmanghelich	University of Pittsburgh/Carnegie Mellon University, USA
Laura Igual	Universitat de Barcelona, Spain
Lauren O'Donnell	Harvard University, USA
Le Lu	Ping An Technology US Research Labs, USA
Li Cheng	A*STAR Singapore, Singapore
Lilla Zöllei	Massachusetts General Hospital, USA
Linwei Wang	Rochester Institute of Technology, USA
Marc Niethammer	University of North Carolina at Chapel Hill, USA
Marius Staring	Leiden University Medical Center, The Netherlands
Marleen de Bruijne	Erasmus MC Rotterdam/University of Copenhagen, The Netherlands/Denmark
Marta Kersten	Concordia University, Canada
Mattias Heinrich	University of Luebeck, Germany
Meritxell Bach Cuadra	University of Lausanne, Switzerland
Miaomiao Zhang	Washington University in St. Louis, USA
Moti Freiman	Philips Healthcare, Israel
Nasir Rajpoot	University of Warwick, UK
Nassir Navab	Technical University of Munich, Germany
Pallavi Tiwari	Case Western Reserve University, USA
Pingkun Yan	Rensselaer Polytechnic Institute, USA
Purang Abolmaesumi	University of British Columbia, Canada
Ragini Verma	University of Pennsylvania, USA
Raphael Sznitman	University of Bern, Switzerland
Sandrine Voros	University of Grenoble, France

Sotirios Tsaftaris	University of Edinburgh, UK
Stamatia Giannarou	Imperial College London, UK
Stefanie Speidel	National Center for Tumor Diseases (NCT) Dresden, Germany
Stefanie Demirci	Technical University of Munich, Germany
Tammy Riklin Raviv	Ben-Gurion University, Israel
Tanveer Syeda-Mahmood	IBM Research, USA
Ulas Bagci	University of Central Florida, USA
Vamsi Ithapu	University of Wisconsin-Madison, USA
Yanwu Xu	Baidu Inc., China

Scientific Review Committee

Amir Abdi
Ehsan Adeli
Iman Aganj
Ola Ahmad
Amr Ahmed
Shazia Akbar
Alireza Akhondi-asl
Saad Ullah Akram
Amir Alansary
Shadi Albarqouni
Luis Alvarez
Deepak Anand
Elsa Angelini
Rahman Attar
Chloé Audigier
Angelica Aviles-Rivero
Ruqayya Awan
Suyash Awate
Dogu Baran Aydogan
Shekoofeh Azizi
Katja Bühler
Junjie Bai
Wenjia Bai
Daniel Balfour
Walid Barhoumi
Sarah Barman
Michael Barrow
Deepti Bathula
Christian F. Baumgartner
Pierre-Louis Bazin
Delaram Behnami
Erik Bekkers
Rami Ben-Ari

Martin Benning
Aïcha BenTaieb
Ruth Bergman
Alessandro Bevilacqua
Ryoma Bise
Isabelle Bloch
Sebastian Bodenstedt
Hrvoje Bogunovic
Gerda Bortsova
Sylvain Bouix
Felix Bragman
Christopher Bridge
Tom Brosch
Aurelien Bustin
Irène Buvat
Cesar Caballero-Gaudes
Ryan Cabeen
Nathan Cahill
Jinzheng Cai
Weidong Cai
Tian Cao
Valentina Carapella
M. Jorge Cardoso
Daniel Castro
Daniel Coelho de Castro
Philippe C. Cattin
Juan Cerrolaza
Suheyla Cetin Karayumak
Matthieu Chabanas
Jayasree Chakraborty
Rudrasis Chakraborty
Rajib Chakravorty
Vimal Chandran

Catie Chang
Pierre Chatelain
Akshay Chaudhari
Antong Chen
Chao Chen
Geng Chen
Hao Chen
Jianxu Chen
Jingyun Chen
Min Chen
Xin Chen
Yang Chen
Yuncong Chen
Jiezhi Cheng
Jun Cheng
Veronika Cheplygina
Farida Cheriet
Minqi Chong
Daan Christiaens
Serkan Cimen
Francesco Ciompi
Cedric Clouchoux
James Clough
Dana Cobzas
Noel Codella
Toby Collins
Olivier Commowick
Sailesh Conjeti
Pierre-Henri Conze
Tessa Cook
Timothy Cootes
Pierrick Coupé
Alessandro Crimi
Adrian Dalca
Sune Darkner
Dhritiman Das
Johan Debayle
Farah Deeba
Silvana Dellepiane
Adrien Depeursinge
Maria Deprez
Christian Desrosiers
Blake Dewey
Jwala Dhamala
Qi Dou
Karen Drukker

Lei Du
Lixin Duan
Florian Dubost
Nicolas Duchateau
James Duncan
Luc Duong
Nicha Dvornek
Oleh Dzyubachyk
Zach Eaton-Rosen
Mehran Ebrahimi
Matthias J. Ehrhardt
Ahmet Ekin
Ayman El-Baz
Randy Ellis
Mohammed Elmogy
Marius Erdt
Guray Erus
Marco Esposito
Joset Etzel
Jingfan Fan
Yong Fan
Aly Farag
Mohsen Farzi
Anahita Fathi Kazerooni
Hamid Fehri
Xinyang Feng
Olena Filatova
James Fishbaugh
Tom Fletcher
Germain Forestier
Denis Fortun
Alfred Franz
Muhammad Moazam Fraz
Wolfgang Freysinger
Jurgen Fripp
Huazhu Fu
Yang Fu
Bernhard Fuerst
Gareth Funka-Lea
Isabel Funke
Jan Funke
Francesca Galassi
Linlin Gao
Mingchen Gao
Yue Gao
Zhifan Gao

Utpal Garain
Mona Garvin
Aimilia Gastounioti
Romane Gauriau
Bao Ge
Sandesh Ghimire
Ali Gholipour
Rémi Giraud
Ben Glocker
Ehsan Golkar
Polina Golland
Yuanhao Gong
German Gonzalez
Pietro Gori
Alejandro Granados
Sasa Grbic
Enrico Grisan
Andrey Gritsenko
Abhijit Guha Roy
Yanrong Guo
Yong Guo
Vikash Gupta
Benjamin Gutierrez Becker
Séverine Habert
Ilker Hacihaliloglu
Stathis Hadjidemetriou
Ghassan Hamarneh
Adam Harrison
Grant Haskins
Charles Hatt
Tiancheng He
Mehdi Hedjazi Moghari
Tobias Heimann
Christoph Hennersperger
Alfredo Hernandez
Monica Hernandez
Moises Hernandez Fernandez
Carlos Hernandez-Matas
Matthew Holden
Yi Hong
Nicolas Honnorat
Benjamin Hou
Yipeng Hu
Heng Huang
Junzhou Huang
Weilin Huang

Xiaolei Huang
Yawen Huang
Henkjan Huisman
Yuankai Huo
Sarfaraz Hussein
Jana Hutter
Seong Jae Hwang
Atsushi Imiya
Amir Jamaludin
Faraz Janan
Uditha Jarayathne
Xi Jiang
Jieqing Jiao
Dakai Jin
Yueming Jin
Bano Jordan
Anand Joshi
Shantanu Joshi
Leo Joskowicz
Christoph Jud
Siva Teja Kakileti
Jayashree Kalpathy-Cramer
Ali Kamen
Neerav Karani
Anees Kazi
Eric Kerfoot
Erwan Kerrien
Farzad Khalvati
Hassan Khan
Bishesh Khanal
Ron Kikinis
Hyo-Eun Kim
Hyunwoo Kim
Jinman Kim
Minjeong Kim
Benjamin Kimia
Kivanc Kose
Julia Krüger
Pavitra Krishnaswamy
Frithjof Kruggel
Elizabeth Krupinski
Sofia Ira Ktena
Arjan Kuijper
Ashnil Kumar
Neeraj Kumar
Punithakumar Kumaradevan

Manuela Kunz
Jin Tae Kwak
Alexander Ladikos
Rodney Lalonde
Pablo Lamata
Catherine Laporte
Carole Lartizien
Toni Lassila
Andras Lasso
Matthieu Le
Maria J. Ledesma-Carbayo
Hansang Lee
Jong-Hwan Lee
Soochahn Lee
Etienne Léger
Beatrice Lentes
Wee Kheng Leow
Nikolas Lessmann
Annan Li
Gang Li
Ruoyu Li
Wenqi Li
Xiang Li
Yuanwei Li
Chunfeng Lian
Jianming Liang
Hongen Liao
Ruizhi Liao
Roxane Licandro
Lanfen Lin
Claudia Lindner
Cristian Linte
Feng Liu
Hui Liu
Jianfei Liu
Jundong Liu
Kefei Liu
Mingxia Liu
Sidong Liu
Marco Lorenzi
Xiongbiao Luo
Jinglei Lv
Ilwoo Lyu
Omar M. Rijal
Pablo Márquez Neila
Henning Müller

Kai Ma
Khushhall Chandra Mahajan
Dwarikanath Mahapatra
Andreas Maier
Klaus H. Maier-Hein
Sokratis Makrogiannis
Grégoire Malandain
Anand Malpani
Jose Manjon
Tommaso Mansi
Awais Mansoor
Anne Martel
Diana Mateus
Arnaldo Mayer
Jamie McClelland
Stephen McKenna
Ronak Mehta
Raphael Meier
Qier Meng
Yu Meng
Bjoern Menze
Liang Mi
Shun Miao
Abhishek Midya
Zhe Min
Rashika Mishra
Marc Modat
Norliza Mohd Noor
Mehdi Moradi
Rodrigo Moreno
Kensaku Mori
Aliasghar Mortazi
Peter Mountney
Arrate Muñoz-Barrutia
Anirban Mukhopadhyay
Arya Nabavi
Layan Nahlawi
Ana Ineyda Namburete
Valery Naranjo
Peter Neher
Hannes Nickisch
Dong Nie
Lipeng Ning
Jack Noble
Vincent Noblet
Alexey Novikov

Ilkay Oksuz
Ozan Oktay
John Onofrey
Eliza Orasanu
Felipe Orihuela-Espina
Jose Orlando
Yusuf Osmanlioglu
David Owen
Cristina Oyarzun Laura
Jose-Antonio Pérez-Carrasco
Danielle Pace
J. Blas Pagador
Akshay Pai
Xenophon Papademetris
Bartlomiej Papiez
Toufiq Parag
Magdalini Paschali
Angshuman Paul
Christian Payer
Jialin Peng
Tingying Peng
Xavier Pennec
Sérgio Pereira
Mehran Pesteie
Loic Peter
Igor Peterlik
Simon Pezold
Micha Pfeifer
Dzung Pham
Renzo Phellan
Pramod Pisharady
Josien Pluim
Kilian Pohl
Jean-Baptiste Poline
Alison Pouch
Prateek Prasanna
Philip Pratt
Raphael Prevost
Esther Puyol Anton
Yuchuan Qiao
Gwénolé Quellec
Pradeep Reddy Raamana
Julia Rackerseder
Hedyeh Rafii-Tari
Mehdi Rahim
Kashif Rajpoot

Parnesh Raniga
Yogesh Rathi
Saima Rathore
Nishant Ravikumar
Shan E. Ahmed Raza
Islem Rekik
Beatriz Remeseiro
Markus Rempfler
Mauricio Reyes
Constantino Reyes-Aldasoro
Nicola Rieke
Laurent Risser
Leticia Rittner
Yong Man Ro
Emma Robinson
Rafael Rodrigues
Marc-Michel Rohé
Robert Rohling
Karl Rohr
Plantefeve Rosalie
Holger Roth
Su Ruan
Danny Ruijters
Juan Ruiz-Alzola
Mert Sabuncu
Frank Sachse
Farhang Sahba
Septimiu Salcudean
Gerard Sanroma
Emine Saritas
Imari Sato
Alexander Schlaefer
Jerome Schmid
Caitlin Schneider
Jessica Schrouff
Thomas Schultz
Suman Sedai
Biswa Sengupta
Ortal Senouf
Maxime Sermesant
Carmen Serrano
Amit Sethi
Muhammad Shaban
Reuben Shamir
Yeqin Shao
Li Shen

Bibo Shi
Kuangyu Shi
Hoo-Chang Shin
Russell Shinohara
Viviana Siless
Carlos A. Silva
Matthew Sinclair
Vivek Singh
Korsuk Sirinukunwattana
Ihor Smal
Michal Sofka
Jure Sokolic
Hessam Sokooti
Ahmed Soliman
Stefan Sommer
Diego Sona
Yang Song
Aristeidis Sotiras
Jamshid Sourati
Rachel Sparks
Ziga Spiclin
Lawrence Staib
Ralf Stauder
Darko Stern
Colin Studholme
Martin Styner
Heung-Il Suk
Jian Sun
Xu Sun
Kyunghyun Sung
Nima Tajbakhsh
Sylvain Takerkart
Chaowei Tan
Jeremy Tan
Mingkui Tan
Hui Tang
Min Tang
Youbao Tang
Yuxing Tang
Christine Tanner
Qian Tao
Giacomo Tarroni
Zeike Taylor
Kim Han Thung
Yanmei Tie
Daniel Toth

Nicolas Toussaint
Jocelyne Troccaz
Tomasz Trzcinski
Ahmet Tuysuzoglu
Andru Twinanda
Carole Twining
Eranga Ukwatta
Mathias Unberath
Tamas Ungi
Martin Urschler
Maria Vakalopoulou
Vanya Valindria
Koen Van Leemput
Hien Van Nguyen
Gijs van Tulder
S. Swaroop Vedula
Harini Veeraraghavan
Miguel Vega
Anant Vemuri
Gopalkrishna Veni
Archana Venkataraman
François-Xavier Vialard
Pierre-Frederic Villard
Satish Viswanath
Wolf-Dieter Vogl
Ingmar Voigt
Tomaz Vrtovec
Bo Wang
Guotai Wang
Jiazhuo Wang
Liansheng Wang
Manning Wang
Sheng Wang
Yalin Wang
Zhe Wang
Simon Warfield
Chong-Yaw Wee
Juergen Weese
Benzheng Wei
Wolfgang Wein
William Wells
Rene Werner
Daniel Wesierski
Matthias Wilms
Adam Wittek
Jelmer Wolterink

Ken C. L. Wong
Jonghye Woo
Pengxiang Wu
Tobias Wuerfl
Yong Xia
Yiming Xiao
Weidi Xie
Yuanpu Xie
Fangxu Xing
Fuyong Xing
Tao Xiong
Daguang Xu
Yan Xu
Zheng Xu
Zhoubing Xu
Ziyue Xu
Wufeng Xue
Jingwen Yan
Ke Yan
Yuguang Yan
Zhennan Yan
Dong Yang
Guang Yang
Xiao Yang
Xin Yang
Jianhua Yao
Jiawen Yao
Xiaohui Yao
Chuyang Ye
Menglong Ye
Jingru Yi
Jinhua Yu
Lequan Yu
Weimin Yu
Yixuan Yuan
Evangelia Zacharaki
Ernesto Zacur

Guillaume Zahnd
Marco Zenati
Ke Zeng
Oliver Zettinig
Daoqiang Zhang
Fan Zhang
Han Zhang
Heye Zhang
Jiong Zhang
Jun Zhang
Lichi Zhang
Lin Zhang
Ling Zhang
Mingli Zhang
Pin Zhang
Shu Zhang
Tong Zhang
Yong Zhang
Yunyan Zhang
Zizhao Zhang
Qingyu Zhao
Shijie Zhao
Yitian Zhao
Guoyan Zheng
Yalin Zheng
Yinqiang Zheng
Zichun Zhong
Luping Zhou
Zhiguo Zhou
Dajiang Zhu
Wentao Zhu
Xiaofeng Zhu
Xiahai Zhuang
Aneeq Zia
Veronika Zimmer
Majd Zreik
Reyer Zwiggelaar

Mentorship Program (Mentors)

Stephen Aylward   Kitware Inc., USA
Christian Barillot   IRISA/CNRS/University of Rennes, France
Kayhan Batmanghelich   University of Pittsburgh/Carnegie Mellon University,
                         USA
Christos Bergeles   King's College London, UK

Sponsors and Funders

Platinum Sponsors

- NVIDIA Inc.
- Siemens Healthineers GmbH

Gold Sponsors

- Guangzhou Shiyuan Electronics Co. Ltd.
- Subtle Medical Inc.

Silver Sponsors

- Arterys Inc.
- Claron Technology Inc.
- ImSight Inc.
- ImFusion GmbH
- Medtronic Plc

Bronze Sponsors

- Depwise Inc.
- Carl Zeiss AG

Travel Bursary Support

- MICCAI Society
- National Institutes of Health, USA
- EPSRC-NIHR Medical Image Analysis Network (EP/N026993/1), UK

Contents – Part I

Image Quality and Artefacts

Conditional Generative Adversarial Networks for Metal Artifact Reduction
in CT Images of the Ear 3
   Jianing Wang, Yiyuan Zhao, Jack H. Noble, and Benoit M. Dawant

Neural Network Evolution Using Expedited Genetic Algorithm for Medical
Image Denoising. 12
   Peng Liu, Yangjunyi Li, Mohammad D. El Basha, and Ruogu Fang

Deep Convolutional Filtering for Spatio-Temporal Denoising and Artifact
Removal in Arterial Spin Labelling MRI 21
   David Owen, Andrew Melbourne, Zach Eaton-Rosen, David L. Thomas,
   Neil Marlow, Jonathan Rohrer, and Sébastien Ourselin

DeepASL: Kinetic Model Incorporated Loss for Denoising Arterial Spin
Labeled MRI via Deep Residual Learning 30
   Cagdas Ulas, Giles Tetteh, Stephan Kaczmarz, Christine Preibisch,
   and Bjoern H. Menze

Direct Estimation of Pharmacokinetic Parameters from DCE-MRI Using
Deep CNN with Forward Physical Model Loss. 39
   Cagdas Ulas, Giles Tetteh, Michael J. Thrippleton, Paul A. Armitage,
   Stephen D. Makin, Joanna M. Wardlaw, Mike E. Davies,
   and Bjoern H. Menze

Short Acquisition Time PET/MR Pharmacokinetic Modelling
Using CNNs. 48
   Catherine J. Scott, Jieqing Jiao, M. Jorge Cardoso, Kerstin Kläser,
   Andrew Melbourne, Pawel J. Markiewicz, Jonathan M. Schott,
   Brian F. Hutton, and Sébastien Ourselin

Can Deep Learning Relax Endomicroscopy Hardware Miniaturization
Requirements? 57
   Saeed Izadi, Kathleen P. Moriarty, and Ghassan Hamarneh

A Framework to Objectively Identify Reference Regions for Normalizing
Quantitative Imaging 65
   Amir Fazlollahi, Scott Ayton, Pierrick Bourgeat, Ibrahima Diouf,
   Parnesh Raniga, Jurgen Fripp, James Doecke, David Ames,
   Colin L. Masters, Christopher C. Rowe, Victor L. Villemagne,
   Ashley I. Bush, and Olivier Salvado

Evaluation of Adjoint Methods in Photoacoustic Tomography
with Under-Sampled Sensors   73
  Hongxiang Lin, Takashi Azuma, Mehmet Burcin Unlu, and Shu Takagi

A No-Reference Quality Metric for Retinal Vessel Tree Segmentation   82
  *Adrian Galdran, Pedro Costa, Alessandro Bria, Teresa Araújo,
  Ana Maria Mendonça, and Aurélio Campilho*

Efficient and Accurate MRI Super-Resolution Using a Generative
Adversarial Network and 3D Multi-level Densely Connected Network   91
  *Yuhua Chen, Feng Shi, Anthony G. Christodoulou, Yibin Xie,
  Zhengwei Zhou, and Debiao Li*

A Deep Learning Based Anti-aliasing Self Super-Resolution Algorithm
for MRI.   100
  *Can Zhao, Aaron Carass, Blake E. Dewey, Jonghye Woo, Jiwon Oh,
  Peter A. Calabresi, Daniel S. Reich, Pascal Sati, Dzung L. Pham,
  and Jerry L. Prince*

Gradient Profile Based Super Resolution of MR Images
with Induced Sparsity   109
  Prabhjot Kaur and Anil Kumar Sao

Deeper Image Quality Transfer: Training Low-Memory Neural Networks
for 3D Images   118
  *Stefano B. Blumberg, Ryutaro Tanno, Iasonas Kokkinos,
  and Daniel C. Alexander*

High Frame-Rate Cardiac Ultrasound Imaging with Deep Learning   126
  *Ortal Senouf, Sanketh Vedula, Grigoriy Zurakhov, Alex Bronstein,
  Michael Zibulevsky, Oleg Michailovich, Dan Adam,
  and David Blondheim*

Image Reconstruction Methods

Phase-Sensitive Region-of-Interest Computed Tomography.   137
  *Lina Felsner, Martin Berger, Sebastian Kaeppler, Johannes Bopp,
  Veronika Ludwig, Thomas Weber, Georg Pelzer, Thilo Michel,
  Andreas Maier, Gisela Anton, and Christian Riess*

Some Investigations on Robustness of Deep Learning in Limited
Angle Tomography   145
  *Yixing Huang, Tobias Würfl, Katharina Breininger, Ling Liu,
  Günter Lauritsch, and Andreas Maier*

Adversarial Sparse-View CBCT Artifact Reduction 154
Haofu Liao, Zhimin Huo, William J. Sehnert, Shaohua Kevin Zhou,
and Jiebo Luo

Nasal Mesh Unfolding – An Approach to Obtaining 2-D Skin Templates
from 3-D Nose Models 163
Hongying Li, Marc Robini, Zhongwei Zhou, Wei Tang, and Yuemin Zhu

Towards Generating Personalized Volumetric Phantom from Patient's
Surface Geometry 171
Yifan Wu, Vivek Singh, Brian Teixeira, Kai Ma, Birgi Tamersoy,
Andreas Krauss, and Terrence Chen

Multi-channel Generative Adversarial Network for Parallel Magnetic
Resonance Image Reconstruction in K-space 180
Pengyue Zhang, Fusheng Wang, Wei Xu, and Yu Li

A Learning-Based Metal Artifacts Correction Method for MRI Using
Dual-Polarity Readout Gradients and Simulated Data. 189
Kinam Kwon, Dongchan Kim, and HyunWook Park

Motion Aware MR Imaging via Spatial Core Correspondence 198
Christoph Jud, Damien Nguyen, Robin Sandkühler, Alina Giger,
Oliver Bieri, and Philippe C. Cattin

Nonparametric Density Flows for MRI Intensity Normalisation. 206
Daniel C. Castro and Ben Glocker

Ultra-Fast T2-Weighted MR Reconstruction Using Complementary
T1-Weighted Information. 215
Lei Xiang, Yong Chen, Weitang Chang, Yiqiang Zhan, Weili Lin,
Qian Wang, and Dinggang Shen

Image Reconstruction by Splitting Deep Learning Regularization
from Iterative Inversion 224
Jiulong Liu, Tao Kuang, and Xiaoqun Zhang

Adversarial and Perceptual Refinement for Compressed Sensing
MRI Reconstruction 232
Maximilian Seitzer, Guang Yang, Jo Schlemper, Ozan Oktay,
Tobias Würfl, Vincent Christlein, Tom Wong, Raad Mohiaddin,
David Firmin, Jennifer Keegan, Daniel Rueckert, and Andreas Maier

Translation of 1D Inverse Fourier Transform of K-space to an Image Based
on Deep Learning for Accelerating Magnetic Resonance Imaging 241
Taejoon Eo, Hyungseob Shin, Taeseong Kim, Yohan Jun,
and Dosik Hwang

Deep Learning Using K-Space Based Data Augmentation for Automated
Cardiac MR Motion Artefact Detection   250
  Ilkay Oksuz, Bram Ruijsink, Esther Puyol-Antón, Aurelien Bustin,
  Gastao Cruz, Claudia Prieto, Daniel Rueckert, Julia A. Schnabel,
  and Andrew P. King

Cardiac MR Segmentation from Undersampled k-space Using Deep
Latent Representation Learning.   259
  Jo Schlemper, Ozan Oktay, Wenjia Bai, Daniel C. Castro,
  Jinming Duan, Chen Qin, Jo V. Hajnal, and Daniel Rueckert

A Comprehensive Approach for Learning-Based Fully-Automated
Inter-slice Motion Correction for Short-Axis Cine Cardiac MR
Image Stacks   268
  Giacomo Tarroni, Ozan Oktay, Matthew Sinclair, Wenjia Bai,
  Andreas Schuh, Hideaki Suzuki, Antonio de Marvao, Declan O'Regan,
  Stuart Cook, and Daniel Rueckert

Automatic View Planning with Multi-scale Deep Reinforcement
Learning Agents   277
  Amir Alansary, Loic Le Folgoc, Ghislain Vaillant, Ozan Oktay,
  Yuanwei Li, Wenjia Bai, Jonathan Passerat-Palmbach,
  Ricardo Guerrero, Konstantinos Kamnitsas, Benjamin Hou,
  Steven McDonagh, Ben Glocker, Bernhard Kainz, and Daniel Rueckert

Towards MR-Only Radiotherapy Treatment Planning: Synthetic CT
Generation Using Multi-view Deep Convolutional Neural Networks   286
  Yu Zhao, Shu Liao, Yimo Guo, Liang Zhao, Zhennan Yan,
  Sungmin Hong, Gerardo Hermosillo, Tianming Liu, Xiang Sean Zhou,
  and Yiqiang Zhan

Stochastic Deep Compressive Sensing for the Reconstruction of Diffusion
Tensor Cardiac MRI   295
  Jo Schlemper, Guang Yang, Pedro Ferreira, Andrew Scott,
  Laura-Ann McGill, Zohya Khalique, Margarita Gorodezky,
  Malte Roehl, Jennifer Keegan, Dudley Pennell, David Firmin,
  and Daniel Rueckert

Automatic, Fast and Robust Characterization of Noise Distributions
for Diffusion MRI.   304
  Samuel St-Jean, Alberto De Luca, Max A. Viergever,
  and Alexander Leemans

An Automated Localization, Segmentation and Reconstruction Framework
for Fetal Brain MRI   313
    Michael Ebner, Guotai Wang, Wenqi Li, Michael Aertsen,
    Premal A. Patel, Rosalind Aughwane, Andrew Melbourne, Tom Doel,
    Anna L. David, Jan Deprest, Sébastien Ourselin, and Tom Vercauteren

Retinal Image Understanding Emerges from Self-Supervised
Multimodal Reconstruction.   321
    Álvaro S. Hervella, José Rouco, Jorge Novo, and Marcos Ortega

Locality Adaptive Multi-modality GANs for High-Quality PET
Image Synthesis   329
    Yan Wang, Luping Zhou, Lei Wang, Biting Yu, Chen Zu,
    David S. Lalush, Weili Lin, Xi Wu, Jiliu Zhou, and Dinggang Shen

Joint PET+MRI Patch-Based Dictionary for Bayesian Random Field
PET Reconstruction.   338
    Viswanath P. Sudarshan, Zhaolin Chen, and Suyash P. Awate

Analysis of 3D Facial Dysmorphology in Genetic Syndromes
from Unconstrained 2D Photographs   347
    Liyun Tu, Antonio R. Porras, Alec Boyle, and Marius George Linguraru

Double Your Views – Exploiting Symmetry in Transmission Imaging   356
    Alexander Preuhs, Andreas Maier, Michael Manhart, Javad Fotouhi,
    Nassir Navab, and Mathias Unberath

Real Time RNN Based 3D Ultrasound Scan Adequacy for Developmental
Dysplasia of the Hip   365
    Olivia Paserin, Kishore Mulpuri, Anthony Cooper, Antony J. Hodgson,
    and Rafeef Garbi

Direct Reconstruction of Ultrasound Elastography Using an End-to-End
Deep Neural Network   374
    Sitong Wu, Zhifan Gao, Zhi Liu, Jianwen Luo, Heye Zhang, and Shuo Li

3D Fetal Skull Reconstruction from 2DUS via Deep Conditional
Generative Networks   383
    Juan J. Cerrolaza, Yuanwei Li, Carlo Biffi, Alberto Gomez,
    Matthew Sinclair, Jacqueline Matthew, Caronline Knight,
    Bernhard Kainz, and Daniel Rueckert

Standard Plane Detection in 3D Fetal Ultrasound Using an Iterative
Transformation Network   392
    Yuanwei Li, Bishesh Khanal, Benjamin Hou, Amir Alansary,
    Juan J. Cerrolaza, Matthew Sinclair, Jacqueline Matthew,
    Chandni Gupta, Caroline Knight, Bernhard Kainz, and Daniel Rueckert

Towards Radiotherapy Enhancement and Real Time Tumor Radiation
Dosimetry Through 3D Imaging of Gold Nanoparticles Using XFCT   401
*Caroline Vienne, Adrien Stolidi, Hermine Lemaire, Daniel Maier,
Diana Renaud, Romain Grall, Sylvie Chevillard, Emilie Brun,
Cécile Sicard, and Olivier Limousin*

Dual-Domain Cascaded Regression for Synthesizing 7T from 3T MRI   410
*Yongqin Zhang, Jie-Zhi Cheng, Lei Xiang, Pew-Thian Yap,
and Dinggang Shen*

Machine Learning in Medical Imaging

Concurrent Spatial and Channel 'Squeeze & Excitation' in Fully
Convolutional Networks.   421
Abhijit Guha Roy, Nassir Navab, and Christian Wachinger

SPNet: Shape Prediction Using a Fully Convolutional Neural Network   430
S. M. Masudur Rahman Al Arif, Karen Knapp, and Greg Slabaugh

Roto-Translation Covariant Convolutional Networks for Medical
Image Analysis.   440
*Erik J. Bekkers, Maxime W. Lafarge, Mitko Veta, Koen A. J. Eppenhof,
Josien P. W. Pluim, and Remco Duits*

Bimodal Network Architectures for Automatic Generation of Image
Annotation from Text   449
*Mehdi Moradi, Ali Madani, Yaniv Gur, Yufan Guo,
and Tanveer Syeda-Mahmood*

Multimodal Recurrent Model with Attention for Automated Radiology
Report Generation.   457
*Yuan Xue, Tao Xu, L. Rodney Long, Zhiyun Xue, Sameer Antani,
George R. Thoma, and Xiaolei Huang*

Magnetic Resonance Spectroscopy Quantification Using Deep Learning.   467
Nima Hatami, Michaël Sdika, and Hélène Ratiney

A Lifelong Learning Approach to Brain MR Segmentation Across Scanners
and Protocols   476
*Neerav Karani, Krishna Chaitanya, Christian Baumgartner,
and Ender Konukoglu*

Respond-CAM: Analyzing Deep Models for 3D Imaging Data
by Visualizations.   485
Guannan Zhao, Bo Zhou, Kaiwen Wang, Rui Jiang, and Min Xu

Generalizability *vs.* Robustness: Investigating Medical Imaging Networks
Using Adversarial Examples.   493
   Magdalini Paschali, Sailesh Conjeti, Fernando Navarro,
   and Nassir Navab

Subject2Vec: Generative-Discriminative Approach from a Set of Image
Patches to a Vector.   502
   Sumedha Singla, Mingming Gong, Siamak Ravanbakhsh, Frank Sciurba,
   Barnabas Poczos, and Kayhan N. Batmanghelich

3D Context Enhanced Region-Based Convolutional Neural Network
for End-to-End Lesion Detection.   511
   Ke Yan, Mohammadhadi Bagheri, and Ronald M. Summers

Keep and Learn: Continual Learning by Constraining the Latent Space
for Knowledge Preservation in Neural Networks.   520
   Hyo-Eun Kim, Seungwook Kim, and Jaehwan Lee

Distribution Matching Losses Can Hallucinate Features in Medical
Image Translation   529
   Joseph Paul Cohen, Margaux Luck, and Sina Honari

Generative Invertible Networks (GIN): Pathophysiology-Interpretable
Feature Mapping and Virtual Patient Generation   537
   Jialei Chen, Yujia Xie, Kan Wang, Zih Huei Wang, Geet Lahoti,
   Chuck Zhang, Mani A. Vannan, Ben Wang, and Zhen Qian

Training Medical Image Analysis Systems like Radiologists.   546
   Gabriel Maicas, Andrew P. Bradley, Jacinto C. Nascimento, Ian Reid,
   and Gustavo Carneiro

Joint High-Order Multi-Task Feature Learning to Predict the Progression
of Alzheimer's Disease   555
   Lodewijk Brand, Hua Wang, Heng Huang, Shannon Risacher,
   Andrew Saykin, and Li Shen for the ADNI

Fast Multiple Landmark Localisation Using a Patch-Based
Iterative Network   563
   Yuanwei Li, Amir Alansary, Juan J. Cerrolaza, Bishesh Khanal,
   Matthew Sinclair, Jacqueline Matthew, Chandni Gupta,
   Caroline Knight, Bernhard Kainz, and Daniel Rueckert

Omni-Supervised Learning: Scaling Up to Large Unlabelled
Medical Datasets.   572
   Ruobing Huang, J. Alison Noble, and Ana I. L. Namburete

Recurrent Neural Networks for Classifying Human Embryonic Stem
Cell-Derived Cardiomyocytes   581
  Carolina Pacheco and René Vidal

Group-Driven Reinforcement Learning for Personalized
mHealth Intervention   590
  *Feiyun Zhu, Jun Guo, Zheng Xu, Peng Liao, Liu Yang,
  and Junzhou Huang*

Joint Correlational and Discriminative Ensemble Classifier Learning
for Dementia Stratification Using Shallow Brain Multiplexes   599
  *Rory Raeper and Anna Lisowska, Islem Rekik, and The Alzheimer's
  Disease Neuroimaging Initiative*

Statistical Analysis for Medical Imaging

FDR-HS: An Empirical Bayesian Identification of Heterogenous Features
in Neuroimage Analysis.   611
  Xinwei Sun, Lingjing Hu, Fandong Zhang, Yuan Yao, and Yizhou Wang

Order-Sensitive Deep Hashing for Multimorbidity Medical
Image Retrieval   620
  Zhixiang Chen, Ruojin Cai, Jiwen Lu, Jianjiang Feng, and Jie Zhou

Exact Combinatorial Inference for Brain Images   629
  *Moo K. Chung, Zhan Luo, Alex D. Leow, Andrew L. Alexander,
  Richard J. Davidson, and H. Hill Goldsmith*

Statistical Inference with Ensemble of Clustered Desparsified Lasso   638
  Jérôme-Alexis Chevalier, Joseph Salmon, and Bertrand Thirion

Low-Rank Representation for Multi-center Autism Spectrum
Disorder Identification   647
  *Mingliang Wang, Daoqiang Zhang, Jiashuang Huang, Dinggang Shen,
  and Mingxia Liu*

Exploring Uncertainty Measures in Deep Networks for Multiple Sclerosis
Lesion Detection and Segmentation   655
  Tanya Nair, Doina Precup, Douglas L. Arnold, and Tal Arbel

Inherent Brain Segmentation Quality Control from Fully ConvNet Monte
Carlo Sampling   664
  *Abhijit Guha Roy, Sailesh Conjeti, Nassir Navab,
  and Christian Wachinger*

Perfect MCMC Sampling in Bayesian MRFs for Uncertainty Estimation
in Segmentation   673
  Saurabh Garg and Suyash P. Awate

On the Effect of Inter-observer Variability for a Reliable Estimation
of Uncertainty of Medical Image Segmentation.   682
   Alain Jungo, Raphael Meier, Ekin Ermis, Marcela Blatti-Moreno,
   Evelyn Herrmann, Roland Wiest, and Mauricio Reyes

Towards Safe Deep Learning: Accurately Quantifying Biomarker
Uncertainty in Neural Network Predictions.   691
   Zach Eaton-Rosen, Felix Bragman, Sotirios Bisdas, Sébastien Ourselin,
   and M. Jorge Cardoso

Image Registration Methods

Registration-Based Patient-Specific Musculoskeletal Modeling Using High
Fidelity Cadaveric Template Model.   703
   Yoshito Otake, Masaki Takao, Norio Fukuda, Shu Takagi,
   Naoto Yamamura, Nobuhiko Sugano, and Yoshinobu Sato

Atlas Propagation Through Template Selection.   711
   Hongzhi Wang and Rui Zhang

Spatio-Temporal Atlas of Bone Mineral Density Ageing   720
   Mohsen Farzi, Jose M. Pozo, Eugene McCloskey, Richard Eastell,
   J. Mark Wilkinson, and Alejandro F. Frangi

Unsupervised Learning for Fast Probabilistic Diffeomorphic Registration. . . .   729
   Adrian V. Dalca, Guha Balakrishnan, John Guttag,
   and Mert R. Sabuncu

Adversarial Similarity Network for Evaluating Image Alignment in Deep
Learning Based Registration.   739
   Jingfan Fan, Xiaohuan Cao, Zhong Xue, Pew-Thian Yap,
   and Dinggang Shen

Improving Surgical Training Phantoms by Hyperrealism: Deep Unpaired
Image-to-Image Translation from Real Surgeries.   747
   Sandy Engelhardt, Raffaele De Simone, Peter M. Full, Matthias Karck,
   and Ivo Wolf

Computing CNN Loss and Gradients for Pose Estimation
with Riemannian Geometry   756
   Benjamin Hou, Nina Miolane, Bishesh Khanal, Matthew C. H. Lee,
   Amir Alansary, Steven McDonagh, Jo V. Hajnal, Daniel Rueckert,
   Ben Glocker, and Bernhard Kainz

GDL-FIRE^{4D}: Deep Learning-Based Fast 4D CT Image Registration.   765
   Thilo Sentker, Frederic Madesta, and René Werner

Adversarial Deformation Regularization for Training Image Registration
Neural Networks.   774
    Yipeng Hu, Eli Gibson, Nooshin Ghavami, Ester Bonmati,
    Caroline M. Moore, Mark Emberton, Tom Vercauteren, J. Alison Noble,
    and Dean C. Barratt

Fast Registration by Boundary Sampling and Linear Programming   783
    Jan Kybic and Jiří Borovec

Learning an Infant Body Model from RGB-D Data for Accurate Full Body
Motion Analysis   792
    Nikolas Hesse, Sergi Pujades, Javier Romero, Michael J. Black,
    Christoph Bodensteiner, Michael Arens, Ulrich G. Hofmann, Uta Tacke,
    Mijna Hadders-Algra, Raphael Weinberger, Wolfgang Müller-Felber,
    and A. Sebastian Schroeder

Consistent Correspondence of Cone-Beam CT Images Using Volume
Functional Maps.   801
    Yungeng Zhang, Yuru Pei, Yuke Guo, Gengyu Ma, Tianmin Xu,
    and Hongbin Zha

Elastic Registration of Geodesic Vascular Graphs   810
    Stefano Moriconi, Maria A. Zuluaga, H. Rolf Jäger, Parashkev Nachev,
    Sébastien Ourselin, and M. Jorge Cardoso

Efficient Groupwise Registration of MR Brain Images via Hierarchical
Graph Set Shrinkage   819
    Pei Dong, Xiaohuan Cao, Pew-Thian Yap, and Dinggang Shen

Initialize Globally Before Acting Locally: Enabling Landmark-Free 3D US
to MRI Registration.   827
    Julia Rackerseder, Maximilian Baust, Rüdiger Göbl, Nassir Navab,
    and Christoph Hennersperger

Solving the Cross-Subject Parcel Matching Problem Using
Optimal Transport.   836
    Guillermo Gallardo, Nathalie T. H. Gayraud, Rachid Deriche,
    Maureen Clerc, Samuel Deslauriers-Gauthier,
    and Demian Wassermann

GlymphVIS: Visualizing Glymphatic Transport Pathways Using
Regularized Optimal Transport   844
    Rena Elkin, Saad Nadeem, Eldad Haber, Klara Steklova, Hedok Lee,
    Helene Benveniste, and Allen Tannenbaum

Hierarchical Spherical Deformation for Shape Correspondence   853
    Ilwoo Lyu, Martin A. Styner, and Bennett A. Landman

Diffeomorphic Brain Shape Modelling Using Gauss-Newton Optimisation . . .   862
    Yaël Balbastre, Mikael Brudfors, Kevin Bronik, and John Ashburner

Multi-task SonoEyeNet: Detection of Fetal Standardized Planes Assisted
by Generated Sonographer Attention Maps.   871
    Yifan Cai, Harshita Sharma, Pierre Chatelain, and J. Alison Noble

Efficient Laplace Approximation for Bayesian Registration
Uncertainty Quantification   880
    Jian Wang, William M. Wells III, Polina Golland, and Miaomiao Zhang

Correction to: Medical Image Computing and Computer Assisted
Intervention – MICCAI 2018 . . . .   C1
    *Alejandro F. Frangi, Julia A. Schnabel, Christos Davatzikos,
    Carlos Alberola-López, and Gabor Fichtinger*

Author Index   889

Image Quality and Artefacts

Conditional Generative Adversarial Networks for Metal Artifact Reduction in CT Images of the Ear

Jianing Wang$^{(\boxtimes)}$, Yiyuan Zhao, Jack H. Noble,
and Benoit M. Dawant

Department of Electrical Engineering and Computer Science,
Vanderbilt University, Nashville, TN 37235, USA
`jianing.wang@vanderbilt.edu`

Abstract. We propose an approach based on a conditional generative adversarial network (cGAN) for the reduction of metal artifacts (RMA) in computed tomography (CT) ear images of cochlear implants (CIs) recipients. Our training set contains paired pre-implantation and post-implantation CTs of 90 ears. At the training phase, the cGAN learns a mapping from the artifact-affected CTs to the artifact-free CTs. At the inference phase, given new metal-artifact-affected CTs, the cGAN produces CTs in which the artifacts are removed. As a preprocessing step, we also propose a band-wise normalization method, which splits a CT image into three channels according to the intensity value of each voxel and we show that this method improves the performance of the cGAN. We test our cGAN on post-implantation CTs of 74 ears and the quality of the artifact-corrected images is evaluated quantitatively by comparing the segmentations of intra-cochlear anatomical structures, which are obtained with a previously published method, in the real pre-implantation and the artifact-corrected CTs. We show that the proposed method leads to an average surface error of 0.18 mm which is about half of what could be achieved with a previously proposed technique.

Keywords: Conditional generative adversarial networks
Metal artifact reduction · Cochlear implants

1   Introduction

Metallic implants in the human body can cause artifacts in computed tomography (CT) scans. Methods for the reduction of metal artifacts (RMA) in CTs have been investigated for nearly 40 years [1]. RMA algorithms can be roughly divided into three groups: physical effects correction, interpolation in the projection domain, and iterative reconstruction [2]. Despite these efforts, developing RMAs for dense metal implants and for multiple metallic objects in the field of view remains challenging and there is no known universal solution [1].

Conditional generative adversarial networks (cGANs) [3, 4] have emerged as a general-purpose solution to image-to-image translation problems. We propose an approach based on cGANs for RMA. At the training phase, a cGAN learns a mapping

© Springer Nature Switzerland AG 2018
A. F. Frangi et al. (Eds.): MICCAI 2018, LNCS 11070, pp. 3–11, 2018.
https://doi.org/10.1007/978-3-030-00928-1_1

from the artifact-affected CTs to the artifact-free CTs. At the inference phase, given an artifact-affected CT, the cGAN produces an artifact-corrected image. We apply our method to CT ear images of cochlear implants (CIs) recipients and get remarkable results.

Compared to the current leading traditional RMA methods, which generally necessitate the raw data from CT scanners [1], our approach is a post reconstruction processing method for which the raw data is not required. Our results also indicate that the post reconstruction processing methods, which have been considered to be ineffective [1], can in fact be effective. To the best of our knowledge, published RMA methods based on machine learning either depend on existing traditional RMA methods or require post-processing of the outputs produced by machine learning models [2, 5, 6]. Ours is unique in being able to synthesize directly an artifact-free image from an image in which artifacts are present.

2 Background

The cochlea is a spiral-shaped cavity that is part of the inner ear. CIs are surgically implanted neural prosthetic devices for treating severe-to-profound hearing loss [7] and are programmed postoperatively by audiologists to optimize outcomes. Accurately localizing the CI electrodes relative to the intra-cochlear anatomy in post-implantation CTs (Post-CTs) can help audiologists to fine-tune and customize the CI programming. This requires the accurate segmentation of the scala-tympani (ST), the scala-vestibuli (SV), and the modiolus (MOD) in these images (Fig. 1). Noble *et al.* have developed an active shape model-based method [8], which we refer to as NM, to segment ST, SV, and MOD in pre-implantation CTs (Pre-CTs). To the best of our knowledge, NM is the most accurate published automatic method for intra-cochlear anatomy segmentation in Pre-CTs. However, NM cannot be directly applied to Post-CTs due to the strong artifacts produced by the electrodes. Reda *et al.* have proposed a library-based method [9], which we refer to as RM, to segment ST, SV, and MOD in Post-CTs but it leads to segmentation errors that are substantially larger than errors obtained with pre-operative images. Here, we propose an alternative. First, we remove the artifacts from the Post-CTs using a novel RMA. Next, we apply NM to the processed images. We show that this novel approach leads to an error that is about half the error obtained with RM.

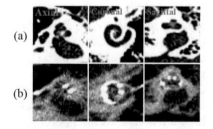

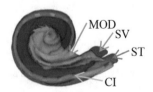

Fig. 1. An illustration of intra-cochlear anatomical structures and CI electrodes.

Fig. 2. Three orthogonal views of (a) the Pre-CT and (b) the Post-CT of an example ear.

3 Dataset

Our dataset consists of Pre- and Post-CT pairs of 164 ears, all these CTs have been acquired with the CIs recipients in roughly the same position. The CTs are acquired with several conventional scanners (GE BrightSpeed, LightSpeed Ultra; Siemens Sensation 16; and Philips Mx8000 IDT, iCT 128, and Brilliance 64) and a low-dose flat-panel volumetric CT scanner (Xoran Technologies xCAT® ENT). The typical voxel size is $0.25 \times 0.25 \times 0.3$ mm^3 for the conventional CTs (cCTs), and $0.4 \times 0.4 \times 0.4$ mm^3 for the low-dose CTs (lCTs). The 164 ears are randomly partitioned into a set of 90 for training and a set of 74 for testing. 82 of the 90 ears used for training have Post-CTs of type lCT and Pre-CTs of type cCT, and the remaining 8 ears have both Post-CTs and Pre-CTs of type cCT. 62 of the 74 ears for testing have Post-CTs of type lCT and Pre-CTs of type cCT, and the remaining 12 ears have both Post-CTs and Pre-CTs of type cCT.

4 Method

4.1 cGAN

In this work we rely on the cGAN framework proposed by Isola *et al.* [4]. A cGAN consists of a generator G and a discriminator D. The total loss can be expresses as

$$L = arg \ \min_G \ \max_D L_{cGAN}(G, D) + \lambda L_{L_1}(G) \tag{1}$$

wherein

$$L_{cGAN}(G, D) = \mathbb{E}_{x,y}[\log(D(x, y))] + \mathbb{E}_{x,z}[\log(1 - D(x, G(x, z)))] \tag{2}$$

is the adversarial loss and $L_{L1}(G)$ is the L1 norm loss. G is tasked with producing an artifact-corrected image from a Post-CT x and a random noise vector z. The image generated by G should not be distinguishable from the real artifact-free Pre-CT y by D, which is trained to do as well as possible to detect G's "fakes". The generated images need to be similar to y in the L1 sense.

We explore two generator architectures: (1) a U-net [10] (UNet), and (2) a network that contains two stride-2 convolutions, 9 residual blocks, and two fractionally strided convolutions with stride $\frac{1}{2}$ [11–14] (ResNet). For the discriminator, we use a 70×70 PatchGAN [4, 15] that aims to determine whether 70×70 overlapping image patches are real or fake. We run the PatchGAN convolutationally across the image, averaging all responses to provide the ultimate output of D.

4.2 Image Pre-processing

The Pre-CTs are registered to the Post-CTs using intensity-based rigid registration techniques. The registrations have been visually inspected and confirmed to be accurate. 3D patch pairs that contain the cochlea are cropped from the Pre- and Post-CTs, i.e., paired patches contain the same cochlea; one patch with and the other without the implant (Fig. 2). These patches are then upsampled to $0.1 \times 0.1 \times 0.1$ mm^3.

We apply a band-wise intensity normalization (BWN) to the Post-CT patches that acts as a piecewise linear stretch. For each 3D patch, we calculate the 2% percentile (p_2), the 98% percentile (p_{98}) and the 99.95% percentile ($p_{99.95}$) of the intensity values. Then the patch is separated into three channels: first, we copy the whole patch into channels 1, 2, and 3; second, the intensity values in channel 1, 2, and 3 are clamped to the ranges p_2 to $(p_2 + p_{98})/2$, $(p_2 + p_{98})/2$ to p_{98}, and p_{98} to $p_{99.95}$, respectively; and finally each channel is normalized to the -1 to 1 range. As discussed later, this heuristic improves some of our results.

For each Pre-CT patch, the intensity values are also clamped to the range between the bottom 1% and the top 1% voxel values. Then the patch is normalized to the -1 to 1 range.

4.3   Evaluation

The quality of the artifact-corrected images is evaluated quantitatively by comparing the segmentations of ST, SV, and MOD obtained with NM applied to the real Pre-CTs with the results obtained when applying NM to the artifact-corrected CTs. The output of NM are surface meshes of ST, SV, and MOD that have a pre-defined number of vertices. There are 3344, 3132, and 17947 vertices on the ST, SV, and MOD surfaces, respectively, for a total of 24423 vertices. Point-to-point errors (P2PEs), computed as the Euclidean distance in millimeter, between the corresponding vertices on the meshes generated from the real Pre-CTs and the meshes generated from artifact-corrected images are calculated to quantify the quality of the artifact-corrected images.

To compare the proposed method to the state of the art, we also segment ST, SV, and MOD using RM in Post-CTs. The output of RM are surface meshes for ST, SV, and MOD that have the same anatomical correspondences as the meshes generated by NM. The P2PEs between the corresponding vertices on the meshes generated from real Pre-CTs by using NM and the meshes generated from Post-CTs by using RM are calculated and serve as baseline for comparison.

To evaluate our BWN approach, we train the cGAN with and without such pre-processing step, and we compare the results that are generated with each strategy.

5   Experiments

The PyTorch implementation of the cGAN provided by Isola et al. [4] is used in our experiments. Since the cGAN is a 2D network, we train our cGAN on the axial view of the CTs. Input images are 2D 3-channel images, each of those is the slice of the 3D 3-channel Post-CT patch. As the current implementation of the cGAN requires the number of input and output channels to be the same, the target images of the cGAN are 2D 3-channel images in which each channel is identical and is the patch's slice in the Pre-CT that matches the patch's slice in the Post-CT used as input. In total 14346 paired Pre- and Post-CT 2D slices are used for training. To augment the number of training pairs, each slice is resized to 256×256 pixels and then padded to 286×286

pixels. Sub-images of 256×256 pixels are randomly cropped at the same location in the paired Pre- and Post-CT slices during the training. Horizontal flipping of the training pairs is also applied during the training to further augment the number of training pairs. The default value of $\lambda = 100$ is used to weigh the L1 distance loss. The cGAN is trained alternatively between one stochastic gradient descent (SGD) step on D, then one step on G, using minibatch size of 1 and the Adam solver [16] with momentum 0.5. The cGAN is trained for 200 epochs in which a fixed learning rate of 0.0002 is applied in the first 100 epochs, and a learning rate that is linearly reduced to zero in the second 100 epochs. The output of D, which is recorded every 100 iterations in each epoch, represents the probability that an image is real rather than fake. D is unable to differentiate between the real and the fake images when the output of D is 0.5 [17]. For each epoch, we calculate the median of the outputs of D and the model that is saved at the epoch in which the median is the closest to 0.5 among the 200 epochs is used as our final cGAN model. At the testing phase, the cGAN processes the testing 3D Post-CTs patches slice by slice, then the artifact-corrected slices are stacked to create 3D patches. These 3D patches are resized to their original sizes and translated back to their original spatial locations in the Post-CTs. Then we use NM to segment ST, SV, and MOD in these images.

6   Results

For each testing ear, we calculate the P2PEs of the 24423 vertices, and we calculate the maximum (Max), mean, median, standard deviation (STD), and minimum (Min) of the P2PEs. Figure 3a shows the boxplots of these statistics for the 74 testing ears, wherein Baseline denotes segmenting the intra-cochlear anatomical structures in Post-CTs using RM, Unet-1 denotes using UNet as the generator of the cGAN but without the BWN, Unet-3 denotes using UNet with BWN, ResNet-1 denotes using ResNet without BWN, and ResNet-3 denotes using ResNet with BWN. The means of Max, median, and STD of the P2PEs of the five approaches are shown in Table 1.

Table 1. The means of Max, median, and STD of the P2PEs of the five approaches (mm).

	ResNet-3	ResNet-1	UNet-3	UNet-1	Baseline
Max	0.575	0.599	0.625	0.660	0.912
Median	0.191	0.211	0.214	0.225	0.409
STD	0.084	0.085	0.091	0.097	0.133

Table 1 and the plots show that the cGAN-based methods substantially reduce the P2PEs obtained with the baseline approach. The median of the baseline method is 0.366 mm, whereas the median of ResNet-3 is 0.173 mm, which is less than the half of that of the baseline method. We perform paired t-tests on the Max, median, and STD

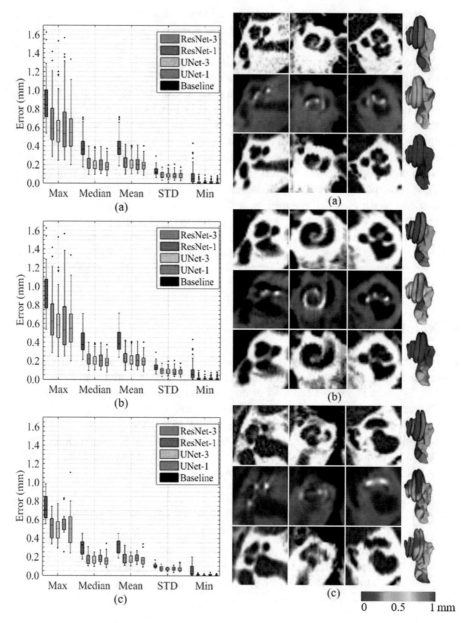

Fig. 3. Boxplot of P2PEs of (a) the 74 ears, (b) the 62 ears scanned by the conventional scanners, (c) the 12 ears scanned by the low-dose scanners.

Fig. 4. Three example cases in which ResNet-3 achieves (a) best, (b) average, and (c) worst performances. The left, middle, and right column of each case show the axial, coronal, and sagittal views of the 3D patches.

values of the baseline method between cGAN-based methods, the results show that the cGAN-based methods significantly reduce the P2PEs compared to the baseline method for Max, median, and STD ($p < 0.05$). We also perform paired t-tests between the four cGAN-based approaches. ResNet-3 leads to the lowest median error among the four. Pairwise t-tests show that the difference is statistically significant ($p < 0.05$). There is a substantial but not statistically significant difference between the Max and STD of ResNet-3 and of the other three approaches ($p > 0.05$). For ResNet, applying BWN results in statistically significant lower point-to-point median errors ($p < 0.05$). There is a visible but not statistically significant difference between the medians of UNet-3 and UNet-1 ($p > 0.05$). These results show that BWN affects the architectures differently but comparing the boxplots of UNet-3 and UNet-1, and those of ResNet-1 and ResNet-3, it is apparent that the interquartile ranges of the distributions is reduced when applying BWN.

Figure 3b shows the boxplots of the 62 lCTs, which show the same trend as Fig. 3a. Figure 3c shows the boxplot of the 12 cCTs, it also shows the same trend except that the interquartile ranges of the distributions are not reduced when applying BWN. It could be that the BWN approach does not generalize well to all image types but we also note that we only have 8 lCTs in the training set and 12 lCTs in the testing set. It is thus difficult to draw hard conclusions at this point. We are acquiring more data to address this issue.

Figure 4 shows three example cases in which our proposed method (ResNet-3) achieves (a) the best, (b) an average, and (c) the worst performances, in the sense of the medians of the P2PEs. For each case, the top row shows three orthogonal views of the Pre-CT and the meshes generated when applying NM to this CT. The ST, SV, and MOD surfaces are shown in red, blue, and green, respectively. The middle row shows the Post-CT and the meshes generated when applying RM to this CT. The bottom row shows the output of cGAN and the meshes generated when applying NM to this image. The meshes in the middle and the bottom rows are color-coded with the P2PE at each vertex on the meshes. These images confirm the results presented in Fig. 3. Notably, even in the worst case, segmentation errors are on the order of 0.2 mm for a large portion of the structures. We also note that the output images of cGAN show good slice-to-slice consistency, i.e., there is no "jaggedness", in the coronal and the sagittal views, although the cGAN is a 2D network and it is trained on the axial view only.

RM has also been applied to these artifact-corrected images. The results are better than with the artifact-affected images but statistically worse than those obtained with NM on the synthetic images.

7 Summary

We have developed a method that is capable of removing metallic artifacts in CT ear images of CI recipients. This new method has been tested on a large dataset, and we show that it permits to significantly reduce the segmentation error for intra-cochlear structures in post-operative images when compared to the current state-of-the-art approach. The technique we propose can be potentially used for RMA in CTs at other body sites. It would also be interesting to explore the possibility of applying such idea to correct various types of artifact in other types of medical images. Although the results we have obtained so far are encouraging, we believe there is room for improvement. It is possible for instance that a 3D network would be better than a 2D network. To test this, we have extended the current architecture to a 3D one. At the time of writing the results obtained with the latter are inferior to those presented herein. Training of and training set size required for a 3D network are issues we are currently addressing.

Acknowledgements. This work has been supported in parts by NIH grants R01DC014037 and R01DC014462 and by the Advanced Computing Center for Research and Education (ACCRE) of Vanderbilt University. The content is solely the responsibility of the authors and does not necessarily represent the official views of this institute.

References

1. Gjesteby, L., et al.: Metal artifact reduction in CT: where are we after four decades? IEEE Access. **4**, 5826–5849 (2016)
2. Zhang, Y., Yu, H.: Convolutional neural network based metal artifact reduction in x-ray computed tomography. arXiv:1709.01581 (2017)
3. Mirza, M., Osindero, S.: Conditional generative adversarial nets. arXiv:1411.1784 (2014)
4. Isola, P., Zhu, J.-Y., Zhou, T., Efros, A.A.: Image-to-image translation with conditional adversarial networks. arXiv:1611.07004 (2017)
5. Park, H.S., et al.: Machine-learning-based nonlinear decomposition of CT images for metal artifact reduction. arXiv:1708.00244 (2017)
6. Gjesteby, L., et al.: Reducing metal streak artifacts in CT images via deep learning: pilot results. In: The 14th International Meeting on Fully Three-Dimensional Image Reconstruction in Radiology and Nuclear Medicine, vol. 14(6), pp. 611–614 (2017)
7. Cochlear Implants. National Institute on Deafness and Other Communication Disorders, No. 11-4798 (2011)
8. Noble, J.H., et al.: Automatic segmentation of intracochlear anatomy in conventional CT. IEEE Trans. Biomed. Eng. **58**(9), 2625–2632 (2011)
9. Reda, F.A., et al.: Automatic segmentation of intra-cochlear anatomy in post-implantation CT. In: Proceedings of the SPIE 8671, Medical Imaging 2013: Image-Guided Procedures, Robotic Interventions, and Modeling, 86710I (2013)
10. Ronneberger, O., Fischer, P., Brox, T.: U-Net: convolutional networks for biomedical image segmentation. arXiv:1505.04597 (2015)
11. Johnson, J., Alahi, A., Fei-Fei, L.: Perceptual losses for real-time style transfer and super-resolution. In: Leibe, B., Matas, J., Sebe, N., Welling, M. (eds.) ECCV 2016. LNCS, vol. 9906, pp. 694–711. Springer, Cham (2016). https://doi.org/10.1007/978-3-319-46475-6_43
12. He, K., Zhang, X., Ren, S., Sun, J.: Deep residual learning for image recognition. arXiv: 1512.03385 (2015)
13. Zhu, J.-Y., Park, T., Isola, P., Efros, A.A.: Unpaired image-to-image translation using cycle-consistent adversarial networks. arXiv:1703.10593 (2017)

14. Li, C., Wand, M.: Precomputed real-time texture synthesis with markovian generative adversarial networks. In: Leibe, B., Matas, J., Sebe, N., Welling, M. (eds.) ECCV 2016. LNCS, vol. 9907, pp. 702–716. Springer, Cham (2016). https://doi.org/10.1007/978-3-319-46487-9_43
15. Ledig, C., et al.: Photo-realistic single image super-resolution using a generative adversarial network. arXiv:1609.04802, (2017)
16. Kingma, D.P., Ba, J.: Adam: a method for stochastic optimization. arXiv:1412.6980 (2014)
17. Goodfellow, I.J., et al.: Generative adversarial networks. arXiv:1406.2661 (2014)

Neural Network Evolution Using Expedited Genetic Algorithm for Medical Image Denoising

Peng Liu, Yangjunyi Li, Mohammad D. El Basha, and Ruogu Fang$^{(\boxtimes)}$

J. Crayton Pruitt Family Department of Biomedical Engineering,
University of Florida, Gainesville, FL, USA
Ruogu.Fang@bme.ufl.edu

Abstract. Convolutional neural networks offer state-of-the-art performance for medical image denoising. However, their architectures are manually designed for different noise types. The realistic noise in medical images is usually mixed and complicated, and sometimes unknown, leading to challenges in creating effective denoising neural networks. In this paper, we present a Genetic Algorithm (GA)-based network evolution approach to search for the fittest genes to optimize network structures. We expedite the evolutionary process through an experience-based greedy exploration strategy and transfer learning. The experimental results on computed tomography perfusion (CTP) images denoising demonstrate the capability of the method to select the fittest genes for building high-performance networks, named EvoNets, and our results compare favorably with state-of-the-art methods.

Keywords: Medical image denoising · Genetic Algorithm
Convolutional neural networks · Evolution · Low-dose imaging

1 Introduction

Medical imaging techniques, such as Computed Tomography (CT), Magnetic Resonance Imaging (MRI), and X-rays are popular diagnostic tools. Nevertheless, these techniques are susceptible to noise. For example, CT perfusion images are often associated with complicated mixed noise due to the photon starvation artifacts. In recent decades, different methods have been widely investigated to solve the problem, ranging from spatial filtering techniques, such as Wiener filters [7], to patch similarity methods, such as BM3D [1]. However, complicated mixed noise in medical images still leads to the unsatisfactory performance of these methods and remains a valuable research direction.

Convolutional Neural Networks (CNN) have shown superior performance over traditional models on denoising tasks. A typical CNN is composed of several stacked layers, including layer connections and hyperparameters (e.g., number of layers, neurons in each layer, type of activation function). RED-Net [5] consists of a chain of 30 convolutional layers and symmetric deconvolutional layers.

© Springer Nature Switzerland AG 2018
A. F. Frangi et al. (Eds.): MICCAI 2018, LNCS 11070, pp. 12–20, 2018.
https://doi.org/10.1007/978-3-030-00928-1_2

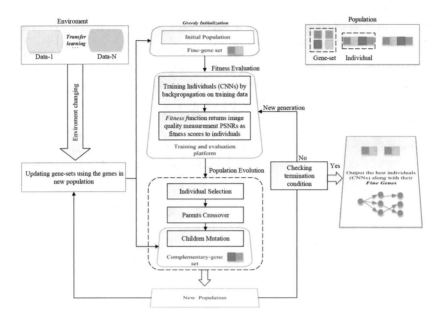

Fig. 1. Overview of the proposed method composing of fitness evaluation and population evolution. The CNN architecture is trained on medical images using a fitness score. The individual networks labeled with the fitness scores are sent to individual selection. The survived individuals are presented as parents for crossover and mutation.

Another state-of-the-art method, DnCNN [10], adopts concise stacked-layer connections but achieves impressive performance via appropriate hyperparameters (e.g., ReLU [6]) selection. Consequently, hyperparameters play a dominant role in optimizing image denoising tasks.

Although these modern networks present promising image restoration performance, they are all manually designed based on empirical knowledge. It is expensive and slow to manually search for the optimal network structures with exponential combinations of hyperparameters and layers connections. To address this issue, it is critical to automatically construct promising CNN-based denoisers with concise layer connections and optimal hyperparameter combinations. Moreover, an efficient algorithm is important to explore the optimal CNN structures within reasonable computational time.

In this work, we construct a CNN-based medical image denoiser, named EvoNet, automatically. To more effectively navigate large search spaces, we formulate an optimized genetic algorithm (GA). Basically, GA initializes candidate solutions (e.g., networks) as an initial generation, and then applies genetic operations to evolve the solutions in each generation. As shown in Fig. 1, for the population evolution process, we define three standard genetic operations: selection, crossover, and mutation. A fitness function is formulated to help us select best individuals (e.g., CNN) in each generation. Each of these solutions is evaluated by fitness scores through a denoising evaluation criteria. The contributions of the paper are as follows:

- It is the first time to propose a GA-based method to construct CNN structures for medical image denoising automatically. This evolution approach provides the flexibility to optimize both CNN parameters and network structures.
- We optimize the standard genetic algorithm to speed up the evolutionary progress. Specifically, we use an experience based greedy strategy on the initialization stage to enrich high-performance individuals in the first generation. In addition, we select an appropriate mutation rate to make a trade-off between the diversity of the population (CNNs) and convergence of optimum generation.
- We dynamically update hyperparameter sets to make the architectures of the population (CNNs) transferable between datasets of different sizes. Particularly, we split all possible hyperparameters into fine-genes and complementary-genes for initialization and mutation respectively.

2   Methodology

Background. Genetic Algorithms (GAs) [2] are inspired by the natural biological evolution. Typically, a GA is composed of a "population" P of N "individuals", and has operations including initialization, individual selection, parents crossover, and children mutation (see Fig. 1). A sequence of operations is referred as an evolutionary "generation". The competition among individuals is simulated by a *fitness* function that selects the fittest individuals over the weaker ones.

GA has been widely utilized as a heuristic search and optimization technique and also has been applied in machine learning approaches, and function optimization. Recently, Xie et al. [8] applied GA to explore CNN architectures automatically for image classification. These methods focus on exploring the structural module blocks and connections among layers. However, the study of an efficient way for building a concise CNN-based denoiser on medical image automatically is still lacking.

A concise but also promising CNN-based denoiser relies on a specific learning strategy (e.g., Residual learning) and one choice of hyperparameter combinations (e.g., DnCNN). Therefore, in this work, we aim at building a simple but effective CNN structure via focusing on exploring the effective combinations of CNN hyperparameters instead of the structural blocks and layer connections. One significant challenge of using GA is how to accelerate the evolutionary process dynamically in a huge search space. To address this issue, we present an *Optimized Genetic Algorithm* (Algorithm 1) with an experience based greedy exploration strategy in the next section.

Gene Splitting. A "gene" is the basic functional unit in a biological body. In an artificial neural network, genes represent hyperparameters, such as the number of layers, the number of neurons, the activation function, and the type

---

Algorithm 1. The Proposed Genetic Algorithm for Exploring CNNs

---

Input: one all-possible-gene set $\theta = \theta_c \cup \theta_f$, initial fine-gene set θ_f, initial complementary-gene set θ_c, initial population size N, initial number of generation G, percentage of selected individuals after each generation σ, number of children of crossed over out O, mutation rate ϵ, termination condition E, small and large training datasets $D = \{D_s, D_l\}$

1: **for** d = 1, 2, ..., length(D) **do**
2:     **for** g = 1, 2, ..., $G - 1$ **do**
3:         **for** i = 1, 2, ..., N **do**
4:             **if** $g = 1$ **then**
5:                 *Initialize* a set of randomized individuals $\{P_i^g\}_{i=1}^N$ based on θ_f
6:             **end if**
7:             Return *trained* individuals $\{P_i^{g,t}\}_{i=1}^N$ by Keras and Tensorflow
8:             Return *fitness scores* $F_i^g = F(P_i^{g,t})$ to individuals
9:         **end for**
10:         $Sort\left\{P_i^{g,trained}\right\}_{i=1}^N$ by F_i^g with descending order
11:         $\Re = \left\{P_i^{g,trained,sorted}\right\}_{i=1}^{N*\sigma}$ *Select the top* $N * \sigma$ *best individuals*
12:         $P_i^{g,new} = P_i^{g,new} + = \varnothing$
13:         **while** $length(P_i^{g,new}) < N - length(\Re)$ **do**
14:             $\Upsilon_{mom}, \Upsilon_{dad} = uniformRandom(\Re)$ Select parents
15:             $\{\Psi_o\}_{o=1}^O = Genome(\Upsilon_{mom}, \Upsilon_{dad})$ Have children with crossover genes
16:             **if** $\epsilon > Random(0,1)$ **then** Mutation with a rate μ
17:                 $\Psi_{selected} = selectRandom(\{\Psi_o\}_{o=1}^O)$ Randomly select one child
18:                 $\theta_{selected} = selectRandom(\theta_{\Psi_{selected}})$ Randomly select one gene
19:                 $\theta_{c,selected} = selectRandom(\theta_c, Genotype(\theta_{selected}))$
20:                 $\{\Psi_o^m\}_{o=1}^O = replace(\Psi_{selected}, \theta_{selected}, \theta_{c,selected})$
21:                 $P_i^{g,new} = P_i^{g,new} + \{\Psi_o^m\}_{o=1}^O$
22:             **else**
23:                 $P_i^{g,new} = P_i^{g,new} + \{\Psi_o\}_{o=1}^O$
24:             **end if**
25:             $P_i^{g,new} = removeDuplicate(P_i^{g,new})$
26:         **end while**
27:         $P_i^{g,new} = P_i^{g,new} + \Re$
28:         **if** $E = True$ **then** May say "the highest fitness score is not changing"
29:             Terminate generation and go to output
30:         **end if**
31:     **end for**
32:     $\theta_f^u = Update(\theta_f, \Re)$ Replace fine-gene set with the genes in $\Re$
33:     $\theta_c^u = \theta - \theta_f$ Update complementary-gene set
34: **end for**

Output: Select the best individuals (CNNs) from $P_i^{g,new}$

---

of optimizers. To speed up the evolution process, let θ be the set of all possible genes, and it is split into a fine-gene set θ_f and a complementary-gene set θ_c. Fine-genes are the hyperparameters selected from those state-of-the-art CNN structures in the literature (e.g., DnCNN) or previous GA generations. The rest genes in θ are the complementary genes. The first population is initialized based on θ_f. The mutation process is solely built upon θ_c. An individual (CNN) is composed of different genes, and N individuals form a population-P.

Our method emphasizes the fittest gene more than the survived individuals (network structures). This strategy ensures the promising genes are passed down to offspring, and the fittest individuals are more likely to be explored effectively in early generations. Therefore, our approach can accelerate the evolution process via optimizing gene search space dynamically. The overview and algorithm details of the proposed method are shown in Fig. 1 and Algorithm 1 respectively.

Experience Based Greedy Exploration. We optimize GA with an experience based greedy exploration strategy, which determines how to update gene sets and terminate evolution process. Experience represents CNN hyperparameters from the last generation, our approach stores and transfers such experience to next generation. In another word, we initialize the fine-gene sets with top-performance CNNs evolved in the previous generations.

Transfer Learning. Another novel contribution of our approach is using a *transfer learning* strategy [9] that allows the explored CNN architectures to be transferable among training data of different sizes. For instance, we may use a small dataset to quickly optimize the gene-set space first, and then explore CNNs on a larger dataset by initializing a new population using the fine genes identified from the small dataset. It further expedites the network evolution process.

Fitness Evaluation. The *fitness* function $F(P_i)$ returns the restored image quality measure as a fitness score to each individual P_i. Fitness score performs the following functions: (1) evaluating individual fitness; (2) updating gene-sets; (3) serving as a stopping rule. Hence, the fitness function is critical for designing an effective GA-based method. Algorithm 1 presents the details of the proposed GA for exploring the promising CNNs to handle with medical image denoising.

3   Experiments

Training and Testing Data. Our dataset is a collection of 10,775 cerebral perfusion CT images, all of which are 512×512 gray-scale images. Training data D consist of randomly selected 250 images from the perfusion CT dataset, all of them are cropped uniformly to the size of 331×363. This pre-processing step removes skull and background from raw CT images and improves feature learning efficiency during training. Testing data are randomly selected 250 images with no overlap with the training data, and they remain as 512×512 grayscale images. Another 100 images with no overlap with the training/testing data are selected as the validation set. We use Peak Signal-to-Noise Ratio (PSNR) as the fitness function in approach.

Transfer Learning. GA requires high computational resources due to the large search space, which leads difficulties to evaluate performance on large datasets directly. Our strategy is to explore promising CNN hyperparameter combinations by training on a small subset D_s. In particular, 35 images from the training data are randomly selected and segmented with patch size 50×50 at a stride of 20. Therein, 8,576 image patches are generated for the initial evolution. We then transfer hyperparameters observed from results on D_s to a large training set D_l. With the same patch size and stride length, 100 images of D_l are segmented into 17,280 patches for further evolution.

Low-Dose Noise Simulation. Repeated scans at different radiation dose on the same patient are not ethical due to increased unnecessary radiation exposure. Therefore, in this paper, low-dose perfusion CT images are stimulated and added to the regular dose perfusion CT images. Specifically, spatially correlated, normally distributed noise is added to both training data and testing data. The added noise has a standard deviation of $\sigma = 17, 22, 32$, which corresponds to the tube current-time product of 30, 20, 10 mAs. The regular dose level is 190 mAs.

Experimental Setup. All possible genes θ are selected from CNN hyperparameters with promising performance reported in the literature [5,10]. In this paper, we consider a constrained case with θ consisting of four sub-genotypes: number of layers = (1, 2, 3, 4, 5, 6, 7), number of neurons in each layer = (16, 32, 64, 96, 128, 256), activation = ('ReLU', 'Tanh', 'SELU', 'ELU', 'Sigmoid'), and optimizers = ('rmsprop', 'sgd', 'adam', 'adamax', 'adadelta', 'adagrad'). During initialization, we set the initial fine-gene set θ_f from set θ as number of layers = (5, 6), number of neurons in each layer = (32, 48), activation = ('ReLU', 'ELU', 'Sigmoid'), and optimizers = ('sgd', 'adam'). We create an initial population size $N = 20$ individuals and perform genetic operations for 10 rounds (generation). For each generation, we set mutation possibility rate $\epsilon = 0.1$. Crossover happens between any two random parents networks. After each crossover and muta-

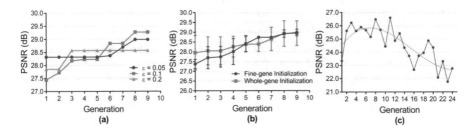

Fig. 2. (a) The performance of best individual with respect to mutation rate $\epsilon = 0.05, 0.1, 0.2$. (b) The average performance over top 5 individuals with respect to the initialization process with a fine-gene set θ_f and whole-gene set θ. (c) The average performance overall individuals with respect to the generation number. All training are processed on large dataset D_l

tion, we check the whole population and eliminate duplicate individuals (see Algorithm 1). Other hyperparameters (e.g., learning rate) follow Tensorflow default settings. Residual learning [4] is adopted to accelerate training process. All GA progresses are processed on Tensorflow platform with GEFORCE GTX TITAN GPUs.

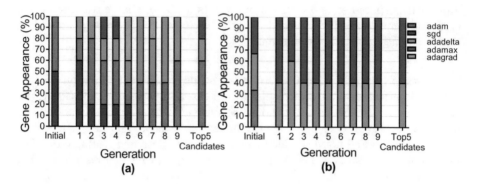

Fig. 3. The activation gene appearance changing during evolutionary progress on the small dataset D_s (a), and the large dataset D_l (b) with transferred initialization set. In each generation, 5 top performed individuals are selected to summarize changes. Top 5 Candidates bar refers to the final optimizer gene distribution after one evolutionary progress.

Parameters Selection. We evaluate the performance of different mutation rate as shown in Fig. 2(a). When the mutation rate is too high, it increases the searching speed in the search space but may not find optimal individuals in each generation. On the other hand, when the mutation rate is too low, it can lead individuals to converge rapidly to local optimum instead of the global optimum. From Fig. 2(a), $\epsilon = 0.1$ gives the optimal performance. We also evaluate different initialization strategies as shown in Fig. 2(b). Fine-gene initialization with selected genes can reach the same performance as the whole gene initialization strategy after 8 generations. While we set fine-genes as greedy initialization set, it helps early generations find high-performance individuals. However, after certain generations, more mutation genes are introduced due to the duplicate individual elimination, which increases population diversity but reduces the average performance. This strategy helps to stop early at an optimal generation and improves search efficiency. This is demonstrated in Fig. 2(c). We use 10 generations as shown in Fig. 2(c).

Gene Evolution. We track the evolution of genes over generations and illustrate the optimizer genes in Fig. 3. We show the top 5 individuals in each generation trained on a small training set and after transferring to a large training set. When training on a small set (Fig. 3(a)), the low-performance genes are eliminated over the generations, such as *sgd* and *adagrad*. At the same time, the high-performance genes are introduced from mutation, such as *adadelta*. After being transferred to a large training set (Fig. 3(b)), the initialization set is transferred from (a), where good "genes" such as *adam, adadelta,* and *adamax* are preserved. Through the evolution, top performance genes such as *adamax* and *adadelta* dominate the optimizer genes. This tracking process demonstrates that our greedy initialization strategy helps to search for high-performance genes efficiently. More importantly, it shows that the learned CNN hyperparameters (genes) and structures are transferable from small datasets to large datasets.

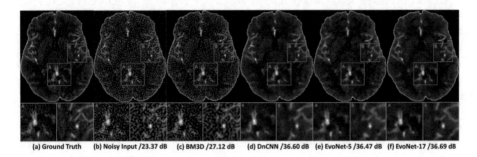

(a) Ground Truth   (b) Noisy Input /23.37 dB   (c) BM3D /27.12 dB   (d) DnCNN /36.60 dB   (e) EvoNet-5 /36.47 dB   (f) EvoNet-17 /36.69 dB

Fig. 4. Visual Results of perfusion CT dataset with noise $\sigma = 22$. A region of Interest (ROI) is selected (red region) and scaled up for better visual comparison.

Comparison with State-of-the-Art Methods. Both quantitative and qualitative comparisons are provided. We compared with state-of-the-art methods including BM3D and DnCNN. DnCNN has been reported to work on medical images [3]. We obtained the EvoNet-5 (5 layers, 64 neurons each layer, *adadelta, ReLu*) from D_s, and EvoNet-17 (17 layers, 64 neurons each layer, *adadelta, ReLu*) from D_l.

In Table 1, we present the summary of quantitative results. The deeper EvoNet-17 outperforms other state-of-the-art methods with PSNR on the testing dataset. The shallow EvoNet-5 achieves comparable performance to DnCNN; however, it is deep (20 layers) while the EvoNet-5 is a compact structure with

Table 1. Average PSNR, SSIM, and computation time of algorithms: BM3D, DnCNN, EvoNet-5, and EvoNet-17 at different noise levels $\sigma = 17, 22, 32$. Best performance is highlighted in bold.

σ	BM3D [1]		DnCNN [10]		EvoNet-5		EvoNet-17	
	PSNR(dB)	SSIM	PSNR(dB)	SSIM	PSNR(dB)	SSIM	PSNR(dB)	SSIM
17	29.07	0.4515	36.64	**0.9158**	36.30	0.9062	**36.65**	0.9074
22	26.98	0.3578	35.87	0.8863	35.66	0.8914	**35.92**	**0.8988**
32	23.95	0.2385	35.03	0.8671	34.35	0.8578	**35.04**	**0.8846**

stacked convolutional layers without regularization technique. Deeper (6, 7 layers) and larger (128, 256 neurons) networks are eliminated due to overfitting on small data. Figure 4 shows visual results. Our method perfectly restores physiological structures, circuit contour and texture of the cerebral cortex and gains high PSNR values. It is matching with quantitative results.

4   Conclusions

In this work, we propose an optimized GA-based strategy to explore CNN structure for medical image denoising. We introduce an experience-based greedy exploration strategy and transfer learning to accelerate GA evolution. We evaluate EvoNets on a perfusion CT dataset and demonstrate promising performance. In the current work, we only consider a constrained case. In future work, the proposed method can be extended to explore more flexible CNN structures for challenging tasks, such as tumor detection.

Acknowledgment. This work is partially supported by NSF IIS-1564892.

References

1. Dabov, K., Foi, A., Katkovnik, V., Egiazarian, K.: BM3D image denoising with shape-adaptive principal component analysis. In: SPARS 2009-Signal Processing with Adaptive Sparse Structured Representations (2009)
2. Holland, J.H.: Genetic algorithms. Sci. Am. **267**(1), 66–73 (1992)
3. Jifara, W., Jiang, F., Rho, S., Cheng, M., Liu, S.: Medical image denoising using convolutional neural network: a residual learning approach. J. Supercomput. pp. 1–15 (2017)
4. Kiku, D., Monno, Y., Tanaka, M., Okutomi, M.: Residual interpolation for color image demosaicking. In: 2013 IEEE International Conference on Image Processing, pp. 2304–2308. IEEE (2013)
5. Mao, X.J., Shen, C., Yang, Y.B.: Image restoration using convolutional auto-encoders with symmetric skip connections. arXiv preprint arXiv:1606.08921 (2016)
6. Nair, V., Hinton, G.E.: Rectified linear units improve restricted boltzmann machines. In: Proceedings of the 27th International Conference on Machine Learning (ICML-10), pp. 807–814 (2010)
7. Wintermark, M., Lev, M.: FDA investigates the safety of brain perfusion CT. Am. J. Neuroradiol. **31**(1), 2–3 (2010)
8. Xie, L., Yuille, A.: Genetic cnn. arXiv preprint arXiv:1703.01513 (2017)
9. Yosinski, J., Clune, J., Bengio, Y., Lipson, H.: How transferable are features in deep neural networks? In: Advances in Neural Information Processing Systems, pp. 3320–3328 (2014)
10. Zhang, K., Zuo, W., Chen, Y., Meng, D., Zhang, L.: Beyond a gaussian denoiser: residual learning of deep cnn for image denoising. IEEE Trans. Image Proc. **26**(7), 3142–3155 (2017)

Deep Convolutional Filtering for Spatio-Temporal Denoising and Artifact Removal in Arterial Spin Labelling MRI

David Owen[1,4]($\boxtimes$), Andrew Melbourne[1,4], Zach Eaton-Rosen[1,4],
David L. Thomas[1,2], Neil Marlow[3], Jonathan Rohrer[2],
and Sébastien Ourselin[1,4]

[1] Translational Imaging Group, University College London, London, UK
rmapdow@ucl.ac.uk
[2] Dementia Research Centre, Institute of Neurology,
University College London, London, UK
[3] Institute for Women's Health, University College London, London, UK
[4] School of Biomedical Engineering and Imaging Sciences,
King's College London, London, UK

Abstract. Arterial spin labelling (ASL) is a noninvasive imaging modality, used in the clinic and in research, which can give quantitative measurements of perfusion in the brain and other organs. However, because the signal-to-noise ratio is inherently low and the ASL acquisition is particularly prone to corruption by artifact, image processing methods such as denoising and artifact filtering are vital for generating accurate measurements of perfusion. In this work, we present a new simultaneous approach to denoising and artifact removal, using a novel deep convolutional joint filter architecture to learn and exploit spatio-temporal properties of the ASL signal. We proceed to show, using data from 15 healthy subjects, that our approach achieves state of the art performance in both denoising and artifact removal, improving peak signal-to-noise ratio by up to 50%. By allowing more accurate estimation of perfusion, even in challenging datasets, this technique offers an exciting new approach for ASL pipelines, and might be used both for improving individual images and to increase the power of research studies using ASL.

1 Introduction

Arterial spin labelling (ASL) is an MR imaging technique that allows quantitative, noninvasive measurements of perfusion in the brain and other organs. ASL has demonstrated its utility in both research and clinical use, and has the potential to be used as a biomarker in several diseases [1]. However, ASL suffers from

Electronic supplementary material The online version of this chapter (https://doi.org/10.1007/978-3-030-00928-1_3) contains supplementary material, which is available to authorized users.

the twin problems of having low signal-to-noise ratio (SNR) and being prone to artifacts from patient motion, RF coil instability and several other sources.

Typically, to address these problems, denoising and artifact filtering are used. Denoising uses statistical properties of the ASL signal to improve the effective SNR, for example by modelling the signal using total variation priors, a wavelet basis, or anatomy-derived spatial correlation [2,3]. Denoising methods tend to assume Gaussian noise, and are not usually robust to non-Gaussian artifacts, for example due to patient motion or hardware instability. Artifact filtering methods, conversely, remove or down-weight parts of the ASL signal that have severe artifacts, allowing subsequent processing to assume Gaussian noise [4–7].

Denoising and artifact removal are usually considered in isolation from one another, but are overlapping problems: noise is often neither strictly Gaussian nor spatially homogeneous, and artifact filtering often results in the rejection of entire image volumes when only a fraction of the image is thoroughly corrupted. In this work, we develop a deep convolutional neural network (CNN) for simultaneous denoising and artifact filtering, making full use of the available data. Inspired by cutting-edge developments in computer vision, we create a novel deep learning architecture that can relate noisy, artifact-corrupted ASL images to the true underlying perfusion. This architecture uses joint convolutional filtering [8] in order to efficiently extract spatio-temporal information from the ASL signal, allowing our method to distinguish artifact from noise. We present results from our method in ASL data from 15 healthy volunteers, showing that our method improves on the state of the art for both artifact filtering and denoising, increasing the peak SNR by up to 50%. These promising initial results show that deep convolutional joint filtering holds great promise for ASL processing, and suggest our approach might be useful both for improving individual subjects' images and for increasing the statistical power of neuroimaging studies.

2   Methods

2.1   Arterial Spin Labelling

ASL images are acquired by tagging blood magnetically – applying inversion pulses at the neck before the blood flows to the brain. Images are acquired with and without this tagging, with the difference between these images being a function of the blood flow. Standard models exist in the literature to relate the measured signal to the underlying perfusion [1,9].

In this work, we use an ASL dataset from 35 healthy 19-year-old volunteers (F/M = 17/18). Images were acquired on a 3T Phillips Achieva with 2D EPI pseudo-continuous ASL using 30 control-label pairs, PLD = $1800\,\text{ms}$ + $41\,\text{ms/slice}$, $\tau = 1650\,\text{ms}$, $3 \times 3 \times 5\,\text{mm}$. We also acquired M_0 images and 3D T_1-weighted volumes at $1\,\text{mm}$ isotropic resolution. All ASL data were motion corrected via rigid registration before being used – note, however, that motion correction often does not fully compensate for subject motion, and this is one of the artifacts that should ideally be filtered when estimating the true perfusion.

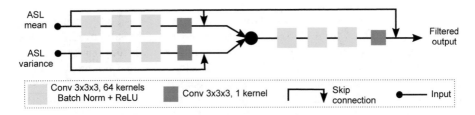

Fig. 1. Architecture diagram for our deep convolutional joint filter. For the mean-only filter, the ASL variance input is not used.

2.2 Deep Convolutional Joint Filtering

Convolutional neural networks (CNNs) are a well-established means of processing images for a variety of tasks. Here, we focus on *pixel-to-pixel* networks: in general terms, we wish to take input images and produce a higher quality output image. Although CNNs show state of the art performance in natural image processing [8], their application to ASL images has, to date, been limited to Hadamard-encoded ASL, and has had limited success [10]. Part of the reason may be the great benefit to ASL processing of *spatio-temporal* models: it is easier to distinguish artifact from perfusion when one is aware of whether a particular part of the signal was transient or permanent [2]. Processing a sequence of several 3D images rapidly becomes computationally expensive, however. Our solution is to explicitly feed in temporal variance information so the network has two inputs: the mean ASL signal, and the ASL signal variance over time.

The naive approach to using spatio-temporal information would be to feed the signal mean and variance maps into the same CNN, similarly to colour channels in a natural image. However, initial testing showed poor performance, as the network was unable to translate voxel-level features into meaningful cross-channel information. To achieve this end, we created a novel *joint convolutional filter* architecture, inspired by image processing approaches to integrating RGB cameras and depth sensors [8]. In our architecture, information is extracted and processed in parallel from the mean ASL image and the ASL temporal variance. These images are combined at a later stage in the network, with several more layers used to extract meaningful features from their combination. Skip connections in the parallel stages improve network convergence and robustness, as well as transferring global information in the learning process [8].

To train our models, we first identified artifact-corrupted volumes using the filtering method of Tan et al. [4]. We generated gold standard high-quality perfusion maps by removing these outlying volumes and using all of the remaining data to fit perfusion according to literature recommendations [1]. These gold standard images were used as ground truth. The inputs to our network were derived by taking 10 random volumes from the ASL series, including artifact-corrupted volumes to train the network to correct for artifacts in addition to denoising. The loss function used was mean squared error within the brain mask.

We implemented our CNNs in Keras, using the Adam optimiser with learning rate 0.01 with 20 subjects for training and 15 subjects for validation. To avoid overfitting and improve generalisation, we augmented with random translations sampled uniformly up to 5 mm in each dimension. We also augmented input images with Gaussian noise, magnitude approximately 1% of the ASL noise as estimated from gold standard data. We trained to convergence (approximately 1000 iterations), which took 12 h using an NVIDIA K80 graphics card.

2.3   Comparison to Pre-existing Methods and Validation

For both denoising and artifact filtering, we compare our method with a state of the art spatial regularisation technique using total generalised variation (TGV), which has been shown to produce reliable and accurate denoising with built-in artifact rejection via robust statistics [2]. For reference, we also compare against voxelwise fitting with no spatial regularisation – this remains a very common way to process ASL data, and acts as a representative baseline.

We evaluate our method, using the full spatio-temporal information as discussed in Sect. 2.2, and we also evaluate a simpler CNN architecture using only spatial information (see Fig. 1), to show the benefit of the joint filter. We evaluate the performance by examining filtered images for residual artifacts, and by producing maps of absolute error relative to the gold standard perfusion map. These are shown in Fig. 2. We show slices from subject 7, where there is extreme artifact; and subject 4, with less severe artifact. Subsequently we perform quantitative validation by calculating the PSNR for each denoising method, again calculated relative to the gold standard[1].

Often, outlier filtering is performed as a separate step prior to denoising; so we also compare against TGV and voxelwise fitting with explicit outlier rejection via z-score filtering [4]. Our validation dataset was chosen such that each subject contains one or more artifact volumes, as identified by z-score filtering on the full dataset. We remove artifact volumes for the reference methods, showing how they would perform in conjunction with z-score filtering. For our joint filter, however, we do not remove the volumes in this comparison, as the purpose of the joint filter was to use the non-artifact information within partially-corrupted images. As before, we evaluate example images from subjects 4 and 7, and then we present quantitative validation over all subjects using PSNR calculations.

3   Results

3.1   Example Images

Figure 2 shows example axial slices from subjects 4 and 7, as well as maps of absolute error. For subject 7, there is a strong hyperintense ring artifact near the front of the brain. Similarly, for subject 4, several artifacts present as extreme

---

[1] $PSNR = 20 \log_{10} (S_{max}/RMSE)$, where S_{max} is the maximum ASL signal over all voxels and $RMSE$ is the root mean square error.

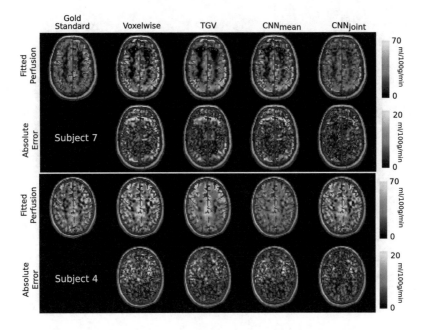

Fig. 2. Example fits and errors, no separate artifact filtering step.

intensity changes, mostly near the edges of the brain. Voxelwise fitting shows these most plainly in both subjects, as the fitting has no implicit artifact removal. TGV results in heavily smoothed images, removing some of the artifact seen in the voxelwise images, but also losing detail in the image. CNN mean-only smooths away even more spatial detail than TGV, and shows a similar pattern of artifact to voxelwise fitting. However, the joint filter produces a significantly less artifact-prone image, as well as improved denoising.

Figure 3 shows example axial slices for subjects 4 and 7 again, this time pre-processed with artifact removal as a separate step. This is a more realistic comparison – certainly for voxelwise smoothing, which has no built-in artifact rejection. Here, the mean-only CNN performs closer to the joint CNN, although the joint CNN continues to produce visibly better denoising. Moreover, the remaining artifacts have been better removed by the joint CNN, despite the joint CNN being the only method to have no explicit artifact rejection before fitting.

3.2 Quantitative Evaluation via PSNR

Figure 4 shows the PSNR for each subject and method, when there is no explicit artifact filtering. Because there are relatively few ASL images, and there is large inter-subject variability in the artifacts and global perfusion, PSNR varies greatly across subjects. To assist comparison between methods, Fig. 4 shows change in PSNR relative to voxelwise fitting for each subject. The joint CNN produces the best result in all subjects except subject 15, where TGV performs marginally

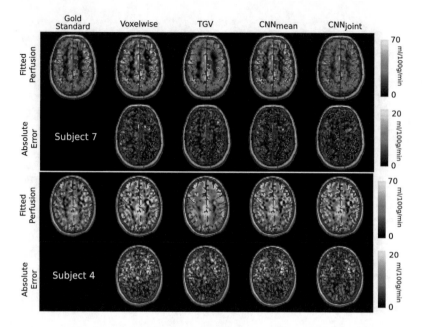

Fig. 3. Example fits and errors, separate artifact filtering performed before fitting.

better. The average per-subject improvement of the joint CNN over TGV is 1.25 dB ($p < 0.01$), although for some subjects with extreme artifact the improvement can be as high as 6 dB. Crucially, while the mean-only CNN is often worse than TGV, the joint filter outperforms it significantly ($p < 0.05$ for each) in 11/15 subjects, marginally in 3/15 subjects, and is marginally worse (0.72 dB, $p = 0.07$) only in subject 15. Although joint filtering does not always produce significantly better results than the mean-only CNN, it is significantly better than the mean-only CNN ($p < 0.05$) in nine subjects.

Figure 5 shows the PSNR for each subject and each method, when there is an explicit artifact filtering step as described in Sect. 2.3. Joint filtering again performs the best, always better than or comparable to the runner-up. Joint filtering is significantly ($p < 0.05$) better than TGV in 13/15 subjects, and marginally superior in subjects 9 and 13. The average improvement over TGV per subject is 1.64 dB ($p < 0.001$). Moreover, the second-best method is typically the mean-only CNN – with this explicit filtering step, even the mean-only CNN consistently outperforms TGV filtering ($p < 0.05$ for 12/15 subjects). This is reasonable: when there is less artifact influence, temporal information is less important and the problem becomes one of spatial regularisation, where CNNs excel. Additionally, TGV often performs worse than voxelwise fitting – over-regularising the fits based on the scarce data remaining after filtering.

4   Discussion and Conclusions

As demonstrated by the visible improvements in image quality (Fig. 2) and the significant increase in PSNR (Fig. 4), our joint filtering approach performs better than state of the art for denoising in the presence of artifact. Of particular note is the filter's strong performance in artifact removal – in subject 7, for example, a prominent edge artifact is removed completely from the output image without any appreciable drop in denoising. The superior performance of the joint filter, compared with a mean-only CNN, shows the value in providing temporal variance information when processing artifact-prone data.

Compared with pipelines involving separate filtering and denoising, our method again outperforms state of the art (Figs. 3 and 5). By retaining parts of a corrupted volume, more information can be used in denoising, meaning the joint filter performs better than mean-only CNN filtering in most subjects. This is evidence the joint filter is able to perform better, on average, than combining a simpler CNN approach with explicit artifact filtering. Moreover, even the mean-only CNN is itself an advance on state of the art: this approach outperforms TGV in 12/15 subjects when filtering is applied separately.

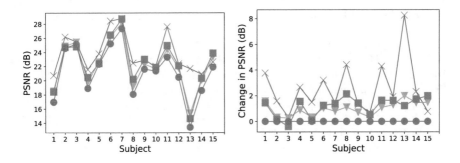

Fig. 4. PSNR for each subject and method, no separate artifact filtering step. Key: × joint CNN, ▼ mean-only CNN, ■ TGV, ● voxelwise.

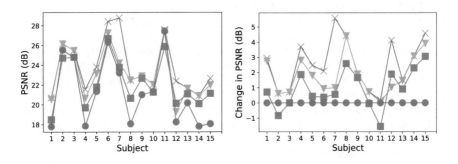

Fig. 5. PSNRs with artifact filtering before denoising as described in Sect. 2.3.

Future work will involve validation across different ASL acquisitions and subject populations, leading the way for use in neuroimaging studies and the clinic. Future work might also explore alternative ways to exploit temporal information, for example through a recurrent-convolutional architecture. More importantly, any method should handle variations in ASL data such as readout and label type. Currently this requires retraining on each new dataset, but it may be possible for a single network to handle these different cases. Finally, a limitation of this work is the necessity for higher-quality data (e.g. more ASL volumes) in a subset of subjects for training; so we wish to explore how cross-validation derived loss functions might ameliorate this. To this end, transfer learning may be helpful to reduce the computational cost of retraining in several cross-validation folds.

The innovative joint approach to denoising and artifact filtering presented here has the potential to substantially increase the quality of ASL images, even salvaging datasets that were previously considered unusable. By fusing temporal variance information with spatial information in a novel network architecture, our deep convolutional joint filter method outperforms state of the art in both denoising and filtering. Our method is applicable to any ASL data, subject to training requirements, and could even be used in other imaging modalities. Consequently, deep convolutional joint filtering presents an exciting future direction for medical image processing in noisy and artifact-prone modalities, and may eventually be used to improve the statistical power of neuroimaging studies.

Acknowledgements. We acknowledge the MRC (MR/J01107X/1), the National Institute for Health Research (NIHR), the EPSRC (EP/H046410/1) and the NIHR University College London Hospitals Biomedical Research Centre (NIHR BRC UCLH/UCL High Impact Initiative BW.mn.BRC10269). The Wellcome Trust (210182/Z/18/Z, 101957/Z/13/Z), the EPSRC (NS/A000027/1). This work is supported by the EPSRC-funded UCL Centre for Doctoral Training in Medical Imaging (EP/L016478/1) and the Wolfson Foundation.

References

1. Alsop, D., et al.: Recommended implementation of arterial spin-labeled perfusion MRI for clinical applications. MRM **73**(1), 102–116 (2015)
2. Spann, S., Kazimierski, K., Aigner, C., et al.: Spatio-temporal TGV denoising for ASL perfusion imaging. Neuroimage **157**, 81–96 (2017)
3. Owen, D., et al.: Anatomy-driven modelling of spatial correlation for regularisation of arterial spin labelling images. In: Descoteaux, M., et al. (eds.) MICCAI 2017. LNCS, vol. 10434, pp. 190–197. Springer, Cham (2017). https://doi.org/10.1007/978-3-319-66185-8_22
4. Tan, H., Maldjian, J.A., Pollock, J.M., et al.: A fast, effective filtering method for improving clinical pulsed arterial spin labeling MRI. JMRI **29**(5), 1134–1139 (2009)
5. Wang, Z.: Improving cerebral blood flow quantification for arterial spin labeled perfusion MRI by removing residual motion artifacts and global signal fluctuations. MRM **30**(10), 1409–1415 (2012)

6. Shirzadi, Z., Crane, D.E., Robertson, A.D., et al.: Automated removal of spurious intermediate cerebral blood flow volumes improves image quality among older patients: a clinical arterial spin labeling investigation. MRM **42**(5), 1377–1385 (2015)
7. Tanenbaum, A.B., Snyder, A.Z., Brier, M.R., et al.: A method for reducing the effects of motion contamination in arterial spin labeling MRI. J. Cereb. Blood Flow Metab. **35**(10), 1697–1702 (2015)
8. Li, Y., Huang, J.B., Narendra, A., Yang, M.H.: Deep joint image filtering. In: European Conference on Computer Vision (2016)
9. Buxton, R., et al.: A general kinetic model for quantitative perfusion imaging with arterial spin labeling. MRM **40**(3), 383–396 (1998)
10. Kim, K.H., Choi, S.H., Park, S.H.: Improving arterial spin labeling by using deep. Radiology **287**, 171154 (2017)

DeepASL: Kinetic Model Incorporated Loss for Denoising Arterial Spin Labeled MRI via Deep Residual Learning

Cagdas Ulas[1]([⊠]), Giles Tetteh[1], Stephan Kaczmarz[2], Christine Preibisch[2], and Bjoern H. Menze[1]

[1] Department of Computer Science,
Technische Universität München, Munich, Germany
cagdas.ulas@tum.de
[2] Department of Neuroradiology,
Technische Universität München, Munich, Germany

Abstract. Arterial spin labeling (ASL) allows to quantify the cerebral blood flow (CBF) by magnetic labeling of the arterial blood water. ASL is increasingly used in clinical studies due to its noninvasiveness, repeatability and benefits in quantification. However, ASL suffers from an inherently low-signal-to-noise ratio (SNR) requiring repeated measurements of control/spin-labeled (C/L) pairs to achieve a reasonable image quality, which in return increases motion sensitivity. This leads to clinically prolonged scanning times increasing the risk of motion artifacts. Thus, there is an immense need of advanced imaging and processing techniques in ASL. In this paper, we propose a novel deep learning based approach to improve the perfusion-weighted image quality obtained from a subset of all available pairwise C/L subtractions. Specifically, we train a deep fully convolutional network (FCN) to learn a mapping from noisy perfusion-weighted image and its subtraction (residual) from the clean image. Additionally, we incorporate the CBF estimation model in the loss function during training, which enables the network to produce high quality images while simultaneously enforcing the CBF estimates to be as close as reference CBF values. Extensive experiments on synthetic and clinical ASL datasets demonstrate the effectiveness of our method in terms of improved ASL image quality, accurate CBF parameter estimation and considerably small computation time during testing.

1 Introduction

Arterial spin labeling (ASL) is a promising MRI technique that allows quantitative measurement of cerebral blood flow (CBF) in the brain and other body organs. ASL-based CBF shows a great promise as a biomarker for many neurological diseases such as stroke and dementia, where perfusion is impaired, and thereby the blood flow alterations need to be investigated [2]. ASL has been increasingly used in clinical studies since it is completely non-invasive and uses

© Springer Nature Switzerland AG 2018
A. F. Frangi et al. (Eds.): MICCAI 2018, LNCS 11070, pp. 30–38, 2018.
https://doi.org/10.1007/978-3-030-00928-1_4

magnetically labeled blood water as an endogenous tracer where the tagging is done through inversion radio-frequency (RF) pulses [2,12]. In ASL, a perfusion-weighted image is obtained by subtracting a label image from a control image in which no inversion pulse is applied. The difference reflects the perfusion, which can be quantified via appropriate modelling [2,11].

Despite its advantages, ASL significantly suffers from several limitations including the low signal-to-noise ratio (SNR), poor temporal resolution and volume coverage in conventional acquisitions [5]. Among these limitations, the low SNR is the most critical one, necessitating numerous repetitions to achieve accurate perfusion measurements. However, this leads to impractical long scanning time especially in multiple inversion time (multi-TI) ASL acquisitions with increased susceptibility to motion artifacts [2,9,12].

To alleviate this limitation, several groups have proposed spatial and spatio-temporal denoising techniques, for instance denoising in the wavelet domain [3], denoising in the image domain using adaptive filtering [13], non-local means filtering combined with wavelet filtering [10], spatio-temporal low-rank total variation [5], and spatio-temporal total generalized variation [12]. Just recently, a deep learning based ASL denoising method [9] has been shown to produce compelling results. All of these methods primarily consider improving the quality of noisy perfusion-weighted images, followed by CBF parameter estimation as a separate step although accurate quantification of CBF is the main objective in ASL imaging.

In this paper, unlike the previous deep learning work [9] which is only data driven, we follow a mixed modeling approach in our denoising scheme. In particular, we demonstrate the benefit of incorporating a formal representation of the underlying process – a CBF signal model – as a prior knowledge in our deep learning model. We propose a novel deep learning based framework to improve the perfusion-weighted image quality obtained by using a lower number of subtracted control/label pairs. First, as our main contribution, we design a custom loss function where we incorporate the Buxton kinetic model [4] for CBF estimation as a separate loss term, and utilize it when training our network. Second, we specifically train a deep fully-convolutional neural network (CNN) adopting the residual learning strategy [7]. Third, we use the images from various noise levels to train a single CNN model. Therefore, the trained model can be utilized to denoise a test perfusion-weighted image without estimating its noise level. Finally, we demonstrate the superior performance of our method by validations using synthetic and clinical ASL datasets. Our proposed method may facilitate scan time reduction, making ASL more applicable in clinical scan protocols.

2 Methods

2.1 Arterial Spin Labeling

In ASL, arterial blood water is employed as an endogenous diffusible tracer by inverting the magnetization of inflowing arterial blood in the neck area by using RF pulses. After a delay for allowing the labeled blood to perfuse into the brain, label and control images are repeatedly acquired with and without tagging respectively [2,11]. The signal difference between control and label images is proportional to the underlying perfusion [2]. The difference images are known as perfusion-weighted images (ΔM), and can be directly used to fit a kinetic model. For CBF quantification in a single inversion-time (TI) ASL, the single-compartment kinetic model (so-called Buxton model [4]) is generally used. According to this model, the CBF in ml/100g/min can be calculated in every individual voxel for pseudo-continuous ASL (pCASL) acquisitions as follows,

$$f(\Delta M) = \text{CBF} = \frac{6000 \cdot \beta \cdot \Delta M \cdot e^{\frac{PLD}{T_{1b}}}}{2 \cdot \alpha \cdot T_{1b} \cdot \text{SI}_{\text{PD}} \cdot \left(1 - e^{-\frac{\tau}{T_{1b}}}\right)}, \tag{1}$$

where β is the brain-blood partition coefficient, T_{1b} is the longitudinal relaxation time of blood, α is the labeling efficiency, τ is the label duration, PLD is the post-label delay, and SI_{PD} is the proton density weighted image [2].

2.2   Deep Residual Learning for ASL Denoising

Formulation. Our proposed CNN model adopts the residual learning formulation [7,8]. It is assumed that the task of learning a residual mapping is much easier and more efficient than original unreferenced mapping [14]. With the utilization of a residual learning strategy, extremely deep CNN can be trained and superior results have been achieved for object detection [7] and image denoising [14] tasks.

The input of our CNN model is a noisy perfusion-weighted image ΔM_n that is obtained by averaging a small number of pairwise C/L subtractions. We denote a complete perfusion-weighted image as ΔM_c estimated by averaging all available C/L subtractions. We can relate the noisy and complete perfusion-weighted image as $\Delta M_n = \Delta M_c + N$, where N denotes the noise image which degrades the quality of the complete image. Following the residual learning strategy, our CNN model aims to learn a mapping between ΔM_n and N to produce an estimate of the residual image $\tilde{N}$; $\tilde{N} = \mathcal{R}(\Delta M_n | \Theta)$, where $\mathcal{R}$ corresponds to the forward mapping of the CNN parameterised by trained network weights Θ. The final estimate of the complete image is obtained by $\Delta \tilde{M}_c = \Delta M_n - \tilde{N}$.

Loss Function Design. In this work, we design a custom loss function to simultaneously control the quality of the denoised image and the fidelity of CBF estimates with respect to reference CBF values. Concretely, given a set of training samples $\mathcal{D}$ of input-target pairs (ΔM_n, N), a CNN model is trained to learn the residual mapping $\mathcal{R}$ for accurate estimation of complete image by minimizing the following cost function,

$$\mathcal{L}(\Theta) = \sum_{(\Delta M_n, N) \in \mathcal{D}} \lambda \|N - \tilde{N}\|_2^2 + (1 - \lambda)\|f_t - f(\Delta M_n - \tilde{N}; \xi)\|_2^2, \tag{2}$$

where λ is regularization parameter controlling the trade-off between the fidelity of the residual image and CBF parameter estimates, f_t represents the reference

CBF values corresponding to an input ΔM_n, and ξ denotes all predetermined variables as given in (1). We emphasize that the second term of our loss function (2) explicitly enforces the consistency of CBF estimates with respect to reference CBF values, computed from the complete perfusion-weighted image through the use of the Buxton kinetic model. This integrates the image denoising and CBF parameter estimation steps into a single pipeline allowing the network to generate better estimates of perfusion-weighted images by reducing noise and artifacts.

Network Architecture. Figure 1 depicts the architecture of our network. The network takes 2D noisy gray image patches as input and residual image patches as output. Our network consists of eight consecutive 2D convolutional layers followed by parametric rectified linear units (PReLU) activation. Although ReLU activation has been reported to achieve good performance in denoising tasks [9, 14], we empirically obtained better results on our ASL dataset using PReLU in which negative activation is allowed through a small non-zero coefficient that can be adaptively learned during training [6]. The number of filters in every convolutional layer is set to 48 with a filter size of 3×3. Following eight consecutive layers, we apply one last convolutional layer without any activation function. The last layer only includes one convolutional filter, and its output is considered as the estimated residual image patch.

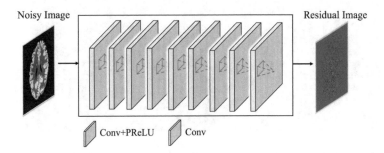

Fig. 1. The architecture of the proposed network used for the estimation of a residual image from the noisy perfusion-weighted image given as input.

Training. Training was performed using 18000 noisy and residual patch pairs of size 40×40. The network was trained using the Adam optimizer with a learning rate of 10^{-4} for 200 epochs and mini-batch size of 500. We trained a single CNN model for denoising the noisy input images from different noise levels. Inference on test data was also performed in a patch-wise manner.

3   Experiments and Results

Datasets. Pseudo-continuous ASL (pCASL) images were acquired from 5 healthy subjects on a 3T MR scanner with a 2D EPI readout using the following acquisition parameters (TR/TE = 5000/14.6 ms, flip angle = $90°$, voxel size $= 2.7 \times 2.7 \times 5$ mm^3, matrix size $= 128 \times 128$, 17 slices, labeling duration $(\tau) = 1800$ ms, post-label delay $(PLD) = 1600$ ms). 30 C/L pairs and one SI$_{PD}$ image were acquired for each subject.

Additionally, high resolution synthetic ASL image datasets were generated for each real subject based on the acquired SI$_{PD}$ and coregistered white-matter (WM) and grey-matter (GM) partial volume content maps. To create a ground-truth CBF map, we assigned the CBF values of 20 and 65 mL/100g/min to the WM and GM voxels respectively, as reported in [12]. To generate synthetic data with a realistic noise level, the standard deviation over 30 repetitions was estimated from the acquired C/L images for each voxel. We subsequently added Gaussian noise with estimated standard deviation to each voxel of the synthetic images. This step was repeated 100 times to create a synthetic data per subject containing 100 C/L pairs. For synthetic data, we set $\tau = 1600$ ms and $PLD = 2200$ ms. All the other constant variables in (1) were fixed based on the recommended values for pCASL given in [2].

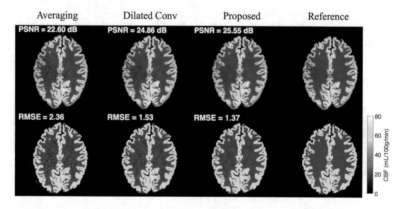

Fig. 2. Visual comparison of denoising results (top) and resulting CBF maps (bottom) on an examplary synthetic data using 20% of 100 pairwise subtractions. Corresponding PSNR and RMSE values calculated with respect to references are also displayed at top-left corner of each image estimate. The proposed method can yield the best results both qualitatively and quantitatively.

Data Preprocessing. Prior to training the network, the standard preprocessing steps (motion correction, co-registration, Gaussian smoothing with 4 mm kernel size) [2] were applied on C/L pairs using our in-house toolbox implementation for ASL analysis. The top and bottom slices of each subject were removed from the analysis due to excessive noise caused by motion correction.

Data augmentation was applied on every 2D image slices using rigid transformations. After augmentation, every image was divided into non-overlapping 2D patches of size 40×40, leading to 5440 patches per subject. This process was repeated for input, target, and other variables required for network training.

For each subject, we consider four different noise levels obtained by averaging randomly selected 20%, 40%, 60% and 80% of all available C/L repetitions, all of which were used during training and also tested on the trained network.

Experimental Setup. All experiments were performed using the leave-one-subject-out fashion. The synthetic and in-vivo models were trained and tested separately. In order to show the benefit of our proposed method, we compare it with the recent deep learning based denoising method [9] for ASL. Throughout the paper we refer to this method as *Dilated Conv*. For this network we use exactly same dilation rates and number of filters as suggested in the paper, and evaluate it using mean-squared-error (MSE) loss during training. We employ the peak signal-to-noise ratio (PSNR) to quantitatively assess the quality of image denoising, and the root-mean-squared error (RMSE) and Lin's concordance correlation coefficient (CCC) to assess the accuracy of CBF parameter estimation. We run the experiments on a NVIDIA GeForce Titan Xp GPU, and our code was implemented using Keras library with TensorFlow [1] backend.

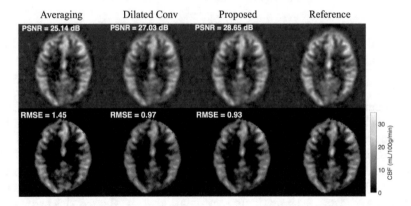

Fig. 3. Visual comparison of denoising results (top) and resulting CBF maps (bottom) on an examplary real data using 40% of 30 pairwise subtractions. Although the estimated images qualitatively look similar, the quantitative metrics calculated inside the brain demonstrates the better performance of the proposed method.

Results. Figure 2 demonstrates the denoised images and corresponding CBF maps of an exemplary slice of a synthetic dataset. Here, only 20% of 100 synthetic C/L subtractions were used. Our proposed model produces the highest quality perfusion-weighted images where noise inside the brain is significantly removed compared to conventional averaging. The resulting CBF map of our proposed method is also closer to the reference CBF map yielding the lowest RMSE score.

In Fig. 3 we present the qualitative results from a real subject's data using 40% of 30 C/L subtractions. Although the proposed method achieves the best PSNR and RMSE for perfusion-weighted image and CBF map respectively, the improvement against conventional averaging is less apparent compared to the

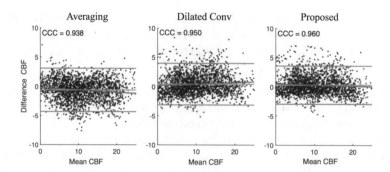

Fig. 4. Bland-Altman plots of different methods obtained in a grey-matter region of a real subject's data. Differences in CBF (y-axis) between the reference and compared method is plotted against the mean (x-axis) values of the two. The unit for horizontal and vertical axes are in ml/100g/min. Solid green lines indicate mean difference. Solid gray lines at top and bottom correspond to upper and lower margins of 95% limits of agreement. Linear regression lines are also shown with red solid lines. Corresponding CCC values are displayed at top-left corner of each plot.

synthetic data. The underlying reason is that as it can be clearly seen in Fig. 3, our reference perfusion-weighted images obtained by averaging all 30 C/L subtractions still suffer from significant noise and artifacts. Since we train our network using these images as target, the network cannot produce results that show better quality beyond the reference images. The Dilated Conv method also faces similar problem for real data. Figure 4 depicts the Bland-Altman plots of CBF values in GM tissue obtained from different methods using a real subject's data. The plots indicate that our proposed method can yield better fidelity of CBF estimation with smaller bias (green solid line) and variance (difference between solid grey lines). The linear regression line (solid red) fitted in the averaging method also shows a systematic underestimation error whereas this error is considerably reduced by the proposed method where the regression line is closer to a straight line, $y = 0$. Note that all three methods contain outlier voxels caused due to excessive noise and artifacts observable in most of the C/L subtractions.

We also quantitatively compare the predicted results in Table 1 in terms of PSNR, RMSE and CCC. Our proposed method outperforms other competing methods in all the metrics when either $\lambda = 0.2$ or $\lambda = 0.5$, which further demonstrates the advantage of the incorporation of CBF estimation model in denoising step. Taking into account data from all subjects, the differences between PR-$\lambda = 0.2$ and the Dilated Conv method on synthetic dataset are statistically significant with $p \ll 0.05$ for all metrics. The differences are also statistically significant on real dataset for PSNR and RMSE, but not significant for CCC with $p = 0.1388$. Finally, we emphasize that image denoising using our trained network takes approximately 5 ms on a single slice of matrix size 128×128.

Table 1. Quantitative evaluation in terms of *mean(std)* obtained by different methods using all the subjects for synthetic and real datasets. The best performances are highlighted in bold font. All the metric values are calculated inside the brain region. Note that PR-$\lambda = x$ denotes our proposed method when λ value is set to x.

Method	Synthetic dataset			Real dataset		
	PSNR	RMSE	CCC	PSNR	RMSE	CCC
Averaging	20.3(4.81)	2.20(2.51)	0.88(0.06)	23.6(6.16)	1.49(0.80)	0.85(0.07)
Dilated Conv	25.2(5.09)	1.48(1.06)	0.93(0.05)	24.2(5.90)	1.41(0.72)	0.87(0.06)
PR-$\lambda = 0.2$	**28.0(3.82)**	**1.33(0.79)**	**0.95(0.04)**	**25.1(5.36)**	**1.37(0.65)**	**0.88(0.05)**
PR-$\lambda = 0.5$	26.9(4.23)	1.40(0.84)	**0.95(0.04)**	24.3(5.35)	1.38(0.67)	**0.88(0.06)**
PR-$\lambda = 0.7$	25.6(6.07)	1.51(1.76)	0.94(0.06)	24.0(5.39)	1.39(0.69)	**0.88(0.06)**
PR-$\lambda = 1.0$	25.3(5.62)	1.49(1.56)	0.93(0.05)	23.9(6.00)	1.42(0.70)	0.87(0.06)

4   Conclusion

We have proposed a novel deep learning based method for denoising ASL images. In particular, we utilize the Buxton kinetic model for CBF parameter estimation as a separate loss term where the agreement with reference CBF values is simultaneously enforced on the denoised perfusion-weighted images. Furthermore, we adopt the residual learning strategy on a deep FCN which is trained to learn a single model for denosing images from different noise levels. We have validated the efficacy of our method on synthetic and in-vivo pCASL datasets. Future work will aim at extending our work to perform denoising on multi-TI ASL data where the estimation of the arterial transit time (ATT) parameter can be also exploited in the loss function.

Acknowledgements. The research leading to these results has received funding from the European Unions H2020 Framework Programme (H2020-MSCA-ITN- 2014) under grant agreement no 642685 MacSeNet. We gratefully acknowledge the support of NVIDIA Corporation with the donation of the Titan Xp GPU used for this research.

References

1. Abadi, M., et al.: TensorFlow: large-scale machine learning on heterogeneous systems (2015). https://www.tensorflow.org/, software available from tensorflow.org
2. Alsop, D.C.: Recommended implementation of arterial spin-labeled perfusion MRI for clinical applications: a consensus of the ISMRM perfusion study group and the European consortium for ASL in dementia. MRM **73**(1), 102–116 (2015)
3. Bibic, A., et al.: Denoising of arterial spin labeling data: wavelet-domain filtering compared with gaussian smoothing. MAGMA **23**(3), 125–137 (2010)
4. Buxton, R.B., et al.: A general kinetic model for quantitative perfusion imaging with arterial spin labeling. MRM **40**(3), 383–396 (1998)
5. Fang, R., et al.: A spatio-temporal low-rank total variation approach for denoising arterial spin labeling MRI data. In: IEEE ISBI, pp. 498–502, April 2015
6. He, K., et al.: Delving deep into rectifiers: surpassing human-level performance on imagenet classification. In: IEEE ICCV, pp. 1026–1034, December 2015

7. He, K., et al.: Deep residual learning for image recognition. In: IEEE CVPR, pp. 770–778, June 2016
8. Kiku, D., et al.: Residual interpolation for color image demosaicking. In: IEEE ICIP, pp. 2304–2308, September 2013
9. Kim, K.H., et al.: Improving arterial spin labeling by using deep learning. Radiology **287**(2), 658–666 (2018)
10. Liang, X.: Voxel-wise functional connectomics using arterial spin labeling functional magnetic resonance imaging: the role of denoising. Brain Connect. **5**(9), 543–53 (2015)
11. Owen, D., et al.: Anatomy-driven modelling of spatial correlation for regularisation of arterial spin labelling images. In: Descoteaux, M., et al. (eds.) MICCAI 2017. LNCS, vol. 10434, pp. 190–197. Springer, Cham (2017). https://doi.org/10.1007/978-3-319-66185-8_22
12. Spann, S.M., et al.: Spatio-temporal TGV denoising for ASL perfusion imaging. Neuroimage **157**, 81–96 (2017)
13. Wells, J.A., et al.: Reduction of errors in ASL cerebral perfusion and arterial transit time maps using image de-noising. MRM **64**(3), 715–724 (2010)
14. Zhang, K.: Beyond a gaussian denoiser: residual learning of deep CNN for image denoising. IEEE Trans. Image Process. **26**(7), 3142–3155 (2017)

Direct Estimation of Pharmacokinetic Parameters from DCE-MRI Using Deep CNN with Forward Physical Model Loss

Cagdas Ulas[1]($\boxtimes$), Giles Tetteh[1], Michael J. Thrippleton[2], Paul A. Armitage[4],
Stephen D. Makin[2], Joanna M. Wardlaw[2], Mike E. Davies[3],
and Bjoern H. Menze[1]

[1] Department of Computer Science, Technische Universität München,
Munich, Germany
cagdas.ulas@tum.de
[2] Department of Neuroimaging Sciences, University of Edinburgh, Edinburgh, UK
[3] Institute for Digital Communications, University of Edinburgh, Edinburgh, UK
[4] Department of Cardiovascular Sciences, University of Sheffield, Sheffield, UK

Abstract. Dynamic contrast-enhanced (DCE) MRI is an evolving imaging technique that provides a quantitative measure of pharmacokinetic (PK) parameters in body tissues, in which series of T_1-weighted images are collected following the administration of a paramagnetic contrast agent. Unfortunately, in many applications, conventional clinical DCE-MRI suffers from low spatiotemporal resolution and insufficient volume coverage. In this paper, we propose a novel deep learning based approach to directly estimate the PK parameters from undersampled DCE-MRI data. Specifically, we design a custom loss function where we incorporate a forward physical model that relates the PK parameters to corrupted image-time series obtained due to subsampling in k-space. This allows the network to directly exploit the knowledge of true contrast agent kinetics in the training phase, and hence provide more accurate restoration of PK parameters. Experiments on clinical brain DCE datasets demonstrate the efficacy of our approach in terms of fidelity of PK parameter reconstruction and significantly faster parameter inference compared to a model-based iterative reconstruction method.

1 Introduction

Dynamic contrast-enhanced (DCE) MRI involves the administration of a T_1-shortening Gadolinium-based contrast agent (CA), followed by the acquisition of successive T_1-weighted images as the contrast bolus enters and subsequently leaves the organ [9]. In DCE-MRI, changes in CA concentration are derived from changes in signal intensity over time, then regressed to estimate pharmacokinetic (PK) parameters related to vascular permeability and tissue perfusion [6]. Since perfusion and permeability are typically affected in the presence of vascular and

© Springer Nature Switzerland AG 2018
A. F. Frangi et al. (Eds.): MICCAI 2018, LNCS 11070, pp. 39–47, 2018.
https://doi.org/10.1007/978-3-030-00928-1_5

cellular irregularities, DCE imaging has been considered as a promising tool for clinical diagnostics of brain tumours, multiple sclerosis lesions, and neurological disorders where disruption of blood-brain barrier (BBB) occurs [4,7].

Despite its effectiveness in quantitative assessment of microvascular properties, conventional DCE-MRI is challenged by suboptimal image acquisition that severely restricts the spatiotemporal resolution and volume coverage [2,3]. The shortest possible scanning time often leads to limited spatial resolution hampering detection of small image features and accurate tumor boundaries. Low temporal resolution hinders accurate fitting of PK parameters. Furthermore, volume coverage is usually inadequate to cover the known pathology, for instance in the case multiple metastatic lesions [3]. Facing such severe constraints, DCE imaging can significantly benefit from undersampled acquisitions.

So far, existing works in [2,6,11] have proposed compressed sensing and parallel imaging based reconstruction schemes to accelerate DCE-MRI acquisitions, mainly targeting to achieve better spatial resolution and volume coverage while retaining the same temporal resolution. These methods are referred to as indirect methods [3] because they are based on the reconstruction of dynamic DCE image series first, followed by a separate step for fitting the PK parameters on a voxel-by-voxel level using a tracer kinetic model [9]. More recently, a model-based direct reconstruction model [3] has been proposed to directly estimate PK parameters from undersampled (k, t) space data. The direct reconstruction method generally poses the estimation of PK maps as an error minimization problem. This approach has been shown to produce superior PK parameter maps and allows for higher acceleration compared to indirect methods. However, the main drawback of this method is that parameter reconstruction of an entire volume requires considerably high computation time.

Motivated by the recent advances of deep learning in medical imaging, in this paper, we present a novel deep learning based approach to directly estimate PK parameters from undersampled DCE-MRI data. First, our proposed network takes the corrupted image-time series as input and *residual* parameter maps, which represent deviations from a kinetic model fitting on fully-sampled image-time series, as output, and aims at learning a nonlinear mapping between them. Our motivation for learning the *residual* PK maps is based on the observation that residual maps are more sparse and topologically less complex compared to target parameter maps. Second, we propose the *forward physical model loss*, a custom loss function in which we exploit the physical relation between true contrast agent kinetics and measured time-resolved DCE signals when training our network. Third, we validate our method experimentally on human *in vivo* brain DCE-MRI dataset. We demonstrate the superior performance of our method in terms of parameter reconstruction accuracy and significantly faster estimation of parameters during testing, taking approximately 1.5 s on an entire 3D test volume. To the best of our knowledge, we present the first work leveraging the machine learning algorithms – specifically deep learning – to directly estimate PK parameters from undersampled DCE-MRI time-series.

2   Methods

We treat the parameter inference from undersampled data in DCE imaging as a mapping problem between the corrupted intensity-time series and *residual* parameter maps where the underlying mapping is learned using deep convolutional neural networks (CNNs). We provide a summary of general tracer kinetic models applied in DCE-MRI in Sect. 2.1, formulate the forward physical model relating the PK parameters to undersampled data in Sect. 2.2, finally describe our proposed deep learning methodology for PK parameter inference in Sect. 2.3.

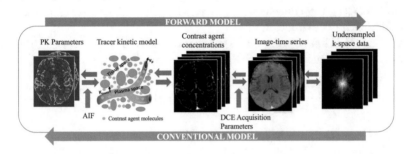

Fig. 1. Computational steps in the forward model and the conventional pipeline of PK parameter estimation in DCE-MRI.

2.1   Tracer Kinetic Modeling in DCE-MRI

Tracer kinetic modeling aims at providing a link between the tissue signal enhancement and the physiological or so-called pharmacokinetic parameters, including the fractional plasma volume (v_p), the fractional interstitial volume (v_e), and the volume transfer rate (K^{trans}) at which contrast agent (CA) is delivered to the extravascular extracellular space (EES). One of the well-established tracer kinetic models is known as Patlak model [8]. This model describes a highly perfused two compartment tissue, ignoring backflux from the EES into the blood plasma compartment. The CA concentration in the tissues is determined by,

$$C(\mathbf{r}, t) = v_p(\mathbf{r})C_p(t) + K^{trans}(\mathbf{r}) \int_0^t C_p(\tau)d\tau, \tag{1}$$

where $\mathbf{r} \in (x, y, z)$ represent image domain spatial coordinates, $C(\mathbf{r}, t)$ is the CA concentration over time, and $C_p(t)$ denotes the arterial input function (AIF) which is usually measured from voxels in a feeding artery.

In this work, we specifically employ the Patlak model for tracer pharmacokinetic modeling and estimation of ground truth tissue parameters. This model is a perfect match for our DCE dataset because it is often applied when the temporal resolution is too low to measure the cerebral blood flow, and it has been commonly used to measure the BBB leakage with DCE-MRI in acute brain stroke and dementia [4,9]. An attractive feature of Patlak model is that the model equation in (1) can be linearized and fitted using linear least squares which has a closed-form solution, hence parameter estimation is fast [9].

2.2 Forward Physical Model: From PK Parameters to Undersampled Data

Figure 1 depicts the conventional and forward model approaches relating the PK parameter estimation to undersampled or fully-sampled k-space data, and vice versa. For direct estimation of PK parameters from the measured k-space data, as proposed in [1,3], a forward model can be formulated by inverting the steps in the conventional model as follows:

1. Given the sets of PK parameter pairs $(K^{\text{trans}}(\mathbf{r}), v_p(\mathbf{r}))$ and arterial input function $C_p(t)$, CA concentration curves over time $C(\mathbf{r}, t)$ are estimated using the Patlak model equation in (1).
2. Dynamic DCE image series $S(\mathbf{r}, t)$ are converted to $C(\mathbf{r}, t)$ through the steady-state spoiled gradient echo (SGPR) signal equation [3], given by

$$S(\mathbf{r}, t) = \frac{M_0(\mathbf{r})\sin\alpha(1 - e^{-(K+L)})}{1 - \cos\alpha e^{-(K+L)}} + \left(S(\mathbf{r}, 0) - \frac{M_0(\mathbf{r})\sin\alpha(1 - e^{-K})}{1 - \cos\alpha e^{-K}}\right) \quad (2)$$

where $K = T_R/T_{10}(\mathbf{r})$, $L = r_1 C(\mathbf{r}, t)T_R$, T_R is the repetition time, α is the flip angle, r_1 is the contrast agent relaxivity taken as $4.2 \text{ s}^{-1}\text{mM}^{-1}$, $S(\mathbf{r}, 0)$ is the baseline (pre-contrast) image intensity, and $T_{10}(\mathbf{r})$ and $M_0(\mathbf{r})$ are respectively the T_1 relaxation and equilibrium longitudinal magnetization that are calculated from a pre-contrast T_1 mapping acquisition.
3. The undersampled raw (k, t)-space data $S(\mathbf{k}, t)$ can be related to $S(\mathbf{r}, t)$ for a single-coil data by an undersampling fast Fourier transform (FFT), F_u,

$$S(\mathbf{k}, t) = F_u S(\mathbf{r}, t), \quad (3)$$

where $\mathbf{k} \in (k_x, k_y, k_z)$ represents k-space coordinates.

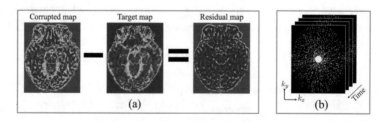

Fig. 2. (a) The relation between a corrupted (θ_u), target (θ_t) and residual (θ_r) PK maps, (b) Exemplary golden-angle sampling scheme in the k_x-k_y plane through time.

By simply integrating the three computation steps in (1–3), we can form a single function f_m modeling the signal evolution in (k-t) space given the PK maps $\theta = \{K^{\text{trans}}(\mathbf{r}), v_p(\mathbf{r})\}$, as $S(\mathbf{k}, t) = f_m(\theta; \boldsymbol{\xi})$, where $\boldsymbol{\xi}$ denotes all the predetermined acquisition parameters as mentioned above.

Given the undersampled (k,t)-space data $S(\mathbf{k}, t)$, the corrupted image series $S_u(\mathbf{r}, t)$ can be obtained by applying IFFT to $S(\mathbf{k}, t)$, i.e. $S_u(\mathbf{r}, t) = F_u^{\mathsf{T}} S(\mathbf{k}, t)$. We further define a new function $\tilde{\boldsymbol{f}}_m$ that integrates only the first two computation steps (1–2) to compute the dynamic DCE image series. We will incorporate $\tilde{\boldsymbol{f}}_m$ in our custom loss function that will be explained in the following section.

2.3   PK Parameter Inference via Forward Physical Model Loss

Formulation. We hypothesize that a direct inversion between corrupted PK parameter maps θ_u and $S_u(\mathbf{r}, t)$ is available through forward model, i.e., $S_u(\mathbf{r}, t) = \tilde{\boldsymbol{f}}_m(\theta_u)$. However, this cannot provide yet sufficiently accurate estimate of target parameter maps θ_t obtained from fully-sampled data $S(\mathbf{r}, t)$. To this end, we estimate a correction or residual map θ_r from the available signal $S_u(\mathbf{r}, t)$ satisfying $\theta_r = \theta_u - \theta_t$. As shown in Fig. 2-(a), we observe that *residual* PK maps involve more sparse representations and exhibit spatially less varying structures inside the brain. The task of learning a residual mapping was shown to be much easier and effective than the original mapping [10]. Following the same approach, we adopt the residual learning strategy using deep CNNs. Our CNN is trained to learn a mapping between $S_u(\mathbf{r}, t)$ and θ_r to output an estimate of residual maps $\tilde{\theta}_r$; $\tilde{\theta}_r = \mathcal{R}(S_u(\mathbf{r}, t)|\mathbf{W})$, where $\mathcal{R}$ represents the forward mapping of the CNN parameterised by $\mathbf{W}$. The final parameter estimate is obtained via $\tilde{\theta}_t = \theta_u - \tilde{\theta}_r$.

Loss Function. We simultaneously seek the signal belonging to the corrected model estimates to be sufficiently close to true signal, i.e., $\tilde{\boldsymbol{f}}_m(\tilde{\theta}_t) \approx S(\mathbf{r}, t)$. Therefore, we design a custom loss function which requires solving the forward model in every iteration of the network training. We refer the resulting loss as *forward physical model loss*. Given a set of training samples $\mathcal{D}$ of input-output pairs $(S_u(\mathbf{r}, t), \theta_r)$, we train a CNN model that minimizes the following loss,

$$\mathcal{L}(\mathbf{W}) = \sum_{(S_u(\mathbf{r},t),\theta_r)\in\mathcal{D}} \lambda\|\theta_r - \tilde{\theta}_r\|_2^2 \; + \; (1-\lambda)\|S(\mathbf{r}, t) - \tilde{\boldsymbol{f}}_m(\theta_u - \tilde{\theta}_r; \boldsymbol{\xi})\|_2^2, \quad (4)$$

where λ is a regularization parameter balancing the trade-off between the fidelity of the parameter and signal reconstruction. We emphasize that the second term in (4) allows the network to intrinsically exploit the underlying contrast agent kinetics in training phase.

Network Architecture. Figure 3 illustrates our network architecture. The network takes a 4D image-time series as input, where time frames are stacked as input channels. The first convolutional layer applies 3D filters to each channel individually to extract low-level temporal features which are aggregated over frames via learned filter weights to produce a single output per voxel. Following the first layer, inspired by the work on brain segmentation [5], our network consists of parallel dual pathways to efficiently capture multi-scale information. The local pathway at the top focuses on extracting details from the local vicinity while the global pathway at the bottom is designed to incorporate more contextual global information. The global pathway consists of 4 dilated convolutional layers with dilation factors of $2, 4, 8, 16$, implying increased receptive field sizes. The filter size of each convolutional layer including dilated convolutions is $3 \times 3 \times 3$, and the rectified linear units (ReLU) activation is applied after each convolution. Local and global pathways are then concatenated to form a multi-scale feature set. Following this, 2 fully-connected layers are used to determine the best possible feature combination that can accurately map the input to output of the network. Finally, the last layer outputs the estimated residual maps.

3   Experiments and Results

Datasets. We perform experiments on fully-sampled DCE-MRI datasets acquired from three mild ischaemic stroke patients. DCE image series were acquired using a 1.5 T clinical scanner with a 3D T1W spoiled gradient echo sequence (TR/TE = 8.24/3.1 ms, flip angle = 12°, FOV = 24×24 cm, matrix = 256×192, slice thickness = 4 mm, 73 s temporal resolution, 21 dynamics). An intravenous bolus injection of 0.1 mmol/kg of gadoterate meglumine (Gd-DOTA) was administered simultaneously. The total acquisition time for DCE-MRI was approximately 24 minutes. Two pre-contrast acquisitions were carried out at flip angles of 2° and 12° to calculate pre-contrast longitudinal relaxation times.

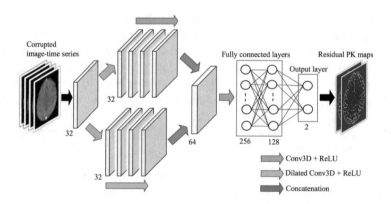

Fig. 3. The network architecture used for the estimation of residual PK maps. The number of filters and output nodes are provided at the bottom of each layer.

Preprocessing. Undersampling was retrospectively applied to the fully-sampled data in the k_x-k_y plane using a randomized golden-angle sampling pattern [12] over time (see Fig. 2-(b)) with a 10-fold undersampling factor. The pre-contrast first frame was fully sampled. Due to the low temporal resolution of our data, we estimated subject-specific vascular input functions (VIFs) extracted by averaging a few voxels located on the superior sagittal sinus where the inflow artefact was reduced compared to a feeding artery [4]. Data augmentation was employed by applying rigid transformations on image slices. We generated random 2D+t undersampling masks to be applied on the images of different orientations. This allows the network to learn diverse patterns of aliasing artifacts. All the subject's data required for network training/testing were divided into non-overlapping 3D blocks of size $52 \times 52 \times 33$, resulting in 64 blocks per subject.

Experimental Setup. All experiments were performed in a leave-one-subject-out fashion. The networks were trained using the Adam optimizer with a learning rate of 10^{-3} (using a decay rate of 10^{-4}) for 300 epochs and mini-batch size of 4. To demonstrate the advantage of the proposed method, we compare it with the state-of-the-art model-based iterative parameter reconstruction method using the MATLAB implementation provided by the authors [3]. We use the concordance correlation coefficient (CCC) and structured similarity metric (SSIM) metrics to quantitatively assess the PK parameter reconstruction, and peak signal-to-noise ratio (PSNR) metric to assess the image reconstruction. Experiments were run on a NVIDIA GeForce Titan Xp GPU with 12 GB RAM.

Results. Figure 4 shows the qualitative PK parameter reconstructions obtained from different methods using 10-fold undersampling. The results indicate that CNN-$\lambda = 0.5$ incorporating two loss terms simultaneously produces better maps and considerably higher SSIM score calculated with respect to fully-sampled PK maps. The model-based iterative reconstruction yields the PK maps where the artifacts caused by undersampling are still observable. In Fig. 5 we present the exemplary reconstructed images obtained by applying the operation $\tilde{f}_m$ to the estimated PK maps. All the reconstruction approaches result in high quality images, however, the model-based reconstruction can better preserve the finer details. Unfortunately, our fully-sampled data suffer from Gibbs artifacts appearing as multiple parallel lines throughout the image. As marked by white arrows, our CNN method can significantly suppress these artifacts whereas they still appear in the image obtained by model-based iterative reconstruction. Finally, Fig. 6 demonstrates the quantitative results of parameter estimation and image reconstruction. The highest CCC and SSIM values for parameter estimation are achieved by our CNN model when both loss terms are incorporated with $\lambda = 0.3$ and $\lambda = 0.5$, yielding an average score of 0.88 and 0.92, respectively. The difference is statistically significant for both CCC ($p = 0.017$) and SSIM ($p = 0.0086$) when compared against model-based reconstruction. The model-based reconstruction performs the highest PSNR for image reconstruction, where it is followed by the proposed CNN with $\lambda = 0.3$. The difference between them is statistically significant with $p \ll 0.05$. The PSNR also shows a decreasing trend with increasing λ as expected.

We emphasize that the parameter inference of our method on a 3D test volume takes around 1.5 s while the model-based method requires around 95 min to reconstruct the same volume, enabling $\approx 4 \times 10^3$ faster computation.

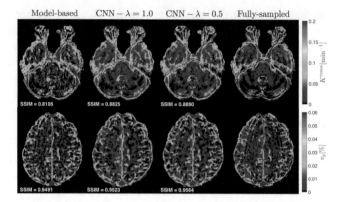

Fig. 4. Reconstructed PK parameter maps of two exemplary slices of a test subject with a 10-fold undersampling. Brain masks are applied to estimated maps. Our CNN model incorporating both loss terms ($\lambda = 0.5$) achieves the best paramater estimates. The resulting SSIM values are provided at the bottom-left corner of each map.

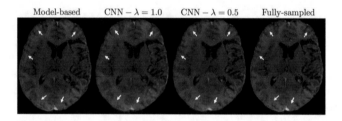

Fig. 5. Visual comparison of the image reconstruction results of an examplary DCE slice. White arrows indicate a few regions where the Gibbs artifacts are observable. Our CNN model with both $\lambda = 0.5$ and 1.0 can significantly suppress the artifacts appearing in fully-sampled image and model-based reconstruction as well.

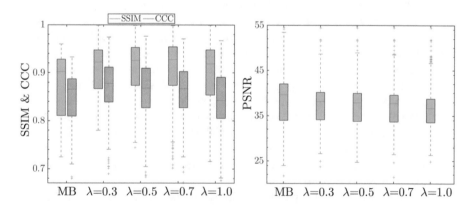

Fig. 6. Parameter estimation (SSIM & CCC) and image reconstruction (PSNR) performances calculated on all test slices for model-based (MB) reconstruction method and our proposed CNN model with different λ settings.

4   Conclusion

We present a novel deep learning based framework for direct estimation of PK parameter maps from undersampled DCE image-time series. Specifically, we design a *forward physical model loss* function through which we exploit the physical model relating the contrast agent kinetics to the time-resolved DCE signals. Moreover, we utilize the residual learning strategy in our problem formulation. The experiments demonstrate that our proposed method can outperform the state-of-the-art model-based reconstruction method, and allow almost instantaneous inference of the PK parameters in the clinical workflow of DCE-MRI.

Acknowledgements. The research leading to these results has received funding from the European Unions H2020 Framework Programme (H2020-MSCA-ITN-2014) under grant agreement no 642685 MacSeNet. We acknowledge Wellcome Trust (Grant 353 088134/Z/09/A) for recruitment and MRI scanning costs. We also gratefully acknowledge the support of NVIDIA Corporation with the donation of the GeForce Titan Xp GPU used for this research.

References

1. Fang, R., et al.: Direct estimation of permeability maps for low-dose CT perfusion. In: IEEE ISBI, pp. 739–742, April 2016
2. Guo, Y., et al.: High-resolution whole-brain DCE-MRI using constrained reconstruction. Med. Phys. **43**(5), 2013–2023 (2016)
3. Guo, Y., et al.: Direct estimation of tracer-kinetic parameter maps from highly undersampled brain dynamic contrast enhanced MRI. MRM **78**(4), 1566–1578 (2017)
4. Heye, A.K., et al.: Tracer kinetic modelling for DCE-MRI quantification of subtle bloodbrain barrier permeability. NeuroImage **125**, 446–455 (2016)
5. Kamnitsas, K., et al.: Efficient multi-scale 3d CNN with fully connected CRF for accurate brain lesion segmentation. Med. Image Anal. **36**, 61–78 (2017)
6. Lebel, R.M., et al.: Highly accelerated dynamic contrast enhanced imaging. MRM **71**(2), 635–644 (2014)
7. O'Connor, J.P.B., et al.: Dynamic contrast-enhanced MRI in clinical trials of antivascular therapies. Nat. Rev. Clin. Oncol. **9**(3), 167–77 (2012)
8. Patlak, C.S., et al.: Graphical evaluation of blood-to-brain transfer constants from multiple-time uptake data. J. Cereb. Blood Flow Metab. **3**(1), 1–7 (1983)
9. Sourbron, S.P., Buckley, D.L.: Classic models for dynamic contrast-enhanced MRI. NMR Biomed. **26**(8), 1004–1027 (2013)
10. Zhang, K., et al.: Beyond a gaussian denoiser: residual learning of deep CNN for image denoising. IEEE Trans. Image Process. **26**(7), 3142–3155 (2017)
11. Zhang, T., et al.: Fast pediatric 3d free-breathing abdominal dynamic contrast enhanced MRI with high spatiotemporal resolution. JMRI **41**(2), 460–473 (2015)
12. Zhu, Y., et al.: GOCART: GOlden-angle CArtesian randomized time-resolved 3D MRI. Magn. Reson. Imag. **34**(7), 940–950 (2016)

Short Acquisition Time PET/MR Pharmacokinetic Modelling Using CNNs

Catherine J. Scott[1(✉)], Jieqing Jiao[1], M. Jorge Cardoso[1,2], Kerstin Kläser[1], Andrew Melbourne[2,3], Pawel J. Markiewicz[1], Jonathan M. Schott[4], Brian F. Hutton[5], and Sébastien Ourselin[2]

[1] Centre for Medical Image Computing, University College London, London, UK
catherine.scott.14@ucl.ac.uk
[2] School of Biomedical Engineering and Imaging Sciences,
King's College London, London, UK
[3] Department of Medical Physics and Biomedical Engineering,
University College London, London, UK
[4] Dementia Research Centre, Institute of Neurology,
University College London, London, UK
[5] Institute of Nuclear Medicine, University College London, London, UK

Abstract. Standard quantification of Positron Emission Tomography (PET) data requires a long acquisition time to enable pharmacokinetic (PK) model fitting, however blood flow information from Arterial Spin Labelling (ASL) Magnetic Resonance Imaging (MRI) can be combined with simultaneous dynamic PET data to reduce the acquisition time. Due the difficulty of fitting a PK model to noisy PET data with limited time points, such 'fixed-R_1' techniques are constrained to a 30 min minimum acquisition, which is intolerable for many patients. In this work we apply a deep convolutional neural network (CNN) approach to combine the PET and MRI data. This permits shorter acquisition times as it avoids the noise sensitive voxelwise PK modelling and facilitates the full modelling of the relationship between blood flow and the dynamic PET data. This method is compared to three fixed-R_1 PK methods, and the clinically used standardised uptake value ratio (SUVR), using 60 min dynamic PET PK modelling as the gold standard. Testing on 11 subjects participating in a study of pre-clinical Alzheimer's Disease showed that, for 30 min acquisitions, all methods which combine the PET and MRI data have comparable performance, however at shorter acquisition times the CNN approach has a significantly lower mean square error (MSE) compared to fixed-R_1 PK modelling ($p = 0.001$). For both acquisition windows, SUVR had a significantly higher MSE than the CNN method ($p \leq 0.003$). This demonstrates that combining simultaneous PET and MRI data using a CNN can result in robust PET quantification within a scan time which is tolerable to patients with dementia.

1 Introduction

For the accurate quantification of tracer target density (BP_{ND}), such as amyloid-β burden in Alzheimer's disease, phamacokinetic (PK) modelling of dynamic

© Springer Nature Switzerland AG 2018
A. F. Frangi et al. (Eds.): MICCAI 2018, LNCS 11070, pp. 48–56, 2018.
https://doi.org/10.1007/978-3-030-00928-1_6

Positron Emission Tomography (PET) data requires the acquisition to cover the delivery, binding and washout of the injected radiotracer. This may take 60 min or more which is not clinically feasible, due to patient discomfort, scanner availability, and increased motion. A framework which reduces the PET acquisition time by incorporating simultaneously acquired arterial spin labelled (ASL) MRI data into the PK model has been proposed [1]. This involves three steps; conversion of ASL cerebral blood flow (CBF) maps into the relative PET tracer delivery parameter (R_1), extrapolation of the PET input function (C_R) to account for the missing time-points, and PK model fitting to the measured PET data using fixed R_1 and extrapolated C_R. We refer to this as the 'fixed R_1 method'. Unlike the clinically used standardised uptake value ratio (SUVR), this method can account for changes in blood flow, which can confound estimates of target density in longitudinal studies [2]. However, due the difficulty of fitting a PK model to noisy PET data with limited time points, this technique is constrained to a 30 min minimum acquisition time, which may still be intolerable for some patients.

The 'fixed-R_1' approach estimates R_1 from ASL-CBF independently from dynamic PET fitting for target density (BP_{ND}) and washout rate (k_2). This implementation cannot explicitly model the known influence of CBF on washout, due to high uncertainty in washout estimation, and the complex relationship which is dependent on the local tissue tracer kinetics [3]. Furthermore, the extrapolation of the input function, C_R, uses scaled population data under the assumption that tracer washout in this region is equal to the average population value. This assumption is violated in the case of disease or blood flow changes.

In this work we propose a deep learning (DL) framework to achieve PET quantification for a short acquisition time in a single step. We avoid the noise sensitive voxelwise PK curve fitting step, through the use of deep convolutional neural networks which enforce spatial regularisation across the receptive field. Our approach negates the need for explicit modelling between CBF, tracer delivery and tracer washout, as these relationships are learnt from the data and modelled in conjunction with the dynamic PET data. This approach also avoids C_R extrapolation, overcoming the limitation of a population tracer washout rate.

To our knowledge, this is the first time in which DL has been applied to PET PK modelling. This is due to the availability of robust models to describe standard data and the lack of one-to-one mapping between model parameters and dynamic PET data. However, the standard models are not sufficient to describe PET data with missing time-points. Furthermore, the incorporation of ASL-CBF constrains the parameter estimation. DL was chosen for its ability to model the underlying relationship between ASL-CBF and the delivery, binding and washout of the PET tracer without explicit feature extraction. By exploiting all of the PET and MRI information, and avoiding voxelwise fitting, this framework provides more robust estimates of target density with a shorter acquisition.

2   Methods

2.1   Deep Learning Framework for BP_{ND} Estimation

The framework performs regression of PET target density (BP_{ND}) from PET and MRI data directly. The network was implemented in NiftyNet [4] using the 'highresnet' convolutional neural network with 20 convolutional layers [5], which uses a stack of residual dilated convolutions with increasingly large dilation factors. For training we used adaptive moment estimation (Adam) with an initial learning rate of 10^{-3}, and a root mean square error loss function. The networks were initialised randomly and trained for a maximum of 50,000 iterations. The training patch size was $56 \times 56 \times 56$ voxels and a smoothed brain mask was used for adaptive sampling. Random rotation and scaling transformations of $\pm 10\%$ were used for training data augmentation. All inputs were 3D image volumes: the ASL-CBF maps, the structural T1 weighted MRI, and the dynamic PET data, which were entered as one frame per channel, see Fig. 1.

2.2   Gold Standard PK Modelling

The linearised simplified reference tissue model (SRTM) is used for gold standard PET quantification (1). Basis functions for $C_R(t) \otimes e^{-\theta t}$ are pre-calculated over a physiologically plausible range of θ [6], where $C_R(t)$ is the tracer concentration in the reference region. $C_R(t)$ is used as an input function since the reference region, cerebellar grey matter, is considered to be devoid of the imaging target. $C_T(t)$ is the measured tracer concentration in the target tissue. The model parameters are: R_1 (the delivery rate constant in the target tissue relative to reference tissue), k_2 (the transfer rate constant from target tissue to blood), and the parameter of interest BP_{ND} (the binding potential which is related to target density and consequently amyloid-β burden). The parameters are estimated via curve fitting to $C_R(t)$ and $C_T(t)$ acquired over $t = 0{:}60\,\text{min}$.

$$C_T(t) = R_1 C_R(t) + \phi C_R(t) \otimes e^{-\theta t}$$
$$\text{where} \quad \phi = k_2 - R_1 k_2/(1 + BP_{ND}), \quad \theta = k_2/(1 + BP_{ND}) \tag{1}$$

2.3   Acquisition Window Definition

For gold standard PK modelling the scan starts at tracer injection, $t_s = 0$, with a duration of $t_d = 60\,\text{min}$. However, for the short acquisition methods $t_s > 0$, and t_d is chosen to fit clinical requirements. We optimise the timing window, $t = t_s{:}t_s + t_d$, for each method at different t_d's. This was performed over $t = 30{:}60\,\text{min}$, as this period is recommended for routine clinical scans using this tracer.

2.4   Comparison Methods for Short Acquisition PET Quantification

We compare the proposed technique to four short PET acquisition methods: three fixed-R_1 methods, and the clinical standard, SUVR.

Fixed R_1 Methods. Two methods are used to derive R_1 from ASL-CBF: the linear regression (LR) method [1], and the image fusion (IF) method [7]. Both methods require a database of subjects with 60 min of PET data and ASL.

The LR method performs linear regression between R_1 and ASL-CBF on the database and the relationship is applied to an unseen ASL-CBF map. For IF, the local similarity between the unseen ASL-CBF map and those in the database is used to weight the propagation of R_1 database values into the subject's space. An additional method using the gold standard R_1 (true R_1) is also included to demonstrate the upper limit of this approach, where R_1 is estimated perfectly from the ASL data.

For all three methods the estimation of BP_{ND} was carried out as previously described [1,7]. Briefly, the reference region, C_R is extrapolated to $t = 0$, at tracer injection, by scaling the mean population C_R

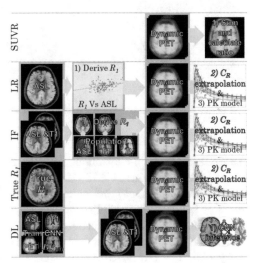

Fig. 1. Overview of methods tested. Blue boxes indicate input subject data and green boxes population data.

to the measured data using a linear least squares fit, then the derived R_1 value and the extrapolated C_R are used in (1) to estimate k_2 and BP_{ND} from the measured PET data.

Standardised Uptake Value Ratio (SUVR). SUVR is calculated by dividing the image (C_T) by the mean value in the reference region (C_R) to yield relative tracer uptake, which can not take blood flow into account. For comparison with BP_{ND}, one is subtracted, as $BP_{ND} \approx \frac{C_T}{C_R} - 1$. SUVR is calculated over different timing windows by first summing the relevant reconstructed frames.

2.5   Data Acquisition and Pre-processing

Database Construction. For each subject the T1 and ASL-CBF MR images were affinely registered into PET space. The subjects were randomly split between training (38, ~70%), validation (6, ~10%) and testing (11, ~20%). The input data used and an overview of each methodology is summarised in Fig. 1, where the dynamic PET data include the frames acquired over $t = t_s : t_s + t_d$.

PET Data. 60 min of PET data were acquired following intravenous injection of an amyloid-β targeting radiotracer, [^{18}F]florbetapir. Dynamic PET data were binned into $15s \times 4$, $30s \times 8$, $60s \times 9$, $180s \times 2$, $300s \times 8$ time frames, such that all frames for $t \geq 20$ min were 5 min long. The data were reconstructed into $2 \times 2 \times 2$ mm voxels, accounting for dead-time, attenuation (using synthetic CT), scatter, randoms and normalisation [8].

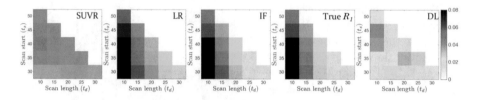

Fig. 2. MSE averaged across subjects for different timing windows and methods

ASL Data. Pseudo-continuous ASL data were acquired at $t = 55{:}60$ min, using a 3D GRASE readout at $3.75 \times 3.75 \times 4$ mm and reconstructed to $1.88 \times 1.88 \times 4$ mm voxels. 10 control-label pairs were acquired with a pulse duration and post labelling delay of 1800 ms. Proton density, S_0, was estimated by fitting saturation recovery images, at three recovery times (1, 2, 4s), for [T1, S_0]. Cerebral blood flow (CBF) maps were then estimated from the ASL and saturation recovery images [9]. The parameter values were 0.9 ml/g for the plasma/tissue partition coefficient, 1650 ms for blood T1, and 0.85 for labelling efficiency.

3   Experiments and Results

Data. Imaging data were collected from 55 cognitively normal subjects participating in Insight 46, a neuroimaging sub-study of the MRC National Survey of Health and Development [10], who underwent simultaneous PET and multi-modal MRI on a Siemens Biograph mMR 3T PET/MRI scanner. 11 subjects were used for testing, with the remaining subjects used in the database for training and validation.

Validation. The proposed deep learning (DL) method was compared to three fixed-R_1 methods (LR, IF and true R_1), and SUVR. BP_{ND} estimation accuracy was assessed using the mean square error: MSE $= 1/v \sum_v (I_v^{est} - I_v^{GS})^2$, where I is intensity, v is the number of voxels, GS is the gold standard and est is the estimate. Statistical tests were performed using the Wilcoxon signed rank test.

3.1   Method Comparison over Different Timing Windows

Figure 2 shows the average MSE across subjects for different data acquisition windows for each method. Here, SUVR shows minimal influence from acquisition timing and length due to the simplicity of the technique. However, since it is not able to account for tracer delivery or washout it has a consistently high MSE. For the three methods which perform kinetic modelling with a fixed R_1 there is a strong time dependence, with the error increasing greatly as the scan time is reduced. Consequently they outperform SUVR for 30 min acquisitions, but for scans of less than 20 min, where the number of datapoints is ≤ 4, they produce a higher error. This is due to the difficulty in fitting the PK model to a few noisy datapoints, and the increased uncertainty in the extrapolation of C_R.

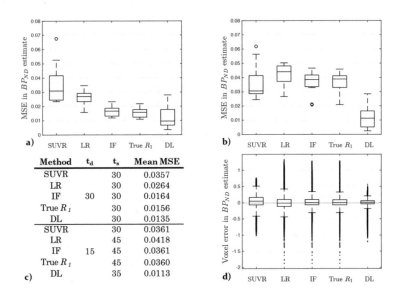

Method	t_d	t_s	Mean MSE
SUVR		30	0.0357
LR		30	0.0264
IF	30	30	0.0164
True R_1		30	0.0156
DL		30	0.0135
SUVR		30	0.0361
LR		45	0.0418
IF	15	45	0.0361
True R_1		45	0.0360
DL		35	0.0113

Fig. 3. Subject MSE for (a) 30 and (b) 15 min scans, summarised in (c). The voxel-wise error for all subjects for a 15 min scan is shown in (d).

The deep learning based method (DL) shows a consistently low MSE across timing windows compared to the other techniques. This is because voxel based PK modelling, and C_R extrapolation, which are acquisition length dependent, are avoided. Furthermore, blood flow information is leveraged to inform both tracer delivery and washout, reducing the acquisition time required relative to the fixed-R_1 PK modelling techniques. For DL there is no clear trend to the acquisition window dependence which makes it more flexible for clinical implementation.

3.2   Optimised Timing Window Method Comparison

Based on the mean MSE, shown in Fig. 2, the best timing window for each method was selected for a 30 min (6 frames) and 15 min (3 frames) scan, representing a long clinical scan and a tolerable scan duration respectively, see Fig. 3c.

30 min Optimised Acquisition. Figure 3(a) shows the MSE across subjects for the 30 min acquisition window. As expected the fixed-R_1 methods have a lower MSE than SUVR due to the more accurate modelling of tracer delivery and washout. For this acquisition length the benefit of using the deep learning approach is limited compared to the fixed R_1 methods, and the difference in MSE did not reach statistical significance. However, DL has a significantly lower MSE compared to SUVR ($p = 0.003$). Figure 4(a) shows an example subject, which highlights the good performance of the IF, true R_1 and DL methods, while SUVR shows a large over estimation. The LR method shows corruption due to artefacts in the ASL-CBF map which propagate directly into the BP_{ND} estimation.

15 min Optimised Acquisition. When the scan time is reduced to 15 min the MSE in the fixed-R_1 methods increases, even when using the true R_1 parameter. By contrast, the DL and SUVR methods maintain their performance levels. Now DL has a significantly lower MSE than both the fixed-R_1 methods ($p \leq 0.001$) and SUVR ($p = 0.001$). The DL method also has a lower bias than all other methods, see Fig. 3(d), but this does not reach statistical significance.

Figure 4(b) shows the estimated BP_{ND} images using a 15 min acquisition for the different methods for an example subject. Here, the noise in the fixed-R_1 methods is a result of the limited timepoints for the fit. SUVR gives a plausible estimate of BP_{ND}, however the image demonstrates a general overestimation of the target density compared to the true image. By contrast, the DL technique yields a low noise image due to the spatial regularisation inherent in the technique, with high accuracy as the model is able to combine the dynamic PET data with the blood flow information from the ASL to accurately estimate BP_{ND}.

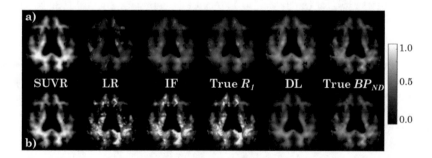

Fig. 4. Example subject BP_{ND} maps optimised for (a) 30 and (b) 15 min acquisition, where the true BP_{ND} is calculated over 60 min for both.

4   Discussion and Conclusion

In this paper we present a deep learning approach to PET target density estimation, by combining dynamic PET data with MRI blood flow and structural images to significantly reduce the acquisition time to just 15 min, compared to the gold standard 60 min. This is applied to amyloid PET data which is used in the diagnosis and monitoring of Alzheimer's disease, as the symptoms of the disease necessitate short scans. This method was compared to the clinical standard, SUVR, as well as previously proposed techniques which fix the tracer delivery parameter R_1 using MRI blood flow data in the PET PK modelling to reduce the acquisition time. This demonstrated that, for a 30 min acquisition, the proposed technique performed comparably to the previously proposed fixed-R_1 techniques, and significantly better than SUVR ($p = 0.003$). When the acquisition window was reduced to 15 min, the fixed-R_1 methods had insufficient data to fit the PK model. However, the deep learning method maintained its low MSE, which was significantly lower than the clinically used SUVR ($p = 0.001$).

This initial work proves the benefit of using deep learning to perform PET quantification where limited PET data means that the standard model fails. In the future we intend to build on this approach by explicitly encoding the PET frame timing information into the model. This would not only give the model more information, but also the potential to cope with discontinuous scans.

Acknowledgements. This work was supported by the EPSRC UCL Centre for Doctoral Training in Medical Imaging (EP/L016478/1), UCL Leonard Wolfson Experimental Neurology Centre (PR/ylr/18575), MRC (MR/J01107X/1), EPSRC (NS/A000027/1), NIHR UCLH Biomedical Research Centre (inc. High Impact Initiative, BW.mn.BRC10269). Insight 1946 receives funding from Alzheimer's Research UK (ARUKPG2014-1946, ARUKPG2014-1946), MRC Dementia Platform UK (CSUB19166), The Wolfson Foundation, and Brain Research Trust. The Florbetapir tracer was kindly supplied by Avid Radiopharmaceuticals, a wholly owned subsidiary of Eli Lilly. We are grateful to the Insight 46 participants for their involvement in this study and to K. Erlandsson for his advice.

References

1. Scott, C.J., et al.: ASL-incorporated pharmacokinetic modelling of PET data with reduced acquisition time: application to amyloid imaging. In: Ourselin, S., Joskowicz, L., Sabuncu, M.R., Unal, G., Wells, W. (eds.) MICCAI 2016. LNCS, vol. 9902, pp. 406–413. Springer, Cham (2016). https://doi.org/10.1007/978-3-319-46726-9_47
2. van Berckel, B.N.M., Ossenkoppele, R., Tolboom, N., et al.: Longitudinal amyloid imaging using 11C-PiB: methodologic considerations. J. Cereb. Blood Flow Metab. **54**(9), 1570–6 (2013)
3. Wu, Y., Carson, R.E.: Noise reduction in the simplified reference tissue model for neuroreceptor functional imaging. J. Cereb. Blood Flow Metab. **22**(12), 1440–1452 (2002)
4. Gibson, E., Li, W., Sudre, C., et al.: Niftynet: a deep-learning platform for medical imaging. arXiv preprint arXiv:1709.03485 (2017)
5. Li, W., Wang, G., Fidon, L., et al.: On the compactness, efficiency, and representation of 3D convolutional networks: brain parcellation as a pretext task. In: Information Processing in Medical Imaging (2017)

6. Gunn, R.N., Lammertsma, A.A., Hume, S.P., et al.: Parametric imaging of ligand-receptor binding in PET using a simplified reference region model. NeuroImage **6**(4), 279–287 (1997)

7. Scott, C., et al.: Short acquisition time PET quantification using MRI-based pharmacokinetic parameter synthesis. In: Descoteaux, M., et al. (eds.) MICCAI 2017. LNCS, vol. 10434, pp. 737–744. Springer, Cham (2017). https://doi.org/10.1007/978-3-319-66185-8_83

8. Markiewicz, P.J., Ehrhardt, M.J., Erlandsson, K., et al.: NiftyPET: a High-throughput Software Platform for High Quantitative Accuracy and Precision PET Imaging and Analysis. Neuroinformatics **16**(1), 95–115 (2017)

9. Melbourne, A., Toussaint, N., Owen, D., et al.: Niftyfit: a software package for multi-parametric model-fitting of 4D magnetic resonance imaging data. Neuroinformatics **14**(3), 319–337 (2016)

10. Lane, C.A., Parker, T.D., Cash, D.M., et al.: Study protocol: Insight 46 - a neuroscience sub-study of the MRC National Survey of Health and Development. BMC Neurol. **17**(1), 75 (2017)

Can Deep Learning Relax Endomicroscopy Hardware Miniaturization Requirements?

Saeed Izadi$^{(\boxtimes)}$, Kathleen P. Moriarty, and Ghassan Hamarneh

School of Computing Science, Simon Fraser University, Burnaby, Canada
{saeedi,kmoriart,hamarneh}@sfu.ca

Abstract. Confocal laser endomicroscopy (CLE) is a novel imaging modality that provides *in vivo* histological cross-sections of examined tissue. Recently, attempts have been made to develop miniaturized *in vivo* imaging devices, specifically confocal laser microscopes, for both clinical and research applications. However, current implementations of miniature CLE components such as confocal lenses compromise image resolution, signal-to-noise ratio, or both, which negatively impacts the utility of *in vivo* imaging. In this work, we demonstrate that software-based techniques can be used to recover lost information due to endomicroscopy hardware miniaturization and reconstruct images of higher resolution. Particularly, a densely connected convolutional neural network is used to reconstruct a high-resolution CLE image, given a low-resolution input. In the proposed network, each layer is directly connected to all subsequent layers, which results in an effective combination of low-level and high-level features and efficient information flow throughout the network. To train and evaluate our network, we use a dataset of 181 high-resolution CLE images. Both quantitative and qualitative results indicate superiority of the proposed network compared to traditional interpolation techniques and competing learning-based methods. This work demonstrates that software-based super-resolution is a viable approach to compensate for loss of resolution due to endoscopic hardware miniaturization.

1   Introduction

Last year, colorectal cancer caused an estimated 50,260 deaths in the United States alone and another 140,030 people are expected to be diagnosed with this disease during 2018 [12,13]. Accordingly, it is the third most commonly diagnosed cancer among both men and women [13]. Early diagnosis and treatment of colorectal cancer is crucial for reducing the mortality rate. Gastroenterologists screen and monitor the status of their patients' digestive systems through specialized endoscopy procedures such as colonoscopy and sigmoidoscopy. During colonoscopy, a flexible video endoscope is guided through the large intestine, capturing images used to differentiate between neoplastic (intraepithelial neoplasia, cancer) and non-neoplastic (e.g., hyperplastic polyps) tissues.

© Springer Nature Switzerland AG 2018
A. F. Frangi et al. (Eds.): MICCAI 2018, LNCS 11070, pp. 57–64, 2018.
https://doi.org/10.1007/978-3-030-00928-1_7

Since the introduction of endoscopy to gastroenterology, many significant advances have been made toward improving the diagnostic and therapeutic yield of endoscopy. Confocal laser endomicroscopy (CLE), first introduced to the endoscopy field in 2004 [5], is an emerging imaging modality that allows histological analysis at cellular and subcellular resolutions during ongoing endoscopy. An endomicroscope is integrated into the distal tip of a conventional video colonoscope, providing an *in vivo* microscopic visualization of tissue architecture and cellular morphology in real-time. Endomicroscopes offer a magnification and resolution comparable to that obtained from *ex vivo* histology imaging techniques, without the need for biopsy (i.e., tissue removal, sectioning and staining).

Despite the promise of confocal laser endomicroscopy, both clinicians and researchers prefer compact instruments with relatively large penetration depth to recognize tissue structures such as the mucosa, the submucosa, and the muscular layers. Compact instruments can also directly benefit the patients, as smaller devices improve early diagnostic procedures by offering greater flexibility during hand-held use, for a quicker and less invasive endoscopy [3]. In this regard, further attempts have been made to design miniaturized confocal scanning lasers capable of capturing images from the tissue subsurface with micron resolution *in vivo*, once installed on top of a flexible fiber bundle. However, miniaturization implies using smaller optical elements, which introduces pixelation artifacts in images. Therefore, there exists a trade-off between miniaturizing the CLE components and the resultant image resolution.

Image super-resolution, transforms an image from low-resolution (LR) to high-resolution (HR) by recovering the high-frequency cues and reconstructing textural information. In the past decade, various learning-based approaches have been proposed to learn the desired LR-to-HR mapping, including dictionary learning [18,19], linear regression [14,17], and random decision forests [10].

In recent years, deep learning models have been applied to various image interpretation tasks. Among such efforts, convolutional neural networks (CNN) have been utilized to resolve the ill-posed inverse problem of super-resolution. Dong et al. [1] demonstrated that a fully convolutional network trained end-to-end can be used to perform the LR-to-HR nonlinear mapping. The same authors extended their previous work by introducing deconvolutional layers at the end of the architecture, such that the mapping between LR and HR images is learned directly without image interpolation [2]. They also slightly increased the depth of the network and adopted smaller kernels for better performance. Instead of HR images, Kim et al. [6] suggested to train deeper neural networks through predicting the residual images, which when summed with an interpolated image gives the desired output. Increasing the network depth by adding weighted layers introduces more parameters, which can lead to overfitting. Kim et al. [7] tackled overfitting by using a deeply-recursive convolutional network. In their work, the same convolutional layers are used recursively without the need for extra parameters. To simplify the training of the network, they suggested recursive supervision and skip connections to avoid the notorious vanishing/exploding gradients.

Given the constraints imposed by CLE hardware miniaturization, we propose to leverage state-of-the-art deep learning super-resolution methods to mitigate the unwanted trade-off between miniaturization and image resolution. In other words, we show that the pixelation artifact, which is a consequence of hardware miniaturization, can be significantly remedied through an efficient and practical use of software-based techniques, particularly machine learning methods. To this end, we employ a densely connected CNN in which extensive usage of skip connections is exploited [15]. Dense connections help information flow in backpropagation algorithms and alleviate the vanishing gradient problem. Furthermore, the low-level features from early layers are efficiently combined with those of later layers. In addition, we use sub-pixel convolutional layers [11] to render the upsampling operation learnable and expedite the reconstruction process.

2   Method

Our main goal in this work is to super-resolve an LR image by passing it through a set of nonlinear transformations to recover high-frequency details and reconstruct the HR image, effectively increasing the number of pixels from $N_{LR} \times N_{LR}$ to $N_{HR} \times N_{HR}$, where $\frac{N_{HR}}{N_{LR}}$ is the scale factor. The proposed architecture consists of dense blocks and upsampling layers which are efficiently designed to combine the features from earlier layers with those of later layers and improve information flow throughout the model. Figure 1 depicts the architecture of the employed model.

Low-level Features. A series of low-level features are extracted from small regions of the LR input image using two successive convolutional layers with kernel size 3×3 and ReLU non-linearity. The number of feature channels for the first and second layer is 64 and 128, respectively. The learned low-level features are used to efficiently represent the intrinsic textural differences between LR and HR images.

High-level Features. The resultant low-level feature maps are used as the input to a fully convolutional DenseNet architecture to provide high-level features. DenseNet, which was first introduced by Huang et al. [4], consists of a set of dense blocks in which any layer is connected to every other layer in a feed-forward fashion. Alternatively stated, the ith layer in a dense block receives the concatenation of outputs by all preceding layers as the input:

$$L_i = relu(\psi_{\theta^i}(L_1 +\!\!+ L_2 +\!\!+ ... +\!\!+ L_{i-1})) \tag{1}$$

where ψ_{θ^i} denotes the transformation of the ith layer parameterized by θ^i and $+\!\!+$ denotes the concatenation operation. Dense skip connections help alleviate the vanishing-gradient problem and improve information flow throughout the network. Counter-intuitively, the number of parameters is also reduced since the previously-generated feature maps are re-used in the subsequent layers, thus minimizing the need for learning redundant features. As depicted in Fig. 1, a single dense block consists of m convolutional layers, each producing k feature maps,

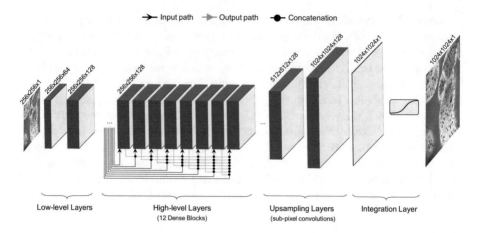

Fig. 1. Overall architecture of the DenseNet model, shown here for $\times 4$ scale factor, i.e., from a 256^2 LR input image to a 1024^2 HR output image. In each dense block, convolutional layers are connected to all subsequent layers.

referred to as the *growth rate*. Accordingly, the final output of each dense block has $m \times k$ features maps. The growth rate regulates how much new information each layer contributes to achieving the final performance. In this study, we set m and k to be 8 and 16, respectively. Thus, each dense block receives and produces 128 feature maps as input and output. We stack 12 dense blocks in a feed-forward fashion to construct the DenseNet part of our proposed architecture.

Upsampling Layers. In some SR methods [1,6,16], the LR image is first resized to match the HR spatial dimensions using bicubic interpolation. Thereafter, several convolution layers are employed to enhance the interpolated input in the HR space. In addition to having a considerable increase in memory usage and computational complexity, these interpolation methods are categorized as non-learnable upsampling techniques, which do not leverage data statistics to bring new information for more accurate reconstruction. As an alternative, deconvolutional layers, which are learnable operations, are utilized to enlarge the spatial dimensions of the LR image. However, the most prominent problem associated with deconvolutional layers is the presence of checkerboard artifacts in the output image. To overcome this, extra post-processing steps or smoothness constraints are required. In this work, we use sub-pixel convolutional layers [11], to upsample the spatial size of the feature maps within the network. Suppose that we desire to spatially upsample c feature maps of size $h \times w \times c$ to size $H \times W \times c$, by a scale factor $r = H/h = W/w$. The LR feature maps would be fed into a convolution layer that increases the number of channels by a factor of r^2, resulting in a volume of size $h \times w \times (c \times r^2)$. Next, the resultant volume is simply re-arranged to be of shape $(h \times r) \times (w \times r) \times c$, which is equal to $H \times W \times c$. Here, we use successive $\times 2$ upsampling layers to gradually increase the spatial dimensionality. Each upsampling block contains a single convolutional layer with 3×3 kernel size and ReLU non-linearity.

Integration Layer. Once the features maps match the spatial dimension in the HR space, an integration layer is used to consolidate the features across the channels into a single channel. The integration layer is a convolutional layer with 3×3 kernel size and a single output channel. Finally, a *sigmoid* activation function is employed to produce the super-resolved image.

3 Experiments

Data. We evaluate our study on the dataset provided by Leong et al. [9]. The dataset contains 181 gray scale confocal images of size 1024×1024 from 31 patients and 50 different anatomical sites. Each patient has undergone a confocal gastroscopy (Pentax EC-3870FK, Pentax, Tokyo, Japan) under conscious sedation. CLE images and forceps biopsies of the same sites were taken sequentially at standardized locations (i.e., sites of the small intestine). Each forceps biopsy was then assessed by 2 experienced blinded histopathologists. Despite our application of interest being colorectal cancer, we used the publicly available CLE celiac dataset as a proof-of-concept. Colorectal cancer images are assessed primarily in the large intestine as opposed to the small intestine used in celiac assessment, however the imaging procedure (CLE) remains the same. This dataset was made publicly available as part of an International Symposium on Biomedical Imaging (ISBI) challenge and we used the provided training and test sets, consisting of 108 and 73 images, respectively.

Implementation Details. We partition the HR images into 64×64 non-overlapping patches. Then, the HR patches are downsampled by bicubic interpolation to construct <LR, HR> pairs for training the model. The network is optimized with Adam [8] optimizer with default parameters, i.e. $\beta_1 = 0.9$, $\beta_2 = 0.999$ and $\epsilon = 10^{-4}$. We set the mini-batch size to 128. The learning rate is first initialized with 0.001 and is multiplied by $\gamma = 10$ at epochs 50 and 200. The network is trained for 300 epochs using L1 loss. For data augmentation, we use random horizontal and vertical flips. The proposed method is implemented in PyTorch and is trained using two Nvidia Titan X (Pascal) GPUs. It takes 2 days to train the networks for each upsampling factor. All hyper-parameters (optimizer, learning rate, batch size, and distance metric) are found via grid search on 20 images from the training set.

Qualitative Results. In Fig. 2, we visually compare our proposed super-resolution method to three traditional interpolation techniques and two learning-based approaches with scale factors of $\times 2$, $\times 4$ and $\times 8$. Evidently, DenseNet produces output images of higher quality by reconstructing high-frequency cues and removing visual artifacts, e.g. over-smoothness and pixelation. Specifically for a $\times 8$ scale factor, the densely connected network can accurately recover high-level textural patterns such as grids and granular patterns. Moreover, a more rigorous examination of smaller regions for $\times 4$ scale factor clearly reveals the superiority of DenseNet model in producing sharper edges and improved contrast for lines and shapes.

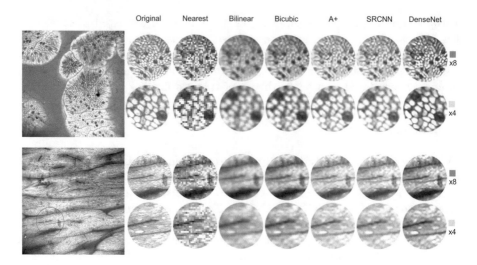

Fig. 2. Qualitative results for two sample images. For each image, the first and second circle rows show the zoomed-in patches for ×4 and ×8, respectively.

From a clinician's point of view, the reconstruction power of the method offers a clear advantage over others. In Fig. 3 we illustrate the trade-off between the amount of lost information after downsampling and the quality of the reconstructed image. As can be seen, a large portion of pixels is discarded in downsampling, restricting the networks to a small fraction of the original image pixels for reconstruction. However, deep learning approaches are clearly capable of generating a sharp image from only 1.6% of pixels (for a scale factor of ×8) with very small L1 distance values which indicates a minimal loss of information.

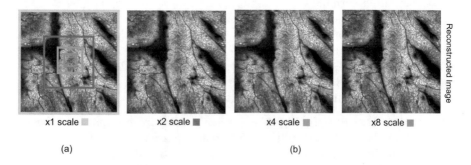

Fig. 3. Reconstruction analysis. (a) visualizes the amount of lost pixels for different scale factors relative to the original size. (b) shows the reconstructed images for scale factors ×2, ×4 and ×8.

Quantitative Results. Table 1 compares our proposed method with three interpolation methods and two learning-based techniques in terms of PSNR

(Peak Signal to Noise Ratio) and SSIM (Structural Similarity). PSNR is a well-known metric for image quality assessment which is inversely proportional to Mean Square Error. SSIM also measures the the similarity between two images and is correlated with quality perception in human visual system. In terms of PSNR, DenseNet yields 2.08, 1.93 and 1.14 average improvements over Nearest, Bilinear and Bicubic interpolation methods across all scale factors, respectively. For learning-based approaches, DenseNet outperforms A+ [14] and SRCNN [1] in terms of average SSIM by 0.020 and 0.019 over all scale factors, respectively.

Table 1. Quantitative results. Average PSNR and SSIM scores for scale factors ×2, ×4 and ×8 on 73 test images.

	Nearest		Bilinear		Bicubic		A+		SRCNN		DenseNet	
	PSNR	SSIM	PSNR	SSIM	PSNR	SSIM	PSNR	SSIM	PSNR	SSIM	PSNR	SSIM
×2	35.32	0.881	34.21	0.849	35.80	0.908	36.21	0.925	35.54	0.930	**38.57**	**0.950**
×4	31.64	0.658	32.38	0.707	32.87	0.755	33.00	0.781	33.01	0.778	**33.32**	**0.801**
×8	30.59	0.528	31.40	0.586	31.70	0.615	31.74	0.636	31.80	0.636	**31.90**	**0.651**

4 Conclusion

Developing smaller hardware for medical imaging devices has several advantages such as increased portability and reduced patient discomfort. However, hardware miniaturization comes at the expense of reduced image quality. In this preliminary study, we obtained encouraging results to support that software-based methods can be used to counteract the loss of image quality due to miniaturized device components. Compared to common interpolation methods, our qualitative and quantitative results indicate that a densely connected convolutional neural network can significantly yield higher PSNR and SSIM scores, resulting in super-resolved images of higher quality. In future work, we will focus on how super-resolved images, compared to low-resolution images, can be advantageous to clinical and research applications. For example, super-resolution images may be used as input to automated machine-learning based disease classification.

Acknowledgments. Thanks to the NVIDIA Corporation for the donation of Titan X GPUs used in this research and to the Collaborative Health Research Projects (CHRP) for funding.

References

1. Dong, C., et al.: Image super-resolution using deep convolutional networks. IEEE PAMI **38**(2), 295–307 (2016)
2. Dong, C., Loy, C.C., Tang, X.: Accelerating the super-resolution convolutional neural network. In: Leibe, B., Matas, J., Sebe, N., Welling, M. (eds.) ECCV 2016, Part II. LNCS, vol. 9906, pp. 391–407. Springer, Cham (2016). https://doi.org/10. 1007/978-3-319-46475-6_25

3. Helmchen, F.: Miniaturization of fluorescence microscopes using fibre optics. Exper. Physiol. **87**(6), 737–745 (2002)
4. Huang, G., et al.: Densely connected convolutional networks. In: IEEE CVPR, pp. 2261–2269 (2017)
5. Kiesslich, R., et al.: Confocal laser endoscopy for diagnosing intraepithelial neoplasias and colorectal cancer in vivo. Gastroenterology **127**(3), 706–713 (2004)
6. Kim, J., et al.: Accurate image super-resolution using very deep convolutional networks. In: IEEE CVPR, pp. 1646–1654 (2016)
7. Kim, J., et al.: Deeply-recursive convolutional network for image super-resolution. In: IEEE CVPR, pp. 1637–1645 (2016)
8. Kingma, D.P., et al.: Adam: A method for stochastic optimization. arXiv:1412.6980 (2014)
9. Leong, R.W., et al.: In vivo confocal endomicroscopy in the diagnosis and evaluation of celiac disease. Gastroenterology **135**(6), 1870–1876 (2008)
10. Schulter, S., et al.: Fast and accurate image upscaling with super-resolution forests. In: IEEE CVPR, pp. 3791–3799 (2015)
11. Shi, W., et al.: Real-time single image and video super-resolution using an efficient sub-pixel convolutional neural network. In: IEEE CVPR, pp. 1874–1883 (2016)
12. Siegel, R.: Colorectal cancer statistics, 2017. CA Cancer J. Clin. **67**(3), 177–193 (2017)
13. Siegel, R.: Cancer statistics, 2018. CA Cancer J. Clin. **68**(1), 7–30 (2018)
14. Timofte, R., De Smet, V., Van Gool, L.: A+: adjusted anchored neighborhood regression for fast super-resolution. In: Cremers, D., Reid, I., Saito, H., Yang, M.-H. (eds.) ACCV 2014, Part IV. LNCS, vol. 9006, pp. 111–126. Springer, Cham (2015). https://doi.org/10.1007/978-3-319-16817-3_8
15. Tong, T., et al.: Image super-resolution using dense skip connections. In: IEEE ICCV, pp. 4809–4817 (2017)
16. Wang, Z., et al.: Deep networks for image super-resolution with sparse prior. In: IEEE ICCV, pp. 370–378 (2015)
17. Yang, C.Y., et al.: Fast direct super-resolution by simple functions. In: IEEE ICCV, pp. 561–568 (2013)
18. Yang, J., et al.: Image super-resolution via sparse representation. IEEE TIP **19**(11), 2861–2873 (2010)
19. Yang, J., et al.: Coupled dictionary training for image super-resolution. IEEE TIP **21**(8), 3467–3478 (2012)

A Framework to Objectively Identify Reference Regions for Normalizing Quantitative Imaging

Amir Fazlollahi[1,2(✉)], Scott Ayton[3,4], Pierrick Bourgeat[1],
Ibrahima Diouf[1], Parnesh Raniga[1], Jurgen Fripp[1], James Doecke[1,2],
David Ames[5], Colin L. Masters[3,4], Christopher C. Rowe[4,5],
Victor L. Villemagne[4,5], Ashley I. Bush[3,4], and Olivier Salvado[1,2]

[1] CSIRO Health and Biosecurity, Brisbane, Australia
fazlollahi@gmail.com
[2] Cooperative Research Centre for Mental Health, Parkville, Australia
[3] Florey Institute of Neuroscience and Mental Health, Parkville, Australia
[4] The University of Melbourne, Parkville, Australia
[5] Austin Health, Heidelberg, Australia

Abstract. The quantitative use of medical images often requires an intensity scaling with respect to the signal from a well-characterized anatomical region of interest. The choice of such a region often varies between studies which can substantially influence the quantification, resulting in study bias hampering objective findings which are detrimental to open science. This study outlines a list of criteria and a statistical ranking approach for identifying normalization region of interest. The proposed criteria include (i) associations between reference region and demographics such as age, (ii) diagnostic group differences in the reference region, (iii) correlation between reference and primary areas of interest, (iv) local variance in the reference region, and (v) longitudinal reproducibility of the target regions when normalized. The proposed approach has been used to establish an optimal normalization region of interest for the analysis of Quantitative Susceptibility Mapping (QSM) of Magnetic Resonance Imaging (MRI). This was achieved by using cross-sectional data from 119 subjects with normal cognition, mild cognitive impairment, and Alzheimer's disease as well as and 19 healthy elderly individuals with longitudinal data. For the QSM application, we found that normalizing by the white matter regions not only satisfies the criteria but it also provides the best separation between clinical groups for deep brain nuclei target regions.

Keywords: Quantification · Reference region · Normalization
QSM

1 Introduction

Emerging quantitative medical imaging techniques have become a promising research tool for investigating metabolic, functional, and molecular properties of tissues. An accurate quantification of neuroimaging data such as Magnetic Resonance Imaging

© Springer Nature Switzerland AG 2018
A. F. Frangi et al. (Eds.): MICCAI 2018, LNCS 11070, pp. 65–72, 2018.
https://doi.org/10.1007/978-3-030-00928-1_8

(MRI), Computed Tomography (CT) or Positron Emission Tomography (PET), often requires intensity scaling or normalization. The intensity normalization aims at accounting for global variations between subjects as well as uncontrolled biological, experimental, and imaging factors that might otherwise bias the results. A ratio of the measured signal to a pre-defined reference region is one common normalization method. Indeed, various normalization regions have been utilized in amyloid PET [1, 2], 18F-FDG PET [3, 4], arterial spin labeling MRI [5–7], quantitative susceptibility mapping (QSM) [8–12] or dynamic susceptibility contrast [13]. An ideal reference region should be spared from pathology in the disorder under study, should have non-specific associations (saturable) to the imaging method and should have a stable measurement. Seldom can a consensus normalization region be established as it depends on the disease, cohort, age, and imaging parameters or tracers, resulting in unwanted variability in reported outcomes [6, 8, 9], even using the same imaging modality and/or pathological cohort.

Intensity normalization methods scale the image by computing the ratio of regions of interest (ROI) values to the average of all voxels within a reference region [1, 2, 5, 9] or a cluster of regions [14, 15]. Intensity normalization aims to reduce measurement variability caused by uncontrolled physiological differences among subjects and imaging techniques. The ideal approach for normalization depends on the underlying source of the variability. Using QSM as an example in this paper, the magnetic susceptibility (i.e. χ) is inferred from a dipole kernel operation, which, due to the zero value in the origin of the kernel in the Fourier domain (DC component), leads to an arbitrary baseline intensity shift in the reconstructed image [16]. Therefore, intensity normalization using a reference region is essential to address this global shift before reporting and comparing QSM findings. Previous studies reported the use of different reference regions including the cerebrospinal fluid (CSF) of the posterior ventricles [8, 11], posterior white-matter (WM) with lower variance across subjects [9], middle frontal WM [17], occipital WM [10], and whole brain or cortical grey-matter [12].

Previous studies established a series of objective criteria for a normalization region which included between- and intra-diagnostic-group differences [3, 11, 13, 17, 18] and associations with age and disease stage in a reference region [11, 17, 19]. However, these analyses were limited to the previously reported list of potential reference regions and the decision was made based on qualitative approaches.

Given the lack of consensus on the choice of the reference region, the existence of a range of imaging modalities and disorders, the current work aims to outline a general framework for identifying objectively a reference region throughout the brain. A series of quantitative criteria are proposed, which were evaluated for QSM-MRI modalities on a cross-sectional and longitudinal cohort of individuals with dementia and normal ageing. The outcome from each criterion was ranked and combined to produce a single rating metric for each region. A power analysis was performed to evaluate the impact of utilizing each reference region on detecting between diagnostic-group differences.

2 Method

2.1 Dataset

Two subsets of data based on the availability of cross-sectional and longitudinal QSM-MRI from the Australian Imaging Biomarkers and Lifestyle (AIBL) were included [20]. For the cross-sectional analysis, 119 QSM scans comprised of 69 cognitively normal (CN), 22 mild cognitive impairment (MCI) and 28 Alzheimer's disease (AD). For longitudinal analysis, a baseline and 18-month follow-up QSM scans for 19 CN subjects without ApoE-ε4 alleles, Clinical Dementia Rating (CDR) = 0, Mini-Mental State Examination (MMSE) > 28 were included. Detailed demographic information is provided in Table 1.

Table 1. Demographic information CDR: Clinical dementia rating, MMSE: Mini-mental state examination

	Cross-sectional					Longitudinal (Age, MMSE and CDR at baseline)				
	#	Age	MMSE	CDR	Sex(F/M)	#	Age	Sex(F/M)	MMSE	CDR
CN	69	74.2 ± 7.3	29 ± 1	0.05 ± 0.2	37/32	19	73.2 ± 6.6	10/9	29.3 + 0.7	0
MCI	22	77.8 ± 5.4	27 ± 2	0.5 ± 0	12/10	–	–	–	–	–
AD	28	74.6 ± 9.3	21 ± 6	1.3 ± 2.1	15/13	–	–	–	–	–

2.2 Image Acquisition

MRI images were acquired on a 3T Siemens Tim Trio scanner with a 12-channel head coil. Subjects underwent anatomical T1-weighted (T1 W), gradient echo (GRE). The T1 W images were acquired using a standard 3D MPRAGE sequence with $1 \times 1 \times 1$ mm^3 resolution, TR/TE/TI = 1900/2.55/900 ms, flip angle 9°, field of view 256×256, and 160 slices. 3D GRE images used for QSM were acquired with 0.93×0.93 mm in-plane resolution and 1.75 mm slice thickness, repetition time/echo time of 27/20 ms, flip angle 20° and field of view 240×256, and 80 slices.

2.3 Image Post-processing

T1-weighted MPRAGE data were segmented into 73 grey-matter (GM) and 32 white-matter (WM) regions by segmentation propagation of an atlas database which had been previously parcellated using the Neuromorphometrics (63 subjects) [21] and FreeSurfer (FS) WM parcellation [22], respectively. The Neuromorphometrics and FS parcellations were then refined by the CSF, GM and WM segmentations obtained using the expectation maximization segmentation algorithm [23] directly applied to the T1-weighted images.

In order to reconstruct QSM images, phase offsets between each channel of the coil were removed by weighting the magnitude of the corresponding channel, and then combined to form a single-phase image. STI Suite software (version 2.2) was used for QSM dipole inversion process [24].

2.4 Reference Region Analysis

For this analysis, 100 reference regions including whole brain, CSF, WM, GM and 65 sub-regions from GM and 31 sub-regions from WM were used. As primary regions neocortex, frontal, parietal, temporal, occipital and hippocampus were considered. For each reference or primary region, a mean value for QSM was computed. To be able to combine statistical models, age and the regional mean values were scaled to zero mean and unit variance. A list of proposed criteria to identify a reliable reference region is as follows:

C1. *Reference region association with subject demographics such as age and sex:* there should be no or minimal association. This criterion was tested based on the β coefficient and standard error (SE) from a linear model with reference region as the dependent variable and subject demographics as covariates (lower β and SE are preferred for each covariate).

C2. *Reference region diagnostic-group separation effect* (e.g. between CN and MCI/AD participants): there should be no or minimal group differences. Any significant group effect in the reference region, e.g. MCI vs. AD, could impose a group difference when looking at the primary regions and therefore bias the normalized values. This was tested based on the β coefficient and SE from a linear model with reference region as the dependent variable, and diagnostic groups (CN, MCI and AD) as a covariate (lower β and SE are preferred for each covariate).

C3. *Reference region correlation with other primary areas of interest e.g. cortical/subcortical regions:* there should be a positive or negative association. The undesired change in the image is a global effect meaning that the measured values (both in the reference and target regions) are dependent. This was tested based on the β coefficient and SE from a linear model with the primary region as the dependent variable and reference region as independent variable while adjusting for age and gender (higher β and lower SE are preferred for the independent variable).

C4. *Reference region signal variations:* there should be a minimum variance. A lower variance in the reference region (of both CN and MCI/AD participants) shows the stability of the measurement as being unaffected by the pathology or a minimal contamination from neighboring structures (e.g. vessels) as well as other physiological or uncontrolled study confounds. This was tested by computing coefficient of variation (CV) where CV = standard deviation/mean (lower CV value is preferred).

C5. *Longitudinal reproducibility of the primary region when normalized:* there should be an improved reproducibility. Linear mixed models were used to assess the relationship between reference and primary regions over the two-time points controlled for age and gender modelled as QSM ~ Age*Gender + Region/Time + (1|ID). A lower β and SE are preferred for the Time (measured in years/months) by region interaction indicating little change between the reference region and the region of interest over time.

To combine all the criteria and obtain a single value representing the goodness-of-reference for normalization, the outcome of each criterion was ranked to 0 to 1 (higher the better) and then averaged to create a composite score. The Cohen's D metric was used as well to compute the overall performance of each reference region in terms of improving the diagnostic accuracy (MCI and AD compared to CN) as previously employed by [3, 4, 19].

3   Results

The top 5 reference regions (out of 100), when used for normalizing the primary regions of interest, are shown in Table 2. The average SE for reference regions (not shown here) were very similar and not significantly different. A comparison of previously reported reference regions and proposed top-ranked regions from Table 2 (first row) is shown in Fig. 1.

Table 2. Top 5 reference regions when used for normalizing regions of interest. GM: gray matter, WM: white-matter, Sup.: superior, Mid.: Middle, Orbi.: Orbital, Front.: Frontal, Post.: Posterior, Ant.: Anterior, Occp.: Occipital

Ranked reference	GM regions of interest					
	Neocortex	Middle frontal	Parietal	Middle temporal	Occipital	Hippocampus
1st	Sup. Temp. GM	Front. Pole WM	Orbi. Gyrus GM	Orbi. Gyrus GM	**Mid. Fron. WM**	**Mid. Fron. WM**
2nd	**Mid. Fron. WM**	**Mid. Fron. WM**	**Mid. Fron. WM**	**Mid. Fron. WM**	Supramaginal WM	Sup. Temp. GM
3rd	Orbi. Gyrus GM	Sup. Temp. GM	Post. Cing. GM	Post. Cing. GM	Insula WM	Occp. Pole GM
4th	Mid. Occp. GM	Supramaginal WM	Supramaginal WM	Ant. Orbi. GM	Postcentral WM	Post. Cing. GM
5th	Supramaginal WM	Angular Gyrus GM	Postcentral WM	Mid. Occp. GM	Lingual gyrus WM	Supramaginal WM

The Middle Frontal White Matter area had the best composite scores and ranked first overall from all the 100 areas considered for the normalization of QSM to study Alzheimer's disease.

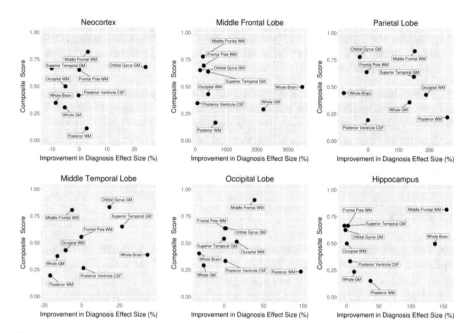

Fig. 1. Performance (in term of effect size) of previously reported reference regions and top-ranked region using the proposed method. A higher composite score (y-axis) represents a more suitable reference region based on the proposed criteria.

4   Discussion

This study proposed an objective framework for identifying a suitable reference region for intensity normalization with the purpose of removing global uncontrolled variations in quantitative images.

We argue in this paper that the selection of a normalization region should be done using objective and open criteria. This would allow fairer comparison between reported results removing doubts about introducing unwanted bias in the processing and interpretation. Furthermore, we also argue that the normalization regions should be dependent on the data acquisition and application. In our example, to study Alzheimer's disease, it would be important that the normalization region does not introduce group difference, and the area that ranked first would be different if another target region (than the neocortex) was under investigation. However, our study shows that one reference region (i.e. Mid Frontal WM) ranked highly overall when investigating multiple brain regions.

Our method is a data-driven approach and as such results ought to be investigated, to avoid spurious selection that would have no justification for the application at hand. Indeed, in our QSM application, the orbital gyrus GM had a better effect size improvement to separate AD from CN, however, in terms of pathophysiology and its lower score for the other criteria do not support it as a suitable choice. This highlights the benefit of having a set of criteria instead of investigating only one (e.g. effect size in this case).

5 Conclusion

Normalization is essential for removing global modulation effects, and consequently improving the sensitivity of quantitative imaging in detecting disease-specific differences. This study proposed a systematic approach to objectively identify a suitable reference region and evaluated it on QSM-MRI data to identify the Mid Frontal WM as the best normalization area for investigating neocortical QSM signal.

References

1. Dore, V., et al.: CapAIBL: automated reporting of cortical PET quantification without need of MRI on brain surface using a patch-based method. In: Wu, G., Coupé, P., Zhan, Y., Munsell, B.C., Rueckert, D. (eds.) Patch-MI 2016. LNCS, vol. 9993, pp. 109–116. Springer, Cham (2016). https://doi.org/10.1007/978-3-319-47118-1_14

2. Brendel, M., et al.: Improved longitudinal [18F]-AV45 amyloid PET by white matter reference and VOI-based partial volume effect correction. NeuroImage **108**, 450–459 (2015)

3. Yakushev, I., et al.: Choice of reference area in studies of Alzheimer's disease using positron emission tomography with fluorodeoxyglucose-F18. Psychiatr. Res. Neuroimaging **164**(2), 143–153 (2008)

4. Dukart, J., et al.: Differential effects of global and cerebellar normalization on detection and differentiation of dementia in FDG-PET studies. NeuroImage **49**(2), 1490–1495 (2010)

5. Mattsson, N., et al.: Association of brain amyloid-β with cerebral perfusion and structure in Alzheimer's disease and mild cognitive impairment. Brain **137**, 1550–1561 (2014)

6. Alsop, D.C., Casement, M., de Bazelaire, C., Fong, T., Press, D.Z.: Hippocampal hyperperfusion in Alzheimer's disease. NeuroImage **42**(4), 1267–1274 (2008)

7. Alsop, D.C., Detre, J.A., Grossman, M.: Assessment of cerebral blood flow in Alzheimer's disease by spin-labeled magnetic resonance imaging. Ann. Neurol. **47**(1), 93–100 (2000)

8. Acosta-Cabronero, J., Williams, G.B., Cardenas-Blanco, A., Arnold, R.J., Lupson, V., Nestor, P.J.: In vivo quantitative susceptibility mapping (QSM) in Alzheimer's disease. PLoS ONE **8**(11), e81093 (2013)

9. Acosta-Cabronero, J., Betts, M.J., Cardenas-Blanco, A., Yang, S., Nestor, P.J.: In vivo MRI mapping of brain iron deposition across the adult lifespan. J. Neurosci. **36**(2), 364–374 (2016)

10. Langkammer, C., et al.: Quantitative susceptibility mapping (QSM) as a means to measure brain iron? a post mortem validation study. Neuroimage **62**(3–2), 1593–1599 (2012)

11. Straub, S., et al.: Suitable reference tissues for quantitative susceptibility mapping of the brain. Magn. Reson. Med. **78**(1), 204–214 (2017)

12. Feng, X., Deistung, A., Reichenbach, J.R.: Quantitative susceptibility mapping (QSM) and R2* in the human brain at 3T: evaluation of intra-scanner repeatability. Z. Med. Phys. **28**(1), 36–48 (2018)

13. Lacalle-Aurioles, M., et al.: Is the cerebellum the optimal reference region for intensity normalization of perfusion MR studies in early Alzheimer's disease? PLoS ONE **8**(12), e81548 (2013)

14. Borghammer, P., Aanerud, J., Gjedde, A.: Data-driven intensity normalization of PET group comparison studies is superior to global mean normalization. NeuroImage **46**(4), 981–988 (2009)

15. Dukart, J., et al.: Reference cluster normalization improves detection of frontotemporal lobar degeneration by means of FDG-PET. PLoS ONE **8**(2), e55415 (2013)

16. Koch, K.M., Papademetris, X., Rothman, D.L., de Graaf, R.A.: Rapid calculations of susceptibility-induced magnetostatic field perturbations for in vivo magnetic resonance. Phys. Med. Biol. **51**(24), 6381–6402 (2006)
17. Fazlollahi, A., et al.: A normalisation framework for quantitative brain imaging; application to quantitative susceptibility mapping. In: 2017 IEEE 14th International Symposium on Biomedical Imaging (ISBI 2017), pp. 97–100 (2017)
18. Schwarz, C.G., et al.: Optimizing PiB-PET SUVR change-over-time measurement by a large-scale analysis of longitudinal reliability, plausibility, separability, and correlation with MMSE. NeuroImage **144**, 113–127 (2017)
19. Yakushev, I., et al.: SPM-based count normalization provides excellent discrimination of mild Alzheimer's disease and amnestic mild cognitive impairment from healthy aging. NeuroImage **44**(1), 43–50 (2009)
20. Ellis, K.A., et al.: The Australian imaging, biomarkers and lifestyle (AIBL) study of aging: methodology and baseline characteristics of 1112 individuals recruited for a longitudinal study of Alzheimer's disease. Int. Psychogeriatr. **21**(4), 672–687 (2009)
21. Tzourio-Mazoyer, N., et al.: Automated anatomical labeling of activations in SPM using a macroscopic anatomical parcellation of the MNI MRI single-subject brain. NeuroImage **15**(1), 273–289 (2002)
22. Salat, D.H., et al.: Regional white matter volume differences in nondemented aging and Alzheimer's disease. NeuroImage **44**(4), 1247–1258 (2009)
23. Leemput, K.V., Maes, F., Vandermeulen, D., Suetens, P.: Automated model-based tissue classification of MR images of the brain. IEEE Trans. Med. Imaging **18**(10), 897–908 (1999)
24. Li, W., Avram, A.V., Wu, B., Xiao, X., Liu, C.: Integrated Laplacian-based phase unwrapping and background phase removal for quantitative susceptibility mapping. NMR Biomed. **27**(2), 219–227 (2014)

Evaluation of Adjoint Methods in Photoacoustic Tomography with Under-Sampled Sensors

Hongxiang Lin[1](✉), Takashi Azuma[2], Mehmet Burcin Unlu[3,4,5], and Shu Takagi[1]

[1] Department of Mechanical Engineering, The University of Tokyo, Tokyo, Japan
hongxianglin@fel.t.u-tokyo.ac.jp
[2] Center for Disease Biology and Integrative Medicine,
The University of Tokyo, Tokyo, Japan
[3] Department of Physics, Bogazici University, Istanbul, Turkey
[4] Global Station for Quantum Medical Science and Engineering,
Global Institution for Collaborative Research and Education,
Hokkaido University, Sapporo, Japan
[5] Department of Radiation Oncology,
Stanford University School of Medicine, Stanford, CA, USA

Abstract. Photo-Acoustic Tomography (PAT) can reconstruct a distribution of optical absorbers acting as instantaneous sound sources in subcutaneous microvasculature of a human breast. Adjoint methods for PAT, typically Time-Reversal (TR) and Back-Projection (BP), are ways to refocus time-reversed acoustic signals on sources by wave propagation from the position of sensors. TR and BP have different treatments for received signals, but they are equivalent under continuously sampling on a closed circular sensor array in two dimensions. Here, we analyze image quality with discrete under-sampled sensors in the sense of the Shannon sampling theorem. We investigate resolution and contrast of TR and BP, respectively in one source-sensor pair configuration and the frequency domain. With Hankel's asymptotic expansion to the integrands of imaging functions, our main contribution is to demonstrate that TR and BP have better performance on contrast and resolution, respectively. We also show that the integrand of TR includes additional side lobes which degrade axial resolution whereas that of BP conversely has relatively small amplitudes. Moreover, omnidirectional resolution is improved if more sensors are employed to collect the received signals. Nevertheless, for the under-sampled sensors, we propose the Truncated Back-Projection (TBP) method to enhance the contrast of BP using removing higher frequency components in the received signals. We conduct numerical experiments on the two-dimensional projected phantom model extracted from OA-Breast Database. The experiments verify our

Electronic supplementary material The online version of this chapter (https://doi.org/10.1007/978-3-030-00928-1_9) contains supplementary material, which is available to authorized users.

A. F. Frangi et al. (Eds.): MICCAI 2018, LNCS 11070, pp. 73–81, 2018.
https://doi.org/10.1007/978-3-030-00928-1_9

theories and show that the proposed TBP possesses better omnidirectional resolution as well as contrast compared with TR and BP with under-sampled sensors.

Keywords: Photoacoustic tomography · Adjoint method
Time-reversal · Back-projection · Hankel asymptotic expansion
Resolution · Contrast

1   Introduction

Photo-Acoustic Tomography (PAT) is a prospective imaging modality that detects optical absorbers in human tissue for noninvasive diagnoses of diseases. When light is absorbed by the tissue and converted to heat, an acoustic wave is generated due to the thermoelastic expansion of the heated volume. Till now, PA microscopy, PA mammography, and PA computed tomography overcome difficulties of achieving rich optical contrast, high spatial resolution of ultrasound, as well as deep penetration depth. Nevertheless, artifacts cause image quality deterioration that significantly impacts the clinical diagnosis based on PA images. Artifacts are always concerned in a research branch called the incomplete PAT problem. In literature, PAT with a limited aperture or an inadequate broadband sensitivity at high frequency has been addressed in a sense of continuous regime. Regarding the discrete spatial sampling, deep learning based PAT can obtain high-quality images with using a training dataset [1].

Adjoint method for photoacoustic wave propagation is a category of mathematical techniques which reverses received signals and refocuses them on source locations. In this work, we consider two typical adjoint methods – Time-Reversal (TR) and Back-Projection (BP). As illustrated in Fig. 1, the TR method is conducted in a cavity and the reversed received waveform signals serve as a dynamic Dirichlet boundary condition. On the other hand, the BP method treats sensor elements as the reversing sources that retransmit circular waves modulated by reversed signals. Compared with some other iteration-based PAT methods, TR and BP possess the explicit imaging functions that illustrate the relative intensity of acoustic source distribution. The article [2] proposes that the two methods are mathematically coincident in a continuous regime with the far-field assumption. However, the numerical study in [3] shows that the limited number of spatially sampled sensor elements inside a finite spatial domain may enlarge the difference between the point spread functions of TR and BP. To investigate the impact of image qualities, we quantitatively analyze resolution and contrast in the under-sampled regime, i.e., the situation where the Shannon sampling theorem is invalid [4].

Here, we focus on establishing a novel methodology to quantitatively analyze resolution and contrast of imaging functions. We unify the forms of TR and BP imaging functions in the frequency domain on one source-sensor pair configuration. Then we decompose the imaging functions as a combination of the Bessel

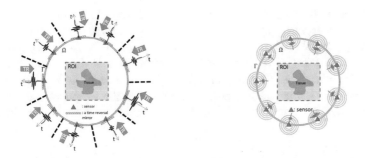

Fig. 1. Schematic diagrams of Time-Reversal (left) and Back-Projection (right).

functions since the free-space Green's function in a homogeneous medium is available. This allows us to see the contribution of main lobe for resolution and the intensity of side lobe corresponding to contrast. We also propose a straightforward variation called Truncated Back-Projection (TBP) to reconstruct the BP imaging function by removing the high-frequency components from the dataset.

2   Mathematical Formulation

Consider that photoacoustic wave excites from optical absorbers and propagates in a two-dimensional lossless homogeneous medium with a speed of sound of c_0; see Fig. 1. The circular boundary Γ of a radius of R is composed by N point-like sensor elements located at $\mathbf{y}_n$ $(n = 1, 2, \cdots, N)$ with equispaced arguments. The photoacoustic signals denoted by $g(\mathbf{y}_n, t)$ are semi-discretized in a time interval $[0, T]$ and sensor elements $\{\mathbf{y}_n\}$ on Γ. The purpose of PAT is to recover the initial pressure distribution p_0 in a region of interest (ROI) given the photoacoustic measurements $g(\mathbf{y}_n, t)$ on $\Gamma \times [0, T]$.

Adjoint methods are derived to approximate p_0 through different treatments for the reversed signals $g(\mathbf{y}_n, T - t)$ as well as refocusing the reversed wavefield on p_0 at the terminal time T. Together with the Green's representation theorem, the boundary-condition treatment for $g(\mathbf{y}_n, T - t)$ yields the semi-discrete TR imaging function:

$$I_{TR}^{<N>}(\mathbf{x}) = h_N \sum_{n=1}^{N} \int_0^T \frac{\partial G_d}{\partial \nu_{\mathbf{y}}}(\mathbf{x}, T | \mathbf{y} = \mathbf{y}_n, t) g(\mathbf{y}_n, T - t) dt + O(h_N^2), \quad (1)$$

where G_d is the Dirichlet Green's function of wave equation, $\nu_{\mathbf{y}}$ an outward unit normal vector at $\mathbf{y}$, and $h_N = 2\pi R/N$ a step size along Γ. On the other hand, the reversing-source treatment for $g(\mathbf{y}_n, T - t)$ infers the semi-discrete BP imaging function:

$$I_{BP}^{<N>}(\mathbf{x}) = \frac{h_N}{c_0} \sum_{n=1}^{N} \int_0^T \frac{\partial G_0}{\partial t}(\mathbf{x}, \tau | \mathbf{y}_n, t = T) g(\mathbf{y}_n, T - \tau) d\tau + O(h_N^2), \quad (2)$$

where G_0 is the free-space Green's function of wave equation. The derivation of Eqs. 1 and 2 is referred to [3] or the supplementary material.

The mathematical analysis is henceforth conducted in the frequency domain. The Fourier transform of a time-history function $f(t)$ is defined as $\hat{f}(\omega) = \int_{-\infty}^{+\infty} f(t)e^{i\omega t}dt$ where ω is an angular frequency and the hat $\wedge$ denotes the Fourier transform. Using the Parseval's identity (see the supplementary material) to Eqs. 1 and 2, we write out the frequency-domain expressions for TR and BP:

$$I_{TR}^{<N>}(\mathbf{x}) = \frac{h_N}{2\pi}\mathbf{Re}\sum_{n=1}^{N}\left\{\int_{-\infty}^{+\infty}\frac{\partial\widehat{G_d}}{\partial\nu_{\mathbf{y}}}(\mathbf{x},\mathbf{y}=\mathbf{y}_n,\omega)\overline{\hat{g}(\mathbf{y}_n,\omega)}d\omega\right\} + O(h_N^2), \quad (3)$$

$$I_{BP}^{<N>}(\mathbf{x}) = -\frac{h_N}{2\pi c_0}\mathbf{Re}\sum_{n=1}^{N}\left\{\int_{-\infty}^{+\infty}i\omega\widehat{G_0}(\mathbf{x},\mathbf{y}_n,\omega)\overline{\hat{g}(\mathbf{y}_n,\omega)}d\omega\right\} + O(h_N^2), \quad (4)$$

where $\mathbf{Re}$ denotes the real part of a complex value and the overline denotes complex conjugate. The free-space Green's function in the frequency domain is written as $\widehat{G_0}(\mathbf{x},\mathbf{y},\omega) = \frac{i}{4}H_0^{(1)}\left(\frac{\omega}{c_0}|\mathbf{x}-\mathbf{y}|\right)$ where $H_0^{(1)}$ is a zeroth-order Hankel function of the first kind.

3   Image Quality Analysis

One source-sensor pair configuration is considered to characterize the image quality of TR and BP images. There is only one acoustic source located at $\mathbf{a}$ in the cavity Ω. The sensor at $\mathbf{y}$ receiving the single-source waveform signal satisfies the frequency-domain expression:

$$\hat{g}(\mathbf{y},\omega) = -i\omega F(\omega)\widehat{G_0}(\mathbf{y},\mathbf{a},\omega), \quad (5)$$

where $F(\omega)$ is a real function of the $\omega_{\max}$-bandlimited spectrum.

3.1   Expansion of Imaging Functions

Substitute Eq. 5 into Eqs. 3 and 4 first, which yields a unified imaging function for the source-sensor pair $(\mathbf{a},\mathbf{y})$ configuration:

$$I_j^{<1>}(\mathbf{x}) = \frac{h_1}{2\pi}\int_{-\infty}^{+\infty}F(\omega)\,\mathrm{Re}[K_j(\mathbf{x},\omega)]d\omega + O(h_1^2), \quad j = \mathrm{TR},\ \mathrm{BP} \quad (6)$$

where the integrands are specified as $K_{TR}(\mathbf{x},\omega) = i\omega\frac{\widehat{\partial G_d}}{\partial\nu_{\mathbf{y}}}(\mathbf{x},\mathbf{y},\omega)\overline{\widehat{G_0}(\mathbf{y},\mathbf{a},\omega)}$, and $K_{BP}(\mathbf{x},\omega) = \frac{\omega^2}{c_0}\widehat{G_0}(\mathbf{x},\mathbf{y},\omega)\overline{\widehat{G_0}(\mathbf{y},\mathbf{a},\omega)}$.

By canceling factors, we reduce K_{TR} and K_{BP} to $\widetilde{K_{TR}}$ and $\widetilde{K_{BP}}$, respectively, such that they share an identical main lobe.[1] Employing Hankel's asymptotic expansion [5], we write out the BP imaging function $I_{BP}^{<1>}$ and the discrepancy function $\Delta I^{<1>}$ between TR and BP in proportion to the integration of $\widetilde{K_{BP}}$ and $\widetilde{K_{TR}} - \widetilde{K_{BP}}$ over the angular frequency domain respectively:

---

[1] In specific, $\widetilde{K_{TR}} = -32\pi c_0^3\frac{|\mathbf{y}-\mathbf{a}|}{|\mathbf{y}|}K_{TR}$ and $\widetilde{K_{BP}} = 32\pi c_0^3 K_{BP}$.

$$I_{BP}^{<1>}(\mathbf{x}) \propto \int_{-\infty}^{+\infty} F(\omega)\, \mathrm{Re}[\widetilde{K_{BP}}](\mathbf{x}, \omega)\mathrm{d}\omega$$

$$\approx \int_{-\infty}^{+\infty} F(\omega) \left[\frac{2\omega c_0}{\pi|\mathbf{y}-\mathbf{a}|} J_0(d_{\mathbf{x},\mathbf{a}}^{(\omega)}) + O((d_{\mathbf{x},\mathbf{a}}^{(\omega)})^3) \right] \mathrm{d}\omega, \qquad (7)$$

$$\Delta I^{<1>}(\mathbf{x}) \propto \int_{-\infty}^{+\infty} F(\omega)\, \mathrm{Re}[\widetilde{K_{TR}} - \widetilde{K_{BP}}](\mathbf{x}, \omega)\mathrm{d}\omega$$

$$\approx e^{i\Theta} \int_{-\infty}^{+\infty} F(\omega) \left[\frac{2c_0^2}{\pi|\mathbf{y}-\mathbf{a}|^2} J_1(d_{\mathbf{x},\mathbf{a}}^{(\omega)}) + O((d_{\mathbf{x},\mathbf{a}}^{(\omega)})^4) \right] \mathrm{d}\omega \qquad (8)$$

where $d_{\mathbf{x},\mathbf{a}}^{(\omega)} = \frac{\omega}{c_0}|\mathbf{x}-\mathbf{a}|$. Θ is the angle corresponding to the opposite side $|\mathbf{x}-\mathbf{y}|$ of the triangle formed by the points $\mathbf{a}$, $\mathbf{x}$ and $\mathbf{y}$. See the derivation in the supplementary material. If ω_c is the angular center frequency and $\Theta = 0$ or π, it yields that the axial pattern of BP is approximately the zeroth-order Bessel function $J_0(d_{\mathbf{x},\mathbf{a}}^{(\omega_c)})$ while that of TR has the same main lobe as BP plus a side lobe of the first-order Bessel function $J_1(d_{\mathbf{x},\mathbf{a}}^{(\omega_c)})$.

3.2   Resolution Analysis

Axial resolution is quantified by Full Width at Half Maximum (FWHM). Based on the axial pattern in Eq. 7, since $J_0(\xi)$ has a maximum at $\xi = 0$ and a half maximum at approximately $\xi = 1.5$, we have FWHM of BP: $W_{\mathrm{BP}}^{\mathrm{FWHM}} \approx 2 \times 1.5/(2\pi/\lambda_c) \approx 0.48\lambda_c$ where λ_c is the wavelength corresponding to the center frequency. Similarly, since the half maximum values of $J_1(\xi)$ are located at $\xi = 0.6$ and 3.1, we have FWHM of the side lobe shown in Eq. 8: $W_{\Delta I}^{\mathrm{FWHM}} \approx (3.1 - 0.6)/(2\pi/\lambda_c) \approx 0.40\lambda_c$. Additionally, for both TR and BP, the lateral resolution degrades by noting that the radial transmission of wavelet implied in Eq. 6 leads to artifact of an arc pattern.

For adjoint methods, the omni-directional resolution of the source point $\mathbf{a}$ can be extended from the axial one through superposition of adjoint wavelets. As shown in Fig. 2, the four wavelets serve as carriers of the same FWHM information oriented from the different directions. In morphology, they partially overlap and form a polygon-like spot approximating a circle. Moreover, the superposed wavefield mitigates the artifact since the amplification at $\mathbf{a}$ significantly inhibits the intensity level of synthesized wavefield in other pixels where there are no sources.

3.3   Contrast Analysis and Truncated Back-Projection

The contrast is discussed in the regime of an under-sampled spatial grid; the full-sampling condition is referred to [4]. Figure 3 shows the profiles of $\widetilde{K_{TR}} - \widetilde{K_{BP}}$ and $\widetilde{K_{BP}}$ along the axial direction with respect to three typical frequencies. The side lobe of the imaging function of TR dominates due to the larger intensity in

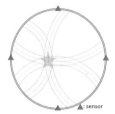

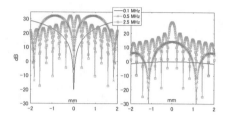

Fig. 2. The sketch of the adjoint wavefield synthesized by four equispaced-sensor signals refocused on the source (star).

Fig. 3. The intensity level of $\widetilde{K_{TR}} - \widetilde{K_{BP}}$ (left) and $\widetilde{K_{BP}}$ (right) on one source-sensor pair configuration along the axial direction. The source **a** is placed at the origin. The reference value is given by $\widetilde{K_{BP}}$ at the central point and at a frequency of 0.1 MHz.

a range of frequency. Therefore, for TR, the intensity level in a prescribed neighborhood of the source spot does not fiercely alter with the change of the spatial sampling rate. Conversely, regrading BP, since we often interpolate the circular-band wavefield on a coarse Cartesian grid, the maximum may occasionally be selected out but the rest of the interpolated grid points have no significantly large values. Their contrast deteriorates after normalization is conducted.

To solve this, we propose the Truncated Back-Projection (TBP) method by means of only exploiting the low frequency components in Eq. 4 given by

$$I_{TBP}^{<N,\mu>}(\mathbf{x}) = -\frac{h_N}{2\pi c_0} \mathbf{Re} \sum_{n=1}^{N} \left\{ \int_{|\omega|<\mu} i\omega \widehat{G_0}(\mathbf{x}, \mathbf{y}, \omega)\overline{\widehat{g}(\mathbf{y}, \omega)}d\omega \right\} + O(h_N^2), \quad (9)$$

where μ is the truncated bound of angular frequency. If we select a μ much smaller than the upper bound $\omega_{\max}$, more large values adjacent to the maximum of $J_0(d_{\mathbf{x},\mathbf{a}}^{(\mu)})$ are attainable in the coarse grid since the larger FWHM proportional to the wavelength has capacity of containing more grid points. We recommend to set $\mu = 2\pi M/(T_M \cdot PPW)$ where M is the number of gird points per side of ROI, T_M acquisition time in ROI, and PPW the number of grid points per wavelength indicating the coarseness of grid.

4   Numerical Experiments

We carry out two numerical experiments with a single source and a breast vasculature phantom model used as initial pressure distributions. The acoustic measurement datasets are synthesized by the K-wave toolbox, a photoacoustic Matlab simulator using the k-space pseudo spectral method [6]. To avoid the inverse crime, the measurement datasets are generated on a fine Cartesian grid but the adjoint methods are conducted on a coarse one.

4.1   Single Source-Sensor Pair Reconstruction

Figure 4 shows the circular-arc wavefields reconstructed by the adjoint methods. All the wavefields are normalized by the maximum absolute values. In terms of axial resolution, the values of FWHM for TR, BP, and TBP are 2.67, 6.19, and 5.58 mm shown in Fig. 4(e). The maximum values, used to assess the contrast, for TR, BP, and TBP are 0.90, 0.089, and 0.78. We observe that the axial profile of the TR image has a fat-tail distribution because of relatively strong side lobe.

In terms of spatial sampling, the maximum is sparsely selected out from a coarse grid. It may lead to the deterioration of contrast in the BP image. The numerical experiment is conducted on a grid of 512-by-512 points, coarse for $PPW = 0.89$, provided $\omega_{\max} = 2.73 \times 10^7$ rad $\cdot$ s^{-1} and $T_M = 1.33 \times 10^{-4}$ s. It requires at least a 2500-by-2500 grid to achieve the regime of full sampling, i.e. $PPW = 4.32$. The truncated bound μ limited to 6.82×10^6 rad $\cdot$ s^{-1} for TBP fulfills the need that the 512-by-512 grid satisfies $PPW = 4.32$ although its point spread function is oscillating.

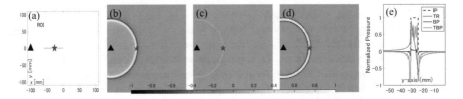

Fig. 4. (a) One source-sensor pair configuration with the source at $(-12.5, 0)$ [mm] and the sensor at $(-100, 0)$ [mm]. The adjoint wavefields reconstructed by (b) TR, (c) BP, and (d) TBP. (e) The normalized pressure distributions of the initial pressure (IP) distribution, TR, BP, and TBP profiles along the red dot line in (a). The black triangles and blue stars represent sensors and sources, respectively.

4.2   Breast Phantom Reconstruction

The breast phantom is extracted from OA-Breast Database [7] and projected to two dimensions. The reconstructed vasculature images with respect to 16, 64, and 256 equispaced sensor elements are shown in Fig. 5, which corresponds to the under sampling, the critical-condition sampling, and the full sampling based on Shannon sampling theorem. The more sensor elements we utilize, the better resolution and contrast will achieve for TR, BP, and TBP, which validates the summary in Sect. 3.2. We demonstrate that whenever the sampling criterion is selected, TR and BP have advantages of contrast and axial resolution, respectively. Moreover, a 256-by-256 grid of $PPW = 1.32$ are used to validate TBP, provided $\omega_{\max} = 1.82 \times 10^7$ rad $\cdot$ s^{-1} and $T_M = 6.67 \times 10^{-5}$ s. The parameter $\mu = 6.82 \times 10^6$ rad $\cdot$ s^{-1} assures high contrast of the TBP image even in the situation of the under-sampled sensors.

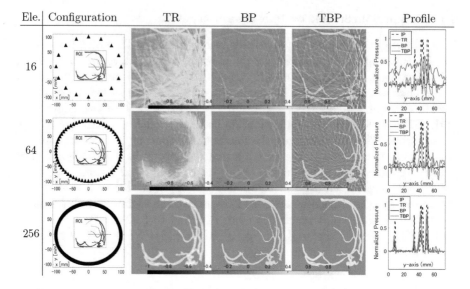

Fig. 5. The breast vasculature images reconstructed by the adjoint methods with the different sampling of sensor elements. ROI is a square centered at the origin with an area of 100×100 mm^2. The reconstructions are carried out on three arrays with equispaced sensor elements (ele.). In the configuration, the black triangles and blue lines represent sensors and sources, respectively. The images reconstructed by TR, BP, and TBP are shown in the middle three columns. The last column shows the profiles along the red dot line in the first column.

5   Conclusions

In this work, we demonstrate that TR and BP possess high contrast and high axial resolution with under-sampled sensors, respectively. Asymptotic expansion technique helps to mathematically specify the intrinsic behaviors of TR and BP in the frequency domain. We propose the TBP method to compensate the contrast issue in the situation of spatial coarse grid. Although all of the analyses and numerical tests are presented in two dimensions, the methodology is possible to be correspondingly extended to high dimensions with the irregular geometry of sensor array and the complex structure of medium [8].

References

1. Antholzer, S., Haltmeier, M., Schwab, J.: Deep learning for photoacoustic tomography from sparse data. arXiv:1704.04587 (2017)
2. Ammari, H., Bretin, E., Garnier, J., Wahab, A.: Time reversal in attenuating acoustic media. Contemp. Math. **548**, 151–163 (2011)
3. Arridge, S.R., Betcke, M.M., Cox, B.T., Lucka, F., Treeby, B.E.: On the adjoint operator in photoacoustic tomography. Inverse Prob. **32**(11), 115012 (2016)
4. Haltmeier, M.: Sampling conditions for the circular radon transform. IEEE Trans. Image Process. **25**(6), 2910–2919 (2016)

5. Abramowitz, M., Stegun, I.: Handbook of Mathematical Functions with Formulas, Graphs, and Mathematical Tables. Dover Publications, New York (1965)
6. Treeby, B.E., Cox, B.T.: k-Wave: MATLAB toolbox for the simulation and reconstruction of photoacoustic wave fields. J. Biomed. Opt. **15**(2), 021314 (2010)
7. Lou, Y., Zhou, W., Matthews, T.P., Appleton, C.M., Anastasio, M.A.: Generation of anatomically realistic numerical phantoms for photoacoustic and ultrasonic breast imaging. J. Biomed. Opt. **22**(4), 041015 (2017)
8. Borcea, L., Papanicolaou, G., Tsogka, C.: Theory and applications of time reversal and interferometric imaging. Inverse Prob. **19**(6), S139 (2003)

A No-Reference Quality Metric
for Retinal Vessel Tree Segmentation

Adrian Galdran[1(✉)], Pedro Costa[1], Alessandro Bria[2], Teresa Araújo[1,3],
Ana Maria Mendonça[1,3], and Aurélio Campilho[1,3]

[1] INESC-TEC - Institute for Systems and Computer Engineering,
Technology and Science, Porto, Portugal
{adrian.galdran,pvcosta,tfaraujo}@inesctec.pt
[2] Università degli studi di Cassino e del Lazio Meridionale, Cassino, Italy
a.bria@unicas.it
[3] Faculdade de Engenharia da Universidade do Porto, Porto, Portugal
{amendon,campilho}@fe.up.pt

Abstract. Due to inevitable differences between the data used for training modern CAD systems and the data encountered when they are
deployed in clinical scenarios, the ability to automatically assess the quality of predictions when no expert annotation is available can be critical.
In this paper, we propose a new method for quality assessment of retinal
vessel tree segmentations in the absence of a reference ground-truth. For
this, we artificially degrade expert-annotated vessel map segmentations
and then train a CNN to predict the similarity between the degraded
images and their corresponding ground-truths. This similarity can be
interpreted as a proxy to the quality of a segmentation. The proposed
model can produce a visually meaningful quality score, effectively predicting the quality of a vessel tree segmentation in the absence of a manually segmented reference. We further demonstrate the usefulness of our
approach by applying it to automatically find a threshold for soft probabilistic segmentations on a per-image basis. For an independent state-
of-the-art unsupervised vessel segmentation technique, the thresholds
selected by our approach lead to statistically significant improvements in
F1-score (+2.67%) and Matthews Correlation Coefficient (+3.11%) over
the thresholds derived from ROC analysis on the training set. The score
is also shown to correlate strongly with F1 and MCC when a reference
is available.

1 Introduction

The ability to automatically assess the quality of the outcomes produced by
CAD systems when they are meant to work in real clinical scenarios is critical. Unfortunately, internal validation data can be contaminated when used for
incremental method development, leading to over-optimistic performance expectations. In addition, differences between the data used for training a model and
the data that such model encounters in practice may lead to relevant failures.

© Springer Nature Switzerland AG 2018
A. F. Frangi et al. (Eds.): MICCAI 2018, LNCS 11070, pp. 82–90, 2018.
https://doi.org/10.1007/978-3-030-00928-1_10

On the other hand, the availability of automatic quality control tools is key for the effective deployment and monitoring of computational tools on large-scale medical image analysis studies or clinical routines. Unfortunately, this aspect of the CAD system design pipeline is seldom addressed in the literature [12].

In the retinal image analysis field, computational models developed for automatic image understanding are ubiquitous. In this context, a task of particular interest is the analysis of the retinal vessel tree. This involves the study of vascular biomarkers that are of great interest as early indicators of potential diseases, like vessel calibers, tortuosity, and fractal dimension. However, in order to reliably extract such biomarkers, the first step is to extract an accurate binary segmentation of the vessels. For this reason, a large body of research has been dedicated to solve this problem [1,15]. In comparison, few research has been addressed to the related task of determining the quality of the extracted segmentations.

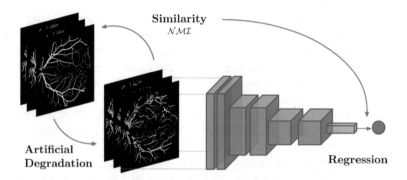

Fig. 1. Representation of the training stage of the proposed method. Similarity between original/degraded vessel maps is measured by Normalized Mutual Information ($\mathcal{NMI}$).

When the task of retinal vessel segmentation is considered as a binary classification problem, standard metrics like accuracy can be applied to measure performance. Nevertheless, due to the sparsity of the vasculature within the retina, vessel segmentation is a highly imbalanced classification problem, and more appropriate performance estimates like sensitivity, specificity, F1 score, or Matthews Correlation Coefficient, are necessary. More advanced techniques have been also proposed, *e.g.* [3] or [14]. In both cases, the overall strategy is to allow for some error margin, in order to compensate also for inter-observer differences in the ground-truth generation stage. This is achieved by analyzing the degree of overlap between a manual reference and a segmentation in an adaptive manner, and also penalizing dissimilarities and disconnections on the vessel skeletons.

All the above approaches belong to the category of full-reference quality metrics, for which a ground-truth image is required. In this paper, a no-reference quality score for the automatic assessment of retinal vessel segmentations is introduced for the first time. The proposed method operates in the absence of a reference image. This is achieved by designing a CNN that predicts the similarity between a manual segmentation and a corresponding artificially degraded transformation, as summarized in Fig. 1. This similarity can be considered as an estimate of the degraded segmentations' quality. The provided experimental results demonstrate that, once trained, the proposed model produces a quality score that correlates well with full-reference quality metrics, and is useful to detect deficient segmentations generated by automatic vessel segmentation techniques.

2   Methodology

In this section we provide a detailed step-by-step technical explanation of the approach proposed to build and train a no-reference retinal vessel quality metric.

2.1   Generating Realistic Degraded Vessel Trees

The first step in our approach is to model an incorrectly segmented vessel tree. The most typical artifacts in this case involve under-segmentations, which often lead to vasculature disconnections and thin vessels vanishing. Another common error source in this case is the presence of the optic disk and retinal lesions, which can be confused with vessels by automatic techniques, leading to over-segmentations.

While the latter class of errors is harder to model due to the wide variability of retinal lesions, under-segmentations can be simulated by local morphological erosions, as shown in Fig. 2. We also include morphological dilations, as well as completely white and dark images degraded with impulse noise on the field-of-view, so as to embed in the model information related to over-segmentations.

The examples generated in this stage are produced from a set of manual expert-delineated binary vessel trees, and they are meant to be supplied later to our model in training time. Hence, they need to be generated in an efficient manner. It is also important to train the model with perfect segmentations so that it can correctly attribute a high score in cases where an algorithm successfully separates the vasculature. For this purpose, given a manual vessel tree v, we produce a synthetically degraded version $\mathbf{deg}(v)$ of it as follows:

$$\mathbf{deg}(v) = \begin{cases} v, & \text{for } 0 \leq p < \frac{1}{5} \\ \mathcal{N}, & \text{for } \frac{1}{5} \leq p < \frac{2}{5} \\ \mathcal{M}(v), & \text{for } \frac{2}{5} \leq p \leq 1, \end{cases} \tag{1}$$

where p is drawn from a uniform probability distribution $\mathcal{U}(0,1)$, $\mathcal{N}$ represents impulse noise, and $\mathcal{M}$ is a stochastic morphological operator that performs a random number of local degradations by first selecting a number n of square image patches $\bar{v}$ of fixed size, extracted from random location on the original vessel image v. Each of these patches undergoes the following transformations:

$$\mathcal{M}(\bar{v}) = \begin{cases} \mathcal{E}_s(\bar{v}), & \text{for } 0 \leq p < \frac{1}{2} \\ \mathcal{D}_s(\bar{v}), & \text{for } \frac{1}{2} < p \leq 1 \end{cases} \tag{2}$$

where $\mathcal{E}_s$ and $\mathcal{D}_s$ are the morphological erosion and dilation operators respectively, specified by a square structuring element s of a size randomly selected to be 3, 5, or 7 at each step. The structuring element is itself randomly built according to a Bernoulli distribution with $p = 0.5$ at each pixel position. Once $\bar{v}$ has been artificially degraded, it is stored back at its original location in v.

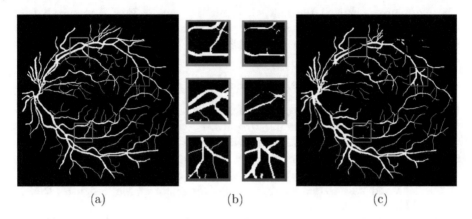

(a)   (b)   (c)

Fig. 2. (a) Manual vessel segmentation. (b) Examples of image patches extracted from (a) with corresponding degraded counterparts. (c) Artificially degraded version of (a). The normalized mutual information between (a) and (c) is $\mathcal{NMI}_{[0,1]} = 0.89$. At the patch level, images in the top row of (b) have $\mathcal{NMI}_{[0,1]} = 0.39$, middle row $\mathcal{NMI}_{[0,1]} = 0.23$, and bottom row $\mathcal{NMI}_{[0,1]} = 0.45$.

2.2 Mutual Information as a Similarity Metric Between Binary Vessel Maps

The next step is to establish a similarity measure between a degraded vessel tree and a manually segmented one. Moreover, since the goal is to build an image quality score, this measure should preferably be bounded a-priori in a finite interval. Among the many possibilities, we select the Normalized Mutual Information in order to analyze the amount of shared information in both images.

Given a manually-segmented vessel tree v and its degraded counterpart $\deg(v)$, Mutual Information considers both the marginal entropies $\mathcal{H}(v)$ and $\mathcal{H}(\deg(v))$ and the entropy of their joint probability distribution $\mathcal{H}(v, \deg(v))$:

$$\mathcal{MI}(v, \deg(v)) = \mathcal{H}(v) + \mathcal{H}(\deg(v)) - \mathcal{H}(v, \deg(v)). \qquad (3)$$

This quantity has been widely used for medical image registration tasks [7]. A derived formulation is the normalized mutual information:

$$\mathcal{NMI}(v, \deg(v)) = \frac{\mathcal{H}(v) + \mathcal{H}(\deg(v))}{\mathcal{H}(v, \deg(v))}, \qquad (4)$$

which is more robust to overlaps in both images, and it is bounded as $1 \leq \mathcal{NMI} \leq 2$, [6]. Finally, in order to obtain a similarity score producing a maximum value of 1 when both images are perfectly aligned, we reparametrize Eq. (4) as follows:

$$\mathcal{NMI}_{[0,1]}(v, \deg(v)) = 2 \cdot [1 - \frac{1}{\mathcal{NMI}(v, \deg(v))}]. \tag{5}$$

The Normalized Mutual Information formula given by Eq. (5) is suitable for the problem of estimating the similarity of a manual vessel segmentation and a degraded version of it, as shown in Fig. 2.

2.3   A Deep Architecture for Vessel Map Similarity Regression

In order to learn a quality score for binary vessel tree images, we proceed as follows: given a dataset of manually segmented vessel maps, we apply the operator defined in Eq. (1) to build degraded versions, which serve as input for the model. The similarity of the input with its manually-segmented counterpart is computed by means of Eq. (5), which is considered as a proxy to the quality of the degraded vessel tree. For regressing this quantity, we design a CNN as specified below.

The proposed architecture consists of a subsequent application of downsampling and convolution layers, specified in Fig. 3. Downsampling was implemented as a convolution with stride of 2. Non-linear activation functions were applied after each layer, specifically Leaky ReLU units with a slope parameter of $\alpha = 0.02$. A Global Average Pooling (GAP) was applied to obtain a uni-dimensional representation of the input vessel tree of size 512. This representation was supplied to two fully-connected layers, and the output was passed through a sigmoid, resulting in a score in $[0, 1]$. This score was compared to the previously computed similarity through an $\mathcal{L}_1$ loss. The weights of the model were then updated by error backpropagation. The loss was minimized via standard mini-batch gradient descent with the Adam optimizer [5] and a learning rate of $2e^{-4}$.

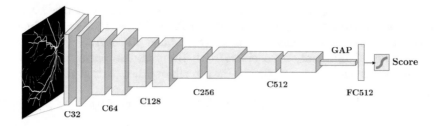

Fig. 3. An architecture for regressing similarity between a degraded vessel tree and a manual segmentation. CN stands for a convolutional layer with N filters of size 3×3.

3   Experimental Results

We provide now a qualitative and quantitative analysis of the performance of the developed No-Reference Quality Metric (NRQM) for retinal vessel segmentation.

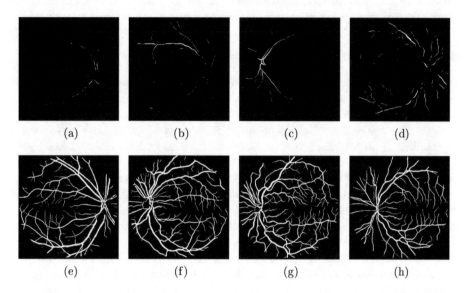

Fig. 4. The four worse and best automatic segmentations extracted from the Messidor dataset with the technique of [9], sorted according to the proposed quality score.

3.1   Qualitative Evaluation

In a first stage, the proposed NRQM is evaluated for the task of detecting when a deficient segmentation is produced by an automatic retinal vessel extraction scheme. The Messidor-1 dataset [2], which contains 1200 images for which no manually-delineated vessel maps are available, is employed. In order to automatically produce segmentations, we apply a U-Net architecture [9]. To train it, we use the DRIVE dataset [11], which has 40 retinal images with vessel ground-truth. The model is trained on 20 images, achieving an area under the Receiver-Operator Curve (ROC) of $97,5\%$ on the remaining images, in line with current methods.

The U-Net model produces grayscale images, referred to as soft segmentations. Each pixel contains its vessel likelihood. In order to generate a binary segmentation that can be used afterwards, $e.g.$ to measure biomarkers related to the retinal vasculature, a binarizing threshold needs to be selected. The only feasible approach when such a system is to be deployed in a clinical scenario is to derive this threshold from the ROC curve as the one that optimizes a certain performance metric. The threshold maximizing the Youden index was selected, for which an accuracy of 95.67% was achieved on the DRIVE test set.

After selecting an optimal threshold, 1200 soft segmentations are generated from the Messidor dataset, and binarized with it. A score is computed for every segmentation, and the segmentations are sorted in descending order relative to it. Figure 4 displays the three best and worst segmentations according to the proposed NRQM. It is important to stress that the identification of these deficient segmentations was performed on a dataset without any reference ground-truth.

3.2 Quantitative Experimental Evaluation

For a quantitative evaluation of our NRQM, we selected the popular COSFIRE unsupervised vessel segmentation technique [1]. To remove any bias in our comparisons, we consider an independent test set, DRiDB [8], composed of 50 retinal images. Our evaluation of the proposed NRQM is twofold. In both cases, vessel segmentation performance will be assessed in terms of F1-score and Matthews Correlation Coefficient (MCC), which are often used within the vessel segmentation literature [1,15] to gain evaluation insight due to the skewed-classes setting.

We compared two binarization strategies. First, ROC analysis was performed on DRIVE soft segmentations produced by COSFIRE to obtain optimal thresholds maximizing F1 score and MCC respectively. These thresholds were used to produce binary segmentations for every DRiDB image. Second, we thresholded DRiDB images at all possible values, and for each image we selected the threshold that led to a binary segmentation maximizing our NRQM. Finally, we performed statistical analysis to compare F1-scores and MCC obtained with the two approaches. Data normality was assessed using the D'Agostino-Pearson test [4]. In all cases, data were not normally distributed. Thus, we performed a nonparametric test to assess whether their population mean ranks differed using the Wilcoxon signed-rank test [13]. F1-scores and MCC of segmentations obtained using our NRQM were statistically significantly higher than those from the other compared approach, with a median difference of 0.03 for both performance metrics.

In a second stage, we investigated whether our NRQM was statistically correlated with the F1-score and MCC metrics. We calculated the F1-score and MCC for 256 uniformly distributed values of the NRQM. Again, we found that data were not normally distributed, thus we performed a nonparametric test to measure the rank correlation between the different metrics using the Spearman's r test [10]. The proposed NRQM was very strongly positively correlated with F1-score ($r = 0.92$) and strongly positively correlated with MCC ($r = 0.68$).

4   Conclusions and Future Work

A no-reference metric for assessing the quality of retinal vessel maps has been introduced. Experimental results demonstrate that this score can capture the nature of deficient segmentations generated by retinal vessel segmentation algorithms, correlating well with full-reference metrics when ground-truth is available.

The approach presented here follows a general idea of modeling the degradation instead of a segmentation goal. If faithful synthetically degraded segmentations can be produced, and a meaningful similarity metric can be defined, a similar model can theoretically be trained to predict the similarity between these degraded examples and the source images. This is independent of the problem at hand, and could be explored on applications beyond retinal vessel tree segmentations.

Acknowledgments. This work is financed by the ERDF – European Regional Development Fund through the Operational Programme for Competitiveness and Internationalisation - COMPETE 2020 Programme, and by National Funds through the FCT - Fundação para a Ciência e a Tecnologia within project CMUP-ERI/TIC/ 0028/2014. Teresa Araújo is funded by the FCT grant contract SFRH/BD/122365/ 2016. The Titan Xp used for this research was donated by the NVIDIA Corporation.

References

1. Azzopardi, G., Strisciuglio, N., Vento, M., Petkov, N.: Trainable COSFIRE filters for vessel delineation with application to retinal images. Med. Image Anal. **19**(1), 46–57 (2015)
2. Decenciére, E., et al.: Feedback on a publicly distributed image database: the messidor database. Image Anal. Stereol. **33**(3), 231–234 (2014)
3. Gegundez-Arias, M.E., Aquino, A., Bravo, J.M., Marin, D.: A function for quality evaluation of retinal vessel segmentations. IEEE Trans. Med. Imaging **31**(2), 231–239 (2012)
4. Ghasemi, A., Zahediasl, S.: Normality tests for statistical analysis: a guide for non-statisticians. Int. J. Endocrinol. Metab. **10**(2), 486 (2012)
5. Kingma, D.P., Ba, J.: Adam: A Method for Stochastic Optimization. arXiv:1412.6980 [cs], December 2014
6. Melbourne, A., Hawkes, D., Atkinson, D.: Image registration using uncertainty coefficients. In: 2009 IEEE International Symposium on Biomedical Imaging: From Nano to Macro, pp. 951–954, June 2009
7. Pluim, J.P.W., Maintz, J.B.A., Viergever, M.A.: Mutual-information-based registration of medical images: a survey. IEEE Trans. Med. Imaging **22**(8), 986–1004 (2003)
8. Prentašić, P., et al.: Diabetic retinopathy image database(DRiDB): a new database for diabetic retinopathy screening programs research. In: 2013 8th International Symposium on Image and Signal Processing and Analysis (ISPA), pp. 711–716, September 2013
9. Ronneberger, O., Fischer, P., Brox, T.: U-Net: convolutional networks for biomedical image segmentation. In: Navab, N., Hornegger, J., Wells, W.M., Frangi, A.F. (eds.) MICCAI 2015. LNCS, vol. 9351, pp. 234–241. Springer, Cham (2015). https://doi.org/10.1007/978-3-319-24574-4_28
10. Spearman, C.: The proof and measurement of association between two things. Am. J. Psychol. **15**(1), 72–101 (1904)
11. Staal, J., Abramoff, M.D., Niemeijer, M., Viergever, M.A.: Ginneken, B.v.: Ridge-based vessel segmentation in color images of the retina. IEEE Trans. Med. Imaging **23**(4), 501–509 (2004)

12. Valindria, V.V., et al.: Reverse classification accuracy: predicting segmentation performance in the absence of ground truth. IEEE Trans. Med. Imaging **36**(8), 1597–1606 (2017)
13. Wilcoxon, F.: Individual comparisons by ranking methods. Biom. Bull. **1**(6), 80–83 (1945)
14. Yan, Z., Yang, X., Cheng, K.T.T.: A skeletal similarity metric for quality evaluation of retinal vessel segmentation. IEEE Trans. Med. Imaging **PP**(99), 1 (2017)
15. Zhang, J., et al.: Robust retinal vessel segmentation via locally adaptive derivative frames in orientation scores. IEEE Trans. Med. Imaging **35**(12), 2631–2644 (2016)

Efficient and Accurate MRI Super-Resolution Using a Generative Adversarial Network and 3D Multi-level Densely Connected Network

Yuhua Chen[1,2]([✉]) [iD], Feng Shi[2] [iD], Anthony G. Christodoulou[2] [iD],
Yibin Xie[2] [iD], Zhengwei Zhou[2] [iD], and Debiao Li[1,2]

[1] University of California, Los Angeles, CA 90095, USA
chyuhua@ucla.edu
[2] Biomedical Imaging Research Institute, Cedars-Sinai Medical Center,
Los Angeles, CA 90048, USA

Abstract. High-resolution (HR) magnetic resonance images (MRI) provide detailed anatomical information important for clinical application and quantitative image analysis. However, HR MRI conventionally comes at the cost of longer scan time, smaller spatial coverage, and lower signal-to-noise ratio (SNR). Recent studies have shown that single image super-resolution (SISR), a technique to recover HR details from one single low-resolution (LR) input image, could provide high quality image details with the help of advanced deep convolutional neural networks (CNN). However, deep neural networks consume memory heavily and run slowly, especially in 3D settings. In this paper, we propose a novel 3D neural network design, namely a multi-level densely connected super-resolution network (mDCSRN) with generative adversarial network (GAN)–guided training. The mDCSRN trains and inferences quickly, and the GAN promotes realistic output hardly distinguishable from original HR images. Our results from experiments on a dataset with 1,113 subjects shows that our new architecture outperforms other popular deep learning methods in recovering 4x resolution-downgraded images and runs 6x faster.

Keywords: MRI · Super-Resolution · Image enhancement · Deep learning

1 Introduction

High spatial resolution MRI produces detailed structural information, benefiting clinical diagnosis, decision making, and accurate quantitative image analysis. However, due to hardware and physics limitations, high-resolution (HR) imaging comes at the cost of long scan time, small spatial coverage, and low signal to noise [1]. The ability to restore an HR image from a single low-resolution (LR) input would potentially overcome these drawbacks. Therefore, single image super-resolution (SISR) is an attractive approach, as it requires only a LR scan to provide an HR output without extra scan time. But SR is a challenging problem because of its underdetermined nature [2]. An infinite number of HR images can produce the same LR image after resolution

© Springer Nature Switzerland AG 2018
A. F. Frangi et al. (Eds.): MICCAI 2018, LNCS 11070, pp. 91–99, 2018.
https://doi.org/10.1007/978-3-030-00928-1_11

degradation. This makes it very difficult to accurately restore texture and structural details. A large portion of previous methods frame SR as a convex optimization problem, to find a plausible HR solution while balancing regularization terms [1, 3]. However, regularization terms require a priori knowledge of the image distribution, often based on experimental assumptions. Popular constraints like total variation implicitly assume that the image is piecewise constant, which is problematic for images with many local details and tiny structures. On the other hand, learning-based approaches do not require such well-defined priors. Especially, deep learning-based techniques have shown great improvement in SISR for images with abundant details, because of its non-linearity and extraordinary ability to imitate accurate transformation between LR and HR in difficult cases. Super-Resolution Convolutional Neural Networks (SRCNNs) [4] and their more recent Faster-SRCNNs (FSRCNNs) [5] draw a lot of attention as they showed that simple structured CNNs can produce outstanding SISR results of 2D natural images.

However, those previous adapted deep-learning approaches do not fully solve the puzzle in the medical image SR problem. First, many medical images are 3D volumes, but previous CNNs only work slice by slice, discarding information from continuous structures in the third dimension. Second, 3D models have far more parameters than 2D models, raising a challenge in memory consumption and computational expenses, making them less practical. Finally, the most widely used optimization objective of CNN is pixel/voxel-wise error like mean squared error (MSE) between model estimation and the reference HR. But as mentioned in [6], MSE and its derivative Peak Signal to Noise Ratio (PSNR) do not directly represent the visual quality of restored images. Thus, using MSE as the only target leads to overall blurring and low perceptual quality.

In this paper, we propose a 3D Multi-Level Densely Connected Super-Resolution Networks (mDCSRN) to fully solve the above problems. By utilizing a densely connected network [7], our mDCSRN is extremely light-weight. When optimized by intensity difference, it provides the state-of-art performance while keeping the model much smaller and faster. Then when trained with a Generative Adversarial Network (GAN), it improves further, outputting sharper and more realistic-looking images.

2 Method

Our proposed SISR neural network model aims to learn the image prior for inversely mapping the LR image to the reference HR image. The model only takes LR images to produce SR images. During the training, HR reference will be used to guide the optimization of the model's parameters. During deployment, SR images can be generated by the model based on the input LR. Details are provided in the followings:

2.1 Background

The resolution downgrading process from an HR image X to a LR image Y can be presented as:

$$Y = f(X), \tag{1}$$

where f is the function causing a loss of resolution. The SISR process is to find an inverse mapping function $g(\cdot) \approx f^{-1}(\cdot)$ to recover HR image $\hat{X}$ from a LR image Y:

$$\hat{X} = g(Y) = f^{-1}(Y) + R, \tag{2}$$

where f^{-1} is the inverse of f and R is the reconstruction residual.

In a CNN SISR approach, three different steps are optimized together: feature extraction, manifold learning, and image reconstruction. During the training, the difference between reconstructed images and ground truth images is not only used to adjust reconstruction layer to restore better images from manifold, but also to guide extraction of accurate image features. This mingling of different components makes it possible for neural network to achieve state-of-art performance among other SISR techniques [4].

2.2 Training a SR Network with GAN

The most intuitive way to optimize the reconstruction is by minimizing the voxel wise difference such as absolute difference (L1 loss) or mean square error (L2 loss). However, minimizing L1 or L2 loss leads to solutions which resemble a voxel-wise average of possible HR candidates, which does not penalize the formation of artificial image features at the neighbor or patch level. Thus, the output tends to be over-blurred and implausible to the human eye. For better optimization, we incorporated the idea from Ledig et al. [6] to use a Generative Adversarial Network (GAN)–based loss function.

The GAN framework has two networks: a generator G and a discriminator D. The basic idea of a GAN is to train a G to produce images with rich details while simultaneously training a D to distinguish the given image as either real or generated. At the end of the training, D will be a very good classifier to separate real and generated images, while the G can generate realistic looking images according to D. The advantage of using GAN is that it can be optimized without a predesigned loss function for a specific task. In SISR, SRGAN was proposed by [6], who showed that adding GAN's D loss to guide the G's training yields high perceptual quality.

However, training of a GAN presents its own challenges. During training, G and D must be balanced to evolve together. If either of them becomes too strong, the training will fail, and G can learn nothing from D. For 2D natural images, a lot of effort have been made to stabilize the training process. However, these approaches greatly rely on the network structure and have yet to be described for newer architectures like DenseNet. To stabilize the training process, the Wasserstein GAN (WGAN) authors [8] observed that the failure of GAN training is due to its optimization toward Kullback-Leibler divergence between real and generated probability. When there is little or no overlap between them, which is very common in the early stage of training, the gradient from the discriminator will vanish and the training will stall. To address this issue, WGAN was proposed. Its loss function approximately optimizes Earth Mover

(EM) distance, which can always guide the generator forward. WGAN enables almost fail-free training and produces quality as good as vanilla GAN. Additionally, the EM distance between real and generated images from D can be regarded an indicator of the image quality. In this work, we used WGAN for additional guiding during training.

2.3 Need for Efficient 3D Super-Resolution Network

It has been shown that 3D super-resolution models outperforming 2D counterparts by a large margin, thanks to the fact that 3D model directly learns the 3D structure of MRI volumetric images [9]. However, one significant drawback of a 3D model is that 3D deep learning model usually has a much larger number of parameters due to the extra dimensions of convolutional filters. For example, a relatively shallow 2D FSRCNN has only 12,000 parameters while its 3D version has 65,000, a > 5x difference. The number of parameters determines the model size and computation cost of a deep learning network, which is a key issue to consider for practical use.

Recently, DenseNet has shown that by using dense skip connections, we can dramatically reduce the network size while maintaining state-of-art performance in natural image classification. Yet, even memory-efficient DenseNets have too many parameters when constructed in 3D. The basic idea of densely connection from DenseNet was applied here, but we also include a new architecture that uses an extra level of skip connections. This not only helps to reduce the parameter number but also speeds up the computation. We discuss the detailed design of mDCSRN in the following section.

2.4 Proposed 3D Multi-level Super-Resolution Network

A recent study [9] shows that Densely Connected Super-Resolution Network (DCSRN) with a single DenseBlock, is already capable of capturing image features and restoring super-resolution images, outperforming other state-of-art techniques. But further improvement of the network performance is required to make use of a deeper model to catch more complex information in SR process. However, the memory consumption of a DenseNet increases dramatically as the number of layers increases, which makes it not feasible to train or deploy a deeper DCSRN.

To address this problem, we propose a multi-level densely connected structure, where a single deep DenseBlock is split into several shallow blocks. As shown in Fig. 1(B), each DenseBlock takes the output from all previous DenseBlock and is directly connected to reconstruction layer, following the same principle of DenseNet. Those skip connections provide direct access to all former layers including the input enables uninterrupted gradient flow, which is proven to be more efficient and less overfit. However, unlike original DenseNet, there is no pooling layer in mDCSRN, so mDCSRN can make full use of information in full resolution.

Another improvement is to add a $1 \times 1 \times 1$ convolutional layer as a compressor before all the following DenseBlocks. One key attribute to empower deep learning models to generalize so well is that the model has an information compression that

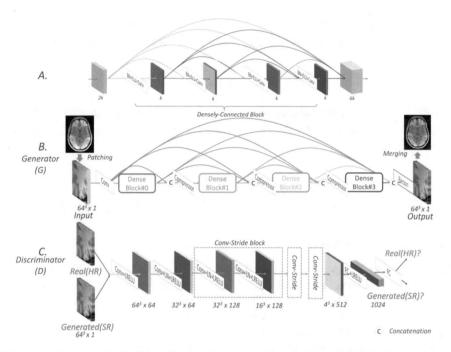

Fig. 1. Architecture of (A) DenseBlock with $3 \times 3 \times 3$ convolutions and (B, C) mDCSRN-GAN Network. The G is b4u4(4 blocks, each has 4 unites) mDCSRN. The first convolutional layer outputs 2k (k = 16) feature maps, and each compressor shrinks down the feature maps to 2k via a $1 \times 1 \times 1$ convolution. The final reconstruction layer is an another 1x1x1 convolution. The D is identical to SRGAN except BatchNorm is replaced by LayerNorm, suggested by WGAN-GP.

forces the model to learn universal features to avoid overfitting. In our design, the compressors bottleneck the network to the same width for each DenseBlock. This is expected to provide at least two benefits: (1) To reduce the memory consumption from hyperbolically to linearly dependent on depth; (2) To equally weight each DenseBlock, preventing later DenseBlocks (which takes care of conceptual level image features) from dominating the network with more parameters, thereby forcing the network not to overlook local image features that are central to the super-resolution task.

2.5 Design of Loss Function

In our work, we utilized gradient penalty variants of WGAN, namely WGAN-GP to speed up the training convergence. Our loss function has two parts: intensity loss $loss_{int}$ and GAN's discriminator loss $loss_{GAN}$:

$$loss = loss_{int} + \lambda loss_{GAN} \qquad (3)$$

where λ is a hyperparameter that we set to 0.001. We used the absolute difference (L1 loss) between network output SR and ground truth HR images as the intensity loss:

$$loss_{int} = loss_{L1}/LHW = \sum_{z=1}^{L} \sum_{y=1}^{H} \sum_{x=1}^{W} \left| I_{x,y,z}^{HR} - I_{x,y,z}^{SR} \right| / LHW \tag{4}$$

where $I_{x,y,z}^{SR}$ is the super-resolution output from the deep learning model and $I_{x,y,z}^{HR}$ is the ground truth HR image patch. We use GAN's discriminator loss as the additional loss to the SR network:

$$loss_{GAN} = loss_{WGAN,D} = -D_{WGAN,\theta}(I^{SR}) \tag{5}$$

where $D_{WGAN,\theta}$ is the discriminator's output digit from WGAN-GP for SR images.

2.6 LR Images Generation

To evaluate an SR approach, we need to generate LR images from ground truth HR images. LR images are generated following the same steps as in [9]: (1) converting HR image into k-space by applying FFT; (2) downgrading the resolution by truncating outer part of 3D k-space with a factor of 2×2; (3) converting back to image space by applying inverse FFT and linearly interpolating to the original image size. This mimics the actual acquisition of LR and HR images by MRI scanners.

3 Experiments

3.1 Dataset and Data Preparation

To better demonstrate the generalization of the deep learning model, we used a large publicly accessible brain structural MRI database, the human connectome project. 3D T1 W images from a total of 1,113 subjects were acquired via Siemens 3T platform using 32-channel head coil on multiple centers. The images come in high spatial resolution as 0.7 mm isotropic in a matrix size of $320 \times 320 \times 256$. These high-quality ground truth images provide detailed small structures, which is a perfect case for SR project. The whole dataset is split into 780 training, 111 validation, 111 evaluation and 111 test samples by subject. No subjects nor image patches appear twice in different subsets. Validation set is used for monitoring training process and evaluation set is used for hyper-parameters selection. We only use test set for final performance evaluation to avoid fine-tuning model favorable to test set data.

The original images were used as ground-truth HR images, and then degraded to LR. We used the exact same process of patching and data augmentation as in [9]. However, we merged the patches without overlapping, which makes model run even faster and results in less blurring. We left a margin of 3 pixels to avoid artifacts on the edge.

3.2 Training Parameters and Experiment Setting

The models were implemented in Tensorflow on a workstation with Nvidia GTX 1080TI GPU. The DenseBlock in mDCSRN setting is similar with DCSRN, where all 3D convolutional layers had filter with size $3 \times 3 \times 3$, growth rate k = 16. For comparison, we picked up relatively small network FSRCNN [9] and more complicated state-of-art SRResNet [6]. We selected the same hyper-parameters according to 2D FSRCNN [5]. And we extended the 2D convolution to 3D for both FSRCNN and SRResNet.

For non-GAN networks, ADAM optimizer with a learning rate 10^{-4} was used to minimize the L1 loss function with a batch size of 2. We trained for 500 k steps as no significant improvement afterward. For GAN experiments, we transfer the weights from well-trained mDCSRN in non-GAN training as the initial G. For the first 10 k steps, we trained the discriminator only. After then for every 7 steps of training discriminator, we trained the generator once; and every 500 steps we train discriminator for an extra 200 step alone, which makes sure that discriminator is always well-trained, as suggested in WGAN. Adam optimizer with 5×10^{-6} is used to optimize both G network for 550 k steps, with little improvement after that.

To demonstrate the effectiveness of mDCSRN compared with DCSRN, we made four different network setups with varied block number(b) and unit number(u). A network with single 8-unit DenseBlock is annotated as *b1u8* and a network with four DenseBlocks each has 4 dense-units is annotated as *b4u4*, respectively. We used three image metrics: subject-wise average structural similarity index (SSIM), peak signal to noise ratio (PSNR), and normalized root mean squared error (NRMSE), to measure the similarity between SR image and reference HR image in the 2×2 down-sampled plane.

3.3 Results

The quantitative results from non-GAN approaches are shown in Table 1. The parameters and running speed of each networks are also listed in Table 1. DCSRN *b1u8* and mDCSRN *b2u4* had the same depth of network, but the later obtained marginally better results and reduce parameters and running time by more than 30%. Among all variants, the largest network *b4u4* has the best performance without too much sacrifice in speed.

Table 1. The results of SSIM, PSNR and NRMSE for different DCSRN architectures. With the same depth, *b2u4* has a slightly better performance than *b1u8* with less number of parameters and computation operation. The deepest network *b4u4* had an average runtime for a whole 3D MRI of a subject just around 20 s while has the best performance.

	DCSRN b1u8			mDCSRN b2u4			mDCSRN b3u4			mDCSRN b4u4		
	SSIM	PSNR	NRMSE	SSIM	PSNR	NRMSE	SSIM	PSNR	NRMSE	SSIM	PSNR	NRMSE
mean	0.9371	35.35	0.0906	*0.9381*	*35.46*	*0.0895*	0.9402	35.56	0.0884	**0.9424**	**35.88**	**0.0852**
std	0.0053	0.79	0.0038	0.0053	0.78	0.0038	0.0052	0.79	0.0038	0.0051	0.78	0.0038
#parm	0.307 M			0.200 M			0.304 M			0.412 M		
#ops	1.247 M			0.813 M			1.236 M			1.672 M		
Time(s)	13.20			**9.74**			15.13			20.87		

mDCSRN *b4u4* was compared with bicubic interpolation as well as other neural networks FSRCNN and SRResNet (Table 2). mDCSRN obtained a large advantage against FSRCNN methods and is slightly better than SRResNet but runs more than 6x faster. Additionally, our mDCSRN-GAN provides much sharpened and visually plausible images compared with non-GAN approaches. Figure 2 demonstrates super-resolution results of one random subject in the 2×2 resolution degrading plane. Among non-GAN methods, the small vessels in mDCSRN are more distinguishable than in other neural networks. However, mDCSRN-GAN provides much better overall image quality: not only does the vessel maintains the same shape and size as in the ground-truth HR image, but the gaps between vessel and gray matter are also much clearer (see red arrows). The mDCSRN-GAN result is almost indistinguishable from the ground truth.

Table 2. Performance comparison between bicubic interpolation, 3D FSRCNN, 3D SRResNet and our proposed mDCSRN *b4u4*. mDCSRN provides similar image quality to SRRestNet but 6x faster and provides much better image quality than bicubic interpolation and FSRCNN. *FSRCNN has large CNN kernels (size: 5 and 9) that are extremely computationally expensive, though small #ops, it takes longer time than mDCSRN which only has small filters (size: 3).

	Bicubic Interpolation			3D FSRCNN*			3D SRResNet			mDCSRN b4u4		
	SSIM	PSNR	NRMSE	SSIM	PSNR	NRMSE	SSIM	PSNR	NRMSE	SSIM	PSNR	NRMSE
mean	0.8377	29.07	0.1873	0.9211	34.11	0.1045	*0.9412*	*35.71*	*0.0869*	**0.9424**	**35.88**	**0.0852**
std	0.0088	0.90	0.0087	0.0059	0.77	0.0042	0.0052	0.79	0.0038	0.0051	0.78	0.0038
#parm	–			0.064 M			2.005 M			0.412 M		
#ops	–			0.261 M*			8.043 M			1.672 M		
Time(s)	–			21.27			*132.71*			**20.87**		

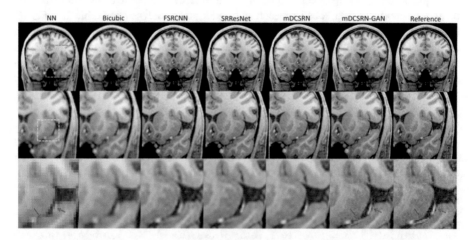

Fig. 2. Illustration of the nearest neighbor(NN) and bicubic interpolation, 3D FSRCNN, 3D SRResNet, mDCSRN, mDCSRN-GAN reconstruction results, and corresponding HR images.

4 Conclusion

We have presented a novel SISR method based on 3D mDCSRN-GAN for MRI. We showed that mDCSRN-GAN can recover local image textures and details more accurately, and 6 times more quickly than current state-of-art deep learning approaches. This new technique would allow 4-fold reduction in scan time while maintaining virtually identical image resolution and quality.

References

1. Plenge, E., et al.: Super-resolution methods in MRI: Can they improve the trade-off between resolution, signal-to-noise ratio, and acquisition time? Magn. Reson. Med. **68**(6), 1983–1993 (2012)
2. Tanno, R., et al.: Bayesian image quality transfer with cnns: exploring uncertainty in dmri super-resolution. In: Descoteaux, M., et al. (eds.) MICCAI 2017. LNCS, vol. 10433, pp. 611–619. Springer, Cham (2017). https://doi.org/10.1007/978-3-319-66182-7_70
3. Shi, F., et al.: LRTV: MR image super-resolution with low-rank and total variation regularizations. IEEE Trans. Med. Imaging **34**(12), 2459–2466 (2015)
4. Dong, C., Loy, C.C., He, K., Tang, X.: Image super-resolution using deep convolutional networks. IEEE Trans. Pattern Anal. Mach. Intell. **38**(2), 295–307 (2016)
5. Dong, C., Loy, C.C., Tang, X.: Accelerating the super-resolution convolutional neural network. In: Leibe, B., Matas, J., Sebe, N., Welling, M. (eds.) ECCV 2016. LNCS, vol. 9906, pp. 391–407. Springer, Cham (2016). https://doi.org/10.1007/978-3-319-46475-6_25
6. Ledig, C., et al.: Photo-realistic single image super-resolution using a generative adversarial network. In: Proceedings of the IEEE Conference on Computer Vision and Pattern Recognition (2017)
7. Huang, G., et al.: Densely connected convolutional networks. In: Proceedings of the IEEE Conference on Computer Vision and Pattern Recognition, vol. 1(2) (2017)
8. Arjovsky, M., Chintala, S., Bottou, L.: Wasserstein gan. arXiv preprint arXiv:1701.07875 (2017)
9. Chen, Y., et al.: Brain MRI super resolution using 3D deep densely connected neural networks. In: Proceedings of 15th International Symposium on Biomedical Imaging (ISBI 2018), pp. 739–742 (2018)

A Deep Learning Based Anti-aliasing Self Super-Resolution Algorithm for MRI

Can Zhao[1]([✉]), Aaron Carass[1,2], Blake E. Dewey[1], Jonghye Woo[3], Jiwon Oh[4], Peter A. Calabresi[4], Daniel S. Reich[5], Pascal Sati[5], Dzung L. Pham[6], and Jerry L. Prince[1,2]

[1] Department of Electrical and Computer Engineering,
The Johns Hopkins University, Baltimore, MD 21218, USA
czhao20@jhu.edu
[2] Department of Computer Science, The Johns Hopkins University,
Baltimore, MD 21218, USA
[3] Department of Radiology, Massachusetts General Hospital,
Boston, MA 02114, USA
[4] Department of Neurology, The Johns Hopkins School of Medicine,
Baltimore, MD 21287, USA
[5] Translational Neuroradiology Unit, National Institute of Neurological Disorders
and Stroke, Bethesda, MD 20892, USA
[6] CNRM, The Henry M. Jackson Foundation for the Advancement
of Military Medicine, Bethesda, MD 20817, USA

Abstract. High resolution magnetic resonance (MR) images are desired in many clinical applications, yet acquiring such data with an adequate signal-to-noise ratio requires a long time, making them costly and susceptible to motion artifacts. A common way to partly achieve this goal is to acquire MR images with good in-plane resolution and poor through-plane resolution (i.e., large slice thickness). For such 2D imaging protocols, aliasing is also introduced in the through-plane direction, and these high-frequency artifacts cannot be removed by conventional interpolation. Super-resolution (SR) algorithms which can reduce aliasing artifacts and improve spatial resolution have previously been reported. State-of-the-art SR methods are mostly learning-based and require external training data consisting of paired low resolution (LR) and high resolution (HR) MR images. However, due to scanner limitations, such training data are often unavailable. This paper presents an anti-aliasing (AA) and self super-resolution (SSR) algorithm that needs no external training data. It takes advantage of the fact that the in-plane slices of those MR images contain high frequency information. Our algorithm consists of three steps: (1) We build a self AA (SAA) deep network followed by (2) an SSR deep network, both of which can be applied along different orientations within the original images, and (3) recombine the multiple orientations output from Steps 1 and 2 using Fourier burst accumulation. We perform our SAA+SSR algorithm on a diverse collection of MR data without modification or preprocessing other than N4 inhomogeneity correction, and demonstrate significant improvement compared to competing SSR methods.

© Springer Nature Switzerland AG 2018
A. F. Frangi et al. (Eds.): MICCAI 2018, LNCS 11070, pp. 100–108, 2018.
https://doi.org/10.1007/978-3-030-00928-1_12

Keywords: Self super-resolution · Deep network · MRI
CNN · Aliasing

1   Introduction

High resolution (HR) magnetic resonance images (MRI) provide more anatomical details and enable more precise analyses, and are therefore highly desired
in clinical and research applications [8]. However, in reality MR images are
usually acquired with high in-plane resolution and lower through-plane resolution (slice thickness) to save acquisition time. Thus in these images, the high
frequency information in the through-plane direction is missing. Some MRI protocols acquire 3D images as stacks of 2D images, which introduce aliasing that
appears as high-frequency artifacts in the images. Interpolation is frequently
used (both on the scanner and in postprocessing) to improve the digital resolution of acquired images, but this process does not restore any high frequency
information. The partial volume artifacts that remain in these images make them
appear blurry and degrade image analysis performance as well [2,8].

To address this problem, a number of super-resolution (SR) algorithms
have been developed, including neighbor embedding regressions [11], random
forests (RF) [9], and convolutional neural networks (CNNs) [5–7]. Generally,
CNN methods need paired atlas images to learn the transformation from low
resolution (LR) to high resolution (HR). They work well with natural images,
but a lack of adequate training data (an LR/HR atlas) is a major problem when
applying these approaches to MRI. There are two reasons for the lack of adequate training data. First, acquisition of HR data with isotropic voxels is time
consuming—potentially taking hours, depending on the desired resolution—in
order to also achieve adequate signal-to-noise ratio. Such long acquisitions are
prohibitive from a subject comfort point of view and are also highly prone to
motion artifacts. Second, MR images have no standardized tissue contrast, so
application of an SR approach trained from a given atlas may not readily apply
to a new subject from scan that has different contrast properties. It is therefore
desirable that any SR approach for MRI not require the use of an external atlas.

To avoid the requirement of external training data, researchers have developed self super-resolution (SSR) methods [3,4,14,16]. SSR methods use the mapping between the high in-plane resolution images and simulated lower resolution
images, to estimate high resolution through-plane images. Previous SSR methods [4,14,16] have achieved good results on medical images. Jog et al. [4] built
an SSR framework that extracts training patches from the LR MRI and blurred
LR_2 images, trains a RF regressor, and applies the trained regressor to LR_2
images in different directions. The resultant images are LR, but have low resolution in different directions. Thus, each of them contributes high frequency
information to a different region of Fourier space. Finally, these images are combined through Fourier burst accumulation (FBA) [1] to obtain an HR image. We
have previously reported [16] a method that replaces the RF framework of Jog
et al. [4] with the state-of-art SR deep network EDSR [7]. This approach applies

the trained network to the original LR image instead of the LR_2 images as in Jog et al. [4]. Weigert et al. [14] reported an SSR method for 3D fluorescence microscopy images based on a U-net and showed improved segmentation. None of these previous works address anti-aliasing (AA).

In this paper, we report an approach for applying both anti-aliasing (AA) and super-resolution (SR) by building the first self AA (SAA) method in conjunction with an SSR deep network. We build upon our own [16] framework and the work of Jog et al. [4], with two major differences. First, the previous approaches constructed the LR_2 data by applying a truncated sinc in k-space simulating the incomplete signal in k-space of LR images for 3D MRI. However, for 2D MRI, this process does not simulate aliasing artifacts and therefore cannot provide training data for removing aliasing. We therefore modify this filtering to suit our desired deep networks. Second, we build two deep networks, one for SAA and one for SSR.

2   Method

Our algorithm needs no preprocessing step other than N4 inhomogeneity correction [12] to make the image intensity homogeneous. The pseudo code is shown in Algorithm 1, and we refer to our algorithm as Synthetic Multi-Orientation Resolution Enhancement (SMORE). Consider an input LR image having slice thickness equal to the slice separation. The spatial resolution (approximate full-width at half-maximum) and voxel separation of this image is assumed to be $a \times a \times b$ where $b > a$. Without loss of generality, we assume that the axial slices are $a \times a$ HR slices. We model this image as a low-pass filtered and downsampled version of the HR image $I(x, y, z)$ which has spatial resolution and voxel separation $a \times a \times a$. Our first step is to apply cubic b-spline (BSP) interpolation to the input image yielding $I_z(x, y, z)$ which has the same spatial resolution $a \times a \times b$ as the input but voxel separation $a \times a \times a$. Aliasing exists in the z direction in this image because the Nyquist criterion is not satisfied (unless the actual frequency content in the z direction is very low, which we assume is not the case in normal anatomies.) We denote the ratio of the resolutions as $k = b/a$, which need not be an integer. Similar to Jog et al. [4], the idea behind the algorithm is that 2D axial slices $I_z(x, y)$ can be thought of as $a \times a$ HR slices, whereas sagittal slices $I_z(z, y)$ and coronal slices $I_z(z, x)$ are $b \times a$ LR slices. Blurring axial slices in the x-direction produces $\tilde{I}_{xz}(x, y)$ with resolution of $b \times a$ which we can use with $I_z(x, y)$ as training data. Any trained system can then be applied to $I_z(z, y)$ or $I_z(z, x)$ to generate HR sagittal and coronal slices. We choose an state-of-art deep network model EDSR [7] as it won the Ntire 2017 super-resolution challenge [10]. We describe the steps of SMORE in details below.

Training Data Extraction: To construct our training data, we desire aliased LR slices $\tilde{I}_{xz}(x, y)$ that accurately simulate the resolution $b \times a$ and have aliasing in the x-axis. For 2D MRI, we need to model the slice selection procedure, thus we use a 1D Gaussian filter $G_\sigma(x)$ in the image domain with a length round(k)

Algorithm 1: SMORE Pseudocode

Data: $I_z(x, y, z)$ with spatial resolution $a \times a \times b$, $k = b/a$
Result: estimate $\hat{I}(x, y, z)$ with spatial resolution $a \times a \times a$

(Step 1) Construct Training Data:
for $n = 0, \ldots, 5$; $\quad \theta := \frac{n\pi}{6}$ **do**

> Rotate image in xy-plane: $I_z^\theta(x, y, z) := R_{xy}(\theta) \circ I_z(x, y, z)$;
> Define a 1D Gaussian filter $G_\sigma(x)$ with length of round (k), FWHM of k;
> Create LR$_2$ images: $I_{xz}^\theta(x, y, z) := I_z^\theta(x, y, z) * G_\sigma(x)$;
> Introduce aliasing in x-axis: $\tilde{I}_{xz}^\theta(x, y, z) := \uparrow_x^k \left(\downarrow_x^k \left(I_{xz}^\theta(x, y, z) \right) \right)$.

end
Feed paired patches into EDSR model:

- from $\left[\tilde{I}_{xz}^\theta(x, y), I_{xz}^\theta(x, y) \right]$ to train a self anti-aliasing network (SAA);
- from $\left[\tilde{I}_{xz}^\theta(x, y), I_z^\theta(x, y) \right]$ to train a self super-resolution network (SSR).

(Step 2) SAA and SSR:
for α *in* $[0, \pi/2]$ **do**

> Rotate image in xy-plane: $I_z^\alpha(x, y, z) := R_{xy}(\alpha) \circ I_z(x, y, z)$;
> Apply trained SAA on xz-plane: $I_z^\alpha(x, z)_{\text{SAA}} := \text{SAA} \circ I_z^\alpha(x, z)$;
> Apply trained SSR on yz-plane: $\hat{I}^\alpha(y, z) := \text{SSR} \circ I_z^\alpha(y, z)_{\text{SAA}}$;
> Stack patches $\hat{I}^\alpha(y, z)$ to reconstruct $\hat{I}^\alpha(x, y, z)$.

end

(Step 3) Apply FBA on the collection of α results:
$$\hat{I}(x, y, z) := \text{FBA} \left(\left\{ \alpha : R_{xy}(-\alpha) \circ \hat{I}^\alpha(x, y, z) \right\} \right)$$

and full-width at half-maximum (FWHM) of k. The filtered image $I_{xz}(x, y, z)$ has the desired LR components without aliasing. To introduce aliasing, the image is downsampled by factor of k using linear interpolation to simulate the large slice thickness. We denote this image as $\downarrow_x^k (I_{xz}(x, y, z))$. To complete the training pair we upsample this image by a factor k using BSP interpolation to generate LR$_2$ which can be represented as $\uparrow_x^k \left(\downarrow_x^k (I_{xz}(x, y, z)) \right)$, but for brevity denoted as $\tilde{I}_{xz}(x, y, z)$. To increase the training samples, we rotate $I_z(x, y, z)$ in the xy-plane by θ and repeat this process to yield $I_z^\theta(x, y, z)$. In this paper we use six rotations where $\theta = n\pi/6$ for $n = 0, \ldots, 5$, but this generalizes for any number and arrangement of rotations.

EDSR Model: We train two networks, one for SAA and one for SSR. (1) To train the SAA network, 32×32 patch pairs are extracted from axial slices in $\tilde{I}_{xz}(x, y, z)$ and $I_{xz}(x, y, z)$ (i.e., aliased LR$_2$ and LR, respectively). We train a deep network SR model, EDSR, to remove this aliasing. We use small patches to enhance edges without structural specificity so that this network can better preserve pathology. Additionally, small patches allow for more training samples. (2) To train our SSR network, 32×32 patch pairs are extracted from axial slices in $\tilde{I}_{xz}(x, y, z)$ and $I_z(x, y, z)$. These patch pairs train another EDSR model to learn how to remove aliasing and improve resolution. Although training needs to be done for every subject, we have found that fine-tuning a pre-trained model is accurate and fast. In practice, training the two models for one subject based on pre-trained models from an arbitrary data set takes less than 40 min in total for a Tesla K40 GPU.

Applying the Networks: Our trained SSR network can be applied to LR coronal and sagittal slices of $I_z(x, y, z)$ to remove aliasing and improve resolution. However, experimentally we discovered that if we apply our SSR network to patches of a sagittal slice $I_z(x, z)$, and subsequently reconstruct a 3D image, then the result only removes aliasing in sagittal slices. To address this, we apply our SAA network to coronal slices to remove aliasing there, and then apply our SSR network to sagittal slices. Subsequently, the aliasing in both the coronal and sagittal planes of our SMORE result are removed. We repeat this procedure by applying SAA in sagittal slices and then SSR to the coronal slices to produce another image. As long as SAA and SSR are applied to orthogonal image planes, we can do this for any rotation α in the xy-plane. The list of SAA and SSR results are finally combined by taking the maximum value for each voxel in k-space for all rotations α. This is the l_∞ variant of Fourier burst accumulation (FBA) [1], which assumes that high values in k-space indicate signal while low values indicate blurring. Since aliasing artifacts appears as high values in k-space, this assumption of FBA necessitates our SAA network. Our presented results use only two α values, 0 and $\pi/2$.

3   Experiments

Evaluation on Simulated LR Data: We compare SMORE to our previous work [16], which uses a different way of training data simulation and uses EDSR to do SSR on MRI without SAA, on T_2-weighted images from 14 multiple sclerosis subjects imaged on a 3T Philips Achieva scanner with acquired resolution of $1 \times 1 \times 1$ mm. These images serve as our ground truth HR images, which are blurred and downsampled by factor $k = \{2, \ldots, 6\}$ in the z-axis to simulate thick-slice MR images. The thick-slice LR MR images, and the results of cubic B-spline interpolation (BSP), our competing MR variant of EDSR [16], and our proposed SMORE algorithm are shown in Fig. 1 for $k = 4$ and 6. Visually, SMORE has significantly better through-plane resolution than BSP and EDSR. For SMORE, the lesions near the ventricle are well preserved when $k = 4$. With $k = 6$, the large lesions are still well preserved but smaller lesions are not as well preserved. The Structural SIMilarity (SSIM) index is computed between each method and the $1 \times 1 \times 1$ mm ground truth. And the mean value masked over non-background voxels is shown in Fig. 2. We also compute the sharpness index S3 [13], a no-reference 2D image quality assessment, along each cardinal axis with the results also shown in Fig. 2. Our proposed algorithm, SMORE, significantly outperforms the competing methods.

Evaluation on Acquired LR Data: We applied BSP, our previous MR variant of EDSR [16], and our proposed SMORE method on eight PD-weighted MR images of marmosets. Each image has a resolution of $0.15 \times 0.15 \times 1$ mm (thus $k \approx 6.667$), with HR in coronal plane. Results are shown in Fig. 3. We observe severe

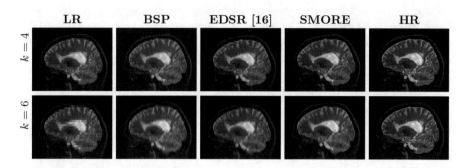

Fig. 1. Sagittal views of the k mm LR image, the cubic B-spline (BSP) interpolated image, an MR variant of EDSR [16], our proposed method SMORE, and the HR ground truth image with lesions anterior and posterior of the ventricle.

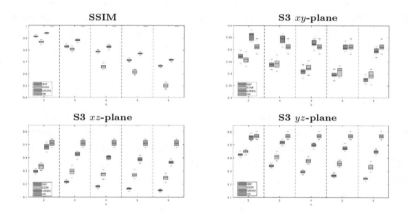

Fig. 2. For $k = 2, \ldots, 6$, we have evaluation of BSP (blue), an MR variant of EDSR [7] (yellow), our proposed method SMORE (red), and the ground truth (green).

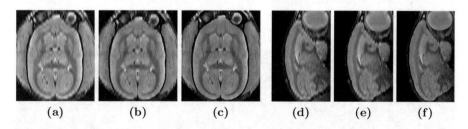

Fig. 3. Experiment on $0.15 \times 0.15 \times 1$ mm LR marmoset PD MRI, showing axial views of (**a**) BSP interpolated image, (**b**) MR variant of EDSR [16], (**c**) SMORE, and sagittal views of (**d**) BSP, (**e**) MR variant of EDSR, and finally (**f**) SMORE.

aliasing on the axial and sagittal plane of the input images, with an example shown in Fig. 3(a) and (d). Although there is no ground truth, visually SMORE removes the aliasing and gives a significantly sharper image (see Figs. 3(c) and (f)). To evaluate the sharpness, we use the S3 sharpness measure [13] on these results (see Fig. 4).

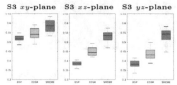

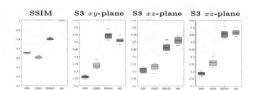

Fig. 4. S3 evaluation for the 0.15 × 0.15 × 1 marmoset data, with BSP (blue), an MR variant of EDSR (yellow), and our proposed method SMORE (red).

Fig. 5. SSIM and S3 for the reconstruction result using three inputs ($k = 6$). We have results from BSP (blue), an MR variant of EDSR (yellow), our proposed method SMORE (red), and the ground truth (green).

Application to multi-view image reconstruction: Woo et al. [15] presented a multi-view HR image reconstruction algorithm that reconstructs a single HR image from three orthogonally acquired LR images. The original algorithm used BSP interpolated LR images as input. We compare using BSP for this reconstruction with the MR variant of EDSR [16] and our proposed method SMORE. We use the same data as in the first experiment, which have ground truth HR images. Three simulated LR images with resolution of $6 \times 1 \times 1$, $1 \times 6 \times 1$, and $1 \times 1 \times 6$ are generated for each data set. Thus $k = 6$ and the input images are severely aliased. We apply each of BSP, EDSR, and SMORE to these three images and then apply our implementation of the reconstruction algorithm [15]. Example results for each of these three approaches are shown in Fig. 6. SSIM is computed for each reconstructed image to its $1 \times 1 \times 1$ mm ground truth HR image, with the mean of SSIM over non-background voxels being shown in

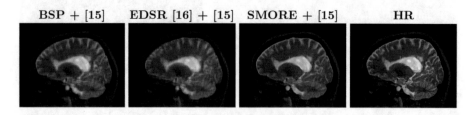

Fig. 6. Sagittal views of the reconstructed image [15] using three inputs ($k = 6$) from results of BSP, MR variant of EDSR [16], our proposed method SMORE, and the HR ground truth image.

Fig. 5. We also compute the sharpness index S3 along each cardinal axis with the results also shown in Fig. 5. Our proposed algorithm, SMORE, significantly outperforms the competing methods.

4   Conclusion and Discussion

This paper presents a self anti-aliasing (SAA) and self super-resolution (SSR) algorithm that can resolve high resolution information from MR images with thick slices and remove aliasing artifacts without any external training data. It needs no preprocessing step other than inhomogeneity correction like N4. The results are significantly better than competing SSR methods, and can be applied to multiple data sets without any modification or parameter tuning. Future work will include an evaluation of its impact on more applications such as skull stripping and lesion segmentation.

Acknowledgments. This work was supported by the NIH/NIBIB under grant R01-EB017743. Support was also provided by the National Multiple Sclerosis Society grant RG-1507-05243 and by the Intramural Research Program of the National Institute of Neurological Disorders and Stroke.

References

1. Delbracio, M., Sapiro, G.: Hand-held video deblurring via efficient Fourier aggregation. IEEE Trans. Comput. Imaging **1**(4), 270–283 (2015)
2. Greenspan, H.: Super-resolution in medical imaging. Comput. J. **52**(1), 43–63 (2008)
3. Huang, J.B., Singh, A., Ahuja, N.: Single image super-resolution from transformed self-exemplars. In: The IEEE Conference on Computer Vision and Pattern Recognition (CVPR), June 2015
4. Jog, A., Carass, A., Prince, J.L.: Self super-resolution for magnetic resonance images. In: Ourselin, S., Joskowicz, L., Sabuncu, M.R., Unal, G., Wells, W. (eds.) MICCAI 2016. LNCS, vol. 9902, pp. 553–560. Springer, Cham (2016). https://doi.org/10.1007/978-3-319-46726-9_64
5. Kim, J., Kwon Lee, J., Lee, K.: Accurate image super-resolution using very deep convolutional networks. In: Proceedings of the IEEE Conference on Computer Vision and Pattern Recognition, pp. 1646–1654 (2016)
6. Ledig, C., et al.: Photo-realistic single image super-resolution using a generative adversarial network. arXiv preprint arXiv:1609.04802 (2016)
7. Lim, B., Son, S., Kim, H., Nah, S., Lee, K.: Enhanced deep residual networks for single image super-resolution. In: The IEEE Conference on Computer Vision and Pattern Recognition (CVPR) Workshops (2017)
8. Lüsebrink, F., Wollrab, A., Speck, O.: Cortical thickness determination of the human brain using high resolution 3 T and 7 T MRI data. Neuroimage **70**, 122–131 (2013)
9. Schulter, S., Leistner, C., Bischof, H.: Fast and accurate image upscaling with super-resolution forests. In: Proceedings of the IEEE Conference on Computer Vision and Pattern Recognition, pp. 3791–3799 (2015)

10. Timofte, R., et al.: Ntire 2017 challenge on single image super-resolution: methods and results. In: IEEE Conference on Computer Vision and Pattern Recognition Workshops (CVPRW), pp. 1110–1121. IEEE (2017)
11. Timofte, R., De Smet, V., Van Gool, L.: A+: adjusted anchored neighborhood regression for fast super-resolution. In: Cremers, D., Reid, I., Saito, H., Yang, M.-H. (eds.) ACCV 2014. LNCS, vol. 9006, pp. 111–126. Springer, Cham (2015). https://doi.org/10.1007/978-3-319-16817-3_8
12. Tustison, N.J., et al.: N4itk: improved N3 bias correction. IEEE Trans. Med. Imaging **29**(6), 1310–1320 (2010)
13. Vu, C.T., Chandler, D.M.: S3: a spectral and spatial sharpness measure. In: First International Conference on Advances in Multimedia, MMEDIA 2009, pp. 37–43. IEEE (2009)
14. Weigert, M., Royer, L., Jug, F., Myers, G.: Isotropic reconstruction of 3D fluorescence microscopy images using convolutional neural networks. In: Descoteaux, M., Maier-Hein, L., Franz, A., Jannin, P., Collins, D.L., Duchesne, S. (eds.) MICCAI 2017. LNCS, vol. 10434, pp. 126–134. Springer, Cham (2017). https://doi.org/10.1007/978-3-319-66185-8_15
15. Woo, J., Murano, E.Z., Stone, M., Prince, J.L.: Reconstruction of high-resolution tongue volumes from MRI. IEEE Trans. Biomed. Eng. **59**(12), 3511–3524 (2012)
16. Zhao, C., Carass, A., Dewey, B.E., Prince, J.L.: Self super-resolution for magnetic resonance images using deep networks. In: IEEE International Symposium on Biomedical Imaging (ISBI) (2018)

Gradient Profile Based Super Resolution of MR Images with Induced Sparsity

Prabhjot Kaur$^{(\boxtimes)}$ and Anil Kumar Sao

Indian Institute of Technology, Mandi, India
prabhjot_kaur@students.iitmandi.ac.in, anil@iitmandi.ac.in

Abstract. Trade-off between resolution and signal to noise ratio(SNR) of magnetic resonance (MR) images can be improved by post processing algorithms to provide high quality MR images required for several medical diagnosis. This paper proposed a constraint to sharpen the gradient profile (GP), typically symbolizes the quality of image, of super-resolved MR images in the framework of sparse representation based super resolution without any external LR (low-resolution)-HR (high resolution) pair images. It has been performed by establishing a piecewise linear relation between GP of LR image up-scaled by Bi-cubic interpolation (UR), and corresponding LR image. The resultant relationship is used to approximate the ground truth HR image such that GP of upsampled LR image is improved. Further, to preserve the details along with its consistency among coronal, sagittal and axial planes, we have learned multiple dictionaries by extracting patches from the same and adjacent slices. The experimental results demonstrate that the proposed approach outperforms qualitatively and quantitatively the existing algorithms of increasing the resolution of MR images.

Keywords: Gradient profile sharpness · MRI super resolution
Sparse representation · Edge preservation · Multiple dictionaries

1 Introduction

The requirement of precise medical diagnosis using MR scanner demands high spatial resolution and signal to noise ratio (SNR) of MR images, which can be achieved either by (i) choosing appropriate parameters of the pulse sequences or (ii) by having expensive materials in the MR scanner [1,2]. However, the spatial resolution which is inversely determined by the voxel size is ultimately lower bounded by the threshold for SNR, and the time requisites in clinical practices also encourages the larger voxel size to speed up the MR scanning [1]. Decreasing the voxel size using pulse sequence parameters results in noisy MR images, which may not be able to serve the clinical purpose. Thus, post-processing algorithms of scanned MR images serve a convenient alternative for improving the trade off between resolution and SNR in order to provide better quality MR images. Moreover, it has been demonstrated experimentally that the application of signal

© Springer Nature Switzerland AG 2018
A. F. Frangi et al. (Eds.): MICCAI 2018, LNCS 11070, pp. 109–117, 2018.
https://doi.org/10.1007/978-3-030-00928-1_13

processing techniques can improve the spatial resolution along with significant increment in the SNR [3] of MR images.

The objective to increase the resolution of MR images can be framed as super resolution problem and various approaches have attempted in literature for the same [4–8]. These approaches can be classified into two broad categories namely - super resolution of MR images (i) using available exemplar HR-LR images [7–9] (ii) without using any external HR or LR images. In the first category of these approaches, the lost fine details of the image to be super resolved are estimated from the external HR MR images. Here, the mapping between LR and HR MR images are learned and the given test LR image is mapped to HR image using learned mapping. These approaches give good reconstruction results but require HR-LR image pairs, which may not be possible to get in real world scenario. This issue is addressed by approaches from the second category, in which the fine image details are estimated using the patches extracted from the same image or same MR image volume itself. This comes from the observation that the same detail structure can be observed in the up and down-sampled versions of the image [10].

Following this, Manajon et.al. [11] exploited the self similarity of MR images with a strategy to construct 3D cube by weighted averaging of the several 3D cubes extracted from the same MR image volume. The averaging operator may smear the fine details of the resultant super resolved image, which otherwise reflect important information of tissue being captured like tissue boundaries in MR images. Moreover, it should be noted that, MR images essentially have many minor details which relate to subparts of the organ and each details' sharpness play its role in clinical practices for e.g., diffused boundary/detail might be interpreted as hemorrhage/deformity. Thus, the preservation of the image details and their profile in super resolved MR images is an important aspect. In single image super resolution, it has been experimented in [5] to preserve the local variations by using total variation (TV) as a regularizer with low rank representation of MR images. The total variation considers the averaged variations in all directions irrespective of the detail's structure, thus it preserves the details but tend to blur and reduce the sharpness of image details.

In this paper, we have proposed a constraint to preserve image details and the corresponding gradient profiles in the super resolved MR images using framework of sparse representation based super resolution without any external LR-HR images. In order to preserve the gradient profile of the details while upsampling, we explore the relation between gradient profile of details in LR image upscaled by bicubic interpolation (UR), and LR image details' profile. It has been observed that the GPS profile of UR and LR images are related by a piecewise linear function, which is used to approximate the gradient profile for HR image estimate. Further, to preserve the details along with its consistency among coronal, sagittal and axial planes, we learn multiple dictionaries by extracting patches from the up-downsampled versions of same and adjacent slices. The experimental results demonstrate that the proposed approach outperforms the existing state-of-the-art single image super resolution algorithms explored to improve resolution of MR images.

The work done in the proposed approach has similarity with the approach in [12], where the super resolution of intensity images is addressed by estimation of gradient map while maintaining the consistency in GPS. Later, estimated gradient map of HR image is fused in intensity image to derive super-resolved HR image. On the contrary, in the proposed work, consistency in GPS is put as a constraint to estimate the MR images. Also it should be noted that, the proposed approach employs the framework of sparse representation based SR, which is completely different from the work in [12].

The rest of the paper is organized as follows: Sect. 2 briefly explains the sparse representation framework for super resolution. The proposed approach for preserving the gradient profile is explained in Sect. 3. Experimental results in Sect. 4 demonstrate that the proposed approach performs better than the existing approaches qualitatively and quantitatively, and the paper is concluded in Sect. 5.

2   Sparse Representation Framework for Super Resolution

Considering the low rank structure and sparse manifold of the MR signal, we use the sparse representation framework for super resolution of MR image ($\mathbf{y}$) with sparsity regularizer [13]. The optimization problem is thus defined as:

$$\hat{\mathbf{x}} = \arg \min_{\mathbf{x}} ||\mathbf{y} - \mathbf{DHA}\boldsymbol{\beta}||_2^2 + ||\boldsymbol{\beta}||_1, \tag{1}$$

where $\mathbf{y} \in \mathbb{R}^m$ is the LR image obtained by degradation with downsampling $\mathbf{D} \in \mathbb{R}^{m \times n}$ and blurring $\mathbf{H} \in \mathbb{R}^{n \times n}$ operators, applied on the HR image $\mathbf{x} \in \mathbb{R}^n, (n >> m)$ which is assumed to be represented as linear combination of columns of the overcomplete dictionary $\mathbf{A}$, which means $\mathbf{x} = \mathbf{A}\boldsymbol{\beta}$. The choice of dictionary $\mathbf{A}$ in Eq. (1) is important and several approaches have been explored to learn $\mathbf{A}$ from the data itself. In this work, PCA based dictionary, as explained in [14] is used to demonstrate the effectiveness of the proposed approach.

3   Proposed Approach

The medical significance of image details in MR images requires the preservation of details along with their gradient profiles. In order to do so, the proposed approach develops a piece-wise linear relation between gradient profile of UR image and LR image, to approximate gradient profile for HR estimate. The estimated gradient profile for HR image is used as constraint to give super resolved images with sharper gradient profiles.

The parameters to model the image details, which mainly describe the edges, can be contrast(h) and width(d) of the edge as shown in Fig. 1(a). These two parameters are computed as explained in [15]. The values of h and d are combined to define the gradient profile sharpness(GPS, $\eta = h/d$), which can be used as a metric for indicating sharpness of image. The higher values of GPS indicate sharper image. To explore the nature of GPS values, HR image is taken randomly from an MR image volume obtained from 7T MR scanner with spatial resolution of 173×173. It is downsampled by factor 2 to obtain LR image, and the histogram of non-zero GPS values for each of UR, LR and HR images is plotted in Fig. 2. It can be seen in Fig. 2(a) that most of the values lie in lower range in case of UR image as compared to LR and HR image. This is due to the upsampling process on LR image, which blurs minor details of image. Blur will account for lower GPS values and zero GPS values are due to various missing details. It is important to note that the HR image is used to observe the behavior of GPS values, but it is not used while estimating the HR image. On the other hand, the percentage of edge pixels in LR and HR image remains almost same, and thus it is reasonable to represent $hist(\boldsymbol{\eta}_H)$ by $hist(\boldsymbol{\eta}_L)$.

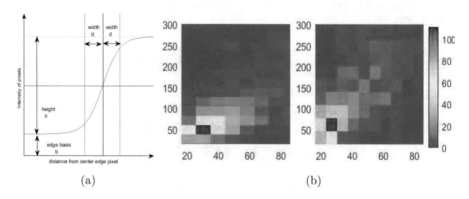

(a)   (b)

Fig. 1. (a) Parameters to characterize the edge; (b) Illustration of 2D histogram for η_U (x-axis) and η_H (y-axis) for upscale factor 2 in left image and for upscale factor 3 in right image.

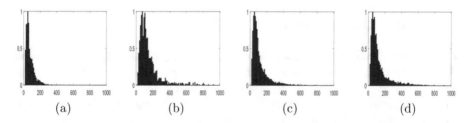

(a)   (b)   (c)   (d)

Fig. 2. Histogram of non-zero GPS values obtained for randomly selected (a) UR image, (b) LR with downsample factor 2, (c) Super resolved HR image, and (d) the corresponding ground truth HR image, from MR image volumes in the dataset. Here x-axis shows the GPS values and y-axis indicates the corresponding count of GPS values scaled in 0 to 1 range.

Table 1. Quantitative comparison of the proposed approach with the existing approaches for upscale factor 2

Subjects		1	2	3	4	5	6	7	8
PSNR	NLM3D	28.53	29.25	28.95	30.07	29.42	29.91	28.87	28.48
		1.29	0.74	1.05	1.05	2.05	2.54	1.22	1.11
	LRTV	30.54	30.97	31.43	31.89	31.61	32.08	30.91	30.67
		1.56	0.87	1.38	1.17	2.53	2.86	1.31	1.39
	Proposed	**31.69**	**32.12**	**32.70**	**33.07**	**32.97**	**33.34**	**32.06**	**32.11**
		2.02	0.94	1.78	1.10	3.45	2.97	1.37	1.85
SSIM	NLM3D	0.53	0.51	0.56	0.53	0.55	0.56	0.54	0.56
		0.0024	0.0012	0.0024	0.0025	0.0019	0.0015	0.0024	0.0017
	LRTV	0.62	0.61	0.64	0.61	0.63	0.66	0.62	0.65
		0.0022	0.0015	0.0028	0.0028	0.0023	0.0018	0.0030	0.0020
	Proposed	**0.67**	**0.65**	**0.69**	**0.67**	**0.69**	**0.70**	**0.68**	**0.70**
		0.0023	0.0015	0.0025	0.0025	0.0022	0.0014	0.0027	0.0019
SNR	NLM3D	20.85	20.39	22.66	22.54	21.55	21.74	21.86	21.06
		0.30	0.46	0.17	0.27	0.29	0.28	0.07	0.21
	LRTV	22.93	22.49	24.90	24.42	23.81	23.99	23.96	23.33
		0.47	0.81	0.33	0.34	0.48	0.32	0.21	0.35
	Proposed	**24.08**	**23.64**	**26.17**	**25.60**	**25.17**	**25.25**	**25.11**	**24.46**
		0.90	1.23	0.55	0.57	0.92	0.67	0.53	0.68

To find the relation between η_U and η_H, we extract the (η_U, η_H) pairs following the spatial distance and gradient distance criteria as described in [12]. The 2D(η_U, η_H) GPS distribution histogram is shown in Fig. 1(b) and Pearson product correlation coefficient(PPCC) is computed to validate the linearity in relation between η_H and η_U. It has been observed that PPCC values is relatively lower for MR images. This can be due to the small details present in MR images which are approximately zero in (η_U) but are non-zero in (η_H). Moreover, as the upscale factor increases, the linearity is distorted. Hence, we divide the GPS values into multiple ranges, and approximate the linear relationship for each range. This results in a piece-wise linear relations of η_U with η_H values. In this work, we have divided the GPS values into four ranges. This linear relation can be modeled by $\eta_H = \alpha\eta_U$, and α can be estimated by minimizing the chi-square distance between histogram of η_L and η_U. For each region, the following optimization cost is used to estimate α.

$$\alpha^* = arg\min \sum_{i=1}^{N} \left(\frac{(f(\eta_L)_i - f(\alpha\eta_U)_i)^2}{(f(\eta_L)_i + f(\alpha\eta_U)_i)} \right), \quad (2)$$

where f(z) represents the histogram of non-zero values of z and N is the number of elements selected in $f(z)$.

3.1   Estimation of HR Image

We transform the gradient profile of UR image in order to define an estimate for gradient profile of high resolution image ($\eta_{Ref} = \alpha^*\eta_U$). This can be used to constrain the solution space further, in order to choose only the solutions with sharper gradient profiles. This in effect reduces the blurring and other artifacts across tissue boundaries which is crucial for medical diagnosis. Thus the cost function with $\mathbf{x} = \mathbf{A}\beta$ can now be:

$$\hat{\mathbf{x}} = \arg\min_{\mathbf{x}} ||\mathbf{y} - \mathbf{DHA}\beta||_2^2 + ||\beta||_1 + ||\eta_x - \eta_{Ref}||_2^2. \tag{3}$$

It can be observed in Fig. 3(c) that the histogram of reconstructed HR image obtained by the proposed approach is similar to that of the ground truth HR image, which demonstrates the preservation of gradient profile of some details.

4   Experimental Results

To compare the performance of proposed algorithm, evaluated metrics(peak signal to noise ratio(PSNR), signal to noise ratio(SNR), structure similarity index

Table 2. Quantitative comparison of the proposed approach with the existing approaches for upscale factor 3

Subjects		1	2	3	4	5	6	7	8
PSNR	NLM3D	24.40	25.70	25.82	26.94	25.36	24.89	25.32	24.57
		2.27	2.96	2.95	3.01	3.07	3.88	3.10	1.64
	LRTV	27.65	28.07	28.39	28.97	28.48	29.08	27.96	27.54
		1.27	0.75	1.13	1.09	2.09	2.74	1.20	1.09
	Proposed	**28.59**	**28.97**	**29.39**	**29.98**	**29.49**	**30.13**	**28.91**	**28.62**
		1.53	0.61	1.34	0.97	3.28	2.75	1.09	1.95
SSIM	NLM3D	0.40	0.42	0.40	0.46	0.43	0.39	0.41	0.45
		0.0028	0.0032	0.0057	0.0036	0.0032	0.0022	0.0028	0.0024
	LRTV	0.49	0.47	0.51	0.48	0.50	0.52	0.49	0.51
		0.0025	0.0011	0.0026	0.0024	0.0022	0.0017	0.0025	0.0019
	Proposed	**0.54**	**0.52**	**0.56**	**0.54**	**0.55**	**0.57**	**0.55**	**0.57**
		0.0027	0.0012	0.0025	0.0026	0.0017	0.0015	0.0023	0.0017
SNR	NLM3D	18.66	17.36	19.00	18.30	19.87	18.82	19.75	17.41
		2.28	4.67	3.60	3.27	4.86	1.67	2.78	4.12
	LRTV	20.02	19.56	21.84	21.48	20.66	20.96	21.00	20.17
		0.27	0.43	0.19	0.23	0.32	0.25	0.08	0.22
	Proposed	**20.96**	**20.46**	**22.85**	**22.50**	**21.67**	**22.02**	**21.94**	**21.25**
		0.61	0.92	0.45	0.54	0.96	0.58	0.25	0.77

measurement(SSIM)) are compared with two existing approaches. - sparse representation based LRTV algorithm [5], weighted averaging based NLM3D [11]. The performance of the proposed algorithm is evaluated using 8 randomly selected MR image volumes scanned by 7 T with $1.05 \times 1.05 \times 1.05\,\mathrm{mm}^3$ from dataset publicly available online [16]. Each volume contains 207 slices out of which we select central 120 slices due to insignificant information in first and last few slices. LR images are formed by first blurring the image with Gaussian kernel with sigma of 1 voxel and downsample the HR image volume in x and y directions with factors 2, and 3.

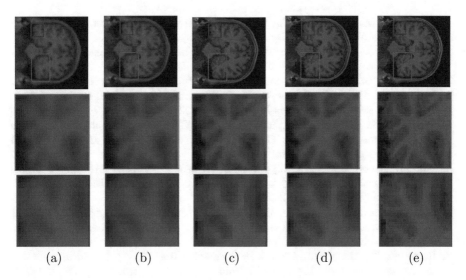

(a)   (b)   (c)   (d)   (e)

Fig. 3. Examples of reconstruction quality of two highlighted windows shown in first row, zoomed in second and third row constructed by various approaches including proposed approach- (a) interpolated image with bicubic spline, (b) upsampled image with NLM3D [11], (c) reconstructed image with LRTV [5], and d) shows the result for proposed algorithm.

Super resolved images for using bicubic spline and NLM3D [11] are displayed in Fig. 3(a,b) which shows the blurry estimates and are not able to distinguish the structures. However, in LRTV [5] shown in Fig. 3(c) the ability to distinguish two distinct tissues is improved, but with blurred gradient profiles and zig-zag artifacts, which are visibly improved in the proposed approach Fig. 3(d) with sharper profiles. Please zoom in the computer screen to appreciate the improvements in the results.

The quality of images for each of the volume constructed using the proposed as well as existing approaches are evaluated quantitatively, and the computed values for metrics are tabulated in Tables 1 and 2 with the corresponding mean and variance values for upscale factor 2 and 3 respectively. It can be observed that the proposed algorithm outperforms the existing algorithms.

5   Conclusion

In the proposed approach, we approximate the piece-wise linear relation of gradient profiles in UR and LR image, in sparse representation framework with multiple dictionaries for restoration as well as for consistency of details in all directions. The proposed approach outperforms the existing approaches qualitatively as well as quantitatively.

References

1. Poldrack, R.A., Mumford, J.A., Nichols, T.E.: Handbook of Functional MRI Data Analysis. Cambridge University Press, Cambridge (2011)
2. Cosmus, T.C., Parizh, M.: Advances in whole-body MRI magnets. IEEE Trans. Appl. Supercond. **21**(3), 2104–2109 (2011)
3. Plenge, E.: Super-resolution methods in MRI: can they improve the trade-off between resolution, signal-to-noise ratio, and acquisition time? Magn. Reson. Med. **68**(6), 1983–1993 (2012). https://doi.org/10.1002/mrm.24187
4. Van Reeth, E., Tham, I.W.K., Tan, C.H., Poh, C.L.: Super-resolution in magnetic resonance imaging: a review. Concepts Magn. Reson. Part A **40A**(6), 306–325 (2012). https://doi.org/10.1002/cmr.a.21249
5. Shi, F., Cheng, J., Wang, L., Yap, P.T., Shen, D.: LRTV: MR image super-resolution with low-rank and total variation regularizations. IEEE Trans. Med. Imaging **34**(12), 2459–2466 (2015)
6. Roy, S., Carass, A., Prince, J.L.: Magnetic resonance image example based contrast synthesis. IEEE Trans. Med. Imaging **32**(12), 2348–2363 (2013). http://www.ncbi.nlm.nih.gov/pmc/articles/PMC3955746/
7. Rousseau, F., Alzheimer's Disease Neuroimaging Initiative: A non-local approach for image super-resolution using intermodality priors. Med. Image Anal. **14**(4), 594–605 (2010). http://www.ncbi.nlm.nih.gov/pmc/articles/PMC2947386/
8. Pham, C.H., Ducournau, A., Fablet, R., Rousseau, F.: Brain MRI super-resolution using deep 3D convolutional networks. In: 2017 IEEE 14th International Symposium on Biomedical Imaging (ISBI 2017), pp. 197–200, April 2017
9. Rueda, A., Malpica, N., Romero, E.: Single-image super-resolution of brain MR images using overcomplete dictionaries. Med. Image Anal. **17**(1), 113–132 (2013). http://dblp.uni-trier.de/db/journals/mia/mia17.html#RuedaMR13
10. Glasner, D., Bagon, S., Irani, M.: Super-resolution from a single image. In: 2009 IEEE 12th International Conference on Computer Vision, pp. 349–356, September 2009
11. Manjón, J.V., Coupé, P., Buades, A., Fonov, V., Louis Collins, D., Robles, M.: Non-local MRI upsampling. Med. Image Anal. **14**(6), 784–792 (2010). https://doi.org/10.1016/j.media.2010.05.010
12. Yan, Q., Xu, Y., Yang, X., Nguyen, T.Q.: Single image superresolution based on gradient profile sharpness. IEEE Trans. Image Process. **24**(10), 3187–3202 (2015)
13. Yang, J., Wright, J., Huang, T.S., Ma, Y.: Image super-resolution via sparse representation. IEEE Trans. Image Process. **19**(11), 2861–2873 (2010)
14. Mandal, S., Bhavsar, A., Sao, A.K.: Noise adaptive super-resolution from single image via non-local mean and sparse representation. Signal Process. **132**, 134–149 (2017). http://www.sciencedirect.com/science/article/pii/S016516841630247X

15. Guan, J., Zhang, W., Gu, J., Ren, H.: No-reference blur assessment based on edge modeling. J. Vis. Commun. Image Represent. **29**, 1–7 (2015). http://www.sciencedirect.com/science/article/pii/S1047320315000085
16. https://www.humanconnectome.org/study/hcp-young-adult/document/1200-subjects-data-release

Deeper Image Quality Transfer: Training Low-Memory Neural Networks for 3D Images

Stefano B. Blumberg[2(✉)], Ryutaro Tanno[2], Iasonas Kokkinos[2], and Daniel C. Alexander[1,2]

[1] Clinical Imaging Research Centre, National University of Singapore, Singapore, Singapore
[2] Department of Computer Science and Centre for Medical Image Computing, University College London (UCL), London, UK
stefano.blumberg.17@ucl.ac.uk

Abstract. In this paper we address the memory demands that come with the processing of 3-dimensional, high-resolution, multi-channeled medical images in deep learning. We exploit memory-efficient backprop-agation techniques, to reduce the memory complexity of network train-ing from being linear in the network's depth, to being roughly constant – permitting us to elongate deep architectures with negligible memory increase. We evaluate our methodology in the paradigm of Image Quality Transfer, whilst noting its potential application to various tasks that use deep learning. We study the impact of depth on accuracy and show that deeper models have more predictive power, which may exploit larger training sets. We obtain substantially better results than the previous state-of-the-art model with a slight memory increase, reducing the root-mean-squared-error by 13%. Our code is publicly available.

1 Introduction

Medical imaging tasks require processing high-resolution (HR), multi-channeled, volumetric data, which produces a large memory footprint. Current graphics pro-cessing unit (GPU) hardware limitations, constrain the range of models that can be used for medical imaging, since only moderately deep 3D networks can fit on common GPU cards during training. Even with moderately deep networks, cur-rent practice in medical imaging involves several compromises, such as utilising a small input volume e.g. patches [1], that forces the network to perform local predictions, or by using a small minibatch size [2], which can destabilise train-ing. Whilst the impact of network depth has been extensively demonstrated to produce improved results in computer vision [3,4], this issue has attracted scant attention in medical image computing, due to the aforementioned limitations.

We introduce memory-efficient backpropagation techniques into medical imaging, where elongating a network produces a negligible memory increase, thus facilitating the training of deeper and more accurate networks. We combine two

© Springer Nature Switzerland AG 2018
A. F. Frangi et al. (Eds.): MICCAI 2018, LNCS 11070, pp. 118–125, 2018.
https://doi.org/10.1007/978-3-030-00928-1_14

memory-efficient learning techniques: checkpointing [5] and reversible networks (RevNets) [6,7], that exchange training speed with memory usage. Deepening an existing architecture, we systematically demonstrate that elongating a network increases its capacity, unleashing the potential of deep learning.

We demonstrate the effectiveness of this technique within the context of Image Quality Transfer (IQT) [8]. IQT is a paradigm for propagating information from rare or expensive high quality images (e.g. from a unique high-powered MRI scanner) to lower quality but more readily available images (e.g. from a standard hospital scanner). We consider the application of IQT to enhance the resolution of diffusion magnetic resonance imaging (dMRI) scans – which has substantial downstream benefits to brain connectivity mapping [1,8].

By studying the impact of network depth on accuracy, we demonstrate that deeper models have substantially more modelling power and by employing larger training sets, we demonstrate that increased model capacity produces significant improvements (Fig. 4). We surpass the previous state-of-the-art model of [1], reducing the root-mean-squared-error (RMSE) by 13% (Fig. 4) – with negligible memory increase (Fig. 6).

We expect that our methods will transfer to other medical imaging tasks that involve volume processing or large inputs, e.g. image segmentation [9], synthesis [10] and registration [11] – therefore our implementation is publicly available at http://mig.cs.ucl.ac.uk/.

2 Memory-Efficient Deep Learning

In this section, we use the concept of a computational graph to explain how the memory consumption of backpropagation increases with deeper networks. We present RevNets and illustrate how to insert them in a pre-defined architecture. Finally we combine checkpointing with this elongated system, to perform manual forward and backward propagation, allowing us to trade memory consumption with computational cost during training.

Memory Usage in Backpropagation. We consider a chain-structured network with sets of neurons organized in consecutive layers $X^1, X^2, \ldots, X^N$, related in terms of non-linear functions, $X^{i+1} = f^i(X^i, \theta^i)$, with parameters θ^i specific to layer i. Training aims at minimizing a loss function, $L(X^N, Y)$, where Y is the target output – in the setting of IQT, the high-quality patch.

Backpropagation recursively computes the gradient of the loss with respect to the parameters θ^i and neuronal activations X_0^i, at layer i. Its computation at layer i takes inputs $\frac{df^i}{dX^i}, \frac{dL}{dX^{i+1}}, X_0^i$ to compute $\frac{dL}{d\theta^i}|_{X_0^i}, \frac{dL}{dX^i}|_{X_0^i}$. Therefore backpropagating from X^N to X^1 requires all intermediate layer activations $X_0^1, \ldots, X_0^N$. This means that memory complexity can scale linearly in the network's depth, which is the case in standard implementations.

Memory-efficient variants of backpropagation trade computational time for training speed without sacrificing accuracy. As an example, when backpropagating at layer i, one can compute X_0^i from scratch, by re-running a forward pass from the input X_0^0 to X_0^i. The memory usage is constant in network depth, but the computational cost is now quadratic in depth. Checkpointing [5] – a method that applies to general graphs, allows the memory cost to scale at square root of the network's depth, whilst increasing the computational cost by a factor of $\frac{3}{2}$. RevNets [6,7], also increase the computational cost by a similar factor, via their invertibility, we may keep the memory consumption constant in the network's depth. In our implementation we use a combination of the two methods, as detailed below.

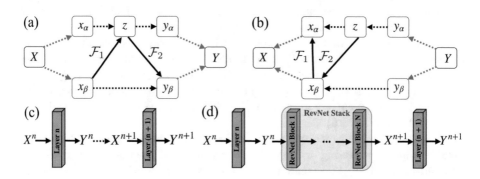

Fig. 1. A RevNet (top) and architecture elongation (bottom). Top: Flowcharts of a RevNet block [6,7], with input and output feature maps respectively X, Y in (a) forward pass and (b) backward pass. Black dotted lines are identity operations, red dotted lines are concatenation and splitting operations, $\mathcal{F}_1, \mathcal{F}_2$ are non-linear functions. Bottom: We elongate a network by inserting N RevNet blocks between layers $n, n+1$ of a neural network. First, as in (c) we split the intermediate activation between layers $n, n+1$ into two computational nodes Y^n, X^{n+1}; then, as in (d), we insert N RevNet blocks between Y^n, X^{n+1}.

Reversible Networks. A RevNet [6,7] is a neural network block containing convolutional layers, where its input activations can be computed from its output activations (Fig. 1b). We use two residual function bottlenecks $\mathcal{F}_1, \mathcal{F}_2$ [4] as its convolutional blocks. When stacking RevNet blocks, we only cache final activations of the entire stack. During backpropagation, we compute intermediate stack activations on-the-fly, via the inversion property. The formulae for the forward and backward (inversion) are:

<table>
<tr><td>**ForwardPass**</td><td>**Inversion**</td></tr>
<tr><td>$X = [x_\alpha, x_\beta]$</td><td>$Y = [y_\alpha, y_\beta]$</td></tr>
<tr><td>$z = x_\alpha + \mathcal{F}_1(x_\beta)$</td><td>$z = y_\alpha$</td></tr>
<tr><td>$y_\beta = x_\beta + \mathcal{F}_2(z)$</td><td>$x_\beta = y_\beta - \mathcal{F}_2(z)$</td></tr>
<tr><td>$y_\alpha = z$</td><td>$x_\alpha = z - \mathcal{F}_1(x_\beta)$</td></tr>
<tr><td>$Y = [y_\alpha, y_\beta]$</td><td>$X = [x_\alpha, x_\beta]$</td></tr>
</table>

Augmenting Deep Neural Networks. Suppose we wish to improve the performance of a neural network architecture by making it deeper [3]. We propose to pick two layers of the architecture and add a stack of RevNets between them (Fig. 1c, d). This refines the intra-layer connection and facilitates a more complicated mapping to be learnt between them.

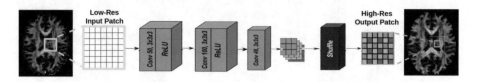

Fig. 2. 2D illustration of the baseline network: 3D ESPCN [1].

Augmenting the ESPCN. We evaluate our procedure with the ESPCN network, which holds the benchmark for HCP data super-resolution (IQT) [1]. The ESPCN (Fig. 2) is a simple four-layer convolutional neural network, followed by a shuffling operation from low-to-high-resolution space: a mapping $H \times W \times D \times r^3C \rightarrow rH \times rW \times rD \times C$, with spatial and channel dimensions respectively H, W, D and C.

We augment the ESPCN (Fig. 3a), by adding N RevNet blocks in a stack, preceding each ESPCN layer. When optimising network weights, we can either perform the forward and backward pass (backpropagation) via the standard implementation i.e. a single computational graph, which we denote as ESPCN-RN-N-Naive; or utilise the reversibility property of RevNets with a variant of checkpointing, denoted by ESPCN-RN-N and illustrated in Fig. 3. Note ESPCN-RN-N-Naive, ESPCN-RN-N have identical predictions and performance (e.g. in Fig. 4), only the computational cost and memory usage differ (Fig. 6). We finally note that this technique is not restricted to the ESPCN or to super-resolution, but may be employed in other neural networks.

3   Experiments and Results

IQT. We formulate super-resolution as a patch-regression, to deal with its large volume, where the input low-resolution (LR) volume is split into overlapping smaller sub-volumes and the resolution of each is sequentially enhanced [1,8]. The HR prediction of the entire 3D brain is obtained by stitching together all the corresponding output patches (Fig. 5).

HCP Data. We follow [1,8] and utilise a set of subjects from the Human Connectome Project (HCP) cohort [12]. This involves healthy adults (22–36 years old), where we specifically vary race, gender and handedness, which effects brain structure. Each subject's scan contains 90 diffusion weighted images (DWIs)

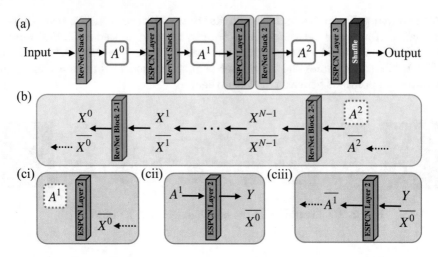

Fig. 3. We augment the ESPCN (Fig. 2) and illustrate (a) the global forward pass, (b, c) the backward pass on part of the network. (a) Augment the ESPCN (1c, d). In the forward pass, we cache (purple squares) activations A^0, A^1, A^2 and create no computational graphs. (b, c) We illustrate backpropagation in the section between the activations A^1, A^2: (b) Load A^2 from the cache (purple dotted square) and receive the loss gradient $\overline{A^2} := \frac{\partial L}{\partial A^2}$ from ESPCN Layer 3 (dotted arrow). Iteratively we pass the activation and gradient backwards per block, deleting redundant values. The final gradient $\overline{X^0}$ is passed to ESPCN Layer 2 (dotted arrow). (c) Backpropagation on ESPCN Layer 2. (ci) Load activation A^1 from the cache (purple dotted square) and $\overline{X^0}$ is passed from RevNet Block 2-1 (dotted arrow) (cii) Create a computational graph through ESPCN Layer 2. (ciii) Combine the computational graph with $\overline{X^0}$ to back-propagate backwards on the ESPCN Layer 2. Finally pass the gradient $\overline{A^1}$ to RevNet Stack 1 (dotted arrow).

of voxel size $1.25^3 \, \text{mm}^3$ with $b = 1000 \, \text{s/mm}^2$. We create the training-and-validation-set (TVS) by sampling HR sub-volumes from the ground truth diffusion tensor images (DTIs, obtained from DWIs) and then down-sampling to generate the LR counterparts. Down-sampling is performed in the raw DWI by a factor of $r = 2$ in each dimension by taking a block-wise mean, where $r = 2$ is the up-sampling rate and then the diffusion tensors are subsequently computed. Lastly all the patch pairs are normalised so the pixel-and-channel-wise mean and variance are 0 and 1. We divide the TVS patches 80%–20% to produce, respectively, training and validation sets. We follow [1,8] in having 8 independent subjects as the test set. As in [1], we evaluate our model separately on the interior region RMSE and exterior (peripheral) region RMSE, of the brain. Furthermore we compare total brain-wise RMSE.

Implementation. As in [1], we extract 2250 patches per subject for TVS, where the central voxel lies within its brain-mask. We utilise PyTorch [13], He parameter initialisation [14], ADAM optimiser [15] with RMSE loss (between the prediction and the inversely-shuffled HR images), decaying learning rate starting at 10^{-4}, ending training either at 100 epochs or when validation set performance fails to improve. Given that results vary due to the random initialisation, we train 4 models for each set of hyperparameters, select the best model from the validation score, to then evaluate on the test set. All our experiments are conducted on a single NVidia Pascal GPU.

Model	Subjects (TVS)	RMSE Interior	RMSE Exterior	RMSE Total
ESPCN	8	6.33 (± 0.30)	14.01 (± 1.12)	9.72 (± 0.64)
ESPCN-best-[1]	8	6.29 (± 0.29)	13.82 (± 0.31)	9.76 (± 0.51)
ESPCN-RN2	8	5.78 (± 0.28)	13.17 (± 1.16)	9.06 (± 0.66)
ESPCN-RN4	8	5.71 (± 0.24)	12.84 (± 1.18)	8.86 (± 0.66)
ESPCN-RN6	8	7.33 (± 1.43)	13.03 (± 1.19)	9.76 (± 0.88)
ESPCN-RN8	8	9.54 (± 4.38)	12.78 (± 1.25)	11.08 (± 2.66)
ESPCN	16	6.12 (± 0.29)	13.42 (± 1.15)	9.33 (± 0.65)
ESPCN-RN4	16	5.51 (± 0.25)	12.40 (± 1.23)	8.56 (± 0.68)
ESPCN	32	6.12 (± 0.29)	13.42 (± 1.15)	9.33 (± 0.65)
ESPCN-RN4	32	5.58 (± 0.25)	12.13 (± 1.24)	8.46 (± 0.67)

Fig. 4. Comparing mean and std RMSE on 8 test subjects, where we first vary number of RevNet blocks per stack, then size of training-validation set (TVS). Network input size 11^3, upsampling rate $r = 2$.

IQT Performance. In Fig. 4, increasing network depth improves accuracy, until the models overfit. Since implementing regularisation deteriorates our results due to the bias-variance tradeoff, we instead utilise larger TVS. Unlike the ESPCN, our extended model registers improvements on both interior and the exterior (peripheral) brain regions, with additional data. To assess statistical significance of our results, we employed a non-parametric Wilcoxon signed-rank test (W statistic) for paired RMSE values of our 8 test subjects, comparing our best model (ESPCN-RN4) over state-of-the-art [1] (Fig. 4), produces $W = 0$, significant with $p = 0.0117$ (critical value for W is 3 at $N = 8$, at significance level alpha $= 0.05$), improvement of the ESPCN-RN4 over ESPCN at 32 subjects also produces $W = 0$, $p = 0.0117$, which is significant as before. We note this improvement occurs with almost identical memory usage (Fig. 6). Comparing the image quality enhancement due to our results in Fig. 4, we observe from Fig. 5 that our augmentation produces sharper recovery of anatomical boundaries between white matter and grey matter, whilst better capturing high-frequency details such as textures on white matter.

Memory Comparison. Despite significantly elongating the ESPCN, our novel procedure performs very well with respect to memory usage – an increase of just 4.0% in Fig. 6 – which also includes caching extra RevNet parameters. Memory consumption is more than halved when using a low memory scheme (ESPCN-RN4), with respect to naively performing backpropagation from a single computational graph and ignoring both checkpointing and the reversibility property of

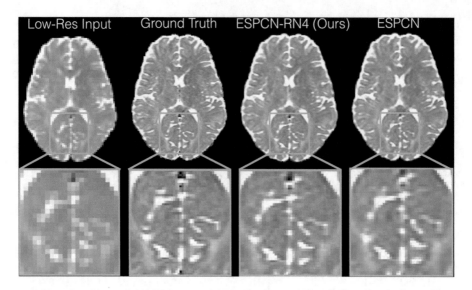

Fig. 5. A visualisation of mean diffusivity maps on an axial slice on a test HCP subject, estimated from: low-resolution input, ground-truth, high-resolution reconstruction from best ESPCN-RN4 (Fig. 4), ESPCN [1].

RevNets (ESPCN-RN4 Naive). Although the computational time tradeoff of the low-memory system is significant, training for each model in Fig. 4 was obtained in under 24 h.

Model	Memory Usage (MB)	Computational Time (s)
ESPCN	523	20
ESPCN-RN4	541	309
ESPCN-RN4 Naive	1091	231

Fig. 6. Comparing the memory usage and computational time on a single epoch with 8 TVS subjects: the original ESPCN, our augmented ESPCN-RN4 and ESPCN-RN4 Naive (ESPCN-RN4 without the low-memory optimisation).

4   Conclusion

Attempts to merge cutting-edge techniques in deep learning with medical imaging data often encounter memory bottlenecks, due to limited GPU memory and large data sets. In this paper, we present how combining checkpointing with RevNets allow us to train long convolutional neural networks with modest computational and memory requirements. Our example – dMRI super-resolution in the paradigm of IQT – illustrates how to improve performance via neural network augmentation, with a negligible increase in memory requirements. However the benefits of this technique extend to many other applications which use deep neural networks, particularly in medical imaging, where large image volumes are the predominant data type.

Acknowledgements. This work was supported by an EPRSC scholarship and EPSRC grants M020533 R006032 R014019. We thank: Adeyemi Akintonde, Tristan Clark, Marco Palombo and Emiliano Rodriguez. Data were provided by the Human Connectome Project, WU-Minn Consortium (PIs: D. V Essen and K. Ugurbil) funded by NiH and Wash. U.

References

1. Tanno, R., et al.: Bayesian image quality transfer with CNNs: exploring uncertainty in dMRI super-resolution. In: MICCAI (2017)
2. Milletari, F., et al.: V-net: fully convolutional neural networks for volumetric medical image segmentation. In: 3DV, pp. 565–571 (2016)
3. Choromanska, A., et al.: The loss surfaces of multilayer networks. In: AISTATS (2015)
4. He, K., et al.: Deep residual learning for image recognition. In: CVPR (2016)
5. Chen, T., et al.: Training deep nets with sublinear memory cost. arXiv preprint arXiv:1604.06174 (2016)
6. Chang, B., et al.: Reversible architectures for arbitrarily deep residual neural networks. In: AAAI (2018)
7. Gomez, A., et al.: The reversible residual network: backpropagation without storing activation. In: NIPS (2017)
8. Alexander, D.: Image quality transfer and applications in diffusion MRI. NeuroImage **152**, 283–298 (2017)
9. Kamnitsas, K.: Efficient multi-scale 3D CNN with fully connected crf for accurate brain lesion segmentation. Med. Image Anal. **36**, 61–78 (2017)
10. Wolterink, J.: Deep MR to CT synthesis using unpaired data. SASHIM **I**, 14–22 (2017)
11. Yang, X., et al.: Fast predictive image registration. In: DLMIA (2016)
12. Sotiropoulos, S.: Advances in diffusion MRI acquisition and processing in the human connectome project. Neuroimage **80**, 125–143 (2013)
13. Paszke, A., et al.: Automatic differentiation in PyTorch (2017)
14. He, K., et al.: Delving deep into rectifiers: surpassing human-level performance on imagenet classification. In: ICCV (2015)
15. Kingma, D., Ba, J.: Adam: a method for stochastic optimization. In: ICLR (2015)

High Frame-Rate Cardiac Ultrasound Imaging with Deep Learning

Ortal Senouf[1(✉)], Sanketh Vedula[1], Grigoriy Zurakhov[1], Alex Bronstein[1],
Michael Zibulevsky[1], Oleg Michailovich[2], Dan Adam[1], and David Blondheim[3]

[1] Technion - Israel Institute of Technology, Haifa, Israel
{senouf,sanketh}@campus.technion.ac.il
[2] University of Waterloo, Waterloo, Canada
[3] Hillel Yaffe Medical Center, Hadera, Israel

Abstract. Cardiac ultrasound imaging requires a high frame rate in order to capture rapid motion. This can be achieved by multi-line acquisition (MLA), where several narrow-focused received lines are obtained from each wide-focused transmitted line. This shortens the acquisition time at the expense of introducing block artifacts. In this paper, we propose a data-driven learning-based approach to improve the MLA image quality. We train an end-to-end convolutional neural network on pairs of real ultrasound cardiac data, acquired through MLA and the corresponding single-line acquisition (SLA). The network achieves a significant improvement in image quality for both 5- and 7-line MLA resulting in a decorrelation measure similar to that of SLA while having the frame rate of MLA.

Keywords: Ultrasound imaging · Machine learning
Multi-line acquisition

1 Introduction

Increasing the frame rate is a major challenge in 2D and 3D echocardiography. Investigating deformations at different stages of the cardiac cycle is crucial for cardiovascular imaging; hence high temporal resolution is highly desired in addition to the spatial resolution. There are several ways to increase the frame rate of ultrasound imaging; one of the most commonly used techniques, which is implemented in many ultrasound scanners, is multi-line acquisition (MLA) [1], often referred to as parallel receive beamforming (PRB) [2].

Single- vs. Multi-line Acquisition. In single-line acquisition (SLA), a narrow-focused pulse is transmitted by introducing transmit time delays through a linear phased array of acoustic transducer elements. Upon reception the obtained signal

Electronic supplementary material The online version of this chapter (https://doi.org/10.1007/978-3-030-00928-1_15) contains supplementary material, which is available to authorized users.

© Springer Nature Switzerland AG 2018
A. F. Frangi et al. (Eds.): MICCAI 2018, LNCS 11070, pp. 126–134, 2018.
https://doi.org/10.1007/978-3-030-00928-1_15

is dynamically focused along the receive (Rx) direction which is identical to the transmit (Tx) direction. The spatial region of interest is raster scanned line-by-line to obtain an ultrasound image.

The need to transmit a large number of pulses sequentially results in a low frame rate and renders SLA inadequate for cardiovascular imaging, where a high frame rate is mandatory, especially for quantitative analysis or during stress tests. For the same reason, SLA is neither useful for scanning large fields of view in real time 3D imaging applications.

In an attempt to overcome the frame rate problem, the MLA method was proposed in [1,3]. The main idea behind MLA is to transmit a weakly focused beam that provides a sufficiently wide coverage for a high number of received lines. On the receiver side, m lines is constructed from the data acquired from each transmit event, thereby increasing the frame rate by m (the latter number is usually referred to as the *MLA factor*). Signal formation in the SLA and MLA modalities is demonstrated in Fig. 1 where 5-MLA is depicted. For a 5-MLA, we construct 5 Rx lines per each Tx thus increasing the frame rate by the factor of 5.

MLA Artifacts. As the Tx and Rx are no longer aligned in the MLA mode, the two-way beam profile is shifted towards the original transmit direction, making the lateral sampling irregular [2]. This *beam warping* effect causes sharp lateral discontinuities that are manifested as block artifacts in the image domain.

The observed block artifacts in the ultrasound images (see, e.g., Fig. 1) tend to be more obvious when the number of transmit events decreases. The MLA artifact can be measured by assessing the correlation coefficient between each two adjacent Rx lines in the in-phase and quadrature (I/Q) demodulated beam-formed data [4]. In SLA or compensated MLA, the averaged correlation values inside MLA groups and between MLA groups are almost the same. In the uncompensated cases, however, the correlation values are different.

Apart from beam warping, there are two other effects caused by the transmit-receive misalignment: *skewing*, where shape of the two-way beam profile becomes asymmetric, and *gain variation*, where the outermost lines inside the group have a lower gain than the innermost lines [4].

Related Work. Several methods have been proposed in literature to decrease MLA artifacts, including transmit sinc apodization [5] and dynamic steering [6], incoherent interpolation [7,8] (applied after envelope detection), and its coherent (before envelope detection) counterparts [2,9]. One of the more prominent methods, synthetic transmit beamforming (STB) [2], creates synthetic Tx lines by coherently interpolating information received from each two adjacent Tx events in intermediate directions. This technique creates highly correlated lines, attenuating block artifacts. A common practice for MLA imaging with focused beams is to create 2-4 Rx lines per each Tx event in cases without overlap, or 4-8 lines in the presence of overlaps from adjacent transmissions, in order to perform the correction [2,4,10]. Thus, creating eight lines with overlaps provides an effective frame rate increase by the factor of 4. In this paper, however, we used odd MLA factors $m = 5, 7$ for the purpose of acquiring data from aligned directions for both SLA and MLA.

Recently, data-driven learning techniques based on convolutional neural networks (CNNs) have been extensively used for solving inverse problems in imaging and in medical imaging in particular, for example, in X-ray CT reconstruction and denoising [11]. Inspired by their success, we propose a data-driven approach to overcome MLA artifacts.

Contributions. We propose an end-to-end CNN-based approach for MLA artifact correction. Our fully convolutional network consists of interpolation layers followed by a trainable apodization layer, and is trained on in-vivo cardiac data to approximate an SLA quality image. We demonstrate the effectiveness of this network both visually and quantitatively using the decorrelation measure (D_c) and SSIM [12] quality criteria. To the best of our knowledge, this is the first study to report good artifact corrections in the case of 5-7-MLA. We show that the trained network generalizes well across patients, as well as to phantom data.

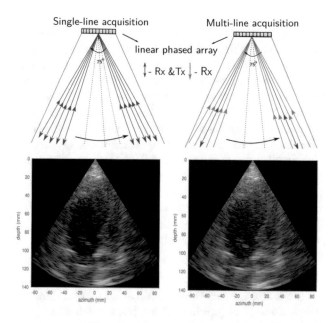

Fig. 1. Single (left) and multi-line (right, with MLA factor $m = 5$) acquisition procedures and their corresponding ultrasound scans. Block artifacts can be seen along the axial direction in MLA. Zooming in is recommended.

2   Methods

2.1   Improving MLA with CNNs

Aiming at providing a general and optimal solution for MLA interpolation achieving SLA quality, we propose to replace MLA artifact correction and apodization phases in the traditional MLA pipeline as shown in Fig. 2 with an end-to-end CNN depicted in Fig. 3. We draw similarities to [10] who showed that combining MLA interpolation with an optimal apodization method produces superior results compared to the traditional approaches. Our network comprises both the interpolation and the apodization stages that are trained jointly.

Interpolation Stage. The interpolation stage consists of our CNN containing 10 convolutional layers with symmetric skip connections [13,14] from each layer in the downsampling track to its corresponding layer in the upsampling track as visualized in Fig. 3. Downsampling is performed using average pooling and strided convolutions are used for upsampling. The number of bifurcations is set to 5 for all the experiments. The interpolation stage takes as an input the time-delayed and phase-rotated element-wise I/Q data from the transducer.

Apodization Stage. Following the interpolation stage, we introduce a convolutional layer to perform apodization. This is performed using point-wise convolutions (1×1) for each element's channel in the network and the results are then added to the learned weights of the convolution. The weights of the channel are initialized with a Hann window.

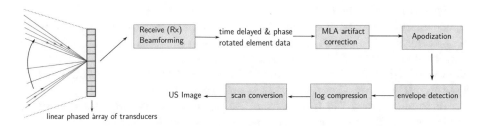

Fig. 2. Traditional MLA ultrasound imaging pipeline.

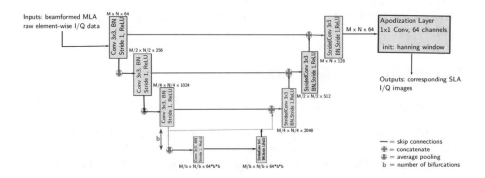

Fig. 3. Proposed CNN-based MLA artifact correction pipeline.

Optimization. We use the L_1 norm training loss to measure the discrepancy between the image predicted by the network and the ground truth SLA images. The loss is minimized using the Adam optimizer [15] with a learning rate of 10^{-4}. We observed that adding the apodization stage accelerates the training process, and makes the network converge faster.

2.2   Data Acquisition and Training

We generated a dataset for training the network using cardiac data from six patients; each patient contributed 4-5 cine loops, containing 32 frames. The data was acquired using a GE experimental breadboard ultrasound system. The same transducer was used for both phantom and cardiac acquisition. Excitation sinusoidal pulses of 1.75 cycles, centered around 2.5 MHz, were transmitted using 28 central elements out of the total 64 element in the probe with a pitch of 0.3 mm, elevation size of 13 mm and elevation focus of 100 mm. The depth focus was set at 71 mm. In order to assess the desired aperture for MLA setup, Field II simulator [16] was used as in [10] using the transducer impulse response and tri-state transmission excitation sequence, requiring a minimal insonification of $-3\,$dB for all MLAs from a single Tx.

On the Rx side, the I/Q demodulated signals were dynamically focused using linear interpolation, with an f-number of 1. The FOV was covered with 140/140 Tx/ Rx lines in SLA mode, 28/140 Tx/Rx lines in the 5-MLA mode, and 20/140 Tx/Rx lines in the 7-MLA mode. For both phantom and cardiac cases, the data were acquired in the SLA mode; 5-MLA and 7-MLA data was obtained by appropriately decimating the Rx pre-beamformed data.

In total, we used 745 frames from five patients for training and validation, while keeping the cine loops from the sixth patient for testing. The data set comprised pairs of beamformed I/Q images with Hann window apodization, and the corresponding 5- and 7-MLA pre-apodization samples with the dimensions of $652 \times 64 \times 140$ (depth $\times$ elements $\times$ Rx lines). The MLA data was acquired by decimation of the Tx lines of the SLA samples by the MLA factor ($m = 5, 7$).

We trained dedicated CNNs for the reconstruction of SLA images from 5- and 7-MLA. Each CNN was trained to a maximum of 200 epochs on mini batches of size 4.

3   Experimental Evaluation

3.1   Settings

In order to assess the performance of our trained networks, we used cine loops from one patient excluded from the training/validation set. From two cine loops, each containing 32 frames, we generated pairs of 5- and 7-MLA samples and their corresponding SLA images the same way as described in Sect. 2.2, resulting in 64 test samples. For quantitative evaluation of the performance of our method we measured the decorrelation (D_c) criterion that evaluates the artifact strength [4], and the SSIM [12] structural similarity criterion with respect to the SLA image. In addition, we tested the performance of our networks on four frames acquired from the GAMMEX Ultrasound 403GS LE Grey Scale Precision Phantom.

3.2 Results

Quantitative results for the cardiac test set are summarized in Table 1. We show a major improvement in decorrelation and SSIM for both 5- and 7-MLA. The corrected 7-MLA performance approaches that of 5-MLA, suggesting the feasibility of larger MLA factors. Figure 4 shows representative images from each imaging modality. We show that the correlation coefficients profile of the corrected 5- and 7-MLA approaches that of SLA.

Table 1. Image reconstruction results on cardiac data: comparison of average decorrelation and SSIM measures between the original and corrected 5- and 7-MLA cardiac images. Decorrelation of SLA is reported in the first column; left and right values in the entry indicate the values calculated for 5- and 7-MLA, respectively.

	SLA	5-MLA		7-MLA	
	Original	Original	Corrected	Original	Corrected
Decorrelation	0.03/−0.04	22.03	0.69	31.7	0.827
SSIM	−	0.75	0.876	0.693	0.826

Table 2. Image reconstruction results on phantom data: Comparison of average decorrelation and SSIM measures between original and corrected 5- and 7-MLA phantom images. Decorrelation of SLA is reported in the first column; left and right values in the entry indicate values calculated for 5- and 7-MLA, respectively.

	SLA	5-MLA		7-MLA	
	Original	Original	Corrected	Original	Corrected
Decorrelation	0.06/−0.089	19.53	0.457	32.34	0.956
SSIM	−	0.815	0.96	0.793	0.935

Similarly, quantitative results for the phantom test set are summarized in Table 2, again showing a significant improvement in the image quality for both 5- and 7-MLA. Visual results with the corresponding correlation coefficients profiles are depicted in Fig. 1 in the Supplementary Material. These results suggest that the networks trained on real cardiac data generalize well to the phantom data without any further training or fine-tuning. For comparison, [4] reported a decorrelation value of −1.5 for a phantom image acquired in a 4−MLA mode with STB compensation, while we report closer to zero D_c values, 0.457 for

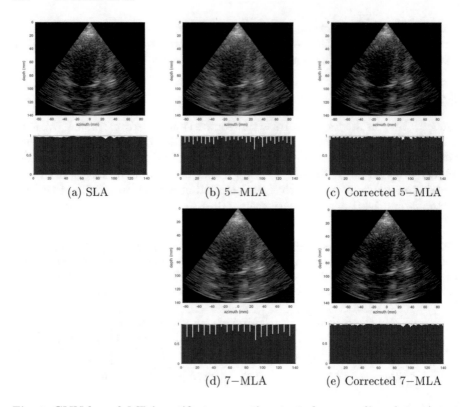

Fig. 4. CNN-based MLA artifact correction tested on cardiac data. A test frame from cardiac sequence demonstrating the performance of the proposed artifact correction algorithm. Each image is depicted along with the plot of the correlation coefficients between adjacent lines.

5-MLA and 0.956 for 7-MLA, which both use a greater decimation rate. The slight dissimilarities in the recovered data can be explained by the acquisition method being used: since the scanned object was undergoing a motion, there is a difference between all but a central line in each MLA group and the matching lines in SLA. We assume that training the network on images of static organs may further improve its performance. Independently, small areas with vertical stripes were observed in several images. In our opinion, the origin of the stripes is a coherent summation of the beamformed lines across the moving object. Since the frame rate of the employed acquisition sequence was slower than of genuine MLA acquisition, the magnitude of this artifact is probably exaggerated.

4   Conclusion

In this paper, we have shown that conventional ultrasound MLA correction can be substituted with an end-to-end CNN performing both optimal interpolation and apodization in order to approximate SLA image quality. In the future, we aim at extending this approach to even earlier stages in multi-line acquisition such as beamforming, assuming it will provide a greater improvement in image quality. Moreover, a similar method could probably be applied for other fast US acquisition modalities, such as multi-line transmission (MLT) [17].

Acknowledgements. The research was partially supported by ERC StG RAPID.

References

1. Shattuck, D.P., Weinshenker, M.D., Smith, S.W., von Ramm, O.T.: Explososcan: a parallel processing technique for high speed ultrasound imaging with linear phased arrays. Acoust. Soc. Am. J. **75**, 1273–1282 (1984)
2. Hergum, T., Bjastad, T., Kristoffersen, K., Torp, H.: Parallel beamforming using synthetic transmit beams. IEEE Trans. Ultrason. Ferroelectr. Freq. Control **54**(2), 271–280 (2007)
3. Ramm, O.T.V., Smith, S.W., Pavy, H.G.: High-speed ultrasound volumetric imaging system. II. parallel processing and image display. IEEE Trans. Ultrason. Ferroelectr. Freq. Control **38**(2), 109–115 (1991)
4. Bjastad, T., Aase, S.A., Torp, H.: The impact of aberration on high frame rate cardiac b-mode imaging. IEEE Trans. Ultrason. Ferroelectr. Freq. Control **54**(1), 32 (2007)
5. Augustine, L.J.: High resolution multiline ultrasonic beamformer. US Patent 4,644,795, 24 February 1987
6. Thiele, K.E., Brauch, A.: Method and apparatus for dynamically steering ultrasonic phased arrays. US Patent 5,322,068, 21 June 1994
7. Holley, G.L., Guracar, I.M.: Ultrasound multi-beam distortion correction system and method. US Patent 5,779,640, 14 July 1998
8. Liu, D.D., Lazenby, J.C., Banjanin, Z., McDermott, B.A.: System and method for reduction of parallel beamforming artifacts. US Patent 6,447,452, 10 September 2002
9. Wright, J.N., Maslak, S.H., Finger, D.J., Gee, A.: Method and apparatus for coherent image formation. US Patent 5,623,928, 29 April 1997
10. Rabinovich, A., Friedman, Z., Feuer, A.: Multi-line acquisition with minimum variance beamforming in medical ultrasound imaging. IEEE Trans. Ultrason. Ferroelectr. Freq. Control **60**(12), 2521–2531 (2013)
11. McCann, M.T., Jin, K.H., Unser, M.: Convolutional neural networks for inverse problems in imaging: a review. IEEE Signal Process. Mag. **34**(6), 85–95 (2017)
12. Wang, Z., Bovik, A.C., Sheikh, H.R., Simoncelli, E.P.: Image quality assessment: from error visibility to structural similarity. IEEE Trans. Image Process. **13**(4), 600–612 (2004)
13. Mao, X., Shen, C., Yang, Y.B.: Image restoration using very deep convolutional encoder-decoder networks with symmetric skip connections. In: Advances in Neural Information Processing Systems, pp. 2802–2810 (2016)
14. Ronneberger, O., Fischer, P., Brox, T.: U-Net: convolutional networks for biomedical image segmentation. In: Navab, N., Hornegger, J., Wells, W.M., Frangi, A.F. (eds.) MICCAI 2015. LNCS, vol. 9351, pp. 234–241. Springer, Cham (2015). https://doi.org/10.1007/978-3-319-24574-4_28
15. Kingma, D.P., Ba, J.: Adam: a method for stochastic optimization. In: Proceedings of the 3rd International Conference on Learning Representations (ICLR) (2015)

16. Jensen, J.A.: Field: a program for simulating ultrasound systems. In: 10th Nordicbaltic Conference on Biomedical Imaging, vol. 4, Supplement 1, Part 1, pp. 351–353. Citeseer (1996)
17. Mallart, R., Fink, M.: Improved imaging rate through simultaneous transmission of several ultrasound beams. In: New Developments in Ultrasonic Transducers and Transducer Systems, vol. 1733, pp. 120–131. International Society for Optics and Photonics (1992)

Image Reconstruction Methods

Phase-Sensitive Region-of-Interest Computed Tomography

Lina Felsner[1](✉), Martin Berger[3], Sebastian Kaeppler[1], Johannes Bopp[1],
Veronika Ludwig[2], Thomas Weber[2], Georg Pelzer[2], Thilo Michel[2],
Andreas Maier[1], Gisela Anton[2], and Christian Riess[1]

[1] Pattern Recognition Lab, Computer Science, University of Erlangen-Nürnberg,
Erlangen, Germany
lina.felsner@fau.de
[2] Erlangen Centre for Astroparticle Physics, University of Erlangen-Nürnberg,
Erlangen, Germany
[3] Siemens Healthcare GmbH, Erlangen, Germany

Abstract. X-Ray Phase-Contrast Imaging (PCI) yields absorption, differential phase, and dark-field images. Computed Tomography (CT) of grating-based PCI can in principle provide high-resolution soft-tissue contrast. Recently, grating-based PCI took several hurdles towards clinical implementation by addressing, for example, acquisition speed, high X-ray energies, and system vibrations. However, a critical impediment in all grating-based systems lies in limits that constrain the grating diameter to few centimeters.

In this work, we propose a system and a reconstruction algorithm to circumvent this constraint in a clinically compatible way. We propose to perform a phase-sensitive Region-of-Interest (ROI) CT within a full-field absorption CT. The biggest advantage of this approach is that it allows to correct for phase truncation artifacts, and to obtain quantitative phase values. Our method is robust, and shows high-quality results on simulated data and on a biological mouse sample. This work is a proof of concept showing the potential to use PCI in CT on large specimen, such as humans, in clinical applications.

1 Introduction

X-ray Phase-Contrast Imaging (PCI) is a novel imaging technique that can be implemented with an X-ray grating interferometer [1]. Such an interferometer provides an X-ray absorption image, and additionally a differential phase-contrast image and a dark-field image. X-ray absorption and phase encode material-specific parameters that are linked to the complex index of refraction n, given as $n = 1 - \delta + i \cdot \beta$. Here, δ relates to the phase shift and β to the attenuation. Since PCI yields high soft tissue contrast [2,3], it is particularly interesting to apply it in Computed Tomography (CT). Figure 1 shows example sinograms for the absorption and phase, and the associated tomographic reconstructions.

© Springer Nature Switzerland AG 2018
A. F. Frangi et al. (Eds.): MICCAI 2018, LNCS 11070, pp. 137–144, 2018.
https://doi.org/10.1007/978-3-030-00928-1_16

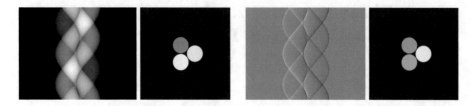

Fig. 1. Sinogram and reconstruction of the absorption (left) and differential phase images (right) of three cylinders with different materials at 82 keV. From the top in clockwise direction: water, PTFE and PVC.

It furthermore shows that their information is complementary, allowing for the distinction of different materials.

One key advantage of a grating-based interferometer is its compatibility with clinical X-ray equipment [1]. For clinical application, several practical challenges were recently addressed. Among these works are significant improvements in acquisition speed [4], higher X-ray energies to penetrate large bodies [5], and system vibrations [6].

However, one major obstacle to clinical implementation lies in the fact that it is not clear whether gratings with a diameter of more than a few centimeters can be integrated in a clinical CT system, due to increasing vibrations sensitivity, production cost and complexity for larger grating sizes. Such a small field of view is a major challenge for medical applications, since it only allows to reconstruct a small region of interest (ROI). This leads to difficult region localization and limited information on surrounding tissue. Furthermore, the object is typically larger than the field of view, which leads to truncation in the projection images.

Truncation is a substantial issue in the reconstruction of conventional projection images, leading to artifacts, such as cupping. Noo *et al.* showed that the reconstruction of a ROI from truncated differential images can be accurately obtained in certain cases [7]. Unfortunately, for the so-called interior problem, where the ROI is completely inside the object, there is no unique solution. Kudo *et al.* [8] found later, that the solution is unique if prior knowledge on the object is available in the form, that the object is known within a small region located inside the region of interest. For differential projection data, the interior problem can be approached iteratively [9,10]. However, these approaches are of limited practical use due to strong assumptions or high computational demand.

In this work, we propose a methodology for phase-sensitive region-of-interest imaging within a standard CT. The key idea is to solve the shortcomings of existing ROI imaging by complementing the small-area phase measurements with the full-field absorption signal, which is similar in spirit to the work by Kolditz *et al.* [11]. To this end, we propose to mount a grating-based system in the center of an absorption CT system. The truncated phase signal can be extrapolated beyond the grating limits using the full absorption information and the phase within the ROI. This mitigates the typical truncation artifacts, and even provides quantitative phase information within the ROI, thereby paving the way towards phase CT in a clinical environment.

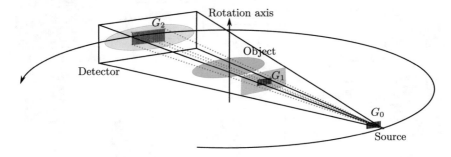

Fig. 2. Setup of the proposed imaging system.

2 Methods

The proposed method consists of a system and a reconstruction algorithm. We describe the system in Sect. 2.1 and the algorithm in Sect. 2.2.

2.1 Realization of the System

A grating-based (Talbot-Lau) interferometer consists of three gratings G_0, G_1, G_2 that are placed between X-ray tube and detector (see Fig. 2). G_0 is placed close to the source to ensure spatial coherence. G_1 is located in front of the object to imprint a periodical phase shift onto the wave front. G_2 is located in front of the detector to resolve sub-resolution wave modulations.

Recently, the implementation of an interferometer into a clinical-like C-arm setup was demonstrated [6]. We propose an embedding of the gratings in a clinical imaging system, such that the gratings cover only a region of interest. An attenuating collimator can be used for mounting the gratings, leading to less dose in the Peripheral Region (PR) outside of the gratings. PCI has a dose advantage compared to attenuation for high-resolution detectors [12], which suggests that it could also be advantageous to perform a high-resolution reconstruction in the ROI and reduce the resolution outside of the grating area to save dose. Figure 2 shows a sketch of the setup.

While the geometry of the full absorption image is a cone-beam, the smaller grating area exhibits approximately parallel beams, simplifying reconstruction. We apply a RamLak filter to the truncation-free absorption signal and a Hilbert filter to the phase-signal.

2.2 Truncation Correction

The pipeline of the proposed algorithm is shown in Fig. 3. We first perform a reconstruction of absorption and truncated phase, and segment the absorption

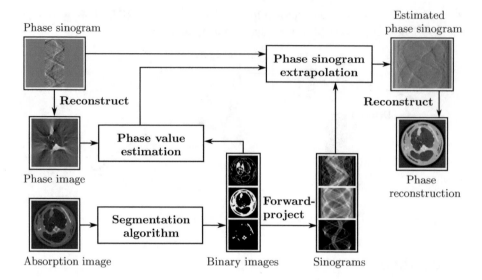

Fig. 3. Overview of the proposed method. A segmentation of the materials allows to obtain an estimate of their respective phase values. A non-truncated sinogram is extrapolated from the truncated sinogram and the extrapolated phase values.

into k materials. This allows to estimate the phase values per material within the ROI, and to extrapolate the phase values across the full area. Reconstructing then the phase from the estimated sinogram gives the non-truncated phase.

Segmentation Algorithm. The absorption signal is decomposed into k materials via segmentation. While in principle any algorithm could be used here, we fitted a Gaussian Mixture Model with k components to the histogram.

Phase Value Estimation. The truncated phase ROI is reconstructed. For each material, we estimate its phase value δ_k by computing the mean over its segmented pixels in the ROI. If a material is not contained in the ROI, we heuristically set it to the mean δ over the ROI. Since the estimated values will be differentiated in a later step, estimation bias is a minor concern.

Phase Sinogram Extrapolation. The phase shift ϕ is

$$\phi = \int \delta \, \mathrm{d}z = \sum_k \left(\delta_k \cdot \int_k \mathrm{d}z \right), \qquad (1)$$

which can be split into k materials. The measured differential phase signal is

$$\varphi = \frac{\lambda \cdot d}{2\pi \cdot p_2} \frac{\partial \phi}{\partial x} = \frac{\lambda \cdot d}{2\pi \cdot p_2} \sum_k \left(\frac{\partial \, \delta_k \int_k \mathrm{d}z}{\partial x} \right), \qquad (2)$$

consisting of sensitivity direction x, wavelength λ, $G_1 - G_2$ distance d, and the G_2 period p_2. The factor $(\lambda \cdot d)/(2\pi \cdot p_2)$ is the setup sensitivity, which is a material-independent scaling factor and can therefore be ignored. Thus, we can obtain the sinogram of the differential phase by applying the derivative to the δ_k-weighted line integrals, given by the forward projections of the segmented materials. That way, the truncated phase sinogram is extrapolated with the missing sinogram information outside the ROI. The extrapolated phase together with the measured ROI allow for a quantitative phase reconstruction.

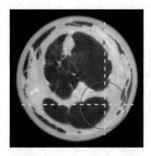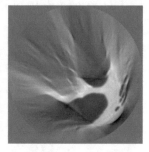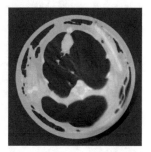

Fig. 4. Mouse sample. Left: ground truth with ROI (red) and line profile (yellow). Center: truncated phase reconstruction. Right: proposed phase reconstruction.

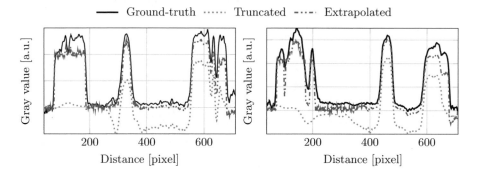

Fig. 5. Line plots of the mouse sample through the region of interest. Left: in horizontal direction; Right: in vertical direction.

3   Experiments

The proposed method is evaluated on a ground-truth reconstruction of the untruncated data after 3×3 pixel smoothing with a median filter. Line plots are obtained in horizontal and vertical direction through the center of the ROI. The quantitative metrics are the Root Mean Square Error (RMSE) and the Structural Similarity (SSIM) inside the ROI.

3.1   Biological Sample

We use a scan of a mouse [13] as biological sample with complex anatomical structures. The scan is manually truncated by cropping the ROI in the sinogram.

This allows us to compare the results to a full reconstruction. The acquisition setup consists of a tungsten anode X-ray tube at 60 kVp and a Varian PaxScan 2520D detector with 127 μm pixel pitch. The grating periods are 23.95 μm, 4.37 μm and 2.40 μm for G_0, G_1, and G_2, respectively. The $G_0 - G_1$ distance is 161.2 cm. Acquisition is done with 8 phase steps with exposures of 3.3 s each and a tube current of 30 mA. The image sequence contains 601 projection images over a full circle. We chose a ROI size of a third of the detector size.

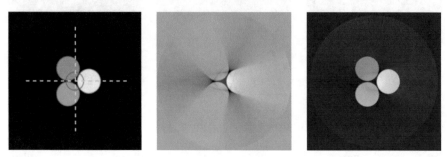

Fig. 6. Simulated sample. Left: ground truth with ROI (red) and line profile (yellow). Center: truncated phase reconstruction. Right: proposed phase reconstruction.

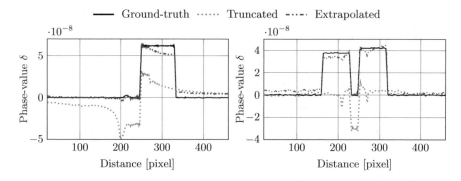

Fig. 7. Line plots on simulated sample in horizontal (left) and vertical direction (right).

We evaluate our method for nine different ROIs on the mouse, with k empirically set to 5. Our algorithm successfully reduces the truncation artifacts for all ROIs. Figure 4 shows example reconstructions of ground truth, truncated phase and estimated phase. The benefit of the truncation correction can be recognized both inside and outside of the ROI. The surrounding tissue of the ROI exhibits slightly sharpened edges due to the segmentation boundaries. The missing structure within the lung is a consequence of the rather simple segmentation. However, this has minimal impact on the quality of the phase information reconstructed within the ROI. The line plots after extrapolation in Fig. 5 are close to the ground truth. Table 1 depicts RMSE and SSIM relative to the ground truth. Our algorithm reduces the RMSE by more than 50%, and SSIM by 64%.

Table 1. Quality metrics with respect to the ground truth inside of the ROIs. Mean and standard deviation over 16 ROIs (simulated data) and 9 ROIs (mouse data).

	Simulation		Mouse	
	RMSE	SSIM	RMSE	SSIM
Truncated	$2.88E - 08 \pm 6.59E - 09$	0.46 ± 0.30	2.08 ± 0.27	0.30 ± 0.33
Estimated	$3.00E - 09 \pm 1.17E - 09$	0.99 ± 0.00	0.66 ± 0.14	0.94 ± 0.05

3.2 Quantitative Evaluation

The quantitative data was created by simulations using reported phase material values for water, polyvinylchlorid (PVC), and polytetrafluorethylen (PTFE) at 82 keV [14]. We used a parallel beam geometry and 360 projection images over a full circle. The size of the ROI is set to 1/8 of the detector width, k is set to 4.

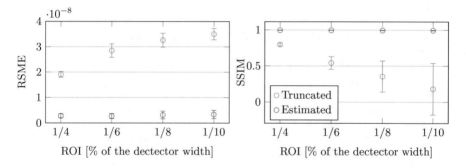

Fig. 8. Performance for simulated data at 82 keV, averaged over different ROI positions for 4 different ROI sizes. Red: truncated reconstruction. Blue: estimated reconstruction.

The absorption and phase reconstructions are shown in Fig. 1. As PTFE and PVC have very similar absorption values, the segmentation erroneously labels them as identical materials. However, the proposed approach is robust to such a missegmentation, which can be recognized by the well distinguishable phase values of PVC and PTFE in Fig. 6. This is supported by the line plots in Fig. 7, where the correctness of the quantitative phase values can also be verified. The measurements in Table 1 support the visual impression, with an average improvement of over 50% for the SSIM and one magnitude decrease for the RMSE. Unfortunately, the phase value of PTFE in Fig. 7 (left) decreases slowly outside the ROI with increasing distance to the ROI.

We also investigate the influence of the ROI size at four different locations, pushing the ROI away from the center. The mean error and standard deviation for RMSE and SSIM are visualized in Fig. 8. The quality of the truncated reconstruction is significantly decreased by a smaller ROI. Contrary, the proposed method is remarkably robust to changes in size and location of the ROI.

4 Conclusion

We propose a system and a method to perform quantitative ROI reconstruction of phase CT. The idea is to embed a grating interferometer into a standard CT, and to extrapolate the phase beyond the ROI with the absorption information to reduce truncation artifacts. Our results on quantitative data and a real biological sample are highly encouraging, and we believe that this is an important step towards using PCI on a clinical setup for larger samples.

Acknowledgments. Lina Felsner is supported by the International Max Planck Research School - Physics of Light (IMPRS-PL).

Disclaimer. The concepts and information presented in this paper are based on research and are not commercially available.

References

1. Pfeiffer, F., Weitkamp, T., Bunk, O., David, C.: Phase retrieval and differential phase-contrast imaging with low-brilliance X-ray sources. Nat. Phys. **2**(4), 258 (2006)
2. Donath, T., et al.: Toward clinical X-ray phase-contrast CT: demonstration of enhanced soft-tissue contrast in human specimen. Inv. Rad. **45**(7), 445–452 (2010)
3. Koehler, T., et al.: Slit-scanning differential x-ray phase-contrast mammography: proof-of-concept experimental studies. Med. Phys. **42**(4), 1959–1965 (2015)
4. Bevins, N., Zambelli, J., Li, K., Qi, Z., Chen, G.H.: Multicontrast x-ray computed tomography imaging using Talbot-Lau interferometry without phase stepping. Med. Phys. **39**(1), 424–428 (2012)
5. Gromann, L.B., et al.: In-vivo x-ray dark-field chest radiography of a pig. Sci. Rep. **7**, 4807 (2017)
6. Horn, F., et al.: Implementation of a Talbot-Lau interferometer in a clinical-like c-arm setup: a feasibility study. Sci. Rep. **8**(1), 2325 (2018)
7. Noo, F., Clackdoyle, R., Pack, J.D.: A two-step hilbert transform method for 2D image reconstruction. Phys. Med. Biol. **49**(17), 3903 (2004)
8. Kudo, H., Courdurier, M., Noo, F., Defrise, M.: Tiny a priori knowledge solves the interior problem in computed tomography. Phys. Med. Biol. **53**(9), 2207 (2008)
9. Cong, W., Yang, J., Wang, G.: Differential phase-contrast interior tomography. Phys. Med. Biol. **57**(10), 2905 (2012)
10. Lauzier, P.T., Qi, Z., Zambelli, J., Bevins, N., Chen, G.H.: Interior tomography in x-ray differential phase contrast CT imaging. Phys. Med. Biol. **57**(9), N117 (2012)
11. Kolditz, D., Kyriakou, Y., Kalender, W.A.: Volume-of-interest (VOI) imaging in C-arm flat-detector CT for high image quality at reduced dose. Med. Phys. **37**(6), 2719–2730 (2010)
12. Raupach, R., Flohr, T.G.: Analytical evaluation of the signal and noise propagation in x-ray differential phase-contrast computed tomography. Phys. Med. Biol. **56**(7), 2219 (2011)
13. Weber, T., et al.: Investigation of the signature of lung tissue in x-ray grating-based phase-contrast imaging. arXiv (2012)
14. Willner, M., et al.: Quantitative X-ray phase-contrast computed tomography at 82 keV. Opt. Expr. **21**(4), 4155–4166 (2013)

Some Investigations on Robustness of Deep Learning in Limited Angle Tomography

Yixing Huang[1(✉)], Tobias Würfl[1], Katharina Breininger[1], Ling Liu[1], Günter Lauritsch[2], and Andreas Maier[1,3]

[1] Friedrich-Alexander Universität Erlangen-Nürnberg, 91058 Erlangen, Germany
yixing.yh.huang@fau.de
[2] Siemens Healthcare GmbH, 91301 Forchheim, Germany
[3] Erlangen Graduate School in Advanced Optical Technologies (SAOT), 91058 Erlangen, Germany

Abstract. In computed tomography, image reconstruction from an insufficient angular range of projection data is called limited angle tomography. Due to missing data, reconstructed images suffer from artifacts, which cause boundary distortion, edge blurring, and intensity biases. Recently, deep learning methods have been applied very successfully to this problem in simulation studies. However, the robustness of neural networks for clinical applications is still a concern. It is reported that most neural networks are vulnerable to adversarial examples. In this paper, we aim to investigate whether some perturbations or noise will mislead a neural network to fail to detect an existing lesion. Our experiments demonstrate that the trained neural network, specifically the U-Net, is sensitive to Poisson noise. While the observed images appear artifact-free, anatomical structures may be located at wrong positions, e.g. the skin shifted by up to 1 cm. This kind of behavior can be reduced by retraining on data with simulated Poisson noise. However, we demonstrate that the retrained U-Net model is still susceptible to adversarial examples. We conclude the paper with suggestions towards robust deep-learning-based reconstruction.

Keywords: Deep learning · Limited angle tomography
Adversarial example

1 Introduction

In practical applications of computed tomography (CT), the gantry rotation of a CT system, particularly an angiographic C-arm device, might be restricted by other system parts or external obstacles. In this case, only limited angle data are acquired. Image reconstruction from an insufficient angular range of data is called limited angle tomography. Due to missing data, artifacts will occur, including distorted boundaries, blurred edges, and biased intensities. These artifacts may

© Springer Nature Switzerland AG 2018
A. F. Frangi et al. (Eds.): MICCAI 2018, LNCS 11070, pp. 145–153, 2018.
https://doi.org/10.1007/978-3-030-00928-1_17

lead to misinterpretation of the images. Therefore, artifact reduction in limited angle tomography has important clinical value.

Many approaches have been investigated to reduce artifacts in limited angle tomography. One approach is to restore missing data using extrapolation/interpolation methods based on the band-limitation property [10] or data consistency conditions [6]. These methods can improve the image quality of simple data, but are not suited for clinical data consisting of complex structures. Another popular approach is iterative reconstruction with total variation [1,13]. Iterative algorithms can reduce artifacts effectively, but are computationally expensive.

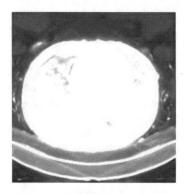

Fig. 1. The fake organ-like structures created by the U-Net, window: $[-1000, -760]$ HU.

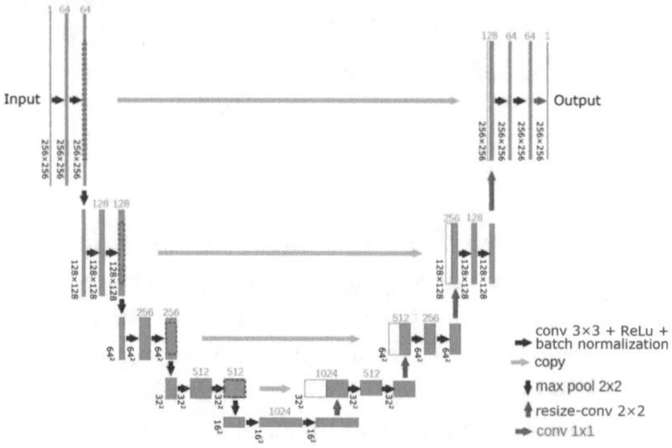

Fig. 2. The modified U-Net architecture for artifact reduction in limited angle tomography with an example of 256×256 input images (modified from [12]).

Recently, deep learning has achieved impressive success in various fields including limited angle tomography [4,5,15]. Würfl et al. [15] propose a neural network to learn the compensation weights for limited angle data based on [11]. Hammernik et al. further add a variational network to eliminate coherent streak artifacts [5]. Gu and Ye adapt the U-Net architecture [12] to learn artifacts from streaky images in the multi-scale wavelet domain [4]. Their work shows a promising prospect of the clinical application of deep learning into limited angle tomography in the near future.

However, the robustness of neural networks in practice is still a concern. It is reported that most neural networks are vulnerable to adversarial examples [16], which are typically generated by adding small perturbations [7,14]. In some cases, the perturbations are too small to be noticed by human eyes. Nevertheless, they will cause a neural network to predict entirely wrong labels. For example, robust physical adversarial examples can be generated to attack an autonomous driving system such that it misclassifies a stop sign as a speed limited sign [2].

Like autonomous driving, clinical applications of deep learning also require a high level of safety and security. In our preliminary experiments on fan-beam limited angle tomography, we observed that the U-Net occasionally creates fake organ-like structures in the background without any attacker model (Fig. 1). This motivates us to look into the robustness of deep learning. In this paper, we aim to investigate whether a trained neural network for limited angle tomography is vulnerable to perturbations. Particularly, the influence of projection-domain Poisson noise, the most common noise existing in real CT data, is investigated. Taking this a step further, we look into trained adversarial examples. We conclude the paper by giving recommendations on how to benchmark deep learning-based approaches.

2   Materials and Methods

2.1   U-Net Architecture

Based on [4,12], we adapt the popular U-Net architecture for artifact reduction in limited angle tomography, as displayed in Fig. 2. The left part is a contraction path which follows the typical architecture of a convolutional network. Each blue arrow represents a 3×3 zero-padded convolution operation, a ReLU operation, and a batch normalization operation. The right side is an expansion path. The green arrow represents an up-sampling operation where we replace the original deconvolution operation by a resize-convolution to avoid checkerboard artifacts [9]. The copy (grey arrow) operation concatenates the up-sampled features with the corresponding features from the contraction path. The last 1×1 convolution operation maps the 64-channel features to a desired output image.

For limited angle tomography, the input images are reconstructed from limited angle data while the output images are the artifact-free images. The Hounsfield scaled images (input and target) are normalized to ensure stable training. An L_2 loss function is used.

2.2   Adversarial Examples

Given a neural network classifier $\mathcal{C}$, an input image $\boldsymbol{f}$, and its true label l, an adversarial example can be described as the following,

$$\text{find } \boldsymbol{f}' \text{ s. t. } ||\boldsymbol{f}' - \boldsymbol{f}|| < \epsilon \text{ such that } \mathcal{C}(\boldsymbol{f}') = l' \text{ and } l' \neq l,$$

where $\boldsymbol{f}'$ is the adversarial example of $\boldsymbol{f}$, l' is the label of $\boldsymbol{f}'$ which is different from l, and ϵ is a parameter to control the difference between $\boldsymbol{f}$ and $\boldsymbol{f}'$. The perturbation is denoted by $\boldsymbol{e}$ where $\boldsymbol{e} = \boldsymbol{f}' - \boldsymbol{f}$. When the new label l' is specified, it is a targeted attack. Otherwise, it is a non-targeted attack.

To the best of our knowledge, adversarial examples have exclusively been reported for classification and segmentation tasks. We intend to investigate the robustness of the U-Net for limited angle tomography, which is a regression neural network. Since no discrete category labels are assigned to the outputs, the influence of a perturbation is evaluated by checking whether the U-Net is able to solve a specific task. In our case, we aim to reconstruct an existing lesion.

We pick a reference image, denoted by f_{ref}. An image reconstructed from its limited angle projection data is denoted by $f_{limited}$. The U-Net predicts an estimation of f_{ref} from $f_{limited}$. The predicted image is denoted by f_{est}. To check the robustness of the U-Net to perturbations, a simulated lesion is added to the reference image. The new reference image is denoted by $f_{ref,L}$ where L is short for "lesion". Its limited angle reconstruction image and the predicted image by the U-Net are denoted by $f_{limited,L}$ and $f_{est,L}$, respectively.

Non-targeted Attack: For non-targeted attacks, the fast gradient sign (FGS) method [7] is the most popular method to generate adversarial examples. However, the perturbations found by the FGS are like "salt-and-pepper" noise, which we do not expect to appear in real CT data. Instead, the most common noise in CT is Poisson noise. Therefore, it is worthwhile to investigate the influence of Poisson noise as the perturbation.

Targeted Attack: For a targeted attack, we try to find a certain perturbation that misleads the U-Net to predict a target image where the lesion is missing. As the target, we use the estimated image without the lesion f_{est}. The perturbation can be generated by the following optimization problem,

$$\arg\min_e J(e) = \arg\min_e ||w_1 \cdot \left(\mathcal{U}(f_{limited,\,L} + e) - f_{est}\right)||_2^2 + \lambda ||w_2 \cdot e||_2^2, \quad (1)$$

where $J(e)$ is the objective function to minimize, $\mathcal{U}$ is the trained U-Net model, w_1 and w_2 are weight vectors which have large weight elements at the lesion area, and λ is a relaxation parameter for the L_2 regularizer. The purpose of w_1 is to penalize the error at the lesion area more than other areas. w_2 further constrains the magnitude of e at the lesion area, otherwise the optimization may result in removing the lesion in the input image. The iterative least-likely class method in [7] is adapted to solve the above optimization problem:

$$e_0 = 0, \qquad e_{i+1} = e_i - \alpha\nabla_e J(e_i), \quad (2)$$

where e_i is an approximation of e at the i-th iteration, $\nabla_e J(e_i)$ is the gradient of $J(e_i)$ w.r.t. the perturbation e and is obtained by back-propagation, and α is the step size for the update.

2.3   Experimental Setup

Experiment (Exp.) 1: In the first experiment, we evaluate the U-Net on lesion detection in cone-beam limited angle tomography without any perturbation as commonly performed in deep learning CT papers. We pick 17 patients from the AAPM Low-Dose CT Grand Challenge data for training and one patient for testing. The limited angle projections are simulated in a 120° angular range scan with an angular step of 1°. The source-to-isocenter distance is 600 mm and the source-to-detector distance is 1200 mm. The detector size is 620 × 480 with an isotropic element size 1.0 mm. Images are reconstructed using FDK with the Ram-Lak kernel from the limited angle projections. The size of the reconstructed images is $256 \times 256 \times 256$ with a pixel size of $1.25\,\mathrm{mm}$, $1.25\,\mathrm{mm}$, and $1\,\mathrm{mm}$ in the X, Y, and Z direction, respectively. For each patient we pick 13 slices from its reconstructed volume. As a result, 221 slices are used as training set. The slices have a distance of $2\,\mathrm{cm}$ in depth between neighbouring slices. Although different slices have different cone angles, the artifacts are mainly caused by the limitation in the scan angle. Therefore, we train on slices instead of volumes.

The U-Net is trained on the above noise-free data using the Adam optimizer. The learning rate is 10^{-3} for the first 100 epochs, 10^{-4} for the $101-130_{\mathrm{th}}$ epochs, and 10^{-5} for the $131-150_{\mathrm{th}}$ epochs. The L_2-norm is applied to regularize the network weights. The regularization parameter is 10^{-4}.

A simulated lesion cylinder is added to the ground truth testing volume. The lesion has a radius of $3\,\mathrm{mm}$ and a contrast of $200\,\mathrm{HU}$. The volume with the lesion is forward projected and reconstructed from its limited angle data. For our lesion attack, we investigate a slice which is $13\,\mathrm{cm}$ away from the center plane for evaluation.

Exp. 2: For the non-targeted attack, Poisson noise is simulated considering an initial exposure of 10^5 photons at each detector pixel before attenuation. A linear attenuation coefficient of $0.02/\mathrm{mm}$ is chosen as $0\,\mathrm{HU}$. Poisson noise is added to the testing volume. The U-Net trained either without or with Poisson noise is evaluated on the selected noisy testing slice.

Exp. 3: For the targeted attack, the weight vectors are set $\boldsymbol{w}_1 = \boldsymbol{w}_2$ in Eq. (1) with a value of 100 at a 15×15 patch (cf. Fig. 5) covering the lesion and a value of 1 for other areas. The L_2 regularizer parameter λ is set to 10. The step size α in Eq. (2) is set to 10^{-3}. 32 iterations are used for the perturbation.

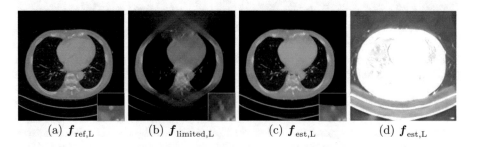

(a) $\boldsymbol{f}_{\mathrm{ref,L}}$ (b) $\boldsymbol{f}_{\mathrm{limited,L}}$ (c) $\boldsymbol{f}_{\mathrm{est,L}}$ (d) $\boldsymbol{f}_{\mathrm{est,L}}$

Fig. 3. The result of lesion detection from $120°$ cone-beam limited angle reconstruction, perturbation/noise-free, window: $[-1000, 1000]\,\mathrm{HU}$. The lesion position is marked by the red arrow and the mispredicted cavity is marked by the blue arrow. A region-of-interest (ROI) at the lesion area is shown at the right bottom corner with a window width of $1000\,\mathrm{HU}$. $\boldsymbol{f}_{\mathrm{est,L}}$ in (c) is re-displayed at a narrow window $[-1000, -760]\,\mathrm{HU}$ in (d).

3   Results and Discussion

Exp. 1: The results of the lesion detection in the perturbation free case are displayed in Fig. 3. Figure 3(b) shows that the limited angle reconstruction $\boldsymbol{f}_{\text{limited,L}}$ suffers from severe artifacts. The body outline is highly distorted at the top and bottom parts. The heart is obscured by streak artifacts. Many vessels in the lung are missing. The lesion (marked by the red arrow) is located at a position where many artifacts appear. $\boldsymbol{f}_{\text{est,L}}$, the estimation of $\boldsymbol{f}_{\text{ref,L}}$ predicted by the U-Net trained from the noise-free data, is shown in Fig. 3(c). The body outline is well restored. Most streaks at the heart are reduced. In addition, most vessel structures in the lung are also recovered. Importantly, the lesion can be clearly seen. These observations indicate a promising prospect of the clinical application of deep learning in the near future.

In contrast to the preliminary fan-beam experiment from Fig. 1, fake organ-like structures are not observed, as shown in Fig. 3(d). However, still not all structures predicted by the U-Net are reliable. For example, the U-Net mispredicts a cavity structure in $\boldsymbol{f}_{\text{est,L}}$, marked by the blue arrow in Fig. 3(c), since this area has a low intensity in $\boldsymbol{f}_{\text{limited,L}}$.

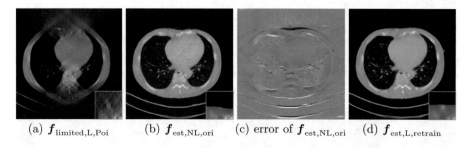

(a) $\boldsymbol{f}_{\text{limited,L,Poi}}$ (b) $\boldsymbol{f}_{\text{est,NL,ori}}$ (c) error of $\boldsymbol{f}_{\text{est,NL,ori}}$ (d) $\boldsymbol{f}_{\text{est,L,retrain}}$

Fig. 4. The influence of Poisson noise in lesion detection: (a) is the reconstruction from the 120° limited angle sinogram with Poisson noise; (b) is the prediction of (a) by the original U-Net model, where the lesion cannot be detected; (c) is the difference image between (b) and the reference image $\boldsymbol{f}_{\text{ref,L}}$ with a window width of 2000 HU; (d) is the prediction of (a) by a retrained U-Net model from the data with Poisson noise, where the lesion is detected again. The lesion position is marked by the red arrow and the "cavity" area is marked by the blue arrow. The window for (a), (b), and (d) is [−1000, 1000] HU and the ROIs have a window width of 1000 HU.

Exp. 2: The influence of projection-domain Poisson noise is shown in Fig. 4. Figure 4(a) is a reconstruction from the 120° limited angle sinogram with Poisson noise, denoted by $\boldsymbol{f}_{\text{limited,L,Poi}}$. Figure 4(b) is an estimation of $\boldsymbol{f}_{\text{ref,L}}$ from $\boldsymbol{f}_{\text{limited,L,Poi}}$ using the original trained U-Net model, denoted by $\boldsymbol{f}_{\text{est,NL,ori}}$. Because of the Poisson noise, the lesion is hardly seen at $\boldsymbol{f}_{\text{est,NL,ori}}$. Although the patient top surface looks realistic, it is severely incorrect, shifting by up to 1 cm. The surface shift area is clearly indicated by the arrow at the difference image between $\boldsymbol{f}_{\text{est,NL,ori}}$ and $\boldsymbol{f}_{\text{ref,L}}$ displayed in Fig. 4(c). These observations demonstrate that the U-Net is sensitive to Poisson noise. In order to make the model robust to Poisson noise, we retrain the U-Net using the data with Poisson noise. The prediction of $\boldsymbol{f}_{\text{limited,L,Poi}}$ using the retrained model, denoted by $\boldsymbol{f}_{\text{est,L,retrain}}$, is shown in Fig. 4(d). The lesion is detected again, although it is smoothed. Interestingly, the "cavity" area marked by the blue arrow in Fig. 4 is predicted well by both U-Nets trained with and without Poisson noise.

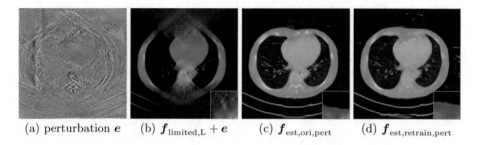

(a) perturbation $\boldsymbol{e}$ (b) $\boldsymbol{f}_{\text{limited,L}} + \boldsymbol{e}$ (c) $\boldsymbol{f}_{\text{est,ori,pert}}$ (d) $\boldsymbol{f}_{\text{est,retrain,pert}}$

Fig. 5. The results of the targeted attack: (a) is the found perturbation $\boldsymbol{e}$; (b) is the adversarial example—the 120° limited angle reconstruction with the perturbation; (c) is the prediction of the adversarial example by the original U-Net model; (d) is the prediction of the adversarial example by the retrained U-Net model with Poisson noise. The patch covering the lesion position is marked by the red box. (a) is displayed at a window width of 200 HU, the window for (b)–(d) is $[-1000, 1000]$ HU, and the ROIs have a window width of 1000 HU.

Exp. 3: The results of the targeted attack are displayed in Fig. 5. Figure 5(a) is the found perturbation which has small magnitude at the marked patch due to weight $\boldsymbol{w}_2$. The limited angle reconstruction with the perturbation is shown in Fig. 5(b). We can still notice the existence of the lesion, and to some extend the perturbation outside the patch. However, the lesion disappears at the predicted image by the original U-Net model (denoted by $\boldsymbol{f}_{\text{est,ori,pert}}$ in Fig. 5(c)). The U-Net retrained with Poisson noise also fails to reconstruct the lesion at the predicted image (denoted by $\boldsymbol{f}_{\text{est,retrain,pert}}$ in Fig. 5(d)).

The nonlinearity and the linear behavior of high-dimensional spaces are the potential causes of adversarial examples [3]. They allow some tiny perturbations or noise to change the outputs of the U-Net drastically. The U-Net has a large perceptive field due to the contraction and expansion path. Therefore, although the perturbation has very small magnitude elements inside the lesion patch, its elements outside the patch still have an influence on the predicted values inside the patch through convolutional layers and make the lesion vanish.

4 Conclusion

In this paper, we investigate the application of the U-Net to limited angle tomography. The U-Net is able to reduce most artifacts. In the predicted image, distorted body outlines are restored, biased intensities are corrected, and missing vessels in the lung come back. The experiments on the robustness of the U-Net to perturbations indicate that training with projection-domain Poisson noise is mandatory for a limited angle reconstruction neural network. However, the retrained neural network is still vulnerable to non-local adversarial examples, despite its resistance to Poisson noise. We believe that the appearance of such adversarial examples in real clinical applications is unlikely, yet their non-localness has to be discussed.

Based on the presented experiments, we suggest that the following recommendations on how to benchmark deep learning CT (DLCT) algorithms should be followed. (1) **DLCT algorithms need to be exposed to accurate physical modelling and evaluated on real measured data.** Evaluation on synthetic data only delivers overly optimistic results. (2) Due to the dependency on training data, we believe that **many DLCT algorithms will be tailored towards specific applications** and not suited for generic image reconstruction. Claims of generality cannot be based on evaluation using a finite dataset. The inclusion of known operators can potentially remedy these problems [8]. (3) DLCT reconstructions appear visually artifact-free. This prevents differentiation between the true signal and image completion solely based on prior knowledge. We demonstrate this quite drastically in our results that produce realistically looking patient surfaces that move by up to 1 cm, simply because the necessary data in the area was not measured. Still these reconstructions may be superior for a specific clinical task. As such **DLCT algorithms must be evaluated task-based**. (4) Additional exploration of **adversarial examples** might be useful to **explore limits of the trained algorithms**. As long as such effects are not sufficiently studied, deep learning-based reconstruction techniques are not yet ready for clinical applications.

Disclaimer: The concepts and information presented in this paper are based on research and are not commercially available.

References

1. Chen, Z., Jin, X., Li, L., Wang, G.: A limited-angle CT reconstruction method based on anisotropic TV minimization. Phys. Med. Biol. **58**(7), 2119–2141 (2013)
2. Evtimov, I., et al.: Robust physical-world attacks on deep learning models. arXiv preprint 1 (2017)
3. Goodfellow, I.J., Shlens, J., Szegedy, C.: Explaining and harnessing adversarial examples. arXiv preprint (2014)
4. Gu, J., Ye, J.C.: Multi-scale wavelet domain residual learning for limited-angle CT reconstruction. In: Proceedings of Fully3D, pp. 443–447 (2017)
5. Hammernik, K., Würfl, T., Pock, T., Maier, A.: A deep learning architecture for limited-angle computed tomography reconstruction. In: Maier-Hein, K.H., Deserno, T.M., Handels, H., Tolxdorff, T. (eds.) Bildverarbeitung für die Medizin 2017. Informatik aktuell, pp. 92–97. Springer, Heidelberg (2017). https://doi.org/10.1007/978-3-662-54345-0_25

6. Huang, Y., et al.: Restoration of missing data in limited angle tomography based on Helgason-Ludwig consistency conditions. Biomed. Phys. Eng. Express **3**(3), 035015 (2017)
7. Kurakin, A., Goodfellow, I., Bengio, S.: Adversarial examples in the physical world. arXiv preprint (2016)
8. Maier, A., et al.: Precision learning: towards use of known operators in neural networks. In: International Conference on Pattern Recognition (2018, to appear). https://arxiv.org/abs/1712.00374
9. Odena, A., Dumoulin, V., Olah, C.: Deconvolution and checkerboard artifacts. Distill **1**(10), e3 (2016)
10. Qu, G.R., Lan, Y.S., Jiang, M.: An iterative algorithm for angle-limited three-dimensional image reconstruction. Acta Math. Appl. Sin. Engl. Ser. **24**(1), 157–166 (2008)
11. Riess, C., Berger, M., Wu, H., Manhart, M., Fahrig, R., Maier, A.: TV or not TV? That is the question. In: Proceedings of Fully3D, pp. 341–344 (2013)
12. Ronneberger, O., Fischer, P., Brox, T.: U-Net: convolutional networks for biomedical image segmentation. In: Navab, N., Hornegger, J., Wells, W.M., Frangi, A.F. (eds.) MICCAI 2015. LNCS, vol. 9351, pp. 234–241. Springer, Cham (2015). https://doi.org/10.1007/978-3-319-24574-4_28
13. Sidky, E., Pan, X.: Image reconstruction in circular cone-beam computed tomography by constrained, total-variation minimization. Phys. Med. Biol. **53**(17), 4777–4807 (2008)
14. Szegedy, C., et al.: Intriguing properties of neural networks. arXiv preprint (2013)
15. Würfl, T., et al.: Deep learning computed tomography: learning projection-domain weights from image domain in limited angle problems. IEEE Trans. Med. Imaging **37**(6), 1454–1463 (2018)
16. Yuan, X., He, P., Zhu, Q., Bhat, R.R., Li, X.: Adversarial examples: attacks and defenses for deep learning. arXiv preprint (2017)

Adversarial Sparse-View CBCT Artifact Reduction

Haofu Liao[1]([⊠]), Zhimin Huo[1], William J. Sehnert[2], Shaohua Kevin Zhou[3],
and Jiebo Luo[1]

[1] Department of Computer Science, University of Rochester,
Rochester, USA
`hliao6@cs.rochester.edu`
[2] Carestream Health Inc., Rochester, USA
[3] Institute of Computing Technology, Chinese Academy of Sciences, Beijing, China

Abstract. We present an effective post-processing method to reduce
the artifacts from sparsely reconstructed cone-beam CT (CBCT) images.
The proposed method is based on the state-of-the-art, image-to-image
generative models with a perceptual loss as regulation. Unlike the traditional CT artifact-reduction approaches, our method is trained in an
adversarial fashion that yields more perceptually realistic outputs while
preserving the anatomical structures. To address the streak artifacts that
are inherently local and appear across various scales, we further propose a
novel discriminator architecture based on feature pyramid networks and
a differentially modulated focus map to induce the adversarial training.
Our experimental results show that the proposed method can greatly correct the cone-beam artifacts from clinical CBCT images reconstructed
using 1/3 projections, and outperforms strong baseline methods both
quantitatively and qualitatively.

1   Introduction

Cone-beam computed tomography (CBCT) is a variant type of computed tomography (CT). Compared with conventional CT, CBCT usually has shorter examination time, resulting in fewer motion artifacts and better X-ray tube efficiency.
One way to further shorten the acquisition time and enhance the healthcare experience is to take fewer X-ray measurements during each CBCT scan. However,
due to the "cone-beam" projection geometry, CBCT images typically contain
more pronounced streak artifacts than CT images and this is even worse when
fewer X-ray projections are used during the CBCT reconstruction [1].

A number of approaches have been proposed to address the artifacts [8,13]
that are commonly encountered in CBCT images. However, to our best knowledge, no scheme has been proposed to correct the cone-beam artifacts introduced
by sparse-view CBCT reconstruction in a post-processing step. Instead of reducing artifacts from the CBCT images directly, many other systems [11,14] propose
to introduce better sparse-view reconstruction methods that yield less artifacts.
Although encouraging improvements have been made, the image quality from the

© Springer Nature Switzerland AG 2018
A. F. Frangi et al. (Eds.): MICCAI 2018, LNCS 11070, pp. 154–162, 2018.
https://doi.org/10.1007/978-3-030-00928-1_18

current solutions are still not satisfactory when only a small number of views are used. This work attempts to fill this gap by refining the sparsely reconstructed CBCT images through a novel cone-beam artifact reduction method.

In relation to this study, there are many works that leverage deep neural networks (DNNs) for low-dose CT (LDCT) denoising. [2] used a residual encoder-decoder architecture to reduce the noise from LDCT images, and achieved superior performance over traditional approaches. More recently, [10] introduced generative adversarial networks (GANs) [3] into their architecture to obtain more realistic outputs, and this work was further improved by [12] where a combination of perceptual loss [5] and adversarial loss was used.

Similarly, this work also proposes to use DNNs for sparse-view CBCT artifact reduction. We train an image-to-image generative model with perceptual loss to obtain outputs that are perceptually close to the dense-view CBCT images. To address the artifacts at various levels, we further contribute to the literature with a novel discriminator architecture based on feature pyramid networks (FPN) [6] and a differentially modulated focus map so that the adversarial training is biased to the artifacts at multiple scales. The proposed approach is evaluated on clinical CBCT images. Experimental results demonstrate that our method outperforms strong baseline methods both qualitatively and quantitatively.

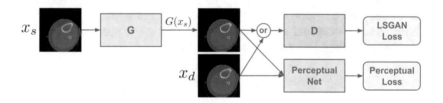

Fig. 1. The overall architecture of the proposed method.

2   Methods

Let x_s be a sparse-view CBCT image, which is reconstructed from a sparse set or low number of projections (or views), and x_d be its dense-view counterpart, which is reconstructed from a dense set or a high number of projections (or views). The proposed method is formulated under an image-to-image generative model as illustrated in Fig. 1 where we train a generator that transforms x_s to an ideally artifact-free image that looks like x_d. The discriminator is used for the adversarial training, and the perceptual network is included for additional perceptual and structural regularization. We use LSGAN [7] against a regular GAN to achieve more stable adversarial learning. The adversarial objective functions for the proposed model can be written as

$$\min_D \mathcal{L}_A(D; G, \Lambda) = \mathbb{E}_{\mathbf{X}_d}[\|\Lambda \odot (D(x_d) - \mathbf{1})\|^2] + \mathbb{E}_{\mathbf{X}_s}[\|\Lambda \odot D(G(x_s))\|^2], \quad (1)$$

$$\min_G \mathcal{L}_A(G; D, \Lambda) = \mathbb{E}_{\mathbf{X}_s}[\|\Lambda \odot (D(G(x_s)) - \mathbf{1})\|^2], \quad (2)$$

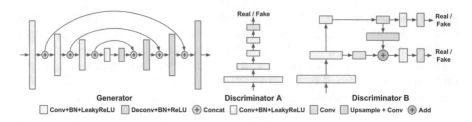

Fig. 2. Detailed network structure of the generator and discriminator.

where Λ is a focus map detailed in Sect. 2.2. Here, we apply a PatchGAN-like [4] design to the discriminator so that the realness is patch based and the output is a score map. The generator G and discriminator D are trained in an adversarial fashion. D distinguishes between x_d and the generated CBCT image $G(x_s)$ (Eq. 1), while G generates CBCT image samples as "real" as possible so that D cannot tell if they are dense-view CBCT images or generated by G (Eq. 2).

Training with the adversarial loss, alone, usually introduces additional artifacts, and previous works often use MSE loss to induce the learning [10]. However, as shown by [12], MSE loss does not handle streak artifacts very well. Therefore, we adopt the choice of [12] by using a perceptual loss to induce the learning and give more realistic outputs. Let $\phi^{(i)}(\cdot)$ denote the feature maps extracted by the i-th layer of the perceptual network ϕ and N_i denote the number of elements in $\phi^{(i)}(\cdot)$, the perceptual loss can be computed by

$$\mathcal{L}_P = \frac{1}{N_i}\|\phi^{(i)}(x_d) - \phi^{(i)}(G(x_s))\|_1. \tag{3}$$

In this work, the perceptual network ϕ is a pretrained VGG16 net [9] and we empirically find that $i = 8$ works well.

2.1   Network Structure

The generator is based on an encoder-decoder architecture [4]. As shown in Fig. 2, the generator has four encoding blocks (in gray) and four decoding blocks (in blue). Each encoding block contains a convolutional layer followed by a batch normalization layer and a leaky ReLU layer. Similarly, each decoding block contains a deconvolutional layer followed by a batch normalization layer and a ReLU layer. Both the convolutional and deconvolutional layers have a 4 × 4 kernel with a stride of 2 so that they can downsample and upsample the outputs, respectively. Outputs from the encoding blocks are shuttled to the corresponding decoding blocks using skip connections. This design allows the low-level context information from the encoding blocks to be used directly together with the decoded high-level information during generation.

A typical discriminator (Fig. 2 Discriminator A) usually contains a set of encoding blocks followed by a classifier to determine the input's realness. In this case, the discrimination is performed at a fixed granularity that is fine when the task is a generative task such as style transfer or image translation, or there is a systematic error to be corrected such as JPEG decompression or super-resolution. For sparse-view CBCT images, the artifacts appear randomly with different scales. To capture such a variation of artifacts, we propose a discriminator that handles the adversarial training at different granularities.

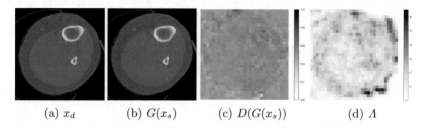

(a) x_d (b) $G(x_s)$ (c) $D(G(x_s))$ (d) Λ

Fig. 3. Saturated (c) score map $D(G(x_s))$ and (d) focus map Λ computed between (a) dense-view CBCT image x_d and (b) generated CBCT image $G(x_s)$.

The core idea is to create a feature pyramid and perform discrimination at multiple scales. As illustrated in Fig. 2 Discriminator B, the network uses two outputs and makes decisions based on different levels of semantic feature maps. We adapt the design from FPN [6] so that the feature pyramid has strong semantics at all scales. Specifically, we first use three encoding blocks to extract features at different levels. Next, we use an upsample block (in purple) to incorporate the stronger semantic features from the top layer into the outputs of the middle layer. The upsample block consists of a unsampling layer and a 3×3 convolutional layer (to smooth the outputs). Because the feature maps from the encoding blocks have different channel sizes, we place a lateral block (in green, essentially a 1×1 convolutional layer) after each encoding block to match this channel difference. In the end, there are two classifiers to make joint decisions on the semantics at different scales. Each classifier contains two blocks. The first block (in yellow) has the same layers as an encoding block, except that the convolutional layer has a 3×3 kernel with a stride of 1. The second block (in green) is simply a 1×1 convolutional layer with stride 1. Let $D_1(x)$ and $D_2(x)$ denote the outputs from the two classifiers, then the new adversarial loss can be given by $\min_D \mathcal{L}_A(D; G, \Lambda_1, \Lambda_2) = \sum_{i=1}^2 \mathcal{L}_A(D_i; G, \Lambda_i)$ and $\min_G \mathcal{L}_A(G; D, \Lambda_1, \Lambda_2) = \sum_{i=1}^2 \mathcal{L}_A(G; D_i, \Lambda_i)$. We also experimented with deeper discriminators with more classifiers for richer feature semantics, but found that they contribute only minor improvements over the current setting.

2.2   Focus Map

When an image from the generator looks mostly "real" (Fig. 3(b)), the score map (Fig. 3(c)) output by the discriminator will be overwhelmed by borderline scores (those values close to 0.5). This saturates the adversarial training as borderline scores make little contribution to the weight update of the discriminator. To address this problem, we propose to introduce a modulation factor to the adversarial loss so that the borderline scores are down-weighted during training. Observing that when a generated region is visually close to the corresponding region of a dense-view image (Fig. 3(a)), it is more likely to be "real" and causes the discriminator to give a borderline score. Therefore, we use a feature difference map (Fig. 3(d)) to perform this modulation.

Let $\phi_{m,n}^{(j)}(\cdot)$ denote the (m,n)-th feature vector of $\phi^{(j)}(\cdot)$, then the (m,n)-th element of the feature difference map Λ between x_d and $G(x_s)$ is defined as

$$\lambda_{m,n} = \frac{1}{Z_j} \|\phi_{m,n}^{(j)}(x_d) - \phi_{m,n}^{(j)}(G(x_s))\|, \tag{4}$$

where Z_j is a normalization term given by

$$Z_j = \frac{1}{N_j} \sum_{m,n} \|\phi_{m,n}^{(j)}(x_d) - \phi_{m,n}^{(j)}(G(x_s))\|. \tag{5}$$

We use the same perceptual network ϕ as the one used for computing the perceptual loss, and j is chosen to match the resolution of $D_1(x)$ and $D_2(x)$. For the VGG16 net, we use $j = 16$ for Λ_1 and $j = 9$ for Λ_2.

3   Experiments

Datasets. The CBCT images were obtained by a multi-source CBCT scanner dedicated for lower extremities. In total, knee images from 27 subjects are under investigation. Each subject is associated with a sparse-view image and a dense-view image that are reconstructed using 67 and 200 projection views, respectively. Each image is processed, slice by slice, along the sagittal direction where the streak artifacts are most pronounced. During the training, the inputs to the models are 256×256 patches that randomly cropped from the slices.

Models. Three variants of the proposed methods as well as two other baseline methods are compared: (i) Baseline-MSE: a similar approach to [10] by combining MSE loss with GAN. 3D UNet[1] and LSGAN is used for fair comparison; (ii) Baseline-Perceptual: a similar approach to [12] by combining perceptual loss with GAN. It is also based on our UNet and LSGAN infrastructure for fair comparison; (iii) Ours-FPN: our method using FPN as the discriminator and setting $\Lambda_1 = \Lambda_2 = \mathbf{1}$; (iv) Ours-Focus: our method using focus map and conventional discriminator (Fig. 2 Discriminator A); (v) Ours-Focus+FPN: our method using focus map as well as the FPN discriminator. We train all the models using Adam optimization with the learning rate $lr = 10^{-4}$ and $\beta_1 = 0.5$. We use $\lambda_a = 1.0$, $\lambda_m = 100$, and $\lambda_p = 10$ to control the weights between the adversarial loss, the

---

[1] Identical to the 2D UNet used in this work with all the 2D convolutional and deconvolutional layers replaced by their 3D counterparts.

MSE loss, and the perceptual loss. The values are chosen empirically and are the same for all models (if applicable). All the models are trained for 50 epochs with 5-fold cross-validation. We perform all the experiments on an Nvidia GeForce GTX 1070 GPU. During testing, the average processing time on $384 \times \times 384 \times 417$ CBCT volumes for the 2D UNet (generator of model (ii)$-$(v)) is 16.05 s, and for the 3D UNet (generator of model (i)) is 22.70 s.

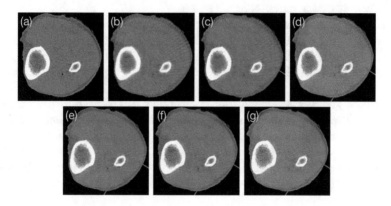

Fig. 4. Qualitative sparse-view CBCT artifact reduction results by different models. The same brightness and contrast enhancement are applied to the images for better and uniform visualization. (a) x_d (b) x_s (c) Baseline-MSE (d) Baseline-Perceptual (e) Ours-Focus (f) Ours-FPN (g) Ours-Focus+FPN

Experimental Results. Figure 4 shows the qualitative results of the models. Although the baseline methods overall have some improvements over the sparse-view image, they still cannot handle the streak artifacts very well. "Baseline-Perceptual" produces less pronounced artifacts than "Baseline-MSE", which demonstrates that using perceptual loss and processing the images slice by slice in 2D give better results than MSE loss with 3D generator. Our models (Fig. 4(e$-$f)) in general produce less artifacts than the baseline models. We can barely see the streak artifacts. They generally produce similar outputs and the result from "Ours-Focus+FPN" is slightly better than"Ours-FPN" and "Ours-Focus". This means that using FPN as the discriminator or applying a modulation factor to the adversarial loss can indeed induce the training to artifacts reduction.

We further investigate the image characteristics of each model in a region of interest (ROI). A good model should have similar image characteristics to the dense-view images in ROIs. When looking at the pixel-wise difference between the dense-view ROI and the model ROI, no structure information should be observed, resulting a random noise map. Figure 5(a) shows the ROI differences of the models. We can see a clear bone structure from the ROI difference map between x_s and x_d (Fig. 5(a) third row), which demonstrates a significant difference in image characteristics between these two images. For "Baseline-MSE", the bone structure is less recognizable, showing more similar image characteristics. For "Baseline-Perceptual" and our models, we can hardly see the structural information and mostly observe random noises. This indicates that these models have very similar image characteristics to a dense-view image. We also measure the mean and standard deviation of the pixel values within the ROI. We can see that our models have very close statistics with x_d, especially the pixel value statistics of "Ours-Focus" and "Ours-Focus+FPN" are almost identical to x_d, demonstrating better image characteristics.

We then evaluate the models quantitatively by comparing their outputs with the corresponding dense-view CBCT image. Three evaluation metrics are used: structural similarity (SSIM), peak signal-to-noise ratio (PSNR), and root mean square error (RMSE). Higher values for SSIM and PSNR and lower values for RMSE indicate better performance. We can see from Table 1 that the baseline methods give better scores than x_s. Similar to the case in the qualitative evaluation, "Baseline-Perceptual" performs better than "Baseline-MSE". Our methods consistently outperform the baseline methods by a significant margin. "Ours-FPN" gives best performance in PSNR and RMSE. However, PSNR and RMSE only measure the pixel level difference between two images. To measure the performance in perceived similarity, SSIM is usually a better choice, and we

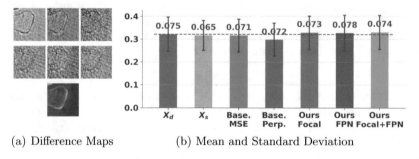

(a) Difference Maps   (b) Mean and Standard Deviation

Fig. 5. ROI characteristics. (a) Patches are obtained by subtracting the corresponding ROI from x_d (third row). First row from left to right: x_s, baseline-MSE, baseline-perceptual. Second row from left to right: Ours-Focus, Ours-FPN, Ours-Focus+FPN. (b) Each bar indicates the mean value of the ROI. The numbers on the top of each bar indicate the standard deviations. The vertical lines indicates the changes of the mean value when ± standard deviations is applied. Pixel values are normalized to [0, 1].

Table 1. Quantitative sparse-view CBCT artifact reduction results of different models.

	x_s	Baseline		Ours		
		MSE	Perc.	Focus	FPN	FPN+Focus
SSIM	0.839	0.849	0.858	0.879	0.871	**0.884**
PSNR (dB)	34.07	34.24	35.39	36.26	**36.38**	36.14
RMSE ($\mathbf{10^{-2}}$)	1.98	1.96	1.70	1.54	**1.52**	1.56

find "Ours-FPN+Focus" has a slightly better performance on this metric. This confirms our observation in qualitative evaluation.

4   Conclusion

We have presented a novel approach to reducing artifacts from sparsely-reconstructed CBCT images. To our best knowledge, this is the first work that addresses artifacts introduced by sparse-view CBCT reconstruction in a post-processing step. We target this problem using an image-to-image generative model with a perceptual loss as regulation. The model generates perceptually realistic outputs while making the artifacts less pronounced. To further suppress the streak artifacts, we have also proposed a novel FPN based discriminator and a focus map to induce the adversarial training. Experimental results show that the proposed mechanism addresses the streak artifacts much better, and the proposed models outperform strong baseline methods both qualitatively and quantitatively.

Acknowledgement. The work presented here was supported in part by New York State through the Goergen Institute for Data Science at the University of Rochester and the corporate sponsor Carestream Health Inc.

References

1. Bian, J., et al.: Evaluation of sparse-view reconstruction from flat-panel-detector cone-beam CT. Phys. Med. Biol. **55**(22), 6575 (2010)
2. Chen, H., et al.: Low-dose CT with a residual encoder-decoder convolutional neural network. IEEE Trans. Med. Imaging **36**(12), 2524–2535 (2017)
3. Goodfellow, I., et al.: Generative adversarial nets. In: Advances in Neural Information Processing Systems, pp. 2672–2680 (2014)
4. Isola, P., Zhu, J.Y., Zhou, T., Efros, A.A.: Image-to-image translation with conditional adversarial networks. arXiv preprint arXiv:1611.07004 (2016)
5. Johnson, J., Alahi, A., Fei-Fei, L.: Perceptual losses for real-time style transfer and super-resolution. arXiv preprint arXiv:1603.08155 (2016)
6. Lin, T.Y., Dollár, P., Girshick, R., He, K., Hariharan, B., Belongie, S.: Feature pyramid networks for object detection. arXiv preprint arXiv:1612.03144 (2016)
7. Mao, X., Li, Q., Xie, H., Lau, R.Y., Wang, Z., Smolley, S.P.: Least squares generative adversarial networks. arXiv preprint arXiv:1611.04076 (2016)
8. Ning, R., Tang, X., Conover, D.: X-ray scatter correction algorithm for cone beam CT imaging. Med. Phys. **31**(5), 1195–1202 (2004)
9. Simonyan, K., Zisserman, A.: Very deep convolutional networks for large-scale image recognition. arXiv preprint arXiv:1409.1556 (2014)
10. Wolterink, J.M., Leiner, T., Viergever, M.A., Išgum, I.: Generative adversarial networks for noise reduction in low-dose CT. IEEE TMI **36**(12), 2536–2545 (2017)
11. Xia, D., et al.: Optimization-based image reconstruction with artifact reduction in C-arm CBCT. Phys. Med. Biol. **61**(20), 7300 (2016)

12. Yang, Q., et al.: Low dose CT image denoising using a generative adversarial network with Wasserstein distance and perceptual loss. arXiv preprint arXiv:1708.00961 (2017)
13. Zhang, Y., Zhang, L., Zhu, X.R., Lee, A.K., Chambers, M., Dong, L.: Reducing metal artifacts in cone-beam CT images by preprocessing projection data. Int. J. Radiat. Oncol. Biol. Phys. **67**(3), 924–932 (2007)
14. Zhang, Z., Han, X., Pearson, E., Pelizzari, C., Sidky, E.Y., Pan, X.: Artifact reduction in short-scan CBCT by use of optimization-based reconstruction. Phys. Med. Biol. **61**(9), 3387 (2016)

Nasal Mesh Unfolding – An Approach to Obtaining 2-D Skin Templates from 3-D Nose Models

Hongying Li[1]([✉]), Marc Robini[2], Zhongwei Zhou[3], Wei Tang[4], and Yuemin Zhu[2]

[1] College of Computer Science, Sichuan University, Chengdu 610065, China
hli@scu.edu.cn
[2] CREATIS (CNRS UMR 5220, Inserm U1206), INSA Lyon,
69621 Villeurbanne Cedex, France
[3] Department of Oral and Maxillofacial Surgery, General Hospital of Ningxia
Medical University, Ningxia 750004, China
[4] West China College of Stomatology, Sichuan University, Chengdu 610065, China
mydrtw@vip.sina.com

Abstract. Nasal reconstruction requires a 2-D template representing the skin area to be taken from the donor site of the patient. We propose a new framework for template design, called *nasal mesh unfolding*, to obtain 2-D skin templates from 3-D nose models. The proposed nasal mesh unfolding framework takes as input a target digital nose model represented by a 3-D triangle mesh and unfolds the nasal mesh under structure constraints using semidefinite programming. The solution of the unfolding problem is in the form of a Gram matrix from which the 2-D representation of the 3-D model, or *embedding*, is extracted. The embedding defines a digital template representing the skin requirement for nasal reconstruction, which can in turn be used to produce a physical 2-D template to apply on the donor site for guiding skin incision. Experiments on synthetic data demonstrate the effectiveness of the proposed unfolding approach, and results on real data show the feasibility of generating physical 2-D skin templates from 3-D nose meshes. The proposed approach efficiently converts 3-D nose models to digital 2-D skin templates for fast easy and accurate preparation of physical templates and can be useful for other plastic surgery tasks.

1 Introduction

Nasal reconstruction aims to restore aesthetics while preserving function. It is a challenging task due to the complexity of nasal anatomy. The nasal cover is of varying thickness and has contours with intersecting concavities and convexities [1]. Its reconstruction requires defining the target nose dimensions and estimating the corresponding skin requirement.

Sultan and Byrne worked with certified anaplastologists and proposed to define target nose dimensions physically by sculpting a wax model according to

© Springer Nature Switzerland AG 2018
A. F. Frangi et al. (Eds.): MICCAI 2018, LNCS 11070, pp. 163–170, 2018.
https://doi.org/10.1007/978-3-030-00928-1_19

patients' expectations [2,3]. Hierl *et al.* [4] defined a 3-D nose shape digitally by an accepted virtual surgery result. When a physical model is available, its shape can be transformed to a 2-D skin template by molding a piece of foil over the model and then by flattening the foil back [3]. Aquaplast can be employed similarly instead of foil, and the resulting 3-D surface template can be converted to a 2-D skin template by releasing cuts [5]. But the precision loss caused by this molding and flattening process still exists and is difficult to quantify. Digital models provide an opportunity to quantify the template accuracy, but at present they do not bring much more information than nose photos, in which case experienced operators are demanded to delineate 2-D skin templates. Optionally we can produce 3-D models, e.g., by 3-D printing, and fall back to the molding and flattening process for 2-D template production.

In this work, we introduce a framework called *nasal mesh unfolding* to bridge the gap between a digital 3-D nose model and a 2-D skin template. We assume that the nose model is a 3-D surface represented by a triangle mesh (obtained for example by scanning a healthy nose) and we focus on unfolding this nasal mesh with the least possible distortion. We propose to unfold the 3-D mesh using a nonlinear dimensionality-reduction technique (see [6] for an overview), namely, semidefinite embedding [7], which positions mesh vertices as far apart as possible under mesh structure constraints. The resulting 2-D embedding is a digital template that can be traced on paper or foil for outlining the skin requirement on the donor site.

2   Materials and Methods

2.1   3-D Nasal Mesh Representation

The nose model is a triangle mesh represented by an ordered list of 3-D vertices $\mathcal{V} := (\boldsymbol{v}_1, \ldots, \boldsymbol{v}_n)$ and an $n \times n$ adjacency matrix $\boldsymbol{A} := [a_{ij}]$ defining the connected vertex pairs, i.e., $a_{ij} = 1$ indicates that there is an edge between vertices $\boldsymbol{v}_i$ and $\boldsymbol{v}_j$, and $a_{ij} = 0$ otherwise. Any three vertices $\boldsymbol{v}_i$, $\boldsymbol{v}_j$, and $\boldsymbol{v}_k$ form a *mesh triangle* if $a_{ij} = a_{ik} = a_{jk} = 1$. We denote the set of mesh triangles by $\mathcal{T}$. Given a vertex $\boldsymbol{v}_i \in \mathcal{V}$, we let $\mathcal{V}(\boldsymbol{v}_i)$ be the set of vertices connected to $\boldsymbol{v}_i$ and $\mathcal{T}(\boldsymbol{v}_i)$ be the set of mesh triangles containing $\boldsymbol{v}_i$, i.e., $\mathcal{V}(\boldsymbol{v}_i) := \{\boldsymbol{v}_j \in \mathcal{V} \,|\, a_{ij} = 1\}$ and $\mathcal{T}(\boldsymbol{v}_i) := \{\boldsymbol{\tau} \in \mathcal{T} \,|\, \boldsymbol{v}_i \in \boldsymbol{\tau}\}$. We call $\mathcal{T}(\boldsymbol{v}_i)$ the *mesh patch* centered on $\boldsymbol{v}_i$, and we denote by $\overline{A}(\boldsymbol{v}_i)$ the average area of the triangles in $\mathcal{T}(\boldsymbol{v}_i)$.

In addition to the adjacency matrix $\boldsymbol{A}$ representing the triangle mesh, we define an $n \times n$ symmetric binary matrix $\boldsymbol{B} := [b_{ij}]$ representing constraints on mesh patches with large areas. Formally, $b_{ij} = 1$ if and only if the following conditions hold: $\boldsymbol{v}_j \notin \mathcal{V}(\boldsymbol{v}_i) \cup \{\boldsymbol{v}_i\}$ and there is a vertice $\boldsymbol{v}_k$ such that $\{\boldsymbol{v}_i, \boldsymbol{v}_j\} \subset \mathcal{V}(\boldsymbol{v}_k)$ and $\overline{A}(\boldsymbol{v}_k) \geqslant \alpha$, where α is a threshold set to the sum of the average and standard deviation of the mesh-triangle areas in the input 3-D mesh in our experiments. The construction of the matrix $\boldsymbol{B}$ is illustrated in Fig. 1 for mesh patches centered on vertices of degree 4 and 5. The purpose of the matrix $\boldsymbol{B}$ is to preserve large-area mesh patches during the unfolding process.

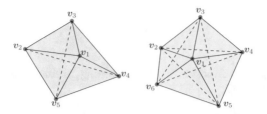

Fig. 1. Illustration of the constraints on large-area mesh patches centered on vertices of degree 4 and 5. The solid line segments are the edges of the triangle mesh represented by the adjacency matrix $\boldsymbol{A}$. The dashed line segments are the mesh-patch constraints added to the triangle mesh if $\overline{A}(\boldsymbol{v}_1) \geqslant \alpha$, where $\overline{A}(\boldsymbol{v}_1)$ is the average area of all the mesh triangles containing $\boldsymbol{v}_1$.

2.2 The Mesh Unfolding Problem

Given the triangle mesh $(\mathcal{V}, \boldsymbol{A})$ modeling the desired nose shape, the unfolding process aims to embed the 3-D vertices $\boldsymbol{v}_1, \ldots, \boldsymbol{v}_n$ in the Euclidean plane while preserving the lengths of the edges encoded in the adjacency matrix $\boldsymbol{A}$ and in the mesh-patch constraint matrix $\boldsymbol{B}$. The correspondence between $\mathcal{V}$ and its 2-D embedding $(\boldsymbol{x}_1, \ldots, \boldsymbol{x}_n)$ is obtained by maximizing the sum of the squared distances between the pairs of 2-D vertices under the edge-length isometry constraints indexed by the binary matrix $\boldsymbol{A} + \boldsymbol{B}$. Let $\| \cdot \|$ denote the standard Euclidean norm, and let $\mathcal{I}$ be the set of index pairs $\{i, j\}$ such that $\{\boldsymbol{v}_i, \boldsymbol{v}_j\}$ is an edge or a mesh-patch constraint, i.e.,

$$\mathcal{I} := \big\{ \{i, j\} \subset \{1, \ldots, n\} \mid a_{ij} + b_{ij} = 1 \big\}. \tag{1}$$

The unfolding problem is the following:

$$\text{maximize} \sum_{i,j=1}^{n} \|\boldsymbol{x}_i - \boldsymbol{x}_j\|^2$$

$$\text{subject to} \begin{cases} \forall \{i, j\} \in \mathcal{I}, \ \|\boldsymbol{x}_i - \boldsymbol{x}_j\| = \|\boldsymbol{v}_i - \boldsymbol{v}_j\| \\ \sum_{i=1}^{n} \boldsymbol{x}_i = \boldsymbol{0}, \end{cases} \tag{2}$$

where the additional constraint $\sum_i \boldsymbol{x}_i = \boldsymbol{0}$ is intended to remove the translational degree of freedom.

2.3 Unfolding by Semidefinite Programming

Given a set of points $\mathcal{X} := (\boldsymbol{x}_1, \ldots, \boldsymbol{x}_n)$ in the Euclidean plane, we let $\boldsymbol{G} := [g_{ij}]$ be the Gram matrix of $\mathcal{X}$; i.e., for every $(i, j) \in \{1, \ldots, n\}^2$, g_{ij} is the dot product of $\boldsymbol{x}_i$ and $\boldsymbol{x}_j$, denoted by $\boldsymbol{x}_i \cdot \boldsymbol{x}_j$. Since $\|\boldsymbol{x}_i - \boldsymbol{x}_j\|^2 = g_{ii} - 2g_{ij} + g_{jj}$ and $\|\sum_i \boldsymbol{x}_i\|^2 = \sum_{i,j} \boldsymbol{x}_i \cdot \boldsymbol{x}_j$, the constraints in (2) are equivalent to

$$g_{ii} - 2g_{ij} + g_{jj} = \|\boldsymbol{v}_i - \boldsymbol{v}_j\|^2 \tag{3}$$

and

$$\sum_{i,j=1}^{n} g_{ij} = 0. \tag{4}$$

Besides, the objective function of the unfolding problem can be expressed in terms of the trace of G:

$$\sum_{i,j=1}^{n} \|x_i - x_j\|^2 = \sum_{i,j=1}^{n} (g_{ii} - 2g_{ij} + g_{jj})$$
$$= 2n \sum_{i=1}^{n} g_{ii} = 2n\mathrm{tr}(G), \tag{5}$$

where the second equality follows from (4). Hence, since a matrix is Gramian if and only if it is positive semidefinite, the unfolding problem is equivalent to the following semidefinite programming problem (we refer to [8] for an introduction to semidefinite programming):

maximize $\mathrm{tr}(G)$ subject to

$$\begin{cases} G \text{ is positive semidefinite} \\ \forall \{i,j\} \in \mathcal{I}, \ g_{ii} - 2g_{ij} + g_{jj} = \|v_i - v_j\|^2 \\ \sum_{i,j=1}^{n} g_{ij} = 0. \end{cases} \tag{6}$$

In our experiments, we use the semidefinite programming solver described in [9]. We now describe how to compute a solution $(x_1^*, \ldots, x_n^*)$ to the original unfolding problem (2) from a solution G^* to (6). Since G^* is positive semidefinite, its eigenvalues $\lambda_1, \ldots, \lambda_n$ are nonnegative and

$$G^* = P \operatorname{diag}(\lambda_1, \ldots, \lambda_n) P^T, \tag{7}$$

where P is the orthogonal matrix whose columns $p_1, \ldots, p_n$ are the eigenvectors of G^* associated with $\lambda_1, \ldots, \lambda_n$. Therefore the coefficients of G^* are given by

$$g_{ij}^* = \sum_{k=1}^{n} \lambda_k p_{ik} p_{jk}, \tag{8}$$

where p_{ik} is the ith component of p_k. Equivalently, G^* is the Gram matrix of the vectors $w_1, \ldots, w_n$ defined by

$$w_i := \left(\sqrt{\lambda_1} p_{i1}, \ldots, \sqrt{\lambda_n} p_{in}\right). \tag{9}$$

Let π be a permutation of $\{1, \ldots, n\}$ that arranges the eigenvalues in decreasing order, i.e., π is a bijection from $\{1, \ldots, n\}$ to itself such that $\lambda_{\pi(1)} \geqslant \cdots \geqslant \lambda_{\pi(n)}$. Let $w_{i,\pi}$ denote the vector obtained by permuting the components of w_i using π. If the triangle mesh $(\mathcal{V}, A)$ lies near a 2-D manifold, then $\lambda_{\pi(2)} \gg \lambda_{\pi(3)}$ [7], and thus

$$w_{i,\pi} \approx \left(\sqrt{\lambda_{\pi(1)}} p_{i\pi(1)}, \sqrt{\lambda_{\pi(2)}} p_{i\pi(2)}, 0, \ldots, 0\right). \tag{10}$$

Hence each point x_i^* is obtained by keeping the first two components of $w_{i,\pi}$, and so the 2-D embedded mesh is $((x_1^*, \ldots, x_n^*), A)$ with

$$x_i^* := \left(\sqrt{\lambda_{\pi(1)}} p_{i\pi(1)}, \sqrt{\lambda_{\pi(2)}} p_{i\pi(2)}\right). \qquad (11)$$

The quality of this embedding depends on the accuracy of the approximation (10) and can be measured via the ratio $\lambda_{\pi(3)}/\lambda_{\pi(2)} \in [0, 1]$; indeed, the smaller this ratio, the closer $(\mathcal{V}, A)$ to a 2-D manifold. Hence the following quality measure:

$$\text{Embedding accuracy (\%)} := 100(1 - \lambda_{\pi(3)}/\lambda_{\pi(2)}). \qquad (12)$$

3 Results

3.1 Synthetic Examples

We start from a 3-D triangle mesh of the volume swept out by moving the 2-D "C" shape shown in Fig. 2(a) along the z-axis. The mesh is displayed in Fig. 2(b) and was generated using the iso2mesh software (available at http://iso2mesh. sourceforge.net) [10]. We consider the mesh subsets shown in Fig. 2(c) and (d), which can be viewed as meshes of simply- and doubly-curved bands and are thus close to 2-D manifolds.

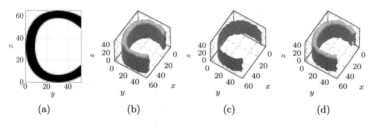

(a)   (b)   (c)   (d)

Fig. 2. Synthetic data: (a) section of the volume used to generate the synthetic mesh; (b) the whole synthetic mesh; (c) simply-curved band (consisting of the outward part of the mesh); (d) doubly-curved band (obtained by removing the vertices located at the extremities of the "C" shape and the vertices with z-coordinate smaller than 10). (The distance unit is arbitrary.)

Simply-Curved Band. Figure 3(a) shows the 2-D embedding of the simply-curved band shown in Fig. 2(c). The color scale reflects the percentage decrease of the triangle areas resulting from the unfolding process. Apart from a few artifacts on the border, the triangle areas are well preserved (the median area-decrease is 3.31%). The embedding accuracy (see (12)) is 99.06%, which confirms that the 3-D mesh has an intrinsic dimensionality of two and is faithfully represented by its embedding.

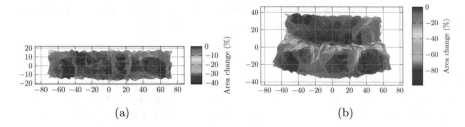

Fig. 3. Embeddings of the simply-curved band and the doubly-curved band shown in Fig. 2(c) and (d). The mesh triangles are colored according to the percentage decrease in area accompanying the unfolding process.

Doubly-Curved Band. The doubly-curved band shown in Fig. 2(d) mimics a high-curvature region of the nasal surface at a subunit junction. Its 2-D embedding is displayed in Fig. 3(b). The median area-decrease, 10.91%, is higher than for the simply-curved band. The shrinking of the triangle areas occurs on or near the junction, which appears as a thin strip in the middle of the unfolded band. The two sides separated by this strip correspond to simply-curved bands and hence are well preserved by the unfolding process. The overall embedding accuracy is 98.99%, confirming the two-dimensionality of the 3-D mesh and the faithfulness of its unfolded representation.

3.2 Unfolding a Real Nasal Surface

Data. The real nose mesh (see Fig. 4(a)) is extracted after imaging the face of a healthy volunteer using an optical 3-D scanner (FaceSCAN[3D], 3D-Shape, Erlangen, Germany). For simplicity, the inner nostril regions are not considered in unfolding. We also printed a 3-D model of the whole nose (see Fig. 4(b)) for physical template quality evaluation.

Embedded Mesh. Figure 5(a) shows the embedding of the 3-D nose mesh. As in Sect. 3.1, the color scale reflects the percentage decrease of the triangle areas accompanying the unfolding process. The median area-decrease, 10.25% $(0.12\,\text{mm}^2)$, is similar to that observed for the doubly-curved band. The shrinking of the triangle areas largely occurs at subunit junctions; the total area-decrease is 14.47% $(435.26\,\text{mm}^2)$. The embedding accuracy is 97.11%, which indicates that the 3-D nose mesh is close to a 2-D manifold and is properly unfolded.

Physical Template. To create a ready-to-use template, we first scale the 2-D embedding in Fig. 5(a) so that its printing has the same area as the input 3-D mesh in Fig. 4(b). The resulting paper template is then used to delineate the contour of an aluminum foil, as illustrated in Fig. 5(b) and (c). The quality of the foil template is evaluated by wrapping it around the 3-D printed nose model (see Fig. 6). The borders of the 2-D template fit with the 3-D nose. A few small regions pointed out by the arrows are not covered by the template. The nostril holes are not covered, which complies with the input 3-D mesh. The foil is slightly broken in the nasion region (blue arrow), which is predictable from the percentage decrease in area visualised in Fig. 5(a). However, this defect and the non-covered locations on the border are small enough to be compensated by skin elasticity.

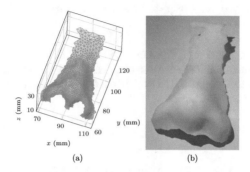

(a)   (b)

Fig. 4. Real nasal data: (a) nose mesh obtained from optical 3-D scanning a volunteer's face; (b) 3-D print of the nose mesh.

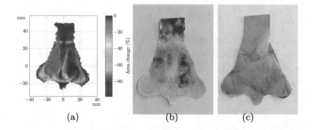

(a)   (b)   (c)

Fig. 5. Templates obtained aftering unfolding the nose mesh shown in Fig. 4(a): (a) digital template; (b) paper print; (c) aluminum foil template delineated from the paper template.

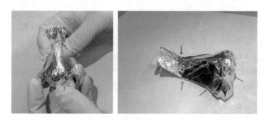

Fig. 6. Template quality evaluation. The aluminum foil template is wrapped around the 3-D printed model; the arrows point out the regions that are not properly covered.

4   Conclusion

A nasal cover of correct shape and dimensions is necessary to give a natural appearance to the reconstructed nose. With this in mind, we have developed a mesh unfolding framework to find optimal 2-D skin templates for nasal reconstruction. Starting from a 3-D nose mesh, our approach generates a digital 2-D skin template that eases the preparation of physical 2-D templates (e.g., paper and foil templates). We demonstrated its effectiveness on both synthetic and real nasal surface meshes.

Acknowledgments. Work supported by NSFC grant 61701325, the Region Auvergne Rhône-Alpes of France under the project CMIRA COOPERA/EXPLORA PRO 2016, the Program PHC-Cai Yuanpei 2016 (No 36702XD), and the French ANR under MOSI-FAH ANR-13-MONU-0009-01.

References

1. Weathers, W.M., Koshy, J.C., Wolfswinkel, E.M., Thornton, J.F.: Overview of nasal soft tissue reconstruction: keeping it simple. Semin. Plast. Surg. **27**(2), 83–89 (2013)
2. Byrne, P.J., Garcia, J.R.: Autogenous nasal tip reconstruction of complex defects: a structural approach employing rapid prototyping. Arch. Fac. Plast. Surg. **9**(5), 358–364 (2007)
3. Sultan, B., Byrne, P.J.: Custom-made, 3D, intraoperative surgical guides for nasal reconstruction. Fac. Plast. Surg. Clin. N. Am. **19**(4), 647–653 (2011)
4. Hierl, T., Arnold, S., Kruber, D., Schulze, F.P., Hümpfner-Hierl, H.: CAD-CAM-assisted esthetic facial surgery. J. Oral Maxillofac. Surg. **71**(1), e15–e23 (2013)
5. Murrell, G.L., Burget, G.C.: Aesthetically precise templates for nasal reconstruction using a new material. Plast. Reconstr. Surg. **112**(7), 1855–1861 (2003)
6. Van Der Maaten, L., Postma, E., Van den Herik, J.: Dimensionality reduction: a comparative. J. Mach. Learn. Res. **10**, 66–71 (2009)
7. Weinberger, K.Q., Saul, L.K.: Unsupervised learning of image manifolds by semidefinite programming. Int. J. Comput. Vis. **70**(1), 77–90 (2006)
8. Vandenberghe, L., Boyd, S.: Semidefinite programming. SIAM Rev. **38**(1), 49–95 (1996)
9. Borchers, B.: CSDP, A C library for semidefinite programming. Optim. Methods Softw. **11**(1–4), 613–623 (1999)
10. Fang, Q., Boas, D.A.: Tetrahedral mesh generation from volumetric binary and grayscale images. In: 2009 IEEE International Symposium on Biomedical Imaging: From Nano to Macro, pp. 1142–1145 (2009)

Towards Generating Personalized Volumetric Phantom from Patient's Surface Geometry

Yifan Wu[1], Vivek Singh[1(✉)], Brian Teixeira[1], Kai Ma[1], Birgi Tamersoy[1], Andreas Krauss[2], and Terrence Chen[1]

[1] Medical Imaging Technologies, Siemens Healthineers, Princeton, NJ, USA
vivek-singh@siemens-healthineers.com
[2] Siemens Healthcare GmbH, Forchheim, Germany

Abstract. This paper presents a method to generate a volumetric phantom with internal anatomical structures from the patient's skin surface geometry, and studies the potential impact of this technology on planning medical scans and procedures such as patient positioning. Existing scan planning for imaging is either done by visual inspection of the patient or based on an ionizing scan obtained prior to the full scan. These methods are either limited in accuracy or result in additional radiation dose to the patient. Our approach generates a "CT"-like phantom, with lungs and bone structures, from the patient's skin surface. The skin surface can be estimated from a 2.5D depth sensor and thus, the proposed method offers a novel solution to reduce the radiation dose. We present quantitative experiments on a dataset of 2045 whole body CT scans and report measurements relevant to the potential clinical use of such phantoms. (This feature is based on research, and is not commercially available. Due to regulatory reasons its future availability cannot be guaranteed.)

1 Introduction

Medical imaging technologies such as Computed Tomography (CT) plays a pivotal role in clinical diagnosis and therapy planning. However, acquisition of CT data exposes patients to potentially harmful ionizing radiation. Several planning methodologies to reduce the radiation dose have been developed [7,13]. However, existing CT scan planning is often performed based on coarse patient measurement estimates from visual inspection by the technician or using scouting scans (topograms). For certain other imaging methods such as emission based tomography (PET/SPECT), a CT scan is obtained prior to the procedure, to be used for attenuation correction [14]. Both these methods expose patients to additional radiation. In this paper, we present an approach to generate a volumetric phantom with density estimates of lungs and bone structures, from the patient's body surface mesh.

With the recent developments in human body shape modeling and simulation, accurate and detailed body models are achievable for a wide range of applications in multimedia, safety, as well as diagnostic and therapeutic healthcare

A. F. Frangi et al. (Eds.): MICCAI 2018, LNCS 11070, pp. 171–179, 2018.
https://doi.org/10.1007/978-3-030-00928-1_20

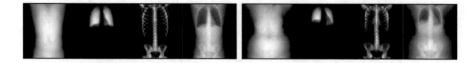

Fig. 1. Illustration of data. From left to right we show the patient's body surface mask, lungs mask, bone mask and phantom respectively, for 2 different patients. All masks and phantoms are volumetric, images displayed here are orthographic projections (averaged along the AP axis).

domains [10,11]. However, existing statistical body shape modeling approaches mainly focus on the skin surface, while the healthcare domain pays more attention to the internal anatomical structures such as organs [5]. Several computational phantoms with internal anatomy have been developed over the years, particularly for the purpose of radiation dosimetry analysis [8]. Attempts have also been made to generate personalized phantoms based on patient's physical attributes, such as body size (height, width), weight, BMI and/or gender [2,14], which reportedly offer benefits over universal phantoms. However, these attribute measurements are often approximate, which limits the degree of personalization, thus, in turn limiting the potential clinical impact.

We present a learning-based framework to generate a volumetric phantom from a detailed mesh representation of the patient's body surface; such body surface representation can be obtained using range sensors [10]. The generated phantom is a 3D volumetric image where the voxel intensity provides an estimate of the physical density based on the statistical distribution over a large dataset of patient scans. Figure 1 illustrates "ground truth" phantoms of different patients which are computed from their whole body CT scans. In this study, we focus on a phantom with lungs and bone structures, which allows evaluating our framework on its ability to generate finer details (on bones structures), while simultaneously attempting to capture the correlation between the body geometry and size/shape of lungs. During the training phase, we utilize the whole body CT scans to obtain the volumetric masks for skin, lungs, and bones, and then train a conditional deep generative network [3,4] to learn a mapping from skin mask to a phantom with lungs and bones. Training is performed using more than 1500 whole body CT scans. Quantitative evaluations are conducted on 133 unseen patients by comparing the generated and ground truth phantoms. We also report several clinically relevant quantitative measures on phantoms which clearly demonstrates the benefits of generating phantoms from the skin surface.

2   Methods

Given the whole body CT scan of a given subject in the training dataset, we obtain the skin surface mask m_s, lungs mask m_l and bone mask m_b using existing CT segmentation algorithms [1], followed by a visual validation. We define the phantom volume p as a weighted combination of these binary masks,

$$p = \alpha \cdot m_s + \beta \cdot m_l + \delta \cdot m_b \tag{1}$$

where α, β, δ are weights for phantom synthesis. For intensity value of the phantom voxels to be comparable to the radiodensity of the respective regions, we set these weights to be proportional to the average Hounsfield units (HU) in those regions relative to the HU of air ($=-1000$). In our experiments, we set $\alpha = 1000$, $\beta = -800$, $\delta = 500$. Figure 1 shows phantoms for different patients.

To model the compositional nature of the phantom, we propose to use a deep network architecture that first estimates the masks for key anatomical regions (in our case, lungs, and bones) from the skin surface and then combines them into the phantom using Eq. 1. While predicting the separate masks for different regions offers the advantage of computing the losses independently and back-propagating them, it suffers from the risk that the masks may not be correlated with each other and result in physically implausible phantoms (e.g. with ribs of spine penetrating the lungs). Thus, the network architecture and training procedure must be appropriately designed to ensure that the generated phantoms are predicted with sufficiently high accuracy while ensuring physical consistency.

To achieve physical consistency, we propose to use Generative Adversarial Networks (GANs) [3]. More specifically, we employ conditional adversarial networks (cGANs) [4] which allows enforcing physical consistency without sacrificing the input output correlation (in our case, the correlation between the skin surface volume and predicted phantom). Figure 2 shows the overview of the proposed framework. In the following sections, we first introduce cGANs and then describe the details on how to adapt them to the phantom generation task.

2.1 Conditional GAN

The cGAN learns a mapping $G : \{x, z\} \rightarrow y$ from an observed image x with additional random noise z to a synthesized image y, where x is referred as a 'real' sample or the condition from the original dataset, y is referred as a 'fake' sample generated by the trained generator G, and z is the random noise to ensure the image variability. The adversarial procedure trains a generator to produce outputs that can hardly be distinguished as a 'fake' by the co-trained discriminator D. Unlike GAN, the discriminator in cGAN utilizes both input x and output y of the generator to determine the 'fake' label based on the joint distribution. The objective function of cGAN is formulated as:

$$\begin{aligned}
\mathcal{L}_{\text{cGAN}}(G, D) = \ &\mathbb{E}_{x,y \sim P_{\text{data}}(x,y)}[\log D(x, y)] \\
&+ \mathbb{E}_{x \sim P_{\text{data}}(x), z \sim P_z(z)}[\log(1 - D(x, G(x, z)))],
\end{aligned} \tag{2}$$

where G is the generator and D is the discriminator. The optimal G^* minimizes this objective against an adversarial D that maximizes it, and it can be solved via a min-max procedure.

2.2 Phantom Generation

The phantom generation is done at two scales. At the coarser scale, the task is formulated as a segmentation task, where network generates a body segmentation into two components - lungs mask and bone mask. At the finer scale within each mask, the network generates as many details as possible. Combining the losses of these two scales, the overall loss function of phantom generation is then defined as the combination of the cGAN loss and the segmentation loss:

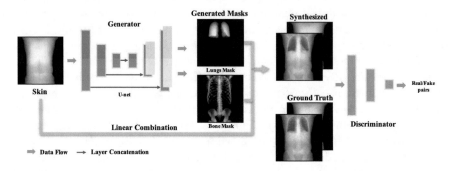

Fig. 2. Overview of the proposed framework for phantom generation. Images displayed here are orthographic projections (averaged along the AP axis).

$$\mathcal{L}_{\text{phantom}}(G, D) = \mathcal{L}_{\text{cGAN}}(G, D) + \mathcal{L}_{\text{seg}}(G) \tag{3}$$

where G is the generator from surface mask to the phantom, and D is the corresponding discriminator to determine whether a pair of skin and phantom are from the ground truth or the synthesis of generated masks. The cGAN loss is adapted as:

$$\begin{aligned}\mathcal{L}_{\text{cGAN}}(G, D) = \ &\mathbb{E}_{m_s, p^{gt} \sim P_{\text{data}}(m_s, p^{gt})}[\log D(m_s, p^{gt})] \\ &+ \mathbb{E}_{m_s \sim P_{\text{data}}(m_s), z \sim P_z(z)}[\log(1 - D(m_s, p^G))]\end{aligned} \tag{4}$$

where z is the random noise, m_s is skin mask, p^{gt} is the ground truth phantom and p^G is the phantom synthesized from the masks m_l^G, m_b^G generated by G using Eq. 1. The segmentation loss that quantifies the similarity between the generated and ground truth segmentation is formulated as:

$$\mathcal{L}_{\text{seg}}(G) = \mathbb{E}_{s, m^{gt} \sim P_{\text{data}}(m_s, m^{gt})} H(m^{gt}, m^G) \tag{5}$$

where $m^{gt} = m_l^{gt}, m_b^{gt}$ is the ground truth mask, $m^G = m_l^G, m_b^G$ is the generated mask from G, and H is the cross entropy function.

This objective function is optimized via the cGAN adversarial procedure to obtain an optimal generator G^*,

$$G^* = \arg \min_G \max_D \mathcal{L}_{\text{phantom}}(G, D) \tag{6}$$

2.3   Architecture

We adapt our generator and discriminator network architectures from the Image-to-Image translation [4]. Both networks use modules consisting of Convolution-InstanceNorm-ReLU. The generator is a "U-Net" [9] with a stride of 2. The size of the embedding layer is $1 \times 1 \times 1$. Two drop-out layers serve as the random noise z. We employ a patch-based discriminator which outputs an $N \times N \times N$ matrix. We set N to 30 with a receptive field of size $34 \times 34 \times 34$.

3   Experiments

3.1   Experimental Setup

To evaluate our approach, we collected 2045 whole body Computed Tomography (CT) scans from patients at several different hospital sites in North America and Europe. Our dataset contains adults with age between 20 and 87, of which 45% are female. The neck to abdomen length varies from 1243 ± 135 mm. We randomly select 133 patients for testing, and use the rest for training and validation. We present a thorough analysis on phantom prediction from ground truth skin surface masks, which serves as an upper bound to what may be achievable with estimated skin surfaces using range sensors [10].

Given the skin masks and phantoms, we normalize all images to a single scale using the neck and pubic symphysis body markers (since these can be estimated from the body surface data with high accuracy <2 cm) and scaled to 128.

We compare the proposed method (referred as *skin2masks+GAN*) with 2 baseline approaches: (i) Use voxelwise L_1-loss, to regress the phantom from skin mask (referred as *skin2phantom*); (ii) Use binary cross entropy loss to generate the lungs and bone masks from the skin mask, and then obtain the phantom using Eq. 1 (referred as *skin2masks*). For all the experiments, we employ the same "U-Net" architecture and train using Adam [6] with mini-batch SGD. Learning rate was set to 10^{-5}.

3.2   Phantom Generation from Skin Surface

Quantitative Analysis. For a quantitative comparison between the proposed methods and baselines, we report the mean MS-SSIM [12] and mean L_1-error in Table 1. The MS-SSIM score, which measures the visual similarity with the ground truth phantom, is much higher for *skin2masks+GAN* (0.9866) compared to 0.9516 for *skin2phantom* and 0.9533 for *skin2masks*. In addition, the proposed method gains the lowest L_1-loss among the three strategies as well. We attribute the improvement in performance to the conditional adversarial training. Our understanding here is that although the two masks are spatially non-overlapping and linearly composed in the phantom, there are contextually correlated. This not only makes it possible to predict organs from surfaces but also indicates the necessity of co-optimization among parts to achieve global consistency.

Table 1. Comparison between different approaches for phantom generation

	skin2phantom	*skin2masks*	*skin2masks+GAN*
L_1-loss	17.3549	17.0599	**16.0404**
MS-SSIM (along SI axis)	0.9516	0.9533	**0.9866**
MS-SSIM (along AP axis)	0.9514	0.9525	**0.9752**

Qualitative Analysis. Figure 4 show images of phantoms, predicted using the 3 methods, for several different patients. Observe that the generated phantoms from the proposed pipeline (in column 3) look visually plausible with excellent details in lungs and bone structures, indicating that the trained model reasonably maintains the underlined structures. In addition, the predicted lungs and bones mostly display adaptive variation in sizes with the ground truth. We can also see that visually neither of the two baseline methods engenders comparable quality of phantoms with the proposed method (column 3). The *skin2phantom* produce less details especially over the bone regions. A closer, more detailed look also reveals several issues. For patient in row 1, spinal curvature is not predicted from his skin surface, which is expected; in general, the predicted spinal columns appear more straight than the real cases. Also, the predictions for relatively larger patients (row 3–4) are not as detailed, especially in the hip region. For patient in row 4, notice that the shape of the right lung in underestimated; we guess that the thicker fat layer increases the difficulty of prediction, thereby, suggesting potential limits of the approach.

3.3 Studying Clinical Relevance of the Synthesized Phantoms

Density Estimation. To study the accuracy of the predicted density estimates, we computed the maximum deviation between the mean slice density profiles (mean intensity for every slice along SI axis) of predicted and ground truth phantoms. Such profile for a patient in testing set is shown in Fig. 3(a). The maximum deviation over testing set has a mean error of 35.73 ± 19.01, which is promising. However, the histogram of the maximum deviations (see Fig. 3(b)) suggests that for 3–4% cases, error may be too high (above 80).

Lungs Estimation. Over the testing data, the distance between lung top and liver top varies between 123 and 195 mm. The lung volume varies significantly with ratio between the smallest to the largest lungs at about 3.2. We obtain the left and right lung masks from the generated phantoms and measure the volume. For volume estimation, the mean percentage error is 21.37 ± 13.24 and 18.75 ± 14.29 for left and right lung respectively. In comparison, the error reported by attribute based phantom [14] is 28 ± 8 and 30 ± 15. We attribute this improvement to using a detailed patient surface.

For potential use in patient positioning for lung scans, we measure the error in estimating the position of the slice that marks the lung bottom. Our method achieves a remarkably low mean error of 17.16 ± 12.81 mm (with *max*: 51,

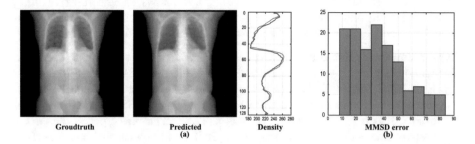

Fig. 3. Density estimation analysis (a) predicted and ground truth phantoms with their corresponding density profiles shown in red and blue respectively, (b) histogram of maximum deviation in mean slice density (MMSD) profile.

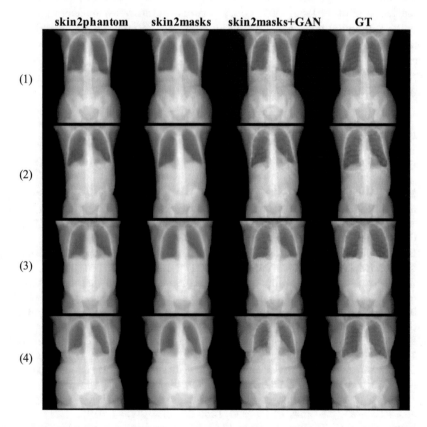

Fig. 4. Phantom generation results. Images displayed here are orthographic projections. Each row shows a different patient from the unseen test dataset; each column is a different method and last column is the ground truth.

90%: 33) and 15.55 ± 11.21 mm (with *max*: 30, 90%: 54) for left and right lung respectively. Although the error is large for 5% of patients, the overall low mean and 90-percentile errors clearly demonstrate the potential for clinical use.

Evaluation from Estimated Skin Surface. We use [10] to estimate complete 3D skin surface mesh and provide results for the cases for which we have both depth and full body CT data (15 cases). The mean surface distance between estimated and CT skin surface is 13.64 ± 4.21 mm. The MS-SSIM of the predicted phantom CT is 0.96 and average L_1 loss is 17.28. The mean percentage error for lung volume estimation increases from 21% to 27% with estimated surface instead of CT surface, which is still better than using patient meta-data [14].

4   Conclusion

In this paper, we present a method to generate a volumetric phantom from the patient's skin surface, and report various quantitative measurements that are achievable with deep learning based methods. While the generated patient specific phantom is still likely to be limited in its ability to predict the internal anatomy, but it may still be clinically more reliable for scan planning compared to technician's visual estimates and have the potential to be used for attenuation correction in emission tomography.

References

1. Birkbeck, N., et al.: Lung segmentation from CT with severe pathologies using anatomical constraints. In: MICCAI (2014)
2. Ding, A., Mille, M.M., Liu, T., Caracappa, P.F., Xu, X.G.: Extension of RPI-adult male and female computational phantoms to obese patients and a Monte Carlo study of the effect on CT imaging dose. Phys. Med. Biol. **57**(9), 2441–2459 (2012)
3. Goodfellow, I., et al.: Generative adversarial nets. In: NIPS (2014)
4. Isola, P., Zhu, J.Y., Zhou, T., Efros, A.A.: Image-to-image translation with conditional adversarial networks. In: CVPR (2017)
5. Khankook, A.E.: A feasibility study on the use of phantoms with statistical lung masses for determining the uncertainty in the dose absorbed by the lung from broad beams of incident photons and neutrons. J. Radiat. Res. **58**(3), 313–328 (2017)
6. Kingma, D., Ba, J.: Adam: a method for stochastic optimization. In: ICLR (2015)
7. McCollough, C.H., Primak, A.N., Braun, N., Kofler, J., Yu, L., Christner, J.: Strategies for reducing radiation dose in CT. Radiol. Clin. **47**, 27–40 (2009)
8. Na, Y.H.: Deformable adult human phantoms for radiation protection dosimetry: anthropometric data representing size distributions of adult worker populations and software algorithms. Phys. Med. Biol. **55**, 3789–3811 (2010)
9. Ronneberger, O., Fischer, P., Brox, T.: U-Net: convolutional networks for biomedical image segmentation. In: Navab, N., Hornegger, J., Wells, W.M., Frangi, A.F. (eds.) MICCAI 2015. LNCS, vol. 9351, pp. 234–241. Springer, Cham (2015). https://doi.org/10.1007/978-3-319-24574-4_28

10. Singh, V., et al.: DARWIN: deformable patient avatar representation with deep image network. In: Descoteaux, M., Maier-Hein, L., Franz, A., Jannin, P., Collins, D.L., Duchesne, S. (eds.) MICCAI 2017. LNCS, vol. 10434, pp. 497–504. Springer, Cham (2017). https://doi.org/10.1007/978-3-319-66185-8_56
11. Tsoli, A., Mahmood, N., Black, M.J.: Breathing life into shape: capturing, modeling and animating 3D human breathing. ACM Trans. Graph. **33**(4), 52 (2014)
12. Wang, Z., Simoncelli, E.P., Bovik, A.C.: Multiscale structural similarity for image quality assessment. In: IEEE Conference Record of the Thirty-Seventh Asilomar Conference on Signals, Systems and Computers, vol. 2, pp. 1398–1402 (2003)
13. Zacharias, C.: Pediatric CT: strategies to lower radiation dose. Am. J. Roentgenol. **200**(5), 950–956 (2013)
14. Zhong, X., et al.: Generation of personalized computational phantoms using only patient metadata. In: IEEE Nuclear Science Symposium and Medical Imaging Conference Record (2017)

Multi-channel Generative Adversarial Network for Parallel Magnetic Resonance Image Reconstruction in K-space

Pengyue Zhang[1,3(✉)], Fusheng Wang[1], Wei Xu[2], and Yu Li[3]

[1] Department of Computer Science, Stony Brook University,
Stony Brook, USA
pengyue.zhang@stonybrook.edu
[2] Computational Science Initiative, Brookhaven National Laboratory,
Upton, USA
[3] Department of Cardiac Imaging, DeMatteis Center for Cardiac Research
and Education, St. Francis Hospital, Greenvale, USA

Abstract. Magnetic Resonance Imaging (MRI) typically collects data below the Nyquist sampling rate for imaging acceleration. To remove aliasing artifacts, we propose a multi-channel deep generative adversarial network (GAN) model for MRI reconstruction. Because multi-channel GAN matches the parallel data acquisition system architecture on a modern MRI scanner, this model can effectively learn intrinsic data correlation associated with MRI hardware from originally-collected multi-channel complex data. By estimating missing data directly with the trained network, images may be generated from undersampled multi-channel raw data, providing an "end-to-end" approach to parallel MRI reconstruction. By experimentally comparing with other methods, it is demonstrated that multi-channel GAN can perform image reconstruction with an affordable computation cost and an imaging acceleration factor higher than the current clinical standard.

1 Introduction

Magnetic Resonance Imaging (MRI) is a powerful tool for disease diagnosis and treatment. However, the clinical applications of MRI are limited by its intrinsically low imaging speed. On a clinical MRI scanner, data are typically collected below the Nyquist sampling frequency for imaging acceleration. As undersampling may introduce aliasing artifacts, image reconstruction is challenging in MRI.

Parallel imaging is a conventional approach to reconstruct images from undersampled data in MRI. This approach requires a radiofrequency coil array for collecting multi-channel images in parallel [2,7,9]. The coil sensitivity differences between channels may be used to remove aliasing artifacts in image reconstruction. Several parallel imaging techniques including GRAPPA [2] and SENSE [9] have been commercialized and are being used as clinical standards. A drawback

© Springer Nature Switzerland AG 2018
A. F. Frangi et al. (Eds.): MICCAI 2018, LNCS 11070, pp. 180–188, 2018.
https://doi.org/10.1007/978-3-030-00928-1_21

of these techniques is that coil sensitivity must be calibrated and the calibration procedure may reduce the effective parallel imaging acceleration factor. Recently, compressed sensing has become an active area of research interest in MRI [6]. This approach relies on a sparsity constraint on MRI data and uses an iterative algorithm to reconstruct images. Although a calibration procedure is not needed, the computation is expensive. In addition, most compressed sensing techniques are sensitive to regularization parameters in image reconstruction and their clinical performance is not as robust as parallel imaging.

Deep learning has made many breakthroughs in the field of computer vision and medical imaging. Recent years have seen a number of research works on its applications in MRI reconstruction. For example, a data-driven scheme based on generative adversarial network (GAN) has been used in combination with compressed sensing [8]. This work, like many other deep learning studies, treats MRI reconstruction as a computer vision problem and removes aliasing from DICOM images in grayscale or RGB magnitude generated by a series of pre- and post-processing procedures [5, 8, 10, 14]. However, it should be known that MRI physically collects multi-channel complex data samples in Fourier space (termed k-space in the field of MRI) with both magnitude and phase information. By transforming complex k-space data into a grey-scale DICOM image with pre- and post-processing, a large amount of information is lost, which introduces low data utility in the network. As a result, image reconstruction may not take full advantage of the data-driven power of deep learning.

Our work aims to develop a deep generative model that can process multi-channel MRI raw data. It is expected that image reconstruction may take advantage of all the information in MRI data. The work is inspired by a well-known fact in parallel imaging: multi-channel coil sensitivity introduces k-space data correlation and every data sample may be represented by the convolution of their neighboring samples with a filter. This filter can be well modelled by convolutional neural networks in k-space. By training a GAN with multi-channel k-space raw data, our model may learn and use parallel imaging mechanisms underlying MRI data to reconstruct images from undersampled data. Herein, we present a multi-channel GAN model for MRI reconstruction from undersampled data in this paper. This model has the following features:

(1) The multi-channel GAN receives multi-channel complex undersampled MRI data at the input and generates multi-channel complex fully-sampled MRI data at the output.
(2) The model provides an "end-to-end" approach to MRI reconstruction, i.e., images can be generated directly from raw MRI data. No pre- or post-processing procedures are needed.
(3) A new loss function is introduced to combine adversarial and perceptual loss for improved artifact suppression in image reconstruction.
(4) The model is trained with multiple sets of multi-channel MRI data. In every training step, all the channels of the network are updated simultaneously with the multi-channel raw data.

(5) The trained model is used as a general reconstructor for all new datasets. This is different from conventional MRI methods that use a different reconstructor for different datasets.

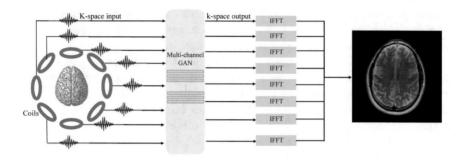

Fig. 1. An overview of the proposed Multi-channel GAN. Multi-channel k-space data are collected simultaneously from multiple coils and fed in to GAN to generate multi-channel outputs for MRI reconstruction.

2   Method

MRI raw data are collected in complex k-space (Fourier spatial-frequency domain) from a multi-channel (typically 8–32 channels) radiofrequency coil array. If data are fully sampled at the Nyquist frequency, an inverse Fourier transform may generate the real images. To accelerate MRI, k-space is usually undersampled, which introduces aliasing artifacts in image-space. Since multi-channel coil sensitivity may introduce k-space data correlation, a parallel imaging technique (e.g., GRAPPA, SPIRiT) may estimate missing data by the linear convolution of partially collected k-space with a filter. In our work, a GAN-based network is used to model the filter used in parallel imaging for image reconstruction. In GAN pipeline, two models are jointly trained: a generator model G which captures the training data distribution and a discriminator model D which justifies if the generated data come from the distribution of the training data. Through the training process, the generator should be trained to estimate the embedding data manifold and generate samples to fool the discriminator. Then after training the generator alone can be used to generate new samples that are similar to real samples.

Here a multi-channel GAN based model (a multi-input and multi-output system) is trained to estimate complex-valued data in k-space. Given a set of data pairs: fully sampled k-space data y and undersampled zero-filling data $x = M_R y$, where M_R is an undersampling mask with an acceleration factor of R, a generator G is trained to generate *fake* samples from x and these *fake* samples should be justified as *real* samples by the discriminator D. The adversarial loss of the generator is given by:

$$L_{adv} = \mathbb{E}_x (1 - D(G(x)))^2 \tag{1}$$

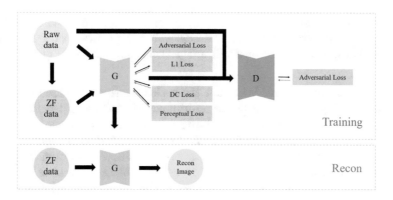

Fig. 2. Multi-channel GAN structure for MRI reconstruction from undersampled k-space data.

To minimize the difference between the generated data and ground truth data, a pixelwise MSE loss is also introduced. Here an l_1 cost term is used for more robust performance in noise and blurring suppression:

$$L_{l_1} = \mathbb{E}_{x,y}||y - G(x)||_1 \tag{2}$$

In addition, a data consistency loss is used to minimize the sum of squared difference between the acquired data samples and their estimates. This loss is formulated as:

$$L_{dc} = \mathbb{E}_{x,y}||M_R y - M_R G(x)||^2 \tag{3}$$

The terms above encourage the generator to generate an output that matches the ground truth at the k-space sampling positions. To suppress artifacts that can not be quantified by Eqs. 1, 2 and 3, we introduce a perceptual loss based on high-level features extracted from pre-trained networks and combine the pixelwise loss with perceptual loss for improved visual quality of the reconstructed image. Here let $\phi_j(\cdot)$ be the j-th layer output of a pre-trained network with shape $C_j \times W_j \times H_j$. We can use $\phi_j(\cdot)$ as a feature extractor which captures high-level image characteristics. The perceptual loss is formulated as:

$$L_{perc} = \mathbb{E}_{x,y} \frac{1}{C_j W_j H_j} ||\phi_j(y) - \phi_j(G(x))||_2^2 \tag{4}$$

By summing the adversarial loss, pixelwise loss, data consistency loss and perceptual loss together, the overall loss functions for generator and discriminator are formed as:

$$L_{gen}(G) = L_{adv} + \alpha L_{l_1} + \beta L_{dc} + \gamma L_{perc} \tag{5}$$

$$L_{dis}(D) = \mathbb{E}_x(D(G(x)))^2 + \mathbb{E}_y(1 - D(y))^2 \tag{6}$$

The parameters α, β and γ are used to balance the adversarial loss, l_1 loss, data consistency loss and perceptual loss. The generator and discriminator are trained with mini-batch stochastic gradient descent and back-propagation algorithms. The two sub-networks are updated alternatively until convergence. The trained generator is then used to reconstruct images from new raw MRI data.

Generator Architecture. We adapt the basic architecture of identity residual network with skip connections [3] for multi-channel MRI reconstruction. During training, multi-channel undersampled and fully sampled complex k-space data are fed into the network. Then 5 residual blocks are stacked sequentially where each block has two convolutional layers and skip connections from block input to output. Each convolutional layer in the residual block consists of 128 feature maps using 3×3 kernels and is followed by batch normalization and ReLU activation. The network is followed by three convolutional layers with kernel size 1×1. A VGG-16 network [11] pre-trained on ImageNet is used as feature extractor and the output of relu2_2 layer is used as perceptual feature.

Discriminator Architecture. A discriminator is connected to the generator output. The discriminator is a regular convolutional network which consists of 7 convolutional layers, each of which is followed by batch normalization and ReLU layers. We use 8, 16, 32, 64, 64, 64 feature maps for the first 6 layers, respectively. We use 3×3 kernels for the first 5 layers and 1×1 kernels for the last 2 layers. The discriminator output is a scaler between 0 and 1 measuring the estimated score of the "realness" of the generated data.

3   Experiment

3.1   Dataset and Training Details

To validate the proposed method, we perform several experiments with 170 2D multi-channel MRI images. These data are collected from the brain anatomy of different human subjects using an 8 channel coil array with a T1/T2 weighted TSE sequences (axial resolution 256×256 and FOV 240×240 **mm**). The data are randomly grouped into a training (127 images) and a test (43 images) set. To replicate the reconstruction process, we use uniform Cartesian masks with various undersampling factors. A Nvidia Tesla V100 GPU is used for training with batch size 4. The learning rate is initially set as 1×10^{-5} and reduced in half every 10,000 iterations. An Adam optimizer is used for optimization. The network is trained for 2,000 epochs, which is about 1,500 min.

3.2   Results and Discussion

The proposed method is used to reconstruct images from undersampled data generated from the 43 test data samples in comparison to GRAPPA [2], SPIRiT [7], Compressive Sensing (CS) [6] and GANCS [8]. GRAPPA, SPIRiT and Compressive Sensing reconstruction uses Berkeley ESPIRiT [12] and BART [13] toolboxes. In GRAPPA and SPIRiT, additional fully-sampled 18×18 k-space areas in central k-space are used as autocalibration signals (ACS). In GANCS [8], the raw k-space data are transformed to image-space and only the magnitude images are used. Figure 3 shows a few examples with an undersampling factor of 5 in reference to the ground truth images and the Zero-filling (ZF) Fourier reconstruction results, which are used to show the spatial distribution of aliasing artifacts. Quantitative results including Structural SIMilarity (SSIM) and PSNR are given in Table 1. It is found that parallel imaging methods (GRAPPA and SPIRiT) gives higher PSNRs. However, they may generate image blurs with noticeable background noise, indicating outer k-space is not reconstructed well. Compressive Sensing gives better image details with less noise, but at a cost of computation time (Table 1) and considerable artifacts near tissue boundaries. GANCS gives apparently worse performance both qualitatively (Fig. 3) and quantitatively (Table 1). In comparison, the proposed method gives high-quality images with a low computation cost. It should be noted that this new method does not need calibration data, implying the net undersampling factor is higher than that in parallel imaging.

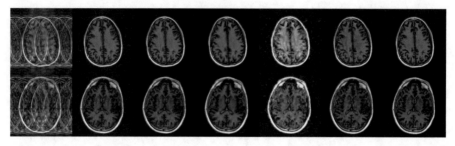

Fig. 3. Representative reconstructed images for two test samples with 5-fold uniform Cartesian undersampling (From left to right): Zero-filling, GRAPPA, SPIRiT, CS, GANCS, our method and ground truth. Contrast and exposure of the images are properly adjusted for better visualization.

Table 1. Comparison of average PSNR (dB), SSIM and Reconstruction time (second) of different methods with 5-fold undersampling

Method	ZF	GRAPPA	SPIRiT	CS	GANCS	our method
SSIM	0.38	0.80	0.83	0.76	0.82	0.88
PSNR	18.80	32.80	35.02	34.27	28.66	32.32
Recon Time	0.05	0.25	9.74	1.10	0.28	0.37

It should be mentioned that the performance of GANCS shown in Fig. 3 is worse than that in the original paper [8]. This should be attributed to the following differences: First, in the previous study, GANCS is used to reconstruct images from radial data. In this study, Cartesian data are used. Compared with radial undersampling, Cartesian undersampling introduces more patterned aliasing artifacts, which cannot be effectively removed with compressed sensing. Second, the previous GANCS study uses a total number of 45,300 training images.

This study uses only 127 training data samples. The significant reduction in training data size should be a major factor that affects the reconstruction performance.

In this study, the proposed method is based on the same GAN structure as GANCS. However, a multi-channel architecture is used to process multi-channel complex k-space data. Because more information in MRI raw data is used, better performance can be achieved with less training data. This is an advantage of the proposed method. It should also be pointed out that the proposed method is practically useful in MRI. Most MRI protocols are running with fixed parameters on daily basis in clinical practice. Once the proposed deep learning network is trained with a certain amount of data collected from different patients using a fixed protocol, it can be directly used to reconstruct images for the upcoming new patients scanned with the same protocol. This is more time efficient than conventional parallel imaging, which always requires a calibration procedure with additional data acquisition in every scan.

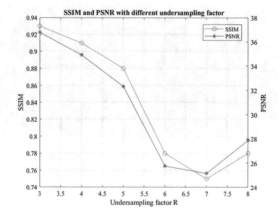

Fig. 4. Average PSNR (dB) and SSIM with various undersampling factor R.

An investigation is also made on the performance of the trained multi-channel GAN with different acceleration factors. As shown in Figs. 4 and 5, the reconstruction performance is not dramatically degraded until the undersampling factor is higher than 5. In previous studies [15], it has been demonstrated that the standard 8-channel head coil used in this work has a maximal parallel imaging acceleration factor of 4 due to hardware limitation. This indicates that the proposed method can learn not only parallel imaging mechanisms but also useful k-space data features from MRI raw data, making it possible to accelerate MRI beyond the parallel imaging limit.

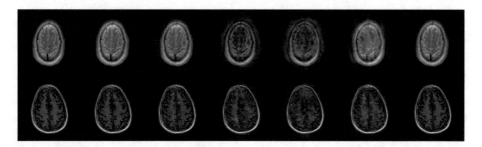

Fig. 5. Representative reconstructed images for two test samples with various under-sampling factor R. From left to right: reconstructed images with $R = 3, 4, 5, 6, 7, 8$ and ground truth images.

4   Conclusion

In this paper, we propose a multi-channel GAN model for parallel MRI recon-struction. Compared to other existing deep learning approaches, the proposed method directly uses multi-channel complex-valued k-space data. Instead of learning anatomy structure in image space, we reformulate MRI reconstruction as a data completion problem and learn physical data relationship in k-space with a multi-channel GAN model. The experimental results demonstrate that the pro-posed method outperforms other state-of-the art MRI reconstruction methods for imaging acceleration.

Acknowledgement. This research is supported in part by grants from NIH R01 EB022405, NSF ACI 1443054 and IIS 1350885.

References

1. Goodfellow, I., et al.: Generative adversarial nets. In: Advances in Neural Infor-mation Processing Systems, pp. 2672–2680 (2014)
2. Griswold, M.A., et al.: Generalized autocalibrating partially parallel acquisitions (GRAPPA). Magn. Reson. Med. **47**(6), 1202–1210 (2002)
3. He, K., Zhang, X., Ren, S., Sun, J.: Identity mappings in deep residual networks. In: Leibe, B., Matas, J., Sebe, N., Welling, M. (eds.) ECCV 2016. LNCS, vol. 9908, pp. 630–645. Springer, Cham (2016). https://doi.org/10.1007/978-3-319-46493-0_38
4. Johnson, J., Alahi, A., Fei-Fei, L.: Perceptual losses for real-time style transfer and super-resolution. In: Leibe, B., Matas, J., Sebe, N., Welling, M. (eds.) ECCV 2016. LNCS, vol. 9906, pp. 694–711. Springer, Cham (2016). https://doi.org/10.1007/978-3-319-46475-6_43
5. Lee, D., Yoo, J., Ye, J. C.: Deep artifact learning for compressed sensing and parallel MRI (2017). arXiv preprint arXiv:1703.01120
6. Lustig, M., Donoho, D., Pauly, J.M.: Sparse MRI: The application of compressed sensing for rapid MR imaging. Magn. Reson. Med. **58**(6), 1182–1195 (2007)
7. Lustig, M., Pauly, J.M.: SPIRiT: Iterative self-consistent parallel imaging recon-struction from arbitrary k-space. Magn. Reson. Med. **64**(2), 457–471 (2010)

8. Mardani, M., et al.: Deep generative adversarial networks for compressed sensing automates MRI (2017). arXiv preprint arXiv:1706.00051
9. Pruessmann, K.P., Weiger, M., Scheidegger, M.B., Boesiger, P.: SENSE: sensitivity encoding for fast MRI. Magn. Reson. Med. **42**(5), 952–962 (1999)
10. Schlemper, J., Caballero, J., Hajnal, J.V., Price, A., Rueckert, D.: A deep cascade of convolutional neural networks for MR Image reconstruction. In: Niethammer, M., Styner, M., Aylward, S., Zhu, H., Oguz, I., Yap, P.-T., Shen, D. (eds.) IPMI 2017. LNCS, vol. 10265, pp. 647–658. Springer, Cham (2017). https://doi.org/10.1007/978-3-319-59050-9_51
11. Simonyan, K., Zisserman, A.: Very deep convolutional networks for large-scale image recognition (2014). arXiv preprint arXiv:1409.1556
12. Uecker, M., et al.: ESPIRiT - an eigenvalue approach to autocalibrating parallel MRI: where SENSE meets GRAPPA. Magn. Reson. Med. **71**(3), 990–1001 (2014)
13. Uecker, M., et al.: Berkeley advanced reconstruction toolbox. In: Proc. Intl. Soc. Mag. Reson. Med., vol. 23, p. 2486 (2015)
14. Yu, S., et al.: Deep De-Aliasing for fast compressive sensing MRI (2017). arXiv preprint arXiv:1705.07137
15. Li, Y., Dumoulin, C.: Correlation imaging for multiscan MRI with parallel data acquisition. Magn. Reson. Med. **68**(6), 2005–2017 (2012)

A Learning-Based Metal Artifacts Correction Method for MRI Using Dual-Polarity Readout Gradients and Simulated Data

Kinam Kwon[1], Dongchan Kim[2], and HyunWook Park[1(✉)]

[1] Korea Advanced Institute of Science and Technology (KAIST),
Daejeon, South Korea
hwpark@kaist.ac.kr
[2] Gachon University, Incheon, South Korea

Abstract. In MRI, metallic implants can generate magnetic field distortions and interfere in the spatial encoding of gradient magnetic fields. This results in image distortions, such as bulk shifts, pile-up and signal-loss artifacts. Three-dimensional spectral imaging methods can reduce the bulk shifts to a single-voxel level, but they still suffer from residual artifacts such as pile-up and signal-loss artifacts. Fully phase encoding methods suppress metal-induced artifacts, but they require impractically long imaging times. In this paper, we applied a deep learning method to correct metal artifacts. A neural network is proposed to map two distorted images obtained by dual-polarity readout gradients into a distortion-free image obtained by fully phase encoding. Simulated data were utilized to supplement and substitute real MR data for training the proposed network. Phantom experiments were performed to compare the quality of reconstructed images from several methods at high and low readout bandwidths.

1 Introduction

Magnetic resonance imaging (MRI) is an essential medical imaging modality for clinical diagnosis because it provides high-quality soft-tissue contrast. However, general MRI sequences are susceptible to metallic implants, whose images are distorted near the metallic implants. The utilization of various metallic implants in the body has increased, for example, in shoulder/hip/knee replacement surgeries, surgical clips, and, so on, and as a result, correcting metal-induced artifacts is essential to properly follow up post surgeries, or to diagnose lesions near the metallic implants.

For MR imaging near metallic implants, three-dimensional multispectral imaging (3D MSI) methods acquire multiple spectral-bin images with different frequency offsets to handle a wide range of off-resonance frequencies induced by the metallic implants [1]. They significantly reduce bulk shifts induced by off-resonance frequencies to a single-voxel level, but they still suffer from residual artifacts induced by the large local gradient of the off-resonance frequencies [2]. On the other hand, fully-phase-encoding (FPE) methods can obtain distortion-free images near metallic implants using phase encoding in all three orthogonal directions [3]. They avoid metal-induced artifacts by substituting phase encoding steps for a frequency encoding, but they require impractically long imaging times.

© Springer Nature Switzerland AG 2018
A. F. Frangi et al. (Eds.): MICCAI 2018, LNCS 11070, pp. 189–197, 2018.
https://doi.org/10.1007/978-3-030-00928-1_22

Meanwhile, deep learning has shown remarkable performances in various medical imaging applications, for classification, segmentation, recognition, and so on [4]. Recently, deep learning has been also applied to medical image reconstruction, such as accelerated MR image reconstruction [5]. Learning-based methods for image reconstruction have advantages, such as data-driven regularization for ill-posed problems and fast reconstruction times, but they require sufficient training data to avoid overfitting problems.

In this paper, we apply deep learning to correct metal-induced artifacts with a relatively short imaging time. A neural network is proposed to map two distorted images obtained with dual-polarity readout gradients into a distortion-free image from the fully phase encoding method. Simulated data are utilized to supplement and substitute real MR data for training the proposed network. Phantom experiments are performed to compare the quality of the reconstructed images from several methods at high and low readout bandwidths.

2   Background

An MR image (I) can be simply formulated as $I(\mathbf{r}) = \rho(\mathbf{r})\Delta R(\mathbf{r})$, where $\rho(\mathbf{r})$ and $\Delta R(\mathbf{r})$ are the average spin density within a voxel and the volume of a voxel at a position, $\mathbf{r} = (x, y, z)$, respectively.

In the presence of off-resonance frequency (δv), an MR image (I) is distorted from a typical spatial encoding mechanism with a frequency-encoding gradient and sequential phase-encoding gradients as follows:

$$I(\mathbf{r}) = I(x, y, z) \xrightarrow{\delta v(r)} I'(\mathbf{r}) = I\left(x - \frac{2\pi\delta v(\mathbf{r})}{\gamma G_x}, y, z\right) \tag{1}$$

where x is an index to represent a frequency-encoding direction, and y and z are indices to represent two phase-encoding directions in an image domain. In (1), γ and G_x are the gyromagnetic ratio of the imaged nuclei and the amplitude of the applied readout gradient (frequency-encoding). Bulk shifts are induced by off-resonance frequency along the frequency-encoding direction unlike the phase-encoding directions.

In the presence of a local gradient of off-resonance frequency ($\frac{\partial \delta v}{\partial r}$), the voxel volume ($\Delta R$) is also affected along the frequency-encoding direction as follows:

$$\Delta R(\mathbf{r}) = \Delta X(\mathbf{r})\Delta Y(\mathbf{r})\Delta Z(\mathbf{r}) \xrightarrow{\frac{\partial \delta v(r)}{\partial r}} \Delta R'(\mathbf{r}) = \frac{\Delta X(\mathbf{r})}{\left|1 + \frac{2\pi}{\gamma G_x}\frac{\partial \delta V(\mathbf{r})}{\partial X}\right|}\Delta Y(\mathbf{r})\Delta Z(\mathbf{r}) \tag{2}$$

where ΔX, ΔY, and ΔZ are voxel sizes in the x, y, and z directions, respectively. The distorted voxel volumes result in local hyper-intensities or hypo-intensities in the images [2].

The conventional 3D MSI methods acquire multispectral-bin images with high readout bandwidth, which reduces the bulk shifts to a single-voxel level [1, 2]. However, they suffer from residual artifacts, so-called pile-up or signal-void, in the presence of the strong local gradients of off-resonance frequencies near metallic implants [2].

To avoid artifacts induced by the frequency encoding, FPE methods utilize phase encoding instead of frequency encoding along the x direction [3]. The FPE methods require N_x times longer imaging time than 3D MSI techniques, where N_x is the number of encoding steps along the x direction.

3 Method

3.1 Proposed Neural Network

The proposed network, shown in Fig. 1, was designed to correct metal-induced arti-facts in a relatively short imaging time. The proposed network maps two distorted images, acquired with dual-polarity readout gradients in the frequency encoding direction, into a corrected image from the FPE method. The proposed network sub-stitutes two readout acquisitions for the N_x phase encoding steps of the FPE method, which reduces imaging time by $N_x/2$ times. Two distorted images have voxel shifts along opposite directions and have pile-up or signal-void in different locations. We assume that a distortion-free image can be estimated from the two distorted images.

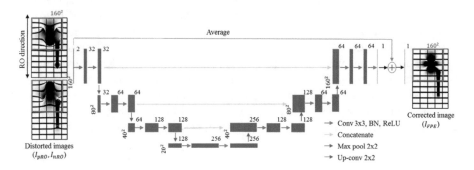

Fig. 1. Schematic diagram of the proposed neural network

The proposed network was modified from U-net [6]. Sub-images of two distorted images and the corresponding corrected image were utilized as the input and output, respectively, of the proposed network (red boxes). The convolutional layers were utilized to consider the bandlimited property of the field perturbation induced by a metallic implant. All convolutional layers used a kernel of 3×3, and the input of each convolution layer was zero-padded to keep the spatial dimensions. Batch normalization (BN) and rectified linear unit (ReLU) were sequentially applied after each convolu-tional layer (red arrows) [7, 8]. A multi-scale architecture using down-sampling and up-sampling operations (blue and green arrows) was utilized to efficiently increase the dependency of neighboring voxels and to consider the dispersed metal-induced arti-facts. Max pooling layers were utilized for down-sampling, and both the kernel size and the stride size of the max pooling layers were 2×2. The transposed convolution operation with a kernel of 3×3 and a stride of 2×2 was utilized for up-sampling, and the transposed convolution operation is represented as 'up-conv 2×2' in Fig. 1. The number of feature channels was doubled after each pooling layer, and was halved after each up-sampling layer. The concatenate layer of each scale (yellow arrows) was utilized to avoid the information loss of multi-scale features. The average layer (black arrow) was utilized to learn the residual values between the average distorted images and a corrected image, which helps keep learning stable and fast.

3.2 Generation of Training Data

To train the proposed network, sufficient training data is required. However, it is unrealistic and difficult to collect training data because too many resources are required, for example, long imaging time, expenses, and inter-scan patient motions. In this paper, training data was generated by simulations considering various conditions, and were then utilized to train the proposed network.

The overall scheme to generate training data for the proposed network is displayed in Fig. 2. We additionally generated susceptibility maps ($\chi(\mathbf{r})$) from the model of a total hip replacement implant [9] by randomly changing susceptibility values and performing erosion, dilation, and rotation operations. The off-resonance maps ($\delta v(\mathbf{r})$) can be computed from the generated susceptibility maps [10]. The average spin density of each spectral bin is computed as $\rho_b(\mathbf{r}) = \rho(\mathbf{r})RF(\delta v_b(\mathbf{r}))$, where RF is the RF excitation profile and $\delta v_b(\mathbf{r})$ is an actual frequency at each bin. Natural images from ImageNet 2012 dataset [11] were utilized for spin density, ρ. Natural images are easier to apply for ρ than real MR images, specifically for handling background regions outside the imaging objects, overfitting issues with imaging objects, and positioning of the metallic implants. For simplification, two dimensions of $\tilde{\mathbf{r}} = (x, y)$ were used rather than three dimensions of $\mathbf{r} = (x, y, z)$. Two distorted images using positive and negative readout gradients (I_{pRO}, I_{nRO}), respectively, were generated as follows:

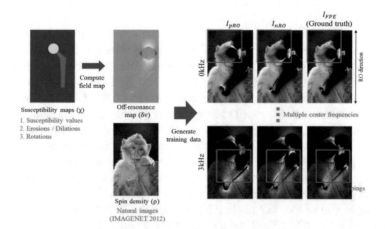

Fig. 2. Overall scheme to generate the training data

$$I_{pRO}(\tilde{\mathbf{r}}) = \rho_b\left(x - \frac{2\pi\delta v_b(\tilde{\mathbf{r}})}{\gamma G_x}, y\right)\frac{\Delta X(\tilde{\mathbf{r}})}{\left|1 + \frac{2\pi}{\gamma G_x}\frac{\partial \delta v_b(\tilde{\mathbf{r}})}{\partial X}\right|}\Delta Y(\tilde{\mathbf{r}}) \tag{3}$$

$$I_{nRO}(\tilde{\mathbf{r}}) = \rho_b\left(x + \frac{2\pi\delta v_b(\tilde{\mathbf{r}})}{\gamma G_x}, y\right)\frac{\Delta X(\tilde{\mathbf{r}})}{\left|1 - \frac{2\pi}{\gamma G_x}\frac{\partial \delta v_b(\tilde{\mathbf{r}})}{\partial X}\right|}\Delta Y(\tilde{\mathbf{r}}) \tag{4}$$

A corresponding corrected image (I_{FPE}) for the desired output of the proposed network was generated as $I_{FPE}(\tilde{\mathbf{r}}) = \rho_b(\tilde{\mathbf{r}})\Delta X(\tilde{\mathbf{r}})\Delta Y(\tilde{\mathbf{r}})$.

3.3 Training of the Proposed Neural Network

The generated images for input and output of the proposed network were normalized by dividing by the maximum value of the input to enable the input and output to have a specific intensity range from 0 to 1. The loss function to train the proposed network was defined as the sum of a typical 2-norm loss and the image gradient difference loss. The image gradient difference loss helps to avoid blurry results in the estimated output [12]. Weight values of the proposed network were initialized by random values with uniform distribution [13]. To minimize the loss function, ADAM optimizer was applied using a learning rate of 0.0005 [14]. The proposed network was implemented using a deep learning package, 'TensorFlow', on a personal computer with an Intel Quad Core i7-3770 3.4 GHz and a NVIDIA Geforce GTX TITAN-x [15]. To train the proposed network, 120,000 sets for input and output were utilized, and 50 thousand back propagations were performed using a learning batch size of 64. It took 8 h in the personal computer environment.

3.4 Metal Artifact Correction Using the Proposed Neural Network

To give the distorted MR images appropriate intensity levels, the distorted MR images were normalized by dividing by the maximum value of the distorted MR images. Two sets of multi-spectral images were acquired using dual-polarity readout gradients. After the normalization, two distorted images of each spectral bin were utilized as the input of the learned network to estimate the corrected image of each spectral bin. A final image using the proposed method was reconstructed using the root-sum-of-squares (RSOS) of the multiple spectral bins.

3.5 Evaluation of the Proposed Methods

Multi-acquisition with variable resonance image combination (MAVRIC), whose spectral-bin images are utilized for the input of the proposed network, was compared with the proposed method. Two MAVRIC images using positive and negative readout gradients were reconstructed using RSOS along the spectral-bins dimension.

To analyze the gains from the deep network and dual-polarity images, an additional network was learned, denoted as 'DL(pRO)', representing deep learning using only the positive readout image. The only difference between DL(pRO) and the proposed method is that DL(pRO) utilizes a distorted image obtained with only the positive readout gradient for input, but the proposed method utilizes two distorted images obtained by positive and negative readout gradients for input.

3.6   Phantom Experiments

Phantom experiments were conducted using the 3T MRI system (Siemens Verio, Germany). Two physical phantoms with different sizes were imaged for validation and test sets, respectively. The phantom for the test set contained a hip joint replacement implant consisting of a femoral head and a femoral stem. The implant was fixed with acryl grids, and filled with CuSO4 solution. The phantom made for the validation set was relatively small in order to reduce the field of view and the imaging time. The small phantom only contained a femoral head, fixed with acryl grids, filled with CuSO4 solution.

To optimize the hyper-parameters, a few validation sets were acquired. Their imaging parameters were as follows: TR/TE = 800/5 ms, the number of spectral bins = 1 (Gaussian RF profiles with 2.25 full-width-half-maximum on resonance frequency), matrix size = $160 \times 160 \times 20$, voxel size = $1 \times 1 \times 5$ mm^3, echo train length (ETL) = 8, and readout bandwidth = 780 Hz/pixel. The imaging times for input and output were 10 m 40 s (2×320 s), and 14 h and 14 m, respectively.

To show the performance of the proposed method, test sets were acquired using dual polarity readout gradients; the corresponding output was not acquired because the imaging time was too long. Their imaging parameters were as follows: TR/TE = 800/5 ms, the number of spectral bins = 25 (Gaussian RF profiles with 2.25 full-width-half-maximum separated by 1 kHz), matrix size = $512 \times 160 \times 20$, voxel size = $1 \times 1 \times 5$ mm^3, and echo train length (ETL) = 8. The imaging time was 4 h 26 m (2×8000 s). The phantom experiments were performed for two cases: high readout bandwidth = 780 Hz/pixel (Fig. 3), and low readout bandwidth = 390 Hz/pixel (Fig. 4).

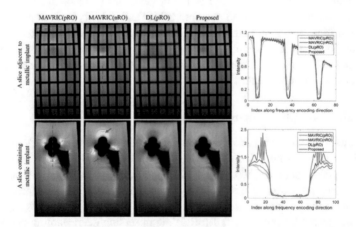

Fig. 3. Corrected images from several methods at high readout bandwidth (780 Hz/pixel), and cut views along the red dotted lines.

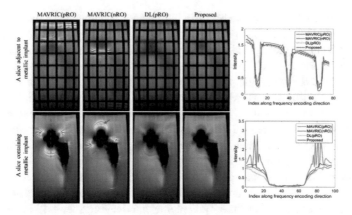

Fig. 4. Corrected images from several methods at low readout bandwidth (390 Hz/pixel), and cut views along the red dotted lines.

4   Experiment Results

Figures 3 and 4 show the corrected images from several methods, which include slices containing and adjacent to metallic implant at high and low readout bandwidths, respectively. As shown in the cut views of Fig. 3, the blurring artifacts of the images from MAVRIC are invisible because bulk shifts are reduced to a single-voxel level. However, the images from MAVRIC have residual pile-up and signal-loss artifacts (blue arrows). The residual artifacts are resolved well in the image from the proposed method. DL(pRO) suppresses the residual artifacts, but the effect is somewhat partial and blurry because of insufficient information.

As the readout bandwidth decreases, the metal-induced artifacts become more severe in the images from MAVRIC as shown in Fig. 4. The size of bulk shifts is in inverse proportion to the amplitude of the applied readout gradient in (1). Although the bulk shifts are limited to a single-voxel level at high readout bandwidth, which is typically utilized in 3D MSI methods, the bulk shifts increase as the readout bandwidth decreases. This effect is easily observed even in locations distant from the metallic implant in Fig. 4 (red arrows). Likewise, pile-up and signal-loss artifacts grow worse as the readout bandwidth decreases. The proposed method significantly suppresses the metal-induced artifacts using deep learning and dual-polarity readout gradients.

5   Discussion and Conclusion

The proposed method suppressed metal-induced artifacts by utilizing deep learning and two images obtained using dual-polarity readout gradients. To save resources needed to collect training data, and to avoid regulation issues for medical data, the proposed network was learned from simulated data, which could be an efficient strategy to supplement insufficient training data. The proposed method estimated a FPE image from two 3D MSI images, which reduced imaging time $N_x/2$ times faster than FPE.

Conventional 3D MSI methods utilize high readout bandwidth to reduce bulk shifts to a single-voxel level. The proposed method significantly suppressed the metal-induced artifacts at the halved readout bandwidth. This means that the proposed method can work at double bandwidth of the RF excitation pulse. Using broad bandwidth of the RF excitation pulse allows the number of spectral bins to be reduced. Of course, we utilized a 3T MRI system in this paper, and the bandwidth of the Gaussian RF pulse was limited by the peak amplitude of the RF, in consideration of the specific absorption rate (SAR). The proposed method would work more efficiently with a lower field MRI system because the bandwidth of the RF pulse could be increased within the SAR limitation.

The proposed method was proven only in phantom experiments. In-vivo experiments would be studied in future works. In addition, the imaging sequence would be optimized to reduce imaging time by applying interleaving spectral bins and parallel imaging.

Acknowledgement. This research was supported by Institute for Information & communications Technology Promotion (IITP) grant funded by the Korea government (MSIT) (No. 2017-0-01778).

References

1. Koch, K.M., et al.: A multispectral three-dimensional acquisition technique for imaging near metal implants. MRM **61**, 381–390 (2009)
2. Koch, K.M., et al.: Imaging near metal: the impact of extreme static local field gradients on frequency encoding processes. MRM **71**, 2024–2034 (2014)
3. Ramos-Cabrer, P., et al.: MRI of hip prostheses using single-point methods: in vitro studies towards the artifact-free imaging of individuals with metal implants. MRI **22**, 1097–1103 (2004)
4. Greenspan, H., et al.: Guest editorial deep learning in medical imaging: overview and future promise of an exciting new technique. IEEE TMI **35**, 1153–1159 (2016)
5. Kwon, K., et al.: A parallel MR imaging method using multilayer perceptron. Med. Phys. **44**, 6209–6224 (2017)
6. Ronneberger, O., Fischer, P., Brox, T.: U-Net: convolutional networks for biomedical image segmentation. In: Navab, N., Hornegger, J., Wells, W.M., Frangi, A.F. (eds.) MICCAI 2015. LNCS, vol. 9351, pp. 234–241. Springer, Cham (2015). https://doi.org/10.1007/978-3-319-24574-4_28
7. Ioffe, S., Szegedy C.: Batch normalization: accelerating deep network training by reducing internal covariate shift. In: ICML, pp. 448–456 (2015)
8. Glorot, X., Bordes, A., Bengio, Y.: Deep sparse rectifier neural networks. In: ICAIS, pp. 315–323 (2011)
9. Shi, X., et al.: Metallic implant geometry and susceptibility estimation using multispectral B0 field maps. MRM **77**, 2402–2413 (2017)
10. Koch, K.M., et al.: Rapid calculations of susceptibility-induced magnetostatic field perturbations for in vivo magnetic resonance. PMB **51**, 6381–6402 (2006)
11. Russakovsky, O., et al.: ImageNet large scale visual recognition challenge. Int. J. Comput. Vis. **115**, 211–252 (2015)

12. Mathieu, M., et al.: Deep multi-scale video prediction beyond mean square error. In: ICLR (2016)
13. Glorot, X., Bengio, Y.: Understanding the difficulty of training deep feedforward neural networks. In: ICAIS, pp. 249–256 (2010)
14. Kingma, D.P., Ba, J.L.: ADAM: a method for stochastic optimization. In: ICLR (2015)
15. Abadi, M, et al.: TensorFlow: a system for large-scale machine learning. In: 12th USENIX Symposium on Operating Systems Design and Implementation, vol. **16**, pp. 265–283 (2016)

Motion Aware MR Imaging via Spatial Core Correspondence

Christoph Jud[1]([⊠]), Damien Nguyen[1,2], Robin Sandkühler[1], Alina Giger[1], Oliver Bieri[1,2], and Philippe C. Cattin[1]

[1] Department of Biomedical Engineering, University of Basel, Allschwil, Switzerland
christoph.jud@unibas.ch
[2] Department of Radiology, Division of Radiological Physics, University Hospital Basel, Basel, Switzerland

Abstract. Motion awareness in MR imaging is essential when it comes to long acquisition times. For volumetric high-resolution or temporal resolved images, sporadic subject movements or respiration induced organ motion has to be considered in order to reduce motion artifacts. We present a novel MR imaging sequence and an associated retrospective reconstruction method incorporating motion via spatial correspondence of the k-space center. The sequence alternatingly samples k-space patches located in the center and in peripheral higher frequency regions. Each patch is transformed into the spatial domain in order to normalize for spatial transformations rigidly as well as non-rigidly. The k-space is reconstructed from the spatially aligned patches where the alignment is derived using image registration of the center patches. Our proposed method assumes neither periodic motion nor requires any binning of motion states to properly compensate for movements during acquisition. As we directly acquire volumes, 2D slice stacking is avoided. We tested our method for brain imaging with sporadic head motion and for chest imaging where a volunteer has been scanned under free breathing. In both cases, we demonstrate high-quality 3D reconstructions.

Keywords: Magnetic Resonance Imaging · Motion correction 4DMRI

1 Introduction

The presence of subject motion during magnetic resonance (MR) imaging is a critical factor particularly for brain, arm and leg imaging. When not explicitly considered, it can results in motion artifacts which render the image acquisition useless. Especially for uncooperative subjects such as pediatric, stroke or Parkinson patients a lot of time is wasted in the clinic with re-scanning. Furthermore, organ movements induced by natural respiration are challenging to handle in chest imaging, as e.g. lung patients cannot be asked for breath holding. Hence, when it comes to longer acquisition times, for volumetric high-resolution or dynamic 3D imaging, motion needs to be taken into account.

© Springer Nature Switzerland AG 2018
A. F. Frangi et al. (Eds.): MICCAI 2018, LNCS 11070, pp. 198–205, 2018.
https://doi.org/10.1007/978-3-030-00928-1_23

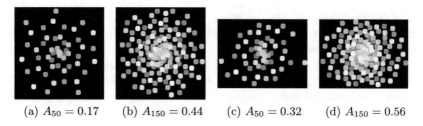

(a) $A_{50} = 0.17$ (b) $A_{150} = 0.44$ (c) $A_{50} = 0.32$ (d) $A_{150} = 0.56$

Fig. 1. Sampling pattern for the first and second phase encoding dimension in the k-space: 128×128 px and 128×96 px with a shift-factor of $b = 16$ and $b = 1$ respectively, at time points $t = 50$ and $t = 150$. Patches at higher time points are visualized brighter. The center patch is colorized in yellow.

In this paper, we present a novel motion aware MR imaging method which can deal with spatial movements, including *rigid* and *non-rigid* ones. The key idea is that the k-space is sampled patch-wise such that each patch can be transformed into the spatial domain. Specifically, patches in the k-space center and patches in higher frequency regions are sampled alternatingly. A high frequency patch can thus be corrected for the relative motion between its simultaneously acquired center patch and a reference one. The spatial transformation between two center patches is obtained using image registration. The k-space at a given time-point is finally reconstructed using the motion corrected patches by accumulating their frequency representation. We demonstrate a high-quality 3D reconstruction of a brain image acquired under sporadic head movements. In addition, we are able to reconstruct a chest image acquiring under free breathing.

Motion correction in MR imaging has been widely studied in the past decades. For a comprehensive review about motion correction methods we refer to [13] and for a focus on prospective methods to [5]. Prospective methods correct the pulse sequence according to the subject motion during acquisition. They generally require additional equipment such as optical tracking systems or active markers and are therefore difficult to implement in the clinic. Methods which rely on k-space or image navigators [12] require unused time in the sequence to acquire accurate motion information and have real-time constraints which restricts the computational budget. Retrospective approaches try to invert the motion affected changes in the acquired data after the acquisition has ended. Most retrospective as well as prospective methods are limited to rigid body motion with up to 6 degrees of freedom. Non-rigid motion remains a major challenge. Approaches which consider non-rigid motion are based on gating/triggering [10], binning of motion states [4], are limited to 2D [1,7] or perform a piece-wise rigid approximation of the non-rigid motion [1,4]. In present 4D approaches, partial image data is acquired over several periodic motion cycles and retrospectively sorted using surrogate signals or image similarity measures in order to reconstruct coherent volumes [11]. It is, however, difficult to validate that the reconstructed partial data yields a valid 3D volume.

Our contributions are the following: our method is able to correct for non-rigid motion, which is derived from low-frequency representations of the imaged object, without the use of rigid approximation techniques. At each time-point a full 3D volume can be reconstructed. The specific k-space sampling pattern of our sequence allows for a gradual increase of the image quality. For our method, neither periodic motion has to be assumed nor binning of motion states or gating is required. As we acquire volumes, 2D slice stacking is avoided.

2   Method

For large 3D volumes, conventional k-space sampling strategies often exceed the time frame given for moving structure. Our idea is therefore, to split the k-space into smaller patches which are sampled at a high-temporal rate where motion artifacts are not dominant. Patches in the k-space center and peripheral patches in higher frequency regions are sampled alternatingly. The center patches, transformed into the spatial domain, are low-frequency representations of the imaged object and are used to estimate relative spatial transformations. Due to the patch-wise sampling not only the center but also high-frequencies can be transformed into the spatial domain where they are rigidly and non-rigidly aligned with the transformation found using the center patches.

2.1   Sequence

For this work, a product sequence for a radio-frequency spoiled gradient echo acquisition with short repetition time and low flip angles [2] was modified in order to alter the sampling of k-space. The full resolution in the readout direction is acquired with a short repetition time. In the first and second phase encoding dimensions circular patches are pseudo-randomly sampled.

Undersampling of the k-space. The patch-wise undersampling should cover the k-space with a variable density which is higher in low-frequency regions to improve the fidelity of the reconstructed images. Furthermore, it should gradually increase the coverage of the k-space such that at any time the acquisition can be stopped while the k-space coverage is maximized. At each time point where a patch is sampled therefore, an image can be flexibly reconstructed using patches of an arbitrary time interval. To this end, frequencies which are sampled multiple times should be averaged which results in a gradual increase of the image quality. To integrate these features into our sequence, the peripheral patch centers are derived by a variant of the radial CIRCUS method [3], a low discrepancy additive recurrence sequence for pseudo-randomly sample the k-space.

We define the sampling sequence in the first two phase encoding dimensions as follows: Let $N_{\min}$ be the number of k-space points of the smaller of the two dimensions. With patch radii r_p we define the patch centers $k_c \in \mathbb{R}^2$ as

$$
\begin{aligned}
k_{c_1} &= \cos\left(2\pi m K^{-1}\right) r \\
k_{c_2} &= \sin\left(2\pi m K^{-1}\right) r
\end{aligned}, \quad
m = \left\lfloor \left(\frac{s+t}{\alpha} \mod 1\right) K \right\rfloor,
\tag{1}
$$

where $\alpha = \frac{1+\sqrt{5}}{2}$ is the golden angle ratio, $K = 1000$ the number of points along a perimeter, $r = \frac{t \cdot N_{\min}}{2\delta}$ is the radius with steps $\delta = \frac{2N_{\min}}{2r_p+1} - 1$, T the number of time points $t \in \{0, 1, 2, \ldots, T\}$ and $s := b \cdot r$ where $b \in \mathbb{N}_+$ is a shift parameter. If the number of points in the two dimensions is not equal, the radius r is adjusted accordingly. We optimize b such that the k-space coverage A_T with T time points is maximized

$$\underset{b \leq 100}{\arg\max} \sum_{T \in \{10,20,\ldots,300\}} \log A_T. \tag{2}$$

In Fig. 1, examples of the patch sampling sequence are visualized with a center patch radius of 6 px and peripheral patch radius of 5 px.

2.2 Reconstruction

For each time point t, a part of the k-space $P_t \subset \mathbb{C}^3$ is sampled consisting of a patch in the center (core) C_t and a high-frequency peripheral patch H_t. The relative spatial motion $u_t : \mathcal{X} \to \mathbb{R}^3$ on the image domain $\mathcal{X} \subset \mathbb{R}^3$ between a reference patch P_r and any other patch P_t is derived via correspondence estimation between the reference core C_r and C_t in the spatial domain:

$$u_t := \underset{u}{\arg\min} \; \mathcal{D}\big(\mathcal{F}^{-1}(C_r) \circ u, \mathcal{F}^{-1}(C_t)\big), \tag{3}$$

where $\mathcal{D}$ is a dissimilarity measure, $\mathcal{F}^{-1}$ is the inverse Fourier transform and $\circ$ the function composition. For the reconstruction of an image I_r at the reference time point we distinguish between rigid and non-rigid transformations u_t.

Rigid Reconstruction. In the special case of a rigid transformation the motion correction can be directly performed in the k-space while the registration is still performed in the spatial domain. The spatial translation $\Delta x_t \in \mathbb{R}^3$ corresponds to a phase shift in the k-space and the spatial rotation with the rotation matrix R_t is equivalent to the same rotation in the k-space:

$$P_t^{\Delta x}(k_x) := e^{i2\pi(k_x^T \Delta x_t)} P_t(k_x) \tag{4}$$

$$\hat{P}_t(k_x) = P_t^{\Delta x}(R_t k_x), \tag{5}$$

where k_x is the k-space coordinate and $\hat{P}_t$ is the rigidly corrected patch of P_t. The reconstruction yields

$$\hat{I}_r = \mathcal{F}^{-1}\left(\hat{W} \sum_{t=1}^{T} \hat{P}_t\right), \tag{6}$$

$$\hat{W}(k_x) = \begin{cases} \frac{1}{\hat{w}_{k_x}} & \hat{w}_{k_x} > 0 \\ 1 & \text{otherwise} \end{cases}, \quad \hat{w}_{k_x} = \sum_{t=1}^{T} \hat{W}^t(k_x), \quad \hat{W}^t(k_x) = \begin{cases} 1 & |\hat{P}_t(k_x)| > 0 \\ 0 & \text{otherwise}, \end{cases}$$

where $\hat{W}$ normalizes overlapping patch regions.

Non-Rigid Reconstruction. For non-rigid transformations, the motion correction is performed in the spatial domain. The reconstruction is

$$\tilde{I}_r = \mathcal{F}^{-1}\left(\widetilde{W}\sum_{t=1}^{T}\mathcal{F}\Big(\mathcal{F}^{-1}(P_t)\circ u_t\Big)\right), \tag{7}$$

where $\mathcal{F}$ is the forward Fourier transform. In the non-rigid case, it is not clear how to derive an exact normalization $\widetilde{W}$ which would correspond to the normalization $\hat{W}$ in the rigid case. This is because the non-rigid transformed patch $\tilde{P}_t = \mathcal{F}\big(\mathcal{F}^{-1}(P_t)\circ u_t\big)$ contains frequencies not present in P_t. To still derive a valid reconstruction of the k-space, we propose to keep only motion corrected points which originally have a non-zero magnitude

$$\bar{I}_r = \mathcal{F}^{-1}\left(W\sum_{t=1}^{T}W^t\mathcal{F}\Big(\mathcal{F}^{-1}(P_t)\circ u_t\Big)\right), \tag{8}$$

$$W(k_x) = \begin{cases} \frac{1}{w_{k_x}} & w_{k_x} > 0 \\ 1 & \text{otherwise} \end{cases}, \quad w_{k_x} = \sum_{t=1}^{T}W^t(k_x), \quad W^t(k_x) = \begin{cases} 1 & |P_t(k_x)| > 0 \\ 0 & \text{otherwise,} \end{cases}$$

where W normalizes overlapping patches. Upcoming frequencies $\tilde{P}_t \cap P_t$ which are masked out by W^t are covered by other patches located at the respective k-space region.

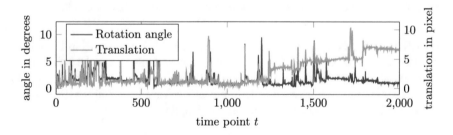

Fig. 2. Measured rigid head motion using the rigid registration.

3   Results

We demonstrate the reconstruction performance of our method on brain MR imaging under sporadic head motion and on dynamic chest MR imaging under free breathing. The volunteers were scanned at 3 T using a Siemens MAGNE-TOM Prisma. We distinguish between three variants of our method: *Static* where no motion correction is performed ($u_t = id$), *Rigid* where the rigid motion correction is performed directly in the k-space cf. Eq. 6 and *Non-rigid* where the motion is corrected non-rigidly using Eq. 8. In all acquisitions, the center and peripheral patch radius was set to 6 and 5 pixels respectively yielding 109 and 69 k-space pixels to sample in the first two phase encoding dimensions per time point. The signals from multiple coils are combined in the spatial domain using the absolute sum of squares method [8].

3.1 Brain Experiment *Rigid* Reconstruction

We asked the volunteer to sporadically move their head during the acquisition of 2000 time points. In Fig. 2, the rotation angle and translation estimated by the rigid registration are plotted. The first two phase encoding dimensions have been set to the traversal plane with a size of 160 × 144 px while the readout direction

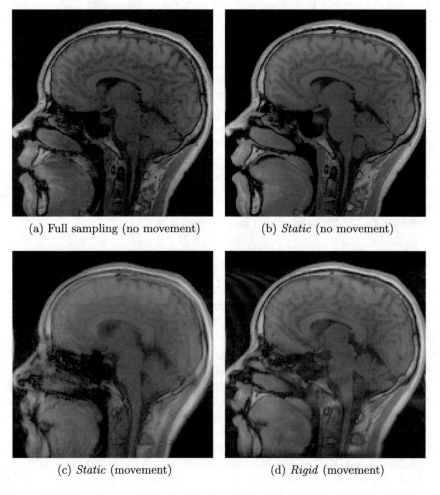

(a) Full sampling (no movement)   (b) *Static* (no movement)

(c) *Static* (movement)   (d) *Rigid* (movement)

Fig. 3. (a) Full k-space sampling (no head motion), (b) *Static* reconstruction (no head motion), (c) *Static* reconstruction (with head motion), (d) *Rigid* motion compensated reconstruction (with head motion).

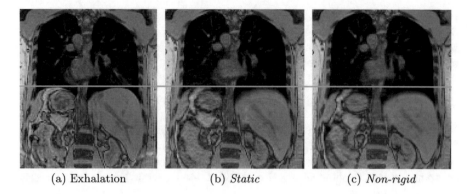

(a) Exhalation   (b) *Static*   (c) *Non-rigid*

Fig. 4. (a) Breath-hold reference exhalation scan, (b) *Static* and (c) *Non-rigid* reconstruction under free-breathing. For comparison, the green line marks the exhalation level of the diaphragm.

was craniocaudal with 160 px. With an echo time of TE = 2.5 ms and a repetition time of TR = 5.9 ms the duration of a time point yields $\sim$ 1 s. In the registration (Eq. 3), the Mattes' mutual information dissimilarity metric [6] has been used. For a reference scan, we repeated the experiment but with the volunteer holding their head still. In Fig. 3, a sagittal slice of the reconstructed volume from the different reconstruction variants are shown. Comparing the reconstruction of the full k-space and the *Static* reconstruction of the reference scan *Static* achieves a better image quality which is the result of the high oversampling. By considering rigid motion, *Rigid* substantially reduces motion artifacts and generally yields better quality and higher contrast than *Static*. Some intensity inhomogeneities remain e.g. in the brain stem and mouth regions.

3.2 Chest Experiment *Non-rigid* Reconstruction

The chest has been acquired under free breathing for 2000 time points. The first two phase encoding dimensions have been set to the sagittal plane with a size of 256 $\times$ 88 px while the readout direction was left-right with 128 px. With an echo time of TE = 1.0 ms and a repetition time of TR = 2.5 ms the duration of a time point yields 445 ms. For the registration, a graph-based method [9] has been used applying the local cross correlation as dissimilarity measure. A reference core in inhalation state was chosen. In its spatial representation, the expected sliding boundaries have been masked and considered in the registration. Figure 4a shows a reference breath-hold scan at exhalation with full k-space sampling. Due to the averaging, *Static* reconstructs a perceived exhalation state, as this is the most frequent respiratory state in natural breathing (Fig. 4b). However, a lot of details are lost and motion lines are visible especially in the liver. With our method (Fig. 4c), the respiratory state of the reconstruction can be controlled by selecting the reference core. Hence, *Non-rigid* reconstructs a high quality image in inhalation state, where the motion lines are disappeared.

4   Conclusion

We have presented a new 3D MR imaging method which corrects for rigid and non-rigid subject motion derived from the k-space center. The introduced sequence samples the k-space patch-wise which allows to correct for non-rigid transformations for each patch separately. We demonstrated the feasibility of the method with a brain acquisition under sporadic movements and a chest acquisition under free-breathing. In both cases, we have achieved high-quality reconstructions. We plan to investigate compressed sensing reconstructions which will allow to drastically improve acquisition time by acquiring fewer time points.

References

1. Batchelor, P., Atkinson, D., Irarrazaval, P., Hill, D., Hajnal, J., Larkman, D.: Matrix description of general motion correction applied to multishot images. Magn. Reson. Med. **54**(5), 1273–1280 (2005)
2. Haase, A., Frahm, J., Matthaei, D., Hanicke, W., Merboldt, K.D.: Flash imaging. rapid NMR imaging using low flip-angle pulses. J. Magn. Reson. **67**(2), 258–266 (1986)
3. Liu, J., Saloner, D.: Accelerated MRI with CIRcular Cartesian UnderSampling (CIRCUS): a variable density cartesian sampling strategy for compressed sensing and parallel imaging. Quant. Imaging Med. Surg. **4**(1), 57 (2014)
4. Luo, J., et al.: Nonrigid motion correction with 3D image-based navigators for coronary mr angiography. Magn. Reson. Med. **77**(5), 1884–1893 (2017)
5. Maclaren, J., Herbst, M., Speck, O., Zaitsev, M.: Prospective motion correction in brain imaging: a review. Magn. Reson. Med. **69**(3), 621–636 (2013)
6. Mattes, D., Haynor, D.R., Vesselle, H., Lewellen, T.K., Eubank, W.: PET-CT image registration in the chest using free-form deformations. IEEE Trans. Med. Imaging **22**(1), 120–128 (2003)
7. Pipe, J.G., et al.: Motion correction with PROPELLER MRI: application to head motion and free-breathing cardiac imaging. Magn. Reson. Med. **42**(5), 963–969 (1999)
8. Roemer, P.B., Edelstein, W.A., Hayes, C.E., Souza, S.P., Mueller, O.: The NMR phased array. Magn. Reson. Med. **16**(2), 192–225 (1990)
9. Sandkühler, R., Jud, C., Pezold, S., Cattin, P.C.: Adaptive graph diffusion regularisation for discontinuity preserving image registration. In: Klein, S., Staring, M., Durrleman, S., Sommer, S. (eds.) WBIR 2018. LNCS, vol. 10883, pp. 24–34. Springer, Cham (2018). https://doi.org/10.1007/978-3-319-92258-4_3
10. Schmidt, J.F., Buehrer, M., Boesiger, P., Kozerke, S.: Nonrigid retrospective respiratory motion correction in whole-heart coronary MRA. Magn. Reson. Med. **66**(6), 1541–1549 (2011)
11. von Siebenthal, M., Szekely, G., Gamper, U., Boesiger, P., Lomax, A., Cattin, P.: 4D MR imaging of respiratory organ motion and its variability. Phys. Med. Biol. **52**(6), 1547 (2007)
12. White, N., et al.: Promo: Real-time prospective motion correction in MRI using image-based tracking. Magn. Reson. Med. **63**(1), 91–105 (2010)
13. Zaitsev, M., Maclaren, J., Herbst, M.: Motion artifacts in MRI: a complex problem with many partial solutions. J. Magn. Reson. Imaging **42**(4), 887–901 (2015)

Nonparametric Density Flows for MRI Intensity Normalisation

Daniel C. Castro$^{(\boxtimes)}$ and Ben Glocker

Biomedical Image Analysis Group, Imperial College London,
London, UK
{dc315,b.glocker}@imperial.ac.uk

Abstract. With the adoption of powerful machine learning methods in medical image analysis, it is becoming increasingly desirable to aggregate data that is acquired across multiple sites. However, the underlying assumption of many analysis techniques that corresponding tissues have consistent intensities in all images is often violated in multi-centre databases. We introduce a novel intensity normalisation scheme based on density matching, wherein the histograms are modelled as Dirichlet process Gaussian mixtures. The source mixture model is transformed to minimise its L^2 divergence towards a target model, then the voxel intensities are transported through a mass-conserving flow to maintain agreement with the moving density. In a multi-centre study with brain MRI data, we show that the proposed technique produces excellent correspondence between the matched densities and histograms. We further demonstrate that our method makes tissue intensity statistics substantially more compatible between images than a baseline affine transformation and is comparable to state-of-the-art while providing considerably smoother transformations. Finally, we validate that nonlinear intensity normalisation is a step toward effective imaging data harmonisation.

1 Introduction

Many medical image analysis methods rely on the hypothesis that corresponding anatomical structures present similar intensity profiles. Unlike computed tomography, magnetic resonance imaging does not produce scans in an absolute standard scale, in general. Even when using the same imaging protocols, there can be significant variation between different scanners. Acquisition parameters have a complex effect on the luminance of the acquired images, therefore a simple linear rescaling of intensities is usually insufficient for effective data harmonisation [5]. Therefore, a crucial factor for enabling the construction of large-scale image databases from multiple sites is accurate nonlinear intensity normalisation.

A number of different approaches have been introduced for this task (cf. [1]), the most widely-adopted of which is that of Nyúl et al. [7]. The authors proposed to normalise intensities by matching a set of histogram quantiles, using these as landmarks for a piecewise linear transformation. Despite its apparent simplicity, it has proven very effective in clinical applications [9].

© Springer Nature Switzerland AG 2018
A. F. Frangi et al. (Eds.): MICCAI 2018, LNCS 11070, pp. 206–214, 2018.
https://doi.org/10.1007/978-3-030-00928-1_24

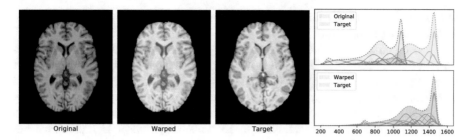

Fig. 1. Comparison of two MRI scans, before and after the proposed NDFLOW normalisation. *Right:* histograms (shaded) and fitted mixture models (*dotted:* likelihood, *solid:* mixture components).

Our proposed method, nonparametric density flows (NDFLOW), is perhaps conceptually closest to [5], which involves matching Gaussian mixture models (GMMs) fitted to a pair of image histograms. The author used a finite mixture to represent a pre-defined set of five tissues classes, whereas we propose to use nonparametric mixtures, focusing on accurately modelling the density rather than discriminating tissue types, and sidestepping the problem of pre-selecting the number of components. A further difference to our work is that, instead of polynomially interpolating between the means of corresponding components, we build a smooth transformation model based on density flows.

2   Method

We begin by justifying and describing the density model used to represent the intensity distributions to be matched. We then introduce the chosen objective function with its gradients for optimisation. Finally, we present our flow-based transformation model, which deforms the data so it conforms to the matched density model. Note that we focus here on single-modality intensity normalisation, although the entire formulation below extends naturally to the multivariate case.

2.1   Intensity Model

In order to be able to match the intensity distributions of a pair of images, a suitable probability density model is required. Typically, finite mixture models are considered for this task [5,8]. However, a well-known limitation of these is the requirement to specify a priori a fixed number of components, which may in addition call for an iterative model selection loop (e.g. [8]).

On the opposite end of the spectrum, another approach is to use kernel density estimation, which is widespread for shape registration (e.g. [4,6]). However, this formulation would result in an unwieldy optimisation problem, involving thousands or millions of parameters and all pairwise interactions. Furthermore, the derived transformation would likely not be satisfactorily smooth without additional regularisation.

To overcome both issues we propose to use Dirichlet process Gaussian mixture models (DPGMMs) [3]. Instead of specifying a fixed number of components, they rely on a vague concentration parameter, which regulates the expected amount of clustering fragmentation and enables them to adapt their complexity to the data at hand. By allowing an unbounded number of components and setting a versatile prior on the mixture proportions, they appear as a parsimonious middle ground for flexibility and tractability.

We fit the DPGMMs to each image's intensities using variational inference [2]. More specifically, we implemented an efficient weighted variant to fit a mixture directly to each 1D histogram.

2.2   Density Matching

The first step is to perform a coarse affine alignment by matching the moving density's first and second moments to the target's, accounting for arbitrary translation and rescaling of the values. This same affine transformation is then also applied to the data before the nonlinear warping takes place.

We quantify the disagreement between two probability density functions q and p on a probability space $\mathcal{X}$ by means of the L^2 divergence:

$$D_{L^2}[q,p] = \tfrac{1}{2}\|q - p\|^2 = \tfrac{1}{2}\|q\|^2 + \tfrac{1}{2}\|p\|^2 - \langle q, p \rangle, \tag{1}$$

where $\langle q, p \rangle = \int q(x)\,p(x)\,\mathrm{d}x$ is the L^2 inner product and $\|q\| = \sqrt{\langle q, q \rangle}$ is its induced norm. Aside from being symmetric, this quantity is positive and reaches zero iff $q \overset{\text{a.e.}}{=} p$. Crucially, unlike the usual Kullback–Leibler divergence, it is expressible in closed form for Gaussian mixture densities.

Let $q = \sum_k \pi_k q_k$ and $p = \sum_m \tau_m p_m$ denote two Gaussian mixtures, with components $q_k(x) = \mathcal{N}(x \mid \mu_k, \lambda_k^{-1})$ and $p_m(x) = \mathcal{N}(x \mid \nu_m, \omega_m^{-1})$. Equation (1) has tractable gradients w.r.t. the parameters of q, which we use to optimise its components' means $\{\mu_k\}_k$ and precisions $\{\lambda_k\}_k$ (cf. extended version).[1]

We have found, in practice, that it is largely unnecessary to adapt the mixing proportions, $\{\pi_k\}_k$, to get an excellent agreement between mixture densities. In fact, changing the mixture weights would require transferring samples *between* mixture components. Although surely possible, we point out that in the context of histogram matching this would imply altering their semantic value (e.g. consider a mixture of two well-separated components representing different tissue types).

2.3   Warping

After matching one GMM to another, we also need a way to transform the data modelled by that GMM so it matches the target data. To this end, we draw

---

[1] Available at: http://arxiv.org/abs/1806.02613.

inspiration from fluid mechanics and define the warping transformation, f, as the trajectories of particles under the effect of a velocity field u over time, taking the probability density q for the mechanical mass density. The key property that such flow must satisfy is *conservation of mass*: $\partial_t q + \partial_x (qu) = 0$, where $t \mapsto q^{(t)}$ is specified directly from the density matching.

Let us first consider the case of warping a single mixture component. A random variable $x \sim \mathcal{N}(\mu_k, \lambda_k^{-1})$ can be expressed via a diffeomorphic reparametrisation of a standard Gaussian, with $x = \psi_k(\epsilon) = \mu_k + \epsilon/\sqrt{\lambda_k}$ and $\epsilon \sim \mathcal{N}(0, 1)$. Assuming its mean and precision are changing with rates $\dot{\mu}_k$ and $\dot{\lambda}_k$, respectively, we can introduce a velocity field $u_k = \dot{\psi}_k \circ \psi_k^{-1}$ for its samples so that they agree with this evolving density. The instantaneous velocity at 'time' t is thus given by

$$u_k^{(t)}(x) = \dot{\mu}_k^{(t)} - \frac{\dot{\lambda}_k^{(t)}}{2\lambda_k^{(t)}} \left(x - \mu_k^{(t)}\right). \tag{2}$$

In the case of a mixture with constant weights $\{\pi_k\}_k$, we can construct a smooth, *mass-conserving* global velocity field u as

$$u^{(t)}(x) = \sum_k \frac{\pi_k q_k^{(t)}(x)}{q^{(t)}(x)} u_k^{(t)}(x), \tag{3}$$

which is simply a point-wise convex combination of each component's velocity field, u_k, weighted by the corresponding posterior assignment probabilities.

Finally, the warping transformation $f^{(t)}$ is given by the solution to the following ordinary differential equation (ODE):

$$\partial_t f^{(t)}(x) = u^{(t)}(f^{(t)}(x)), \quad f^{(0)}(x) = x. \tag{4}$$

With f defined as above, we can prove that $q^{(t)}$ is indeed the density of samples from $q^{(0)}$ transformed through $f^{(t)}$, i.e. $q^{(0)} = |\partial_x f^{(t)}| q^{(t)} \circ f^{(t)}$ (cf. extended version). Crucially, the true solution to Eq. (4) is diffeomorphic by construction, and can be numerically approximated (and inverted) with arbitrary precision. In particular, we employ the classic fourth-order Runge–Kutta ODE solver (RK4).

Now assume we obtain optimal parameter values $\{\mu_k^*\}_k$ and $\{\lambda_k^*\}_k$ after matching q to p. We can then warp the data using the above approach, for example linearly interpolating the intermediate parameter values, $\mu_k^{(t)} = t\mu_k^* + (1-t)\mu_k^{(0)}$ and $\lambda_k^{(t)} = t\lambda_k^* + (1-t)\lambda_k^{(0)}$, hence setting the rates in Eq. (2) to constant values, $\dot{\mu}_k = \mu_k^* - \mu_k^{(0)}$ and $\dot{\lambda}_k = \lambda_k^* - \lambda_k^{(0)}$, and integrating Eq. (4) for $t \in [0, 1]$.

2.4   Practical Considerations

Since each medical image in a dataset can have millions of voxels, computing the posteriors and flows for every voxel individually can be too expensive for batch processing. To mitigate this issue, we can compute the end-to-end transformation on a mesh in the range of interest, which is then interpolated for the intensities in the entire volume. In the reported experiments, we have used a uniformly-spaced mesh of 200 points, which has proven accurate enough for normalisation purposes.

Note that the transformation could also be computed on the histogram of discrete intensity values and built into a look-up table. However, this would not scale well to two or more dimensions for multi-modal intensity normalisation, whereas a mesh would not need to be very fine nor require a regular grid layout.

3   Experiments

3.1   Dataset

Our experiments were run on 581 T1-weighted MRI scans from the IXI database, collected from three imaging centres with different scanners.[2] Each scan was bias field-corrected using SPM12[3] with default settings and rigidly registered to MNI space. SPM12 was further used to produce grey matter (GM), white matter (WM) and cerebrospinal fluid (CSF) tissue probability maps. We obtained brain masks by adding the three probability maps and thresholding at 0.5. The statistics reported below were weighted by the voxel-wise tissue probabilities to account for partial-volume effects and segmentation ambiguities.

3.2   Setup

We firstly fitted the nonparametric mixture models to the full integer-value histograms of the raw images (inside the brain masks), as described in Sect. 2.1. We set the DP's concentration parameter to 2 and used data-driven Normal–Gamma priors for the components. As an ad-hoc post-processing step, we pruned the leftover mixture components with weights smaller than 10^{-3}. In the absence of one global reference distribution, we affinely aligned these DPGMMs and the corresponding data to zero mean and unit variance (cf. Fig. 2, middle).

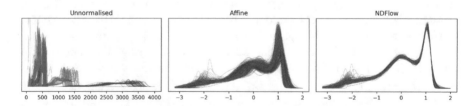

Fig. 2. Population densities, colour-coded by imaging centre

After this rough alignment, global and centre-wise average densities were computed. These were then considered as histograms to which we fitted global and centre-wise reference DPGMMs.

---

[2] http://brain-development.org/ixi-dataset/.

[3] http://www.fil.ion.ucl.ac.uk/spm/software/spm12/.

For normalisation, we consider two scenarios. The first is to normalise each centre's reference distribution to the global target, then to apply this same transformation to all subjects in that centre. In the other approach, each subject's image is individually normalised to the global target density. These scenarios reflect different practical applications where the centre-wise normalisation aims to preserve intra-centre variation, which might be desired. On the other hand, the individual normalisation aims to make all scans as similar as possible.

We compare our technique to Nyúl et al.'s prevalent quantile-based, piecewise linear histogram matching method [7], considered state-of-the-art for intensity normalisation and referred here as NYUL. We acquired the default 11 landmarks (histogram deciles and upper/lower percentiles) from the affine-aligned data for all subjects, then normalised each subject to this set of average landmarks.

3.3 Results

Histogram Fitness. Fig. 3 illustrates the results of normalisation between the pair of images in Fig. 1, which have a notable dissimilarity in the CSF region of the histograms. We observe that both our NDFLOW- and NYUL-transformed histograms present substantially lower mean absolute and root mean squared errors (MAE and RMSE) than the affine-aligned one, and our method performed best by a small margin. This is confirmed in a number of trials with other images.

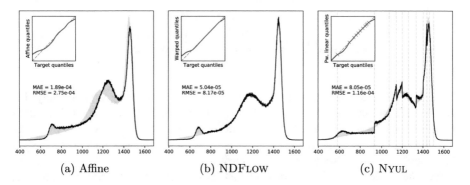

(a) Affine   (b) NDFLOW   (c) NYUL

Fig. 3. Histograms and Q–Q plots of each of the methods against the target histogram. The shading shows the discrepancy between the transformed (black) and target histogram (light red). In the rightmost plot, the landmarks are indicated by vertical lines in the histogram and ticks in the Q–Q plot.

A noteworthy artefact of NYUL are abrupt jumps produced at the landmark values (e.g. Fig. 3c), which appear because interval are uniformly compressed or dilated by different factors, and may be detrimental to downstream histogram-based tasks (e.g. mutual information registration). NDFLOW causes no such discontinuities due to the smoothness of the mass-conserving flows.

Tissue Statistics. In Table 1 we report the WM, GM and CSF intensity statistics for different normalisations. Firstly, we see that the centre-wise normalisation had a small but significant effect on the overall distribution statistics. More importantly, the variances of the statistics after individual NDFLOW and NYUL transformations were typically similar, and both were almost always substantially smaller than the variance after only affine alignment, with the exception of CSF.

Table 1. Tissue statistics after normalisation (mean ± std. dev., $N = 581$)

	Method	1st Quartile	Median	3rd Quartile
WM	Affine	0.900 ± 0.040	1.024 ± 0.045	1.126 ± 0.055
	NDFLOW: Centre	0.898 ± 0.040	1.020 ± **0.040**	1.121 ± **0.043**
	NDFLOW: Indiv.	0.890 ± **0.029**	1.014 ± **0.018**	1.120 ± **0.016**
	NYUL	0.897 ± **0.029**	1.023 ± **0.015**	1.126 ± **0.008**
GM	Affine	−0.296 ± 0.142	0.025 ± 0.117	0.344 ± 0.080
	NDFLOW: Centre	−0.297 ± **0.139**	0.025 ± **0.114**	0.344 ± **0.076**
	NDFLOW: Indiv.	−0.312 ± **0.094**	0.027 ± **0.065**	0.351 ± **0.058**
	NYUL	−0.309 ± **0.106**	0.027 ± **0.070**	0.350 ± **0.064**
CSF	Affine	−2.036 ± 0.145	−1.486 ± 0.140	−1.024 ± 0.156
	NDFLOW: Centre	−2.035 ± **0.143**	−1.480 ± 0.142	−1.018 ± 0.160
	NDFLOW: Indiv.	−2.031 ± **0.136**	−1.484 ± 0.170	−1.028 ± 0.191
	NYUL	−2.025 ± **0.111**	−1.474 ± 0.178	−1.029 ± 0.207

Bold: $p < .01$, one-tailed Brown–Forsythe test for lower variance than 'Affine'

It is known that the amount of intra-cranial fluid can vary substantially due to factors such as age and some neurodegenerative conditions, and this reflects on the distributions of intensities in brain MRI scans, which is evident in Fig. 2. As a result, normalising all subjects to a 'mean' distribution fails to identify a consistent reference range for CSF intensities.

A fundamental limitation of any histogram matching scheme is that it is unclear how to proceed when the distributions are *genuinely* different. Intensity distributions can be strongly affected by anatomical differences; for example, we can observe large variations in the amounts of fluid and fat in brain or whole-body scans, which may heavily skew the overall distributions (moderate example in Fig. 3). The underlying assumption of these methods (including ours) is that the distributions are similar enough up to an affine rescaling and a mild nonlinear deformation of the values, thus handling histograms of truly different shapes remains an open challenge. For images with different fields of view, it may be beneficial to perform image registration before applying intensity normalisation.

Centre Classification. To evaluate the effectiveness of intensity normalisation for data harmonisation, we conducted a centre discrimination experiment with random forest classifiers trained on the full images. We report the pooled test results from two-fold cross validation (detailed results in extended version).

Relative to affine normalisation, centre-wise and individual NDFLOW and NYUL showed a slight drop in overall classification accuracy (94.1% vs. 92.7%, 93.6%, 92.9%, resp.). On the other hand, the uncertainty, as measured by the entropy of the predictions, was significantly higher (paired t-test, all $p < .01$). Nonlinear intensity normalisation therefore seems to successfully remove some of the biasing factors which are discriminative of the origin of the images.

4   Conclusion

In this paper, we have introduced a novel method for MRI intensity normalisation, called *nonparametric density flows* (NDFLOW). It is based on fitting and matching Dirichlet process Gaussian mixture densities, by minimising their L^2 divergence, and on mass-conserving flows, which ensure that the empirical intensity distribution agrees with the matched density model.

We demonstrated that our normalisation approach makes tissue intensity statistics significantly more consistent across subjects than a simple affine alignment, and compares favourably to the state-of-the-art method of Nyúl et al. [7]. We have additionally verified that NDFLOW is able to accurately match histograms without introducing spurious artefacts produced by the competing method. Finally, we argued that both normalisation techniques can reduce some discriminative scanner biases, in a step toward effective data harmonisation.

By employing nonparametric mixture models, we are able to represent arbitrary histogram shapes with any number of modes. In addition, our formulation has the flexibility to match only part of the distributions, by freezing the parameters of some mixture components. This may be useful for ignoring lesion-related modes (e.g. multiple sclerosis hyperintensities), if the corresponding components can be identified (e.g., via anomaly detection). Evaluating this approach and its robustness against lesion load is a compelling direction for further research.

Acknowledgements. This project was supported by CAPES, Brazil (BEX 1500/2015-05), and by the European Research Council under the EU's Horizon 2020 programme (grant agreement No 757173, project MIRA, ERC-2017-STG).

References

1. Bergeest, J.P., Jäger, F.: A comparison of five methods for signal intensity standardization in MRI. In: Tolxdorff, T., Braun, J., Deserno, T.M., Horsch, A., Handels, H., Meinzer, H.P. (eds.) Bildverarbeitung für die Medizin, pp. 36–40. Springer, Heidelberg (2008)
2. Blei, D.M., Jordan, M.I.: Variational inference for Dirichlet process mixtures. Bayesian Anal. **1**(1), 121–144 (2006)
3. Ferguson, T.S.: Bayesian density estimation by mixtures of normal distributions. Recent Adv. Stat. **24**(1983), 287–302 (1983)

4. Hasanbelliu, E., Giraldo, L.S., Principe, J.C.: A robust point matching algorithm for non-rigid registration using the Cauchy-Schwarz divergence. In: IEEE International Workshop on Machine Learning for Signal Processing, pp. 1–6. IEEE (2011)
5. Hellier, P.: Consistent intensity correction of MR images. In: Proceedings of the 2003 International Conference on Image Processing (ICIP 2003). IEEE (2003)
6. Jian, B., Vemuri, B.C.: Robust point set registration using Gaussian mixture models. IEEE Trans. Pattern Anal. Mach. Intell. **33**(8), 1633–1645 (2011)
7. Nyúl, L.G., Udupa, J.K., Zhang, X.: New variants of a method of MRI scale standardization. IEEE Trans. Med. Imaging **19**(2), 143–150 (2000)
8. Roy, A.S., Gopinath, A., Rangarajan, A.: Deformable density matching for 3D non-rigid registration of shapes. In: Ayache, N., Ourselin, S., Maeder, A. (eds.) MICCAI 2007. LNCS, vol. 4791, pp. 942–949. Springer, Heidelberg (2007). https://doi.org/10.1007/978-3-540-75757-3_114
9. Shah, M., Xiao, Y., Subbanna, N., Francis, S., Arnold, D.L., Collins, D.L., Arbel, T.: Evaluating intensity normalization on MRIs of human brain with multiple sclerosis. Med. Image Anal. **15**(2), 267–282 (2011)

Ultra-Fast T2-Weighted MR Reconstruction Using Complementary T1-Weighted Information

Lei Xiang[1], Yong Chen[2], Weitang Chang[2], Yiqiang Zhan[1],
Weili Lin[2], Qian Wang[1(✉)], and Dinggang Shen[2(✉)]

[1] Institute for Medical Imaging Technology, School of Biomedical Engineering,
Shanghai Jiao Tong University, Shanghai, China
wang.qian@sjtu.edu.cn
[2] Department of Radiology and BRIC, University of North Carolina
at Chapel Hill, Chapel Hill, NC, USA
dgshen@med.unc.edu

Abstract. T1-weighted image (T1WI) and T2-weighted image (T2WI) are the two routinely acquired Magnetic Resonance Imaging (MRI) protocols that provide complementary information for diagnosis. However, the total acquisition time of ~ 10 min yields the image quality vulnerable to artifacts such as motion. To speed up MRI process, various algorithms have been proposed to reconstruct high quality images from under-sampled k-space data. These algorithms only employ the information of an individual protocol (e.g., T2WI). In this paper, we propose to combine complementary MRI protocols (i.e., T1WI and under-sampled T2WI particularly) to reconstruct the high-quality image (i.e., fully-sampled T2WI). To the best of our knowledge, this is the first work to utilize data from different MRI protocols to speed up the reconstruction of a target sequence. Specifically, we present a novel deep learning approach, namely Dense-Unet, to accomplish the reconstruction task. The Dense-Unet requires fewer parameters and less computation, but achieves better performance. Our results have shown that Dense-Unet can reconstruct a 3D T2WI volume in less than 10 s, i.e., with the acceleration rate as high as 8 or more but with negligible aliasing artefacts and signal-noise-ratio (SNR) loss.

1 Introduction

Magnetic Resonance Imaging (MRI) is widely applied for numerous clinical applications, as it can provide non-invasive, reproducible and quantitative measurements of both anatomical and functional information that are essential for disease diagnosis and treatment planning. MRI can better measure different soft tissue contrasts than many other medical imaging modalities, e.g., Computed Tomography (CT). It also avoids exposing patients to harmful ionizing radiation, implying higher safety. However, MRI acquisitions need to sample full k-space for orthogonal encoding of the spatial information if no acceleration scheme is employed, therefore limiting acquisition speed. The k-space data that encode spatial-frequency information are commonly acquired line-by-

The original version of this chapter was revised: an Acknowledgements section has been added. The correction to this chapter is available at https://doi.org/10.1007/978-3-030-00928-1_100

line with a fixed interval (repetition time). During MR acquisition, patient movement or physiological motion, e.g., respiration, cardiac motion, and blood flow, could result in significant artefacts in the MR images. Long scan time also increases the healthcare cost and limits the availability of MR scanner for patients.

In clinical routines, T1WI and T2WI images are the two basic MR sequences for assessing anatomical structure and pathology, respectively. T1WI is useful for assessing the cerebral cortex, identifying fatty tissue, characterizing focal liver lesions and in general for obtaining morphological information, as well as for post-contrast imaging. T2WI is useful for detecting edema and inflammation, revealing white matter lesions and assessing zonal anatomy in the prostate and uterus. These two sequences provide complementary information to each other and help characterize the abnormalities of the patients. Typical scanning time for T1WI and T2WI is ~ 10 min, in which T2WI takes the majority due to its longer repetition time (TR) and echo time (TE). In clinical practice, further acceleration in MR acquisition is desired to (1) scan more patients and (2) reduce motion artefacts. Since image acquisition time for a given sequence depends on the number of sampled lines in the k-space, many methods focus on the reduction of the k-space sampling rate, i.e., under-sampling the k-space. These approaches capitalize the inherent redundancy in MRI, where individually sampled points in the k-space do not arise from distinct spatial locations.

Recently, deep learning techniques have been applied to accelerate MRI acquisition. Wang et al. [1] proposed to train a CNN model to learn the mapping between the MR image obtained from zero-filled under-sampled and fully-sampled k-space data, and then use the reconstruction result either as an initialization or a regularization term in the classical CS MRI process. Lee *et al.* [2] further introduced a deep multi-scale residual learning algorithm to reconstruct the under-sampled MR image by formulating the CS MRI problem as a residual regression problem. Schlemper *et al.* [3] developed a deep cascade of CNNs to reconstruct the aggressive Cartesian under-sampled MR image. When the frames of the sequences are reconstructed jointly, they demonstrated to learn the spatiotemporal correlation efficiently by leveraging convolution and data sharing layers together.

Although T1WI and T2WI have different contrasts, these two protocols contain highly related information. White matter in T1WI is of high signal intensity, while it becomes dark in T2WI. Similarly, grey matter is of low signal intensity in T1WI, while it appears white in T1WI. Two lesion examples are labeled in the red circle and green box in Fig. 1. These two lesions are both clear in T2WI, while only one lesion in green box can be noted in the T1WI. In 1/8 under-sampled T2WI, the lesions can still be found, but the boundary details are mostly missing. The reduced image quality in 1/8 T2WI is also prevalent in normal areas as indicated by the blue arrows. These observations inspire us to design a deep learning approach that achieves ultra-fast T2WI reconstruction by combining T1WI with highly under-sampled T2WI.

Several studies [4, 5] attempt to reconstruct T2WI from T1WI. However, to the best of our knowledge, this is the *first work* that intends to reconstruct T2WI using both T1WI and under-sampled T2WI. Our method can leverage the complex relation between T1WI and T2WI and utilize the unique information in under-sampled T2WI to reconstruct the fully-sampled T2WI. We adapt the deep fully convolutional neural network, i.e., the Unet architecture [6] that consists of a contracting (or encoding) path and a symmetric expanding (decoding), to leverage the context information from multi-

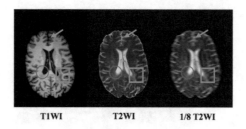

T1WI   T2WI   1/8 T2WI

Fig. 1. Examples of the pairs of T1WI, T2WI and 1/8 under-sampled T2WI data from the same patient. Multiple sclerosis lesions are marked by circles and boxes in the figure.

scale feature maps. In this way, we can combine T1WI and T2WI through the network. We particularly select multiple corresponding 2D slices from T1WI and under-sampled T2WI, and concatenate them as multi-channel input to the network. We further develop the Dense-Unet architecture by introducing dense blocks, which significantly reduces the parameters of the network while boosts the reconstruction quality. Experimental results suggest that the acceleration rate can be as high as 8 or more with negligible aliasing artefacts and signal-noise-ratio (SNR) loss.

2 Method

Overview. The framework for accelerating the T2WI reconstruction with T1WI and under-sampled T2WI is shown in Fig. 2(a). First, the original T2WI is retrospectively under-sampled and only the center part of the k-space with the ratio R, e.g., $R = 1/2, 1/4, 1/8, \ldots$, is utilized to reconstruct the under-sampled T2WI. The under-sampled T2WI is then concatenated with the fully-sampled T1WI, and fed together into the Dense-Unet architecture. To be specific, we implement the input as two groups of consecutive axial slices (N from fully-sampled T1WI and N corresponding ones from under-sampled T2WI). These $2N$ slices are jointly considered as part of the feature maps of the first convolutional layer in the network. The output of the network consists of N consecutive axial slices that correspond to the input. In testing, we synthesize every N consecutive axial slices for the reconstructed T2WI, and combine the outputs into the final 3D volume of T2WI by simple averaging. We regard this joint synthesis of the N consecutive slices as a quasi-3D mapping.

Pre-feature Extraction Layer. Dense-Unet first extracts feature maps from the concatenated pair of T1WI and under-sampled T2WI by a convolutional layer. These feature maps are forwarded to the latter dense blocks for further feature extraction. Denoting the concatenated input as (x_{T2}, y_{T1}), we can compute the output of the first layer as

$$F_1 = \sigma(W_1 * [x_{T2}, y_{T1}] + B_1) \tag{1}$$

where W_1 and B_1 represent the kernels associated with the first convolutional layer, and '$*$' denotes the convolution operator.

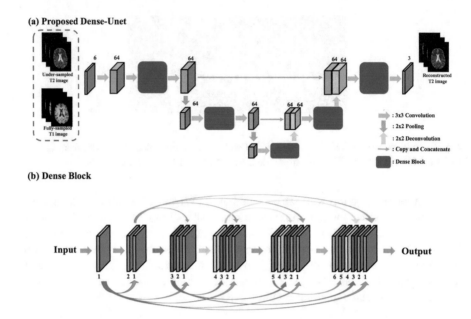

Fig. 2. Illustration of (a) the framework for T2WI reconstruction with T1WI and under-sampled T2WI and (b) the detailed configuration of dense block.

Dense Block. Dense connectivity has been proposed in [7] to further improve the information flow between layers. We adopt this new convolutional network architecture in our model so that we can increase the depth of the whole network to dozens of layers with feasible optimization. Moreover, the dense block requires substantially fewer parameters and less computation, which makes the model more efficient and costs less memory. Figure 2(b) illustrates the layout of the dense block. Consequently, the mth layer receives the feature maps of all preceding layers as the input:

$$z_l = \boldsymbol{H}_l([z_0, \ldots, z_{l-1}]) \tag{2}$$

where $[z_0, \ldots, z_{l-1}]$ refers to the concatenation of the feature maps from previous layers $0, \ldots, l-1$. $\boldsymbol{H}_l(*)$ is defined as a composite function of three consecutive operations: batch normalization (BN), followed by rectified linear unit (ReLU) and a 3×3 convolution (Conv). The hyper-parameters for dense block are the growth rate (GR) and the number of convolution layers (NC). Figure 2(b) gives an example of dense block with $GR = 16$ and $NC = 5$.

Transition Layers. We refer the convolution (or deconvolution) layers following the dense block as the transition layers, which include batch normalization, convolution and pooling (if in the contracting path), or just batch normalization and deconvolution (if in the expanding path). The transition layer in the contracting path used in our experiments consists of a BN layer and a 1×1 Conv layer followed by a 2×2 average pooling layer. In our experiment, the feature map number is always set to 64. On the expanding path, the dense block is followed by batch normalization and deconvolution layer consisting of 64 filters of size 3×3.

Reconstruction Layer. The proposed Dense-Unet model ends with the reconstruction layer that reconstructs fully-sampled T2WI from the feature maps outputted by the last dense block. The reconstruction can be attained by a single convolutional layer as

$$\tilde{\boldsymbol{y}}_{T2} = \boldsymbol{W}_R * \boldsymbol{F}_D + \boldsymbol{B}_R. \tag{3}$$

Here, $\boldsymbol{F}_D$ is the feature maps outputted by the last dense block, and $\tilde{\boldsymbol{y}}_{T2}$ is the T2WI estimated by the reconstruction layer. Note that there is no activation function employed in the reconstruction layer. We use mean squared error (MSE) as loss function.

3   Experimental Result

3.1   Dataset

We utilized the dataset from the MICCAI Multiple Sclerosis (MS) segmentation challenge 2016 [8] to demonstrate the capability of proposed Dense-Unet. We selected 5 subjects with paired T1WI and T2WI. These subjects were scanned by the same Philips Ingenia 3T scanner. The voxel size is $0.7 \times 0.744 \times 0.744$ mm^3. Multiple pre-processing steps are applied, including: (1) denoising with the NL-means algorithm of each image; (2) rigid registration of each image; (3) brain extraction using the volBrain platform from T1WI and then being applied on the other modalities with sinc inter-polation; (4) bias correction using the N4 algorithm; (5) intensity normalization to range (0,1) by dividing the maximum intensity. The final matrix size of the images is $336 \times 336 \times 261$. We used consecutive 2D slices to train our model. In this way, each subject can provide hundreds of samples, which is sufficient for the training of the network.

3.2   Experimental Setting

In this paper, PyTorch was used to implement the Dense-Unet architecture. In the training phase, we extracted 2D whole slices from the 3D image, and each 3D image could contribute ~ 200 samples. We excluded the slices without any brain tissue. The leave-one-out cross-validation strategy was employed for evaluation. Also, data aug-mentation of left-right flipping was applied. Therefore, we prepared enough samples for training our deep model. We adopted Adam optimization with momentum of 0.9 and performed 100 epochs in training stage. The batch size was set to 4 and the initial learning rate was set to 0.0001, which was divided by 10 after 50 epochs. We used zero-padding during every convolution layer to make sure that the size of the output is the same as the input. To quantitatively evaluate the reconstruction performance, we used the standard metric of peak signal-noise ratio (PSNR) and normalized mean absolute error (MAE).

3.3   Contribution of Adding T1WI

To demonstrate the effectiveness of integrating T1WI data for the reconstruction of under-sampled T2WI, we compare the performance achieved (1) by using under-sampled T2WI as the only input and (2) by using the combination of T1WI and under-sampled T2WI. When dealing with the only input of under-sampled T2WI, we employed the same setting as in Fig. 2, but the input layer only includes the under-sampled T2WI. The under-sample ratio was 1/8 for this experiment. Averaged PNSRs and MAEs are listed in Table 1. '1/8 T2' indicates the PSNR/MAE scores computed by comparing the input 1/8 under-sampled T2WI with the ground-truth T2WI directly. 'Reconstructed T2 with T1 (or 1/8 T2)' represents the reconstructed T2WI results using only T1WI (or only 1/8 T2WI) as input. 'Reconstructed T2 with T1 and 1/8 T2' represents the reconstructed T2WI using combined inputs of T1WI and 1/8 T2WI.

Table 1. The evaluation of the reconstructed T2WI using different input settings.

	1/8 T2	Reconstructed T2 with T1	Reconstructed T2 with 1/8 T2	Reconstructed T2 with T1 and 1/8 T2
PSNR	32.5	30.6	33.9	36.9
MAE	0.023	0.033	0020	0.014

We can see that the results of 'Reconstructed T2 with T1 and 1/8 T2' are superior than both 'Reconstructed T2 with T1' and 'Reconstructed T2 with 1/8 T2'. The image quality of 'Reconstructed T2 with 1/8 T2' (PSNR: 33.9 dB) improves just a little compared to '1/8 T2' (PSNR: 32.5 dB), which implies that over under-sampled T2WI is difficult to be reconstructed. However, with T1WI added, the reconstructed results of 'Reconstructed T2 with T1 and 1/8 T2' (PSNR: 36.9 dB) demonstrate a clear improvement compared to that of 'Reconstructed T2 with 1/8 T2' (PSNR: 33.9 dB). This verifies the idea that different image contrasts have complementary information to each other in reconstruction. And, with the additional contrast information of T1WI, we can achieve better reconstruction of T2WI.

We also provide one example in Fig. 3 for visual observation, where our method yields satisfying reconstruction result regarding the ground-truth by keeping high contrast of tissue boundaries. For 'Reconstructed T2 with T1', it has predicted the common tissue structure correctly, e.g., white matter and gray matter in the red circle, but it misses the lesion part (green box). This is because there are no enough cues in T1WI to show the whole lesion information. When it comes to 'Reconstructed T2 with 1/8 T2', we can see that lesion part (green box) is preserved and reconstructed, but it has fuzzy boundary. Moreover, other contrast details (red circle) have become blurred because they are all recovered from only the under-sampled T2WI. Based on the experimental results above, we design the proposed model that takes advantages of both T1WI (for detailed and clear common structure) and under-sampled T2WI (for the unique information that only appears in the T2WI). So we combine the T1WI and 1/8 T2WI together as the input of our proposed Dense-Unet. Finally, 'Reconstructed T2 with T1 and 1/8 T2' gives the most satisfying reconstruction result with high perceptive quality. Note that most of the current compressed sensing methods can only handle reconstruction of under-sample ratio around 1/4. Our proposed method pushes this limitation to a new level, i.e., for even under-sample 1/8 we can still reconstruct correct image details, which further accelerates the speed of scanning T2WI by twice faster while preserving image quality. Moreover, our proposed quasi-3D mapping preserves the consistency in the third view, as shown in both coronal and sagittal views.

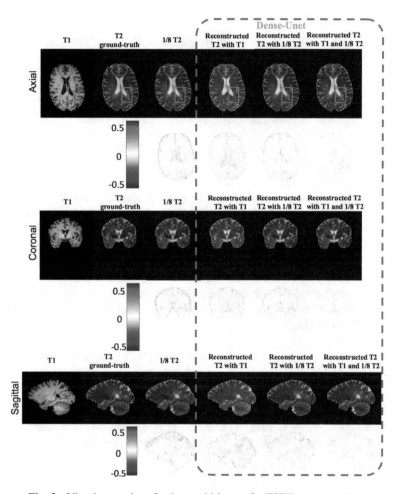

Fig. 3. Visual examples of using multi-inputs for T2WI reconstruction.

3.4   Comparison with Unet

In the literature, there are many studies that successfully reconstruct fully-sampled MR image from under-sampled images. But none of them attempted to solve this problem by utilizing information from another contrast, e.g., T1WI. This is the *first work* that utilizes T1WI and under-sampled T2WI to reconstruct the fully-sampled T2WI. In this section, we mainly compare our method with the popular neural network architecture, Unet, which can handle two inputs naturally. Quantitative results of average PSNRs and MAEs are summarized in Table 2. We compare their performance in different under-sampled ratios. Dense-Unet clearly outperforms the Unet under all comparisons. Note that Unet has 9.5 M parameters, while Dense-Unet only has 3.2 M parameters. Thus, Dense-Unet consumes 3 times less storage than Unet. Also, the running-time for Dense-Unet is 9.5 s for a 3D volume ($336 \times 336 \times 260$), which is highly efficient.

Table 2. The reconstruction comparison of Unet and Dense-Unet.

	T1 + 1/4 T2		T1 + 1/8 T2		T1 + 1/16 T2	
	PSNR	MAE	PSNR	MAE	PSNR	MAE
Unet	37.6	0.013	36.6	0.015	33.8	0.020
Dense-Unet	**39.1**	**0.011**	**36.9**	**0.014**	**34.3**	**0.019**

4 Conclusion

In this paper, we propose a novel Dense-Unet model to reconstruct the T2WI from the T1WI and under-sampled T2WI. The added T1WI makes the reconstruction of T2WI from 1/8 under-sample ratio in k-space possible, which leads to 8 times speed-up. The dense block, which requires substantially fewer parameters and less computation, is integrated within Unet architecture in our work. This enables our model to further improve the quality of the reconstructed T2WI. Comprehensive experiments showed superior performance of our method, including the perceptive quality and the running speed. This work thus can potentially improve the acquisition efficiency and image quality in clinical settings.

Acknowledgement. This work was supported in part by NIH grant EB006733.

References

1. Wang, S., Su, Z., Ying, L., Peng, S., Liang, F., Feng, D., Liang, D.: Accelerating magnetic resonance imaging via deep learning. In: IEEE 13th International Symposium on Biomedical Imaging (ISBI), pp. 514–517. IEEE (2016)
2. He, K., Zhang, X., Ren, S., Sun, J.: Deep residual learning for image recognition. In: Proceedings of the IEEE Conference on Computer Vision and Pattern Recognition, pp. 770–778 (2016)
3. Schlemper, J., Caballero, J., Hajnal, J.V., Price, A., Rueckert, D.: A Deep Cascade of Convolutional Neural Networks for Dynamic MR Image Reconstruction. arXiv preprint arXiv:1704.02422 (2017)
4. Alkan, C., Cocjin, J., Weitz, A.: Magnetic Resonance Contrast Prediction Using Deep Learning (2017)
5. Vemulapalli, R., Van Nguyen, H., Kevin Zhou, S.: Unsupervised cross-modal synthesis of subject-specific scans. In: Proceedings of the IEEE International Conference on Computer Vision, pp. 630–638 (2015)

6. Ronneberger, O., Fischer, P., Brox, T.: U-Net: convolutional networks for biomedical image segmentation. In: Navab, N., Hornegger, J., Wells, W.M., Frangi, Alejandro F. (eds.) MICCAI 2015. LNCS, vol. 9351, pp. 234–241. Springer, Cham (2015). https://doi.org/10. 1007/978-3-319-24574-4_28
7. Huang, G., Liu, Z., Weinberger, K.Q., van der Maaten, L.: Densely connected convolutional networks. arXiv preprint arXiv:1608.06993 (2016)
8. Commowick, O., Cervenansky, F., Ameli, R.: MSSEG challenge proceedings: multiple sclerosis lesions segmentation challenge using a data management and processing infrastructure. In: MICCAI (2016)

Image Reconstruction by Splitting Deep Learning Regularization from Iterative Inversion

Jiulong Liu, Tao Kuang, and Xiaoqun Zhang[✉]

Institute of Natural Sciences and School of Mathematical Sciences and MOE-LSC,
Shanghai Jiao Tong University, 800 Dongchuan Road, Shanghai 200240, China
xqzhang@sjtu.edu.cn

Abstract. Image reconstruction from downsampled and corrupted measurements, such as fast MRI and low dose CT, is mathematically ill-posed inverse problem. In this work, we propose a general and easy-to-use reconstruction method based on deep learning techniques. In order to address the intractable inversion of general inverse problems, we propose to train a network to refine intermediate images from classical reconstruction procedure to the ground truth, i.e. the intermediate images that satisfy the data consistence will be fed into some chosen denoising networks or generative networks for denoising and removing artifact in each iterative stage. The proposed approach involves only techniques of conventional image reconstruction and usual image representation/denoising deep network learning, without a specifically designed and complicated network structures for a certain physical forward operator. Extensive experiments on MRI reconstruction applied with both stack auto-encoder networks and generative adversarial nets demonstrate the efficiency and accuracy of the proposed method compared with other image reconstruction algorithms.

Keywords: Inverse problems · MRI reconstruction · Deep learning
Regularization

1 Introduction

Image reconstruction problems arisen in medical imaging area such as fast MRI and low dose CT are mathematically ill-posed inverse problems. We often consider a linear imaging system with a forward operator A, for example partial 2D Fourier transform for MRI and X-ray transform for CT. The measurement y is given as $y = Ax$ for x being the underlying image in the perfect noise free case. The linear operator A is ill-posed for most applications; therefore some statistical priors are necessary to make these problems invertible. Sparsity priors such as total variation (TV) [1] and wavelet tight frame [2] have been among those popular regularization and studied extensively in the literature. 5 In practice, the measurements are often corrupted by noise, i.e.

$$y = Ax + \epsilon \tag{1}$$

© Springer Nature Switzerland AG 2018
A. F. Frangi et al. (Eds.): MICCAI 2018, LNCS 11070, pp. 224–231, 2018.
https://doi.org/10.1007/978-3-030-00928-1_26

if we assume it is i.i.d additive Gaussian noise. Derived by a maximum-likelihood estimator of the physical process and sparsity prior distribution of the original image, it is common to solve the following unconstrained model

$$\min_x \frac{1}{2}\|Ax - y\|_2^2 + \mu\|\mathcal{D}x\|_1, \tag{2}$$

where $\mathcal{D}$ is a sparsity transform, for example, the mentioned spatial gradient operator ∇ (total variation) and a tight frame transform $\mathcal{W}$.

However, some side effects will also be involved by sparsity regularization due to the predefined sparsity transform, for example, the staircasing effects are introduced by TV. Deep networks have been successfully applied to many image restoration tasks such as image denoising, inpainting, super resolution [3–5]. It is shown in these work that those delicately designed deep networks achieved state-of-the-art performance for these image processing problems. However, despite their superior performance, it is still challenging to adapt the network for medical image reconstruction problems as the networks are specifically designed for those particular forward operators. Most of the emerged deep learning based medical image reconstruction are based on the sparsity optimization algorithms such as primal dual methods and Alternating Direction of Multiplier methods (ADMM). For example, ADMM-net [6] and the learned variational network in [7] aim to mimic the optimization algorithms for solving the sparse regularization model (2) and build a network to learn the sparsity transform $\mathcal{D}$. In [6,8,9], analytic solutions are obtained for the inversion layers and a proximal operator is learned for the denoising/anti-artifact layers. In the work [10,11], the authors carefully designed a MRI reconstruction network to enhance data consistence. These networks achieve state-of-the-art reconstruction results and at the same time are usually more complicated compared to common neural networks, especially for derivative computing.

Because of the intractability of inversion of an ill-posed operator with partial and corrupted measurements, we do not intend to learn an end-to-end inversion mapping from the measurements to the reconstructed image as previous work. Inspired by regularization based image reconstruction methods, we propose to split the task of inversion of a known forward operator from learning an image representation network. In order to feed the inputs into networks implicitly, we establish a data consistence constrained network loss function and then apply ADMM to split the tasks of solving the inversion and learning a network. The problem is solved through simple iterations of existing techniques of conventional inversion and usual image representation/denoising deep network learning. We note that our method is different from ADMM-net, as ADMM-net considered the solution of the sparsity optimization algorithms ADMM as the network output and the sparsity transform $\mathcal{D}$ is considered as network parameters to be learned. Our method does not intend to design a new network structure but integrate existing ones in the ADMM algorithm to solve the proposed model. The prior of to-be-reconstructed images is obtained by the learned network, which can be easily used for the inference process. Finally, data consistence is maintained through iteration for the reconstruction, which is usually not the case for most of learning based reconstruction methods.

2   Our Approach

The Stacked Auto-Encoder (SAE) deep network has shown to be a useful image representation method for denoising [12], where a greedy layerwise approach is proposed for pretraining. Stacked Convolutional Auto-Encoder (SCAE) [13] was further proposed to preserve frequently repeated local image features. And some improvement has been achieved by the Stacked Non-Local Auto-Encoder (SNLAE) in [14] by using a nonlocal collaborative stabilization. In recent years, more and more networks emerge for image restoration problems. For example, it has been demonstrated that generative adversarial network (GAN) model is powerful for medical or natural image restoration problems such as super-resolution [4] and deburring [15].

In the following, we propose our image reconstruction learning model based on a denoising network or GAN model. We denote the input dataset for a network $x = \{x_k\}_{k=1}^m$ with the corresponding ground truth $\tilde{x} = \{\tilde{x}_k\}_{k=1}^m$ where m is the number of samples. In image reconstruction inverse problems, we denote the corresponding measurements $y = \{y_k\}_{k=1}^m$ for $y_k = Ax_k$ where A is a known forward operator. Here we use the boldface to denote the vectors of all the input and output images in the training procedure and we use the regular characters for their counterparts for the inference.

The learning procedure of a denoising network is designed to minimize a cost function $L_H(x, \theta)$, for example the quadratic function

$$\min_\theta L_H(x, \theta) := \|f(x, \theta) - \tilde{x}\|_2^2 \tag{3}$$

where $f(x, \theta)$ is the output and θ is the set of network parameters. For GAN model, the following min-max problem is considered

$$\max_{\theta_d} \min_{\theta_g} L_G(x, \theta_g, \theta_d) = \frac{1}{m} \sum_{i=1}^m [\log(D(\tilde{x}_i, \theta_d))] + \frac{1}{m} \sum_{i=1}^m [\log(1 - D(G(x_i, \theta_g), \theta_d))] \tag{4}$$

where θ_g and θ_d are the parameter sets for the generative and discriminative networks respectively, and $G(\cdot, \theta_g)$ and $D(\cdot, \theta_d)$ are the outputs of the two networks.

Let

$$J(x) = \eta \left(\sum_{i=1}^m \|Ax_i - y_i\|_2^2 + \mu \|\mathcal{D}x_i\|_1 \right) \tag{5}$$

be the conventional data consistency term with sparse regularization. The formulation can be easily generalized for other data fidelity derived from max-likelihood of a posteriori estimation, and with other regularization term in $J(x)$. The regularization parameter μ can be very small or even zero.

Being motivated by the fact that many powerful networks are available for removing noise and artifact, we now attempt to propose to integrate deep learning network in the image reconstruction. Our basic idea is to use the variable $\boldsymbol{x}$ which meets the data consistence implicitly to fed into the to-be-learned networks, by solving the following problem with a deep learning regularization

$$\min_{\boldsymbol{x},\theta} L_H(\boldsymbol{x},\theta) + J(\boldsymbol{x}), \tag{6}$$

and

$$\max_{\theta_d} \min_{\theta_g,\boldsymbol{x}} L_G(\boldsymbol{x},\theta_g,\theta_d) + J(\boldsymbol{x}) \tag{7}$$

for L_H and L_G being the cost function for a denoising network and GAN model respectively.

The above two models can be solved by adapting ADMM algorithm [16]. Taking (6) as an example, we reformulate it as

$$\begin{aligned} \min_{\boldsymbol{x},\theta,\boldsymbol{z}} \quad & L_H(\boldsymbol{x},\theta) + J(\boldsymbol{z}) \\ s.t. \quad & \boldsymbol{x} = \boldsymbol{z}. \end{aligned} \tag{8}$$

The augmented Lagrangian for the problem (8) is given as

$$L_\rho(\boldsymbol{x},\theta,\boldsymbol{z},\boldsymbol{p}) = L_H(\boldsymbol{x},\theta) + J(\boldsymbol{z}) + \boldsymbol{p}^T(\boldsymbol{x}-\boldsymbol{z}) + \frac{\rho}{2}\|\boldsymbol{x}-\boldsymbol{z}\|_2^2 \tag{9}$$

for a parameter $\rho > 0$.

The idea of the ADMM algorithm for solving the optimization problem (8) is to alternatingly update the primal variables $\boldsymbol{x},\theta,\boldsymbol{z}$ by minimizing the augmented Lagrangian function (9) and update the dual variable $\boldsymbol{p}$ with a dual ascent step, which leads to the following scheme

$$\begin{cases} \boldsymbol{z}^{k+1} = \arg\min_{\boldsymbol{z}} J(\boldsymbol{z}) + \frac{\rho}{2}\|\boldsymbol{x}^k - \boldsymbol{z} + \boldsymbol{b}^k\|_2^2 \\ \theta^{k+1} = \arg\min_{\theta} L_H(\boldsymbol{x}^k,\theta) \\ \boldsymbol{x}^{k+1} = \arg\min_{\boldsymbol{x}} L_H(\boldsymbol{x},\theta^{k+1}) + \frac{\rho}{2}\|\boldsymbol{x} - \boldsymbol{z}^{k+1} + \boldsymbol{b}^k\|_2^2 \\ \boldsymbol{b}^{k+1} = \boldsymbol{b}^k + (\boldsymbol{x}^{k+1} - \boldsymbol{z}^{k+1}) \end{cases} \tag{10}$$

for $\boldsymbol{p}^k = \rho\boldsymbol{b}^k$. The variables $\boldsymbol{x}^0$ and $\boldsymbol{z}^0$ are initialized by

$$\boldsymbol{x}^0 = \boldsymbol{z}^0 = \arg\min_{\boldsymbol{z}} J(\boldsymbol{z}). \tag{11}$$

For the first subproblem in (10), we can solve this conventional reconstruction problem with a classical reconstruction method, such as ADMM again if there is a sparse regularization term present in J; For the second subproblem in (10), it is a typical loss function minimization for a deep learning network with the input $\boldsymbol{x}^k$, and a stochastic gradient descent method built in the neural network tools can be applied; For the third subproblem in (10), we can also use a stochastic gradient descent method.

The similar alternating scheme as (10) can be obtained for solving the GAN training model (7) by replacing the second step in (10) by

$$(\theta_g^{k+1}, \theta_d^{k+1}) = \arg\max_{\theta_d} \min_{\theta_g} L_G(\boldsymbol{x}^k, \theta_g, \theta_d). \tag{12}$$

Here we need to alternatingly apply gradient descent for updating θ_g^{k+1} and gradient ascent for updating θ_d^{k+1} as the general GAN methods do.

After we obtain the network parameter set θ^*, the learned network is ready to be used for mapping a given input image $\hat{x}$ to an estimated ground truth image x by $x = f(\hat{x}, \theta^*)$. More precisely, given a measurement y, we obtain the reconstructed image x through the following scheme

$$\begin{cases} z^{k+1} = \arg\min_z J(z) + \frac{\rho}{2}\|x^k - z + b^k\|_2^2 \\ \hat{x}^{k+1} = f(x^k, \theta^*) \\ x^{k+1} = \frac{1}{1+\rho}(\hat{x}^{k+1} + \rho(z^{k+1} - b^k)) \\ b^{k+1} = b^k + (\hat{x}^{k+1} - z^{k+1}). \end{cases} \tag{13}$$

The initialization of $\boldsymbol{x}^0$ and $\boldsymbol{z}^0$ are performed similarly as (11). For the GAN based reconstruction model, we can use the similar scheme to (13) by replacing $f(\boldsymbol{x}^{k+1}, \theta^*)$ with $G(\boldsymbol{x}^{k+1}, \theta_g^*)$ in the second step to obtain the reconstructed image x from a measurement.

3   Experiments

In this section, we perform the experiments on MRI reconstruction from downsampled measurements. The MRI data are generated by partial Fourier transform with Gaussian noise corruption, i.e. $y = K\mathcal{F}(x + l*(\xi_1 + \xi_2 * i))$ where l is the noise level, ξ_1, ξ_2 obey i.i.d normal distribution, x is the ground truth image, and K is the downsample operator. In our experiments, the MRI image dataset is from ADNI (Alzheimer's Disease Neuroimaging Initiative) of which 300 slices of size 192×160 are used for training and 21 slices are used for inferring, and three different downsampling patterns with three downsamping rates are used for simulating the measurements. To speed up the training process and alleviate the ill-conditionness when the sampling rate is severely low, we use TV term in the reconstruction functional $J(x)$ (5), but its weight μ is decreasing by outer loops of our method. As μ gets smaller and smaller, the contribution of TV is eventually much smaller than what is used for sparsity regularized reconstruction. In order to demonstrate the flexibility of our approach, we implement three kinds of networks for MRI reconstruction, i.e. SCAE [13], SNLAE [14] and GAN [5]. The basic setup and training/test time on a PC with an Intel i7 and a Nvidia GPU GTX1060 for the three networks SCAE, SNLAE and GAN are listed in Table 1. To demonstrate the convergence of the proposed method, the intermediate training results and inferring results by SCAE of one slice are shown in Fig. 1, in which we can see that the images trend to be of good quality and higher PSNR.

Table 1. Network setup and computation time

Parameters	SCAE/GAN Gen.	SNLAE	GAN Discri.
Dataset size	$(300, 192, 160)$	$(300, 192, 160)$	$(300, 192, 160)$
Number of layers	6	6	8
Filter size in hidden layers	$[3, 3, 3, 3, 3, 3]$	–	$[3, 3, 3, 3, 3, 1, 1]$
Stride in hidden layers	$[1, 1, 1, 1, 1, 1]$	–	$[2, 2, 2, 2, 2, 1, 1]$
Number of neurons/filters in hidden layers	$[2^5, 2^6, 2^7, 2^6, 2^5]$	$[2^9, 2^{10}, 2^{11}, 2^{10}, 2^9]$	$[2^3, 2^6, 2^6, 2^6, 2^6, 2^6, 2^6]$
Outer loops	5	5	5
Train time(h)	11	16	36
Test time(sec)	3.2/3.3	4.1	–

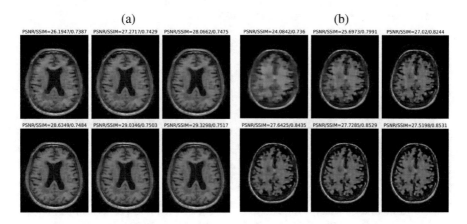

Fig. 1. Intermediate results $[f(x^0, \theta^0), f(x^1, \theta^1), \cdots, f(x^5, \theta^5)]$ for MRI reconstruction with 25% radial downsampling by SCAE. (a) training step; (b) inferring step

In Fig. 2, we show the comparison of our methods with the zero-filling method (ZF) [17], TV regularization based reconstruction [18], and ADMM-net [6] for the case with 1D random downsampling pattern and 25% downsampling rate (the results for the other sampling patterns and rates are provided in the Supplementary file). For the three downsampling patterns, we observe that in the case of noise-free, the reconstructed images by our proposed methods including SCAE, SNLAE and GAN, and by ADMM-net have better spatial resolution. In the case of noise level 10% and with measurements of very low sampling rate, our method with the four networks still achieve good performance. Specially, for the case with 1D random downsampling pattern, we can find our methods have alleviate both noise and artifact. Visually, our methods generally achieved cleaner images compared to ADMM-net for noisy data. To assess reconstruction image quality quantitatively, we further show the results of PSNR and SSIM in Table 2. All the best PSNR are scattered at the methods with learned regularization.

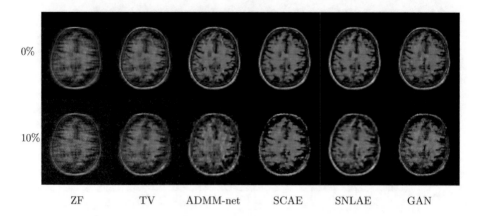

Fig. 2. MRI reconstruction results. Sampling pattern and rate: 1D random with 25%; The first row: noise free; The second row: 10% noise.

Table 2. MRI reconstruction quality (PSNR/SSIM)

Method	Noise	Rate	ZF	TV	ADMM-net	SCAE	SNLAE	GAN
Radial	0%	1/5	24.36/0.47	30.73/0.86	**32.31**/0.92	32.00/0.92	30.47/0.83	30.13/0.84
		1/4	25.45/0.51	32.32/0.90	33.67/0.93	**33.94**/0.94	32.53/0.88	32.26/0.90
		1/3	27.25/0.56	34.60/0.94	35.27/0.94	**36.37**/0.96	35.15/0.92	34.49/0.94
	10%	1/5	22.18/0.35	24.69/0.49	25.44/0.59	25.52/0.73	**25.98**/0.68	25.02/0.73
		1/4	22.38/0.36	25.16/0.49	25.96/0.61	26.13/0.70	**26.38**/0.66	25.53/0.74
		1/3	22.37/0.37	25.28/0.49	26.50/0.60	26.64/0.74	26.70/0.65	**26.71**/0.75
2D random	0%	1/5	24.91/0.49	31.69/0.89	33.81/0.93	**34.24**/0.94	31.95/0.86	31.79/0.89
		1/4	25.30/0.50	32.79/0.90	34.97/0.94	**35.61**/0.95	32.85/0.86	32.94/0.91
		1/3	26.32/0.53	34.93/0.93	36.31/0.95	**37.71**/0.96	35.33/0.91	35.10/0.94
	10%	1/5	22.37/0.37	24.97/0.51	25.42/0.61	**25.90**/0.73	25.97/0.67	25.78/0.75
		1/4	22.38/0.36	24.92/0.49	25.84/0.60	26.06/0.74	26.15/0.67	**26.31**/0.75
		1/3	22.37/0.37	24.91/0.47	26.14/0.56	26.38/0.72	26.41/0.62	**26.48**/0.76
1D random	0%	1/5	22.78/0.61	25.22/0.75	28.53/0.85	**28.79**/0.87	28.73/0.86	27.21/0.81
		1/4	23.06/0.62	25.77/0.76	28.99/0.87	**29.37**/0.88	29.06/0.86	27.47/0.82
		1/3	23.86/0.65	27.34/0.81	**32.18**/0.91	31.25/0.91	30.98/0.89	30.09/0.86
	10%	1/5	20.72/0.27	22.38/0.39	22.59/0.40	22.22/0.61	**24.52**/0.60	22.76/0.67
		1/4	20.37/0.26	22.25/0.37	22.98/0.44	22.72/0.63	**24.39**/0.56	23.32/0.69
		1/3	20.37/0.28	22.59/0.37	23.96/0.47	23.75/0.62	**24.98**/0.58	23.93/0.70

4   Conclusion

We developed a variational image reconstruction method which integrates image representation network and classical image reconstruction method. The proposed model exhibits flexibility of choosing classical reconstruction method and powerful deep representation network. The application on MRI image reconstruction shows the effectiveness of the proposed method and it is also clear that the proposed method can be easily extended to other applications.

References

1. Rudin, L.I., Osher, S., Fatemi, E.: Nonlinear total variation based noise removal algorithms. Phys. D Nonlinear Phenom. **60**(1–4), 259–268 (1992)
2. Cai, J.F., Dong, B., Osher, S., Shen, Z.: Image restoration: total variation, wavelet frames, and beyond. J. Am. Math. Soc. **25**(4), 1033–1089 (2012)
3. Xie, J., Xu, L., Chen, E.: Image denoising and inpainting with deep neural networks. In: Advances in Neural Information Processing Systems, pp. 341–349 (2012)
4. Ledig, C., et al.: Photo-realistic single image super-resolution using a generative adversarial network. arXiv preprint (2016)
5. Goodfellow, I., et al.: Generative adversarial nets. In: Advances in Neural Information Processing Systems, pp. 2672–2680 (2014)
6. Sun, J., Li, H., Xu, Z., et al.: Deep ADMM-Net for compressive sensing MRI. In: Advances in Neural Information Processing Systems, pp. 10–18 (2016)
7. Hammernik, K., et al.: Learning a variational network for reconstruction of accelerated MRI data. Magn. Reson. Med. **79**(6), 3055–3071 (2018)
8. Adler, J., Öktem, O.: Learned primal-dual reconstruction. arXiv preprint arXiv:1707.06474 (2017)
9. Adler, J., Öktem, O.: Solving ill-posed inverse problems using iterative deep neural networks. arXiv preprint arXiv:1704.04058 (2017)
10. Mardani, M., et al.: Deep generative adversarial networks for compressed sensing automates MRI. arXiv preprint arXiv:1706.00051 (2017)
11. Schlemper, J., Caballero, J., Hajnal, J.V., Price, A.N., Rueckert, D.: A deep cascade of convolutional neural networks for dynamic mr image reconstruction. IEEE Trans. Med. Imaging **37**(2), 491–503 (2018)
12. Bengio, Y., Lamblin, P., Popovici, D., Larochelle, H.: Greedy layer-wise training of deep networks. In: Advances in Neural Information Processing Systems, pp. 153–160 (2007)
13. Masci, J., Meier, U., Cireşan, D., Schmidhuber, J.: Stacked convolutional autoencoders for hierarchical feature extraction. In: Honkela, T., Duch, W., Girolami, M., Kaski, S. (eds.) ICANN 2011. LNCS, vol. 6791, pp. 52–59. Springer, Heidelberg (2011). https://doi.org/10.1007/978-3-642-21735-7_7
14. Wang, R., Tao, D.: Non-local auto-encoder with collaborative stabilization for image restoration. IEEE Trans. Image Process. **25**(5), 2117–2129 (2016)
15. Fan, K., Wei, Q., Wang, W., Chakraborty, A., Heller, K.: InverseNet: Solving inverse problems with splitting networks. arXiv preprint arXiv:1712.00202 (2017)
16. Fortin, M., Glowinski, R.: Augmented Lagrangian Methods: Applications to the Numerical Solution of Boundary-Value Problems. North-Holland Publishing Company, Amsterdam (1983)
17. Bernstein, M.A., Fain, S.B., Riederer, S.J.: Effect of windowing and zero-filled reconstruction of mri data on spatial resolution and acquisition strategy. J. Magn. Reson. Imaging **14**(3), 270–280 (2001)
18. Lustig, M., Donoho, D., Pauly, J.M.: Sparse MRI: the application of compressed sensing for rapid MR imaging. Magnetic resonance in medicine **58**(6), 1182–1195 (2007)

Adversarial and Perceptual Refinement for Compressed Sensing MRI Reconstruction

Maximilian Seitzer[1,2(✉)], Guang Yang[3,4], Jo Schlemper[2], Ozan Oktay[2], Tobias Würfl[1], Vincent Christlein[1], Tom Wong[3,4], Raad Mohiaddin[3,4], David Firmin[3,4], Jennifer Keegan[3,4], Daniel Rueckert[2], and Andreas Maier[1]

[1] Pattern Recognition Lab, Friedrich-Alexander-Universität, Erlangen, Germany
maximilian.seitzer@fau.de
[2] Biomedical Image Analysis Group, Imperial College, London, UK
[3] National Heart and Lung Institute, Imperial College, London, UK
[4] Cardiovascular Research Centre, Royal Brompton Hospital, London, UK

Abstract. Deep learning approaches have shown promising performance for compressed sensing-based Magnetic Resonance Imaging. While deep neural networks trained with mean squared error (MSE) loss functions can achieve high peak signal to noise ratio, the reconstructed images are often blurry and lack sharp details, especially for higher undersampling rates. Recently, adversarial and perceptual loss functions have been shown to achieve more visually appealing results. However, it remains an open question how to (1) optimally combine these loss functions with the MSE loss function and (2) evaluate such a perceptual enhancement. In this work, we propose a hybrid method, in which a visual refinement component is learnt on top of an MSE loss-based reconstruction network. In addition, we introduce a semantic interpretability score, measuring the visibility of the region of interest in both ground truth and reconstructed images, which allows us to objectively quantify the usefulness of the image quality for image post-processing and analysis. Applied on a large cardiac MRI dataset simulated with 8-fold undersampling, we demonstrate significant improvements ($p < 0.01$) over the state-of-the-art in both a human observer study and the semantic interpretability score.

1 Introduction

Compressed sensing-based Magnetic Resonance Imaging (CS-MRI) is a promising paradigm allowing to accelerate MRI acquisition by reconstructing images from only a fraction of the normally required k-space measurements. Traditionally, sparsity-based methods and their data-driven variants such as dictionary learning [9] have been popular due to their mathematically robust formulation for perfect reconstruction. However, these methods are limited in acceleration

---

G. Yang and J. Schlemper/D. Rueckert and A. Maier share second/last coauthorship.

© Springer Nature Switzerland AG 2018
A. F. Frangi et al. (Eds.): MICCAI 2018, LNCS 11070, pp. 232–240, 2018.
https://doi.org/10.1007/978-3-030-00928-1_27

factor and also suffer from high computational complexity. More recently, several deep learning-based architectures have been proposed as an attractive alternative for CS-MRI. The advantages of these techniques are their computational efficiency, which enables real-time application, and that they can learn powerful priors directly from the data, which allows higher acceleration rates. The most widely adopted deep learning approach is to perform an end-to-end reconstruction using multi-scale encoding-decoding architectures [7,14]. Alternative approaches carry out the reconstruction in an iterative manner [15], conceptually extending traditional optimization algorithms. Most previous studies focus on exploring the network architecture; however, the optimal loss function to train the network remains an open question.

Recently, as an alternative to the commonly used MSE loss, adversarial [2] and perceptual losses [5] have been proposed for CS-MRI [14]. As these loss functions are designed to improve the visual quality of the reconstructed images, we refer to them as *visual loss functions* in the following. So far, approaches using visual loss functions still rely on an additional MSE loss for successful training of the network. Directly combining all these losses in a joint optimization leads to a suboptimal training process resulting in reconstructions with lower peak signal to noise ratio (PSNR) values. In this work, we propose a two-stage architecture that avoids this problem by separating the reconstruction task from the task of refining the visual quality. Our contributions are the following: (1) we show that the proposed refinement architecture improves visual quality of reconstructions without compromising PSNR much, and (2) we introduce the semantic interpretability score as a new metric to evaluate reconstruction performance, and show that our approach outperforms competing methods on it.

2   Background

Deep Learning-Based CS-MRI Reconstruction. Let $x \in \mathbb{C}^N$ denote a complex-valued MR image of size N to be reconstructed, and let $y \in \mathbb{C}^M$ ($M \ll N$) represent undersampled k-space measurements obtained by $y = F_u x + \varepsilon$, where F_u is the undersampling Fourier encoding operator and ε is complex Gaussian noise. The linear inversion $x_u = F_u^H y$, also called zero-filled reconstruction, is fundamentally ill-posed and generates an aliased image due to violation of the Nyquist-Shannon sampling theorem. Therefore, it is necessary to add prior knowledge into the reconstruction to constrain the solution space, traditionally formulated as the following optimization problem:

$$\arg\min_{x} \mathcal{R}(x) + \lambda \|y - F_u x\|_2^2 \qquad (1)$$

Here, $\mathcal{R}$ expresses a regularization term on x (e. g. ℓ_0/ℓ_1-norm for CS-MRI), and λ is a hyper-parameter reflecting the noise level. In deep learning approaches, one learns the inversion mapping directly from the data. However, rather than learning the mapping from Fourier directly to image domain, it is common to formulate this problem as *de-aliasing* the zero-filled reconstructions x_u in the image domain [12,14]. Let $\mathcal{D}$ be our training dataset of pairs (x, x_u) and $\hat{x} = R(x_u)$ be the image generated by the reconstruction network R. Given $\mathcal{D}$, the network is trained by minimizing the empirical risk $\mathcal{L}(R) = \mathbb{E}_{(x,x_u)\sim\mathcal{D}} \, d(x, \hat{x})$, where d is a distance function measuring the dissimilarities between the reference fully-sampled image and the reconstruction.

For the choice of the reconstruction network R, most previous approaches [7, 14] relied on an encoder-decoder structure (e.g. U-Net [10]), but our preliminary experiments showed that these architectures performed subpar in terms of PSNR. Instead, we use the architecture proposed in [12], as it performed well even for high undersampling rates. This network consists of n_c consecutive de-aliasing blocks, each containing n_d convolutional layers. Each de-aliasing block takes an aliased image $x^{(i)} \in \mathbb{R}^{2N}$ as the input and outputs the de-aliased image $x^{(i+1)} \in \mathbb{R}^{2N}$, with $i \in \{0, \ldots n_c - 1\}$ and $x^0 = x_u = F_u^H y$ being the zero-filled reconstruction. Interleaved between the de-aliasing blocks are data consistency (DC) layers, which enforce that the reconstruction is consistent with the acquired k-space measurements by replacing frequencies of the intermediate image with frequencies retained from the sampling process. This process can be seen as an unrolled iterative reconstruction where de-aliasing blocks and DC layers perform the role of the regularization step and data fidelity step, respectively [12].

Loss Functions for Reconstruction. In deep learning-based approaches to inverse problems, such as MR reconstruction and single image super-resolution, a frequently used loss function [7,15] is the MSE loss $\mathcal{L}_{\mathrm{MSE}}(R) = \mathbb{E}_{(x,x_u)\sim\mathcal{D}}\|x - \hat{x}\|_2^2$. Though networks trained with MSE criterion can achieve high PSNR, the results often lack high frequency image details [1]. Perceptual loss functions [5] are an alternative to the MSE loss. They minimize the distance to the target image in some feature space. A common perceptual loss is the VGG loss $\mathcal{L}_{\mathrm{VGG}}(R) = \mathbb{E}_{(x,x_u)\sim\mathcal{D}}\|f_{\mathrm{VGG}}(x) - f_{\mathrm{VGG}}(\hat{x})\|_2^2$, where f_{VGG} denotes VGG feature maps [13].

Another choice is an adversarial loss based on Generative Adversarial Networks (GANs) [2,3]. A discriminator and a generator network are setup to compete against each other such that the discriminator is trained to differentiate between real and generated samples, whereas the generator is encouraged to deceive the discriminator by producing more realistic samples. For us, the discriminator D learns to differentiate between fully-sampled and reconstructed images, and the reconstruction network, playing the role of the generator, reacts by changing the reconstructions to be more similar to the fully-sampled images. The discriminator loss is then given by $\mathcal{L}_{\mathrm{GAN}}(D) = -\mathbb{E}_{(x,x_u)\sim\mathcal{D}} \log(D(x)) + \log(1 - D(R(x_u)))$. During training, the reconstruction network minimizes $\mathcal{L}_{\mathrm{adv}}(R) = -\mathbb{E}_{(x,x_u)\sim\mathcal{D}} \log(D(R(x_u)))$, which has the effect of pulling the reconstructed images closer towards the distribution of the training data.

Perceptual losses are known to increase textural details [6], but also to introduce high frequency artifacts [2], whereas adversarial losses can produce realistic, high frequency details [6]. As perceptual and adversarial losses complement each other, it is sensible to combine them into a single visual loss $L_{\mathrm{vis}}(R) = \mathcal{L}_{\mathrm{adv}}(R) + \mathcal{L}_{\mathrm{VGG}}(R)$. For MR reconstruction, previous attempts [14] further combined adversarial and/or perceptual loss with the MSE loss to stabilize the training. This simultaneous optimization yields acceptable solutions, typically however with low PSNR. We argue this is because the different training objectives compete with each other, leading to the network ultimately converging to a suboptimal local maximum.

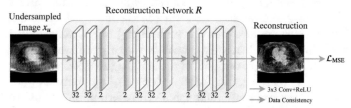

(a) Stage 1: training of reconstruction network using $\mathcal{L}_{\mathrm{MSE}}(R)$.

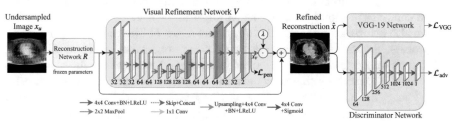

(b) Stage 2: training of visual refinement network using $\mathcal{L}_{\mathrm{vis}}(V)$.

Fig. 1. Overview of proposed method.

3   Method

The observation above motivates our approach: instead of directly training a reconstruction network with all loss functions jointly, we use a two-stage procedure, detailed in Fig. 1. In the first stage, the reconstruction network R is trained with $\mathcal{L}_{\mathrm{MSE}}(R)$. In the second stage, we fix the reconstruction network and train a visual refinement network V on top of R by optimizing $\mathcal{L}_{\mathrm{vis}}(V)$. The final reconstruction is then given by $\hat{x} = R(x_u) + V(R(x_u))$, i.e. V learns an additive mapping which refines the base reconstruction. In this setup, discriminator and VGG network still receive the full reconstruction $\hat{x}$ as input.

The decoupling of the refinement step from the reconstruction task has several benefits. The discriminator begins training by seeing reasonably good reconstructions, which avoids overfitting it to suboptimal solutions during the training process. Furthermore, compared to training from scratch, the optimization is easier as it starts closer to the global optimum. Finally, the visual refinement step always starts out from the best possible MSE solution achievable with R, whereas this guarantee is not given when jointly training R with $\mathcal{L}_{\mathrm{MSE}}$ and $\mathcal{L}_{\mathrm{vis}}$.

The choice of the architecture for the visual refinement network is flexible, and in this work we use a U-Net architecture. Within V, we gate the output of the network by a trainable scalar λ, which improves the adversarial training dynamics during the early stages of training. If we initialize $\lambda = 0$, the discriminator receives $\hat{x} = R(x_u)$, and the gradient signal to V is forced to zero. This allows the discriminator to initially only learn on clean reconstructions from R, untainted by the randomly initialized output of V. For the refinement network, the impact of less useful gradients is reduced while the discriminator has not yet learned to correctly differentiate between the ground truth (i. e. fully-sampled data) and the reconstructions. We also scale $R(x_u)$ to the range of $(-1, 1)$ before using it as V's input and then scale $\hat{x}$ back to the original range after adding the refinement. In accordance to our goal of reaching high PSNR values, we constrain the output x_V of V (before gating with λ) with an ℓ^1-penalty $\mathcal{L}_{\mathrm{pen}}(V) = \|x_V\|_1$. This guides V to learn the minimal sparse transformation needed to fulfill the visual loss, i. e. to change the MSE-optimal solution only in areas important for visual quality. In practice, this means that our approach yields higher PSNR values compared to joint training, as we show in Sect. 4.

We also utilize a couple of techniques known to stabilize the adversarial learning process. For the discriminator network, we use one-sided label smoothing [11] of 0.1, and an experience replay buffer [8] of size 80 with probability $p = 0.5$ to draw from it. For the refinement network, we add a feature matching loss [11] $\mathcal{L}_{\mathrm{feat}}(V) = \mathbb{E}_{(x,x_u)\sim\mathcal{D}} \frac{1}{N} \sum_{i=1}^{N} \|f_D^{(i)}(x) - f_D^{(i)}(\hat{x})\|_1$, where $f_D^{(i)}$ denotes the i'th of N feature maps of the discriminator. The total loss for V is given by

$$\mathcal{L}(V) = \frac{1}{2}\left(\frac{\mathcal{L}_{\mathrm{adv}}(V)}{M} + \frac{\mathcal{L}_{\mathrm{feat}}(V)}{N}\right) + \frac{\mathcal{L}_{\mathrm{VGG}}(V)}{O} + \alpha\mathcal{L}_{\mathrm{pen}}(V) \qquad (2)$$

with α being the penalty strength, and M, N, O constants set such that $\frac{\mathcal{L}_{\mathrm{adv}}}{M} = \frac{\mathcal{L}_{\mathrm{feat}}}{N} = \frac{\mathcal{L}_{VGG}}{O} = 1$ in the first iteration of training, which amounts to assigning the two adversarial loss terms the same initial importance as $\mathcal{L}_{\mathrm{VGG}}$. The penalty strength α is important for training speed and stability. Choosing α such that $\mathcal{L}_{\mathrm{pen}} \approx 0.1$ in the first training iteration gave us sufficiently good results.

Semantic Interpretability Score. The most commonly used metrics to evaluate reconstruction quality are PSNR and the structural similarity index (SSIM). It has been shown that those two metrics do not necessarily correspond to visual quality for human observers, as e. g. demonstrated by human observer studies in [1,6]. Therefore, PSNR and SSIM alone are not sufficient in the evaluation of image reconstructions. This poses the question on how to evaluate reconstruction quality taking human perception into account. One possibility is to let domain experts (e.g. clinicians and MRI physicists) rate the reconstructions and average the results to form a mean opinion score (MOS). Obtaining opinion scores from expert observers is costly, hence cannot be used during the development of new models. However, if expert-provided segmentation labels are available, we can design a metric indicating how visible the segmented objects are in the reconstructed images, in the following referred to as *semantic interpretability score* (SIS). This metric is motivated by Inception scores [11] in GANs, which tells how well an Inception network can identify objects in generated images.

SIS is defined as the mean Dice overlap between the ground truth segmentation and the segmentation predicted by a pre-trained segmentation network from the reconstructed images. The scores are normalized by the average Dice score on the ground-truth images to obtain a measure of segmentation performance relative to the lower error-bound. We only consider images in which at least one instance of the object class is present, and ignore the background class. We argue that if a pre-trained network is able to produce better segmentations, the regions of interest are better visible (e.g. have clearly defined boundaries) in the images. Implementing SIS requires a segmentation network trained on the same distribution of images as the reconstruction dataset. In practice, the segmentation network is trained on the fully-sampled images used for training the reconstruction method. We trained an off-the-shelf U-Net architecture to segment the left atrium, achieving a Dice score of 0.796 on the ground truth images.

4   Experiments

Datasets. We evaluated our method on 3D late gadolinium enhanced cardiac MRI datasets acquired in 37 patients. We split the 2D axial slices of the 3D volumes into 1248 training images, 312 validation images, and 364 testing images of size 512×512 pixels. For training, we generated random 1D-Gaussian masks keeping 12.5% of raw k-space data, which corresponded to an $8\times$ speed-up. During testing, we randomly generated a mask for each slice, which we kept the same for all evaluated methods.

Training Details and Parameters. For the reconstruction network, we used $n_c = 3$ de-aliasing blocks, and $n_d = 3$ convolutional layers with 32 filters of size 3×3. For the refinement network, we used a U-Net with 32, 64, 128 encoding filters and 64, 32 decoding filters of size 4×4, batch normalization and leaky ReLU with slope 0.1. The discriminator used a PatchGAN [4] architecture with 64, 128, 256, 512, 1024, 1024 filters of size 4×4, and channelwise dropout after the last 3 layers. The VGG loss used the final convolutional feature maps of a VGG-19 network pre-trained on ImageNet. The reconstruction network was trained for 1500 epochs with batch size 20, the refinement network for 200 epochs with batch size 5, both using the Adam optimizer with learning rate 0.0002, $\beta_1 = 0.5$, $\beta_2 = 0.999$. We found that the training is sensitive to the network's initialization. Thus, we chose orthogonal initialization for the refinement network and Gaussian initialization from $\mathcal{N}(0, 0.02)$ for the discriminator.

Evaluation Metrics. We use PSNR and SIS as evaluation metrics. To further evaluate our approach and assess how useful SIS is as a proxy for visual quality, we also asked a domain expert to rate all reconstructed images in which the left atrium anatomy and the atrial scars are visible. The rating ranges from 1 (poor) to 4 (very good), and is based on the overall image quality, the visibility of the atrial scar and occurrence of artifacts. To obtain an unbiased rating, the expert was shown all images from all methods in randomized order.

Results. We compared our approach against three other reconstruction methods: RecNet [12] (i.e. the proposed approach without refinement step), DAGAN[1] [14] using both adversarial and perceptual loss, and DLMRI[2] [9], a dictionary learning based method. No data augmentation was used for any of the methods.

Table 1. Quantitative results for 8-fold undersampling. Highest measures in bold.

Method	PSNR (dB)	MOS	SIS
Ground truth	∞	3.78 ± 0.45	1
RecNet [12]	$\mathbf{32.46} \pm 2.26$	2.75 ± 0.78	0.801
DLMRI [9]	31.45 ± 2.40	1.09 ± 0.29	0.842
DAGAN [14]	28.41 ± 1.91	2.61 ± 0.83	0.812
Proposed method	31.89 ± 2.18	$\mathbf{3.24} \pm 0.63$	$\mathbf{0.941}$

We show the results of our evaluation in Table 1, and a sample reconstruction in Fig. 2. RecNet performed best in terms of PSNR, which is expected as its training objective directly corresponds to this metric, but its reconstructions were over-smoothed. DLMRI had the lowest MOS, with its reconstructions showing heavy oil paint artifacts. DAGAN, combining MSE loss with a visual loss function without any further precautions, suffered from low PSNR. While its reconstructions also looked sharp, they were noisy and often displayed aliasing artifacts, which was reflected in a lower MOS compared to our method. Our proposed approach achieved significantly[3] higher mean opinion score than all other methods, while still maintaining high PSNR. Reconstructions obtained by our method appeared sharper with better contrast. Moreover, our method achieved the highest SIS close to segmentation performance on the ground truth data, which indicated that the segmented objects were clearly visible in the reconstructed images.

These results further demonstrate that PSNR alone is a subpar indicator for reconstruction quality, making our SIS a useful supplement to those metrics. For our method, SIS agreed with the quality score given by the expert user. Somewhat surprising is that the SIS of DLMRI is slightly higher than RecNet and DAGAN although DLMRI has the worst MOS. We conjecture this is because, although DLMRI reconstructed images lack textural details, areas belonging to the same organ have similar intensity values, which helps the segmentation task. While scoring through an expert user is thus still the safest way to evaluate reconstructions, we believe that in conjunction with PSNR, SIS is a helpful tool to quickly judge image quality during the development of new models.

---

[1] https://github.com/nebulaV/DAGAN.
[2] http://www.ifp.illinois.edu/~yoram/DLMRI-Lab/DLMRI.html.
[3] Significance determined by a two-sided paired Wilcoxon signed-rank test at $p < 0.01$.

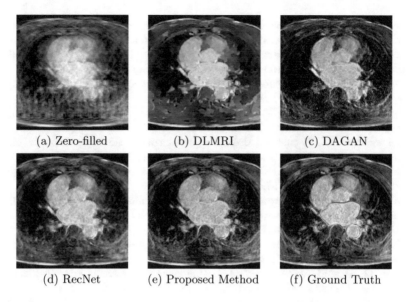

(a) Zero-filled   (b) DLMRI   (c) DAGAN

(d) RecNet   (e) Proposed Method   (f) Ground Truth

Fig. 2. Qualitative visualization for 8-fold undersampling. Contour of predicted segmentation of left atrium in yellow, contour of ground truth segmentation in red.

5   Conclusion

In this work, we highlighted the inadequacy of previously proposed deep learning based CS-MRI methods using MSE loss functions in direct combination with visual loss functions. We improved on them by proposing a new refinement approach, which incorporates both loss functions in a harmonious way to improve the training stability. We demonstrated that our method can produce high quality reconstructions with large undersampling factors, while keeping higher PSNR values compared to other state-of-the-art methods. We also showed that the reconstruction obtained by our method can provide the best segmentation of the ROIs among all compared methods.

References

1. Dahl, R., et al.: Pixel recursive super resolution. In: ICCV, pp. 5449–5458 (2017)
2. Dosovitskiy, A., Brox, T.: Generating images with perceptual similarity metrics based on deep networks. In: NIPS (2016)
3. Goodfellow, I.J., et al.: Generative adversarial nets. In: NIPS (2014)
4. Isola, P., et al.: Image-to-image translation with conditional adversarial networks. In: IEEE CVPR, pp. 5967–5976 (2017)
5. Johnson, J., Alahi, A., Fei-Fei, L.: Perceptual losses for real-time style transfer and super-resolution. In: Leibe, B., Matas, J., Sebe, N., Welling, M. (eds.) ECCV 2016. LNCS, vol. 9906, pp. 694–711. Springer, Cham (2016). https://doi.org/10.1007/978-3-319-46475-6_43

6. Ledig, C., et al.: Photo-realistic single image super-resolution using a generative adversarial network. In: IEEE CVPR, pp. 105–114 (2017)
7. Lee, D., et al.: Deep residual learning for compressed sensing MRI. In: IEEE 14th International Symposium on Biomedical Imaging, pp. 15–18 (2017)
8. Pfau, D., Vinyals, O.: Connecting generative adversarial networks and actor-critic methods. arXiv preprint arXiv:1610.01945 (2016)
9. Ravishankar, S., Bresler, Y.: MR image reconstruction from highly undersampled k-space data by dictionary learning. IEEE TMI **30**, 1028–1041 (2011)
10. Ronneberger, O., Fischer, P., Brox, T.: U-Net: convolutional networks for biomedical image segmentation. In: Navab, N., Hornegger, J., Wells, W.M., Frangi, A.F. (eds.) MICCAI 2015. LNCS, vol. 9351, pp. 234–241. Springer, Cham (2015). https://doi.org/10.1007/978-3-319-24574-4_28
11. Salimans, T., et al.: Improved Techniques for Training GANs. In: NIPS (2016)
12. Schlemper, J., et al.: A deep cascade of convolutional neural networks for dynamic MR image reconstruction. IEEE TMI (2017)
13. Simonyan, K., Zisserman, A.: Very deep convolutional networks for large-scale image recognition. In: ICLR (2015)
14. Yang, G., et al.: DAGAN: deep de-aliasing generative adversarial networks for fast compressed sensing MRI reconstruction. IEEE TMI (2018)
15. Yang, Y., et al.: Deep ADMM-net for compressive sensing MRI. In: NIPS (2016)

Translation of 1D Inverse Fourier Transform of K-space to an Image Based on Deep Learning for Accelerating Magnetic Resonance Imaging

Taejoon Eo, Hyungseob Shin, Taeseong Kim, Yohan Jun,
and Dosik Hwang[✉]

School of Electrical and Electronic Engineering,
Yonsei University, Seoul, Republic of Korea
dosik.hwang@yonsei.ac.kr

Abstract. To reconstruct magnetic resonance (MR) images from undersampled Cartesian k-space data, we propose an algorithm based on two deep-learning architectures: (1) a multi-layer perceptron (MLP) that estimates a target image from 1D inverse Fourier transform (IFT) of k-space; and (2) a convolutional neural network (CNN) that estimates the target image from the estimated image of the MLP. The MLP learns the relationship between 1D IFT of undersampled k-space which is transformed along the frequency-encoding direction and the target fully-sampled image. The MLP is trained line by line rather than by a whole image, because each frequency-encoding line of the 1D IFT of k-space is not correlated with each other. It can dramatically decrease the number of parameters to be learned because the number of input/output pixels decrease from N^2 to N. The next CNN learns the relationship between an estimated image of the MLP and the target fully-sampled image to reduce remaining artifacts in the image domain. The proposed deep-learning algorithm (i.e., the combination of the MLP and the CNN) exhibited superior performance over a single MLP and a single CNN. And it outperformed the comparison algorithms including CS-MRI, DL-MRI, a CNN-based algorithm (denoted as Wang's algorithm), PANO, and FDLCP in both qualitative and quantitative evaluation. Consequently, the proposed algorithm is applicable up to a sampling ratio of 25% in Cartesian k-space.

Keywords: Magnetic resonance imaging · Undersampling
Multi-layer perceptron · Convolutional neural networks · 1D Fourier transform

1 Introduction

Magnetic resonance imaging (MRI) is an imaging technique that can provide various contrast mechanisms for visualizing anatomical structures and physiological functions in human body. However, MRI is relatively slow because it is not possible to

---

Electronic supplementary material The online version of this chapter (https://doi.org/10.1007/978-3-030-00928-1_28) contains supplementary material, which is available to authorized users.

© Springer Nature Switzerland AG 2018
A. F. Frangi et al. (Eds.): MICCAI 2018, LNCS 11070, pp. 241–249, 2018.
https://doi.org/10.1007/978-3-030-00928-1_28

simultaneously sample multiple data points in the raw data domain (i.e. 2D Fourier domain of an image, which is referred to as k-space).

To accelerate MRI acquisition, k-space can be subsampled at a frequency that is lower than the Nyquist rate (i.e., it can be undersampled) instead of acquiring the fully-sampled k-space (i.e., sampling the data at the Nyquist rate). However, a simple reconstruction (i.e., 2D inverse Fourier transform) from the undersampled k-space brings out aliasing artifacts in the image domain and obscures many anatomical and physiological information. To reduce the aliasing artifacts and recover the missing information in images, various reconstruction algorithms such as compressed sensing (CS) [1] and parallel imaging (PI) [2] have been developed. The CS algorithms have been developed to the combination with low-rank constraint terms [3] and to image-adaptive algorithms that enforce sparsity on image patches [4].

In recent, deep-learning based reconstruction algorithms have been introduced and regarded as alternatives of CS. The first deep-learning algorithm applied to MRI reconstruction comprises a 3-layer convolutional neural network (CNN) that learns the relationship between undersampled images and fully-sampled images, and the conventional CS is followed at the end (hereafter denoted as Wang's algorithm) [5]. After the study, various deep-learning algorithms such as CNN-based sparse residual (artifacts) learning algorithm [6], a cascaded CNN with interleaved data fidelity [7], multi-layer perceptron (MLP)-based parallel imaging (PI) algorithms have been introduced [8]. Especially, the automated transform by manifold approximation (AUTOMAP) algorithm provided a new perspective for reconstruction algorithm by directly translating k-space to the target image with neural networks [9].

In this study for accelerating MRI, we propose an algorithm that can efficiently translate 1D inverse Fourier transform (IFT) of undersampled k-space in data-acquisition direction (i.e., frequency-encoding direction) to the target fully-sampled images using two different deep-learning architectures: (1) a multi-layer perceptron (MLP) that estimates a target image from 1D inverse Fourier transform of k-space; and (2) a convolutional neural network (CNN) that reduces remaining artifacts in the output of the MLP. The proposed algorithm can utilize the maximum possible extent of the raw k-space while reducing the number of optimizing parameters dramatically compared with existing deep-learning algorithms, which enables efficient learning and results in better reconstructions than comparison algorithms.

2   Methods

2.1   Problem Formulation

Let $\mathbf{y} \in \mathbb{C}^{n_{kx} \times n_{ky}}$, where n_{kx} and n_{ky} represent the number of horizontal and vertical pixels of k-space respectively, denote a 2D complex-valued MR k-space. Our purpose is to reconstruct a fully-sampled image $\mathbf{x} \in \mathbb{C}^{n_x \times n_y}$, where n_x and n_y represent the number of horizontal and vertical pixels of $\mathbf{x}$, from the undersampled k-space, $\mathbf{y_u}$, obtained by multiplication of a binary undersampling mask $\mathbf{U}$ and $\mathbf{y}$ as follows:

$$\mathbf{y_u} = \mathbf{U} \circ \mathbf{y} = \mathbf{U} \circ \mathcal{F}_{2D}(\mathbf{x}) = \mathbf{y}_{u,r} + i\mathbf{y}_{u,i} \tag{1}$$

$$\mathbf{x_u} = \mathcal{F}_{2D}^{-1}(\mathbf{y_u}) = \mathbf{x}_{u,r} + i\mathbf{x}_{u,i} \tag{2}$$

where $\mathbf{y_u} \in \mathbb{C}^{n_{kx} \times n_{ky}}$ denotes the undersampled k-space; $\mathbf{U} \in \mathbb{R}^{n_{kx} \times n_{ky}}$ denotes the binary undersampling mask; $\circ$ denotes element-wise multiplication; $\mathcal{F}_{2D}$ and $\mathcal{F}_{2D}^{-1}$ denote the 2D Fourier transform (FT) and IFT, respectively; $\mathbf{y}_{u,r} \in \mathbb{R}^{n_{kx} \times n_{ky}}$ and $\mathbf{y}_{u,i} \in \mathbb{R}^{n_{kx} \times n_{ky}}$ denote the real and imaginary channels of $\mathbf{y_u}$, respectively; $\mathbf{x_u}$ denotes the undersampled image; and $\mathbf{x}_{u,r}$ and $\mathbf{x}_{u,i}$ denote the real and imaginary channels of $\mathbf{x_u}$, respectively.

To estimate $\mathbf{x}$ from a small number of samples in the k-space, $\mathbf{y_u}$, we introduce an algorithm comprising two deep-learning architectures, one is MLP that translates 1D IFT of undersampled k-space to an image, and the other is CNN that removes remaining artifacts in image domain. The objective function to optimize the parameters of the MLP, Θ_{MLP}, is

$$\mathrm{argmin}_{\Theta_{MLP}} \|\mathbf{x} - H_{MLP}(\mathbf{z_u}; \Theta_{MLP})\|_2^2 \tag{3}$$

where $\mathbf{z_u} = \mathcal{F}_{1D}^{-1}(\mathbf{y_u}) \in \mathbb{C}^{n_x \times n_{ky}}$ denotes the 1D IFT of $\mathbf{y_u}$ along the frequency-encoding (horizontal) direction; and H_{MLP} denotes the hypothesis function that estimates fully-sampled image $\mathbf{x}$ from 1D IFT of undersampled k-space, $\mathbf{z_u}$, by the MLP. The other objective function to optimize the parameters of the CNN for artifacts removal, Θ_{CNN}, is

$$\mathrm{argmin}_{\Theta_{CNN}} \|\mathbf{x} - H_{CNN}(\hat{\mathbf{x}}_{MLP}; \Theta_{CNN})\|_2^2 + \lambda \|\mathbf{y_u} - \mathbf{U} \circ \mathcal{F}_{2D}(H_{CNN}(\hat{\mathbf{x}}_{MLP}; \Theta_{CNN}))\|_2^2 \tag{4}$$

where H_{CNN} denotes the hypothesis function for reducing the remaining artifacts in the image reconstructed by the MLP, $\hat{\mathbf{x}}_{MLP} = H_{MLP}(\mathbf{z_u}; \Theta_{MLP})$; and λ is the regularization parameter for data fidelity. The combined equation of Eqs. (3) and (4) to optimize Θ_{MLP} and Θ_{CNN}, which is the final objective function of this study, can be represented as

$$\mathrm{argmin}_{\Theta_{MLP}, \Theta_{CNN}} \begin{matrix} \|\mathbf{x} - H_{CNN}(H_{MLP}(\mathcal{F}_{1D}^{-1}(\mathbf{y_u}); \Theta_{MLP}); \Theta_{CNN})\|_2^2 \\ + \lambda \|\mathbf{y} - \mathbf{U} \circ \mathcal{F}_{2D}(H_{CNN}(H_{MLP}(\mathcal{F}_{1D}^{-1}(\mathbf{k_u}); \Theta_{MLP}); \Theta_{CNN}))\|_2^2 \end{matrix} \tag{5}$$

In Fig. 1, the proposed deep-learning frameworks to solve Eq. (5) are presented.

2.2 The Proposed MLP: Translation from 1D IFT of K-space to an Image

The proposed MLP learns the relationship between 1D IFT of the undersampled Cartesian k-space which is transformed along the frequency-encoding (horizontal) direction, $\mathbf{z_u}$, and the target fully-sampled image $\mathbf{x}$. The proposed MLP is trained line by line rather than by a whole image, because each phase-encoding (vertical) line of the 1D IFT of k-space is not correlated with each other. Then, the estimation of a vertical

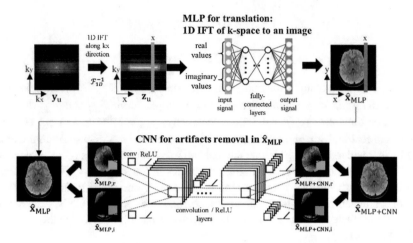

Fig. 1. The proposed reconstruction algorithm based on the MLP for translating 1D IFT of k-space to an image and the CNN for artifacts removal in the output of the MLP

line of the fully-sampled image **x** from the corresponding line of the 1D IFT of undersampled k-space, $\mathbf{z}_u$, using the MLP can be represented as

$$\widehat{\mathbf{X}}_{MLP}(x) = \mathbf{w}_{NFL}(\dots \sigma(\mathbf{w}_2 \sigma(\mathbf{w}_1 \mathbf{Z}_u(x) + \mathbf{b}_1) + \mathbf{b}_2)\dots) + \mathbf{b}_{NFL} \qquad (6)$$

where

$$\widehat{\mathbf{X}}_{MLP}(x) = [\hat{\mathbf{x}}_{MLP}(x, 1), \hat{\mathbf{x}}_{MLP}(x, 2), \cdots, \hat{\mathbf{x}}_{MLP}(x, y)]^{\mathbf{T}} \in \mathbb{C}^{1 \times n_y} \qquad (7)$$

$$\mathbf{Z}_u(x) = [\mathbf{z}_u(x, 1), \mathbf{z}_u(x, 2), \cdots, \mathbf{z}_u(x, n_{k_y})]^{\mathbf{T}} \in \mathbb{C}^{1 \times n_{ky}} \qquad (8)$$

where x and y denote horizontal and vertical indices in the image domain, respectively; $\mathbf{w}_n$ and $\mathbf{b}_n$ are weight and bias matrices of the MLP, respectively, where n = 1, 2, 3, ..., NFL; σ is the activation function; and NFL denotes the number of fully-connected layers of the MLP. As depicted in Eq. (9), The loss function for training the MLP is defined as the mean-squared error between $\mathbf{Z}(x)$ and the estimation of $\mathbf{Z}(x)$ (i.e., $H_{MLP}(\mathbf{Z}_u(x); \boldsymbol{\theta}_{MLP}) = \widehat{\mathbf{X}}_{MLP}(x)$).

$$L_{MLP}(\boldsymbol{\theta}_{MLP}) = \frac{1}{2M} \sum_{m=1}^{M} \|\mathbf{x}(x_m) - H_{MLP}(\mathbf{Z}_u(x_m); \boldsymbol{\theta}_{MLP})\|_2^2 \qquad (9)$$

where

$$\boldsymbol{\theta}_{MLP} = \{(\mathbf{w}_1, \mathbf{b}_1), (\mathbf{w}_2, \mathbf{b}_2), \dots, (\mathbf{w}_{NFL}, \mathbf{b}_{NFL})\} \qquad (10)$$

where $\mathbf{x}(x_m)$ and $\mathbf{Z}_u(x_m)$ denote the m-th vertical line of the fully-sampled image and the m-th vertical line of 1D IFT of the undersampled k-space, respectively; and M denotes the batch size. This line-by-line training can dramatically decrease the number of parameters to be learned because the number of input/output pixels (i.e., $\mathbf{Z}_u(x)$ and $\widehat{\mathbf{X}}_{MLP}(x)$) decrease from $n_x n_{ky}$ to n_{ky}. Finally, the hypothesis function and the parameters (i.e., weight and bias matrices) of the MLP that estimates the 2D fully-sampled image $\mathbf{x}$ from $\mathbf{z}_u$ can be represented as

$$H_{MLP}(\mathbf{z}_u; \mathbf{\Theta}_{MLP}) = \hat{\mathbf{x}}_{MLP} = \mathbf{W}_{NFL}(\ldots \sigma(\mathbf{W}_2 \sigma(\mathbf{W}_1 \mathbf{z}_u + \mathbf{B}_1) + \mathbf{B}_2) \ldots) + \mathbf{B}_{NFL} \quad (11)$$

where

$$\mathbf{\Theta}_{MLP} = \{(\mathbf{W}_1, \mathbf{B}_1), (\mathbf{W}_2, \mathbf{B}_2), \ldots, (\mathbf{W}_{NFL}, \mathbf{B}_{NFL})\} \quad (12)$$

where $\mathbf{W}_n = \mathbf{1}\mathbf{w}_n$, $\mathbf{B}_n = \mathbf{1}\mathbf{w}_n$, $\mathbf{1} = [1, 1, \cdots, 1]^T \in \mathbb{R}^{1 \times n_{ky}}$, and n = 1, 2, 3, ..., NFL.

More details for the MLP, including optimizer parameters, network specifications, including network depths, the number of outputs, activation function, deep-learning libraries, and training/testing times, are provided in the supporting information.

2.3 The Proposed CNN with Data Fidelity: Artifacts Removal in the MLP Output

The proposed CNN aims to remove the artifacts remaining in the output images of the previous MLP. The hypothesis function of H_{CNN} that estimates the fully-sampled image $\mathbf{x}$ from the output of the MLP, $\hat{\mathbf{x}}_{MLP}$, using CNN can be represented as

$$H_{CNN}(\hat{\mathbf{x}}_{MLP}; \mathbf{\Theta}_{CNN}) = \boldsymbol{\omega}_{NCL} * (\ldots \sigma(\boldsymbol{\omega}_2 * \sigma(\boldsymbol{\omega}_1 * \hat{\mathbf{x}}_{MLP} + \boldsymbol{\beta}_1) + \boldsymbol{\beta}_2) \ldots) + \boldsymbol{\beta}_{NCL} \quad (13)$$

where

$$\mathbf{\Theta}_{CNN} = \{(\boldsymbol{\omega}_1, \boldsymbol{\beta}_1), (\boldsymbol{\omega}_2, \boldsymbol{\beta}_2), \ldots, (\boldsymbol{\omega}_{NCL}, \boldsymbol{\beta}_{NCL})\} \quad (14)$$

where $\boldsymbol{\omega}_n$ and $\boldsymbol{\beta}_n$ are convolution and bias matrices in each convolution layer, respectively, where $n = 1, 2, 3, \ldots, NCL$; $*$ denotes the convolution operator; and NCL denotes the number of convolution layers. The loss function used for training the CNN is

$$L_{CNN}(\mathbf{\Theta}_{CNN}) = \frac{1}{2M} \sum_{m=1}^{M} \left\| \mathbf{x}_m - H_{CNN}(\hat{\mathbf{x}}_{MLP,m}; \mathbf{\Theta}_{CNN}) \right\|_2^2 \quad (15)$$

where $\mathbf{x}_m$ and $\hat{\mathbf{x}}_{MLP,m}$ denote the m-th fully-sampled image and the m-th estimated image of the MLP in the training dataset, respectively; and M denotes the batch size.

The final data fidelity is performed in k-space as a closed form solution [4] as

$$\hat{\mathbf{y}}_f(k_x, k_y) = \begin{cases} \frac{\hat{\mathbf{y}}_{MLP+CNN}(k_x, k_y) + \lambda \mathbf{y}_u(k_x, k_y)}{1+\lambda} & \text{if } \mathbf{U}(k_x, k_y) = 1 \\ \hat{\mathbf{y}}_{MLP+CNN}(k_x, k_y) & \text{if } \mathbf{U}(k_x, k_y) = 0 \end{cases} \quad (16)$$

where

$$\hat{\mathbf{y}}_{\mathbf{MLP+CNN}} = \mathcal{F}_{2D}(\hat{x}_{\mathbf{MLP+CNN}}) = \mathcal{F}_{2D}(H_{CNN}(\hat{\mathbf{x}}_{\mathbf{MLP}}; \mathbf{\Theta}_{CNN})) \qquad (17)$$

where k_x and k_y are horizontal and vertical indices of k-space, respectively. Then, the final solution of the proposed algorithm is obtained by IFT of $\hat{y}_f$ as $\hat{x}_f = \mathcal{F}_{2D}^{-1}(\hat{y}_f)$.

More details for the CNN, including optimizer parameters, network specifications, including network depths, filter sizes, activation function, deep-learning libraries, and training/testing times, are provided in the supporting information.

2.4   Experimental Frameworks

All experiments conducted in the present study were approved by the institutional review board. Written informed consent was obtained from all human subjects. Two MR datasets were used: T_2-fluid attenuated inversion recovery (T_2-FLAIR) brain real-valued dataset provided by the Alzheimer's Disease Neuroimaging Initiative (ADNI) [10], and T_2-weighted complex-valued dataset acquired at our local institute. Details of data acquisition, including scanner information, sequence parameters, and the number of slices used for training and testing, are provided in the supporting information.

Undersampled k-space data were retrospectively obtained by subsampling the fully-sampled k-space data. Before undersampling, all MR images were normalized to a maximum magnitude of 1. A Cartesian undersampling scheme in a phase encoding direction (1D random) was used for generating undersampled k-space dataset. The sampling ratio for the undersampling was 25%. The binary undersampling masks is presented in the supporting information (Supporting Figure S1).

The proposed algorithm was compared with the following six algorithms: baseline zero-filling, CS-MRI [1], DL-MRI [4], a CNN-based algorithm by Wang et al. [5] (denoted as Wang's algorithm), PANO [11], and FDLCP [12]. The parameters of the comparison algorithms are provided in the supporting information. Peak signal-to-noise ratio (PSNR) and structure similarity (SSIM) [13] were used for quantitative metrics. The patch size used to calculate SSIM was 11.

3   Results

3.1   The Conventional Image-to-Image MLP vs. the Proposed MLP

In Fig. 2, we evaluated the two different MLPs: The conventional MLP introduced in [8] which translates each vertical line of the 2D IFT of the undersampled k-space (i.e., the undersampled image) to the corresponding line of the target image and the proposed MLP which translates each vertical line of 1D IFT of the undersampled k-space to the corresponding line of the target image. Variables such as the number of outputs and the network depths in MLPs were exactly same. In Fig. 2, the proposed MLP (h) showed better reconstructions than the conventional image-to-image MLP (g) in terms of restoring details and reducing aliasing artifacts.

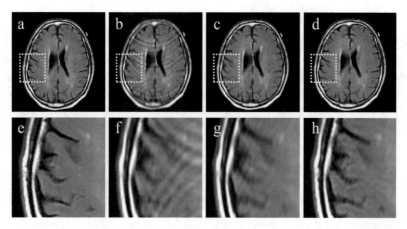

Fig. 2. (a) the fully-sampled image in T_2-FLAIR (ADNI) dataset, (b) the zero-filling image at the sampling ratio = 25%, the reconstructed images by (c) the image-to-image MLP and (d) the proposed MLP. (e–h) are the magnified images of boxed region of interests (ROIs) in (a–d).

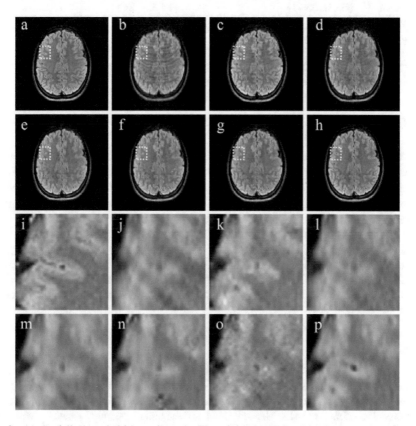

Fig. 3. (a) the fully-sampled image from the T_2-weighted (our local institute) dataset, (b) zero-filling image with the sampling ratio = 25%, and the images reconstructed with (c) CS-MRI, (d) DL-MRI, (e) Wang's algorithm, (f) PANO, (g) FDLCP, and (h) the proposed algorithm. (i–p) are the magnified images of the boxed ROIs in (a–h).

3.2   Comparison Study with Conventional Algorithms

Qualitative and quantitative comparisons are provided for the six conventional algorithms and the proposed algorithm. Figure 3 depicts the resultant images from the complex-valued T_2-weighted dataset (from our local institute). The results of the real-valued T_2-FLAIR dataset are provided in the supporting information (Supporting Figure S3). Table 1 depicts quantitative results for the two data sets. The proposed algorithm outperformed the six comparison algorithms in both qualitative and quantitative tests.

Table 1. Quantitative results of comparison algorithms and the proposed algorithm. Average PSNR/SSIMs for the sampling ratio = 25% on the two datasets (real-valued T_2-FLAIR and complex-valued T_2-weighted)

Algorithm	T_2-FLAIR ADNI (real-valued data)	T_2-weighted (complex-valued data)
Zero filling	29.05/0.8675	23.62/0.8191
CS-MRI	29.77/0.9360	25.01/0.8477
DL-MRI	35.18/0.9477	25.62/0.8487
Wang's	36.03/0.9454	24.84/0.8436
PANO	38.36/0.9670	27.16/0.8803
FDLCP	38.88/0.9655	26.78/0.8720
Proposed	**40.07/0.9773**	**31.72/0.9320**

4   Conclusion

The current study presents a domain-transform algorithm comprising two deep-learning architectures (MLP and CNN) for reconstructing MR images from undersampled Cartesian k-space. Experimental results on the two different datasets demonstrated that the proposed algorithm outperforms the comparison state-of-the-art reconstruction algorithms. More discussion is provided in the supporting information.

Acknowledgements. This research was supported by the National Research Foundation of Korea (NRF) grant funded by the Korean government (MSIP) (2016R1A2B4015016) and was partially supported by the Graduate School of YONSEI University Research Scholarship Grants in 2017 and the Brain Korea 21 Plus Project of Dept. of Electrical and Electronic Engineering, Yonsei University in 2018.

References

1. Lusting, M., Donoho, D., Pauly, J.M.: The application of compressed sensing for rapid MR imaging. Magn. Reson. Med. **58**(6), 1182–1195 (2007). https://doi.org/10.1002/mrm.21391
2. Griswold, M.A., et al.: Generalized autocalibrating partially parallel acquisitions (GRAPPA). Magn. Reson. Med. **247**(6), 1202–1210 (2002). https://doi.org/10.1002/mrm.10171

3. Otazo, R., Candès, E., Sodickson, D.K.: Low-rank plus sparse matrix decomposition for accelerated dynamic MRI with separation of background and dynamic components. Magn. Reson. Med. **73**(3), 1125–1136 (2015). https://doi.org/10.1002/mrm.25240

4. Ravishankar, S., Bresler, Y.: MR image reconstruction from highly undersampled k-space data by dictionary learning. IEEE Trans. Med. Imaging **30**(5), 1028–1041 (2015). https://doi.org/10.1109/TMI.2010.2090538

5. Wang, S., et al.: Accelerating magnetic resonance imaging via deep learning. In: Proceedings of the IEEE 13th International Symposium on Biomedical Imaging (ISBI), pp. 514–517 (2016)

6. Lee, D., Yoo, J., Ye, J.: Deep residual learning for compressed sensing MRI. In: Proceedings of the IEEE 14th International Symposium on Biomedical Imaging (ISBI), pp. 15–18 (2017)

7. Schlemper, J., Caballero, J., Hajnal, J.V., Price, A., Rueckert, D.: A deep cascade of convolutional neural networks for mr image reconstruction. In: Niethammer, M., et al. (eds.) IPMI 2017. LNCS, vol. 10265, pp. 647–658. Springer, Cham (2017). https://doi.org/10.1007/978-3-319-59050-9_51

8. Kwon, K., Kim, D., Park, H.: A parallel MR imaging method using multilayer perceptron. Med. Phys. **44**(12), 6209–6224 (2017). https://doi.org/10.1002/mp.12600

9. Zhu, B., Liu, J.Z., Rosen, R.B., Rosen, M.S.: Image reconstruction by domain transform manifold learning. Nature **555**(7697), 487–492 (2018). https://doi.org/10.1038/nature25988

10. Jack, C.R., et al.: The Alzheimer's disease neuroimaging initiative (ADNI): MRI methods. J. Magn. Reson. Imaging **27**(4), 685–691 (2008). https://doi.org/10.1002/jmri.21049

11. Qu, X., Hou, Y., Lam, F., Guo, D., Zhong, J., Chen, Z.: Magnetic resonance image reconstruction from undersampled measurements using a patch–based nonlocal operator. Med. Image Anal. **18**(6), 843–856 (2014). https://doi.org/10.1016/j.media.2013.09.007

12. Zhan, Z., Cai, J.-F., Guo, D., Liu, Y., Chen, Z., Qu, X.: Fast multiclass dictionaries learning with geometrical directions in MRI reconstruction. IEEE Trans. Biomed. Eng. **63**(9), 1850–1861 (2016). https://doi.org/10.1109/TBME.2015.2503756

13. Wang, Z., Bovik, A.C., Sheikh, H.R., Simoncelli, E.P.: Image quality assessment: from error visibility to structural similarity. IEEE Trans. Image Process. **13**(4), 600–612 (2004). https://doi.org/10.1109/TIP.2003.819861

Deep Learning Using K-Space Based Data Augmentation for Automated Cardiac MR Motion Artefact Detection

Ilkay Oksuz[1](✉), Bram Ruijsink[1,2], Esther Puyol-Antón[1], Aurelien Bustin[1], Gastao Cruz[1], Claudia Prieto[1], Daniel Rueckert[3], Julia A. Schnabel[1], and Andrew P. King[1]

[1] School of Biomedical Engineering and Imaging Sciences,
King's College London, London, UK
ilkay.oksuz@kcl.ac.uk
[2] Guy's and St Thomas' Hospital NHS Foundation Trust, London, UK
[3] Biomedical Image Analysis Group, Imperial College London, London, UK

Abstract. Quality assessment of medical images is essential for complete automation of image processing pipelines. For large population studies such as the UK Biobank, artefacts such as those caused by heart motion are problematic and manual identification is tedious and time-consuming. Therefore, there is an urgent need for automatic image quality assessment techniques. In this paper, we propose a method to automatically detect the presence of motion-related artefacts in cardiac magnetic resonance (CMR) images. As this is a highly imbalanced classification problem (due to the high number of good quality images compared to the low number of images with motion artefacts), we propose a novel k-space based training data augmentation approach in order to address this problem. Our method is based on 3D spatio-temporal Convolutional Neural Networks, and is able to detect 2D+time short axis images with motion artefacts in less than 1 ms. We test our algorithm on a subset of the UK Biobank dataset consisting of 3465 CMR images and achieve not only high accuracy in detection of motion artefacts, but also high precision and recall. We compare our approach to a range of state-of-the-art quality assessment methods.

Keywords: Cardiac MR · Image quality assessment
Motion artefacts · UK Biobank · Convolutional Neural Networks

1 Introduction

High diagnostic accuracy of image analysis pipelines requires high quality medical images. Misleading conclusions can be drawn when the original data are of

Electronic supplementary material The online version of this chapter (https://doi.org/10.1007/978-3-030-00928-1_29) contains supplementary material, which is available to authorized users.

© Springer Nature Switzerland AG 2018
A. F. Frangi et al. (Eds.): MICCAI 2018, LNCS 11070, pp. 250–258, 2018.
https://doi.org/10.1007/978-3-030-00928-1_29

low quality, in particular for cardiac magnetic resonance (CMR) imaging. CMR images can contain a range of image artefacts [3], and assessing the quality of images acquired on MR scanners is a challenging problem. Traditionally, images are visually inspected by one or more experts, and those showing an insufficient level of quality are excluded from further analysis. However, visual assessment is time consuming and prone to variability due to inter-rater and intra-rater differences.

The UK Biobank is a large-scale study with all data accessible to researchers worldwide, and will eventually consist of CMR images from 100,000 subjects [11]. To maximize the research value of this and other similar datasets, automatic quality assessment tools are essential. One specific challenge in CMR is motion-related artefacts such as mistriggering, arrhythmia and breathing artefacts. These can result in temporal and/or spatial blurring of the images, which makes subsequent processing difficult [3]. For example, this type of artefact can lead to erroneous quantification of left ventricular (LV) volumes, which is an important indicator for cardiac functional assessment. Examples of a good quality image and an image with blurring motion artefacts are shown in Fig. 1a–b for a short-axis view CINE CMR scan.

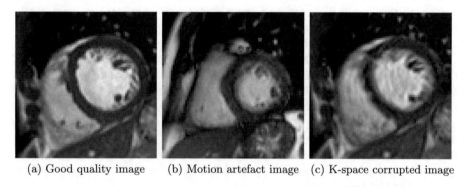

(a) Good quality image   (b) Motion artefact image   (c) K-space corrupted image

Fig. 1. Examples of a good quality CINE CMR image (a), an image with blurring motion artefacts (b), and a k-space corrupted image (c). The k-space corruption process is able to simulate realistic motion-related artefacts. (Please see videos in supplementary material.)

2 Background

Convolutional Neural Networks (CNNs) have been utilized for image quality assessment in the computer vision literature with considerable success [4], especially for image compression detection. This success has motivated the medical image analysis community to utilize CNNs on multiple image quality assessment challenges such as fetal ultrasound [15] and echocardiography [1]. CNNs have also been utilized for real-time scan plane detection for ultrasound with high accuracy [2]. Relevant work in motion artefact detection includes Meding et al. [8], who proposed a technique to detect motion artefacts caused by patient movement for brain MR using a simple CNN architecture. Their algorithm used training data from fruit images and artificial motion data. Also, Kustner et al. [6] proposed a patch-based motion artefact detection method for brain and abdomen MR images, but they made their tests on a small dataset of 16 MR images with significant motion artefacts. Motion artefacts in CMR imaging are largely caused by ECG mistriggering and pose a significantly different problem.

In the context of CMR, recent work on image quality assessment has targeted the detection of missing apical and basal slices [16]. Missing slices adversely affect the accurate calculation of the LV volume and hence the derivation of cardiac functional metrics such as ejection fraction. Tarroni et al. [13] addressed the same problem using multiple view CMR images and decision trees for landmark localization. One other image quality issue is off-axis acquisition of 4-chamber view CMR, which was detected with a simple CNN in [10]. CMR image quality was also linked with automatic quality control of image segmentation in [12]. In the context of detection of CMR motion artefacts, Lorch et al. [7] investigated synthetic motion artefacts. In their work, they used histogram, box, line and texture features to train a random forest algorithm to detect motion artefacts for different artefact levels. However, their algorithm was tested only on artificially corrupted synthetic data and aimed only at detecting breathing artefacts.

In this paper, we aim to accurately detect motion artefacts in large CMR datasets. We use a CNN for the detection of such cases and evaluate our method on a dataset of 3465 2D+time CMR sequences from the UK Biobank. There are two major contributions of this work. First, we address the problem of fully automatic motion artefact detection in a real large-scale CMR dataset for the first time. Second, we introduce a realistic k-space based data augmentation step to address the class imbalance problem. We generate artefacts from good quality images using a k-space corruption scheme, which results in highly realistic artefacts as visualized in Fig. 1c.

3   Methods

The proposed framework of using a spatio-temporal CNN for motion artefact detection consists of two stages; (1) image preprocessing consisting of normalization and region-of-interest (ROI) extraction; (2) CNN image classification of motion artefacts and good quality images.

3.1   Image Preprocessing

Given a 2D CINE CMR sequence of images we first normalize the pixel values between 0 and 1. Since the image dimensions vary from subject to subject, instead of image resizing we propose to use a motion information based ROI extraction to 80×80 pixels. Avoiding image resizing is of particular importance for image quality assessment, because resizing can influence the image quality significantly. The ROI is determined by using an unsupervised technique based on motion as proposed in [5]. Briefly, the ROI is determined by performing a Fourier analysis of the sequences of images, followed by a circular Hough transform to highlight the center of periodically moving structures.

3.2 Network Architecture

The proposed CNN consists of eight layers as visualized in Fig. 2. The architecture of our network follows a similar architecture to [14], which was originally developed for video classification using a spatio-temporal 3D CNN. In our case we use the third dimension as the time component and use 2D+time mid-ventricular sequences for classification. The input is an intensity normalized 80×80 cropped CMR image with 50 time frames. The network has 6 convolutional layers and 4 pooling layers, 2 fully-connected layers and a softmax loss layer to predict motion artefact labels. After each convolutional layer a ReLU activation is used. We then apply pooling on each feature map to reduce the filter responses to a lower dimension. We apply dropout with a probability of 0.5 at all convolutional layers and after the first fully connected layer to enforce regularization. All of these convolutional layers are applied with appropriate padding (both spatial and temporal) and stride 1, thus there is no change in terms of size from the input to the output of these convolutional layers.

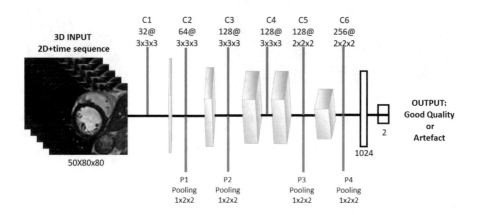

Fig. 2. The CNN architecture for motion artefact detection.

3.3 K-Space Corruption for Data Augmentation

We generate k-space corrupted data in order to increase the amount of motion artefact data for our under-represented low quality image class. The UK Biobank dataset that we use was acquired using Cartesian sampling and we follow a

Cartesian k-space corruption strategy to generate synthetic but realistic motion artefacts. We first transform each 2D short axis sequence to the Fourier domain and change 1 in z Cartesian sampling lines to the corresponding lines from other cardiac phases to mimic motion artefacts. We set $z = 3$ for generating realistic corruptions. In Fig. 3 we show an example of the generation of a corrupted frame i from the original frame i using information from the k-space data of other temporal frames. We add a random frame offset j when replacing the lines. In this way the original good quality images from the training set are used to increase the total number of low quality images in the training set. This is a realistic approach as the motion artefacts that occur from mistriggering arise from similar misallocations of k-space lines.

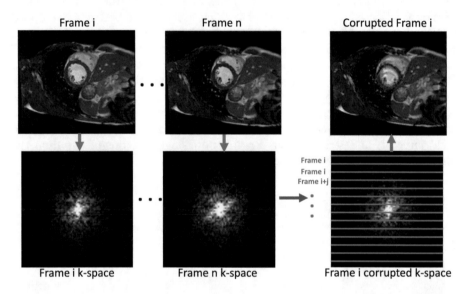

Fig. 3. K-space corruption for motion artefact generation in k-space. We use the Fourier transformation of each frame to generate the k-space of each image and replace k-space lines with lines from different temporal frames to generate corruptions.

3.4   Data Augmentation

Data augmentation was applied to achieve a more generalized model. Translational invariance is ensured with random shifts in both the horizontal and vertical directions in the range of [W/5, H/5], where W and H represent the width and height of the image respectively (i.e. W = H = 80 pixels in our case). Rotations are not used due to their influence on image quality caused by the necessary interpolation. Balanced classes are ensured using augmentation with the k-space corrupted data (see Sect. 3.3) for the under-represented motion artefact class. Note that none of the augmented data were used for testing. They were only used for increasing the total number of training images.

3.5   Implementation Details

The training of a CNN can be viewed as a combination of two components, a loss function or training objective, and an optimization algorithm that minimizes this function. In this study, we use the Adadelta optimizer to minimize the binary cross entropy. The cross entropy represents the dissimilarity of the approximated output distribution from the true distribution of labels after a softmax layer. The training ends when the network does not significantly improve its performance on the validation set for a predefined number of epochs (50). An improvement is considered sufficient if the relative increase in performance is at least 0.5%.

During training, a batch-size of 50 2D+time sequences was used. The learning rate of the optimizer was 0.0001. The parameters of the convolutional and fully-connected layers were initialized randomly from a zero-mean Gaussian distribution. In each trial, training was continued until the network converged. Convergence was defined as a state in which no substantial progress was observed in the training loss. We used the Keras Framework with Tensorflow backend for implementation and training the network took around 4 h on a NVIDIA Quadro 6000P GPU. Classification of a single image sequence took less than 1 ms.

4   Experimental Results

We evaluated our algorithm on a subset of the UK Biobank dataset consisting of 3360 good quality acquisitions and 105 short axis acquisitions containing arrythmia, mistriggering and breathing artefacts. This subset was chosen to be free of other types of image quality issues such as missing axial slices and was visually verified by an expert cardiologist. The details of the acquisition protocol of the UK Biobank dataset can be found in [11]. 50 temporal frames of each subject at mid-ventricular level were used to detect the motion artefacts.

We tested four different training configurations of our proposed CNN technique to evaluate its performance in more detail: (1) training using only real data without any data augmentation, (2) training using data augmentation with translations only, (3) training using data augmentation with k-space corrupted data only, (4) training using data augmentation with both translations and k-space corrupted data. In each setup, the real motion artefact data is used.

We compared our algorithm with a range of alternative classification techniques: K-nearest neighbours, Support Vector Machines (SVMs), Decision Trees, Random Forests, Adaboost and Naive Bayesian. The inputs to all algorithms were the cropped intensity-normalized data as described in Sect. 3.1. We optimized the parameters of each algorithm using a grid search. We also tested two techniques developed for image quality assessment in the computer vision literature: the NIQE metric [9] is based on natural scene statistics and is trained using a set of good quality CMR images to establish a baseline for good image quality; and the Variance of Laplacians is a moving filter that has been used to detect the blur level of an image. For both of these techniques we used a SVM for classification of the final scores.

We used a 10-fold stratified cross validation strategy to test all algorithms, in which each image appears once in the test set over all folds. Due to the high class imbalance, over 0.9 accuracy is achieved by most of the techniques in Table 1. We do not rely only on accuracy in our results due to the bias introduced by the imbalanced classes. The interesting comparison for the methods lies in the recall numbers, which quantify the capability of the methods to identify images with artefacts. The results show that the CNN-based technique is capable of identifying the presence of motion artefacts with high recall compared to other techniques. Note in particular that introducing the data with k-space corruption increases the recall number from 0.466 to 0.642. Additional data augmentation improves the recall further to 0.652. All state-of-the-art classification methods reach high accuracy, but Adaboost is capable to reach comparable recall to CNNs without data augmentation. However, the precision of Adaboost is lower compared to the CNN results. Moreover, the F1-score illustrates the improvement of performance using CNN-based methods compared to state-of-the-art machine learning approaches. The F1-score reaches 0.704 with k-space corrupted data and achieves 0.722 with additional data augmentation.

Table 1. Mean accuracy, precision, recall and F1 score results of image classification for motion artefacts. 10-fold cross validation is used and each image is labelled once over all folds.

Methods	Accuracy	Precision	Recall	F1-score
K-nearest neighbours	0.952	0.074	0.268	0.116
Linear SVM	0.968	0.721	0.385	0.502
Decision Tree	0.951	0.250	0.385	0.303
Random Forests	0.958	0.320	0.315	0.317
Adaboost	0.960	0.230	0.567	0.327
Naive Bayesian	0.801	0.527	0.183	0.111
Variance of Laplacian	0.958	0.113	0.161	0.133
NIQE [9]	0.958	0.210	0.248	0.227
CNN-no augmentation [14]	0.968	0.700	0.466	0.560
CNN-translational augmentation	0.974	0.750	0.600	0.667
CNN-k-space augmentation	0.977	0.779	0.642	0.704
CNN-k-space+translational augmentation	**0.982**	**0.809**	**0.652**	**0.722**

5   Discussion and Conclusion

In this paper, we have proposed a CNN-based technique for identifying motion-related artefacts in a large 2D CINE CMR dataset with high accuracy and recall. We have addressed the issue of high class imbalance by proposing the use of a k-space corruption data generation scheme for data augmentation, which clearly outperforms the basic data augmentation due to its capability to generate realistic artefact images. We have shown that a 3D CNN based neural network architecture developed for video classification is capable of classifying motion artefacts, outperforming other state-of-the-art techniques. To the best knowledge of the authors, this is the first paper to have tackled this clinical problem for a real CMR dataset. Our work brings fully automated evaluation of ventricular function from CMR imaging a step closer to clinically acceptable standards, enabling analysis of large imaging datasets such as the UK Biobank.

In future work, we plan to validate our method on the entire UK Biobank cohort, which is eventually expected to be 100,000 CMR images. Moreover, our current technique focuses only on mid-ventricular slices and in future we will use other slices in order to perform a more thorough image quality assessment.

Acknowledgments. This work was supported by an EPSRC programme Grant (EP/P001009/1) and the Wellcome EPSRC Centre for Medical Engineering at the School of Biomedical Engineering and Imaging Sciences, King's College London (WT 203148/Z/16/Z). This research has been conducted using the UK Biobank Resource under Application Number 17806. The GPU used in this research was generously donated by the NVIDIA Corporation.

References

1. Abdi, A.H., et al.: Quality assessment of echocardiographic cine using recurrent neural networks: feasibility on five standard view planes. In: Descoteaux, M., Maier-Hein, L., Franz, A., Jannin, P., Collins, D.L., Duchesne, S. (eds.) MICCAI 2017, Part III. LNCS, vol. 10435, pp. 302–310. Springer, Cham (2017). https://doi.org/10.1007/978-3-319-66179-7_35

2. Baumgartner, C.F., Kamnitsas, K., Matthew, J., Smith, S., Kainz, B., Rueckert, D.: Real-time standard scan plane detection and localisation in fetal ultrasound using fully convolutional neural networks. In: Ourselin, S., Joskowicz, L., Sabuncu, M.R., Unal, G., Wells, W. (eds.) MICCAI 2016, Part II. LNCS, vol. 9901, pp. 203–211. Springer, Cham (2016). https://doi.org/10.1007/978-3-319-46723-8_24

3. Ferreira, P.F.: Cardiovascular magnetic resonance artefacts. JCMR **15**(1), 1–41 (2013)

4. Kang, L., et al.: Convolutional neural networks for no reference image quality assessment. In: CVPR, vol. 18, pp. 1733–1740 (2014)

5. Korshunova, F.N., et al.: Diagnosing heart diseases with deep neural networks (2016). http://irakorshunova.github.io/2016/03/15/heart.html

6. Kustner, T., et al.: Automated reference-free detection of motion artifacts in magnetic resonance images. MR Mater. Phys. Biol. Med. **31**(2), 1–14 (2017)

7. Lorch, B.: Automated detection of motion artefacts in MR imaging using decision forests. J. Med. Eng. **2017**, 9 (2017)

8. Meding, K., et al.: Automatic detection of motion artifacts in MR images using CNNS. In: ICASSP, pp. 811–815 (2017)

9. Mittal, A.: Making a completely blind image quality analyzer. IEEE Signal Process. Lett. **22**(3), 209–212 (2013)

10. Oksuz, I., et al.: Automatic left ventricular outflow tract classification for accurate cardiac MR planning. In: ISBI (2018)

11. Petersen, S.E.: UK biobank's cardiovascular magnetic resonance protocol. JCMR **18**(1), 1–8 (2016)
12. Robinson, R., et al.: Automatic quality control of cardiac MRI segmentation in large-scale population imaging. In: Descoteaux, M., Maier-Hein, L., Franz, A., Jannin, P., Collins, D.L., Duchesne, S. (eds.) MICCAI 2017, Part I. LNCS, vol. 10433, pp. 720–727. Springer, Cham (2017). https://doi.org/10.1007/978-3-319-66182-7_82
13. Tarroni, G., et al.: Learning-based heart coverage estimation for short-axis cine cardiac MR images. In: Pop, M., Wright, G.A. (eds.) FIMH 2017. LNCS, vol. 10263, pp. 73–82. Springer, Cham (2017). https://doi.org/10.1007/978-3-319-59448-4_8
14. Tran, D., et al.: Learning spatiotemporal features with 3D convolutional networks. In: ICCV, pp. 4489–4497 (2015)
15. Wu, L.: FUIQA: fetal ultrasound image quality assessment with deep convolutional networks. IEEE Trans. Cybern. **47**(5), 1336–1349 (2016)
16. Zhang, L., Gooya, A., Frangi, A.F.: Semi-supervised assessment of incomplete LV coverage in cardiac MRI using generative adversarial nets. In: Tsaftaris, S.A., Gooya, A., Frangi, A.F., Prince, J.L. (eds.) SASHIMI 2017. LNCS, vol. 10557, pp. 61–68. Springer, Cham (2017). https://doi.org/10.1007/978-3-319-68127-6_7

Cardiac MR Segmentation from Undersampled k-space Using Deep Latent Representation Learning

Jo Schlemper[1(✉)], Ozan Oktay[1], Wenjia Bai[1], Daniel C. Castro[1],
Jinming Duan[1], Chen Qin[1], Jo V. Hajnal[2], and Daniel Rueckert[1]

[1] Biomedical Image Analysis Group, Imperial College London, London, UK
{js3611,o.oktay13,w.bai,dc315,j.duan,c.qin15,d.rueckert}@imperial.ac.uk
[2] Imaging and Biomedical Engineering Clinical Academic Group,
King's College London, London, UK
jo.hajnal@kcl.ac.uk

Abstract. Reconstructing magnetic resonance imaging (MRI) from undersampled k-space enables the accelerated acquisition of MRI but is a challenging problem. However, in many diagnostic scenarios, perfect reconstructions are not necessary as long as the images allow clinical practitioners to extract clinically relevant parameters. In this work, we present a novel deep learning framework for reconstructing such clinical parameters directly from undersampled data, expanding on the idea of *application-driven* MRI. We propose two deep architectures, an end-to-end synthesis network and a latent feature interpolation network, to predict cardiac segmentation maps from extremely undersampled dynamic MRI data, bypassing the usual image reconstruction stage altogether. We perform a large-scale simulation study using UK Biobank data containing nearly 1000 test subjects and show that with the proposed approaches, an accurate estimate of clinical parameters such as ejection fraction can be obtained from fewer than 10 k-space lines per time-frame.

1 Introduction

Cardiovascular MR (CMR) imaging enables accurate quantification of cardiac chamber volume, ejection fraction and myocardial mass, which are crucial for diagnosing, assessing and monitoring cardiovascular diseases (CVDs), the leading cause of death globally. However, one limitation of CMR is the slow acquisition time. A routine CMR protocol can take from 20 to 60 min, which makes the tool costly and less accessible to worldwide population. In addition, CMR often requires breath-holds which can be difficult for patients; therefore, accelerating the CMR acquisition is essential. Over the last decades, numerous approaches have been proposed for accelerated MR imaging, including parallel imaging, compressed sensing [7] and, more recently, deep learning approaches [6].

Reconstructing images from accelerated and undersampled MRI is an ill-posed problem and, essentially, all approaches must exploit some type of redundancies or assumptions on underlying data to resolve the aliasing caused by

A. F. Frangi et al. (Eds.): MICCAI 2018, LNCS 11070, pp. 259–267, 2018.
https://doi.org/10.1007/978-3-030-00928-1_30

sub-Nyquist sampling. In the case of dynamic cardiac cine reconstruction, high spatiotemporal redundancy and sparsity can be exploited, however, the acceleration factor for a near perfect reconstruction is currently limited up to 9 [10]. We argue that one effective way of pushing the acceleration factor even higher is to move to the concept of *application-driven MRI* [2]. The key insight is that in many cases, the images are not an end in themselves, but rather means of accessing clinically relevant parameters which are obtained as post-processing steps, such as segmentation or tissue characterisation. Therefore, it is more effective to instead combine the reconstruction and post-processing steps and tailor the acquisition protocol to obtain the final results as accurately and efficiently as possible. In particular, if the end-goal is significantly more compressible than the original image, then one can expect further acceleration and still obtain satisfactory results [3,5]. This work focuses on a scenario where we obtain cardiac segmentation maps directly from heavily undersampled dynamic MR data.

Our contribution is the following: firstly, we propose two network architectures to learn such a mapping. The first model, *Syn-net*, exploits the spatiotemporal redundancy of the input to directly generate the segmentation map. However, under heavy aliasing artefact, the extracted features may not be useful for segmentation. To address the latter case, we propose the second model, *LI-net*, which first predicts the low dimensional latent code of the corresponding segmentation map, which is subsequently decoded. Secondly, we extensively evaluate the two models with large-scale simulation studies to demonstrate the effectiveness of the proposed approaches for various acceleration factors. In particular, we show that for the case where undersampled image contains sufficient geometrical information, Syn-net outperforms LI-net but in a more challenging scenario where only one line of k-space is sampled per frame, LI-net outperforms Syn-net. Finally, we study the latent space structure of these architectures to demonstrate that the models learn useful representations of the data. This work potentially enables interesting future works in which reconstruction, post-processing and analysis stages are integrated to yield smarter imaging protocols.

2   Proposed Methods

End-to-End Synthesis Network (Syn-net): Let $\mathcal{D} \subseteq \mathcal{X} \times \mathcal{Y}$ be dataset of fully-sampled complex valued (dynamic) images $x = \{x_i \in \mathbb{C} \,|\, i \in S\}$, where S denotes indices on a pixel grid, and the corresponding segmentation labels $y = \{y_i \,|\, i \in S\}$ representing different tissue types with $y_i \in \{1, 2, \ldots C\}$. Let $u = \{u_i \in \mathbb{C} \,|\, u = F_u^H F_u x\}$ denote an undersampled image, where F_u is the undersampling Fourier encoding matrix. Let $p(y_i \,|\, x)$ be the true distribution of i-th pixel label given an image, and $r(u \,|\, x, \mathcal{M})$ represent the sampling distribution of the undersampled images given an image x and a (pseudo) random undersampling mask generator $\mathcal{M}$. We aim to learn a synthesis network $q(y_i \,|\, u, \theta)$, termed *Syn-net*, which uses a convolutional neural network (CNN) to model the probability distribution of segmentation maps given the undersampled image parameterised by θ. We train the network by the following modified cross-entropy (CE) loss:

$$\mathcal{L}(\theta) = \sum_{(x,y)\in\mathcal{D}} \mathbb{E}_{u\sim r} \left[\sum_{i\in S} p(y_i \mid x_i) \log q(y_i \mid u_i, \theta) \right], \tag{1}$$

where we take the expectation over differently undersampled images. In practice, we generate one different undersampling pattern on-the-fly for each mini-batch training as an approximation to the expectation. For the network architecture, we use an architecture inspired by the state-of-the-art segmentation network, *U-net* [9], shown in Fig. 1.

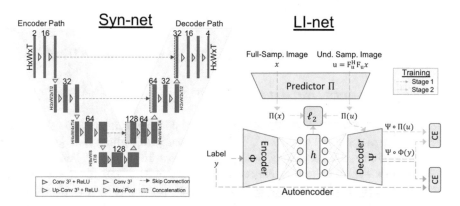

Fig. 1. *(Left)* The detailed architecture of Syn-net: the changes in the number of features are shown above the tensor. *(Right)* For LI-net, the two-stage training strategy is outlined. The same encoder and decoder as Syn-net can be used for LI-Net

Latent Feature Interpolation Network (LI-net): Syn-net assumes that the input data contains sufficient geometrical information to generate the target segmentation. For heavily undersampled (and therefore aliased) images, this assumption may not be valid as the aliasing could mislead the network from identifying the correct boundaries. In the latter case, synthesis is still possible as long as the target domain has a compact, discriminative latent representation $h \in \mathcal{H}$ that can be predicted, an approach motivated by *TL-network* [4]. Such a network can be trained in following steps. In stage 1, one trains an auto-encoder (AE) in the target domain $y = \Psi(\Phi(y; \theta_{enc}); \theta_{dec})$, $y \in \mathcal{Y}$, which is a composition of encoder $\Phi : \mathcal{Y} \to \mathcal{H}$ and decoder $\Psi : \mathcal{H} \to \mathcal{Y}$, parameterised by θ_{enc} and θ_{dec} respectively and $\mathcal{H}$ is a low-dimensional latent space. The AE can be trained using the ℓ_2 norm or CE loss. In stage 2, one trains a predictor network $\Pi : \mathcal{X} \to \mathcal{H}$, parameterised by θ_{pred}. For a given input-target pair (x, y), the predictor attempts to predict the latent code $h = \Phi(y; \theta_{enc})$ from x. This is trained using the ℓ_2 norm in the latent space: $d_{\mathcal{H}}(y, x) = \|\Phi(y; \theta_{enc}) - \Pi(x; \theta_{pred})\|_2$. Once the predictor is trained, one can obtain an input-output mapping by the composition $\hat{y} = \Psi(\Pi(x; \theta_{dec}); \theta_{pred})$.

In our work, the AE is trained to learn the compact representation of segmentations and the predictor is trained to interpolate these from dynamic undersampled images, hence termed a *latent feature interpolation network (LI-net)*.

In stage 1, we train the AE using CE loss. In stage 2, we modify our objective to further encourage the network to produce a *consistent* prediction for differently undersampled versions of the same reference image. This constraint is implemented by forcing the network to produce the same latent code for undersampled images as for the fully-sampled image. Furthermore, we add a CE term $d_{\mathrm{CE}}(y, \Psi \circ \Pi(u))$ to ensure that an accurate segmentation can be obtained from the code. Therefore, our objective term is as follows (here λ_i's are hyperparameters to be adjusted based on the preferred end-goal):

$$\mathcal{L}(\theta_{pred}) = \sum_{(x,y)\in\mathcal{D}} \mathbb{E}_{u\sim r}\Big[d_{\mathcal{H}}(y, u) + \lambda_1 d_{\mathcal{H}}(y, x)$$

$$+ \lambda_2 \|\Pi(x) - \Pi(u)\|_2 + \lambda_3 d_{\mathrm{CE}}(y, \Psi \circ \Pi(u))\Big]. \quad (2)$$

3   Experiments and Results

Dataset and Undersampling: Experiments were performed using 5000 short-axis cardiac cine MR images from the UK Biobank study [8], which is acquired using bSSFP sequence, matrix size $N_x \times N_y \times T = 208 \times 187 \times 50$, a pixel resolution of $1.8 \times 1.8 \times 10.0\,\mathrm{mm}^3$ and a temporal resolution of $31.56\,\mathrm{ms}$. Since the manual annotations are only available at end-systolic (ES) and end-diastolic (ED) frames but we are interested in segmenting the entire time sequence, we use [1], which well agrees with the manual segmentations, to generate the labels for the left-ventricular (LV) cavity, the myocardium and the right-ventricular (RV) cavity for all time-frames including apical, mid and basal slices, which were then treated as the ground truth labels for this work. We split the data into 4000 training subjects and 1000 test subjects, and we simulated random undersampling using variable density 1D undersampling masks. These masks were generated on-the-fly. As only the magnitude images were available we synthetically generated the phase maps (smoothly varying 2D sinusoid waves) on-the-fly to make the simulation more realistic by removing the conjugate symmetry in k-space. Different levels of acceleration factors ($1/n_l$) were considered, $n_l \in [1, 100]$ where n_l is the number of lines per time-frame. Note for fully-sampled image, $n_l = 168$.

Model and Parameters: The input to the network is 2D+t undersampled data and the output is a sequence of segmentation map. Note that z-slices were processed separately due to large slice thickness. The detail of the Syn-net is shown in Fig. 1. To make a fair comparison between the two architectures, we used the encoding path of Syn-net as both encoder Φ and predictor Π, and the decoding path as decoder Ψ. The size of the latent code was set to be $|h| = 1024$. Note that fully-connected layers are used to join the encoder, the latent code and the decoder. They were trained with mini-batch size 8 using Adam with initial learning rate 10^{-4}, which was reduced by a factor of 0.8 every 2 epochs. The AE in LI-net was trained for 30 epochs to ensure that the Dice scores for each class reached 0.95. For both models, we first trained the network to perform segmentation from fully-sampled data as a warm start. The number of lines was gradually reduced and by 10th epoch, we uniformly sampled n_l from $[0, 168]$. The training error for both models plateaued within 50 epochs. For LI-net, the hyper-parameters for the loss function were empirically chosen to be $\lambda_1 = 1$, $\lambda_2 = 10^{-4}$, $\lambda_3 = 10$, which we found to work sufficiently. For data augmentation, we generated affine transformations on-the-fly. We used PyTorch for implementation.

Evaluation: We first took the trained models and evaluated their Dice scores for LV, myocardium (Myo) and RV for $n_l \in [1, 100]$. For each subject, we only included ES and ED frames but aggregated the results across all short-axis slices. The Dice scores versus the number of acquired k-space lines are shown in Fig. 2. The networks maintained the performance up to about 20 lines per frame, demonstrating the capability of the models to directly interpolate the anatomical boundary even in the presence of the aliasing artefact. In general, Syn-net showed superior performance, indicating that the extracted spatiotem-poral features are directly useful for segmentation. In particular, we report that the LI-net underperformed as it does not employ the skip-connection as Syn-net does, which limits how accurately it can delineate the boundaries. We specu-late, however, increasing the capacity of network is likely to improve the results. Interestingly, LI-net outperformed Syn-net for the case of segmentation from 1 line, suggesting that in more challenging domains the approach of LI-net to interpolate the latent code is still a viable option.

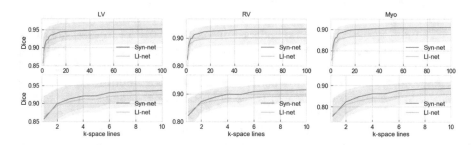

Fig. 2. Dice scores of Syn-net vs LI-net. The second row expands $n_l \in [1, 10]$, the solid lines and the shaded areas show the mean and the standard deviation respectively.

In the second experiment, the models were further fine-tuned for a fixed number of lines for $n_l \in \{1, 10, 20\}$ separately. From the obtained segmentation maps, we computed LV ES/ED volumes (ESV/EDV) RV ESV/EDV, LV mass (LVM) and ejection fraction (EF). The mean percentage errors across all test subjects were reported in Table 1. Syn-net consistently performs better than LI-net and has relatively small errors ($<7.7\%$) for all values for $n_l \in \{10, 20\}$. Both models showed low error for EF, where the correlation coefficient was 0.81 for both models for $n_l = 20$. The examples of the segmentation maps are shown in Fig. 3. Note that due to heavy aliasing artefact of the input image, we instead visualised the temporally averaged image for x-y plane, which was obtained by combining all k-space lines across the temporal axis into a single k_x-k_y grid.

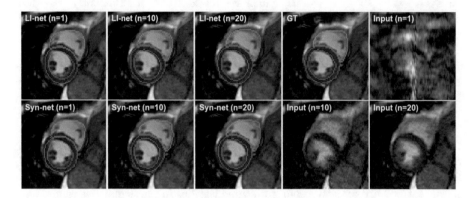

Fig. 3. Visualisation of the ground truth image overlaid with the obtained segmentations. LI-net produced more anatomically regularised, consistent segmentations. Syn-net produced segmentations that are occasionally anatomically implausible but more faithful to the boundary.

Although in theory we expect the reconstructed segmentation maps to be independent of the aliasing artefact present in the input, this is not always the case (Fig. 3). To measure such variability, we define *within subject distances*: given a fully-sampled image, we undersample it differently for $n_{\text{trial}} = 100$ times. From the predicted segmentation maps given by a model, we computed the mean shape, to which we then calculated mean contour distance (MD) and Hausdorff distance (HD) of individual predictions. Small distances indicate that the segmentation is consistent. However, if the network simply produces a *population mean shape* independent of the input, then the above distances can be very low even without producing useful segmentations. To get a better picture, we also measured the *between subject distances*, which computes MD and HD between the population mean shape (a mean predicted shape across *all* subjects) and the individual subject mean shapes. For both experiments, $n_{\text{subject}} = 100$ subject were used and the averaged distances are shown in Table 2. Indeed, we see that LI-net shows lower values for *within subject* distances, indicating that it produces more consistent segmentations than Syn-net ($p \ll 0.01$, Wilcoxon

Table 1. Average percentage errors (%) for each clinical parameter

n_l	LV ESV			LV EDV			RV ESV			RV EDV			LVM			EF		
	1	10	20	1	10	20	1	10	20	1	10	20	1	10	20	1	10	20
LI-net	7.9	3.6	3.2	15.8	7.9	7.0	11.7	6.5	6.6	18.4	10.5	10.6	25.0	13.7	12.9	8.8	5.5	4.9
Syn-net	9.0	4.2	3.4	14.6	7.2	6.1	9.9	4.9	4.1	13.4	7.7	6.5	11.4	6.8	5.8	8.2	5.5	4.6

rank-sum). High *between subject* distances indicate that both models are generating segmentation maps closer to subject-specific means than to the population mean.

Table 2. The *within-subject* and *between-subject* distances of the segmentations

n_l	HD (Within)				MD (Within)				HD (Between)				MD (Between)			
	Myo		RV		Myo		RV		Myo		RV		Myo		RV	
	1	10	1	10	1	10	1	10	1	10	1	10	1	10	1	10
LI-net	3.63	2.58	4.68	3.67	1.47	0.92	1.71	1.14	9.69	10.30	12.55	14.31	4.40	4.94	5.02	5.91
Syn-net	6.47	3.23	6.96	5.05	1.83	0.99	2.15	1.34	10.62	10.34	11.56	15.22	4.16	4.81	4.78	6.03

Finally, we investigate the latent space of the models. For 5 subjects, we generated 50 undersampled images for each number of lines $n_l \in \{1, 5, 10, 15, 20\}$. Here all undersampled images have the same target segmentation per subject. For LI-net, we plotted the predicted latent code $h \in \mathcal{H}$ for these images. For Syn-net, we plotted the activation map before the first upsampling layer to see whether the network exploits any latent space structure for generating the segmentations. We visualised them using Principal Component Analysis (PCA) and t-distributed stochastic neighbour embedding (t-SNE) with $d = 2$, as shown in Fig. 4, where subjects are colour-coded and brighter means higher acceleration factor.

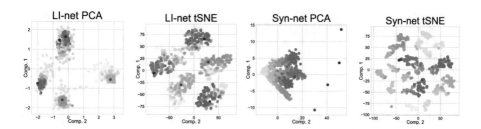

Fig. 4. Visualising the distribution of the latent representations of LI-net and Syn-net. *(Left to right)* LI-net PCA, LI-net t-SNE, Syn-net PCA, Syn-net t-SNE. The darkest points are the latent representations of the fully sampled images, for reference.

For LI-net, both for PCA and t-SNE, the latent space is clearly clustered by individual subjects, indicating that the predictions are indeed consistent for different undersampling patterns. In addition, as the latent code is discriminative for each subject, it enables fitting a classifier for subject-based prediction tasks. On the other hand, for Syn-net, although there are per-subject clusters, there is also a clear tendency to favour clustering the points by the acceleration factors, as seen in the t-SNE plot. Note that since Syn-net also exploits skip connections, one can conclude that the network exploits different reconstruction strategies for different acceleration factors. Another interesting observation is that in Syn-net PCA, the distances between all the points are reduced as the acceleration factor is increased. This means that the latent features for Syn-net are less discriminative when images are heavily aliased. However, the extracted features become gradually more discriminative as more lines are sampled.

4   Conclusion and Discussion

In this work we explored an application-driven MRI, where our end-goal was to extract segmentation maps directly from extremely undersampled data, bypassing image reconstruction. Remarkably, when at least 10 lines per frame are acquired, we showed that we could already compute clinical parameters within 10% error. Even though Syn-net provided better performance overall, and LI-net exhibited more well-behaved latent-space structure. In future work, the latent code of LI-net could be used as a feature for classification tasks, where we may be able to classify whether a patient is abnormal, directly from a few lines of k-space. This work opens a huge avenue for future research where joint pipelines can be exploited for smarter MR imaging that is both fast and accurate.

Acknowledgements. JS is partially funded by EPSRC Grant (EP/P001009/1).

References

1. Bai, W., et al.: Human-level CMR image analysis with deep fully convolutional networks (2017). arXiv preprint: arXiv:1710.09289
2. Caballero, J., Bai, W., Price, A.N., Rueckert, D., Hajnal, J.V.: Application-driven MRI: joint reconstruction and segmentation from undersampled MRI data. In: Golland, P., Hata, N., Barillot, C., Hornegger, J., Howe, R. (eds.) MICCAI 2014, Part I. LNCS, vol. 8673, pp. 106–113. Springer, Cham (2014). https://doi.org/10.1007/978-3-319-10404-1_14
3. Gaur, P., Grissom, W.A.: Accelerated MRI thermometry by direct estimation of temperature from undersampled k-space data. Magn. Reson. Med. **73**(5), 1914–1925 (2015)
4. Girdhar, R., Fouhey, D.F., Rodriguez, M., Gupta, A.: Learning a predictable and generative vector representation for objects. In: Leibe, B., Matas, J., Sebe, N., Welling, M. (eds.) ECCV 2016, Part VI. LNCS, vol. 9910, pp. 484–499. Springer, Cham (2016). https://doi.org/10.1007/978-3-319-46466-4_29
5. Guo, Y., Lingala, S.G., Zhu, Y., Lebel, R.M., Nayak, K.S.: Direct estimation of tracer-kinetic parameter maps from highly undersampled brain dynamic contrast enhanced MRI. Magn. Reson. Med. **78**(4), 1566–1578 (2017)
6. Hammernik, K., et al.: Learning a variational network for reconstruction of accelerated MRI data. Magn. Reson. Med. (2017)
7. Lustig, M., Donoho, D., Pauly, J.M.: Sparse MRI: the application of compressed sensing for rapid MR imaging. Magn. Reson. Med. **58**(6), 1182–1195 (2007)
8. Petersen, S.E., et al.: UK Biobank's cardiovascular magnetic resonance protocol. J. Cardiovasc. Magn. Reson. **18**(1), 8 (2016)

9. Ronneberger, O., Fischer, P., Brox, T.: U-Net: convolutional networks for biomedical image segmentation. In: Navab, N., Hornegger, J., Wells, W.M., Frangi, A.F. (eds.) MICCAI 2015, Part III. LNCS, vol. 9351, pp. 234–241. Springer, Cham (2015). https://doi.org/10.1007/978-3-319-24574-4_28
10. Schlemper, J., Caballero, J., Hajnal, J.V., Price, A., Rueckert, D.: A deep cascade of convolutional neural networks for dynamic MR image reconstruction. IEEE Trans. Med. Imaging **37** (2017)

A Comprehensive Approach for Learning-Based Fully-Automated Inter-slice Motion Correction for Short-Axis Cine Cardiac MR Image Stacks

Giacomo Tarroni[1(✉)], Ozan Oktay[1], Matthew Sinclair[1], Wenjia Bai[1], Andreas Schuh[1], Hideaki Suzuki[2], Antonio de Marvao[3], Declan O'Regan[3], Stuart Cook[3], and Daniel Rueckert[1]

[1] BioMedIA Group, Department of Computing,
Imperial College London, London, UK
g.tarroni@imperial.ac.uk
[2] Division of Brain Sciences, Department of Medicine,
Imperial College London, London, UK
[3] MRC London Institute of Medical Sciences, Imperial College London, London, UK

Abstract. In the clinical routine, short axis (SA) cine cardiac MR (CMR) image stacks are acquired during multiple subsequent breathholds. If the patient cannot consistently hold the breath at the same position, the acquired image stack will be affected by inter-slice respiratory motion and will not correctly represent the cardiac volume, introducing potential errors in the following analyses and visualisations. We propose an approach to automatically correct inter-slice respiratory motion in SA CMR image stacks. Our approach makes use of probabilistic segmentation maps (PSMs) of the left ventricular (LV) cavity generated with decision forests. PSMs are generated for each slice of the SA stack and rigidly registered in-plane to a target PSM. If long axis (LA) images are available, PSMs are generated for them and combined to create the target PSM; if not, the target PSM is produced from the same stack using a 3D model trained from motion-free stacks. The proposed approach was tested on a dataset of SA stacks acquired from 24 healthy subjects (for which anatomical 3D cardiac images were also available as reference) and compared to two techniques which use LA intensity images and LA segmentations as targets, respectively. The results show the accuracy and robustness of the proposed approach in motion compensation.

1 Introduction

Cardiovascular magnetic resonance (CMR) imaging is the reference technique regarding several applications for the anatomical and functional assessment of the heart [1]. While fast SSFP sequences allow the direct acquisition of an anatomical 3D image (A3D) of the whole heart, they are usually limited by

© Springer Nature Switzerland AG 2018
A. F. Frangi et al. (Eds.): MICCAI 2018, LNCS 11070, pp. 268–276, 2018.
https://doi.org/10.1007/978-3-030-00928-1_31

either relatively poor image quality or low temporal resolution, making them often unsuitable for accurate functional assessment. The most common CMR sequence currently used in the clinical practice is still the short axis (SA) SSFP cine, consisting of 10–14 parallel slices and 20–30 frames per cardiac cycle. SA cine stacks are generated during multiple breath-holds (i.e. 1–3 slices acquired per each breath-hold). Although the subjects are instructed to hold their breath at the same breath-hold position, in practice the heart location can vary considerably. If the differences between the breath-hold positions are large, the acquired image stack will be affected by inter-slice motion and not correctly represent the cardiac volume, introducing potential errors in the following analyses and visualisations.

Related Work. Several approaches for SA stack motion correction (MC) have been proposed in the literature. Among the techniques that make use of routinely acquired CMR images, Lotjonen et al. [2] proposed to perform in-plane rigid registration of each SA slice to LA images, used as target. Sinclair et al. [3] implemented a similar approach using LV segmentations (obtained using a fully-convolutional neural network, FCN) instead of the actual images. A very similar technique was also developed by Yang et al. [4], which also included a shape model to better retrieve the actual motion of the myocardium throughout the cardiac cycle. An alternative approach, which has the advantage of being applicable even if LA images are not available, consists in implicitly incorporating correct representations of the heart into a model trained from motion-free stacks, and in using it to perform motion correction. For instance, Oktay et al. [5] proposed to associate each SA slice with a set of probabilistic edge maps (PEMs) outlining the myocardial contours in the same slice as well as in the adjacent one, and to then perform rigid registration between the obtained PEMs.

Contributions. In this paper, we propose a comprehensive approach to automatically correct inter-slice respiratory motion in SA CMR image stacks. Our approach makes use of probabilistic segmentation maps (PSMs) of the left ventricular (LV) cavity generated with hybrid decision forests. PSMs are generated for each slice of the SA stack and rigidly registered in-plane to a target PSM. The main contributions of the paper are the following:

- The proposed approach includes two different techniques: if LA images are available, PSMs are generated from them and combined to create the target PSM. If not, the target PSM is produced from the same stack using a 3D model trained from motion-free stacks;
- If LA images are available, the hybrid forests estimate from them at once both PSMs and landmarks locations for the apex and the mitral valve, which are used to restrict motion correction to the slices of the SA stack between them, thus limiting potential spurious results especially in the basal region;
- The proposed approach was tested on a dataset acquired from 24 healthy subjects (for which anatomical 3D cardiac images were also available as reference) and compared to two techniques which use LA intensity images and LA segmentations (generated using FCNs) as targets, respectively. Testing was also performed after training the techniques on a different dataset to assess their generalisation properties.

2 Methods

Hybrid Decision Forests. A decision tree consists in the combination of split and leaf nodes arranged in a tree-like structure [6]. Decision trees route a sample $x \in \mathcal{X}$ (in our case an image patch) by recursively branching left or right at each split node j until a leaf node k is reached. Each leaf node is associated with a posterior distribution $p(y|x)$ for the output variable $y \in \mathcal{Y}$. Each split node j is associated with a binary split function $h(x, \theta_j) \in \{0, 1\}$, defined by the set of parameters θ_j. During training, at each node the goal is to find the set of parameters θ_j which maximizes a previously defined *information gain* I_j, that is usually defined as $I_j = H(S_j) - \sum_{i \in \{0,1\}} |S_j^i|/|S_j| \cdot H(S_j^i)$, where S_j, S_j^0 and S_j^1 are respectively the training set arriving at node j, leaving the node to the left and to the right. $H(S)$ is the entropy of the training set, whose construction depends on the task at hand (e.g. classification, regression). Different types of nodes (maximizing different information gains) can be interleaved within a single tree structure, thus called hybrid. In the present technique structured classification nodes (aiming at the generation of a PSM of the LV cavity) and regression nodes (aiming at landmark localisation) are combined [7]. During testing, the posterior distributions of the different trees are combined using an ensemble model.

Structured classification nodes associate to each image patch x a label $y \in \mathcal{Y}$ consisting of a segmentation of the LV cavity within x. Structured labels at each split node can be clustered into two subgroups depending on some similarity measure between them following a two-step procedure [8]. First, $\mathcal{Y}$ is mapped to an intermediate space $\mathcal{Z}$ by means of the function $\Pi : \mathcal{Y} \rightarrow \mathcal{Z}$ where the distance between labels can be computed. Then, PCA is applied to the vectors z to map the associated labels y into a binary set of labels $c \in \mathcal{C} = \{0, 1\}$: this is achieved by applying a binary quantization to the principal component of each z vector. Finally, the Shannon entropy $H_{SC}(S) = -\sum_{c \in \mathcal{C}} p(c) log(p(c))$ can be adopted, with $p(c)$ indicating the empirical distribution extracted from training set at the each node. Differently from [7], in which edge maps were generated, to estimate segmentation maps we adopted the mapping

$$\Pi : z = [y(j_1) = y(j_2) = 0] \oplus [y(j_1) = y(j_2) = 1] \qquad \forall j_1 \neq j_2,$$

where j_1 and j_2 are indices spanning every pixel in y. This mapping encodes for each pair of pixels in y whether they are both equal to 0 and whether they are both equal to 1, allowing the correct clustering of the labels at each node based on their similarity. At testing time, each sample patch of the test image is sent down each tree of the forest, and the segmentation maps stored at each selected leaf node are averaged producing a smooth segmentation map (PSM) of the LV cavity. The values in the PSM are proportional to the certainty in LV cavity detection, and can be used to assess the reliability of the prediction.

Regression nodes associate to each image patch x a label $\mathcal{D} = (d^1, d^2, \ldots, d^L)$, where d^l represents for each of the L landmarks (LMs) the N-dimensional displacement vector from the patch centre to the landmark location [7]. The information gain used for regression nodes minimizes the determinant of the full covariance matrix $|\Lambda(S)|$ defined by the landmark displacement vectors: $H_R(S) = \frac{1}{2}log((2\pi e)^d |\Lambda(S)|)$. The regression information is stored at each leaf node k using a parametric model following a $N \cdot L$-dimensional multivariate normal distribution with $\overline{d_k^l}$ and Σ_k^l mean and covariance matrices, respectively. At testing time, for each landmark, Hough vote maps are generated by summing up the regression posterior distributions obtained from each tree for each patch [7]. Finally, the locations of the landmarks are determined by identifying the pixel with the highest value on each of the L Hough vote maps.

For training, the extracted features are multi-resolution image intensity, histogram of gradients (HoG) and gradient magnitude, exactly as in [7]. The described hybrid random forest approach is used to build several models: three for LA images (extracting at once PSMs and landmarks for the apex and the mitral valve) and two for the SA stacks (extracting 2D and 3D PSMs, respectively). These models are then used to perform motion correction with two different possible pipelines, depending on the availability of LA images.

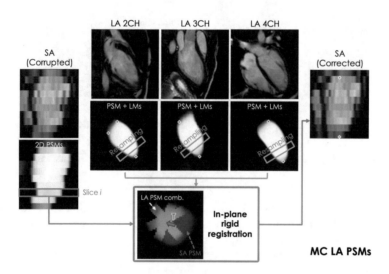

Fig. 1. Pipeline for motion correction using LA PSMs as target.

Motion Correction with LA PSMs (MC LA PSMs). This method relies on 2D SA PSMs generated from the motion-corrupted stack and on LA PSMs (together with landmarks), which are used as target (see Fig. 1). First, LA PSMs are rigidly registered (by 3D translation only, using normalized cross-correlation, NCC, as similarity metric) to the SA PSM stack to compensate for potential motion between different acquisitions. Then, for each slice of the SA PSM stack, the three registered LA PSMs are resampled and combined into a single image (referred to as LA PSM combined) containing the sections of the LA PSMs with respect to a specific slice. Finally, in-plane rigid registration (by translation only, using NCC) is performed between each SA PSM slice and the associated LA PSM combined, and the estimated translation is applied to the SA slice, thus performing the correction. These two steps (LA PSMs registration to the SA PSMs stack, and slice-by-slice SA PSMs registration to LA PSMs combined) are iterated until the maximum translation estimated within the stack is less than two pixels, which usually happens within the first 4 iterations. While this iterative registration scheme is similar to previously published ones [3], a major novelty is that not all the slices of the SA stack actually undergo motion correction: a slice is corrected only if (a) its peak PSM value is above a threshold T_m and (b) it lies between the median apex and median mitral valve points (defined as medians of the landmark sets identified on the LA images). This allows the exclusion of slices outside the LV or with unreliable LV cavity detection.

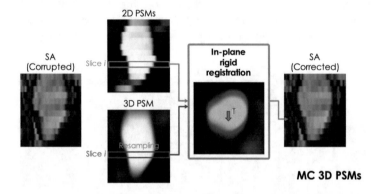

Fig. 2. Pipeline for motion correction using a 3D SA PSM as target.

Motion Correction with 3D SA PSMs (MC 3D PSMs). This method relies only on the information extracted from the motion-corrupted SA stack: 2D SA PSMs and a 3D SA PSM, which is used as target (see Fig. 2). While the models presented so far are trained using 2D patches x and labels y, the 3D SA PSM one is trained using 3D patches encompassing 5 slices in the z direction. Training is performed on a set of high-resolution A3D images (inherently motion-free) with accompanying 3D segmentations, setting the patch thickness equal to that of 5 SA slices combined. This forces the model to learn representations of motion-free stacks. At testing, the model is applied to the SA stack (after an up-sampling step in the z direction to mimic the resolution of A3D images), generating a virtually motion-free 3D PSM which are used as a target for slice-by-slice in-plane registration (by translation only) of the 2D PSMs. The estimated translations are applied to the SA slices, thus performing the correction.

3   Experiments and Results

Image Acquisition. Two distinct CMR image datasets (obtained with different scanners, cardiac array coils and acquisition parameters) were used to test the proposed approach. The first dataset consists of 350 full CMR scans (including also A3D images) of healthy subjects, while the second one consists of 500 scans from the UK Biobank[1]. Only end-diastolic frames were considered.

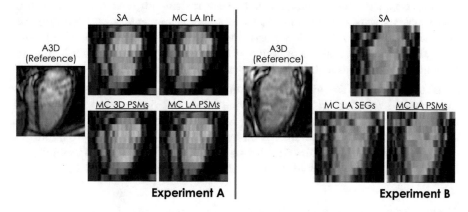

Fig. 3. Results obtained for two different subjects, one per experiment. The proposed techniques are underlined.

Performance Evaluation. Both datasets were annotated (either manually or automatically with subsequent manual corrections) to provide LV cavity segmentations for SA stacks, LA and A3D images as well as landmarks positions for the LA images alone. Two experiments were devised. For experiment A, 24 scans from the first dataset were extracted based on presence of visually-detected inter-slice motion and used as testing, while training was performed on the remaining scans of the same dataset. For this experiment, the proposed approach (with its two methods) was tested against an intensity-based technique (MC LA Int.) which iteratively registers SA slices to LA images (using normalized mutual information as similarity metric), essentially as in [2]. For experiment B, testing was performed on the same 24 scans of experiment A, but training was performed on the whole second dataset. In this case, the proposed approach (using only MC LA PSMs) was tested against a technique (MC LA SEGs) which iteratively registers SA "hard" segmentations to LA segmentations generated with FCNs (trained on images randomly extracted from the same database), essentially as in [3]. To compare the accuracy of the implemented techniques, in both experiments the corrective translations estimated for each slice were applied to the provided SA segmentations. Then, the segmentation of the A3D images, considered as reference, were rigidly registered to the initial SA segmentation stack as well as to the those produced by each technique. Slice-by-slice in-plane registration was performed between reference and initial segmentation stack to identify motion corrupted slices, and those with

---

[1] http://www.ukbiobank.ac.uk/.

more than 3 mm of misalignment were selected, for a total of 74. The evaluation of the accuracy of the implemented techniques was performed on these slices computing mean absolute distances (MAD), Hausdorff distances (HD) and Dice coefficients (DSC) between the LV cavity reference contours and before or after motion correction. The average slice-by-slice relative improvements for each of these metrics were also computed, as well as the percentage of improved values (where 100% would ideally mean that all of the corrupted slices improved their alignment). Of note, in experiment B, the testing set underwent histogram normalisation to match the intensity distributions of the training set.

Implementation Details. For training, standard data augmentation was implemented (random rescaling following a normal distribution with mean 1 and std 0.1, random rotation following a normal distribution with mean 0° and std 30°). Image patch size was 48×48 px for LA models and 32×32 px for SA ones, segmentation label size 16×16 px, number of samples $4 \cdot 10^6$, number of trees 8. Finally, the threshold T_m was set to 0.4 (on a scale from 0 to 1).

Table 1. Error metrics for experiment A (top) and experiment B (bottom). The proposed techniques are underlined.

Motion correction	MAD		HD		DSC		Ratio of
	Mean (mm)	Mean Impr.	Mean (mm)	Mean Impr.	Mean (a.u.)	Mean Impr.	improved slices
Experiment A							
None	3.1		6.9		0.83		
MC LA Int.	2.7	14%	6.2	12%	0.85	2%	77%
MC 3D PSMs	2.6	19%	6.0	15%	0.86	2%	80%
MC LA PSMs	**1.9**	**38%**	**4.9**	**29%**	**0.89**	**7%**	**92%**
Experiment B							
MC LA SEGs	2.3	23%	5.7	16%	0.88	**7%**	88%
MC LA PSMs	**2.1**	**33%**	**5.2**	**26%**	**0.89**	6%	**91%**

Results. Approximate time to perform motion correction of one SA stack on a 6-core CPU is 25 s for MC 3D PSMs and 36 s for MC LA PSMs. The results for both experiment A and B are reported in Table 1 and displayed for two cases in Fig. 3. Experiment A assesses the accuracy of the proposed approach in the scenario of training and testing performed in the same dataset. The results show that the intensity-based method performs worse than the others, and that MC 3D PSMs obtains lower errors even without using LA images. MC LA PSMs is clearly the best method within this batch and is able to improve most (92%) of the motion-corrupted slices. The fact that this method outperforms MC 3D PSMs was expected: while MC 3D PSMs can produce a smoothly aligned stack, more robustly than an intensity-based approach, it does not have any strong target for the realignment and relies only on the implicit model for the LV shape learned from the training set. Experiment B evaluates the accuracy of MC LA PSMs against a state-of-the-art approach like MC LA SEGs in a realistic scenario where motion correction has to be performed on a dataset completely different from the one used for training. Remarkably, MC LA PSMs produces results very similar to the ones obtained when trained on the same dataset. As expected given the similitudes between the two techniques, MC LA SEGs and MC LA PSMs perform similarly (no statistically significant differences were highlighted using a paired t-test). However, MC LA PSMs produces better mean results due to a higher robustness in the basal slices (see Fig. 3, right side): in fact, hard segmentation techniques have no safety mechanism to refrain from aligning slices in the basal region (usually beyond the actual basal slice) for which the FCN has produced spurious segmentations. On the contrary, the proposed approach has two: the check on the peak probability of the PSM and the comparison with the identified landmarks. As a result, the obtained motion correction tends to be more robust to this effect (see again Fig. 3, right side).

4   Conclusion

A comprehensive approach for fully-automated inter-slice motion correction for SA stacks has been presented. This approach relies on the generation of probabilistic segmentation maps of the LV cavity to drive slice-by-slice in-plane registration. It is able to handle cases in which no LA images are provided with a higher accuracy than common intensity-based methods that exploit them. When LA images are instead available, the proposed approach achieves results on par with methods based on hard segmentations while producing fewer outliers thanks to the simultaneous identification of landmarks to constrain the correction.

Acknowledgments. This research has been conducted using the UK Biobank Resource under Application Number 18545. The first author benefited from a Marie Sklodowska-Curie Fellowship.

References

1. Zhuang, X., et al.: A framework combining multi-sequence MRI for fully automated quantitative analysis of cardiac global and regional functions. In: Metaxas, D.N., Axel, L. (eds.) FIMH 2011. LNCS, vol. 6666, pp. 367–374. Springer, Heidelberg (2011). https://doi.org/10.1007/978-3-642-21028-0_47
2. Lötjönen, J., Pollari, M., Kivistö, S., Lauerma, K.: Correction of movement artifacts from 4-D cardiac short- and long-axis MR data. In: Barillot, C., Haynor, D.R., Hellier, P. (eds.) MICCAI 2004, Part II. LNCS, vol. 3217, pp. 405–412. Springer, Heidelberg (2004). https://doi.org/10.1007/978-3-540-30136-3_50
3. Sinclair, M., Bai, W., Puyol-Antón, E., Oktay, O., Rueckert, D., King, A.P.: Fully automated segmentation-based respiratory motion correction of multiplanar cardiac magnetic resonance images for large-scale datasets. In: Descoteaux, M., Maier-Hein, L., Franz, A., Jannin, P., Collins, D.L., Duchesne, S. (eds.) MICCAI 2017, Part II. LNCS, vol. 10434, pp. 332–340. Springer, Cham (2017). https://doi.org/10.1007/978-3-319-66185-8_38

4. Yang, D., Wu, P., Tan, C., Pohl, K.M., Axel, L., Metaxas, D.: 3D motion modeling and reconstruction of left ventricle wall in cardiac MRI. In: Pop, M., Wright, G.A. (eds.) FIMH 2017. LNCS, vol. 10263, pp. 481–492. Springer, Cham (2017). https:// doi.org/10.1007/978-3-319-59448-4_46
5. Oktay, O., et al.: Respiratory motion correction for 2D cine cardiac MR images using probabilistic edge maps. In: Computing in Cardiology, pp. 129–132 (2016)
6. Criminisi, A., Shotton, J., Konukoglu, E.: Decision forests: a unified framework for classification, regression, density estimation, manifold learning and semi-supervised learning. Found. Trends® Comput. Graph. Vis. **7**(2–3), 81–227 (2011)
7. Oktay, O., et al.: Stratified decision forests for accurate anatomical landmark localization in cardiac images. IEEE Trans. Med. Imaging **36**(1), 332–342 (2017)
8. Dollar, P., Zitnick, C.L.: Fast edge detection using structured forests. IEEE Trans. Pattern Anal. Mach. Intell. **37**(8), 1558–1570 (2015)

Automatic View Planning
with Multi-scale Deep Reinforcement
Learning Agents

Amir Alansary$^{(\boxtimes)}$, Loic Le Folgoc, Ghislain Vaillant, Ozan Oktay, Yuanwei Li,
Wenjia Bai, Jonathan Passerat-Palmbach, Ricardo Guerrero,
Konstantinos Kamnitsas, Benjamin Hou, Steven McDonagh, Ben Glocker,
Bernhard Kainz, and Daniel Rueckert

Imperial College London, London, UK
a.alansary14@imperial.ac.uk

Abstract. We propose a fully automatic method to find standardized
view planes in 3D image acquisitions. Standard view images are important in clinical practice as they provide a means to perform biometric
measurements from similar anatomical regions. These views are often
constrained to the native orientation of a 3D image acquisition. Navi-
gating through target anatomy to find the required view plane is tedious
and operator-dependent. For this task, we employ a multi-scale reinforcement learning (RL) agent framework and extensively evaluate several
Deep Q-Network (DQN) based strategies. RL enables a natural learning paradigm by interaction with the environment, which can be used
to mimic experienced operators. We evaluate our results using the distance between the anatomical landmarks and detected planes, and the
angles between their normal vector and target. The proposed algorithm is
assessed on the mid-sagittal and anterior-posterior commissure planes of
brain MRI, and the 4-chamber long-axis plane commonly used in cardiac
MRI, achieving accuracy of 1.53 mm, 1.98 mm and 4.84 mm, respectively.

1 Introduction

In medical imaging, obtaining accurate biometric measurements that are comparable across populations is essential for diagnosis and supporting critical decision
making. For this purpose, standard view planes through a defined anatomy are
commonly used in clinical practice to establish comparable metrics. Finding
these planes in an imaging examination through a 3D volume is slow and suffers
from inter-observer variability. The neuro-imaging community defines a standard
(axial) image plane by adopting the anterior-posterior commissure (ACPC) line.
Transforming an image to the ACPC coordinate system includes a number of
steps: (i) marking the AC point, (ii) obtaining the optimal view of the ACPC
and the mid-sagittal plane, and (iii) marking the PC point. Accurate detection
of the mid-sagittal plane is useful for the initial step in image registration [1].

© Springer Nature Switzerland AG 2018
A. F. Frangi et al. (Eds.): MICCAI 2018, LNCS 11070, pp. 277–285, 2018.
https://doi.org/10.1007/978-3-030-00928-1_32

It is also used in evaluation of pathological brains by estimating the departures from bilateral symmetry in the cerebrum [12]. Similarly, in cardiac MRI standard views are used to assess anomalies. Because of the complexity of cardiac anatomy, the appearance of relevant structures can exhibit large variance according to the positioning of the imaging plane. During conventional cardiac MRI acquisition, the localization of short and long-axis of the heart requires a multi-step approach that involves double-oblique slices, exhibiting both inter and intra-observer variance [6]. These steps include: (i) whole 3D pilot image acquisition, (ii) left ventricle (LV) localization, (iii) short axis orientation, (iv) 3-chamber view calculation, (v) landmark detection in mid-ventricular slices, and (vi) 4- and 2-chamber view calculation.

In this work, we aim to automate the view planning process by using reinforcement learning (RL) where an agent learns to make comprehensive and sensible decisions by mimicking navigation processes as outlined above, in a manner that allows medical experts to gain confidence in fully automatic methods. RL constitutes a sub-field of machine learning concerned with how agents take actions in an environment. In contrast to supervised learning, RL involves learning by interacting with an environment instead of using a set of labeled examples that is typically provided by a knowledgeable supervisor. This learning paradigm allows RL agents to learn complex tasks that may need several steps to find a solution [13]. Mnih et al. [9] adopted a deep convolution network for RL function approximation, known as the Deep Q-Network (DQN), achieving human-level performance in a suite of Atari games. Recently, DQN has shown promising results when employed in related applications in the medical imaging domain. Ghesu et al. [3] introduced an automatic landmark detection approach using a DQN-agent to navigate in 3D images with fixed step actions. Maicas et al. [7] proposed a similar method for breast lesion detection using actions to control the location and size of the bounding box. Liao et al. [5] presented an image registration approach using actions to explore transformation parameters. We adopt different DQN-based architectures as a solution for the proposed RL formulation of the view planning task.

Related Work: Ardekani et al. [1] proposed a method to automatically detect the mid-sagittal plane in 3D brain images by maximizing the cross-correlation between the two image sections on either side of the sought plane. Stegmann et al. [12] proposed to use a sparse set of profiles in the plane normal direction and maximize the local symmetry around them. In [4,6], they proposed an automatic view planning algorithm for cardiac MRI acquisition. Their methods are based on learning the anatomy segmentation and detecting anchor landmarks in order to calculate standard cardiac views. These methods require prior knowledge of the whole 3D image for the purpose of plane detection. This involves manual annotation of anatomical landmarks, which is a tedious and time-consuming task. In our method, we use the acquired standardized views for cardiac scans in training without any manual labeling.

Contribution: We propose a novel RL-based approach for fully automatic standard view plane detection from volumetric MRI data. The proposed model follows a multi-scale search strategy with hierarchical action steps in a coarse-to-fine fashion. By sequentially updating plane parameters, our algorithm is able to reach the target plane. We run extensive experiments for evaluating different DQN baselines on detecting 3 different planes. Applications of our method to brain and cardiac MRI data show a target plane detection in real time with accuracy around 2 and 5 mm, respectively.

2   Background

An RL agent learns by interacting with an environment, E. At every state, s, a single decision is made to choose an action, a, from a set of multiple discrete actions, A. Each valid action choice results in an associated scalar reward, defining the reward signal, R. The agent attempts to learn a policy to maximize both immediate and subsequent future rewards (optimal policy).

Q-Learning: The optimal action-selection policy can be identified by learning a state-action value function, $Q(s, a)$ [16]. The Q-function is defined as the expected value of the accumulated discounted future rewards $E[r_{t+1} + \gamma r_{t+2} + \cdots + \gamma r_{t+n} | s, a]$. $\gamma \in [0, 1]$ is a discount factor that represents the uncertainty in the agent's environment and is used to weight future rewards accordingly. This value function can be unrolled recursively (using the Bellman Equation [2]) and can thus be solved iteratively: $Q_{i+1}(s, a) = E\left[r + \gamma \max_{a'} Q_i(s', a')\right]$.

Deep Q-Learning: Mnih et al. [9] proposed the Deep Q-Network (DQN) and implemented a standard Q-learning algorithm with the addition of approximating the Q-function using a ConvNet, $Q(s, a) \approx Q(s, a; \omega)$, where ω represents the network's parameters. The DQN loss function is defined as:

$$L(\omega) = E\left[\left(r + \gamma \max_{a'} Q_{target}(s', a'; \omega^-) - Q_{net}(s, a; \omega)\right)^2\right],$$

Approximating the Q-function in this manner allows to learn from larger data sets using mini-batches. The DQN uses $Q_{target}(\omega^-)$, a fixed version of $Q_{net}(\omega)$, that is periodically updated. This is used to stabilize rapid policy changes, due to the quick variations in Q-values and the distribution of the data. Another problem that may cause divergence is successive data sampling. To avoid this, an experience replay memory that stores transitions of $(s_t, a_t, r_{t+1}, s_{t+1})$ is randomly sampled to create the mini-batches used for training. We outline below two recent state-of-the-art improvements to the standard DQN.

Double DQN (DDQN): It has been shown that DQN is susceptible to bias in noisy environments, where the target network may cause upward bias due to delayed updates. Van Hasselt et al. [14] proposed a solution that replaces the maximum approximated action from $Q_{target}(s', a'; \omega^-)$ with an action selected from the $Q_{target}(s', Q_{net}(s', a', \omega); \omega^-)$. This strategy is able to mitigate bias by decoupling the selected action from Q_{target}. DDQN improves the stability of learning, which can translate to the ability to learn more complicated tasks but may not necessarily improve the performance [14].

Duel DQN: Wang et al. [15] showed improved performance over the original DQN by defining two separate channels: *(i)* an action-independent value function $V(s)$ to provide an estimate of the value of each state, and *(ii)* an action-dependent advantage function $A(s, a)$ to calculate potential benefits of each action. Both functions are then combined into a single action-advantage Q-function, $Q(s, a) = A(s, a) + V(s)$. Duel DQN may achieve more robust estimates of state value by decoupling it from specific actions, so s could be more explicitly modelled, which yields higher performance in general.

3 Method

A plane P, in the Cartesian coordinate frame of the 3D image, is defined as: $ax + by + cz + d = 0$. Where (a, b, c) represent the normal direction (cosine) to this plane and d is the distance of the plane from the origin. To automate standard view planning, we aim to find the appropriate parameterization of the target plane. We formulate our RL framework by defining the following elements:

– **States:** Our Environment E is represented by a 3D scan and s is a 3D region of interest that contains P. A frame history buffer is used for storing the last planes from previous steps to stabilize search trajectories and prevent getting stuck in repeated cycles. We choose a history size of 4 frames similar to [9].
– **Actions:** The agent interacts with E by taking action steps $a \in A$ to modify the position parameters of the plane. The action space consists of eight actions, $\{\pm a_{\theta_x}, \pm a_{\theta_y}, \pm a_{\theta_z}, \pm a_d\}$, which update the plane parameters $a = cos(\theta_x + a_{\theta_x})$, $b = cos(\theta_y + a_{\theta_y})$, $c = cos(\theta_z + a_{\theta_z})$ and $d = d + a_d$.

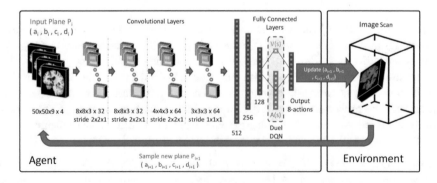

Fig. 1. The pipeline of the proposed multi-scale RL agent. Initially, the environment samples a plane: $ax + by + cz + d = 0$, from the 3D image scan. The agent selects an action to update a single parameter for sampling the next plane. This process is repeated till the agent reaches a terminal state (oscillation).

- **Reward:** The RL reward function forms a proxy for the true task goal and care must be taken to capture exactly what this goal entails. In our problem instance, the difficulty comes from designing a reward that encourages the agent to move towards the target plane while still being learnable. With these considerations, we define the reward $R = \mathrm{sgn}(D(P_{i-1}, P_t) - D(P_i, P_t))$, where D is a function to take the Euclidean distance between plane parameters. We further denote P_i as the current predicted plane at step i, with P_t the target ground truth plane. The difference of the parameter distances, between the previous and current steps, signifies whether the agent is moving closer to or further away from the desired plane parameters. $R \in \{+1, 0, -1\}$ provide the agent with a per step (non-sparse) reward signal, with zero-valued R presents plane oscillations around the correct solution.
- **Terminal State:** The final state is defined as the state in which the agent finds the target plane P_t. A trigger action can be used to signal when the target state is reached [7]. However, adding extra actions increases the action space size, which may in turn increase the complexity of the task to be learned. The maximum number of interactions should also be defined in such a setting. We found that terminating the episode when oscillation is detected heuristically works in practice without the need to expand the action space. However, in contrast to [3], we choose the terminating action with the lower Q-value. We find that Q-values are lower when the target plane is closer. Intuitively, the DQN encourages awarding higher Q-values to actions when the current plane is far from the target.

Multi-scale Agent: In order to provide more structural information, we introduce a novel multi-resolution approach in a coarse-to-fine fashion with hierarchical action steps. In this scenario, E samples a grid of a fixed plane size (P_x, P_y, P_z) of voxels around the plane origin P_o and initial spacing (S_x, S_y, S_z) mm. Initially, the agent searches for the plane with higher action steps. Once the target plane is found, E samples the new planes with smaller spacing and the agent uses smaller action steps. Coarser levels in the hierarchy provide additional guidance to the optimization process by enabling the agent to see larger context of the image. Whereas, finer scales provide sharper adjustments for the final estimation of the plane. Similarly, larger step actions speed up the solution towards the target plane, while smaller steps fine tune the final estimation of plane parameters. The same DQN is shared between all levels in the hierarchy, see Fig. 1. The next section exhibits results of utilizing this multi-scale approach.

4   Experiments and Results

The proposed algorithm is assessed using 12 different experiments; a combination of four different DQN-based methods with three target planes. We evaluate our results using the distance between anatomical landmarks and the detected planes. We also measure the orientation error by calculating the angle between normal vectors of the detected and target planes.

Datasets: A set of 832 isotropic 1 mm MR scans were obtained from the ADNI database [10] to evaluate the proposed method. While, a subset of 728 and 104 images are used for training and testing. All brain images were skull stripped and affinely aligned to the MNI space, thus allowing ground truth planes to be extracted in the standard directions. For cardiac images, we use 455 short-axis cardiac MR of resolution $(1.25 \times 1.25 \times 2)$ mm obtained from the UK Digital Heart Project [8]. A subset of 364 and 91 images are used for training and testing. ACPC planes are evaluated using the AC and PC landmarks for the distance error calculation. Similarly, we use the outer aspect, inferior tip and inner aspect points of splenium of corpus callosum for mid-sagittal planes. For cardiac MRI, we use six landmarks projected on the 4-chamber plane; the two right ventricle (RV) insertion points, right and left ventricles (LV) lateral wall turning points, apex, and the center of the mitral valve, See Fig. 2.

 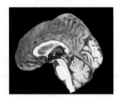

     (a) Axial ACPC plane   (b) Mid-sagittal plane   (c) 4-Chamber plane

Fig. 2. Ground truth planes from brain and cardiac MRI scans. (a) ACPC axial plane marking AC (red) and PC (yellow) points. (b) Mid-sagittal plane with outer aspect (green), inferior tip (yellow) and inner aspect (red) points of splenium of corpus callosum. (c) 4-Chamber view with the projected two RV insertion points (violet, green), RV and LV lateral wall turning points (blue, lime), apex (orange), and the center of the mitral valve (red).

Experiments: During training, a random point is sampled from the 3D input image. The initial random plane is then defined using the normal vector between the center of the image and the random point. The origin of this plane is the projected point of the center of the input image. Finally, a plane of size $(50, 50, 9)$ voxels is sampled around the plane origin with initial spacing $3 \times 3 \times 3$ mm. Initial $a_{\theta_x}, a_{\theta_y}, a_{\theta_z}$ equal 8 and a_d equals 4. With every new scale $a_{\theta_x}, a_{\theta_y}, a_{\theta_z}$ decrease by a factor of 2 and a_d decrease 1 unit. 3-levels of scale with spacing from 3 to 1 mm are used for the brain experiments, and 4-levels of scale from 5 to 2 mm for the cardiac experiment. For experiments on cardiac images, initial planes are sampled randomly from the 3D input image within 20% around the center of the image, to avoid sampling outside the field of view.

Results: During inference, the environment samples a plane and the agent updates sequentially new plane's parameters until reaching the terminal state.

In order to have a fair comparison between different variants of the proposed method, we fix the initial plane for all models during evaluation. Table 1 shows the results from these comparative experiments. All methods share similar performance including speed and accuracy, and there is no unique winner for the best overall method. Best performing agents for detecting the mid-sagittal and ACPC planes achieve accuracy of 1.53 ± 2.2 mm and $2.44 \pm 5.04°$, and 1.98 ± 2.23 mm and $4.48 \pm 14.0°$, respectively. Where in cardiac, the task is more complex due to the lower quality and higher variability between different scans. The agent has to navigate in a bigger field of view compared to brain images. Thus Duel DQN-based architectures achieve the best results for detecting the 4-chamber plane with 4.84 ± 3.03 mm and $8.86 \pm 12.42°$ accuracy, as a result from learning a better state value function by decoupling it from action-value function. These results are better than the state-of-the-art [6], which achieves an accuracy of 5.7 ± 8.5 mm and $17.6 \pm 19.2°$. Unlike [6], our method does not require manual annotation of landmarks. More visualization results are published on our github.

Table 1. Results of our multi-scale RL agent detecting 3 different MRI planes.

Model	Mid-sagittal brain		ACPC brain		4-Chamber cardiac	
	$e_d(mm)$	$e_\theta(°)$	$e_d(mm)$	$e_\theta(°)$	$e_d(mm)$	$e_\theta(°)$
DQN	1.65 ± 1.99	2.42 ± 5.27	2.61 ± 5.44	$\mathbf{3.23 \pm 6.03}$	5.61 ± 4.09	10.16 ± 10.62
DDQN	2.08 ± 2.58	3.44 ± 7.46	$\mathbf{1.98 \pm 2.23}$	4.48 ± 14.00	5.79 ± 4.58	11.20 ± 14.86
Duel DQN	1.69 ± 1.98	3.82 ± 7.15	2.13 ± 1.99	5.24 ± 13.75	$\mathbf{4.84 \pm 3.03}$	8.86 ± 12.42
Duel DDQN	$\mathbf{1.53 \pm 2.20}$	$\mathbf{2.44 \pm 5.04}$	5.30 ± 11.19	5.25 ± 12.64	5.07 ± 3.33	$\mathbf{8.72 \pm 7.44}$

Implementation. Training times are around 12–24 h for the brain experiments and 2–4 days for the cardiac experiments using an NVIDIA GTX 1080Ti GPU. During inference, the agent finds the target plane using iterative steps, where each step takes ~ 0.02 s. The details of the our proposed network for DQN are in Fig. 1. The source code of our implementation is publicly available on github https://git.io/vhuMZ.

5   Discussion and Conclusion

We proposed a novel approach based on multi-scale reinforcement learning agents for automatic standard view extraction. Our approach is capable of finding standardized planes in real time, which in turn enables accelerated image acquisition. Consequently, it can alleviate the comparison between different imaging examinations using anatomically standardized biometric measurements. We extensively evaluated several DQN based strategies for the detection of three different planes. Our approach achieved good results for the automatic detection of the ACPC and mid-sagittal planes from brain MRI with distance error less than 2 mm, and for the detection of the 4-chamber plane from cardiac MRI with distance error around 5 mm.

Limitations: Our results show that the optimal algorithm for achieving the best performance is environment-dependant. In general, reinforcement learning is a difficult problem that needs a careful formulation of its elements such as states, rewards and actions. For example, RL tends to overfit to the reward signals, which may cause unexpected behaviours. Therefore the design of the reward function has to capture exactly the desired task, and still be learnable.

Future Work: we will investigate using a continuous action space to improve the performance through reduction of quantization errors introduced by fixed action steps. We will also explore the use of either competitive or collaborative multi-agents to detect the same or different anatomical planes. Another future direction is inspired by AlphaGo [11], where an RL agent could mimic the moves of a human expert and accumulate this experience, thus learning from experienced operators during real time observation.

References

1. Ardekani, B.A., Kershaw, J., Braun, M., Kanuo, I.: Automatic detection of the mid-sagittal plane in 3-D brain images. TMI **16**(6), 947–952 (1997)
2. Bellman, R.: Dynamic programming. Courier Corporation (2013)
3. Ghesu, F.C., et al.: Multi-scale deep reinforcement learning for real-time 3D-landmark detection in CT scans. PAMI (2017)
4. Le, M., Lieman-Sifry, J., Lau, F., Sall, S., Hsiao, A., Golden, D.: Computationally efficient cardiac views projection using 3D convolutional neural networks. In: Cardoso, M.J., et al. (eds.) DLMIA/ML-CDS 2017. LNCS, vol. 10553, pp. 109–116. Springer, Cham (2017). https://doi.org/10.1007/978-3-319-67558-9_13
5. Liao, R., et al.: An artificial agent for robust image registration. In: AAAI, pp. 4168–4175 (2017)
6. Lu, X., et al.: Automatic view planning for cardiac MRI acquisition. In: Fichtinger, G., Martel, A., Peters, T. (eds.) MICCAI 2011, Part III. LNCS, vol. 6893, pp. 479–486. Springer, Heidelberg (2011). https://doi.org/10.1007/978-3-642-23626-6_59
7. Maicas, G., Carneiro, G., Bradley, A.P., Nascimento, J.C., Reid, I.: Deep reinforcement learning for active breast lesion detection from DCE-MRI. In: Descoteaux, M., Maier-Hein, L., Franz, A., Jannin, P., Collins, D.L., Duchesne, S. (eds.) MICCAI 2017, Part III. LNCS, vol. 10435, pp. 665–673. Springer, Cham (2017). https://doi.org/10.1007/978-3-319-66179-7_76
8. de Marvao, A., et al.: Population-based studies of myocardial hypertrophy: high resolution cardiovascular magnetic resonance atlases improve statistical power. J. Cardiovasc. Magn. Reson. **16**(1), 16 (2014)
9. Mnih, V., Kavukcuoglu, K., Silver, D., et al.: Human-level control through deep reinforcement learning. Nature **518**(7540), 529 (2015)
10. Mueller, S.G., et al.: The Alzheimer's disease neuroimaging initiative. Neuroimaging Clin. **15**(4), 869–877 (2005)
11. Silver, D., et al.: Mastering the game of go with deep neural networks and tree search. Nature **529**(7587), 484–489 (2016)
12. Stegmann, M.B., Skoglund, K., Ryberg, C.: Mid-sagittal plane and mid-sagittal surface optimization in brain MRI using a local symmetry measure. In: Medical Imaging: Image Processing, vol. 5747, pp. 568–580 (2005)

13. Sutton, R.S., Barto, A.G.: Reinforcement Learning: An Introduction, vol. 1. MIT Press, Cambridge (1998)
14. Van Hasselt, H., Guez, A., Silver, D.: Deep reinforcement learning with double Q-learning. In: AAAI, vol. 16, pp. 2094–2100 (2016)
15. Wang, Z., Schaul, T., Hessel, M., Van Hasselt, H., Lanctot, M., De Freitas, N.: Dueling network architectures for deep reinforcement learning (2015). arXiv preprint: arXiv:1511.06581
16. Watkins, C.J., Dayan, P.: Q-learning. Mach. Learn. **8**(3–4), 279–292 (1992)

Towards MR-Only Radiotherapy Treatment Planning: Synthetic CT Generation Using Multi-view Deep Convolutional Neural Networks

Yu Zhao[1], Shu Liao[2], Yimo Guo[2], Liang Zhao[2], Zhennan Yan[2],
Sungmin Hong[3], Gerardo Hermosillo[2], Tianming Liu[1],
Xiang Sean Zhou[2], and Yiqiang Zhan[2(✉)]

[1] The University of Georgia, Athens, GA 30605, USA
[2] Siemens Medical Solutions, Malvern, PA 19355, USA
yiqiang@gmail.com
[3] New York University, New York, NY 10003, USA

Abstract. Recently, Magnetic Resonance imaging-only (MR-only) radiotherapy treatment planning (RTP) receives growing interests since it is radiation-free and time/cost efficient. A key step in MR-only RTP is the generation of a synthetic CT from MR for dose calculation. Although deep learning approaches have achieved promising results on this topic, they still face two major challenges. First, it is very difficult to get perfectly registered CT-MR pairs to learn the intensity mapping, especially for abdomen and pelvic scans. Slight registration errors may mislead the deep network to converge at a sub-optimal CT-MR intensity matching. Second, training of a standard 3D deep network is very memory-consuming. In practice, one has to either shrink the size of the training network (sacrificing the accuracy) or use a patch-based sliding-window scheme (sacrificing the speed). In this paper, we proposed a novel method to address these two challenges. First, we designed a max-pooled cost function to accommodate imperfect registered CT-MR training pairs. Second, we proposed a network that consists of multiple 2D sub-networks (from different 3D views) followed by a combination sub-network. It reduces the memory consumption without losing the 3D context for high quality CT synthesis. We demonstrated our method can generate high quality synthetic CTs with much higher runtime efficiency compared to the state-of-the-art as well as our own benchmark methods. The proposed solution can potentially enable more effective and efficient MR-only RTPs in clinical settings.

Keywords: Cross modality synthesis · Deep learning · Synthetic CT
Radiotherapy

Y. Zhao and S. Hong—This work was mainly accomplished during Yu Zhao, Sungmin Hong's internship at Siemens Medical Solutions.

© Springer Nature Switzerland AG 2018
A. F. Frangi et al. (Eds.): MICCAI 2018, LNCS 11070, pp. 286–294, 2018.
https://doi.org/10.1007/978-3-030-00928-1_33

1 Introduction

Medical imaging plays an important role in radiotherapy treatment planning (RTP) [1] by providing critical information for organ/tumor localization and dose calculation. Currently computed tomography (CT) is the primary modality, which provides electron density information for dose calculation. Since Magnetic Resonance (MR) imaging is more valuable in organ/tumor localization due to its superior soft tissue contrast, it has received more and more interests in RTP. In traditional workflow, MR will be registered to a principal CT dataset [1, 2] so that its superior soft tissue contrast information can be fused with the CT image. However, due to the imperfectness of the current image registration techniques, registration error will bring systematic spatial uncertainty [3], hence, influencing the accuracy of RTP. Recently MR-only RTP receives growing interests since it is radiation-free and time/cost efficient. A key step in MR-only RTP is the generation of a synthetic CT (sCT) from MR for dose calculation.

The major challenge in CT synthesizing is the intensity ambiguity of different tissues, such as bone and air which both appear dark on MR. Traditional approaches for CT synthesis from MR can be divided into two categories: atlas-based [4] and segmentation-based [5]. For the atlas-based approaches, the focus is to register the MR atlas to the patient MR, and then apply the registration transformation on the corresponding CT atlas to generate the synthetic CT [6]. Segmentation-based methods [5] segment different types of tissues from MR. A synthetic CT is then generated by filling a constant CT intensity for each type of tissue. The main obstacles for these approaches are the synthesis speed and registration or segmentation accuracy. Recently, some context-aware deep learning based models are proposed [7–9] and they achieved promising results. However, they still face two major challenges. First, standard deep learning requires a set of perfectly registered CT-MR pairs to learn the intensity mapping from MR to CT. However, since MR and CT images are acquired at different time with different patient positionings and table shapes, it is very difficult to perfectly register them, especially for abdomen and pelvic scans [10]. Thus most works [7–9] focused on brain regions. Slight registration errors may induce large mis-matching in the intensity space, hence, misleading the deep network to converge at a sub-optimal CT-MR intensity matching. Second, training of a standard 3D deep network is very memory-consuming. In practice, even with a high-end deep learning server, one has to simplify the 3D network structure or using a patch-based sliding-window scheme [7, 9] to accommodate large volumes of training data. The simplified network may not model the MR-CT intensity mapping well and sliding-window scheme may sacrifice the speed significantly.

In this work, we proposed a novel method to tackle the aforementioned challenges. First, we designed a maxpooling loss function allowing the network to search optimal intensity matching not only between the corresponding CT-MR patches but across their neighborhood. This kind of "matching freedom" makes the network robust to imperfect CT-MR registration. Second, we proposed a network consisting of multiple 2D sub-networks (from different 3D views) followed by a 3D combination sub-network. It dramatically reduces the memory consumption without losing the 3D context for high quality CT synthesis. Our method generated high quality sCTs with much higher runtime efficiency compared to the state-of-the-art and our own benchmark method.

2   Materials and Methods

2.1   Overview of Multi-view Multi-channel U-Net Structure

U-Net [11] is a deep network originally proposed for image segmentation. It has a symmetric hierarchical structure that enables precise voxel-wise classification by modeling cross-scale anatomical context. In our study, the U-Net is adapted to a regression network, i.e., the output is an image with synthetic CT values. The original U-Net has a 2D fully convolutional structure, which needs to be extended to handle the 3D nature of MR and CT images. In order to train on 3D volumes without reducing network size and speed, we adopt a 2.5D framework (Fig. 1). Our framework consists of two 2D-centric U-Nets (Fig. 2) corresponding to sagittal and axial views, respectively. The stacked output 3D features from these two sub-nets are further combined by a 3D combination sub-net (Fig. 5). Moreover, to deal with the unpreventable misalignments between MR-CT training pairs for accurate model training, a max-pooling hinge-like Huber function is designed as training loss (Fig. 3). Technical details are explained next.

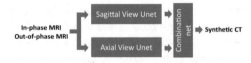

Fig. 1. Multi-channel multi-view U-Net based deep fully convolutional network framework.

2.2   Multi-channel MR Inputs for Information Enhancement

The input of our method is the In-Phase and Out-of-phase images generated by MR Dixon method. These images capture complementary fat and water information for tissue differentiation. As shown in Fig. 2, for single view 2D U-Net inputs, instead of stacking these two images at the input layer, we keep two independent channels for each of them. In this way, the network can capture features from different MR sequences independently for information enhancement.

2.3   Maxpooling and Hinge-like Huber Loss Function

In order to learn the intensity transformation from MR to CT, a set of registered MR-CT pairs are needed for training. However, it is very difficult to perfectly register MR and CT due to organ deformations, different table sizes, etc. To address this problem, an effective loss function is proposed for the network in Fig. 2. Instead of calculating the voxel-wise intensity differences directly between the output slice and the ground-truth slice, a maxpooling process (Fig. 3(a)) is applied to accommodate the slight

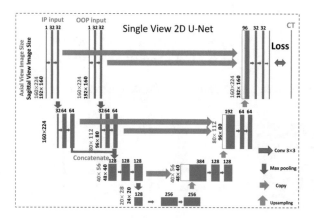

Fig. 2. Single view 2D U-Net (sagittal view and axial view). Multi-channel 2D MR slices (In-phase (IP) and Out-of-phase(OOP)) are network inputs. Loss is designed as maxpooling and hinge-like Huber loss.

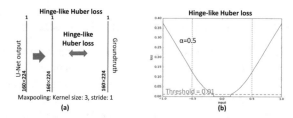

Fig. 3. (a) Maxpooling hinge-like Huber loss function for U-Net structure training. (b) Hinge-like Huber loss function.

misalignment in a translation invariant fashion [12]. A schematic example is presented in Fig. 4. If I_1 and I_2 are perfectly registered, it is easy to learn a consistent mapping function F that maps the intensities of pixel a, b and c to a′, b′ and c′, i.e., $F(I_1(a)) = I_2$ (a′), $F(I_1(b)) = I_2$ (b′), $F(I_1(c)) = I_2$ (c′); However, if I_1 and I_2 are not perfectly registered due to deformable or rigid registration errors, it is very difficult to learn a common mapping function that maps the intensities of a, b and c to a′, b′ and c′, since the intensity transformation becomes inconsistent. By adding max-pooling in the loss function, we essentially give some spatial freedom to the mapping function, allowing it to map the intensity to its neighborhood, i.e., $F(I_1(a)) = I_2$ (a′ + Δa′), $F(I_1(b)) = I_2$ (b′ + Δb′), $F(I_1(c)) = I_2$ (c′ + Δc′). Thus, a consistent mapping function can be learned. Note that the max-pooling allows different voxels to have different small Δ, which address the non-systematic registration errors. The hinge-like function is also adopted with Huber loss as the final loss function (Fig. 3(b)), also shown in Eq. (1). It accommodates major loss and ignores minor ones.

$$L(a) = \begin{cases} 0, |a| < 0.01 \\ \frac{1}{2}a^2, 0.01 < |a| < \alpha \\ \alpha\left(|a| - \frac{1}{2}\alpha\right), otherwise \end{cases} \quad (1)$$

where a is the 2D image slice difference between output and ground-truth CT images.

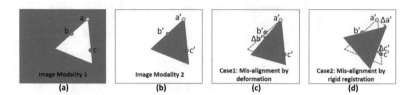

Fig. 4. A schematic explanation of the impact of mis-registration to intensity transformation. (a) Image 1 (Modality 1), (b) Perfectly registered Image modality 2, (c) Image 2 with rigid mis-alignment, (d) Image 2 with non-rigid mis-alignment. Triangles in (a)–(d) represent the same object. Dashed lines in (c) and (d) denote the locations of the perfectly registered Image 2.

2.4   Multi-view Combination of the 2D U-Net Like Structures

Our network includes two 2D U-Nets followed by a combination network (Fig. 5). This design is important to deal with memory limitations. With an 8 GB GPU memory, we cannot fit a 3D 192 * 224 * 168 volume with a 3D network for training. Therefore, we decompose the 3D volume into 2D axial and sagittal slices, respectively, which can be easily fit into two 2D U-Nets. However, since the 2D U-Net ignores the 3D context across neighboring slides, the output may have stitching blurring effect. (c.f. Fig. 7), To remove the blurring effect, output feature maps of 2D U-Nets are stacked into 3D volumes before feeding into a 3D convolution layer with kernel size $1 \times 1 \times 1$. This 3D convolution layer effectively removes the 2D stitching blurring effect.

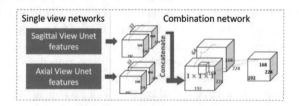

Fig. 5. Combination Network. Single view networks include 2D U-Net structures for both axial and sagittal view. 3D combination network takes 32 channels output 3D features from 2 single view networks as input and output a 3D synthetic CT volume.

The overall loss function is a (empirically-set) weighted mean of maxpooling hinge-like Huber loss from two views and a Huber loss of the 3D synthetic volume with the ground-truth volume (2).

$$L(v) = 0.6L(v)_{sagittal} + 0.33L(v)_{axial} + 0.07Huber(v) \tag{2}$$

where v is the 3D volume difference between the final output synthetic CT of the combination net and the ground-truth CT volumes; 3D $L(v)_{sagittal}$ and $L(v)_{axial}$ are the hinge-like Huber loss maxpooled from sagittal view and axial view 2D slices respectively; $Huber(v)$ is the voxel-wise Huber loss of the 3D volume difference.

2.5 Network Training

Our network training has two stages. First, the two 2D U-Nets of axial and sagittal views are trained independently. Then the feature maps extracted from the second last layers of each 2D U-Net are stacked into 3D volumes and saved as input for further training of the 3D combination network.

3 Results

Due to the lack of perfectly aligned scanned MR and CT pairs, the ground-truth CTs are generated by a multi-atlas-based regression method [13]. The quality of the ground-truth synthetic CT image is confirmed and accepted by experienced oncologists. However, since the multi-atlas-based regression method [13] takes extensive time (i.e., more than 15 min on average) to generate the synthetic CT image, it has limitation in the real world RTP clinical workflow. An Nvidia Quadro M4000 GPU with 8 GB memory was utilized for all the training steps. For the first training stage, training time for each 2D U-Net like structure is dependent on the input size of the images at the corresponding view, 21 h and 95 h for axial view and sagittal view, respectively. For the second training stage, combination net, 7 h was taken. A total time of 123 h was used for the 2-stage training procedure. The testing phase only cost less than 8 s for each subject 3D CT volume synthesis.

3.1 Effectiveness of the Proposed Framework

In the experiment, we have 34 MR-CT pairs, where 27 pairs are used for training and the rest 7 pairs for testing. Our proposed method showed significant improvements at 2D slice level compared to the benchmark U-Net structure Fig. 6. The multi-view combination of the 2D U-Net structures also showed effectiveness on removing the 2D slice stitching blurs across the 3D volume and avoided sacrificing synthetic image quality by shrinking the size of 3D training network (Fig. 7). Comparisons between sCTs generated using our proposed method and ground-truth CTs are discussed in the following sections.

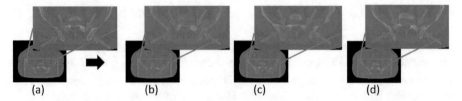

Fig. 6. Improved quality of the bone area synthesis compared to benchmark U-Net schemes. (a) Ground-truth sCT used for training; (b) Bench mark result using original U-Net; (c) Result using benchmark U-Net with maxpooling function; (d) Proposed result.

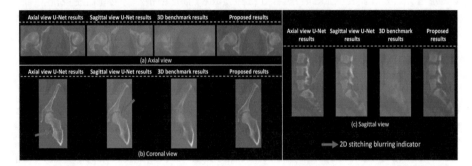

Fig. 7. Removed 2D slice stitching blurring effects (red arrow) by combining multi-view U-Net and improved image quality compared to results from a shrunk size 3D benchmark network.

3.2   Synthetic CT Quality Improvement

We can clearly see the small misalignment deficits from the multi-atlases-based sCTs [13] used for our training by comparing input MRs in Fig. 8. However, our proposed method will compensate these slight misalignments by predicting both the bone edge and soft tissue actual locations, which outperformed the state-of-art multi-atlas-based algorithm.

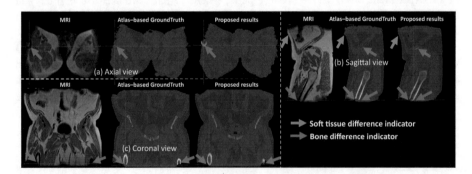

Fig. 8. Improved synthetic quality compared to the ground-truth CTs in 3 different views. Each column is a comparison among the input MR, ground-truth image and proposed predictions.

3.3   Synthetic CT Evaluation

To quantitatively measure the reliability and accuracy of the synthetic CT outputted by our framework and the ground-truth CT images, Mean Absolute Error (MAE) (also used in [1, 10]) was utilized:

$$MAE = \frac{1}{N} \sum_{x,y,z \in V_1, V_2} |V_1(x, y, z) - V_2(x, y, z)| \tag{3}$$

where V_1, V_2 represent the synthetic CT and ground-truth volumes, and N represents total number of the voxels.

As for the 7 pure testing cases, the MAE values are very low (average 16.9 HU) (Table 1). Compared to the state-of-art results (average 58 HU in [10] and around 40 HU in most of works [1]), our method achieves higher accuracy. Compared with 3 benchmark U-Net-based methods, the proposed scheme achieved the best performance (Table 1), demonstrating the effectiveness of our specific design. Besides, the stunning CT synthesis speed (less than 8 s) significantly outperformed the state-of-art multi-atlas-based framework used to generate ground-truth synthetic CTs (more than 10 min), which paves the way for applying the proposed framework to real clinical settings.

Table 1. MAE values comparison for 7 purely testing subjects

MAE[HU]	Sub 1	Sub 2	Sub 3	Sub 4	Sub 5	Sub 6	Sub 7	Mean
Proposed	**14.8**	**9.0**	**21.9**	**16.1**	**16.4**	**13.2**	27.1	**16.9**
Sagittal benchmark U-Net	51.4	32.1	45.4	43.6	42.4	49.9	53.9	45.5
Axial benchmark U-Net	26.0	16.2	28.0	23.6	25.2	25.4	29.7	24.9
Multi-view benchmark	18.3	11.7	20.0	17.0	21.8	18.0	**21.1**	18.3

4   Discussion

In this work, we explored a deep learning framework for CT synthesis from MR. An average MAE of 19.6 HU and ~ 10 s synthesis speed outperform state-of-the-art methods. It shows the potency of the proposed deep learning framework in cross modality synthesis. Compared to other methods, the proposed method also showed significant improvement in sCT quality. In order to evaluate if our method is sufficient for MR-only RTP, it is important to evaluate the dose calculated from sCTs, which is part of our future work. This work gives us a new insight into tackling imperfect training pairs and 3D network training memory efficiency problem and the superior results also gives the promise to our framework for other applications.

References

1. Edmund, J.M., Nyholm, T.: A review of substitute CT generation for MRI-only radiation therapy. Radiat. Oncol. **12**, 28 (2017)
2. Edmund, J.M., et al.: SP-0510: dose planning based on MRI as the sole modality: why, how and when? Radiother. Oncol. **115**, S248–S249 (2015)
3. Paulson, E.S., Erickson, B., Schultz, C., Allen Li, X.: Comprehensive MRI simulation methodology using a dedicated MRI scanner in radiation oncology for external beam radiation treatment planning. Med. Phys. **42**, 28–39 (2014)
4. Sjölund, J., Forsberg, D., Andersson, M., Knutsson, H.: Generating patient specific pseudo-CT of the head from MR using atlas-based regression. Phys. Med. Biol. **60**, 825–839 (2015)
5. Delpon, G., et al.: Comparison of automated atlas-based segmentation software for postoperative prostate cancer radiotherapy. Front. Oncol. **6**, 178 (2016)
6. Dowling, J.A., et al.: An Atlas-based electron density mapping method for magnetic resonance imaging (MRI)-alone treatment planning and adaptive MRI-based prostate radiation therapy. Int. J. Radiat. Oncol. **83**, e5–e11 (2012)
7. Nie, D., et al.: Medical image synthesis with context-aware generative adversarial networks. In: Descoteaux, M., Maier-Hein, L., Franz, A., Jannin, P., Collins, D.L., Duchesne, S. (eds.) MICCAI 2017, Part III. LNCS, vol. 10435, pp. 417–425. Springer, Cham (2017). https://doi.org/10.1007/978-3-319-66179-7_48
8. Wolterink, J.M., Dinkla, A.M., Savenije, M.H.F., Seevinck, P.R., van den Berg, C.A.T., Išgum, I.: Deep MR to CT synthesis using unpaired data. In: Tsaftaris, S.A., Gooya, A., Frangi, A.F., Prince, J.L. (eds.) SASHIMI 2017. LNCS, vol. 10557, pp. 14–23. Springer, Cham (2017). https://doi.org/10.1007/978-3-319-68127-6_2
9. Nie, D., Cao, X., Gao, Y., Wang, L., Shen, D.: Estimating CT image from MRI data using 3D fully convolutional networks, 1 January 2016
10. Andreasen, D., et al.: Computed tomography synthesis from magnetic resonance images in the pelvis using multiple random forests and auto-context features. In: Styner, M.A., Angelini, E.D. (eds.) SPIE Medical Imaging, p. 978417. International Society for Optics and Photonics (2016)
11. Ronneberger, O., Fischer, P., Brox, T.: U-Net: convolutional networks for biomedical image segmentation. In: Navab, N., Hornegger, J., Wells, W.M., Frangi, A.F. (eds.) MICCAI 2015, Part III. LNCS, vol. 9351, pp. 234–241. Springer, Cham (2015). https://doi.org/10.1007/978-3-319-24574-4_28
12. Scherer, D., Müller, A., Behnke, S.: Evaluation of pooling operations in convolutional architectures for object recognition. In: Diamantaras, K., Duch, W., Iliadis, L.S. (eds.) ICANN 2010, Part III. LNCS, vol. 6354, pp. 92–101. Springer, Heidelberg (2010). https://doi.org/10.1007/978-3-642-15825-4_10
13. Liao, S., et al.: Automatic lumbar spondylolisthesis measurement in CT images. IEEE Trans. Med. Imaging **35**, 1658–1669 (2016)

Stochastic Deep Compressive Sensing for the Reconstruction of Diffusion Tensor Cardiac MRI

Jo Schlemper[1], Guang Yang[2,3](✉), Pedro Ferreira[2,3], Andrew Scott[2,3],
Laura-Ann McGill[2,3], Zohya Khalique[2,3], Margarita Gorodezky[2,3],
Malte Roehl[2,3], Jennifer Keegan[2,3], Dudley Pennell[2,3], David Firmin[2,3],
and Daniel Rueckert[1]

[1] Department of Computing, Imperial College London, London, UK
jo.schlemper11@imperial.ac.uk
[2] National Heart and Lung Institute, Imperial College London, London, UK
[3] Cardiovascular Research Centre, Royal Brompton Hospital, London, UK
g.yang@imperial.ac.uk

Abstract. Understanding the structure of the heart at the microscopic scale of cardiomyocytes and their aggregates provides new insights into the mechanisms of heart disease and enables the investigation of effective therapeutics. Diffusion Tensor Cardiac Magnetic Resonance (DT-CMR) is a unique non-invasive technique that can resolve the microscopic structure, organisation, and integrity of the myocardium without the need for exogenous contrast agents. However, this technique suffers from relatively low signal-to-noise ratio (SNR) and frequent signal loss due to respiratory and cardiac motion. Current DT-CMR techniques rely on acquiring and averaging multiple signal acquisitions to improve the SNR. Moreover, in order to mitigate the influence of respiratory movement, patients are required to perform many breath holds which results in prolonged acquisition durations (e.g., ~30 min using the existing technology). In this study, we propose a novel cascaded Convolutional Neural Networks (CNN) based compressive sensing (CS) technique and explore its applicability to improve DT-CMR acquisitions. Our simulation based studies have achieved high reconstruction fidelity and good agreement between DT-CMR parameters obtained with the proposed reconstruction and fully sampled ground truth. When compared to other state-of-the-art methods, our proposed deep cascaded CNN method and its stochastic variation demonstrated significant improvements. To the best of our knowledge, this is the first study using deep CNN based CS for the DT-CMR reconstruction. In addition, with relatively straightforward modifications to the acquisition scheme, our method can easily be translated into a method for online, at-the-scanner reconstruction enabling the deployment of accelerated DT-CMR in various clinical applications.

J. Schlemper has been funded by the EPSRC Programme Grant (EP/P001009/1) and G. Yang has been funded by the British Heart Foundation (PG/16/78/32402). D. Firmin and D. Rueckert are the co-last senior authors.

A. F. Frangi et al. (Eds.): MICCAI 2018, LNCS 11070, pp. 295–303, 2018.
https://doi.org/10.1007/978-3-030-00928-1_34

1   Introduction

Diffusion Tensor Cardiovascular Magnetic Resonance (DT-CMR) is a unique non-invasive technique, which provides rich structural and functional information on the myocardium at a microscopic scale, including parameters relating to the alignment and integrity of cardiomyocytes and aggregates of cardiomyocytes, known as sheetlets. Despite a long history of *in vivo* DT-CMR and great efforts to drive the method towards a clinically usable technique [15], its clinical use remains limited to research studies in a few specialist centres. These limited studies have produced a number of interesting findings in detection and diagnosis of ischemic heart disease, hypertrophic and dilated cardiomyopathies [2,3,14].

In comparison to the well established application of diffusion tensor imaging (DTI) in the brain, DT-CMR faces a number of additional challenges, including: (1) the intrinsically low signal-to-noise ratio (SNR) of typical acquisition methods, which means that multiple signal acquisitions must be acquired and averaged to improve the net SNR; (2) signal loss caused by respiratory and cardiac motion during the application of diffusion sensitising gradients, means that these gradients must be short with respect to the motion and strong gradients must be used to provide sufficient sensitivity to the small diffusive movement of water molecules (on the order of microns) [1]; (3) the transverse relaxation time (T_2) is substantially shorter in the myocardium than in the brain ($\sim$40 ms for the myocardium vs. $\sim$80 ms for the white matter of the brain). In contrast to neurological DTI, this dramatically limits the possible echo time (TE) that can be used in DT-CMR [13]; (4) the increased B_0 inhomogeneity in the thorax may also result in more susceptibility-related distortions in the echo planar imaging (EPI) technique typically used for the DT-CMR [13], which also limits spatial resolution. Some of these challenges have been partially addressed or have benefited from parallel imaging techniques for the in-plane acceleration, e.g., using SENSE (sensitivity encoding) and GRAPPA (generalized autocalibrating partially parallel acquisitions), or simultaneous multislice imaging [9]. However, typical acceleration factors are normally limited to 2–3 [13].

Compressive sensing (CS) is a promising technique for fast MRI [11] that circumvents the Nyquist-Shannon sampling criteria and can achieve a more aggressive acceleration. Comprehensive reviews of CS based fast MRI (CS-MRI) can be found elsewhere [6]. Essentially, CS-MRI can obtain a *perfect* reconstruction by using a *nonlinear optimisation* on *randomly undersampled* raw data, assuming the data or its transformation is *compressible*. Although CS-MRI have been widely investigated [6], most previous studies have focused on the acceleration of the structural MRI, and only very few research studies have been conducted on DT-CMR [8,12,22]. These CS based fast DT-CMR methods demonstrated promising reconstruction results; however, the iterative nonlinear optimisation used in these methods requires a lengthy reconstruction procedure that could prevent their widespread usage, where there is a clinical need to view images immediately at the scanner. Therefore, a CS-based on-the-fly reconstruction of DT-CMR data would be highly desirable.

More recently, deep learning approaches have shown intriguing results in solving various medical image segmentation, registration and reconstruction problems. In particular, there are several deep learning based architectures that have been proposed for reconstruction of MRI data. The most widely used architecture is named U-Net [18], which is used to perform an end-to-end reconstruction [5,10], and often combined with a residual learning [10,23] or generative adversarial networks [23]. Alternative approaches have also been proposed, which modified the deep network architectures to embed traditional optimisation algorithms. These include gradient descent [4], alternating direction method of multipliers (ADMM) [21] or optimisation algorithms inspired by variable splitting techniques [16]. In addition, various clinical applications have been explored including knee imaging [4], brain imaging [23], and dynamic cardiac imaging [19].

In this study, a novel cascaded Convolutional Neural Networks (CNN) based CS technique has been proposed to simulate an efficient reconstruction of highly undersampled DT-CMR data. The proposed architecture improves upon the previously proposed networks by introducing dilated convolution instead of pooling to efficiently increase the receptive field. In addition, we introduce a novel *stochastic* architecture, which is formulated by dropping the subnetworks at training. We show that this approach provides multifold benefits, including accelerated learning, improved robustness and an additional uncertainty estimate of the prediction. The following sections present the details of the proposed methodology, experimental set-up, achieved results and followed by discussions and conclusion.

2   Method

Let $\mathbf{x} \in \mathbb{C}^N$ denote a complex-valued MR image to be reconstructed, represented as a vector with $N = N_x N_y$ where N_x and N_y are width and height of the image. Let $\mathbf{y} \in \mathbb{C}^M$ ($M << N$) represent the undersampled k-space measurements. Our problem is to reconstruct $\mathbf{x}$ from $\mathbf{y}$, formulated as an unconstrained optimisation:

$$\underset{\mathbf{x}}{\text{argmin}} \quad \mathcal{R}(\mathbf{x}) + \lambda \|\mathbf{y} - \mathbf{F}_u \mathbf{x}\|_2^2 \tag{1}$$

Here $\mathbf{F}_u$ is an undersampling Fourier encoding matrix, $\mathcal{R}$ expresses regularisation terms on $\mathbf{x}$ and λ is a hyper-parameter often associated to the noise level.

Deep Cascaded CNN. In general, the regularisation terms $\mathcal{R}$ in Eq. 1 can be non-convex (such as ℓ_0 in the sparsifying domain). Therefore, traditionally, one introduces an auxiliary variable $\mathbf{z}$ as variable splitting technique and solves the following penalty functional:

$$\underset{\mathbf{x},\mathbf{z}}{\text{argmin}} \; \mathcal{R}(\mathbf{z}) + \lambda \|\mathbf{y} - \mathbf{F}_u \mathbf{x}\|_2^2 + \mu \|\mathbf{x} - \mathbf{z}\|_2^2 \tag{2}$$

where μ is a penalty parameter. By applying alternating minimisation over $\mathbf{x}$ and $\mathbf{z}$, Eq. 2 can be solved via the following iterative procedures:

$$\mathbf{z}^{(i)} = \underset{\mathbf{z}}{\operatorname{argmin}}\ \mathcal{R}(\mathbf{z}) + \mu\|\mathbf{x}^{(i)} - \mathbf{z}\|_2^2 \tag{3a}$$

$$\mathbf{x}^{(i+1)} = \underset{\mathbf{x}}{\operatorname{argmin}}\ \lambda\|\mathbf{y} - \mathbf{F}_u\mathbf{x}\|_2^2 + \mu\|\mathbf{x} - \mathbf{z}^{(i)}\|_2^2 \tag{3b}$$

where $\mathbf{x}^{(0)} = \mathbf{x}_u = \mathbf{F}_u^H y$ is the zero-filled (ZF) reconstruction taken as an initialisation and $\mathbf{z}$ can be seen as an intermediate state of the optimisation process. For MRI reconstruction, Eq. 3b is often regarded as a *data consistency* (DC) step where we could obtain the following closed-form solution [20]:

$$\mathbf{x}^{(i+1)} = \mathrm{DC}(\mathbf{z}^{(i)}; \mathbf{y}, \lambda_0, \Omega) = \mathbf{F}^H \mathbf{\Lambda} \mathbf{F} \mathbf{z}^{(i)} + \frac{\lambda_0}{1+\lambda_0} \mathbf{F}_u^H \mathbf{y}, \mathbf{\Lambda}_{kk} = \begin{cases} 1 & \text{if } k \notin \Omega \\ \frac{1}{1+\lambda_0} & \text{if } k \in \Omega \end{cases} \tag{4}$$

which $\mathbf{F}$ is the full Fourier encoding matrix (a discrete Fourier transform in this case), $\lambda_0 = \lambda/\mu$ is a ratio of regularization parameters from Eq. 4, Ω is an index set of the acquired k-space samples and $\mathbf{\Lambda}$ is a diagonal matrix. Equation 3a is the proximal operator of the prior $\mathcal{R}$, and instead of explicitly determining the form of the regularisation term, one can learn the proximal operator by using the CNN directly. In so doing, iterative reconstruction with a cascaded CNN and DC steps is performed. The whole framework can be optimized end-to-end, yielding one cascaded deep network. This network is referred to as *DC-CNN*.

Stochastic DC-CNN. Inspired by [7], we extend the DC-CNN framework into a *stochastic DC-CNN* (s-DC-CNN)—during the training, the i-th subnetwork is dropped with a probability of $p = (i-1)/2n_c$, where n_c is the total number of the cascaded CNN. During the testing (inference), we can use all of the subnetworks to perform the reconstruction, which is expected to provide the best performance as the most depths are used. Alternatively, we could sample the network configurations θ using the distribution P from the above strategy, and then reconstruct the image as an ensemble of the sampled model $\bar{x} = \mathbb{E}_{\theta \sim P}(f(x_u|\theta))$. In so doing, the variance of the predicted value can be used as an *uncertainty estimate* given the ensemble. This alternative approach provides several benefits: (1) it accelerates the learning because the expected depth of the network is much shorter; (2) this simultaneously helps the error terms to be backpropagated better as the depth is shortened, allowing us to train deeper networks if desired; (3) due to the stochastic connection, each subnetwork can see different levels of residual noise that help the network learn better and become more robust.

In addition, we used dilated convolution to efficiently increase the receptive field. In the original DC-CNN framework, each denoising subnetwork only consists of 5 layers of 3×3 2D convolution layers, which has a limited receptive field of size 11. In our new s-DC-CNN framework, we employed the dilated convolution except for the first and the last convolution that has a receptive field of size 23. It is of note that compared to pooling operation, the dilated convolution can avoid the needs of upsampling, and subsequently prevents information loss and interpolation artefacts, and also keeps the network more compact. Furthermore, we employed batch-normalisation to improve the training and applied leaky rectified linear unit with $\alpha = 0.01$.

3   Results

Experimental Settings. In order to test the efficacy of our proposed DC-CNN method for the DT-CMR reconstruction, we performed the following simulation based studies. First, we simulated undersampled DT-CMR datasets using *in vivo* DT-CMR data acquired at peak-systole or in diastasis in healthy volunteers. The data were acquired using a breath hold stimulated echo acquisition mode EPI sequence [15], with diffusion encoded over 1 complete cardiac cycle (detailed scanning parameters in Supplementary Materials). Evaluation has been carried out using 178 DT-CMR scans.

The image data were firstly converted into k-space data using an inverse Fourier transform and undersampled by a pseudo-random 1D undersampling mask. Each line was sampled from a Gaussian distribution with mean centred at the origin of k-space and variance proportional to the extent of k-space. We applied various random undersampling patterns to the data acquired for different diffusion weighting directions and different signal averages in order to make the trained network generalise better on various aliasing artefacts. Note that in this work, the magnitude images were used. However, the effectiveness of the method to complex-valued data has been previously verified in [20].

The studied scans were split into independent training, validation and test sets containing 142, 17 and 19 cases, respectively. In the training stage, both information from fully-sampled data and undersampled data were used. In the testing (inference) stage, the zero-filled undersampled data were input to the trained network to yield a reconstruction.

Comparison Studies. To compare with other state-of-the-art conventional CS-MRI and recently proposed deep learning based methods, we re-implemented the following methods for the DT-CMR reconstruction, including a dictionary learning based CS-MRI (i.e., *DLMRI* [17]) and a U-Net based method (*UNET-CS*). For the proposed approach, we selected to use 6-layer subnetwork with $n_c = 15$ that yields a 105-layer network including the DC layers. Note that the hyperparameters were chosen from a grid search at a coarse scale but is by no means optimal. We performed an ablation study to test the benefits of the proposed improvements. The original network without and with dilated convolution are denoted as *DC-CNN* [19] and *DC-CNN-d*. The proposed stochastic version without and with dilated convolution are referred as *s-DC-CNN* and *s-DC-CNN-d* (the detailed network architectures are described in the supplementary materials). For the stochastic networks, we used all subnetworks for reconstruction except for when generating the uncertainty map.

Training Settings. Each network was trained for 100 epochs using mean squared error loss between the network reconstruction and the ground truth. In the first 50 epochs, the network was trained on various undersampling factors (UF) of (0–12×). For the last 50 epochs, the network was fine-tuned for the UF of $\{2\times, 5\times, 8\times\}$ individually for each experiment. We used the Adam optimiser with a learning rate of 10^{-4}, that was subsequently reduced by a factor of 10 for every 20 epochs during the fine-tuning.

Results. Table 1 tabulates mean and standard deviation (std) of the peak signal-to-noise ratio (PSNR) we obtained by various CS-MRI methods. For the three different UF we tested, the proposed s-DC-CNN-d obtained the best performance, and all our DC-CNN variations outperformed the DLMRI and the UNET-CS. This has been further confirmed by the root mean-squared-error (RMSE) calculated from the computed fractional anisotropy (FA), mean diffusivity (MD) and helix angle (HA) of the 5× undersampling cases.

Table 1. Quantitative results [mean (std)] of the 19 independent testing subjects.

UF	Model	s-DC-CNN-d	s-DC-CNN	DC-CNN-d	DC-CNN	UNET-CS	DLMRI	Zero-Filled
2×	**PSNR**	**37.747 (2.41)**	37.667 (2.35)	37.64 (2.33)	37.73 (2.36)	33.16 (2.14)	33.62 (2.26)	27.89 (2.08)
5×	**PSNR**	**30.96 (2.10)**	30.85 (2.13)	30.88 (2.08)	30.8 (2.1)	28.40 (2.44)	28.40 (2.44)	23.71 (1.72)
8×	**PSNR**	**28.81 (2.00)**	28.50 (2.01)	28.79 (1.97)	28.62 (2.00)	27.35 (2.00)	25.88 (2.36)	22.71 (1.64)
5×	**FA RMSE**	**0.08 (0.03)**	**0.08 (0.03)**	0.09 (0.03)	0.09 (0.03)	0.11 (0.05)	0.11 (0.04)	0.18 (0.04)
	MD RMSE	**0.11 (0.05)**	0.12 (0.05)	**0.11 (0.05)**	0.12 (0.05)	0.16 (0.08)	0.15 (0.07)	0.19 (0.10)
	HA RMSE	**13.34 (2.93)**	13.97 (3.11)	13.68 (2.91)	14.04 (3.04)	16.29 (3.27)	17.88 (2.9)	26.87 (3.31)

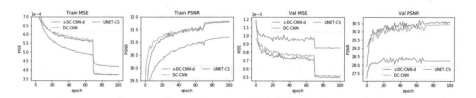

Fig. 1. Convergence analysis of the s-DC-CNN-d compared to the DC-CNN and the UNET-CS.

Convergence analysis (Fig. 1) shows that the proposed s-DC-CNN-d learned slower, but eventually generalised better. The fact that UNET-CS was quickly overfitted may be due to low SNR in the original images that hamper the network to learn a meaningful end-to-end mapping. Compared to the DC-CNN, the proposed s-DC-CNN-d obtained a better PSNR with less epochs during the validation that can be attributed to the fact that the proposed s-DC-CNN-d has an accelerated learning.

Qualitative visualisation (Fig. 2) demonstrates that perceptually both DLMRI and the UNET-CS are over-smoothed in their reconstructed results with clearly larger errors, and the textural details were better preserved in the results

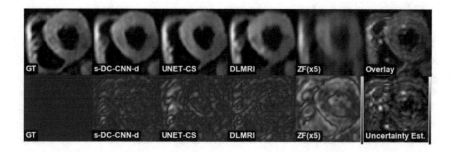

Fig. 2. Qualitative comparison of the reconstructions and error maps for the 5× undersampling.

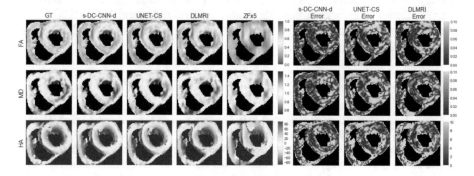

Fig. 3. Comparison of the diffusion tensor parameters and error maps. From top to bottom: fractional anisotropy (FA), mean diffusivity (MD) ($10^{-3}\mathrm{mm}^2\mathrm{s}^{-1}$) and Helix-angle (HA) (degrees).

obtained by the proposed s-DC-CNN-d. From a qualitative analysis, we found that the generated uncertainty estimate using our s-DC-CNN-d highlighted the most challenging area for our algorithms to reconstruct, e.g., the edges of the ventricle and the highly blurred areas in the undersampled input.

Figure 3 shows the computed FA, MD and HA for the 5× undersampling. Overall, our proposed s-DC-CNN-d achieved better calculated diffusion tensor parameters compared to the ones obtained by other methods. In particular, results obtained by the s-DC-CNN-d have a more smooth transition of the HA from epicardial to endocardial surface in the normal left ventricular free wall that resembles the HA calculated by the fully sampled ground truth data.

Finally, we timed the reconstruction of each algorithm (on a GeForce GTX 1080 GPU) and obtained (1) s-DC-CNN-d: 0.065 ± 0.03 s per frame, (2) s-DC-CNN: 0.04 ± 0.02 s per frame, (3) DC-CNN-d: 0.052 ± 0.02 s per frame, (4) DC-CNN: 0.04 ± 0.02 s per frame and (5) UNET-CS: 0.003 ± 0.04 s per frame. The DLMRI method has only a CPU implementation and takes ≈60 s per iteration, and we used 400 iterations per image (>6 h).

4 Discussion and Conclusion

In this study, we proposed a novel deep cascaded CNN based CS-MRI and its stochastic variation for the DT-CMR reconstruction. To the best of our knowledge, it is the first work to consider such application to DT-CMR although the current study is nevertheless simulation based. In addition, we are the first to consider such a stochastic formulation to take the variance of the reconstruction models into account that can be visualised via an uncertainty map. Compared to other state-of-the-art methods using dictionary learning or U-Net based deep learning architecture, our proposed method incorporated dilated convolution and achieved significantly superior reconstruction fidelity with very efficient computation that can be translated into a real-time reconstruction scheme working directly on the scanner. As a future direction, we will carry on further development from on our current simulation based study to accelerate DT-CMR reconstruction and improve its spatial resolution and we can envisage its deployment in various clinical applications.

References

1. Axel, L.: Faster diffusion-weighted MR imaging of cardiac microstructure. Radiology **282**(3), 622–626 (2017)
2. von Deuster, C.: Studying dynamic myofiber aggregate reorientation in dilated cardiomyopathy using in vivo magnetic resonance diffusion tensor imaging. Circ. Cardiovasc. Imaging **9**(10), e005018 (2016)
3. Ferreira, P.F., et al.: In vivo cardiovascular magnetic resonance diffusion tensor imaging shows evidence of abnormal myocardial laminar orientations and mobility in hypertrophic cardiomyopathy. J. Cardiovasc. Magn. Reson. **16**, 87 (2014)
4. Hammernik, K., et al.: Learning a variational network for reconstruction of accelerated MRI data. arXiv preprint arXiv:1704.00447 (2017)
5. Han, Y.: Magn. Reson. Med. Deep learning with domain adaptation for accelerated projection-reconstruction MR **80**(3), 1189–1205 (2018)
6. Hollingsworth, G.: Phys. Med. Biol. Reducing acquisition time in clinical MRI by data undersampling and compressed sensing reconstruction **60**(21), 297–322 (2015)
7. Huang, G., et al.: Deep networks with stochastic depth. arXiv preprint arXiv:1603.09382 (2017)
8. Huang, J.: Cardiac diffusion tensor imaging based on compressed sensing using joint sparsity and low-rank approximation. Technol. Health Care **24**(s2), S593–S599 (2016)
9. Lau, A.Z., et al.: Accelerated human cardiac diffusion tensor imaging using simultaneous multislice imaging. Magn. Reson. Med. **73**(3), 995–1004 (2015)
10. Lee, D., et al.: Deep residual learning for compressed sensing MRI. In: International Symposium on Biomedical Imaging, pp. 15–18. IEEE (2017)
11. Lustig, M.: Sparse MRI: the application of compressed sensing for rapid MR imaging. Magn. Reson. Med. **58**(6), 1182–1195 (2007)
12. Ma, S., et al.: Accelerated cardiac diffusion tensor imaging using joint low-rank and sparsity constraints. IEEE Trans. Biomed. Eng. (2017)
13. Mekkaoui, C.: Diffusion MRI in the heart. NMR Biomed. **30**(3), e3426 (2017)

14. Nielles-Vallespin, S., et al.: Assessment of myocardial microstructural dynamics by in vivo diffusion tensor cardiac magnetic resonance. J. Am. Coll. Cardiol. **69**(6), 661–676 (2017)
15. Nielles-Vallespin, S., et al.: In vivo diffusion tensor MRI of the human heart: reproducibility of breath-hold and navigator-based approaches. Magn. Reson. Med. **70**(2), 454–65 (2013)
16. Qin, C., et al.: Convolutional recurrent neural networks for dynamic MR image reconstruction. arXiv preprint arXiv:1712.01751 (2017)
17. Ravishankar, S., Bresler, Y.: MR image reconstruction from highly undersampled k-space data by dictionary learning. IEEE Trans. Med. Imaging **30**(5), 1028–1041 (2011)
18. Ronneberger, O., Fischer, P., Brox, T.: U-Net: convolutional networks for biomedical image segmentation. In: Navab, N., Hornegger, J., Wells, W.M., Frangi, A.F. (eds.) MICCAI 2015. LNCS, vol. 9351, pp. 234–241. Springer, Cham (2015). https://doi.org/10.1007/978-3-319-24574-4_28
19. Schlemper, J.: A deep cascade of convolutional neural networks for dynamic MR image reconstruction. IEEE Trans. Med. Imaging **37**(2), 491–503 (2018)
20. Schlemper, J., Caballero, J., Hajnal, J.V., Price, A., Rueckert, D.: A deep cascade of convolutional neural networks for MR image reconstruction. In: Niethammer, M. (ed.) IPMI 2017. LNCS, vol. 10265, pp. 647–658. Springer, Cham (2017). https://doi.org/10.1007/978-3-319-59050-9_51
21. Sun, J., et al.: Deep ADMM-Net for compressive sensing MRI. In: NIPS, pp. 10–18 (2016)
22. Wu, Y., et al.: Accelerated MR diffusion tensor imaging using distributed compressed sensing. Magn. Reson. Med. **71**(2), 763–772 (2014)
23. Yang, G., et al.: DAGAN: deep de-aliasing generative adversarial networks for fast compressed sensing MRI reconstruction. IEEE Trans. Med. Imaging, 1310–1321 (2018)

Automatic, Fast and Robust Characterization of Noise Distributions for Diffusion MRI

Samuel St-Jean$^{(\boxtimes)}$, Alberto De Luca , Max A. Viergever,
and Alexander Leemans

Center for Image Sciences, University Medical Center Utrecht,
Utrecht, The Netherlands
samuel@isi.uu.nl

Abstract. Knowledge of the noise distribution in magnitude diffusion MRI images is the centerpiece to quantify uncertainties arising from the acquisition process. The use of parallel imaging methods, the number of receiver coils and imaging filters applied by the scanner, amongst other factors, dictate the resulting signal distribution. Accurate estimation beyond textbook Rician or noncentral chi distributions often requires information about the acquisition process (e.g.coils sensitivity maps or reconstruction coefficients), which is not usually available. We introduce a new method where a change of variable naturally gives rise to a particular form of the gamma distribution for background signals. The first moments and maximum likelihood estimators of this gamma distribution explicitly depend on the number of coils, making it possible to estimate all unknown parameters using only the magnitude data. A rejection step is used to make the method automatic and robust to artifacts. Experiments on synthetic datasets show that the proposed method can reliably estimate both the degrees of freedom and the standard deviation. The worst case errors range from below 2% (spatially uniform noise) to approximately 10% (spatially variable noise). Repeated acquisitions of *in vivo* datasets show that the estimated parameters are stable and have lower variances than compared methods.

1 Introduction

Diffusion magnetic resonance imaging (dMRI) is a non invasive imaging technique which allows probing the microstructure of the brain. Recent advances in parallel imaging techniques and accelerated acquisitions have greatly reduced the inherently long scan time in dMRI. While it is known that the noise distribution found in magnitude dMRI data depends on the reconstruction algorithm used [1] and the number of channels in the receiver coils [2,3], noise correlation effects in adjacent channels change the noise distribution from its theoretical formulation. Assumption of the Rician or more general noncentral chi distributions with degrees of freedom equal to the number of receiver coils deviate due to these effects and other filtering applied by the scanner. The resulting

© Springer Nature Switzerland AG 2018
A. F. Frangi et al. (Eds.): MICCAI 2018, LNCS 11070, pp. 304–312, 2018.
https://doi.org/10.1007/978-3-030-00928-1_35

distribution usually exhibits a lower number of degrees of freedom N than the number of receiver coils and higher noise variance σ_g depending on the spatial location [2,4]. Correcting deviations from the theoretical noise distributions is challenging and oftentimes requires coils correlation maps or information about the complex signal combination process, which is not readily available on most scanners. While some recent algorithms for dMRI are developed to include information about the noise distribution [5,6], there is no method, to the best of our knowledge, providing a fully automatic way to characterize the noise distribution using information from the magnitude data itself only. Due to this gap between the physical acquisition process and noise estimation theory, noise distributions are either assumed as Rician or noncentral chi with N already known and concentrate in estimating the noise standard deviation σ_g [7–9]. We propose to estimate both σ_g and N from the magnitude data only by using a change of variable to a gamma distribution $\Gamma(N, 1)$ [8], whose first moments directly depend on N. This makes the proposed method fast and easy to apply on existing data without additional information, while being robust to artifacts by only considering voxels adhering to the created gamma distribution.

2   Theory and Methods

Signal Distributions in Parallel MRI. To account for uncertainty in the acquisition process, the complex signal measured in k-space by the receiver coil can be modeled with a separate additive zero mean Gaussian noise for each channel, but assumed to have identical variance σ_g^2. When converted to the commonly used magnitude images, the resulting noise distribution follows a Rician or noncentral chi distribution, whose parameters depend on the employed reconstruction algorithm [2]. To account for signal correlations introduced by parallel imaging techniques, the case of the noncentral chi distribution is still valid with spatially varying parameters [4].

Parameter Estimation Using the Method of Moments and Maximum Likelihood. When the underlying signal intensity η is zero, the magnitude signal m reduces to a Rayleigh distribution or in the general case to a chi distribution. The pdf of magnitude noise over zero signal is given by $pdf(m|\eta = 0, \sigma_g, N) = (m^{2N-1})/(2^{N-1}\sigma_g^{2N}\Gamma(N)) \exp\left(-m^2/(2\sigma_g^2)\right)dm$ where $\Gamma(x)$ is the gamma function. With the change of variable $t = m^2/(2\sigma_g^2)$, the pdf can be rewritten as a gamma distribution $\Gamma(N, 1)$ [8]. The pdf of the gamma distribution $\Gamma(\alpha, \beta)$ is defined as $pdf(t|\alpha, \beta) = 1/(\Gamma(\alpha)\beta^\alpha)t^{\alpha-1} \exp\left(-t/\beta\right)dt$ and has theoretical mean $\mu_{gamma} = \alpha\beta$ and variance $\sigma_{gamma}^2 = \alpha\beta^2$. For a gamma distribution $\Gamma(N, 1)$, we obtain that the mean and the variance are equal with a value of N. Another useful identity is that the sum of gamma distributions is a gamma distribution such that if $t_i \sim \Gamma(\alpha_i, \beta)$, then $\sum_{i=1}^{K} t_i \sim \Gamma(\sum_{i=1}^{K} \alpha_i, \beta)$. We can therefore estimate the Gaussian noise standard deviation σ_g and the number of coils N from the moments of the magnitude image themselves where no signal from the imaged object is present. Any method suitable for computing σ_g can be used, or it can also be estimated from the moments once again with the relationship

$$\sigma_g = \frac{1}{\sqrt{2}} \sqrt{\frac{\sum_{k=1}^{K} m_k^4}{\sum_{k=1}^{K} m_k^2} - \frac{1}{K} \sum_{k=1}^{K} m_k^2} \tag{1}$$

where m_k is the magnitude signal for voxel k and K is the number of identified noise only voxels. Once σ_g is known, N can be estimated from the moments with

$$N = \frac{1}{K} \sum_{k=1}^{K} t_k = \frac{1}{2K\sigma_g^2} \sum_{k=1}^{K} m_k^2 \tag{2}$$

where $t_k = m_k^2/(2\sigma_g^2)$ is the change of variable for voxel k. Estimation based on the method of maximum likelihood yields two equations for estimating α and β. Rearranging the equations for a gamma distribution $\Gamma(N,1)$ [10] will give the same expression as Eq. (1) and a second implicit equation for N that is given by

$$\psi(N) = \frac{1}{K} \sum_{k=1}^{K} \log(m_k^2/2\sigma_g^2) \tag{3}$$

where $\psi(x)$ is the digamma function and can be numerically inverted using Newton's method to obtain N.

Estimating σ_g and N. For simplicity, we assume that each 2D slice with the same spatial location belongs to the same distribution throughout each 3D volume. This practical assumption allows selecting a large number of noise only voxels for computing statistics as well as discarding acquisition artifacts such as ghosting. Following a methodology similar to [8], it is possible to identify voxels belonging to the gamma distribution by checking if they fall inside a predefined probability threshold of the inverse cumulative distribution function (cdf). Taking the sum of all MRI volumes can therefore be used to separate the background signal belonging to the gamma distribution $\Gamma(KN,1)$ from the rest of the volume with a rejection step using the inverse cdf. In the particular case $\Gamma(\alpha,1)$ at a probability level p, the inverse cdf is $icdf(\alpha,p) = P^{-1}(\alpha,p)$ where P^{-1} is the inverse lower incomplete regularized gamma function. For the first iteration, initial bounds are set on the value of N and σ_g as they are unknown. We set a lower bound $N_{min} = 1$ and an upper bound $N_{max} = 12$ for the first iteration, noting that [2] reported values of N between 3 and 12 for a 32 channels receiver coil. Similar to [8], an upper bound of σ_g is given by $\sigma_{g_{max}} = median/\sqrt{2\,icdf(N_{max},1/2)}$ where $median$ is the median of the whole 4D dMRI dataset. From this upper bound $\sigma_{g_{max}}$, a search interval with a values is created, where we chose $a = 50$ as in [8]. Each point of the interval $\Phi = [1\sigma_{g_{max}}/a, 2\sigma_{g_{max}}/a, \ldots, a\sigma_{g_{max}}/a]$ is used as an initial value of σ_g in the change of variable $t = m^2/2\sigma_g^2$. With these initial values, an iterative search for σ_g and N is made as follow. The value of Φ which identifies the largest number of voxels between the lower bound given by $\lambda_- = icdf(KN_{min},p/2)$ and the upper bound given by $\lambda_+ = icdf(KN_{max},1-p/2)$ is accepted as σ_g. From those voxels, new values of σ_g are computed with Eq. (1) and N with Eq. (2) or Eq. (3). For the next iteration, we set $\Phi = [0.95\sigma_g, 0.96\sigma_g, \ldots, 1.05\sigma_g]$ and recompute the *icdf* bounds λ_-, λ_+ with the new value of N. Voxels between λ_- and λ_+ belong to the distribution $\Gamma(KN, 1)$ and are recomputed until the values of σ_g and N reach convergence.

Synthetic Phantom Datasets. We generated synthetic datasets based on the ISBI 2013 HARDI challenge[1] with phantomas[2]. Two noiseless single shell phantoms with 64 gradient directions were generated at b = 1000 s/mm² and b = 3000 s/mm² with one b = 0 s/mm² each. The datasets were then corrupted with Rician ($N = 1$) and noncentral chi noise ($N = 4$, 8 and 12), both stationary and spatially varying, at a signal-to-noise ratio (SNR) of 30. The noisy data was generated according to $\hat{I} = \sqrt{\sum_{i=0,j=0}^{N} \left(\frac{I}{\sqrt{N}} + \tau\epsilon_i \right)^2 + \tau\epsilon_j^2}$, where $\hat{I}$ is the resulting noisy volume ϵ_i, ϵ_j are Gaussian distributed with mean 0 and variance $\sigma_g^2 = (mean(b0)/SNR)^2$. In the constant noise case, τ is set to 1 so that the noise is uniform. For the spatially varying noise case, τ is a sphere with a value of 1 in the center up to a value of 1.75 at the edges of the phantom, thus generating a stronger noise profile *outside* the phantom than for the stationary (constant) noise case. This noise profile mimics receiver coils disposed around the surface of the phantom, with an increase in the noise profile near each receiver. One important observation arising from choosing a single SNR level is that the noise standard deviation σ_g is the same for all datasets, while the magnitude standard deviation σ_{m_N} depends on the value of N and we have $\sigma_{m_N} < \sigma_g$.

In Vivo Datasets. We obtained four repetitions of a freely available dMRI dataset of a single subject[3] to assess the reproducibility of noise estimation without *a priori* knowledge. The acquisition was performed on a GE MR750 3T scanner at Stanford university, where a 3x slice acceleration with blipped-CAIPI shift of FOV/3 was used, partial Fourier 5/8 and a minimum TE of 81 ms. Two acquisitions were made in the anterior-posterior phase encoded direction and the two others in the posterior-anterior direction. The voxelsize was 1.7 mm isotropic with 7 b = 0 s/mm² images, 38 volumes at b = 1500 s/mm² and 38 volumes at b = 3000 s/mm².

Noise Estimation Algorithms for Comparison. To assess the performance of the proposed method, we used three other noise estimation algorithms [7–9] previously used in the context of diffusion MRI with their default parameters. The local adaptive noise estimation (LANE) algorithm [9] was designed to estimate the noise standard deviation over tissue for both Rician and noncentral chi noise while also taking into account the structure of the data for adaptive estimation. Since the method works on a 3D volume, we only used the b = 0 s/mm² image for all of the experiments as the signal does not vary spatially for the

---

[1] http://hardi.epfl.ch/static/events/2013_ISBI/.

[2] https://github.com/ecaruyer/phantomas.

[3] https://openfmri.org/dataset/ds000031.

same type of tissue in such image. We used the Marchenko-Pastur (MP) distribution fitting on the principal component analysis (PCA) decomposition of the diffusion data [7]. MPPCA estimates the magnitude noise standard deviation σ_{m_N} in small local windows by finding an optimal threshold in PCA space which separates the signal from the noise. This value of σ_{m_N} is slightly underestimated due to the discrete nature of the PCA decomposition. Finally, we compared our proposed method with the Probabilistic Identification and Estimation of Noise (PIESNO) [8], which originally proposed the change of variable to the gamma distribution that is at the core of our proposed method. PIESNO requires the value of N, which is used to iteratively estimate σ_g until convergence by removing voxels which do not belong to the distribution $\Gamma(N, 1)$ for a given slice. For our proposed algorithm, we set the probability level at $p = 0.05$ and initial values of $a = 50$, $N_{min} = 1$ and $N_{max} = 12$. To the best of our knowledge, ours is the first method which makes it possible to estimate both σ_g and N jointly without requiring any information about the reconstruction process of the MRI scanner. Finally, we quantitatively assessed the performance of each method on the synthetic datasets by measuring the percentage error inside the phantom against the known value of σ_g, where the error is computed as $percentage\,error = 100(\sigma_{g_{estimated}} - \sigma_{g_{true}})/\sigma_{g_{true}}$. We also show the estimated values of N using our method for each dataset.

3 Results

As MPPCA and LANE are designed to estimate σ_g over data, we report the estimation error computed only inside a mask excluding the background for all methods. Figure 1 shows the percentage error of each method on the synthetic datasets. The correct value of N was given to both LANE and PIESNO when σ_g was constant. All methods performed generally well, with our proposed method and PIESNO making less than 2% of errors for all cases. MPPCA and LANE commit larger errors (around 5% and 20% on average respectively) with increasing values of N, where LANE error is the largest when $N = 12$. For the case of spatially varying σ_g, we assumed N to be unknown and set $N = 1$ for LANE and PIESNO. Due to a misspecification of N, PIESNO errors are several orders of magnitude larger than the other methods except for the Rician noise case. MPPCA and LANE both underestimate σ_g (around 20% and between 10 to 15% respectively) while our proposed method resulted in the lowest error, which is around 10%. Figure 2 shows the estimated values of N by the proposed method for all cases of the synthetic datasets. Even when σ_g is underestimated, values of N are close to the real value. Estimating N using Eq. (2) or Eq. (3) gave similar results in both cases, so we used Eq. (2) in the present work. As limited information is available for the *in vivo* datasets, we assumed a Rician distribution for LANE and set $N = 1$ as suggested by [9]. For PIESNO, setting a Rician distribution with $N = 1$ returned less than 10 voxels identified per datasets. We instead assumed $N = 0.5$ since it corresponds to a half Gaussian distribution [2], which is the closest theoretical distribution estimated by our method.

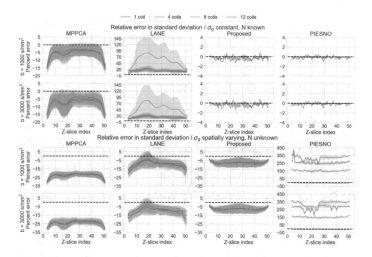

Fig. 1. Percentage of error in estimating the noise standard deviation for each slice along the Z axis with the mean (solid line) and standard deviation (shaded area). In the top image, $\sigma_g = 171$ is constant and N is known while in the bottom image σ_g varies spatially and N is unknown or assumed Rician distributed.

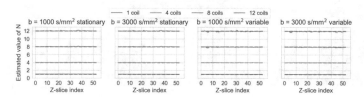

Fig. 2. Estimated value of N by the proposed method. Even for the spatially variable case where σ_g is slightly underestimated, the estimated values of N are stable and correspond to the real values used in the synthetic simulations in every case.

Figure 3 shows the mean (and standard deviation) value of σ_g on the *in vivo* datasets for each methods along axial slices. The value of N as computed by our proposed method is also reported and is stable across datasets. All methods recovered average stable values of σ_g on the four repetitions of the same subject. However, LANE recovered the highest values of σ_g amongst all methods with a large variance, which might indicate overestimation in some areas. Figure 4 shows an axial slice around the cerebellum corrupted by acquisition artifacts likely due to parallel imaging. Voxels containing artifacts were automatically discarded by our method. The values of N and σ_g computed from these voxels also offer a better qualitative fit than assuming a Rayleigh distribution or selecting non brain data. We also timed each method to estimate σ_g on one of the *in vivo* datasets using a standard desktop computer with a 3.5 GHz Intel Xeon processor. All methods were multi threaded while PIESNO was only single threaded. The runtime to estimate σ_g (and N) was around 10 secs for our proposed method, 11 secs for PIESNO, 3 min for MPPCA and 18 min for LANE.

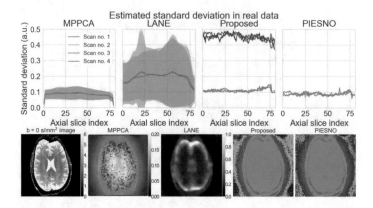

Fig. 3. At the top, estimated values of σ_g for the 4 *in vivo* datasets. For the proposed method, estimated values of N are shown in darker hues for each dataset. On the bottom, an axial slice of a b = 0 s/mm^2 image from one dataset and the estimated values of σ_g for MPPCA and LANE. For the proposed method and PIESNO, a mask of the identified background voxels (in yellow) overlaid on the data.

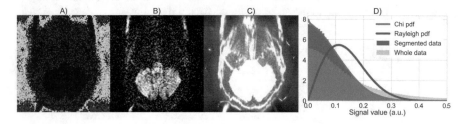

Fig. 4. An axial slice in the cerebellum from one of the *in vivo* datasets. Voxels identified in (A) as noise only (yellow) are free of artifacts in a single slice in (B) or along the sum of all volumes in (C). In (D), the normalized density histogram using the selected voxels from (A) (blue) fits well a chi distribution with $N = 0.47$ and $\sigma_g = 0.11$, while assuming a Rayleigh distribution (green) or using all non brain voxels (orange) leads to a worse visual fit.

4   Discussion and Conclusion

We have shown how a change of variable to a gamma distribution $\Gamma(N, 1)$ can be used to robustly and automatically identify background voxels. Once identified, the moments and maximum likelihood equations (Eqs. (1)–(3)) of the gamma distribution can be used iteratively to compute the number of degrees of freedom N and the Gaussian noise standard deviation σ_g relating to the original noise distribution. The presented equations are also fast to compute (around 10 s on *in vivo* data). Results on the synthetic datasets show that we can reliably estimate both parameters from the magnitude data itself. While the method we have presented assumes that each 2D slice contains a single noise distribution, N can be computed reliably on spatially varying noise and σ_g with an error between 5 and 10%, which is less than the compared methods. On the *in vivo* datasets, our method is stable across the four repetitions and can automatically discard voxels corrupted by acquisition artifacts due to parallel acceleration. From the identified background voxels, without any specific assumption, the recovered distribution parameters fit well the histogram of the data. This distribution is close to a half Gaussian distribution ($N = 0.5$) while the Rician noise assumption would not be adequate in this case. Our method is also the first to identify any type of noise distribution from the magnitude data itself without requiring external information about the scanner or the reconstruction process. Interestingly, while we have shown results on dMRI datasets, the theory we presented applies to any other MRI weighting using large samples of magnitude data e.g.functional MRI. If measurements from the scanner without any object signals are acquired (i.e.noise maps), a local window estimation of our proposed method could be used to overcome the shortcoming of assuming stationary 2D noise distributions. Noise maps measurements could also be used for cases such as body or cardiac imaging where background voxels are usually not available in large quantities. Automatic identification of the noise distribution parameters could help multicenter studies which may not currently collect information about the acquisition and reconstruction process [4] or methods harmonizing data between different scanners and acquisition protocols [11]. Our method can also be used to provide prior knowledge beyond the textbook Rician distribution when computing local diffusion models [5,6].

References

1. Brown, R.W., et al.: Magnetic resonance imaging: physical principles and sequence design. Wiley, New York (2014)
2. Dietrich, O., et al.: Influence of multichannel combination, parallel imaging and other reconstruction techniques on MRI noise characteristics. Magn. Reson. Imaging **26**(6), 754–762 (2008)
3. Sotiropoulos, S.N., et al.: Effects of image reconstruction on fiber orientation mapping from multichannel diffusion MRI: reducing the noise floor using SENSE. Magn. Reson. Med. **70**(6), 1682–1689 (2013)
4. Aja-Fernández, S., Vegas-Sánchez-Ferrero, G., Tristán-Vega, A.: Noise estimation in parallel MRI: GRAPPA and SENSE. Magn. Reson. Imaging **32**(3), 281–290 (2014)
5. Collier, Q., et al.: Diffusion kurtosis imaging with free water elimination: a Bayesian estimation approach. Magn. Reson. Med. **80**(2), 802–813 (2018)
6. Sakaie, K., Lowe, M.: Retrospective correction of bias in diffusion tensor imaging arising from coil combination mode. Mag. Reson. Imaging **37**, 203–208 (2017)
7. Veraart, J., Fieremans, E., Novikov, D.S.: Diffusion MRI noise mapping using random matrix theory. Magn. Reson. Med. **76**(5), 1582–1593 (2016)
8. Koay, C.G., Özarslan, E., Pierpaoli, C.: Probabilistic identification and estimation of noise (PIESNO): a self-consistent approach and its applications in MRI. J. Magn. Reson. **199**(1), 94–103 (2009)
9. Tabelow, K., Voss, H.U., Polzehl, J.: Local estimation of the noise level in MRI using structural adaptation. Med. Image Anal. **20**(1), 76–86 (2015)

10. Thom, H.C.S.: A note on the gamma distribution. Mon. Weather Rev. **86**(4), 117–122 (1958)
11. Mirzaalian, H., et al.: Inter-site and inter-scanner diffusion MRI data harmonization. NeuroImage **135**, 311–323 (2016)

An Automated Localization, Segmentation and Reconstruction Framework for Fetal Brain MRI

Michael Ebner[1](✉) , Guotai Wang[1](✉) , Wenqi Li[1] , Michael Aertsen[2] ,
Premal A. Patel[1] , Rosalind Aughwane[1,3], Andrew Melbourne[1], Tom Doel[1] ,
Anna L. David[3,4], Jan Deprest[1,3,4] , Sébastien Ourselin[1,5],
and Tom Vercauteren[1,4,5]

[1] Translational Imaging Group, WEISS, University College London, London, UK
{michael.ebner.14,guotai.wang.14}@ucl.ac.uk
[2] Department of Radiology, University Hospitals KU Leuven, Leuven, Belgium
[3] Institute for Women's Health, University College London, London, UK
[4] Department of Obstetrics and Gynaecology,
University Hospitals KU Leuven, Leuven, Belgium
[5] School of Biomedical Engineering and Imaging Sciences,
King's College London, London, UK

Abstract. Reconstructing a high-resolution (HR) volume from motion-corrupted and sparsely acquired stacks plays an increasing role in fetal brain Magnetic Resonance Imaging (MRI) studies. Existing reconstruction methods are time-consuming and often require user interaction to localize and extract the brain from several stacks of 2D slices. In this paper, we propose a fully automatic framework for fetal brain reconstruction that consists of three stages: (1) brain localization based on a coarse segmentation of a down-sampled input image by a Convolutional Neural Network (CNN), (2) fine segmentation by a second CNN trained with a multi-scale loss function, and (3) novel, single-parameter outlier-robust super-resolution reconstruction (SRR) for HR visualization in the standard anatomical space. We validate our framework with images from fetuses with variable degrees of ventriculomegaly associated with spina bifida. Experiments show that each step of our proposed pipeline outperforms state-of-the-art methods in both segmentation and reconstruction comparisons. Overall, we report automatic SRR reconstructions that compare favorably with those obtained by manual, labor-intensive brain segmentations. This potentially unlocks the use of automatic fetal brain reconstruction studies in clinical practice.

1 Introduction

Fetal Magnetic Resonance Imaging (MRI) has become increasingly important for prenatal diagnosis as a complementary tool to prenatal sonography. To mitigate the effect of fetal (and maternal) motion, fast imaging methods such as

---

M. Ebner and G. Wang — Contributed equally

© Springer Nature Switzerland AG 2018
A. F. Frangi et al. (Eds.): MICCAI 2018, LNCS 11070, pp. 313–320, 2018.
https://doi.org/10.1007/978-3-030-00928-1_36

Single-Shot Fast Spin Echo (SSFSE) are used to acquire thick, low-resolution (LR) 2D slices that can largely freeze in-plane motion. However, in order to assess and quantify fetal pathology, it is highly desirable to reconstruct a single isotropic, high-resolution (HR) volume. Existing reconstruction toolkits generally rely on an iterative motion-correction/reconstruction approach [3,6,9]. Since the position and orientation of the fetal brain vary significantly between patients in relation to maternal structures, localizing the fetal brain and obtaining a segmented mask to exclude the surrounding tissues is crucial for achieving accurate motion-correction. At present, this usually requires manual localization of the fetal brain and uses manual or semi-automatic methods to obtain fetal brain masks, which is laborious and time consuming. To avoid this, [1] reconstructs the entire field-of-view by breaking each slice into patches. However, in addition to increased computational requirements, this leads to non-rigid motion-correction and therefore suboptimal outcomes for rigidly moving regions such as the fetal brain. We believe that a fully automatic reconstruction pipeline based on *automatic* brain localization, extraction (segmentation) and *robust* reconstruction steps is favored to achieve accurate fetal brain reconstructions and potential clinical translation.

Several works investigate automatic fetal brain localization and segmentation. In [7], these are performed by an automatic reconstruction pipeline using a Support Vector Machine and Random Forests, but these are limited by hand-crafted features and testing inefficiency. The template-based automatic method proposed in [11] takes hours for localization. Convolutional Neural Networks (CNN) are used in in [10] for fast slice-based fetal brain segmentation but can easily obtain false positives and show poor performance for challenging cases.

Robust super-resolution reconstruction (SRR) methods for fetal MRI have been proposed previously to prevent slice misregistrations from affecting the SRR outcome [3,6]. However, in [3] no complete outlier rejection is achieved and the method in [6] relies on multiple hyperparameters to be tuned in order to achieve optimal reconstructions while both require time-consuming optimization methods due to their resulting non-convex problem formulation.

We propose a novel framework for automatic fetal brain reconstruction from fetal MRI as shown in Fig. 1. First, we propose a coarse segmentation-based localization using a CNN. Second, we use a multi-scale loss function for training a second CNN to obtain a fine segmentation of the fetal brain. Third, we introduce an effective complete outlier-rejection approach for robust SRR that relies only on a single hyperparameter and retains a linear least-squares formulation. The proposed framework is validated by producing HR 3D volumes from MR images of fetuses with spina bifida (SB) aperta who were assessed prior to and after in-utero open surgical repair. This procedure is performed in selected fetuses and improves neurological outcome compared to a postnatal repair [8].

2   Methods

Localization Based on Coarse Segmentation. Differently from traditional top-down object localization methods using sliding window classification or

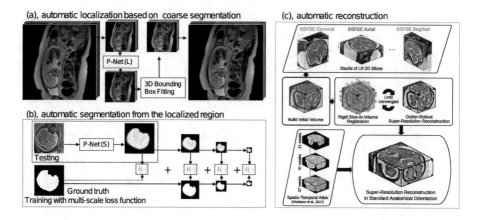

Fig. 1. The proposed fully automatic framework for fetal brain reconstruction.

bounding box regression, we use a bottom-up strategy for fetal brain localization based on a coarse segmentation by a CNN with pixel-level prediction. The framework is theoretically applicable to different CNN models, and we select P-Net [12] for its compactness and efficiency. We refer to this localization task network as **P-Net (L)**. Let I denote a stack of slices and I_i represent the i-th 2D slice of I. To reduce the inference time in this stage, we down-sample I_i to I'_i with a given size 96×96. We use I' to denote the whole down-sampled stack. As shown in Fig. 1(a), to get a 3D bounding box of the fetal brain, we first use the P-Net (L) to obtain a segmentation of I' by stacking the 2D segmentations, i.e., a coarse segmentation, which is smoothed by morphological closing and opening. Then we fit a 3D bounding box to the largest connected component of the smoothed segmentation. The 3D bounding box is rescaled to the original space of I and expanded by a margin of 5 mm, and used as the localization result.

Fine Segmentation. After localization, we use a second CNN to obtain a fine segmentation of the fetal brain. We consistently use the P-Net structure [12] for the fine segmentation and refer to it as **P-Net (S)**. As shown in Fig. 1(b), P-Net (S) works on the extracted region of I based on the localization result, rather than the entire image of I, to reduce false positives. The commonly adopted logistic loss and Dice loss function for image segmentation use a sum of pixelwise losses, without considering the relationship between neighboring pixels. This can result in noise and spatial inconsistency in the prediction. To alleviate this problem, we propose a training loss function across multiple scales $L_S(Y, \hat{Y}) := \frac{1}{S} \sum_{s=1}^{S} l(Y_s, \hat{Y}_s)$ where Y is the prediction of an image given by the segmentation CNN, $\hat{Y}$ is the corresponding ground truth and S is the number of scales. Y_s and $\hat{Y}_s$ are the rescaled versions of Y and $\hat{Y}$ at scale s, respectively. Here, the rescale operation at scale s is implemented by average pooling with a kernel size $2^{s-1} \times 2^{s-1}$. $l(\cdot)$ is a basic loss function, e.g, logistic or Dice loss. When $S > 1$, $l(\cdot)$ encourages the prediction to be close to the ground truth at a higher level.

Outlier-Robust Super-Resolution Reconstruction. Taking advantage of these brain segmentations, we deploy a mask-guided rigid motion correction for all masked slices $\mathbf{y}_k$ followed by an outlier-robust SRR step to recover the most likely HR volume $\mathbf{x}^i$ which satisfies the slice acquisition model $\mathbf{y}_k^i \approx \mathbf{A}_k^i \mathbf{x}^i$ [3] with a linear slice-acquisition operator $\mathbf{A}_k^i$ for reasonably well motion-corrected slices $\mathbf{y}_k^i$ at iteration i. The SRR is solved using a maximum a-posteriori formulation

$$\mathbf{x}^i := \arg\min_{\mathbf{x}} \left(\sum_{k \in \mathcal{K}_\sigma^i} \frac{1}{2} \|\mathbf{y}_k^i - \mathbf{A}_k^i \mathbf{x}\|_{\ell^2}^2 + \frac{\alpha}{2} \|\nabla \mathbf{x}\|_{\ell^2}^2 \right) \quad \text{s. t.} \quad \mathbf{x} \geq 0 \qquad (1)$$

for a slice-index set $\mathcal{K}_\sigma^i := \{1 \leq k \leq K : \text{Sim}(\mathbf{y}_k^i, \mathbf{A}_k^i \mathbf{x}^{i-1}) \geq \sigma\}$ containing only slices in high agreement with their simulated counterparts projected from the previous HR iterate according to a similarity measure Sim and parameter $\sigma > 0$. $\alpha \geq 0$ denotes a regularization parameter and ∇ the differential operator. We thus have a convex SRR problem with complete outlier removal in a linear least-squares formulation that is efficiently solvable using matrix-free operations [2].

3   Experiments and Results

Data and Implementation. The automatic reconstruction framework was applied to a cohort of 16 fetuses with SB, scanned at University Hospitals KU Leuven before (B1) and after (B2) surgical treatment at the gestational age (GA) of 23.47 ± 0.92 weeks and 25.73 ± 1.28 weeks, respectively. For each study, 3 to 10 SSFSE stacks in different planes were collected, with pixel size 0.63 mm to 1.58 mm and slice thickness 3 mm to 6 mm.

For detection and segmentation, separate cohorts of 30 healthy and 16 fetuses with SB (before treatment) with GA 29.51 ± 4.46 weeks and GA 23.60 ± 3.11, respectively, were used for training (126 stacks) and validation (12 stacks). The groups B1 (119 stacks) and B2 (105 stacks) were used for testing. Manual segmentations of the fetal brains were used as the ground truth for the segmentation task. The bounding box of the manual segmentation was extended by 5 mm and used as the ground truth for fetal brain localization. Stack intensities were normalized by its mean and standard deviation. Our CNNs were implemented in TensorFlow using NiftyNet [5]. We used $S = 4$ scales for L_S and used Dice loss as the basic loss function. We used Adaptive Moment Estimation (Adam) for training, with initial learning rate 10^{-3}, weight decay 10^{-7} and $10k$ iterations.

The SRR algorithm was applied to the B1 and B2 cases using the obtained automatic segmentations for the rigid slice-to-volume registrations. The image data was preprocessed using ITK bias field and linear intensity correction. Three two-step rigid slice-to-volume registration and outlier-robust SRR iterations were performed whereby Sim was set to be normalized cross-correlation (NCC) and σ was empirically set to be 0.6, 0.65 and 0.7 per iteration to account for increasing accuracy in (1), respectively. The regularization parameter $\alpha = 0.02$ was determined using L-curve studies. Final SRRs were reconstructed in the standard anatomical space by using a brain-volume matched template from a

Table 1. Quantitative evaluation of different methods for fetal brain localization with * denoting significant differences based on a paired t-test ($p < 0.05$).

	IoU (%)		Centroid distance (mm)		Stack-level runtime(s)
	Group B1	Group B2	Group B1	Group B2	
Keraudren et al. [7]	72.87±10.37	69.18±11.73	7.31±4.58	7.68±2.83	15.03±3.54
P-Net (L)	**84.74±5.55***	**83.67±5.04***	**3.70±2.10***	**4.51±2.45***	**2.35±1.02***

Table 2. Quantitative evaluation of fetal brain segmentation with * denoting significant better performance compared with P-Net (S) based on a paired t-test ($p < 0.05$).

	Dice (%)		Hausdorff (mm)		Stack-level runtime(s)
	Group B1	Group B2	Group B1	Group B2	
Salehi et al. [10]	90.12±4.19	88.57±4.24	14.75±7.51	12.08±6.63	**1.98±0.76**
P-Net (S)	91.56±3.33	90.93±4.95	10.93±5.66	9.83±5.29	3.65±1.34
P-Net (S) + ML	**93.87±2.79***	**92.94±4.14***	**6.94±4.29***	**7.84±3.26***	3.66±1.33

spatiotemporal atlas [4]. The outlier-robust SRR part was implemented in Python using ITK and the LSMR solver for (1). It is made open-source on GitHub[1].

Localization and Segmentation Results. Table 1 summarises the localization results of P-Net (L) compared against the method of Keraudren et al. [7] using the Intersection over Union (IoU) score and the centroid distance between the localized and the ground truth bounding box. A visual comparison is provided in the supplementary material. P-Net (L) was trained using the manual segmentations as pixel-wise annotations. Figure 2 presents a visual comparison of three methods for fetal brain segmentation applied to Group B1 and Group B2 respectively: (1) Salehi et al.[2] [10], applying the U-Net to the whole input image for segmentation without a localization stage, (2) P-Net (S) trained with the basic Dice loss function (at a single scale), and (3) P-Net (S) + ML where P-Net (S) was trained with our proposed multi-scale loss function. Both P-Net (S) and P-Net (S) + ML were applied to the output of P-Net (L). The method of Salehi et al. [10] has a lower performance than our coarse-to-fine segmentation methods. P-Net (S) + ML achieves a better spatial consistency with reduced noises in the segmentation than P-Net (S). Quantitative evaluation of these segmentation methods is presented in Table 2, which shows that the proposed multi-scale loss for training leads to higher segmentation accuracy than P-Net (S).

---

[1] https://github.com/gift-surg/NiftyMIC.
[2] We followed the implementation at https://bitbucket.org/bchradiology/u-net/src and re-trained the model with our own training images.

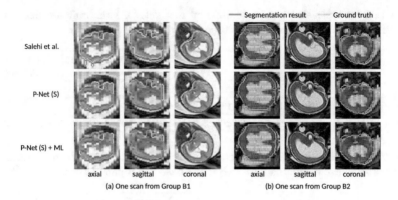

Fig. 2. Visual comparison of different methods for fetal brain segmentation.

Table 3. Slice similarities $\text{Sim}(\mathbf{y}_k^i, \mathbf{A}_k^i \mathbf{x}^i)$ for the respective $\mathcal{K}_{0.7}^i$-slices, $i = 3$.

	NCC		RMSE		SSIM	
	Group B1	Group B2	Group B1	Group B2	Group B1	Group B2
SRR (M)	**0.94±0.06**	**0.94±0.05**	**23.93±8.18**	**30.25±26.03**	**0.71±0.10**	**0.71±0.11**
SRR (S)	**0.94±0.05**	**0.94±0.06**	**24.05±8.54**	**30.80±26.28**	**0.71±0.10**	**0.70±0.12**
SRR (L)	0.87±0.15	0.87±0.14	29.50±14.07	38.56±35.23	0.60±0.16	0.60±0.17

Outlier-Robust SRR Results. Out of the 32 performed reconstructions, six were discarded[3] from the final evaluation leaving 13 cases for each B1/B2 group. For each reconstruction 3/5.7/6/8 (min/mean/median/max) stacks were used. Three different configurations were tested to analyze the input-mask-sensitivity of our proposed SRR algorithm: Reconstructions were performed using the output rectangular masks of P-Net (L), the output masks of P-Net (S) + ML and the manual segmentations which we refer to as SRR (L), SRR (S) and SRR (M), respectively. Table 3 shows the slice similarities $\text{Sim}(\mathbf{y}_k^i, \mathbf{A}_k^i \mathbf{x}^i)$ for the final iteration $i = 3$ using NCC, root mean squared error (RMSE) and structural similarity (SSIM). The proposed SRR (S) algorithm achieves reconstructions of almost identical self-consistency as SRR (M). In absence of a ground-truth, an additional subjective quality assessment in a clinical context was made where two blinded pediatric radiologists assessed all reconstructions side-by-side. We compared this to reconstructions obtained by the state-of-the-art toolkit developed by Kainz et al. [6] using the manual segmentations as input masks. Table 4 underlines that SRR (S) and SRR (M) achieve reconstructions of high quality that are subjectively almost indistinguishable. The comparison against Kainz et al. [6] confirms the effectiveness of our proposed outlier-robust SRR framework which is also illustrated in Fig. 3.

---

[3] Four cases with successful SRRs failed at final template-space alignment step; two failed at SRR due to heavy motion that could not be corrected for by any method.

Table 4. Summary of clinical evaluation. Anatomical clarity was assessed on the cerebellar structure, the aqueduct and the interhemispheric fissure. SRR quality rates introduced artifactual structures and edge uncertainty. The respective average scoring range is shown in square brackets (the higher, the better). Radiologists' preference ranks subjectively from least (0) to most preferred (3) reconstruction. A * denotes a significant difference compared to SRR (M) based on a Wilcoxon signed-rank test ($p < 0.05$).

	Anat. Clarity [0...4]		SRR Quality [0...2]		Radiologists' Pref.	
	Group B1	Group B2	Group B1	Group B2	Group B1	Group B2
SRR (M)	2.32±0.55	**3.01±0.68**	**0.88±0.30**	1.10±0.35	**1.96±0.75**	**2.04±0.69**
SRR (S)	**2.36±0.52**	**3.01±0.75**	0.81±0.51	1.10±0.42	1.54±0.85	1.58±0.81
SRR (L)	1.92±0.69*	2.69±0.84*	0.54±0.43*	0.85±0.43*	0.58±0.64*	0.77±0.67*
Kainz et al. [6]	2.01±0.75*	2.92±0.77	0.83±0.33	**1.15±0.36**	1.92±1.02	1.62±0.79

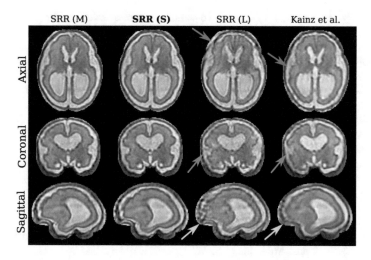

Fig. 3. Visual comparison for one single case showing the SRR (M)/(S) similarity and the effectiveness of the proposed outlier-robust SRR algorithm to prevent artifactual structures such as shown with arrows.

4   Discussion and Conclusion

In this work, we present a fully automated pipeline for fetal brain MRI reconstruction benefiting from deep-learning based automatic fetal brain localization and segmentation. We propose CNN-based coarse segmentation for robust localization and training with a multi-scale loss function for a fine segmentation of the fetal brain. Compared with Keraudren et al. [7], our localization method does not need prior information such as gestational age and achieved superior performance in less time. Unlike [10] which takes a whole image input to a CNN, our segmentation method follows a coarse-to-fine way, and leads to higher segmentation accuracy. Moreover, we propose an alternative robust-outlier rejection method during the SRR step which, in contrast to [3,6], leads to a simple, yet effective, linear least-squares formulation with a single hyperparameter. Overall, our experiments show automatic fetal brain MRI reconstructions that are comparable to manual segmentation-based reconstructions, effectively eliminating the need of any manual intervention. In the future, we aim to apply this framework to quantify the impact of spina bifida repair surgeries by measuring the resolution of the Chiari type II malformation and the degree of ventriculomegaly.

Acknowledgements. This work is supported by Wellcome Trust [WT101957; 203145Z/16/Z], EPSRC [EP/L016478/1; NS/A000027/1; NS/A000050/1], and the NIHR UCLH BRC.

References

1. Alansary, A., et al.: PVR: patch-to-volume reconstruction for large area motion correction of fetal MRI. IEEE Trans. Med. Imaging **36**(10), 2031–2044 (2017)
2. Ebner, M., et al.: Point-spread-function-aware slice-to-volume registration: application to upper abdominal MRI super-resolution. In: Zuluaga, M.A., Bhatia, K., Kainz, B., Moghari, M.H., Pace, D.F. (eds.) RAMBO/HVSMR -2016. LNCS, vol. 10129, pp. 3–13. Springer, Cham (2017). https://doi.org/10.1007/978-3-319-52280-7_1
3. Gholipour, A., Estroff, J.A., Warfield, S.K.: Robust super-resolution volume reconstruction from slice acquisitions: application to fetal brain MRI. IEEE Trans. Med. Imaging **29**(10), 1739–1758 (2010)
4. Gholipour, A., et al.: A normative spatiotemporal MRI atlas of the fetal brain for automatic segmentation and analysis of early brain growth. Sci. Rep. **7**(1), 476 (2017)
5. Gibson, E., et al.: NiftyNet: a deep-learning platform for medical imaging. Comput. Methods Programs Biomed. **158**, 113–122 (2018)
6. Kainz, B., et al.: Fast volume reconstruction from motion corrupted stacks of 2D slices. IEEE Trans. Med. Imaging **34**(9), 1901–1913 (2015)
7. Keraudren, K., et al.: Automated fetal brain segmentation from 2D MRI slices for motion correction. Neuroimage **101**, 633–643 (2014)
8. Ovaere, C., et al.: Prenatal diagnosis and patient preferences in patients with neural tube defects around the advent of fetal surgery in Belgium and Holland. Fetal Diagn. Ther. **37**(3), 226–234 (2015)
9. Rousseau, F., et al.: Registration-based approach for reconstruction of high-resolution in Utero Fetal MR Brain images. Acad. Radiol. **13**(9), 1072–1081 (2006)
10. Salehi, S.S.M., et al.: Real-time automatic fetal brain extraction in fetal MRI by deep learning. arXiv Preprint. arXiv1710.09338 (2017)
11. Tourbier, S., et al.: Automated template-based brain localization and extraction for fetal brain MRI reconstruction. Neuroimage **155**, 460–472 (2017)
12. Wang, G., et al.: Interactive medical image segmentation using deep learning with image-specific fine-tuning. IEEE Trans. Med. Imaging **37**(7), 1562–1573 (2018)

Retinal Image Understanding Emerges from Self-Supervised Multimodal Reconstruction

Álvaro S. Hervella[1,2(✉)], José Rouco[1,2], Jorge Novo[1,2], and Marcos Ortega[1,2]

[1] CITIC-Research Center of Information and Communication Technologies,
University of A Coruña, A Coruña, Spain
[2] Department of Computer Science, University of A Coruña, A Coruña, Spain
{a.suarezh,jrouco,jnovo,mortega}@udc.es

Abstract. The successful application of deep learning-based methodologies is conditioned by the availability of sufficient annotated data, which is usually critical in medical applications. This has motivated the proposal of several approaches aiming to complement the training with reconstruction tasks over unlabeled input data, complementary broad labels, augmented datasets or data from other domains. In this work, we explore the use of reconstruction tasks over multiple medical imaging modalities as a more informative self-supervised approach. Experiments are conducted on multimodal reconstruction of retinal angiography from retinography. The results demonstrate that the detection of relevant domain-specific patterns emerges from this self-supervised setting.

Keywords: Self-supervised · Multimodal · Retinography Angiography

1 Introduction

Nowadays, deep learning-based solutions are commonly used for a significant variety of computer vision applications. Deep Neural Networks (DNN) are able to recognize complex patterns from raw input images and signals, and to hierarchically learn suitable representations of the underlying information at different levels [1]. In order to do so, DNNs train a large number of parameters using also large datasets that include representative annotated data. While large datasets exist for many computer vision applications, they are a scarce resource in clinical environments. The size of annotated medical imaging datasets is usually limited given the significant cost of hand labeling the data. Annotations must be performed by expert clinicians, whose time and expertise is not efficiently used if it is invested in tedious and time-consuming tasks like manual labeling large datasets. Besides, expert-annotated images are better used for the clinical validation of the resulting medical image analysis methods. In contrast, a large amount of unlabeled medical images is readily available from the daily clinical

A. F. Frangi et al. (Eds.): MICCAI 2018, LNCS 11070, pp. 321–328, 2018.
https://doi.org/10.1007/978-3-030-00928-1_37

practice, along with the patient clinical condition, which can be used as a broad label for the image. However, detailed marking of the images is still needed to provide relevant information for the detection and classification of lesions and anatomical structures in the images.

Several approaches have been proposed to alleviate the scarcity of annotated data, some of which have been applied to medical imaging. A common approach is the application of transfer learning, which consists in the reuse of trained models from different domains of application. For example, pretrained networks for ImageNet classification are usually employed for this purpose, either using the first layers as feature extractors or using the whole network as initialization [2]. However, this approach is limited by the differences between natural and medical images. Self-supervised reconstruction of unlabeled input images, e.g., with stacked autoencoders, is used for the same initialization and feature extraction purposes [3]. The advantage is that the image domain remains the same, but it is not guaranteed that the reconstruction relies on relevant features for the target application. A possible solution to this is the simultaneous training of the auxiliary task, i.e. the self-supervised reconstruction, along with the target task [4]. Although other multitask learning settings are also possible [5]. For example, the simultaneous learning of several supervised tasks over the same input, some of which may be based on global labels, augments the labeled data improving the performance on all the tasks [6]. This latter approach allows a more efficient use of the labeled data, but may further benefit from auxiliary self-supervised tasks that are relevant for the target application. A different approach consists in artificially increasing the dataset with synthetic images and labels. This data augmentation is usually performed through basic spatial and intensity transformations. However, the use of generative deep learning models has also been explored to create new plausible sample images [7].

In this work, we explore an innovative source of additional self-supervised learning information for medical environments, which has not been previously used to complement scarce datasets. In many medical environments, it is common that the diagnosis and follow-up of a disease involves the use of multiple image modalities. This eases the gathering of multimodal image datasets. Multimodal image reconstruction, from one image modality to another, using aligned images of the same patient, is a self-supervised task that can provide information about the relevant image objects. On the one hand, each modality provides a complementary view of the same real world object, without a trivial reconstruction path between them. Training the reconstruction may give rise to rich representations involving the joint properties of the imaged objects. On the other hand, some modalities may be more informative about some specific anatomical contents through, e.g., the use of injected contrasts. Our idea is to use these invasive modalities as the target output for the reconstruction from a non-invasive alternative. Thus, the contrast can be seen as a pseudo-label, and the trained network can be used as a non-invasive estimator of the invasive modality.

The proposed experiments in the work herein described are focused on two ophthalmological image modalities: retinography and fluorescein angiography. These two modalities offer complementary information about the structures and pathological lesions of the retina. The angiography is an invasive technique as it requires the injection of fluorescein to the patient, limiting its use to cases with clear symptoms or patients that are already diagnosed. The contrast enhances the visualization of the retinal vasculature and makes the angiography a more suitable modality for the diagnosis and follow-up of cardiovascular diseases. In contrast, the retinography is an affordable and non-invasive modality, suitable for screening programs and regular check-ups. The self-supervised multimodal reconstruction of angiography from retinography can be used to extract relevant retinal patterns and produce a non-invasive estimation of the angiography. Experiments performed in this work focus on this self-supervised reconstruction without adding additional tasks or training data. A rough segmentation of the retinal vasculature shows, nonetheless, an important improvement due to the self-supervised training. Both qualitative and quantitative evaluations demonstrate that retinal image understanding emerges from the multimodal reconstruction.

2   Materials and Methods

2.1   Dataset Preparation

The publicly available Isfahan MISP dataset [8] is used. It contains 59 retinography/angiography pairs divided in healthy and pathological cases. The pathological images correspond to patients with diabetic retinopathy. The images have a resolution of 720×576 pixels.

Multimodal Registration. Each of the eye fundus images displays the retina in a different pose. The registration of the retinography-angiography pairs is needed for building a pixel-wise correspondence. The multimodal registration is performed following the methodology proposed in [9]. An initial registration is estimated using domain-specific landmarks that consist of bifurcations and crossovers of the vessel tree, followed by the application of a RANSAC matching algorithm. Afterwards, a refined transformation is computed using an image-domain similarity metric based on a multiscale enhancement of the vessel regions.

Multimodal ROI. Eye fundus photographies display the retina in a circular region of interest (ROI). The multimodal registration aligns the ROI contents of both images but not the ROI shapes that may no completely overlap. Thus, a multimodal ROI is computed as the intersection of the individual ROIs.

2.2   Network Architecture

For the proposed multimodal reconstruction setting, we adapted the U-Net architecture proposed in [10]. The U-Net model is a fully convolutional network that heavily relies on downsampling and upsampling operations to obtain dense predictions. The core of the model is a convolutional autoencoder with a contractive and a expansive part. In the contractive part, spatial max pooling operations

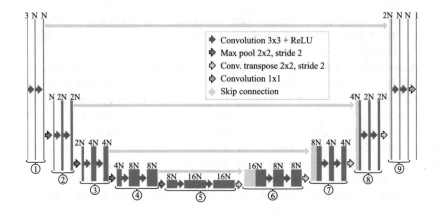

Fig. 1. U-Net architecture, where N is the number of base channels.

are interleaved between convolutional blocks, leading to an internal space with high depth and reduced width. This contraction of the space forces the model to learn high level representations. Conversely, the expansive part has upsampling operations in between convolutional blocks. The expansive decoder allows to generate the output image from the internal space representation. The convolutions are followed by ReLU activations except the last layer that is linear. As the contractive part performs spatial pooling, the precise location of the patterns in the input image is compromised. The U-Net solves this by creating skip connections between layers of the same resolution in the contractive and expansive parts. This allows to bypass the spatial information, improving structural correspondence between the input and output image spaces. Figure 1 shows the U-Net architecture that we used with the default value of $N = 64$ base channels.

Multimodal Reconstruction Loss. Three different metrics are considered for the network loss: L1 norm , L2 norm and Structural Similarity (SSIM) index [11]. L1 and L2 norms are commonly used in deep learning image generation and reconstruction applications. On the contrary, SSIM is commonly used for image quality assessment. It evaluates the structural differences between images comparing local statistics instead of measuring pointwise distances, which leads to a better correlation with the human visual perception [11]. As SSIM measures similarity, the negative SSIM is used as loss. The value of the three losses is computed over the multimodal ROI. The remaining pixels are not considered given they do not contain multimodal information.

Network Training. Network parameters are initialized using the He et al. [12] method, and the optimization is performed using the Adam algorithm [13]. The multimodal dataset was randomly divided into training and validation sets using a 4 to 1 ratio. Early stopping is performed based on the validation loss. The high number of free parameters in the model in relation to the number of samples in the dataset makes it easy for the model to overfit. To resolve this situation we use dropout, with a rate of 0.5, after the convolutional blocks 4 and 5 (see Fig. 1), as

well as data augmentation. The applied data augmentation consists of random
small elastic and affine transformations over the images. No other preprocessing
is applied.

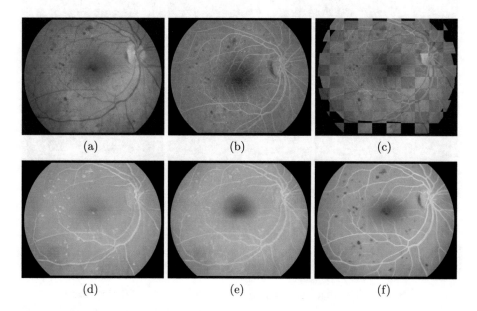

Fig. 2. Examples of generated pseudo-angiography after training with the different
losses: (a) input retinography; (b) corresponding angiography; (c) registered images;
(d), (e), (f) pseudo-angiography results with L1(d), L2(e) and SSIM(f).

3   Results and Discussion

3.1   Qualitative Evaluation

Figure 2 shows an example of a registered image pair and the generated images
with the networks using L1, L2 and SSIM losses. These images are part of the
validation set. It is observed that SSIM generates sharper images with a greater
presence of thin vessels. L1 and L2 losses offer similar visual appearances and
tend to over enhance the vessel borders.

Figure 3 shows more examples from the validation set using the SSIM loss.
Each image is accompanied by the original retinography and angiography. The
network learned different transformations for the vasculature, fovea, optic disc,
pathological structures and retinal background. This provides evidence of an
underlying understanding of important retinal patterns. The vasculature is
enhanced with respect to the retinographies and more small vessels are present.
This visual improvement is also present for vessels with poor visibility as, e.g.,
Fig. 3(b). Bright color pathologies are absent in the reconstruction, as in the
actual angiography (e.g., Fig. 3(e)). Red pathologies are reconstructed with low
intensity values, despite that they may have different appearance in classical
angiographies (Figs. 2(f) and 3(e)).

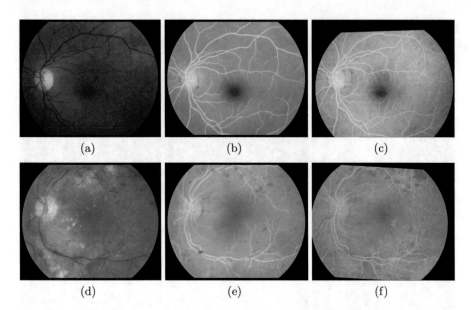

Fig. 3. Two examples of pseudo-angiography generation after training with SSIM: (a), (d) retinography; (b), (e) pseudo-angiography; (c), (f) registered angiography.

Table 1. Training loss comparison in terms of the validation loss.

Training	Validation loss		
loss	L1	L2	1−SSIM
L1	0.0914	0.0125	0.3411
L2	0.0895	0.0121	0.3310
1−SSIM	0.0856	0.0110	0.2768

3.2 Quantitative Evaluation

Table 1 shows the validation losses after training the network with L1, L2 and SSIM losses. The model trained with SSIM outperforms the others even when the comparison is based on the L1 or L2 losses, indicating that SSIM helps training the network.

In order to quantify the complexity of the transformation achieved by the self-supervised multimodal reconstruction we proposed an additional experiment. As the angiography enhances the vasculature, a rough vessel segmentation can be obtained through plain thresholding with an appropriate threshold value. This is not the case with retinography. Thus, it would be expected that a Receiver Operating Characteristic (ROC) analysis of this segmentation provides a higher Area Under Curve (AUC) for the angiography than for the retinography. We apply this ROC analysis comparison to both the retinography and the estimated pseudo-angiography. This evaluation is performed using the DRIVE image database [14], which consists of 40 retinographies of size 565×584 including

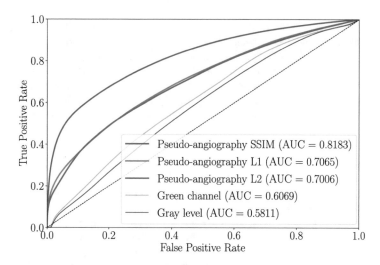

Fig. 4. ROC curves of the quantitative evaluation.

ground truth vasculature segmentations. As the evaluated models are trained in a self-supervised way in the Isfahan dataset, the whole DRIVE dataset is used as test set for this analysis. Figure 4 shows the ROC curves for retinography and pseudo-angiography. Both green channel and grayscale image are compared for retinography, as they are common choices for vessel segmentation. Pseudo-angiography curves correspond to the models trained with L1, L2 and SSIM losses. These results show that the pseudo-angiography provides additional information about the vessel structures and the network is not providing a trivial solution. Thus, the model has learned to recognize relevant patterns in the retina.

4   Conclusions

Motivated by the scarcity of annotated medical imaging datasets and the common availability of multiple imaging modalities, in this work we proposed the use of self-supervised multimodal reconstruction as a more informative alternative to self-supervised reconstruction of the input images. Experiments were performed on retinal angiography reconstruction from aligned retinographies, giving rise to a pseudo-angiography estimator that enhances the vascular structures of the retina. Quantitative and qualitative results indicate that the obtained transformation provides additional understanding of the relevant retinal patterns, noting that it is not a mere intensity mapping. Apart from the potential applications of the self-supervised task on multitask and transfer learning, the generated pseudo-angiography may have important clinical applications as it simulates the angiography enhancement without the need of the invasive contrast injection.

Acknowledgments. This work is supported by I.S. Carlos III, Government of Spain, and the ERDF of the EU through the DTS15/00153 research project, and by the MINECO, Government of Spain, through the DPI2015-69948-R research project. The authors of this work also receive financial support from the ERDF and ESF of the EU, and the Xunta de Galicia through Centro Singular de Investigación de Galicia, accreditation 2016–2019, ref. ED431G/01 and Grupo de Referencia Competitiva, ref. ED431C 2016-047 research projects, and the predoctoral grant contract ref. ED481A-2017/328.

References

1. Shen, D., Wu, G., Suk, H.I.: Deep learning in medical image analysis. Annu. Rev. Biomed. Eng. **19**, 221–248 (2017)
2. Karri, S.P.K., Chakraborty, D., Chatterjee, J.: Transfer learning based classification of optical coherence tomography images with diabetic macular edema and dry age-related macular degeneration. Biomed. Opt. Express **8**(2), 579–592 (2017)
3. Shin, H., Orton, M.R., Collins, D.J., Doran, S.J., Leach, M.O.: Stacked autoencoders for unsupervised feature learning and multiple organ detection in a pilot study using 4D patient data. IEEE Trans. PAMI **35**(8), 1930–1943 (2013)
4. Rasmus, A., Berglund, M., Honkala, M., Valpola, H., Raiko, T.: Semi-supervised learning with ladder networks. Adv. Neural Inf. Process. Syst. **28**, 3546–3554 (2015)
5. Ruder, S.: An overview of multi-task learning in deep neural networks. CoRR abs/1706.05098 (2017)
6. Tan, J.H., Acharya, U.R., Bhandary, S.V., Chua, K.C., Sivaprasad, S.: Segmentation of optic disc, fovea and retinal vasculature using a single convolutional neural network. J. Comput. Sci. **20**, 70–79 (2017)
7. Costa, P., Galdran, A., Meyer, M.I., Niemeijer, M., Abràmoff, M., Mendonça, A.M., Campilho, A.: End-to-end adversarial retinal image synthesis. IEEE Trans. Med. Imaging **37**(3), 781–791 (2018)
8. Alipour, S.H.M., Rabbani, H., Akhlaghi, M.R.: Diabetic retinopathy grading by digital curvelet transform. Comput. Math. Methods Med. (2012)
9. Hervella, A.S., Rouco, J., Novo, J., Ortega, M.: Multimodal registration of retinal images using domain-specific landmarks and vessel enhancement. In: International Conference on Knowledge-Based and Intelligent Information and Engineering Systems (KES) (2018)
10. Ronneberger, O., Fischer, P., Brox, T.: U-Net: convolutional networks for biomedical image segmentation. In: Navab, N., Hornegger, J., Wells, W.M., Frangi, A.F. (eds.) MICCAI 2015. LNCS, vol. 9351, pp. 234–241. Springer, Cham (2015). https://doi.org/10.1007/978-3-319-24574-4_28
11. Wang, Z., Bovik, A.C., Sheikh, H.R., Simoncelli, E.P.: Image quality assessment: from error visibility to structural similarity. IEEE Trans. Image Proc. **13**(4), 600–612 (2004)
12. He, K., Zhang, X., Ren, S., Sun, J.: Delving deep into rectifiers: Surpassing human-level performance on imagenet classification. In: IEEE International Conference on Computer Vision (ICCV), pp. 1026–1034, December 2015
13. Kingma, D.P., Ba, J.: Adam: A method for stochastic optimization. In: International Conference on Learning Representations (ICLR), May 2015
14. Staal, J., Abramoff, M., Niemeijer, M., Viergever, M., van Ginneken, B.: Ridge based vessel segmentation in color images of the retina. IEEE Trans. Med. Imaging **23**(4), 501–509 (2004)

Locality Adaptive Multi-modality GANs for High-Quality PET Image Synthesis

Yan Wang[1], Luping Zhou[2(✉)], Lei Wang[3], Biting Yu[3], Chen Zu[3],
David S. Lalush[4], Weili Lin[5], Xi Wu[6], Jiliu Zhou[1,6],
and Dinggang Shen[5(✉)]

[1] School of Computer Science, Sichuan University, Chengdu, China
[2] School of Electrical and Information Engineering,
University of Sydney, Sydney, Australia
luping.zhou.jane@googlemail.com
[3] School of Computing and Information Technology,
University of Wollongong, Wollongong, Australia
[4] Joint Department of Biomedical Engineering, University of North Carolina
at Chapel Hill and North Carolina State University, Raleigh, NC, USA
[5] Department of Radiology and BRIC, University of North Carolina
at Chapel Hill, Chapel Hill, USA
dgshen@med.unc.edu
[6] School of Computer Science,
Chengdu University of Information Technology, Chengdu, China

Abstract. Positron emission topography (PET) has been substantially used in recent years. To minimize the potential health risks caused by the tracer radiation inherent to PET scans, it is of great interest to synthesize the high-quality full-dose PET image from the low-dose one to reduce the radiation exposure while maintaining the image quality. In this paper, we propose a locality adaptive multi-modality generative adversarial networks model (LA-GANs) to synthesize the full-dose PET image from both the low-dose one and the accompanying T1-weighted MRI to incorporate anatomical information for better PET image synthesis. This paper has the following contributions. First, we propose a new mechanism to fuse multi-modality information in deep neural networks. Different from the traditional methods that treat each image modality as an input channel and apply the same kernel to convolute the whole image, we argue that the contributions of different modalities could vary at different image locations, and therefore a unified kernel for a whole image is not appropriate. To address this issue, we propose a method that is locality adaptive for multi-modality fusion. Second, to learn this locality adaptive fusion, we utilize $1 \times 1 \times 1$ kernel so that the number of additional parameters incurred by our method is kept minimum. This also naturally produces a fused image which acts as a pseudo input for the subsequent learning stages. Third, the proposed locality adaptive fusion mechanism is learned jointly with the PET image synthesis in an end-to-end trained 3D conditional GANs model developed by us. Our 3D GANs model generates high quality PET images by employing large-sized image patches and hierarchical features. Experimental results show that our method

The original version of this chapter was revised: an Acknowledgements section has been added. The correction to this chapter is available at https://doi.org/10.1007/978-3-030-00928-1_100

outperforms the traditional multi-modality fusion methods used in deep networks, as well as the state-of-the-art PET estimation approaches.

1 Introduction

As a nuclear imaging technology, positron emission topography (PET) has been increasingly used in clinics for disease diagnosis and intervention. It enables the visualization of metabolic processes of human body by detecting pairs of gamma rays emitted indirectly from the radioactive tracer injected into the human body. However, the radioactive exposure inevitably raises concerns for potential health hazards. Nevertheless, lowering the tracer dose will introduce noises and artifacts, thus degrading the PET image quality to a certain extent. Therefore, it is of great interest to synthesize the high-quality full-dose PET (F-PET) image from the low-dose PET (L-PET) image to reduce the radiation exposure while maintaining the image quality. Modern PET scans are usually accompanied by other modalities, such as computed tomography (CT) and magnetic resonance imaging (MRI). By combining functional and morphologic information, PET/MRI system could increase diagnostic accuracy for various malignancies. Previous research also indicates the benefit brought by multi-modality data to PET image quality enhancement [1–3].

There have been some works for F-PET image synthesis. Most of them, however, are based on voxel-wise estimation methods, e.g., random forest regression method [1], mapping-based sparse representation method [2], semi-supervised tripled dictionary learning method [4], and multi-level canonical correlation analysis (CCA) framework [5]. These methods are all based on small patches and the final estimation of each voxel is determined by averaging the overlapped patches, resulting in over-smoothed images that lack the texture of a typical F-PET image.

In recent years, deep learning has been used to improve image synthesis. Dong et al. [6] proposed a convolutional neural networks (CNNs) model for image super-resolution. With the similar architecture, Li et al. [7] estimated the missing PET image from MRI for the same subject. More recently, generative adversarial networks (GANs) have also showed their superior performance in many image synthesis tasks [8]. In the literature, the incorporation of multi-modality data in deep learning models is usually conducted in a global manner. For example, in CNN-based deep learning models such as two recent multi-channel GANs models [9], multi-modalities are treated as multiple input channels, and for each channel a unified kernel (invariant to image locations) is applied for the convolution over the whole image. Such a kind of multi-modality fusion is referred to as the multi-channel method in this paper. However, we argue that *the contributions of different modalities could vary at different image locations, and therefore a unified kernel for a whole image is not appropriate*.

In this paper, inspired by the appealing success of GANs and also motivated to tackle the limitation of the current multi-channel deep architectures, we propose a "locality adaptive" multi-modality GANs (LA-GANs) model to synthesize the F-PET image from both the L-PET and the accompanying T1-weighted MRI images. The contributions of our method are as follows. (1) We propose a new mechanism to fuse multi-modality information in deep neural networks. The weight of each imaging modality varies with image locations to better serve the synthesis of F-PET. (2) Using multi-modality (especially making it locality adaptive) may induce many additional parameters to learn. We therefore propose to utilize $1 \times 1 \times 1$ kernel to learn such locality adaptive fusion mechanism to minimize the increase on the number of parameters. Doing so also naturally leads to a fused image that acts as a pseudo input for the subsequent learning stages. (3) We develop a 3D conditional GANs model for PET image synthesis, and jointly learn the proposed locality adaptive fusion with the synthesis process in an end-to-end trained manner. Our 3D GANs model generates high quality PET images by employing large-sized image patches and hierarchical features.

2 Methodology

The proposed LA-GANs model is illustrated in Fig. 1, which consists of three parts: (1) the locality adaptive fusion network, (2) the generator network, and (3) the discriminator network. Concretely, the locality adaptive fusion network takes both an L-PET and a T1-MRI as input and generates a fused image by learning different convolutional kernels at different image locations. After that, the generator network produces a synthesized F-PET from the fused image, and the discriminator network subsequently takes a pair of images as input, i.e., the L-PET and the real or synthetic F-PET, and aims to distinguish between the real and synthetic pairs. When the discriminator can easily distinguish between them, it means that the synthesized F-PET has not well resembled the real one, and that the fusion network and the generator network should be further improved to produce more realistic synthesis. Otherwise, the discriminator should be enhanced instead. Therefore, the three networks are trained jointly with the discriminator network trying to correctly distinguish between the real and synthetic F-PET, while the fusion and generator networks trying to produce realistic images that can fool the discriminator. Please note that, we use 3D operations for all the networks to better model the 3D spatial information.

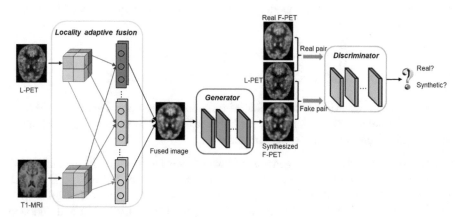

Fig. 1. Overview of the proposed pipeline for full-dose PET (F-PET) synthesis from low-dose counterpart (L-PET) and the accompanying T1-MRI image.

2.1 Architecture

Locality Adaptive Fusion Network: This is a module for multi-modality information fusion. As mentioned before, in most multi-channel based networks, image convolution is performed in a global manner, i.e., for each modality the same filter is applied to all image locations to generate the feature maps that will be combined in higher layers. This could not effectively handle the location-varying contributions from different imaging modalities. To tackle this problem, locality adaptive convolution should be enforced. However, if the locality adaptive convolution is simply conducted in the multi-channel framework, many additional parameters will have to be learned due to adding new imaging modalities. This is not favorable for medical applications where the number of the training samples is often limited. Therefore, we propose to add a module that produces a fused image from multi-modality images and use the fused image as the pseudo input to the generator network. In this way, the increase of the number of modalities will not cause any increase on the number of parameters in the generator. Moreover, we propose to utilize $1 \times 1 \times 1$ kernel for locality adaptive convolution to minimize the number of necessary parameters to learn in this fusion module. The fusion network will be jointly learned with the generator and the discriminator to ensure that they can effectively negotiate with each other to achieve the best possible performance on image synthesis. Specifically, the entire L-PET and T1-MRI images are partitioned, respectively, into N non-overlapping small patches, i.e., P_i^L and $P_i^{T1} (i = 1, \ldots, N)$, as indicated by the patches in different colors in Fig. 1. Then, the two patches at the same location (indicated by using the same color) from the two modalities, i.e., P_i^L and P_i^{T1}, are convolved, respectively, using two different $1 \times 1 \times 1$ filters with parameters w_i^L and w_i^{T1}. For instance, in the fusion block in Fig. 1, the two gray filters are respectively operated on the two gray patches of the L-PET and T1-MRI images to generate their corresponding combined patch. Formally, the combined patch P_i^C is obtained as follows:

$$P_i^C = w_i^L * P_i^L + w_i^{T1} * P_i^{T1},$$
$$\text{s.t.} \, w_i^L + w_i^{T1} = 1; w_i^L > 0; w_i^{T1} > 0, i = 1, \ldots, N \tag{1}$$

In this way, we will learn N pairs of different convolution kernels for N local patches. The outputs of the fusion are further assembled to form an entire fused image as the input of the following generator network.

Generator Network: In our generator network, we adopt both the convolutional layers and de-convolutional layers to ensure the same size of the input and output. Since the L-PET and F-PET images belong to the same modality, there is a lot of low-level information shared between them. As such, we follow the U-Net and add skip connections between the convolutional and de-convolutional layers, thus combining hierarchical features for better synthesis. Also, the skip connection strategy mitigates the vanishing gradient issue, allowing the network architecture to be much deeper.

Our network architecture (more details in the supplementary) contains multiple Convolution-BatchNormalization-LeakyRelu components. Specifically, it constitutes

12 3D convolutional layers. In the encoder part which includes the first 6 convolutional layers, we use $4 \times 4 \times 4$ filters and a stride of 2 for convolution, and 0.2 negative slope for the leaky ReLu. The number of feature maps increases from 64 in the 1st layer to 512 in the 6th layer. In the decoder part, we perform up-sampling with a factor of 2.

Discriminator Network: The discriminator network is a typical CNN architecture consisting of 4 convolutional layers, and each of them uses $4 \times 4 \times 4$ filters with a stride of 2, similar to the encoder structure of the generator. The first convolution layer produces 64 feature maps, and this number is doubled at each of the following convolutional layers. On top of the convolutional layers, a fully connected layer is applied and followed by a sigmoid activation to determine whether the input is the real pair or the synthetic one.

2.2 Objective Functions

Let us denote x_L an L-PET image, x_{T1} the accompanying T1-MRI image, and y_F the corresponding real F-PET image (i.e., the ground truth annotation). In this study, we learn three function mappings. The first mapping $F_\alpha : (x_L \in \mathbb{R}_{Low}, x_{T1} \in \mathbb{R}_{T1-MRI}) \rightarrow \bar{y}_F \in \mathbb{R}_{Fused}$ is for the locality adaptive fusion network, which produces a fused image $\bar{y}_F$ from x_L and x_{T1}. The second mapping $G_\beta : \bar{y}_F \in \mathbb{R}_{Fused} \rightarrow \bar{\bar{y}}_F \in \mathbb{R}_{Synthetic}$ is for the generator network, which maps the fused image $\bar{y}_F$ to a synthetic F-PET image $\bar{\bar{y}}_F$. The third mapping corresponds to the discriminator network function $D_\gamma : (x_L \in \mathbb{R}_{Low}, x_{T1} \in \mathbb{R}_{T1-MRI}, Y_F \in \mathbb{R}_{Full}) \rightarrow d \in [0,1]$, whose task is to distinguish the synthetic pair $Y_F := (x_L, \bar{\bar{y}}_F)$ (ideally $d \rightarrow 0$) from the real pair $Y_F := (x_L, y_F)$ (ideally $d \rightarrow 1$). The symbols α, β and γ denote the parameter sets of the three networks, respectively, and are automatically learned from a training set $\{(x_L^i, x_{T1}^i, y_F^i)\}_{i=1}^m$. Formally, we solve the following optimization problem

$$\min_\alpha \min_\beta \max_\gamma V(F_\alpha, G_\beta, D_\gamma) =$$
$$\mathbb{E}[\log D_\gamma(x_L, y_F)] + \mathbb{E}[\log(1 - D_\gamma(x_L, G_\beta(F_\alpha(x_L, x_{T1}))))] + \lambda V_{L1}(F_\alpha, G_\beta), \tag{2}$$

with $\lambda > 0$ being a trade-off constant. The last term is an L1 loss, used to ensure that the synthetic F-PET image stays close to its real counterpart. The L1 loss is defined as

$$V_{L1}(F_\alpha, G_\beta) = \mathbb{E}\left[\left\|y_F - G_\beta(F_\alpha(x_L, x_{T1}))\right\|_1\right]. \tag{3}$$

Please note that, the fusion network F and the generator network G, in a sense, can be regarded as a whole network whose goal is to synthesize realistic-looking F-PET images that can fool the discriminator network D. Following the approximation scheme in [10], the term $\log(1 - D_\gamma(x_L, G_\beta(F_\alpha(x_L, x_{T1}))))$ can be replaced by minimizing a simpler form $-\log D_\gamma(x_L, G_\beta(F_\alpha(x_L, x_{T1})))$. Therefore, training the fusion network F and generator network G equals minimizing

$$L_{\mathcal{F},\mathcal{G}}(F_\alpha, G_\beta) = -\sum_i \log D_\gamma(x_L^i, G_\beta(F_\alpha(x_L^i, x_{T1}^i))) + \lambda \sum_i \left(\left\| y_F - G_\beta(F_\alpha(x_L^i, x_{T1}^i)) \right\|_1 \right). \quad (4)$$

On the other hand, the discriminator network D tries to tell the real pair (x_L, y_F) from the synthetic pair $(x_L, \bar{\bar{y}}_F)$ by maximizing Eq. (2). Therefore, training the discriminator network corresponds to maximizing

$$L_D(D_\gamma) = \sum_i \left(\left[\log D_\gamma(x_L^i, y_F^i) \right] + \log\left(1 - D_\gamma(x_L^i, G_\beta(F_\alpha(x_L^i, x_{T1}^i)))\right) \right). \quad (5)$$

2.3   Training LA-GANs

The fusion network F together with the generator network G and the discriminator network D are trained in an alternating manner as [10]. Specifically, we first fix F and G to train D, and then fix D to train F and G. As shown in Eq. (2), the training of F, G and D is just like playing a min-max game: F and G try to minimize the loss function while D tries to maximize it, until an equilibrium is reached. In the test stage, only the fusion and generator networks are needed for synthesis. All networks are trained by Adam solver with mini-batch stochastic gradient descent (SGD) and the mini-batch size is 128. The training process runs for 200 epochs, and the learning rate is set to 0.0002 for the first 100 epochs, and then linearly decays to 0 in the second 100 epochs.

3   Experiments and Results

We validate our proposed method on a real human brain dataset consisting of 8 normal control (NC) subjects and 8 mild cognitive impairment (MCI) subjects, each with an L-PET image, a T1-MRI image and an F-PET image. Subjects were administered an average of 203 MBq of $[^{18}F]$FDG. The PET scans were acquired by a Siemens Biograph mMR PET-MR scanner. For each subject, the PET images are aligned to its T1-MRI to build the voxel-level correspondence via affine transformation. Each aligned image has the resolution of $2.09 \times 2.09 \times 2.03$ mm^3 and the image size of $128 \times 128 \times 128$. Considering the small number of the training samples, we extract 125 large 3D image patches of size $64 \times 64 \times 64$ from each image, rather than directly using the entire 3D image, to train the deep model. In addition, to make full use of available samples, we follow the widely used "Leave-One-Subject-Out" strategy. To train the proposed locality adaptive convolution network, we further partition each large image patch into 4096 non-overlapping $4 \times 4 \times 4$ regions for fusion. Our method is implemented by PyTorch, and all the experiments are carried out on an NVIDIA GeForce GTX 1080 Ti with 11 GB memory.

Comparison with the State-of-the-Art PET Estimation Methods: We compare our method with the following state-of-the-art multi-modality based PET estimation methods: (1) mapping based sparse representation method (m-SR) [2], (2) tripled dictionary learning method (t-DL) [4], (3) multi-level CCA method (m-CCA) [5], and (4) auto-context CNN method [3]. The averaged PSNR are given in Fig. 2(a), from where we can see that our proposed method outperforms all the other competing methods, demonstrating its effectiveness and advantages. In Fig. 2(b), we show an example visual result of our method compared with two methods (m-CCA and auto-context CNN) which produce the top two results in the literature. As observed, the estimated images by the m-CCA method are over-smoothed compared with the real F-PET images due to the averaging of the overlapping patches to construct the final output images. Compared with the auto-context CNN network, our model tends to better preserve the detailed information in the estimated F-PET images, as indicated by the red arrows. We argue that this is because the adversarial training network used in our model constrains the synthesized images to be similar to the real ones.

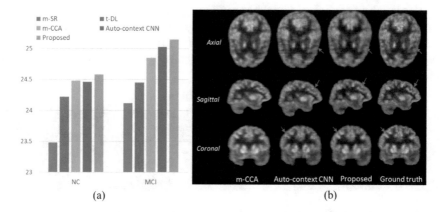

Fig. 2. Comparison with the state-of-the-art PET estimation methods.

Comparison with our method using single-modality or multi-channel strategy: To study the contribution of the anatomical information from MRI for PET synthesis and evaluate the effectiveness of the locality adaptive fusion network of our proposed model, we further conduct experiments to compare our method with its two variants: one using only single modality of L-PET [11], and the other using the common multi-channel strategy [9] for multi-modality. The results are reported in Table 1. First, we can see that our method obtains higher PSNR than the single-modality L-PET variant (p-value in paired t-test: 0.0092 for NC and 0.0036 for MCI), indicating that the anatomical information from MRI yields important cues for PET synthesis. Second, compared with the multi-channel variant, our method boosts the averaged PSNR approximately 0.28 and 0.2 for NC and MCI groups, respectively. The standard deviation of our method is also smaller than that of the multi-channel GANs while the median is higher. Also, the paired t-test indicates that our improvement from the multi-channel one is statistically significant ($p < 0.05$). Moreover, it is found that the number of increased learning parameters induced by adding T1-MRI is 4096 for our method and 8192 for the multi-channel GANs, suggesting that our model produces better performance with less parameters to learn.

Table 1. Quantitative comparison with two variants of our method (single-modality GANs and multi-channel GANs) in terms of PSNR. Here, Med. means median.

Method	NC subjects			MCI subjects		
	Mean (std.)	Med.	p-value	Mean (std.)	Med.	p-value
L-PET	19.88 (2.34)	20.68	7.7E–05	21.33 (2.53)	21.62	2.3E–04
Single-modality	23.94 (2.04)	24.78	0.0092	24.37 (1.95)	24.85	0.0036
Multi-channel	24.31 (1.91)	24.59	0.0391	24.95 (2.01)	25.30	0.0071
Proposed	**24.58 (1.78)**	**25.21**	–	**25.15 (1.97)**	**25.49**	–

We also provide a visual comparison in Fig. 3, where the two leftmost images are the input T1-MRI and L-PET images and the rightmost image is the ground-truth F-PET. We can clearly see that the synthesized F-PET image of our proposed model has less artifacts than those of the single-modality method and the multi-channel method, as indicated by the red arrows.

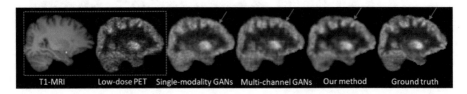

Fig. 3. Visual comparison with single-modality and multi-channel GANs methods.

4   Conclusion

In this work, we proposed a 3D locality adaptive multi-modality GANs model for synthesizing high-quality PET images from the L-PET and T1-MRI images. Both qualitative and quantitative results demonstrate that our method significantly outperforms the traditional multi-modality fusion methods used in deep networks, as well as the state-of-the-art PET estimation approaches. Our model could also be applied to other related applications such as mapping one or two modalities to another modality. In the future, we will investigate the potential of our model for general synthesis tasks as well.

Acknowledgement. This work was supported in part by NIH grant EB006733.

References

1. Kang, J., Gao, Y., Shi, F., et al.: Prediction of standard-dose brain PET image by using MRI and low-dose brain [18F] FDG PET images. Med. Phys. **42**(9), 5301–5309 (2015)

2. Wang, Y., Zhang, P., An, L., et al.: Predicting standard-dose PET image from low-dose PET and multimodal MR images using mapping-based sparse representation. Phys. Med. Biol. **61** (2), 791–812 (2016)
3. Xiang, L., Qiao, Y., Nie, D., et al.: Deep auto-context convolutional neural networks for standard-dose PET image estimation from low-dose PET/MRI. Neurocomputing **267**, 406–416 (2017)
4. Wang, Y., Ma, G., An, L., et al.: Semi-supervised tripled dictionary learning for standard-dose PET image prediction using low-dose PET and multimodal MRI. IEEE Trans. Biomed. Eng. **64**(3), 569–579 (2017)
5. An, L., Zhang, P., Adeli, E., et al.: Multi-level canonical correlation analysis for PET image estimation. IEEE Trans. Image Process. **25**(7), 3303–3315 (2016)
6. Dong, C., Loy, C.C., He, K., Tang, X.: Image super-resolution using deep convolutional networks. IEEE Trans. Pattern Anal. Mach. Intell. **38**(2), 295–307 (2016)
7. Li, R., Zhang, W., Suk, H.-I., Wang, L., Li, J., Shen, D., Ji, S.: Deep learning based imaging data completion for improved brain disease diagnosis. In: Golland, Polina, Hata, Nobuhiko, Barillot, Christian, Hornegger, Joachim, Howe, Robert (eds.) MICCAI 2014. LNCS, vol. 8675, pp. 305–312. Springer, Cham (2014). https://doi.org/10.1007/978-3-319-10443-0_39
8. Zhang, H., Xu, T., Li, H., Zhang, S., Huang, X., Wang, X., Metaxas, D.: StackGAN: text to photo-realistic image synthesis with stacked generative adversarial networks. In: IEEE International Conference on Computer Vision (ICCV), pp. 5907–5915 (2017)
9. Bi, L., Kim, J., Kumar, A., Feng, D., Fulham, M.: Synthesis of positron emission tomography (PET) images via multi-channel generative adversarial networks (GANs). In: Cardoso, M.J., Arbel, T., Gao, F., Kainz, B., van Walsum, T., Shi, K., Bhatia, K.K., Peter, R., Vercauteren, T., Reyes, M., Dalca, A., Wiest, R., Niessen, W., Emmer, B.J. (eds.) CMMI/SWITCH/RAMBO -2017. LNCS, vol. 10555, pp. 43–51. Springer, Cham (2017). https://doi.org/10.1007/978-3-319-67564-0_5
10. Goodfellow, I., Pouget-Abadie, J., Mirza, M.: Generative adversarial nets. In: Advances in Neural Information Processing Systems, pp. 2672–2680 (2014)
11. Wang, Y., Yu, B., Wang, L., Zu, C., Lalush, D., Lin, W., Wu, X., Zhou, J., Shen, D., Zhou, L.: 3D conditional generative adversarial networks for high-quality PET image estimation at low dose. Neuroimage **174**, 550–562 (2018)

Joint PET+MRI Patch-Based Dictionary for Bayesian Random Field PET Reconstruction

Viswanath P. Sudarshan[1,2,3(✉)], Zhaolin Chen[3,4], and Suyash P. Awate[1]

[1] Computer Science and Engineering Department, Indian Institute of Technology
(IIT) Bombay, Mumbai, India
psvish@cse.iitb.ac.in
[2] IITB-Monash Research Academy, Indian Institute of Technology (IIT) Bombay,
Mumbai, India
[3] Department of Electrical and Computer Systems Engineering, Monash University,
Melbourne, Australia
[4] Monash Biomedical Imaging, Monash University, Melbourne, Australia

Abstract. Multimodal imaging combining positron emission tomography (PET) and magnetic resonance imaging (MRI) provides complementary information about metabolism and anatomy. While the appearances of MRI and PET images are distinctive, there are fundamental inter-image dependencies relating structure and function. In PET-MRI imaging, typical PET reconstruction methods use priors to enforce PET-MRI dependencies at the very fine scale of image gradients and, so, cannot capture larger-scale inter-image correlations and intra-image texture patterns. Some recent methods enforce statistical models of MRI-image patches on PET-image patches, risking infusing anatomical features into PET images. In contrast, we propose a novel *patch-based joint dictionary model* for PET and MRI, learning regularity in individual patches and correlations in spatially-corresponding patches, for *Bayesian* PET reconstruction using expectation maximization. Reconstructions on simulated and *in vivo* PET-MRI data show that our method gives better-regularized images with smaller errors, compared to the state of the art.

Keywords: PET-MRI · Reconstruction · Joint generative model
Joint dictionary model · Patches · Sparsity
Bayesian Markov random field · EM

1 Introduction and Related Work

Multimodal imaging systems [14,19] incorporating positron emission tomography (PET) and magnetic resonance imaging (MRI) acquire both functional and anatomical information to improve clinical diagnosis, therapy, and scientific studies in the human body (e.g., neurology and oncology). PET and MRI images

S. P. Awate—We thank IIT Bombay Seed Grant 14IRCCSG010, Reignwood Cultural Foundation and Australian Research Council Linkage grant LP170100494.

© Springer Nature Switzerland AG 2018
A. F. Frangi et al. (Eds.): MICCAI 2018, LNCS 11070, pp. 338–346, 2018.
https://doi.org/10.1007/978-3-030-00928-1_39

have *distinctive appearances*. The intrinsic spatial resolution of radioactivity in PET, typically 4–6 mm [1], is far lower than the anatomical resolution in MRI, typically 1–1.5 mm. Spatial resolution in PET is limited by positron range, non-collinearity of the annihilation photons, scatter inside the scintillation crystals, finite crystal dimension, interaction depth, etc. In PET-MRI, PET reconstruction is challenged by the stochasticity in gamma-ray emission and the reliability of attenuation-map estimation without the computed tomography (CT) images; thus, it typically relies on *statistical prior* models on the MRI and PET images.

After expectation maximization (EM) based maximum-likelihood (ML) estimation for PET reconstruction [15], edge-preserving smoothness priors and other gradient based penalties within the EM framework were exploited [7]. The method in [4] relies on hierarchical image segmentation, while that in [11] uses voxel-reweighted fidelity based on Fisher information. Some methods use *edge* information in the associated *anatomical* image through edge locations [5,6,8,9] or mutual information of voxel intensities [16]. However, all these priors [5–9,11,16] use *very local neighborhoods* to enforce piecewise-smooth images and cannot capture larger-scale inter-image (structure-function) correlations and intra-image texture patterns in PET images or associated MRI images. In contrast, we propose a framework to model *regularity within* and *statistical dependencies across* spatially-corresponding *patches* in PET and MRI.

For dynamic PET, recent methods [12,13] use hidden Markov random field (MRF) label priors with a Gaussian mixture model for intensities. Some methods [20] use spatially-varying smoothing using kernel similarity on time curves and others [10] use a Bowsher prior to capture edge information from the anatomical image. However, these methods [10,12,13,20] do *not* capture spatial dependencies across PET and MRI. So, we propose a *joint patch-based dictionary* as a *MRF prior* on the PET-MRI image pair for Bayesian PET reconstruction. Early works on patch-based (multimodal) medical image denoising are in [2,3].

Very recent works [17,18] on PET reconstruction use a patch dictionary learned from MRI images, but this strategy risks over/underfitting the functional features of PET images by the anatomical features of MRI. In contrast, we propose a *joint generative model*, based on joint patch regularity, for the pair of PET and MRI images and leverage the joint model to reconstruct PET images. Our model subsumes learning PET image patch statistics by jointly learning statistics of PET image patches and spatially-corresponding MRI patches.

We propose a novel *joint generative model* for the pair of images of PET radiotracer activity and MRI magnitude. We rely on a *joint patch-based sparse dictionary* model formulated as a *MRF prior* for Bayesian PET reconstruction using EM. While our model learns the fine-scale and larger-scale regularity in patches in PET and MRI images individually, it also learns correlations between spatially-corresponding patches in MRI and PET images. Reconstructions on simulated and *in vivo* PET-MRI show that our method produces (i) qualitatively better regularity and (ii) quantitatively lower errors and higher structural similarity (SSIM), over the state of the art.

2   Methods

We describe our novel generative model on joint PET-MRI, relying on a sparse joint-dictionary model, and our Bayesian PET image reconstruction using EM.

2.1   Generative Model for PET-MRI Using a Joint Sparse Dictionary

We propose a joint MRF-based sparse dictionary model for the pair of MRI magnitude and PET activity images. Let X model the MRI image and Y model the PET activity image, in a common spatial coordinate frame. Let (X, Y) be a MRF with a neighborhood system $\mathcal{N} := \{\mathcal{N}_i\}_{i=1}^I$, where $\mathcal{N}_i$ is the neighbors of voxel i. For any voxel i in the MRI or PET images, its neighbors include all other voxels in the MRI image within a distance d_X and all other voxels in the PET image within a distance d_Y. This paper sets $d_X := 4$ mm, $d_Y := 8$ mm. This neighborhood system allows us to model the MRF's Gibbs energy in terms of square-shaped cliques (patches) $\mathcal{P}_i$ of width 5 mm ($d_X + 1$) in the MRI image and patches $\mathcal{Q}_i$ of width 9 mm ($d_Y + 1$) in the PET image. We model the PET-MRI joint patch ($X_{\mathcal{P}_i}, Y_{\mathcal{Q}_i}$), at each voxel i, as a sparse linear combination of template patches in the joint dictionary A with J atoms, where the j-th atom comprises a MRI template patch A_j^X paired with a PET template patch A_j^Y. Because the PET and MRI images are non-negative, we model the components of atoms A_j^X, A_j^Y as non-negative and we enforce non-negativity on the coefficients in the dictionary fit. The prior $P(X, Y | A) := \eta \exp(-G(X, Y, A))$, where the Gibbs energy $G(X, Y, A) := \sum_{i=1}^I \min_{c_i \succeq 0} \beta \|X_{\mathcal{P}_i} - A^X c_i\|_2^2 + (1 - \beta)\|Y_{\mathcal{Q}_i} - A^Y c_i\|_2^2 + \lambda\|c_i\|_1$, c_i is the common coefficient vector used for fitting patches in both MRI and PET images at voxel i, $c_i \succeq 0$ constraints each coefficient within c_i to be non-negative, and η is the normalizing constant. Free parameter $\beta \in [0, 1]$ balances the quality of fit in the MRI and PET images, adapted to their relative noise levels. Free parameter $\lambda \in \mathbb{R}^+$ controls the sparsity of the dictionary coefficients. We tune free parameters β, λ using cross validation.

Learning a Joint PET-MRI Dictionary. We learn the joint dictionary A, comprising atom pairs $\{(A_j^X, A_j^Y)\}_{j=1}^J$, from a training set of T high-quality PET-MRI images $\{(\mathring{X}^t, \mathring{Y}^t)\}_{t=1}^T$, as the maximum-a-priori estimate $\arg\max_A \prod_{t=1}^T P(\mathring{X}^t, \mathring{Y}^t | A)$ subject to scale constraints on the atoms $\|A_j^X\|_2^2 + \|A_j^Y\|_2^2 \leq 1, \forall j$, positivity constraints on the atoms $A_j^X \succeq 0, A_j^Y \succeq 0, \forall j$, and positivity constraints on the coefficients $c_i \succeq 0$. Our design of the dictionary learning (and coding) formulation leads to *smooth convex* problems for optimizing (i) A given c and (ii) c given A; both involve quadratic objective functions and convex constraint sets. We solve by iterative alternating optimization of A and c, where each update uses projected gradient descent with an adaptive step size to ensure improvement in the objective function value. We initialize atoms through (i) k-means++ on the subset of joint patches ($\mathring{X}_{\mathcal{P}_i}, \mathring{Y}_{\mathcal{P}_i}$) with variance significantly higher than the noise variance, excluding constant patches, and

(ii) adding two constant atoms each modeling patches in MRI or PET that are constant or have the minimum intensity as positive.

2.2   MAP Reconstruction of PET with Joint-Dictionary Prior, EM

Likelihood Model for PET. Given Y_i as the rate of gamma-ray emission counts at each voxel i, let $\alpha_{i,d}$ be the emission fraction reaching detector d in a ring of D detectors. We model $\alpha_{i,d}$ as voxel strip integrals, as in STIR (github.com/UCL/STIR). At detector d, let the emission rate coming from voxel i be $Y_{i,d} := Y_i \alpha_{i,d}$ and let the total emission rate be $\sum_{i=1}^{I} Y_{i,d}$. Let the observed emission at detector d be $Z_d \sim \text{Poisson}(\sum_{i=1}^{I} Y_{i,d})$. Equivalently, let the part of the observed emission at detector d coming from voxel i be $Z_{i,d} \sim \text{Poisson}(Y_{i,d})$. Then, the likelihood $P(Z|Y) := \prod_{d=1}^{D} P(Z_d | \sum_{i=1}^{I} Y_{i,d}) = \prod_{d=1}^{D} \prod_{i=1}^{I} P(Z_{i,d}|Y_{i,d})$.

Given the observed PET data $\{z_d\}_{d=1}^{D}$, the observed MRI image X, and the joint dictionary A, our reconstructed PET activity image Y is the MAP estimate: $\arg\max_Y P(Y|z, x, A) = \arg\max_Y P(z|Y)P(Y, x|A)$.

EM for PET Image Reconstruction. We propose to solve the MAP estimation problem for parameter Y, given observations $\{z_d\}_{d=1}^{D}$, using EM. We model $Z_{i,d}$ as the hidden variable. We initialize the iterative EM optimization with the PET image estimate based on filtered back-projection followed by standard EM [15] without any priors. At iteration m, let the current estimate of the PET image be y^m. The E step designs the function $Q(Y; y^m) := E_{P(\{Z_{i,d}\}_{i=1,d=1}^{I,D}|y^m, \{z_d\}_{d=1}^{D}; X, A)}[\log P(z|Y) + \log P(Y, x|A)]$, where the expectand is the sum of the complete-data log likelihood and the log prior. The M step maximizes the $Q(Y; y^m)$ function to produce the updated reconstruction estimate y^{m+1} using the update rule based on the one-step-late modified-EM [7] strategy adapted to our PET-MRI joint-dictionary modeling framework. Thus, the M step updates the reconstruction estimate, for each voxel i, as

$$y_i^{m+1} := \left(\sum_{d=1}^{D} \frac{y_i^m \alpha_{i,d} z_d}{\sum_{i=1}^{I} y_i^m \alpha_{i,d}} \right) \bigg/ \left(\frac{\partial G(y, x, A)}{\partial y_i} \bigg|_{y_i = y_i^m} + \sum_{d=1}^{D} \alpha_{i,d} \right), \forall i, \quad (1)$$

where we evaluate $\partial G(y, x, A)/\partial y_i$ at $y_i = y_i^m$ by (i) fitting the dictionary A to the image pair (x, y^m), as dictated within $G(y, x, A)$, to produce optimal coefficients $\{c_i^*\}_{i=1}^{I}$ (our formulation makes this is a quadratic programming problem having efficient solvers leading to global optima) and then (ii) taking the partial derivative of $(1 - \beta) \sum_{i=1}^{I} \|Y_{Q_i} - A^Y c_i^*\|_2^2$ with respect to y_i. EM iterations stop when the relative change in the estimates y^m and y^{m+1} is small.

3   Evaluation, Results, and Discussion

We compare our method with 5 other reconstruction methods: (i) EM without priors (MLEM) [15], (ii) EM with edge-preserving Huber-loss based MRF prior (HuberMRF), (iii) joint total variation (JTV) prior [6], (iv) parallel level set (PLS) [5,6] prior, (v) MRI-patch dictionary prior for PET reconstruction (MRI-Dict) [18]. For all methods relying on the information in the MRI image, including JTV and PLS, we fix the acquired MRI image to the ground truth. For all methods we tune the underlying free parameters to give the best results qualitatively and quantitatively. We evaluate on 3 datasets: (i) simulated phantom used in [5,6], (ii) simulated BrainWeb used in [5,6], and (iii) *in vivo* PET-MRI. For quantitative evaluation we use SSIM [21] and relative root mean squared error (RRMSE), i.e., ratio of RMSE between y^{true} and y^{estimate} to RMS of y^{true}.

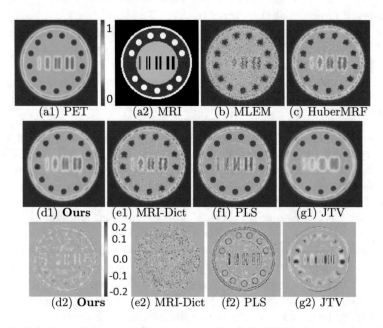

Fig. 1. Validation: Simulated Phantom. (a1)–(a2) PET-MRI ground truth. **(b), (c), (d1)–(g1)** PET reconstructions using various methods. **(d2)–(g2)** Residual (reconstructed - truth) images for the results in (d1)–(g1). **RRMSE: Ours 0.06**, MRI-Dict 0.10, PLS 0.09, JTV 0.08, HuberMRF 0.09, MLEM 0.18. **SSIM: Ours 0.92**, MRI-Dict 0.81, PLS 0.86, JTV 0.90, HuberMRF 0.84, MLEM 0.61.

Validation: Simulated Phantom. For the simulated phantom (Fig. 1(a1)–(a2)), we sufficiently blur the PET image to reproduce the *lower resolution in PET* [1], relative to MRI. The EM reconstruction without any prior (Fig. 1(b)) retains a lot of the noise compared to prior-based methods. EM with the HuberMRF prior (Fig. 1(c)) gets rid of most of the random noise. JTV and PLS (Fig. 1(g1), (f1)) leverage the anatomical structure in the MRI, encouraging edges in the PET reconstruction to occur at the same spatial locations as the edges in the MRI image. They improve over HuberMRF, but the gradient-based penalty limits the quality of reconstruction of the (i) blue circular blobs,

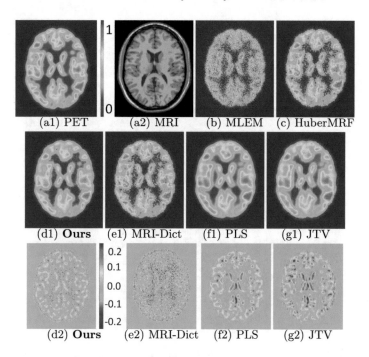

Fig. 2. Validation: BrainWeb-based Phantom. (a1)–(a2) PET and MRI ground truth. **(b), (c), (d1)–(g1)** PET image reconstructions using various methods. **(d2)–(g2)** Residual (truth - reconstructed) images for the results shown in (d1)–(g1).

(ii) red circular outside rim, and (iii) red parallel bars in the center. Using a MRI-patch statistical model to reconstruct PET images (PET patch intensities being significantly smoother than MRI patch intensities) results in overfitting of the dictionary to the noise (Fig. 1(e1)). Our reconstruction (Fig. 1(d1)) using a joint patch-based dictionary model maintains both fine-scale regularity, in the form of smoothness, and larger-scale regularity by preservation of structures like the straightness and separability of the red bars, circularity of the blue blobs, and the continuity in the red outer ring. Our reconstruction has much smaller residual magnitudes (Fig. 1(d2)–(g2)) compared to all other methods, and is closest to the ground truth qualitatively and quantitatively (Fig. 1).

Validation: BrainWeb-Based Phantom. We simulated PET-MRI from BrainWeb MRI and segmentation, akin to the scheme in [5], but our PET image is much smoother than the MRI image, as exhibited in *in vivo* imaging. We learn our joint dictionary A on patches from five slices and reconstruct 50 slices. Our reconstructions (i) better preserve fine-scale and larger-scale structure (Fig. 2) and (ii) have better RRMSE and SSIM (Fig. 4(c)), over all other methods.

Results: *In vivo* Brain PET-MRI. We collected data for 5 subjects using a 3T PET-MRI Siemens scanner (PET slice thickness 2 mm and T1 MRI 1 mm³ voxels). We learn the joint patch dictionary from one subject and reconstruct

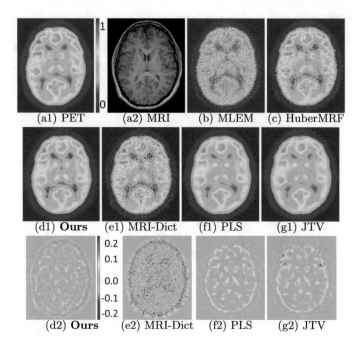

Fig. 3. Results on *in vivo* Brain PET-MRI. (a1)–(a2) PET and MRI ground truth. (b), (c), (d1)–(g1) PET image reconstructions using various methods. (d2)–(g2) Residual (truth - reconstructed) images for the results shown in (d1)–(g1).

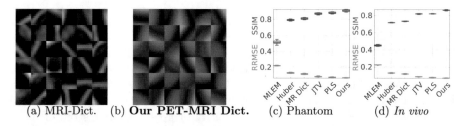

Fig. 4. Results: Quantitative Evaluation. (a) Dictionary of MRI patches, used by [18] (MR-Dict). (b) Our joint dictionary of PET-MRI patches (MRI patch appears as red channel; corresponding PET patch as green channel). (c)–(d) Box plots for RRMSE and SSIM for 50 slices from BrainWeb simulation and 4 subjects *in vivo*.

50 slices from the other subjects. Unlike the dictionary of MR patches in MRI-Dict (Fig. 4(a)), our joint dictionary (Fig. 4(b)) captures regularity in individual patches (which is distinctive for PET and MRI) and PET-MRI correlations in spatially-corresponding patches. Our reconstructions are qualitatively (Fig. 3) and quantitatively (Fig. 4(d)) better than all other methods.

Conclusion. We propose a novel *joint generative model* for the PET-MRI image pair, relying on a *joint patch-based dictionary model*, formulated as a *MRF prior* for Bayesian PET reconstruction using EM. While our model learns the fine-scale and larger-scale regularity in patches in PET and MRI images individually, it also learns structure-function correlations between spatially-corresponding patches in MRI and PET images. Our reconstructions on simulated and *in vivo* PET-MRI improve qualitatively and quantitatively over the state of the art.

References

1. Aklan, B., et al.: Impact of point-spread function modeling on PET image quality in integrated PET/MR hybrid imaging. J. Nucl. Med. **57**(1), 78–84 (2016)
2. Awate, S.P., Whitaker, R.T.: Nonparametric neighborhood statistics for MRI denoising. In: Christensen, G.E., Sonka, M. (eds.) IPMI 2005. LNCS, vol. 3565, pp. 677–688. Springer, Heidelberg (2005). https://doi.org/10.1007/11505730_56
3. Awate, S.P., Whitaker, R.T.: Feature-preserving MRI denoising: a nonparametric empirical-Bayes approach. IEEE Trans. Med. Imag. **26**(9), 1242–55 (2007)
4. Bowsher, J., Johnson, V., Turkington, T., Jaszczak, R., Floyd, C., Coleman, R.: Bayesian reconstruction and use of anatomical a priori information for emission tomography. IEEE Trans. Med. Imag. **15**(5), 673–86 (1996)
5. Ehrhardt, M., et al.: PET reconstruction with an anatomical MRI prior using parallel level sets. IEEE Trans. Med. Imag. **35**(9), 2189–99 (2016)
6. Ehrhardt, M., et al.: Joint reconstruction of PET-MRI by exploiting structural similarity. Inverse Probl. **31**(1), 015001 (2014)
7. Green, P.: Bayesian reconstructions from emission tomography data using a modified EM algorithm. IEEE Trans. Med. Imag. **9**(1), 84–93 (1990)
8. Knoll, F., Holler, M., Koesters, T., Otazo, R., Bredies, K., Sodickson, D.: Joint MR-PET reconstruction using a multi-channel image regularizer. IEEE Trans. Med. Imag. **36**(1), 1–16 (2017)
9. Leahy, R., Yan, X.: Incorporation of anatomical MR data for improved functional imaging with PET. In: Colchester, A.C.F., Hawkes, D.J. (eds.) IPMI 1991. LNCS, vol. 511, pp. 105–120. Springer, Heidelberg (1991). https://doi.org/10.1007/BFb0033746
10. Loeb, R., Navab, N., Ziegler, S.: Direct parametric reconstruction using anatomical regularization for simultaneous PET/MRI data. IEEE Trans. Med. Imag. **34**(11), 2233–47 (2015)
11. Nuyts, J., Fessler, J.: A penalized-likelihood image reconstruction method for emission tomography, compared to post-smoothed maximum-likelihood with matched spatial resolution. IEEE Trans. Med. Imag. **22**(9), 1042–52 (2003)
12. Pedemonte, S., Bousse, A., Hutton, B.F., Arridge, S., Ourselin, S.: 4-D generative model for PET/MRI reconstruction. In: Fichtinger, G., Martel, A., Peters, T. (eds.) MICCAI 2011. LNCS, vol. 6891, pp. 581–588. Springer, Heidelberg (2011). https://doi.org/10.1007/978-3-642-23623-5_73
13. Pedemonte, S., Cardoso, M.J., Arridge, S., Hutton, B.F., Ourselin, S.: Steady-state model of the radio-pharmaceutical uptake for MR-PET. In: Ayache, N., Delingette, H., Golland, P., Mori, K. (eds.) MICCAI 2012. LNCS, vol. 7510, pp. 289–297. Springer, Heidelberg (2012). https://doi.org/10.1007/978-3-642-33415-3_36
14. Pichler, B., Wehrl, H., Kolb, A., Judenhofer, M.: PET/MRI: the next generation of multi-modality imaging? Semin. Nucl. Med. **38**(3), 199–208 (2008)
15. Shepp, L., Vardi, Y.: Maximum likelihood reconstruction for emission tomography. IEEE Trans. Med. Imag. **1**(2), 113–22 (1982)

16. Somayajula, S., Panagiotou, C., Rangarajan, A., Li, Q., Arridge, S., Leahy, R.: PET image reconstruction using information theoretic anatomical priors. IEEE Trans. Med. Imag. **30**(3), 537–49 (2011)
17. Tahaei, M., Reader, A.: Patch-based image reconstruction for PET using prior-image derived dictionaries. Phys. Med. Biol. **61**(18), 6833 (2016)
18. Tang, J., Wang, Y., Yao, R., Ying, L.: Sparsity-based PET image reconstruction using MRI learned dictionaries. In: IEEE 11th International Symposium on Biomedical Imaging (ISBI), p. 1087 (2014)
19. Vandenberghe, S., Marsden, P.: PET-MRI: a review of challenges and solutions in the development of integrated multimodality imaging. Phys. Med. Biol. **60**, R115 (2015)
20. Wang, G., Qi, J.: PET image reconstruction using kernel method. IEEE Trans. Med. Imag. **34**(1), 61–71 (2015)
21. Wang, Z., Bovik, A., Sheikh, H., Simoncelli, E.: Image quality assessment: from error visibility to structural similarity. IEEE Trans. Imag. Proc. **13**(4), 600 (2004)

Analysis of 3D Facial Dysmorphology in Genetic Syndromes from Unconstrained 2D Photographs

Liyun Tu[1], Antonio R. Porras[1], Alec Boyle[1],
and Marius George Linguraru[1,2(✉)]

[1] Sheikh Zayed Institute for Pediatric Surgical Innovation,
Children's National Health System, Washington DC, USA
MLingura@childrensnational.org
[2] School of Medicine and Health Sciences, George Washington University,
Washington DC, USA

Abstract. The quantification of facial dysmorphology is essential for the detection and diagnosis of genetic conditions. Facial analysis benefits from 3D image data, but 2D photography is more widely available at clinics. The aim of this paper is to analyze 3D facial dysmorphology using unconstrained (uncalibrated) 2D pictures at three orientations: frontal, left and right profiles. We estimate a unified 3D face shape by fitting a 3D morphable model (3DMM) to all the images by minimizing the differences between the 2D projected position of the selected 3D vertices in the 3DMM and their corresponding position in the 2D pictures. Using the estimated 3D face shape, we compute a set of facial dysmorphology measurements and train a classifier to identify genetic syndromes. Evaluated on a set of 48 subjects with and without genetic conditions, our method reduced the landmark detection errors obtained by using a single photograph by 44%, 48%, and 49% on the frontal photograph, left profile, and right profile, respectively. We achieved a point-to-point projection error of $1.98 \pm 0.38\%$ normalized to the size of face, significantly improving ($p \leq 0.01$) the error obtained with state-of-the-art methods of $4.17 \pm 2.83\%$. In addition, the geometric features calculated from the 3D reconstructed face obtained an accuracy of 73% in the detection of facial dysmorphology associated to genetic syndromes, compared with the error of 58% using state-of-the-art methods from 2D pictures. That accuracy increased to 96% when we included local texture information. Our results demonstrate the potential of this framework to assist in the earlier and remote detection of genetic syndromes throughout the world.

Keywords: Facial dysmorphology · 3D face reconstruction · 2D photographs
Statistical shape model · Morphable model

© Springer Nature Switzerland AG 2018
A. F. Frangi et al. (Eds.): MICCAI 2018, LNCS 11070, pp. 347–355, 2018.
https://doi.org/10.1007/978-3-030-00928-1_40

1 Introduction

Each year, nearly one million children are born with a genetic condition. The pheno-type variability among genetic syndromes and among populations with different age and/or ethnical background often causes delays and errors in their identification and diagnosis, which can translate into irreversible injuries and even death. The reported average accuracy in the detection of one of the most studied genetic syndromes (Down syndrome) by a trained pediatrician is as low as 64% [1], so methods for their early detection are critical [2].

New developments in the analysis of facial dysmorphology from photographic data have shown promising results in genetic syndrome detection [3, 4]. However, two-dimensional (2D) photography only provides a projection of the patient's face in one plane, and therefore quantification of dysmorphology from 2D photography is sensitive to the orientation of the patient's face with respect to the camera. To overcome these limitations, some works [5, 6] have explored the use of three-dimensional (3D) pho-tography to quantify facial dysmorpholgy. However, the use of 3D photography to screen children in routine clinics is not practical because of the need for a dedicated area in the clinics, the cost of the equipment, and the limited access to it in developing countries.

To address this challenge, we propose a novel method to use the 3D shape of the face estimated from three views: one frontal and two profiles (left and right) uncon-strained 2D photographs (uncalibrated images acquired using a smartphone).

Recent works on 3D face shape estimation from 2D pictures use a variety of techniques, such as landmark-based [7], shape-from-shading-based [8] and learning-based [9, 10] methods. Although these methods have revolutionized 3D face recon-struction using a single image, they struggle to accurately locate feature points at the face boundaries and the ears. The work [11] tried to mitigate this problem by using large data collections including multiple images acquired at different poses, which only focused on the frontal part of the face and optimized each picture independently.

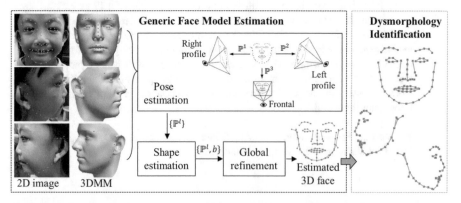

Fig. 1. Workflow of the proposed method to identify facial dysmorphology associated to genetic syndromes from unconstrained frontal and profile photographs of a patient. Note the landmarks used on the frontal and profile photographs. The pose parameters $\mathbb{P}^l, l \in \{1, 2, 3\}$, for the lth 2D photograph, and the shape coefficients b are iteratively optimized.

In this paper, we estimate the 3D face shape by integrating information from three views of the same subject. First, we use a unified 3D morphable model (3DMM) [12] to estimate the 3D locations of a set of landmarks from the 2D images by minimizing the difference between the observed positions of the landmarks in the 2D images and the projections of their corresponding predicted 3D positions. Then, from the reconstructed 3D face, we calculate a set of geometric features, and we use them together with the texture information around those landmarks to train a classifier to quantify facial dysmorphology and to detect genetic syndromes.

2 Methods

2.1 Generic Face Model Estimation

To reconstruct the 3D face shape of a subject from different 2D pictures, we used the 3DMM Basel Face Model (BFM) [12], which was built from 3D scans of 100 male and 100 female faces using principal components analysis. We selected a set of vertices on the 3DMM corresponding to the landmarks defined on the 2D face images as shown in Fig. 1. In addition to the 68 automatic landmarks detected in the frontal images based on [13], we incorporated a set of 8 manual landmarks to better describe the nose region. We also placed 25 landmarks on each profile image.

We used a scaled orthographic perspective transformation to fit the 3DMM to the 2D pictures, similar to the approach presented in [7] for a single image. With this approach, the 2D projections of the 3D vertices do not depend on the distance from the camera, but only on a uniform scale $s \in \mathbb{R}^+$. That scale is given by the ratio of the focal length of the camera and the mean distance from the camera to the object. Thus, the projected 2D position of a 3D point $v = (x, y, z)^T$ from the 3DMM is

$$p = s\left(\begin{bmatrix} 1 & 0 & 0 \\ 0 & 1 & 0 \end{bmatrix} R_{rot} v + t\right), \qquad (1)$$

where $R_{rot} \in \mathbb{R}^{3\times3}$ is the 3D rotation matrix and $t \in \mathbb{R}^2$ is the 2D translation. The coordinates of vertex v in the 3DMM can be expressed as $v = Pb + \bar{u}$, where $b \in \mathbb{R}^S$ are the shape parameters, $\bar{u} \in \mathbb{R}^{3n}$ is the mean shape with n vertices, and $P \in \mathbb{R}^{3n\times S}$ are the S principal components.

The 3DMM was fitted to each 2D image l by minimizing the projection error (E_l),

$$E_l = \frac{1}{n}\sum_{i=1}^{n} \|q_i^l - s^l(R^l v_i^l + t^l)\|_F^2, \qquad (2)$$

where $l \in \{1, 2, 3\}$ represents the frontal (index 1) and two profile 2D images (indices 2 and 3), $\|\cdot\|_F$ is the Frobenius norm, q_i^l represent the 2D landmarks on the image, and $v_i^l = P_i^l b + \bar{u}_i^l$ are the selected corresponding vertices on the 3DMM, R^l represents the rotation which holds the first two rows in R_{rot} (Eq. 1), and t^l and s^l are the translation, and scaling of the lth image, respectively.

Since the optimization of Eq. 2 for the three images is not a convex problem, we solved it in three steps: (A) first we estimated the pose parameters (R^l, t^l, s^l) for each 2D image; (B) then we estimated the shape coefficients (b) as a linear least squares problem; and (C) we refined the pose parameters and shape coefficients simultaneously as a nonlinear least squares problem.

(A) Pose Estimation

We made an initial estimation of the pose parameters R^l, t^l, and s^l using the constrained pose from the orthography and scaling method [7]. With this approach, we approximated the perspective projection with a scaled orthographic projection (Eq. 1) by solving the following linear system

$$\underset{R^l, t^l, s^l}{\arg\min} \frac{1}{2} \|C\phi - \mathcal{H}\|_2^2, \tag{3}$$

where $C = s^l R^l P_i^l$ is the projected position of the selected vertices on the 3DMM in homogeneous coordinates, $p_i = (x_i, y_i)^T$ are the observed landmarks in the 2D images, $\mathcal{H} = p_i^l - s^l (R^l \bar{u}_i^l + t^l)$ is the concatenated position of the n landmarks on the l [th] 2D image in corresponding to the 3D vertices, and $\bar{u}_i^l$ is the selected 3D vertices. ϕ represents the estimated coefficients, which are used to extract our pose parameters R^l, t^l, s^l. This model allows for 6 degrees of freedom, with 3 coefficients for 3D rotation, 2 for translation in the 2D projection plane, and 1 for isotropic scaling.

Unlike our formulation from Eq. 2, in Eq. 3, we represent the rotation about each axis as a different scalar angle, instead of one single matrix representing all rotations. We used singular value decomposition to ensure that the estimated R^l was a valid rotation matrix. After the initial pose estimation using Eq. 3, we refined the pose parameters by minimizing the projection errors E_l in Eq. 2 with respect to themselves using the trust-region reflective algorithm [14].

(B) Shape Estimation

Once the pose parameters were calculated, we estimated the shape coefficients b by concatenating the locations of the observed landmarks in the 2D images of the 3 views of a subject, and minimizing the difference between these locations and the 2D projections of their corresponding vertices in the 3DMM iteratively using $\sum_{l=1}^{3} E_l$ with respect to b. During optimization, the shape parameters were constrained to the range $[-3\lambda, 3\lambda]$ to ensure a plausible shape, where λ is the eigenvalue associated to each principal component in the 3DMM. The 2D projections for the l [th] image were computed using their own pose parameters $(R^l, t^l, \text{and } s^l)$, while the shape coefficients for each of the 3 images was estimated simultaneously.

(C) **Global Refinement**

Since different pose parameters were optimized for the different 2D images, we performed a bundle adjustment to iteratively align the 3 views (frontal and two profile images). We used the trust-region reflective algorithm to solve the following non-linear optimization:

$$\arg\min_{b,R^l,t^l,s^l} \left(\sum_{l=1}^{3} w_l E_1 + \delta \sum_{i=1}^{k} \left(\frac{b_i}{\sqrt{\lambda_i}} \right)^2 \right), \tag{4}$$

where $\sum_{i=1}^{k} \left(b_i/\sqrt{\lambda_i} \right)^2$ is the shape prior adopted from [7] to ensure the plausibility of the solution, k is the number of principal components of the 3DMM, λ is the eigenvalue of the 3DMM, w_l is the weight of the lth image calculated as a function of the number of landmarks in the image similar to [7], and δ is the weight for the shape prior as used in [7]. Both the pose parameters and the shape coefficients were estimated simultaneously using Eq. 4, thus obtaining the final face shape estimation given by the shape parameters b.

2.2 Identification of Dysmorphology Associated to Genetic Syndromes

Once we estimated the 3D shape of the face, our goal was to detect facial dysmorphology associated to genetic syndromes. To that end, we first computed the set of 24 facial features as shown in Fig. 2, which have been shown to be relevant to identify genetic syndromes in [3, 4]. Unlike these previous works, our approach used the estimated 3D geometric measurements instead of their projection in 2D.

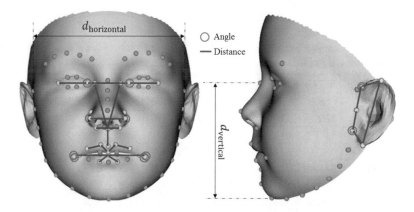

Fig. 2. Geometric measurements used to identify facial dysmorphology. $d_{horizontal}$ and $d_{vertical}$ were used to normalize horizontal and vertical distances, respectively.

As presented in [3, 4], appearance information around each landmark provides meaningful information to detect genetic syndromes. For that reason, we followed the approach described in [4] to quantify the texture around each landmark in the 2D photographs. In summary, we calculated the local binary pattern (LBP) of the patch around each landmark. Then, we used a 2D extension of linear discriminant analysis [4] to convert this LBP to a single score at each landmark (Fig. 2, yellow points), which describes how likely the appearance is to describe dysmorphology.

From all the geometric and texture features, we first selected the most discriminative ones using recursive feature elimination, thus training a linear support vector machine classifier and recursively eliminating the features with the lowest weight. Then, we evaluated the accuracy of our approach to identify facial dysmorphology associated to genetic syndromes using a leave-one-out cross-validation.

2.3 Datasets

We collected 3 2D photographs (frontal, left and right profile) from a group of 48 subjects (22 male and 26 female, average age 4 ± 3 years, age range 1 month to 12 years) of diverse ancestry, using an in-house smartphone app. Twenty-four subjects presented genetic syndromes (including Down, Noonan, Turner, Wolf-Hirschorn syndromes, etc.), and the other 24 cases were healthy. The subjects of both groups were matched by age, ethnicity, and gender.

3 Experimental Results and Discussion

To evaluate the accuracy estimating the 3D shape of the face, we computed the point-to-point root mean square error (RMSE) and the standard deviation (SD) between the 2D projected position of the vertices in the estimated 3D face shape and their corresponding locations observed on the 2D images. We normalized all differences by the face size, similar to [3, 13].

Table 1. Errors obtained by estimating the 3D face using different combination of the fontal (F), left (L), and right (R) profile images. Lower value is desirable.

Data	RMSE $\pm$ SD (%)			
	Frontal	Right profile	Left profile	Average of all views
F	**1.92 $\pm$ 0.59**	9.02 $\pm$ 1.97	8.93 $\pm$ 1.62	4.72 $\pm$ 0.89
R	5.00 $\pm$ 1.05	**3.25 $\pm$ 2.09**	7.90 $\pm$ 2.93	5.23 $\pm$ 1.45
L	4.96 $\pm$ 1.31	7.89 $\pm$ 2.48	**2.92 $\pm$ 1.58**	5.13 $\pm$ 1.33
R+L	4.68 $\pm$ 0.72	3.49 $\pm$ 0.91	3.35 $\pm$ 0.82	4.18 $\pm$ 0.61
F+L	2.41 $\pm$ 0.52	7.32 $\pm$ 1.15	3.79 $\pm$ 0.87	3.66 $\pm$ 0.53
F+R	2.52 $\pm$ 0.53	4.14 $\pm$ 1.04	7.11 $\pm$ 1.02	3.75 $\pm$ 0.54
F+R+L	1.98 $\pm$ 0.38	3.84 $\pm$ 1.02	3.53 $\pm$ 0.74	**2.66 $\pm$ 0.43**

Table 1 shows the RMSE for the face shape estimated using one photograph, 2 photographs, or 3 photographs. We obtained an average reconstruction error of $2.66 \pm 0.43\%$ using the 3 photographs simultaneously, improving by 44%, 49%, and

48% the results obtained on all 3 views using only the frontal, right, and left profile photographs, respectively. These improvements were statistically significant (p-value < 0.001 for all) as determined by the Wilcoxon signed-rank test. As it may be expected, the lowest error at each individual view (frontal or profile) was obtained when using only the photograph of that view. Unsurprisingly, results using the 3 views are slightly worse than using a single view because of the simultaneous fitting to all views, but there is a substantial decrease in standard deviation, which indicated better stability of the method.

Table 2. Comparisons of RMSE between the proposed and the state-of-the-art methods. (%)

	Bas et al. [7]	Zhu et al. [10]	Proposed
RMSE±SD	4.17 ± 2.83	5.27 ± 2.81	**1.98 ± 0.38**

Furthermore, we compared the estimated faces resulting from our proposed method with those obtained using state-of-the-art methods [7, 10]. Since those methods were designed to work only with single images, for a fair comparison, only the frontal image of each subject was used. In addition, the method from Bas et al. [7] was revised to use our landmark correspondence. As shown in Table 2, our method outperforms the state-of-the-art methods. An example of the landmarks estimated with the proposed method is shown in Fig. 3, where we can observe low differences between the estimated landmark position projected on the 2D photographs and their true location. Results show that the proposed method provides a closer face shape reconstruction to the observations from the 2D photographs.

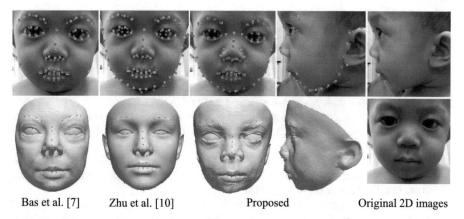

Bas et al. [7]   Zhu et al. [10]   Proposed   Original 2D images

Fig. 3. The faces reconstructed using different methods. The right column shows the acquired 2D photographs. Top row: the 2D projected location (red) of the vertices of the estimated 3D face shape and the ground truth (green) in the 2D photographs. Bottom row: the estimated 3D face shapes. The red dots indicate the corresponding vertices to the 2D photographs.

Finally, cross-validation of the classifier trained using the geometric measurements estimated from our 3D reconstructed face shape reported an accuracy of 73%, compared to the results of 58% that we obtained using the geometric measurements from the 2D photographs (p-value < 0.001). Our accuracy increased to 96% (with sensitivity 96%, specificity 100%) when we combined our estimated 3D measurements with the local texture information.

A potential limitation is the use of a statistical model built from an older population, which is a parameter that will be easily fixed when more data are available. However, the innovation in our method and formulation is independent on what statistical model is used. Even with such limitation, our method outperformed state-of-the-art approaches.

4 Conclusions

We presented a method for an accurate reconstruction of the 3D shape of the face from unconstrained 2D photographs using a statistical 3D morphable model. Our method achieved the lowest reconstruction error compared with other state-of-the-art approaches on single photographs. Moreover, we showed that the 3D measurements estimated with our framework outperformed the results obtained using 2D measurements for the quantification of facial features used to assess dysmorphology associated to genetic syndromes. Importantly, the proposed framework does not require camera calibration, which allowed us to acquire these pictures using a standard mobile phone. This makes our technology easily translatable to the clinics, with the potential to assist in earlier detection of genetic syndromes.

References

1. Sivakumar, S., Larkins, S.: Accuracy of clinical diagnosis in Down's syndrome. Arch. Dis. Child. **89**(7), 691 (2004)
2. Kruszka, P., et al.: 22q11.2 deletion syndrome in diverse populations. Am. J. Med. Genet. Part A **173**(4), 879–888 (2017)
3. Zhao, Q., et al.: Digital facial dysmorphology for genetic screening: hierarchical constrained local model using ICA. Med. Image Anal. **18**(5), 699–710 (2014)
4. Cerrolaza, J.J., et al.: Identification of dysmorphic syndromes using landmark-specific local texture descriptors. In: 2016 IEEE 13th International Symposium on Biomedical Imaging (ISBI), pp. 1080–1083 (2016)
5. Weinberg, S.M., et al.: The 3D facial norms database: part 1. a web-based craniofacial anthropometric and image repository for the clinical and research community. Cleft Palate-Craniofacial J. **53**(6), e185–e197 (2016)
6. Liang, S., et al.: Improved detection of landmarks on 3D human face data. In: 2013 35th Annual International Conference of the IEEE Engineering in Medicine and Biology Society (EMBC), 6482–6485 (2013)
7. Bas, A., et al.: Fitting a 3D morphable model to edges: a comparison between hard and soft correspondences. In: Asian Conference on Computer Vision (ACCV) Workshops, pp. 377–391 (2016)

8. Roth, J., et al.: Adaptive 3D face reconstruction from unconstrained photo collections. In: 2016 IEEE Conference on Computer Vision and Pattern Recognition (CVPR), pp. 4197–4206 (2016)
9. Kemelmacher-Shlizerman, I., Basri, I.: 3D face reconstruction from a single image using a single reference face shape. IEEE Trans. Pattern Anal. Mach. Intell. **33**(2), 394–405 (2011)
10. Zhu, X., et al.: Face alignment across large poses: a 3D solution. In: 2016 IEEE Conference on Computer Vision Pattern Recognition, pp. 146–155 (2016)
11. Piotraschke, M., Blanz, V.: Automated 3D face reconstruction from multiple images using quality measures. In: 2016 IEEE Conference on Computer Vision and Pattern Recognition (CVPR), pp. 3418–3427 (2016)
12. Blanz, V., Vetter, T.: Face recognition based on fitting a 3D morphable model. IEEE Trans. Pattern Anal. Mach. Intell. **25**(9), 1063–1074 (2003)
13. Zhu, X., Ramanan, D.: Face detection, pose estimation, and landmark localization in the wild. In: IEEE Conference on Computer Vision and Pattern Recognition (CVPR), pp. 2879–2886 (2012)
14. Coleman, T.F., Li, Y.: An interior trust region approach for nonlinear minimization subject to bounds. SIAM J. Optim. **6**(2), 418–445 (1996)

Double Your Views – Exploiting Symmetry in Transmission Imaging

Alexander Preuhs[1(✉)], Andreas Maier[1], Michael Manhart[2], Javad Fotouhi[3],
Nassir Navab[3], and Mathias Unberath[3]

[1] Pattern Recognition Lab, Friedrich-Alexander-Universität Erlangen-Nürnberg,
Erlangen, Germany
`Alexander.Preuhs@fau.de`
[2] Siemens Healthcare GmbH, Forchheim, Germany
[3] Computer Aided Medical Procedures, Johns Hopkins University, Baltimore, USA

Abstract. For a plane symmetric object we can find two views—mirrored at the plane of symmetry—that will yield the exact same image of that object. In consequence, having one image of a plane symmetric object and a calibrated camera, we can automatically have a second, virtual image of that object if the 3-D location of the symmetry plane is known. In this work, we show for the first time that the above concept naturally extends to transmission imaging and present an algorithm to estimate the 3-D symmetry plane from a set of projection domain images based on Grangeat's theorem. We then exploit symmetry to generate a virtual trajectory by mirroring views at the plane of symmetry. If the plane is not perpendicular to the acquired trajectory plane, the virtual and real trajectory will be oblique. The resulting X-shaped trajectory will be data-complete, allowing for the compensation of in-plane motion using epipolar consistency. We evaluate the proposed method on a synthetic symmetric phantom and, in a proof-of-concept study, apply it to a real scan of an anthropomorphic human head phantom.

Keywords: Consistency conditions · Cone-beam CT
Motion compensation · Data completeness
Tomographic reconstruction

1 Introduction

Symmetry is a powerful concept with applications ranging from art to physics and mathematics [1]. This manuscript is concerned with symmetry in computer vision where we consider a theoretically sound yet surprisingly little known property of symmetric objects: when imaging a symmetric object using a calibrated camera, knowledge of the 3-D symmetry plane yields a second, virtual camera that corresponds to a mirrored version of the image seen by the true camera. This circumstance enables metric 3-D stereo reconstruction of symmetric objects using a single calibrated camera [2–4].

© Springer Nature Switzerland AG 2018
A. F. Frangi et al. (Eds.): MICCAI 2018, LNCS 11070, pp. 356–364, 2018.
https://doi.org/10.1007/978-3-030-00928-1_41

For the first time, we demonstrate that the above property naturally extends to transmission imaging, i.e. X-ray fluoroscopy, and devise image-based algorithms that exploit this circumstance to estimate intra-scan motion in circular C-arm cone-beam computed tomography (CBCT). In CBCT imaging, all camera positions are calibrated suggesting that a virtual source trajectory becomes available once the 3-D symmetry plane is known. We show that (1) this plane can be estimated efficiently from multiple projective images and (2) circular trajectories in a plane oblique to the plane of symmetry contain information that substantially benefits motion detection using recent consistency conditions.

2 Methods

2.1 Epipolar Consistency Conditions

Theory: In CBCT an X-ray source radially emits photons, that—after attenuation—are registered at a detector. The attenuation process for a ray is described by an integral. However, due to the radial structure of the rays, integrating along a detector line does not result in the Cartesian plane integral of the underlying object f but differs by a radial weighting.

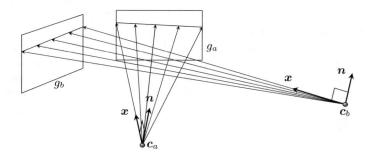

Fig. 1. Schematic drawing of a scene including two projections.

Grangeat's theorem describes the connection between this weighted integral and a plane integral—i.e. the 3-D radon value $\mathcal{R}f(\boldsymbol{n}, d)$ describing the integral along a plane with normal $\boldsymbol{n} \in \mathcal{S}^2$ at distance d. Using a derivative operation the radial weighting can be canceled out. Grangeat defined an intermediate function $S_\lambda(\boldsymbol{n})$ that is calculated from projection data and is related to the derivative of the 3-D radon transform

$$S_\lambda(\boldsymbol{n}) = \int_{\mathcal{S}^2} \delta'(\boldsymbol{x}^\top \boldsymbol{n}) g_\lambda(\boldsymbol{x}) d\boldsymbol{x} = \frac{\partial}{\partial d}\mathcal{R}f(\boldsymbol{n}, d)|_{d=c_\lambda^\top \boldsymbol{n}}, \qquad (1)$$

where $\delta'(\cdot)$ describes the derivative of the Dirac delta distribution, $g_\lambda(\boldsymbol{x})$ describes a single value on the detector with λ the projection index, $\boldsymbol{c}_\lambda$ the source position and x a vector from the source to a detector pixel. The geometry for two projections is visualized in Fig. 1. A detailed derivation of Eq. (1) can be found in [5], and some simplifications are discussed in [6]. From Eq. (1) it directly follows that two projections a, b must satisfy

$$S_a(n) = S_b(n) \qquad \forall n \in \mathcal{S}^2 : c_b^\top n = c_a^\top n. \tag{2}$$

If the geometric calibration is wrong, e. g. due to object motion, Eq. (2) will not hold. Thus, we can use it as a measure of inconsistency. The global indexing by the plane normal n can be replaced by a local projection-pair-dependent indexing per the epipolar geometry. This particular sampling of the intermediate function is commonly denoted as epipolar consistency (EC) [6] and allows to efficiently evaluate redundant values only based on the corresponding projection matrices P_a and P_b, allowing the reformulation of Eq. (2) to

$$S_a(P_a, P_b) = S_b(P_b, P_a), \tag{3}$$

where S denotes the array of intermediate values computed from S.

Short Scans and the Circular Trajectory: State of the art head imaging protocols for CBCT consist of a circular trajectory of 496 projections. Hereby the source detector gantry rotates around the patient covering a 200° segment. All source positions within the trajectory lie on a plane, typically referred to as trajectory plane. We define this plane coincident with the x, y-plane.

Rigid patient motion or geometry misalignment can be estimated and compensated for using EC [7–9]. This is achieved by finding a rigid transformation T_i for each projection matrix P_i, accounting for the patient motion at acquisition of projection i. The motion is expected to be compensated, when the inconsistency between all projections is minimal. The result of motion estimation is a set of rigid transformations $T = [T_1, \ldots T_{496}]$ that satisfy

$$\hat{T} = \arg\min_{T} \sum_{a,b=1}^{496} \|S_a(P_a T_a, P_b T_b) - S_b(P_b T_b, P_a T_a)\|_2. \tag{4}$$

However, there are theoretical limitations due to the geometry of the circular trajectory. Most radon planes of the object that include two source positions are almost parallel to the trajectory plane. As the consistency is based on the radon value, only motion that steps out of the radon plane is detectable. As a consequence only out-plane motion (r_x, r_y, t_z) can be estimated well, while in-plane motion (t_x, t_y, r_z) cannot be estimated robustly [7]. In the following, we show that we can exploit symmetry to generate a short scan-like trajectory which is data complete and, thus, beneficial for estimation of in-plane motion.

2.2   Symmetric View Augmentation

Symmetry in Transmission Imaging: Consider a plane-symmetric scene as depicted in Fig. 2. The two points $x_a \in \mathbb{P}^3$ and $x_b \in \mathbb{P}^3$ are symmetric to the

z, y-plane. This bilateral symmetry relation can be expressed by an involutive isometric transformation F—i. e. a reflection matrix—as

$$x_a = F\,x_b \qquad\qquad x_b = F\,x_a, \tag{5}$$

where $F \in \mathbb{R}^{4\times4}$ only flips the sign of the x component. Since F is an isometric transformation we find the mirrored projection matrix as PF (cf. Fig. 2). The resulting image on the right detector will be the projection of the points x_a and x_b under P and the resulting image on the left detector will be the projected points x_a and x_b under PF giving

$$u_a = Px_a \qquad u_b = Px_b \qquad u'_a = PFx_a \qquad u'_b = PFx_b. \tag{6}$$

Inserting the symmetry relation given by Eq. (5) in the two leftmost equations of Eq. 6 gives the relation

$$u_a = Px_a = PFx_b = u'_b \qquad\qquad u_b = Px_b = PFx_a = u'_a. \tag{7}$$

This result allows to conclude that both detector images will exhibit the exact same image. Note that this only holds since the reflection of the projection matrix also flips the u and v axis. Consequently, a transmission image of a plane symmetric object can be interpreted as acquired under either the projection P or PF. This observation allows to effectively double the views of an acquisition if the symmetry plane is known.

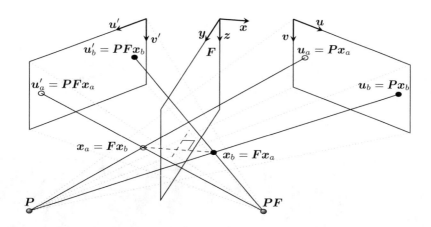

Fig. 2. Visualization of a plane symmetric scene.

Symmetry Plane Estimation: We apply EC (cf. Eq. (4)) to find the reflection F' that represents the most consistent transformation, which is—by definition—the reflection at the symmetry plane. To optimize for a certain symmetry plane, we need to find the transformation describing F', which is given by $F' = TFT^{-1}$, with T being a rigid transformation. The reflection F' is then found by optimizing for $\hat{T}$ minimizing the inconsistency defined as

$$\hat{T} = \arg\min_{T} \sum_{a,b=1}^{N} \left\| S_a(P_a TFT^{-1}, P_b) - S_b(P_b, P_a TFT^{-1}) \right\|_2, \qquad (8)$$

where N is the number of projections used for finding the symmetry plane.

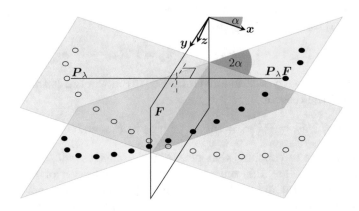

Fig. 3. Visualization of X-trajectory. The acquired trajectory is embedded in the blue trajectory plane (blank dots) and the mirrored virtual trajectory is embedded in the red trajectory plane (solid dots).

The X-Trajectory: If the symmetry plane of the scanned object is oblique to the trajectory plane of a short scan by an angle α as visualized in Fig. 3, the mirrored trajectory plane will be rotated to the acquired trajectory plane by 2α. Thus, for adequate angles α, the combined trajectory fulfills Tuy's condition and the short scan becomes data complete. This in turn enables the use of Grangeat's theorem to detect in-plane motion.

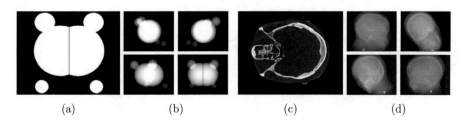

Fig. 4. (a): Slice through the symmetric phantom. (b): Digitally rendered radiographs (DRR) of the phantom. (c): Aligned reconstruction of anthropomorphic head phantom. (d): raw projection data from a short scan of the head phantom.

2.3   Experiments

Data: To evaluate our method we synthetically generated a plane symmetric phantom, consisting of four small balls, and two half spheres (cf. Fig. 4a). From this phantom, a short scan is simulated *in silico* (cf. Fig. 4b). The second dataset is a short scan acquired from a real anthropomorphic human head phantom using a robotic C-arm system (Artis zeego, Siemens Healthcare GmbH, Germany). The phantom is placed, such that the expected symmetry plane is oblique to the trajectory plane. As expected in a real clinical case, the head phantom does not exhibit a perfect plane symmetry. A slice through the reconstruction and projections from the acquired short scan of the head are shown in Figs. 4c and 4d, respectively.

Estimation of Symmetry Plane: Using the synthetic and real datasets, we first estimate the symmetry plane. The plane is found from projection domain images only by minimizing Eq. (8) using the Nelder-Mead method. The optimization searches for the symmetry plane parameters described by three DoF.

Application to Rigid Motion: To study the impact of the X-trajectory in dependence of α on in- and out-plane motion, we add a rigid spline motion to each motion parameter. The motion amplitude is in the range of ± 0.3 mm or degree, respectively, and distributed only in the central part of the trajectory, where no opposing views are available. Then we compute combined consistency grids of the motion affected trajectory using the synthetic phantom. The grid is build up by a $(N \times N)$ matrix C, where each element c_{ab} denotes the consistency between views a and b. The lower-left triangle of the consistency grid denotes the conventional EC (CEC) computed from two views on the circular trajectory. The upper-right triangle is computed as the EC between an acquired view a and a mirrored view b, which we denote as mirrored EC (MEC).

In addition we inspect the inconsistency induced by an r_z motion pulse distributed over view 238–288 on the acquired human head phantom consisting of 496 views. We compare the CEC solely computed from the short scan, epipolar consistency between mirrored and acquired view (MEC) and a combination of both (combined CEC and MEC).

3   Results and Discussion

Estimation of Symmetry Plane: The estimated and ground truth symmetry plane parameters for the synthetic phantom are listed in Table 1. Estimation succeeded with very high accuracy.

The head phantom, while not perfectly symmetric, exhibits a well defined symmetry plane that was estimated very robustly. A reconstruction aligned w.r.t. the symmetry plane is depicted in Fig. 5.

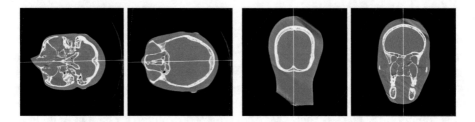

Fig. 5. Reconstruction of acquired head phantom. The volume is aligned to the symmetry plane (white line) and shown from an axial and coronal view.

Table 1. Ground truth symmetry plane parameters (normal and signed distance from origin) of synthetic phantom and estimated symmetry plane parameters.

	n_x	n_y	n_z	d
Ground truth	0	1	0	0
Estimation	0.0000926	0.9999999	0.0000005	0.0000822

Application to Rigid Motion: Comparing upper and lower row of Fig. 6 that correspond to $\alpha = 0°$ and $\alpha = 30°$, respectively, the impact of the X-trajectory is evident. The CEC (lower left triangle of the grid) detects inconsistency within out-plane parameters (three rightmost columns) while in-plane motion (three leftmost columns) is not detected well. Using MEC and an angle $2\alpha = 60°$ between the acquired and mirrored trajectory plane, prominently reveals in-plane motion.

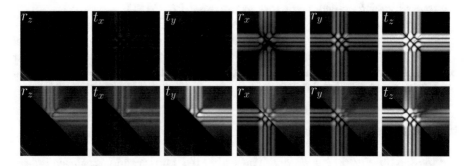

Fig. 6. Inconsistency due to motion in the trajectory using the synthetic phantom. Bright pixels encode a high inconsistency and dark regions encode consistent view pairs. Upper row: $\alpha = 0°$, lower row: $\alpha = 30°$.

Figure 7 shows the different consistency measures (CEC, MEC, combined CEC and MEC) responding to a motion impulse on the acquired data. All measures are able to detect large scale motion. However, using CEC the global

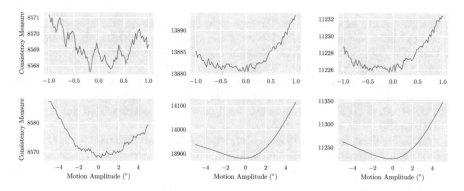

Fig. 7. Sensitivity of consistency measure to motion impulse. Left column: CEC. Middle column: MEC. Right column: combined CEC and MEC.

optimum is displaced by 0.2°. The MEC optimum is displaced by 0.03°, combined CEC and MEC shows a displacement of 0.06°, suggesting that, in this setup, MEC is more accurate than CEC by a factor of 10.

4   Conclusion

We presented the concept of plane symmetry for transmission imaging and provided an algorithm to estimate the 3-D plane of symmetry based on projection images only. In combination with a short scan trajectory oblique to the symmetry plane, an X-shaped trajectory arises that is associated with several benefits. For adequate angles α, both in- and out-of-plane motion directions are detectable using Grangeat's theorem. This property naturally arises from the observation that the X-trajectory is Tuy-complete. We have evaluated the proposed algorithm on a real scan of an anthropomorphic head phantom. Despite being only partially symmetric, the proposed concept of exploiting symmetry was still found applicable. Future research is needed to find effective optimization strategies to estimate complex motion patterns. We conclude that symmetry is a powerful concept in transmission imaging with the potential to benefit diverse imaging problems that make use of consistency condition such as calibration, beam hardening- and truncation-correction.

Disclaimer: The concepts and information presented in this paper are based on research and are not commercially available.

References

1. Field, M., Golubitsky, M.: Symmetry in Chaos: A Search for Pattern in Mathematics, Art, and Nature. SIAM (2009)
2. Rothwell, C., Forsyth, D.A., Zisserman, A., Mundy, J.L.: Extracting projective structure from single perspective views of 3D point sets. In: ICV, pp. 573–582 (1993)

3. François, A.R., Medioni, G.G., Waupotitsch, R.: Reconstructing mirror symmetric scenes from a single view using 2-view stereo geometry. In: ICPR, pp. 12–16 (2002)
4. François, A.R., Medioni, G.G., Waupotitsch, R.: Mirror symmetry 2-view stereo geometry. Image Vis. Comput. **21**(2), 137–143 (2003)
5. Defrise, M., Clack, R.: A cone-beam reconstruction algorithm using shift-variant filtering and cone-beam backprojection. TMI **13**(1), 186–195 (1994)
6. Aichert, A., et al.: Epipolar consistency in transmission imaging. TMI **34**(11), 2205–2219 (2015)
7. Frysch, R., Rose, G.: Rigid motion compensation in interventional C-arm CT using consistency measure on projection data. In: Navab, N., Hornegger, J., Wells, W.M., Frangi, A.F. (eds.) MICCAI 2015. LNCS, vol. 9349, pp. 298–306. Springer, Cham (2015). https://doi.org/10.1007/978-3-319-24553-9_37
8. Maass, N., Dennerlein, F., Aichert, A., Maier, A.: Geometrical jitter correction in computed tomography. In: CT-Meeting, pp. 338–342 (2014)
9. Preuhs, A., Manhart, M., Maier, A.: Fast epipolar consistency without the need for pseudo matrix inverses. In: CT-Meeting, pp. 202–205 (2018)

Real Time RNN Based 3D Ultrasound Scan Adequacy for Developmental Dysplasia of the Hip

Olivia Paserin[✉], Kishore Mulpuri, Anthony Cooper, Antony J. Hodgson, and Rafeef Garbi

BiSICL, University of British Columbia, Vancouver, Canada
opaserin@ece.ubc.ca

Abstract. Acquiring adequate ultrasound (US) image data is crucial for accurate diagnosis of developmental dysplasia of the hip (DDH), the most common pediatric hip disorder affecting on average one in every one thousand births. Presently, the acquisition of high quality US deemed adequate for diagnostic measurements requires thorough knowledge of infant hip anatomy as well as extensive experience in interpreting such scans. This work aims to provide rapid assurance to the operator, automatically at the time of acquisition, that the data acquired are suitable for accurate diagnosis. To this end, we propose a deep learning model for a fully automatic scan adequacy assessment of 3D US volumes. Our contributions include developing an effective criteria that defines the features required for DDH diagnosis in an adequate 3D US volume, proposing an efficient neural network architecture composed of convolutional layers and recurrent layers for robust classification, and validating our model's agreement with classification labels from an expert radiologist on real pediatric clinical data. To the best of our knowledge, our work is the first to make use of inter-slice information within a 3D US volume for DDH scan adequacy. Using 200 3D US volumes from 25 pediatric patients, we demonstrate an accuracy of 82% with an area under receiver operating characteristic curve of 0.83 and a clinically suitable runtime of one second.

Keywords: Pediatric · Ultrasound · Hip · Bone imaging
Developmental dysplasia of the hip · DDH · CNN · RNN
US scan adequacy

1 Introduction

Developmental dysplasia of the hip (DDH) is a congenital condition representing a range of disorders involving a partial or complete dislocation of the hip joint. DDH is the most common pediatric hip disorder, affecting on average one in every one thousand births [1]. Failure to diagnose DDH in its early stages often gives rise to serious adverse outcomes affecting the hip such as painful early

© Springer Nature Switzerland AG 2018
A. F. Frangi et al. (Eds.): MICCAI 2018, LNCS 11070, pp. 365–373, 2018.
https://doi.org/10.1007/978-3-030-00928-1_42

adult osteoarthritis and significant difficulties in future treatment that typically includes expensive corrective surgical procedures [2].

Ultrasound (US) imaging is currently considered the gold standard for DDH diagnosis during early childhood development as it is low cost, portable, and does not use potentially harmful ionizing radiation [3]. Although 2D US is the present clinical standard, several works have recently shown that using 3D US gives a more comprehensive measure of the anatomical deformity and is less prone to probe orientation related errors [6–8]. Our group has pioneered the use of 3D US for DDH diagnosis and shown that it markedly improves the reliability of dysplasia metric measurements compared to 2D US [8]. However, current analysis processes are computationally expensive, with runtimes of three minutes, limiting clinical relevance. Furthermore, the introduction of 3D US poses increased difficulty on operators who may not have experience with volumetric scans. The acquisition of high quality US volumes that are adequate for diagnostic measurements remains an especially challenging task as it requires thorough knowledge of infant hip anatomy and extensive experience in interpreting scans. Such challenges exist even when 2D US is used, e.g. when the quality of hip sonograms across 8 German states was studies in 2011, up to 43% of tested hip sonographers had their licenses revoked because they could not demonstrate sufficient adherence to the imaging guidelines [4]. The top reasons for misdiagnoses were: (1) US probe orientation errors; (2) incorrect anatomical interpretation; and (3) lack of adequacy checks [5]. To improve clinical usability of 3D US, our work aims to provide rapid assurance at the time of acquisition that the US data acquired is suitable for diagnosis.

US standard plane detection, an issue similar to that of US scan adequacy, has been addressed in other fields such as fetal abnormality screening [9–11] and cardiac imaging [12,13] in an effort to provide feedback to sonographers. Maraci et al. [9], Chen et al. [11], Baumgartner et al. [12], and Abdi et al. [13] each proposed classifiers for categorisation of 2D slices from US video data, and Rahmatullah et al. [10] proposed a method based on the AdaBoost learning algorithm for US volume data. In an earlier work [14], our group proposed a technique for automatic 2D US scan adequacy detection in DDH but applying that approach sequentially to slices of a 3D US volume would require a long processing time hampering clinical use. We subsequently developed a fast approach for automatic 3D US scan adequacy [15] but the classified adequacy remained slice-by-slice based thus did not make use of rich, and often very informative, inter-slice information when considering the spatial relationship of the responses from sequential frames within a volume.

In this paper, we propose a deep learning model for fully automatic scan adequacy assessment of 3D US volumes. We design a recurrent neural network (RNN) architecture to incorporate inter-slice information within a 3D US volume for DDH screening. More specifically, our contributions include: (1) developing a list of criteria that defines the features required in an adequate 3D US volume for DDH diagnosis, (2) proposing a neural network architecture, trained end-to-end, comprising convolutional layers and recurrent layers that robustly classify

US scan adequacy, and (3) validating our model's agreement with classification labels from an expert radiologist on real pediatric clinical data.

2   Materials and Method

2.1   Dataset

As part of a larger collaboration with pediatric orthopedic surgeons at British Columbia Children's Hospital, including a multi-year DDH clinical study conducted by our research team, we acquired 200 3D B-mode US volumes from 25 pediatric patients (acquired by two pediatric orthopedic surgeons). The data were obtained as part of routine clinical care under appropriate institutional review board approval using a SonixTouch Q+ scanner (Analogic Inc., Peabody, MA, USA) with a 4DL14-5/38 linear 4D transducer set at 7 MHz and positioned in the coronal plane. Each acquired volume comprised 200 slices with an axial resolution of 0.17 mm. In order to harmonise the input image dimensions to our neural network, we resized the images to 256×256 pixels corresponding to a x-dimension of 38 mm and variable y-dimension of a minimum of 38 mm.

2.2   3D US Scan Adequacy Criteria

It is important to note that a gold standard for clinical classification of US volumes does not yet exist, since 2D assessment is currently the clinical standard for DDH screening. Together with an expert radiologist, we thus developed a list of criteria that defines the features required in an adequate 3D US volume for proper subsequent extraction of the commonly used DDH metrics, namely the α angle (angle between the plane of the ilium and the acetabulum), β angle (angle between the plane of the ilium and the labrum), and femoral head coverage (the percentage area of the femoral head medial to the ilium) [8]. Therefore, anatomical features required to be present within the scan include the ilium, acetabulum, labrum, ischium and entire femoral head as illustrated in Fig. 1. When a volume properly captures the entire hip joint, the femoral head, a hypo-echoic spherical structure, should be seen growing and shrinking in size across the encompassing slices. Additionally, the ilium must appear as a straight, horizontal hyper-echoic line and the acetabulum must appear continuous with the iliac bone. Notably, although these features should be collectively present within an adequate volume, they do not necessarily all need to be present within any single slice of the volume, hence a slice-by-slice analysis is not ideal and compromises accuracy.

2.3   Proposed CNN-RNN Network Architecture

In order to leverage spatial inter-slice information within a volume, we propose a neural network architecture composed of convolutional layers to extract hierarchical features from a scan, followed by recurrent layers to capture the spatial

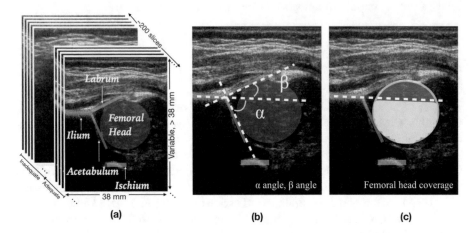

Fig. 1. (a) An annotated frame from an adequate US volume demonstrating the anatomical features required for accurate diagnostic interpretation: the ilium, acetabulum, labrum, ischium and femoral head. (b) Illustration of the α and β angle diagnostic measurements. (c) Illustration of the femoral head coverage diagnostic measurement.

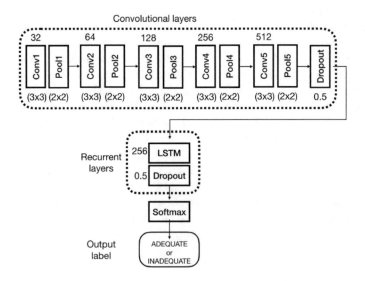

Fig. 2. Overview of our CNN-RNN neural network architecture. The number of filters in each layer are presented above each block and their corresponding filter sizes are presented below each block.

relationship of their responses. An overview of the network is shown in Fig. 2. We designed and implemented our model in Keras [16], a Python API with a TensorFlow [17] backend.

Extracting Hierarchical Features. Due to the relatively small sample size, we deployed a simple Convolutional Neural Network (CNN) architecture to avoid overfitting to the training dataset despite regularisation. Specifically, we used a CNN inspired by the VGG architecture [19] as it has proven to generalise well to other datasets. We include five convolutional layers, increasing the feature maps by a factor of two at each layer. In order to limit the number of parameters in our model, each convolutional layer has small 3×3-sized kernels with their number of kernels increasing by a factor of two as well. Using Keras' TimeDistributed wrapper to process sequential frames as a sequence, we apply convolutions to all the frames of an US volume (sequence of frames). To reduce the feature maps to half their size as well as to decrease feature variance for improved generalisability in our model, we employ Rectified Linear Units (ReLUs) as nonlinear activation functions between layers and 2×2 max-pooling operations with a stride of 2. Lastly, to prevent co-adaptation of features and overfitting to the training dataset, we include a dropout layer with a dropout probability of 0.5.

Leveraging Spatial Inter-slice Information. Long Short-Term Memory (LSTM) [18] networks are Recurrent Neural Networks (RNNs) with an architecture designed for sequence processing. Since we have a relatively small dataset, we propose the use of an RNN over 3D convolutions since they require less parameters for training and are therefore better suited. LSTMs comprise gates that solve the problem of vanishing and exploding gradients, allowing them to store information over long time intervals, well suited for sequences. To analyse inter-slice information, we apply this sequential-learning strategy by inputting a sequence of features extracted from the time-distributed CNN into our LSTM layer. The LSTM uses a system of memory gated functions to process each frame of a sequence while learning to store only the important features from each frame. Our LSTM layer has 256 units and is followed by a dropout probability of 0.5 for improved generalisability.

2.4   Training

In our experiments, we split the available data by patients rather than by volumes in order to avoid mixing similar volume samples between training, validation, and testing data. We split our 25 patients into 60% training, 20% validation, and 20% testing. This resulted in 135 volumes from 15 patients for training and 45 volumes from 5 patients for validation. Additionally, we saved 20 raw US volumes from 5 patients for testing our final model and for cross checking the results with those of our expert radiologist. Each data subset had approximately equal number of adequate and inadequate volumes.

To prepare adequate and inadequate labels for sequences from our volumes, let $S = \{F_1, F_2, ..., F_n\}$ denote a sequence of n frames in which F_A and F_B are the first and last frames with any diagnostic features present, respectively. All frames $F_A, ..., F_B$ are thus grouped as a sequence and labeled adequate. The remaining frames $F_1, ..., F_{A-1}$ and $F_{B+1}, ..., F_n$ are labeled inadequate sequences. The resulting sequence lengths varied from 40–50 frames. Additionally, sequences from US volumes with missing diagnostic features were labeled inadequate.

During training, we used mini-batches of size 32 for 50 epochs and the cost function we minimised was the mean of the binary cross-entropy loss between the output prediction p and the true label vector y, calculated as

$$\mathcal{L}(\theta) = -\frac{1}{n} \sum_{i=1}^{n} \left[y_i \log\left(p_i\right) + \left(1 - y_i\right) \log\left(1 - p_i\right) \right], \tag{1}$$

where i indexes samples and n is the number of samples. We used Adam [20] as our optimizer for minimizing the objective function with a learning rate of 1e–5 and learning rate decay of 1e–6.

3   Results and Discussion

Our collaborating expert radiologist was asked to provide clinical classification labels for 20 test US volumes (new, unseen by our network during training and validation), which we treated as gold standard. In this experiment, we purposely included scans in this test dataset that we expected to be challenging to interpret, for example the volume shown in Fig. 3.

Testing on the sequences from 20 test volumes, our proposed approach achieved an accuracy of 82% and area under receiver operating characteristic curve of 0.83. In order to output a single label for each test volume, we passed sequences of length 50 frames at a time into the network (as in the training) until all 200 frames had been processed. Volumes were labeled as adequate by the network when an adequate sequence was found within a volume. Using this strategy, our network's output labels agreed with our radiologist's manual labels for 16 of the 20 challenging test scans. We further compared results with our previous method [15] and found that it correctly classified only 14 of our 20 test volumes. Since that method was based on a slice by slice analysis, it failed to identify any adequate volumes in which there was not a series of slices that each had all the required anatomy. For example, as illustrated in Fig. 3(c) and (d), frame 23 is missing the acetabulum and frame 51 is missing the ischium, so our previous method classified these slices as inadequate. In comparison, our new method analyses the frames collectively as a sequence and correctly classified this volume as adequate since the all the required features are present across the sequence of frames.

Runtime. Leveraging the GPU-based implementation of neural networks by TensorFlow, the trained model was able to perform a classification of an input

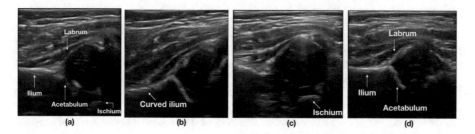

Fig. 3. Selected frames from test volumes. (a) Frame 25 from an optimal volume, capturing all the required features for adequacy. (b) Frame 45 from an inadequate volume, showing a curved ilium. (c) and (d) are frames 23 and 51 from one adequate volume, demonstrating an example of how the required features are not all found in a single frame.

US volume in one second, a time suitable for clinical workflow. This time was achieved on a Intel(R) Core(TM) i7-7800X 3.50 GHz CPU, with a NVIDIA TITAN Xp GPU and 64 GB of RAM. For comparison, our expert radiologist (experienced in DDH diagnosis with 2D scans) took an average of 10–40 s to classify one volume.

4   Conclusions

We presented a technique for fully automatic scan adequacy assessment of 3D US volumes for DDH. We developed a list of criteria defining the features required for diagnosis, proposed a neural network architecture comprising convolutional recurrent layers for robust classification, and validated our model on real pediatric data. Our volume classification agrees well with an expert's manual classification with an average processing time of one second, which is suitable for clinical use. Considering the small size of the training data, we expect better performance as our dataset continues to grow with scans from more patients and a variety of US machines. Future work will include expanding the size of our training set and investigating the differences in reliability and task time between novice and experienced sonographers/surgeons using our setup. We expect real time automatic US scan adequacy assessment to have significant clinical impact with the potential to help in imaging standardisation of 3D US for DDH. Currently, there is no universal screening for DDH in North America due to the high cost of experienced personnel needed for scan acquisition. In future, an automatic assessment tool may potentially reduce DDH screening costs by allowing personnel other than highly trained radiologists or surgeons to obtain reliable 3D US scans suitable for diagnosis and thus make universal DDH screening possible.

References

1. Committee on Quality Improvement, Subcommittee on Developmental Dysplasia of the Hip: Clinical practice guideline: early detection of developmental dysplasia of the hip. Pediatrics **105**(4), 896 (2000)
2. Hoaglund, F.T., Steinbach, L.S.: Primary osteoarthritis of the hip: etiology and epidemiology. JAAOS **9**(5), 320–327 (2001)
3. Atweh, L., Kan, J.: Multimodality imaging of developmental dysplasia of the hip. Pediatr. Radiol. **43**(1), 166–171 (2013)
4. Tschauner, C., Matthissen, H.: Hip sonography with Graf-method in newborns: checklists help to avoid mistakes. OUB **1**, 7–8 (2012)
5. Graf, R., Mohajer, M., Florian, P.: Hip sonography update: quality-management, catastrophes - tips and tricks. Med. Ultrason. J. **15**(4), 299–303 (2013)
6. Jaremko, J., Mabee, M., Swami, V., Jamieson, L., Chow, K., Thompson, R.: Potential for change in US diagnosis of hip dysplasia solely caused by changes in probe orientation: patterns of alpha-angle variation revealed by using three-dimensional US. Radiology **273**(3), 870–878 (2014)
7. Hareendranathan, A., Mabee, M., Punithakumar, K., Noga, M., Jaremko, J.: A technique for semiautomatic segmentation of echogenic structures in 3D ultrasound, applied to infant hip dysplasia. Int. J. Comput. Assist. Radiol. Surg. **11**(1), 31–42 (2016)
8. Quader, N., Hodgson, A., Mulpuri, K., Cooper, A., Abugharbieh, R.: Towards reliable automatic characterization of neonatal hip dysplasia from 3D ultrasound images. In: Ourselin, S., Joskowicz, L., Sabuncu, M.R., Unal, G., Wells, W. (eds.) MICCAI 2016. LNCS, vol. 9900, pp. 602–609. Springer, Cham (2016). https://doi.org/10.1007/978-3-319-46720-7_70
9. Maraci, M., Bridge, C., Napolitano, R., Papageorghiou, A., Noble, A.: A framework for analysis of linear ultrasound videos to detect fetal presentation and heartbeat. Med. Image Anal. **37**, 22–36 (2017)
10. Rahmatullah, B., Papageorghiou, A., Noble, J.A.: Automated selection of standardized planes from ultrasound volume. In: Suzuki, K., Wang, F., Shen, D., Yan, P. (eds.) MLMI 2011. LNCS, vol. 7009, pp. 35–42. Springer, Heidelberg (2011). https://doi.org/10.1007/978-3-642-24319-6_5
11. Chen, H.: Ultrasound standard plane detection using a composite neural network framework. IEEE Trans. Cybern. **47**(6), 1576–1586 (2017)
12. Baumgartner, C.F., Kamnitsas, K., Matthew, J., Smith, S., Kainz, B., Rueckert, D.: Real-time standard scan plane detection and localisation in fetal ultrasound using fully convolutional neural networks. In: Ourselin, S., Joskowicz, L., Sabuncu, M.R., Unal, G., Wells, W. (eds.) MICCAI 2016. LNCS, vol. 9901, pp. 203–211. Springer, Cham (2016). https://doi.org/10.1007/978-3-319-46723-8_24
13. Abdi, A.H., et al.: Quality assessment of echocardiographic cine using recurrent neural networks: feasibility on five standard view planes. In: Descoteaux, M., Maier-Hein, L., Franz, A., Jannin, P., Collins, D.L., Duchesne, S. (eds.) MICCAI 2017. LNCS, vol. 10435, pp. 302–310. Springer, Cham (2017). https://doi.org/10.1007/978-3-319-66179-7_35
14. Quader, N., Hodgson, A.J., Mulpuri, K., Schaeffer, E., Abugharbieh, R.: Automatic evaluation of scan adequacy and dysplasia metrics in 2-D ultrasound images of the neonatal hip. Ultrasound Med. Biol. **43**, 1252–1262 (2017)

15. Paserin, O., Mulpuri, K., Cooper, A., Hodgson, A.J., Abugharbieh, R.: Automatic near real-time evaluation of 3D ultrasound scan adequacy for developmental dysplasia of the hip. In: Cardoso, M.J., et al. (eds.) CARE/CLIP -2017. LNCS, vol. 10550, pp. 124–132. Springer, Cham (2017). https://doi.org/10.1007/978-3-319-67543-5_12
16. Chollet, F.: Keras (2015). https://github.com/fchollet/keras
17. TensorFlow: Large-scale machine learning on heterogeneous systems (2015). tensorflow.org
18. Hochreiter, S., Schmidhuber, J.: Long short-term memory. Neural Comput. $9(8)$, 1735–1780 (1997)
19. Simonyan, K., Zisserman, A.: Very deep convolutional networks for large-scale image recognition. In: International Conference on Learning Representations, pp. 1–14 (2015)
20. Kingma, D.P., Ba, J.L.: Adam: a method for stochastic optimization. In: International Conference on Learning Representations, pp. 1–15 (2015)

Direct Reconstruction of Ultrasound Elastography Using an End-to-End Deep Neural Network

Sitong Wu[1,2], Zhifan Gao[1], Zhi Liu[3], Jianwen Luo[3(✉)], Heye Zhang[1(✉)], and Shuo Li[4]

[1] Shenzhen Institutes of Advanced Technology,
Chinese Academy of Sciences, Shenzhen, China
hy.zhang@siat.ac.cn
[2] Shenzhen College of Advanced Technology,
University of Chinese Academy of Sciences, Shenzhen, China
[3] Tsinghua University, Beijing, China
luo_jianwen@mail.tsinghua.edu.cn
[4] University of Western Ontario, London, Canada

Abstract. In this work, we developed an end-to-end convolutional neural network (CNN) to reconstruct the ultrasound elastography directly from radio frequency (RF) data. The novelty of this network is able to infer the distribution of elastography from real RF data by only using computational simulation as the training data. Moreover, this framework can generate displacement and strain field respectively both from ultrasound RF data directly. We evaluated the performance of this network on 50 simulated RF datasets, 42 phantom datasets, and 4 human datasets. The best results of signal-to-noise ratio (SNR) and contrast-to-noise ratio (CNR) in simulated data, phantom data, and human data are 39.5 dB and 69.64 dB, 32.64 dB and 48.76 dB, 23.24 dB and 46.22 dB, respectively. Furthermore, we also compare the performance of our method to the state-of-art ultrasound elastography using normalized cross-correlation (NCC) technique. From this comparison, it shows that that our method can effectively compute the strain field robustly and accurately in the this paper. These results might imply great potential of this deep learning method in ultrasound elastography application.

Keywords: Ultrasound elastography · Convolutional neural network
Tissue displacement and strain · RF data

1 Introduction

The mechanical behaviour of healthy and pathological tissue are different under external compression because the stiffness of tissue will be changed by the diseases [6]. Ultrasound elastography has been one popular technique in clinical practice to examine the distribution of tissue strain in the suspected lesion area,

© Springer Nature Switzerland AG 2018
A. F. Frangi et al. (Eds.): MICCAI 2018, LNCS 11070, pp. 374–382, 2018.
https://doi.org/10.1007/978-3-030-00928-1_43

according to the tissue displacement derived from the two-dimensional radio frequency (2D RF) data. Many studies have tried to develop varieties of feature extractors, such as normalized cross-correlation [2] and optical flow [3], for estimating the tissue displacement from 2D RF data and then predicting the tissue strain. However, these attempts are always disturbed by the noises or insufficient feature information. Moreover, most of features in previous works only provide low-level information related to local variation of 2D RF data, rather the high-level semantic information related to the tissue strain.

From the viewpoint of computer vision, ultrasound elastography can be considered to explore the key visual information (tissue strain), which attracts the human attention, in the complex environment (noise-corrupted RF data). Extracting high-level semantic image features from RF data can help to robustly reconstruct the elastography. Recently popular deep neural networks have shown its effectiveness in medical image analysis, as it can effectively extract, represent, and integrate highly semantic features without manual intervention.

In this paper, we develop an end-to-end deep neural network to predict the strain and displacement fields directly from RF data under the condition that tissue compressed by the constant external force (i.e. quasi-static ultrasound elastography). The architecture of our framework includes two convolutional neural networks to extract high-level features without manual intervention, for predicting the tissue displacement and strain, respectively. Furthermore, the novelty of our work is that only the simulated data are used in training this deep neural network. The performance of our approach is validated on simulated data (50 cases), phantom data (42 cases) and real clinical data (4 patients), by comparing with the ground truth (in simulated data) and a state-of-the-art ultrasound elastography method. Our experimental results have proved the generalization of our proposed framework in the reconstruction of elastography. To the best of our knowledge, it is the first time to reconstruct the ultrasound elastography using the deep learning method with only simulated training data.

2   Methodology

Network Architecture. The architecture of our network is composed of two stages: one is to estimate tissue displacement from 2D RF data; the other is to predict tissue strain from the tissue displacement. The network architecture is illustrated in Fig. 1. The deformation of soft tissue can be measured by ultrasound technique. We collect two sets of 2D RF data (denoted by I_1 and I_2) before and after compressing the soft tissue. The phase time interval between these two 2D RF data are highly related to the tissue displacement. We get I_1 and I_2 as the input of our network after giving a small global elongation to the post- compression RF data.

In the displacement estimation stage, we firstly use the separable convolution to extract and concatenate the hybrid features of I_1 and I_2. Then we construct a five-layer convolution network to extract the contextual information of the difference between I_1 and I_2. We adopt the locally-connected convolution,

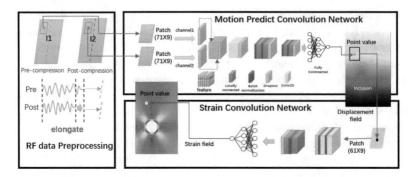

Fig. 1. The flowchart of our approach. The 2D RF data are represented by the first stage of our network after the preprocessing. Then the tissue strain field are computed from the displacement field by the second stage of our network. Note our approach can directly compute both of tissue displacement field and strain field.

instead of the commonly-used fully-connected convolution, to remove the spatial correlation, for increasing the ability of the convolutional kernel to express the high-level information related to spatial location. This will help to differentiate the phase time intervals of tissues with different elasticity. The components to further process the output feature maps in all layers include (from low level to high level) dropout, batch normalization, batch normalization + dropout, batch normalization, batch normalization + dropout, respectively. Then the feature maps generated by the above convolution network are resized into a vector for the subsequent fully-connected network with three layers (64, 32 and 1 units). This fully connected network can get a distribution of the tissue displacements resulting from the compression.

In the strain prediction stage, we use another convolution network with three layers to extract the high-level semantic information of the tissue displacement. The feature maps produced from these three layers are further processed by batch normalization, batch normalization + dropout, batch normalization, and dropout, respectively. Similar to the displacement estimation, a fully-connected network is used to predict the strain from the vectorized feature maps derived from the local displacement field.

Implementation Details. All input images are resized to 2608×128 (pixels) in both training and testing. The patch sizes in the displacement estimation stage and strain prediction stage are 71×9 and 61×9, respectively. In the training process, we use ADAM with the momentum 0.9 as the optimization algorithm. The iteration number is 30 epochs. The learning rate is $10e-4$. The loss function is the absolute mean error. All input images are resized to 2608×128 for training and testing.

3   Experiments and Results

3.1   Datasets and Evaluation Indices

We evaluated the performance our approach on simulation data, phantom data and real data. The training set only contains the 40 simulation data. The testing set is composed of the remaining simulation, all phantom data and patient data. All of the codes for model training and testing were implemented by TensorFlow on a NIVDIA GTX1070 GPU.

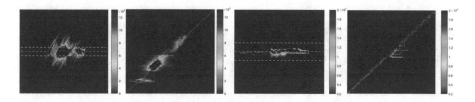

Fig. 2. The results of the Bland-Altman analysis and linear regression (LR) between the ground truth (x-axis in LR) and our approach (y-axis in LR) in all simulation data. The left two plots correspond to the tissue displacement, and the right two plots correspond to the strain percentage with respect to the tissue size. Note that the color indicates the density or the frequency of the scatter points in the two-dimensional BA and LR plane

Table 1. Comparing with the state-of-the-art method in simulation data.

Simulation data	Displacement		Strain		
	SNR_d	RMSE	SNR_e	CNR_e	RMSE
Our approach	96.0746 ± 8.8622	0.2450	28.6832 ± 6.800	62.3249 ± 10.8053	0.2938
AM-Kalman	104.6249 ± 5.3247	0.0852	15.1824 ± 4.1605	31.4127 ± 7.1706	0.9783

Simulation data. We produced 50 simulation tissues with 3 cm width and 5 cm depth, each of which contains with 10000 scatter points with pre-specified locations and an inclusion with random number of scatter points. The Young's module of the background in tissue was set by 25 kPa and the inclusions were set as four different values (8 kPa, 14 kPa, 45 kPa and 80 kPa). Then, we used finite element method (by commercially available software COMSOL 5.1) to compute the positions of all scattering points after compressing the tissue, and moreover the ground truth of tissue displacement field and strain field. Finally, we computed the 2D RF data of the tissue before and after compression by an ultrasound simulation system (Field II) [1] with 6 MHz central frequency and 40 MHz sampling frequency.

Phantom data. We collected the phantom data from a commercially available elasticity QA phantom (CIRS 049, Norfolk, VA, USA) using a VerasonicsVantage 256 system (Verasonics Inc., WA, USA) equipped with an L12-5 transducer. This transducer was applied to image 42 regions of the phantom with four different inclusions (Young's module are 8 kPa, 14 kPa, 45 kPa and 80 kPa) and the background region (25 kPa). The central frequency and sampling frequency of the scanning were 6.25 MHz and 40 MHz, respectively.

Patient data. We acquired the four real clinical data (one is liver and three are breast) from the public dataset [4].

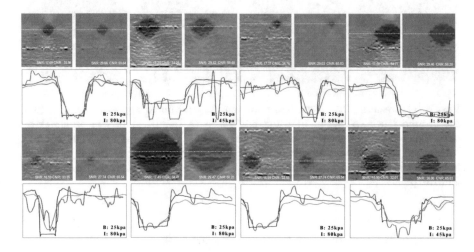

Fig. 3. Sample results of strain estimation in eight simulation data with different Young's module ("B": background; "I": inclusion). In each pair of images, the left is the previous method and the right is our approach. The strain profile in the second and fourth rows corresponds to the white dotted line of the strain field showed in the first and third rows. In the strain profile, the blue, green and red curves corresponds to the ground truth, our approach and AM-Kalman, respectively.

Evaluation Indices. We used the RMSE and displacement signal-to-noise ratio to measure the quality of the displacement estimate. The SNR is defined by $SNR_d = 10\log(l_d - l_g)^2/l_g^2$, where l_d and l_g are displacement profiles generated by our approach and the ground truth, respectively [5]. Then we

Table 2. Comparing with the state-of-the-art method in phantom and patient data.

	Phantom data		Patient data	
	SNR_e	CNR_e	SNR_e	CNR_e
Our approach	30.4339±4.0308	43.2689±10.7117	23.2628±3.2032	40.3475±18.3785
AM-Kalman	17.9304±3.3346	29.5817±7.7203	9.6330±12.8452	36.2232±24.2978

apply elastographic signal-to-noise ratio (SNR$_e$) and elastographic contrast-to-noise ratio (CNR$_e$) to measure the quality of the strain estimate [5], i.e. $SNR_e = 10 \log e_i/\sigma_i$, $CNR_e = 10 \log(2(e_b - e_i)^2)/(\sigma_b^2 + \sigma_i^2)$, where e_b and σ_b are the mean value and variance of the background, and e_i and σ_i the mean value and variance of the inclusion.

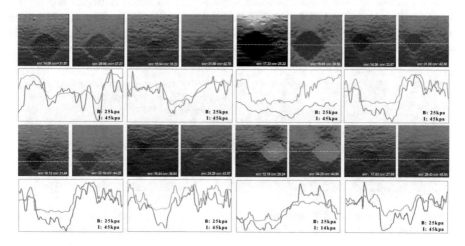

Fig. 4. Sample results of strain estimation in eight phantom data with different Young's module ("B": background; "I": inclusion). The green and red curves shows the strain profile of our approach and AM-Kalman, respectively.

3.2   Comparison with Ground Truth and Other Methods

Simulation Results. Table 1 shows the performance of our approach in the tissue displacement estimation and the strain prediction. In the displacement, the values of SNR$_d$ and RMSE are 96.0746 $\pm$ 8.8622 dB and 0.245, respectively. This indicates the very small difference between the displacement field computed by our approach and the ground truth. In the strain prediction, the value of RMSE (=0.2938) indicates the error of the strain field produced by our approach is at a low level. Besides, the values of SNR$_e$ (28.6832 $\pm$ 6.800 dB) and CNR$_e$ (62.3249 $\pm$ 10.8053 dB) shows not only the strain field in the inclusion less disturbed by noise, but also the strain contrast between the inclusion and background has the high-level signal-to-noise ratio. Then, Fig. 2 shows the results of the Bland-Altman analysis (BA) and linear regression (LR) between the ground truth (x-axis in LR) and our approach (y-axis in LR) in all simulation data. The left two plots correspond to the tissue displacement, and the right two plots correspond to the strain percentage with respect to the tissue size. Note that the color indicates the density or the frequency of the scatter points in the two-dimensional BA and LR plane.

Furthermore, we have compared our framework with the a state-of-the-art method proposed by Rivaz et al. [4] (denoted by AM-Kalman). This method applied 2D analytic minimization to obtain the tissue displacement from RF data and then used the Kalman filter to calculate the smooth strain field. The results in Table 1 shows the displacement estimation of our approach is slightly worse than AM-Kalman (our approach is 8.5503 dB lower for SNR_d and 0.1598 higher for RMSE), but our approach shows much better performance than AM-Kalman in the strain prediction (our approach is 13.5008 dB higher for SNR_e, 30.9122 dB higher for CNR_e, and 0.6845 lower for RMSE). The strain is the important parameter concerned in clinical practice, and thus our framework is superior to AM-Kalman in the simulation data.

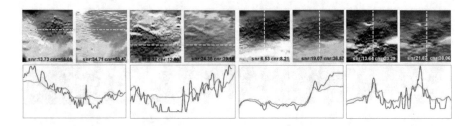

Fig. 5. Sample results of strain estimation in four patient data. The green and red curves shows the strain profile of our approach and AM-Kalman, respectively.

Table 3. Comparing with variants of our network in the displacement estimation.

		Simulation				Phantom		Patient data	
		SNR_d	SNR_e	CNR_e	RMSE	SNR_e	CNR_e	SNR_e	CNR_e
Pooling (max)	Avg	66.01 ± 6.08	8.95 ± 0.65	6.26 ± 1.11	0.65	5.48 ± 1.04	9.58 ± 8.36	3.58 ± 10.59	7.47 ± 4.45
Conv layers(5)	4	66.79 ± 5.00	7.94 ± 1.57	11.53 ± 0.52	0.85	7.39 ± 1.34	14.55 ± 4.06	4.45 ± 2.59	11.13 ± 4.71
	6	$65.43 \pm 7{,}25$	7.67 ± 3.68	8.46 ± 3.00	1.04	8.23 ± 4.69	3.73 ± 2.68	0.68 ± 1.64	0.14 ± 2.54
FC layers (3)	2	60.09 ± 5.62	3.74 ± 1.74	5.06 ± 4.28	1.17	3.42 ± 1.95	3.89 ± 2.73	2.00 ± 2.95	1.95 ± 0.94
	4	50.43 ± 3.83	3.20 ± 0.58	3.82 ± 1.65	2.13	1.45 ± 0.93	4.04 ± 4.64	1.35 ± 1.24	4.50 ± 1.11
Dilation rate (1)	2	65.82 ± 3.66	8.58 ± 1.57	13.16 ± 3.90	0.74	6.28 ± 4.23	17.60 ± 6.06	8.05 ± 3.49	9.45 ± 6.56
	3	75.92 ± 3.96	13.34 ± 2.67	25.45 ± 7.02	0.80	14.33 ± 1.49	24.56 ± 10.27	12.37 ± 4.93	15.57 ± 1.50
Patch_size (71x9)	71 × 5	$89.43 \pm 8{,}86$	15.35 ± 1.57	29.37 ± 12.48	0.39	19.16 ± 2.08	34.83 ± 19.12	12.59 ± 2.26	29.51 ± 7.53
	45 × 9	94.33 ± 7.25	16.45 ± 3.35	36.42 ± 9.23	0.27	34.96 ± 4.22	39.16 ± 9.09	19.83 ± 5.11	37.63 ± 14.20
	31 × 9	55.18 ± 5.10	2.72 ± 0.94	3.78 ± 1.87	1.24	5.56 ± 1.34	3.453 ± 5.39	0.45 ± 1.43	11.46 ± 5.83
Our		96.07 ± 8.86	28.68 ± 6.80	62.32 ± 10.80	0.24	30.43 ± 4.03	43.26 ± 10.71	23.26 ± 3.20	40.34 ± 18.37

Figure 3 shows the sample results from eight simulation data for the comparison between our approach and AM-Kalman in the strain estimation. These sample results indicate that our approach can predict the strain field (green curve) closer to the ground truth (blue curve) than AM-Kalman (red curve).

Phantom Results. Because no ground truth in the phantom experiments, we evaluate the performance of our approach by comparing SNR_e and CNR_e

with AM-Kalman. Table 2 shows the performance of our approach is better than with AM-Kalman (SNR$_e$: 30.4339 dB vs. 17.9304 dB; CNR$_e$: 43.2689 dB vs. 29.5817 dB). Figure 4 shows the sample results from eight phantom data for the comparison between our approach and AM-Kalman in the strain estimation. These sample results indicate that our approach can predict the strain field with higher SNR$_e$ and CNR$_e$ than AM-Kalman.

Patient Data Results. Similar to the phantom experiments, we also compared the values of SNR$_e$ and CNR$_e$ with AM-Kalman in the patient data experiments. Table 2 shows the performance of our approach is superior to with AM-Kalman (SNR$_e$: 23.2628 dB vs. 9.6330 dB; CNR$_e$: 40.3475 dB vs. 36.2232 dB). Figure 5 shows the results of all four patient data for the comparison between our approach and AM-Kalman in the strain estimation. These sample results show the higher SNR$_e$ and CNR$_e$ of the strain field estimated by our approach than AM-Kalman.

Table 4. Comparing with variants of our network in the strain prediction.

		Simulation			Phantom		Patient data	
		SNR$_e$	CNR$_e$	RMSE	SNR$_e$	CNR$_e$	SNR$_e$	CNR$_e$
Pooling (max)	Avg	28.58 ± 5.08	62.07 ± 15.53	0.35	28.37 ± 5.33	47.59 ± 16.69	15.15 ± 9.19	33.91 ± 15.25
Conv layers (5)	3	30.51 ± 3.71	66.99 ± 13.02	0.37	32.64 ± 3.63	48.76 ± 10.06	20.37 ± 3.44	40.65 ± 21.46
	4	30.67 ± 2.13	69.39 ± 14.30	0.37	29.66 ± 3.12	45.39 ± 17.64	23.24 ± 5.97	40.59 ± 22.14
FC layers (3)	2	39.50 ± 4.28	69.64 ± 15.79	0.37	27.5 ± 6.58	44.92 ± 17.77	19.87 ± 3.76	38.76 ± 23.43
	4	30.69 ± 5.24	65.93 ± 16.66	0.35	30.91 ± 2.49	45.46 ± 18.06	16.66 ± 2.82	46.22 ± 15.20
Dilation rate (1)	2	30.17 ± 5.22	65.88 ± 21.74	0.36	28.60 ± 4.67	45.00 ± 13.84	17.39 ± 3.66	43.79 ± 15.73
	3	34.84 ± 6.24	68.86 ± 14.49	0.37	28.34 ± 4.23	46.00 ± 17.85	21.49 ± 5.37	40.85 ± 18.40
Patch_size (71 × 9)	(61 × 5)	32.42 ± 3.02	67.25 ± 10.44	0.34	27.12 ± 7.69	43.56 ± 19.17	16.96 ± 2.99	40.17 ± 18.34
	(41 × 9)	30.56 ± 4.87	60.76 ± 15.58	0.35	27.83 ± 6.26	40.15 ± 23.58	14.29 ± 1.15	40.17 ± 18.34
	(31 × 9)	29.06 ± 7.00	62.34 ± 18.94	0.39	27.02 ± 6.67	45.18 ± 18.43	16.79 ± 1.25	39.17 ± 19.44
Our		28.68 ± 6.80	62.32 ± 10.80	0.29	30.43 ± 4.03	43.26 ± 10.71	23.26 ± 3.20	40.34 ± 18.37

3.3 Comparisons Between Different Configurations of Our Network

The ablation analysis aims to investigate the effectiveness of our network architecture. Table 3 shows the results of the network components for displacement estimation in simulation, phantom and patient data, Table 4 displays those for strain prediction. The digits within the parentheses in the first column shows the configuration of our network architecture. The results in these two tables indicate the effectiveness of current configurations of the architecture in the pooling strategy, layer number, dilated rate of the convolution kernel, and patch size.

4 Conclusion

In this study, we have developed an end-to-end deep learning approach to recover the tissue displacement and strain in ultrasound elastography directly from radio frequency (RF) data. The performance of our approach was tested on 50 simulation data, 42 phantom data and 4 patient data, by comparing with the gold standard and a state-of-the-art method. Experimental results show that our method is effective in calculating the strain field, and moreover implies great potential of this deep learning method in ultrasound elastography application.

References

1. Jensen, J.A.: FIELD: a program for simulating ultrasound systems. In: 10th Nordic-Baltic Conference On Biomedical Imaging, pp. 351–353 (1996)
2. Luo, J., Konofagou, E.E.: A fast normalized cross-correlation calculation method for motion estimation. IEEE Trans. Ultrason. Ferroelectr. Freq. Control **57**(6), 1347–1357 (2010)
3. Pellot-Barakat, C., Frouin, F., Insana, M.F., Herment, A.: Ultrasound elastography based on multiscale estimations of regularized displacement fields. IEEE Trans. Med. Imaging **23**(2), 153–163 (2004)
4. Rivaz, H., Boctor, E.M., Choti, M.A., Hager, G.D.: Real-time regularized ultrasound elastography. IEEE Trans. Med. Imaging **30**(4), 928–945 (2011)
5. Srinivasan, S., Righetti, R., Ophir, J.: Trade-offs between the axial resolution and the signal-to-noise ratio in elastography. Ultrasound Med. Biol. **29**(6), 847–866 (2003)
6. Zaleska-Dorobisz, U., Kaczorowski, K., Pawluś, A., Puchalska, A., Inglot, M.: Ultrasound elastography - review of techniques and its clinical applications. Adv. Clin. Exp. Med. **23**(4), 645–655 (2014)

3D Fetal Skull Reconstruction from 2DUS via Deep Conditional Generative Networks

Juan J. Cerrolaza[1]([✉]), Yuanwei Li[1], Carlo Biffi[1], Alberto Gomez[2],
Matthew Sinclair[1], Jacqueline Matthew[2], Caronline Knight[2], Bernhard Kainz[1],
and Daniel Rueckert[1]

[1] Biomedical Image Analysis Group, Imperial College London, London, UK
`j.cerrolaza-martinez@imperial.ac.uk`
[2] Division of Imaging Sciences and Biomedical Engineering,
King's College London, London, UK

Abstract. 2D ultrasound (US) is the primary imaging modality in ante-natal healthcare. Despite the limitations of traditional 2D biometrics to characterize the true 3D anatomy of the fetus, the adoption of 3DUS is still very limited. This is particularly significant in developing countries and remote areas, due to the lack of experienced sonographers and the limited access to 3D technology. In this paper, we present a new deep conditional generative network for the 3D reconstruction of the fetal skull from 2DUS standard planes of the head routinely acquired during the fetal screening process. Based on the generative properties of conditional variational autoencoders (CVAE), our reconstruction architecture (REC-CVAE) directly integrates the three US standard planes as conditional variables to generate a unified latent space of the skull. Additionally, we propose HiREC-CVAE, a hierarchical generative network based on the different clinical relevance of each predictive view. The hierarchical structure of HiREC-CVAE allows the network to learn a sequence of nested latent spaces, providing superior predictive capabilities even in the absence of some of the 2DUS scans. The performance of the proposed architectures was evaluated on a dataset of 72 cases, showing accurate reconstruction capabilities from standard non-registered 2DUS images.

Keywords: Generative model · Variational autoencoder
Fetal ultrasound

1 Introduction

Ultrasound (US) screening is the primary imaging modality for the prenatal evaluation of growth, gestational age estimation, and early structural abnormalities detection. Thanks to its non-ionizing nature, relative low-cost, and real-time visualization, a detailed mid-trimester morphology US scan is routinely performed at 18–22 weeks of gestation in most countries. As part of the examination, the quantification of 2D biometrics is extensively used to evaluate the

© Springer Nature Switzerland AG 2018
A. F. Frangi et al. (Eds.): MICCAI 2018, LNCS 11070, pp. 383–391, 2018.
https://doi.org/10.1007/978-3-030-00928-1_44

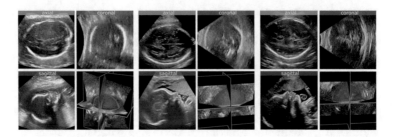

Fig. 1. Fetal standard US scans of the head. Example of the axial (green), sagittal (blue), and coronal (red) standard planes of three patients acquired in freeheand 2DUS during the routine mid-trimester US examination. The image also shows a 3D representation of the skull manually segmented from the corresponding 3DUS volume.

growth and well-being of the fetus. However, the detection rates of fetal abnormalities often remain below the recommended values [1], showing significant differences between industrialized and developing countries. Recently, new technological solutions have been proposed to assist in the acquisition of standard views in freehand 2DUS scans [2], improving reproducibility and reducing operator bias. However, the screening process is still constrained by the inherent limitation of 2D-based biometry to accurately characterize the true 3D anatomy of the fetus. Recent studies have reported on the advantages of 3DUS in the evaluation of fetal anatomy [3], and the superior diagnostic potential of 3D shape analysis over traditional 2D biometrics for the early detection and characterization of cranial deformations [4] (e.g., dolichocephaly, or craniosynostosis). Moreover, studies on 3DUS perception by medical professionals showed their interest in having access to 3D-based information during prenatal screening [5]. However, despite the reported advantages, there are three main factors that have notably hampered the adoption of 3D-based biometry by the obstetric community: (1) the lack of experience with 3DUS often slows down the acquisition process as compared to traditional 2DUS; (2) the need for new image processing solutions that enable efficient real-time analysis, visualization and reconstruction of volumetric information [6]; and (3) the limited access to 3D transducers, especially in developing countries [7]. Aware of these limitations, this paper presents a new practical approach for 3D head biometry, the 3D reconstruction of the fetal skull from standard planes in 2DUS, the current gold standard in obstetric radiology (see Fig. 1).

The reconstruction of 3D anatomical structures from a limited number of 2D views was previously studied as a strategy to reduce cost and radiation exposure to patients: e.g. reconstruction of the femur, pelvic bone, or vertebrae from X-ray images as alternative to 3D computed tomography [8,9]. Typically, these methods rely on deformable statistical models to incorporate *a priori* anatomical constraints to the generation process. Using contour- or registration-based strategies, these approaches often require complex density models of the bones to create virtual X-ray images that guide the generation process [8]. However, these simulation-based strategies are impractical in the less controlled environment of fetal sonography. Fetal US is arguably one of the most challenging imaging modalities, suffering from low signal-to-noise ratio, signal attenuation and dropout, as well as random shadows and occlusions frequently caused by unpredictable movements of the fetus.

With the advent of deep learning-based techniques, convolutional neural networks (CNNs) have become the current state-of-the-art for many medical imaging tasks, including semantic segmentation, and object recognition [2]. However, the prediction of 3D structures remains a relatively unexplored area, with only a few works using deep networks to address the mapping from 2D images to 3D volumes. Of special interest to our work is the TL-embedding network (TL-net) [10]. In this architecture, the authors use a 3D convolutional autoencoder (ConvAE) to generate a latent space of the 3D structures, using a second CNN to map 2D images to the corresponding coordinates in the latent space. Similarly, Wang and Fang [11] also used a common latent vector space between the 2D and the 3D image domains, combining ConvAE with adversarial learning to control the matching process in an unsupervised manner. Alternatively, Choy et al. [12] proposed a recurrent network to incrementally refine the reconstruction as more views of the object are provided. However, the proposed architectures normally rely on the availability of large-scale datasets, and/or the artificial generation of realistic 2D images from 3D synthetic models, both an important limitation when working with medical images.

In this paper, we present a new architecture to address the problem of fetal skull reconstruction from multiple 2DUS standard views of the head. First we propose a deep generative network using the conditional variational autoencoder (CVAE) formulation. Additionally, we present an alternative hierarchical framework, based on the different clinical relevance of each view. Imposing a specific hierarchy on the 2DUS standard views, the model learns a sequence of nested latent spaces, which allows the network to operate effectively even in the absence of any of the predictive views.

2   Method

In this paper, we formulate the 3D reconstruction problem in the form of a conditional manifold learning task. We use the CVAE framework [13] to create deep generative networks able to reconstruct the fetal skull, using freehand 2DUS standard views as predictive variables. These predictors are incorporated in the optimization model in the form of conditional variables, thus modulating the latent space of 3D skulls learned by the network.

Suppose $\mathbf{Y}$ represents a 3D parameterization of the fetal skull (e.g., a binary voxel map of the skull), with $\mathbf{X}_1$, $\mathbf{X}_2$ and $\mathbf{X}_3$ representing the corresponding 2DUS standard views acquired in the coronal, sagittal, and axial plane, respectively (see Fig. 1). For simplicity of notation we denote $\{\mathbf{X}_1, \mathbf{X}_2, \mathbf{X}_3\}$ as $\mathbf{X}_{1,2,3}$. We seek a generative model that learns the conditional distribution $P(\mathbf{Y}|\mathbf{X}_{1,2,3})$, so it produces a close approximation of $\mathbf{Y}^i$, for a given observation $\mathbf{X}_{1,2,3}^i$. In the context of variational autoencoders, the generative process is modeled by means of a latent d-dimensional variable, $\mathbf{z}$, with some known simple distribution (typically $\mathbf{z} \sim \mathcal{N}(\mathbf{0}, \mathbf{I})$). Thanks to this latent variable, the model can generate new instances of the target structure (i.e., the fetal skull) by randomly sampling values of $\mathbf{z}$. However, it would be very difficult in practice to directly infer $P(\mathbf{Y}|\mathbf{X}_{1,2,3})$ without sampling a large number of $\mathbf{z}$ values. Alternatively, we introduce a new function Q (e.g., a high-capacity function here parameterized in the form of a CNN), which can generate values of $\mathbf{z}$ likely to produce $\mathbf{Y}$s. Using Bayes' rule, we have $E_{\mathbf{z} \sim Q}\,[logP(\mathbf{Y}|\mathbf{z}, \mathbf{X}_{1,2,3})]$ $= E_{\mathbf{z} \sim Q}[logP(\mathbf{z}|\mathbf{Y}, \mathbf{X}_{1,2,3}) - logP(\mathbf{z}|\mathbf{X}_{1,2,3}) + logP(\mathbf{Y}|\mathbf{X}_{1,2,3})]$. Rearranging and subtracting $E_{z \sim Q}[logQ(\mathbf{z})]$ from both sides yields

$$logP(\mathbf{Y}|\mathbf{X}_{1,2,3}) - \mathcal{D}_{KL}[Q(\mathbf{z})\|P(\mathbf{z}|\mathbf{Y}, \mathbf{X}_{1,2,3})] =$$
$$E_{\mathbf{z} \sim Q}[logP(\mathbf{Y}|\mathbf{z}, \mathbf{X}_{1,2,3})] - \mathcal{D}_{KL}[Q(\mathbf{z})\|P(\mathbf{z}|\mathbf{X}_{1,2,3})], \tag{1}$$

where $\mathcal{D}_{KL}[a\|b] = E_{\mathbf{z} \sim Q}[log(a) - log(b)]$ represents the Kullback-Leibler (KL) divergence. Typically, the function Q is defined as $Q(\mathbf{z}|\mathbf{Y}, \mathbf{X}_{1,2,3}) = \mathcal{N}(\mathbf{z}|\mu(\mathbf{Y}, \mathbf{X}_{1,2,3}), \Sigma(\mathbf{Y}, \mathbf{X}_{1,2,3}))$ where μ and Σ are arbitrary, deterministic functions learned from the data, and parameterized in the form of CNNs (Σ is constrained to be a diagonal matrix). Since $P(\mathbf{z}|\mathbf{X}_{1,2,3})$ is still $\sim \mathcal{N}(\mathbf{0}, \mathbf{I})$ (i.e., assuming $\mathbf{z}$ is sampled independently of $\mathbf{X}_{1,2,3}$ at test time), this choice of Q allows us to compute $\mathcal{D}_{KL}[Q(\mathbf{z})\|P(\mathbf{z}|\mathbf{X}_{1,2,3})]$ as the KL-divergence between two Gaussians, which has a closed-form solution [13]. Optimizing the right hand side via stochastic gradient descent, and assuming Q is a high-capacity function which can approximate $P(\mathbf{z}|\mathbf{Y}, \mathbf{X}_{1,2,3})$, the KL-term on the left hand side of (1) will tend to 0. That is, we will be directly optimizing $P(\mathbf{Y}|\mathbf{X}_{1,2,3})$. At training time, we make the sampling of $\mathbf{z}$ differentiable with respect to μ and Σ by using the "reparameterization trick" [13], and defining $\mathbf{z}^i = \mu(\mathbf{Y}^i, \mathbf{X}^i_{1,2,3}) + \eta * \Sigma(\mathbf{Y}^i, \mathbf{X}^i_{1,2,3})$, where $\eta \sim \mathcal{N}(\mathbf{0}, \mathbf{I})$.

Based on equation (1), the reconstruction network can be implemented using CNNs, whose structure, at training time, resembles a traditional ConvAE. The function Q takes the form of the encoder, "encoding" $\mathbf{Y}$ and $\mathbf{X}_{1,2,3}$ into a d-dimensional latent space $\mathbf{z}$, via μ and Σ. In the proposed architecture, we use a multi-branch CNN to model Q, using 3D convolutional filters for $\mathbf{Y}$, and a separate view-specific bank of 2D filters for each standard view. The outputs of each branch are concatenated and mapped to two separate fully-connected layers to generate $\mu(\mathbf{Y}, \mathbf{X}_{1,2,3})$ and $\Sigma(\mathbf{Y}, \mathbf{X}_{1,2,3})$, which will be combined with η to create $\mathbf{z}$. Finally, the decoder of the network, modeled also as a CNN, reconstructs $\mathbf{Y}$ given $\mathbf{z}$ and $\mathbf{X}_{1,2,3}$. The conditional dependency on $\mathbf{X}_{1,2,3}$ is explicitly modeled by the concatenation of $\mathbf{z}$ with the vector representation of $\mathbf{X}_{1,2,3}$ (see Fig. 2(a)). At test time, the decoder operates as a generative reconstruction network given the coronal, $\mathbf{X}_1$, sagittal, $\mathbf{X}_2$, and axial, $\mathbf{X}_3$ 2DUS views, generating valid 3D skulls by sampling $\mathbf{z} \sim \mathcal{N}(\mathbf{0}, \mathbf{I})$. In particular, we generate the highest-confidence prediction with $\mathbf{z} = \mathbf{0}$.

With this configuration, the reconstruction network requires the three standard views to approximate the 3D fetal skull. However, it is common in clinical practice that not all the standard views of the head are routinely acquired,

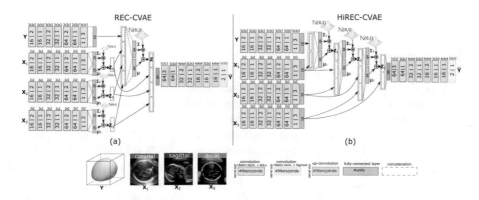

Fig. 2. Deep generative networks for the reconstruction of the fetal skull. (a) REC-CVAE: Reconstruction network based on the conditional variational autoencoder framework. (b) HiREC-CVAE: Hierarchical reconstruction network.

thus limiting the potential utility of our model in retrospective studies. During the mid-trimester examination, axial views of the head (i.e., X_3) are routinely acquired and used for 2D biometrics measurements (e.g., head circumference and biparietal diameter). Additionally, a sagittal view (X_2) is also normally acquired to ensure there is a normal face/head shape. However, coronal planes (X_1) are usually only included as part of a dedicated scan, used to clarify suspicious findings. To make the reconstruction network more flexible and operative in the absence of some of the standard views, we propose two alternative architectures. In the first model, we define the conditional variables as three multidimensional Gaussians $\mathcal{N}(\mathbf{0}, \mathbf{I})$, $\mathbf{z}_1$, $\mathbf{z}_2$, and $\mathbf{z}_3$. Thus, if X_1, or X_2 are missing at test time, we still can approximate $\mathbf{Y}$ with the same network, by sampling $\mathbf{z}_1$, or $\mathbf{z}_2$. The resulting objective function is $CE(\mathbf{Y}, \widehat{\mathbf{Y}}) - \nu(\mathcal{D}_{KL}[\mathbf{z}\|\mathcal{N}(\mathbf{0}, \mathbf{I})] + \sum_{i=i,2,3} \mathcal{D}_{KL}[\mathbf{z}_i\|\mathcal{N}(\mathbf{0}, \mathbf{I})])$, where the first term represents the cross-entropy (CE) between $\mathbf{Y}$ and the reconstructed $\widehat{\mathbf{Y}}$, and ν is a constant set to 0.01. See Fig. 2(a) for a detailed description of the proposed reconstruction network using CVAE (REC-CVAE). While REC-CVAE represents a more direct implementation of the CVAE formulation, we propose a second configuration that explicitly incorporates the predefined hierarchy of the conditional variables as a cascade of conditional blocks, HiREC-CVAE (see Fig. 2(b)). In the first block, only X_1 is used as conditional variable for $\mathbf{Y}$, thus defining a latent space, $\mathbf{z}_1$, for $\mathbf{Y}|X_1$. The sagittal and axial planes are incorporated in the second and third blocks, producing $\mathbf{z}_2$, and $\mathbf{z}_3$, respectively. Unlike REC-CVAE, where a single generative latent space is defined, $\mathbf{z}_1, \mathbf{z}_2, \mathbf{z}_3$ can be interpreted as a set of nested latent spaces. Now, in the absence of one of the views, we are sampling from the corresponding latent-spaces, that effectively integrate the missing components into a manifold of fetal skulls. The resulting objective function is $CE(\mathbf{Y}, \widehat{\mathbf{Y}}) - \nu(\sum_{i=i,2,3} \mathcal{D}_{KL}[\mathbf{z}_i\|\mathcal{N}(\mathbf{0}, \mathbf{I})])$.

3 Results

Both approaches for fetal skull reconstruction were evaluated on a dataset of 72 cases. For each case, one 3DUS volume of the head, and at least one image from each of the standard views in the coronal, sagittal, and transventricular axial planes were acquired by an experienced obstetric sonographer during routine mid-trimester examination (i.e., more than one image per standard view were available for some cases). The mean gestational age was 24.7 weeks, ranging from 20 to 36 weeks. The images were acquired using a Philips Epiq7G US system, with a X6-1 xMatrix array transducer. The data were preprocessed using non-local means filtering, and resampled to isotropic size of 0.50 mm per dimension; the 3D volumes and the 2D standard planes were resized to $96 \times 96 \times 96$ voxels, and to 96×96 pixels, respectively, using cropping and zero-padding if needed. For each volume, the skull was manually delineated under the supervision of an expert radiologist. In this study, we consider a smooth reconstruction of the cranial region located above the transthalamic plane, including the parietal and frontal bones, and excluding the facial bones, sutures and fontanels. The set of manual segmentations were aligned and used as ground-truth for skull reconstruction. No registration was used for the standard planes, using only flipping or mirroring to provide orientation consistency (e.g., the fetus is approximately looking up in the sagittal views as shown in Fig. 1). The patients were randomly divided in two groups, using 58 cases for training and 14 for testing. This process was repeated three times, always using a different subset for testing. During training, data augmentation was applied to the ground-truth volumes, applying random anisotropic scaling in the three orthogonal axes. This strategy allowed us, not only to expand the training set, but also to replicate potential fetal skull anomalies, such as dolichocephaly or trigonocephaly. One image for each standard view was randomly selected, if more than one scan were available, and deformed independently using the corresponding anisotropic scaling, and random translation and rotation. The reconstruction capability of REC-CVAE and HiREC-CVAE was compared with the TL-net, a CNNs-based state-of-the-art architecture for 2D-to-3D reconstruction [10] (see Sect. 1). The TL-net configuration is depicted in Fig. 3(a). All the networks were trained for 1000 epochs on an NVIDIA® GeForce® 1080 Ti (approx. 12 hours per network), using stochastic gradient descent with momentum (Adam with learning rate $= 0.001$, $\beta_1 = 0.9$, and $\beta_2 = 0.995$) in Theano, using a small batch size of 1.

Table 1. The table presents the average and standard deviation for the Dice's coefficient (DC), sensitivity (SEN.), and precision (PPV) of the reconstruction of the fetal skull, and the effect of using three, two, or one standard US views as predictors.

	axial + sagittal + coronal			axial + sagittal			axial		
	DC	SEN.	PPV	DC	SEN.	PPV	DC	SEN.	PPV
REC-CVAE	0.91 ± 0.02	0.91 ± 0.05	0.91 ± 0.06	0.86 ± 0.05	0.88 ± 0.13	0.87 ± 0.09	0.83 ± 0.06	0.86 ± 0.15	0.84 ± 0.13
HiREC-CVAE	0.91 ± 0.04	0.89 ± 0.06	0.93 ± 0.06	0.89 ± 0.05	0.90 ± 0.10	0.91 ± 0.08	0.86 ± 0.05	0.86 ± 0.11	0.90 ± 0.08
TL-net	0.89 ± 0.03	0.93 ± 0.05	0.86 ± 0.07	0.89 ± 0.05	0.90 ± 0.11	0.90 ± 0.06	0.85 ± 0.04	0.88 ± 0.05	0.80 ± 0.09

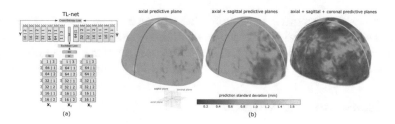

Fig. 3. (a) TL-net architecture (see Fig. 2 for a description of the constituent blocks). The network assumes the three views are used for the reconstruction. A separate network with two $(\mathbf{X}_2, \mathbf{X}_3)$ or one $(\mathbf{X}_3)$ predictors is defined if any of the views are missing. (b) Prediction uncertainty in HiREC-CVAE for a varying number of predictors. The images represent the standard deviation of $N = 50$ different predictions randomly generated from the latent spaces.

Table 1 shows the reconstruction accuracy for the three architectures when using three (coronal, sagittal, and axial), two (sagittal and axial) or one (axial) US standard views as predictors. During testing, the 3D encoder branch was disabled, setting the latent variables $\mathbf{z}$ and $\mathbf{z}_1$ to $\mathbf{0}$, in REC-CVAE and HiREC-CVAE, respectively. In the absence of the coronal or also the sagittal view, the corresponding latent variables, $\mathbf{z}_1$ and $\mathbf{z}_2$ in REC-CVAE, and $\mathbf{z}_2$ and $\mathbf{z}_3$ in HiREC-CVAE, were also set to $\mathbf{0}$ (see Fig. 2). For TL-net, three different case-specific configurations of the network were trained in order to deal with a varying number of available standard views. When using the three planes, REC-CVAE and HiREC-CVAE showed slightly higher (although not statistically significant) performance than the TL-net (e.g., $DC_{REC-CVAE} = 0.91 \pm 0.02$, $DC_{HiREC-CVAE} = 0.91 \pm 0.04$, and $DC_{TL-net} = 0.89 \pm 0.03$). However, the performance of REC-CVAE was significantly affected when one or two of the views were missing ($DC_{REC-CVAE} = 0.86 \pm 0.05$, and 0.83 ± 0.06, respectively). One important limitation in REC-CVAE is the independent Gaussian encoding of the predictors. While this allows the network to operate in the absence of any of the views by automatically generating a valid input from the predefined distributions, the resulting semi-optimal code passed to the decoder (e.g., $(\mathbf{0}, \mathbf{0}, \mathbf{0}, \mathbf{z}_3)$) can produce an inaccurate reconstruction of the skull. In HiREC-CAE, the potential correlation between the predictors is effectively encoded through a three-level nested space of latent variables, showing good reconstruction capabilities even when the coronal, or also the sagittal planes are absent ($DC_{HiREC-CVAE} = 0.89 \pm 0.05$, and 0.86 ± 0.05, respectively). Similar performance was obtained with the dedicated case-specific TL-nets ($DC_{TL-net} = 0.89 \pm 0.05$ and 0.85 ± 0.04), although a separate case-specific network is needed for each scenario. Moreover, the TL-nets require a three-stage training process [10], instead of the end-to-end approach used in REC-CVAE and HiREC-CVAE.

Finally, the generative capability of HiREC-CVAE can be exploited to generate a confidence map of the reconstructed skull. Here, we define the confidence maps as the standard deviation of N ($N = 50$ in Fig. 3(b)) different predictions, randomly generated by sampling z_1, z_2, or z_3 from $\mathcal{N}(0, I)$. These maps can be generated in real-time (each prediction is generated in ~ 0.04 sec.), and used as an indirect indicator of the reconstruction accuracy, thus informing the sonographer about the need of additional views for a more accurate result.

4   Discussion and Conclusion

This paper presents the first deep conditional generative network for the 3D reconstruction of the fetal skull from freehand non-aligned 2D scans of the head. We propose two different models, REC-CVAE, based on the CVAE formulation, and HiREC-CVAE, an alternative configuration that effectively encodes a predefined hierarchy of the predictive variables. Both networks learn a low-dimensional embedding representation of the skull, which guarantees the anatomical consistency of the reconstructions. Moreover, the use of a predefined distribution model for the latent space allows the networks to operate even when some of the 2DUS images are missing. The results demonstrate the potential of the networks for the 3D reconstruction and characterization of the fetal skull from 2DUS standard planes. This framework can contribute significantly to the popularization of 3D-based fetal screening, allowing for large-scale 3D-based biometrics studies that include a wide and varied demographic representation, including cases from developing countries with limited access to 3D transducer technology. In the near future, we will continue exploring the clinical value of the proposed framework and its potential for the early detection and characterization of congenital deformations. We also plan to explore the potential of deep conditional generative networks for 3D cardiac reconstruction from cardiac cine MRI.

Acknowledgement. This research was supported in part by the Marie Sklodowska-Curie Actions of the EU Framework Programme for Research and Innovation, under REA grant agreement 706372.

References

1. Springett, A., et al.: Congenital Anomaly Statistics, 2012. England and Wales. Technical report, British Isles Network of Congenital Anomaly Registerss (2014)
2. Baumgartner, C., et al.: Sononet: real-time detection and localisation of fetal standard scan planes in freehand ultrasound. IEEE TMI **36**, 2204–2215 (2017)
3. Lima, J., et al.: Biometry and fetal weight estimation by two-dimensional and three-dimensional ultrasonography: an intraobserver and interobserver reliability and agreement study. Ultrasound Obstet. Gynecol. **40**, 186–93 (2012)
4. Matthew, J., et al. Novel 3D ultrasound-based metric to assess the fetal skull: a pilot study. In: BMUS Annual Meeting (2017)
5. Lee, S., et al.: Prenatal three-dimensional ultrasound: perception of sonographers, sonologists and undergraduate students. Ultrasound Obstet. Gynecol. **1**(30), 77–80 (2007)
6. Cerrolaza, J.J.: Fetal skull segmentation in 3D ultrasound via structured geodesic random forest. In: Cardoso, M.J. (ed.) FIFI/OMIA -2017. LNCS, vol. 10554, pp. 25–32. Springer, Cham (2017). https://doi.org/10.1007/978-3-319-67561-9_3

7. Shah, S., et al.: Perceived barriers in the use of ultrasound in developing countries. Crit. Ultrasound J. **7**(1), 7–11 (2015)
8. Whitmarsh, T., et al.: Reconstructing the 3D shape and bone mineral density distribution of the proximal femur from dual-energy x-ray absorptiometry. IEEE TMI **12**(30), 2101–2114 (2011)
9. Ehlke, M., et al.: Fast generation of virtual x-ray images for reconstruction of 3D anatomy. IEEE TVCG **19**(12), 2673–2682 (2013)
10. Girdhar, R., Fouhey, D.F., Rodriguez, M., Gupta, A.: Learning a predictable and generative vector representation for objects. In: Leibe, B., Matas, J., Sebe, N., Welling, M. (eds.) ECCV 2016. LNCS, vol. 9910, pp. 484–499. Springer, Cham (2016). https://doi.org/10.1007/978-3-319-46466-4_29
11. Wang, L., Fang, Y.: Unsupervised 3D reconstruction from a single image via adversarial learning (2017). CoRR, abs/1711.09312
12. Choy, C.B., Xu, D., Gwak, J.Y., Chen, K., Savarese, S.: 3D-R2N2: a unified approach for single and multi-view 3D object reconstruction. In: Leibe, B., Matas, J., Sebe, N., Welling, M. (eds.) ECCV 2016. LNCS, vol. 9912, pp. 628–644. Springer, Cham (2016). https://doi.org/10.1007/978-3-319-46484-8_38
13. Kingma, D.P., Welling, M.: Auto-encoding variational bayes. In: ICLR 2014 (2014)

Standard Plane Detection in 3D Fetal Ultrasound Using an Iterative Transformation Network

Yuanwei Li[1]([✉]), Bishesh Khanal[2], Benjamin Hou[1], Amir Alansary[1],
Juan J. Cerrolaza[1], Matthew Sinclair[1], Jacqueline Matthew[2], Chandni Gupta[2],
Caroline Knight[2], Bernhard Kainz[1], and Daniel Rueckert[1]

[1] Biomedical Image Analysis Group, Imperial College London, London, UK
yuanwei.li09@imperial.ac.uk
[2] School of Biomedical Engineering and Imaging Sciences,
King's College London, London, UK

Abstract. Standard scan plane detection in fetal brain ultrasound (US) forms a crucial step in the assessment of fetal development. In clinical settings, this is done by manually manoeuvring a 2D probe to the desired scan plane. With the advent of 3D US, the entire fetal brain volume containing these standard planes can be easily acquired. However, manual standard plane identification in 3D volume is labour-intensive and requires expert knowledge of fetal anatomy. We propose a new Iterative Transformation Network (ITN) for the automatic detection of standard planes in 3D volumes. ITN uses a convolutional neural network to learn the relationship between a 2D plane image and the transformation parameters required to move that plane towards the location/orientation of the standard plane in the 3D volume. During inference, the current plane image is passed iteratively to the network until it converges to the standard plane location. We explore the effect of using different transformation representations as regression outputs of ITN. Under a multi-task learning framework, we introduce additional classification probability outputs to the network to act as confidence measures for the regressed transformation parameters in order to further improve the localisation accuracy. When evaluated on 72 US volumes of fetal brain, our method achieves an error of 3.83 mm/12.7° and 3.80 mm/12.6° for the transventricular and transcerebellar planes respectively and takes 0.46 s per plane.

1 Introduction

Obstetric ultrasound (US) is conducted as a routine screening examination between 18–24 weeks of gestation. US imaging of the fetal head enables clinicians to assess fetal brain development and detect growth abnormalities. This

Electronic supplementary material The online version of this chapter (https:// doi.org/10.1007/978-3-030-00928-1_45) contains supplementary material, which is available to authorized users.

A. F. Frangi et al. (Eds.): MICCAI 2018, LNCS 11070, pp. 392–400, 2018.
https://doi.org/10.1007/978-3-030-00928-1_45

requires the careful selection of standard scan planes such as the transventricular (TV) and transcerebellar (TC) plane that contain key anatomical structures [6]. However, it is challenging and time-consuming even for experienced sonographers to manually navigate a 2D US probe to find the correct standard plane. The task is highly operator-dependent and requires a great amount of expertise. With the advent of 3D fetal US, a volume of the entire fetal brain can be acquired quickly with little training. But the problem of locating diagnostically required standard planes for biometric measurements remains. There is a strong need to develop automatic methods for 2D standard plane extraction from 3D volumes to improve clinical workflow efficiency.

Related work: Recently, deep learning approaches have shown successes in many medical image analysis applications. Several works have applied deep learning techniques to standard plane detection in fetal US [1–3,7]. Baumgartner et al. [1] use a convolutional neural network (CNN) for categorisation of 13 fetal standard views. Chen et al. [3] adopt a CNN-based image classification approach for detecting fetal abdominal standard planes, which they later combined with a recurrent neural network (RNN) that takes into account temporal information [2]. However, these methods identify standard planes from 2D US videos and not 3D volumes. Ryou et al. [7] attempt to detect fetal head and abdominal planes from 3D fetal US by breaking down the 3D volume into a stack of 2D slices which are then classified as head or abdomen using a CNN.

Plane detection is considered an image classification problem in the above works. In contrast, we approach the plane detection problem by regressing rigid transformation parameters that define the plane position and orientation. There are several works on using CNN to predict transformations. Kendall et al. [5] introduce PoseNet for regressing 6-DoF camera pose from RGB image with a loss function that uses quaternions to represent rotation. Hou et al. [4] propose SVRNet for predicting transformation from 2D image to 3D space and use anchor points as a new representation for rigid transformations. These works predict absolute transformation with respect to a known reference coordinate system with one pass of CNN. Our work is different as we use an iterative approach with multiple passes of CNN to predict relative transformation with respect to current plane coordinates, which change at each iteration. Relative transformation is used as our 3D volumes are not aligned to a reference coordinate system.

Contributions: In this paper, we propose the Iterative Transformation Network (ITN) that uses a CNN to detect standard planes in 3D fetal US. The network learns a mapping between a 2D plane and the transformation required to move that plane towards the standard plane within a 3D volume. Our contributions are threefold: **(1)** ITN is a general deep learning framework built for 2D plane detection in 3D volumes. The iterative approach regresses transformations that bring the plane closer to the standard plane. This reduces computation cost as ITN selectively samples only a few planes in the 3D volume unlike classification-based methods that require dense sampling [1–3,7]. **(2)** We study the effect on plane detection accuracy using different transformation representations (quaternions, Euler angles, rotation matrix, anchor points) as CNN regression outputs. **(3)** We

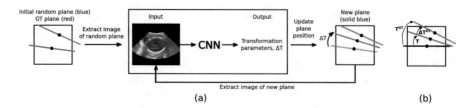

(a)   (b)

Fig. 1. (a) Overall plane detection framework using ITN. (b) Composition of transformations. Red: GT plane. Blue: Arbitrary plane. Black: Identity plane.

improve ITN performance by incorporating additional classification probability outputs as confidence measures of the regressed transformation parameters. At inference, the classification probabilities are used as confidence scores to yield more accurate localisation. During training, regression and classification outputs are learned in a multi-task learning framework, which improves the generalisation ability of the model and prevents overfitting.

2   Method

Overall Framework: Fig. 1a presents the overall ITN framework for plane detection. Given a 3D volume V, the goal is to find the ground truth (GT) standard plane (red). Starting with a random plane initialisation (blue), the 2D image of the plane is extracted and input to a CNN which then predicts a 3D transformation ΔT that will move the plane to a new position closer to the GT plane. The image extracted at the new plane location is then passed to the CNN and the process is repeated until the plane reaches the GT plane.

Composition of Transformations: Transformation is defined with respect to a reference coordinate system. In Fig. 1b, we define an identity plane (black) with origin at the volume centre. T and T^{GT} are defined in the coordinate system of the identity plane and they move the identity plane to the arbitrary plane (blue) and GT plane (red) respectively. ΔT^{GT} is defined in the coordinate system of the arbitrary plane and ΔT^{GT} moves the arbitrary plane to the GT plane. Note that our ITN predicts ΔT^{GT} which is a relative transformation from the point of view of the current plane, and *not* from the identity plane. We compute these transformations from each other using $T^{GT} = T \oplus \Delta T^{GT}$ and $\Delta T^{GT} = T^{GT} \ominus T$ where $\oplus$ and $\ominus$ are the composition and inverse composition operators respectively. The computations defined by the operators are dependent on the choice of the transformation representation.

Network Training: During training, an arbitrary plane is randomly sampled from a volume V by applying a random transformation T to the identity plane. The corresponding 2D plane image X is then extracted. We define $X = I(V, T, s)$ where $I(\cdot)$ is the plane extraction function and s is the length of the square plane. We sample T such that the plane centre falls in the middle 60% of V and the rotation of the plane is within an angle of $\pm 45°$ about each coordinate axis.

Algorithm 1. Iterative Inference of Transformation

1: **procedure** PLANE TRANSFORMATION(V, s, N)
2:     Initialise random plane with T_1
3:     **for** $i = 1$ **to** N **do**
4:         $X_i \leftarrow I(V, T_i, s)$ ▷ Sample plane image
5:         $\Delta T \leftarrow \text{CNN}(X_i)$ ▷ CNN predicts relative transformation
6:         $T_{i+1} \leftarrow T_i \oplus \Delta T$ ▷ Update plane position
7:     **return** T_N

Table 1. Representations of rigid transformations and their loss functions.

Representation (Parameter count)	Loss function
Translation t (3) + Quaternion q (4)	$L = \alpha\left\|t^{GT} - t\right\|_2^2 + \beta\left\|q^{GT} - \frac{q}{\|q\|}\right\|_2^2$
Translation t (3) + Euler angles θ (3)	$L = \alpha\left\|t^{GT} - t\right\|_2^2 + \beta\left\|\theta^{GT} - \theta\right\|_2^2$
Translation t (3) + Rotation matrix R (9)	$L = \alpha\left\|t^{GT} - t\right\|_2^2 + \beta\left\|R^{GT} - R\right\|_2^2$
Anchor points (A_1, A_2, A_3) (9)	$L = \sum_{i=1}^{3}\left\|A_i^{GT} - A_i\right\|_2^2$

This avoids sampling of planes at the edges of the volume where there is no informative image data due to regions falling outside of the US imaging cone.

A training sample is represented by $(X, \Delta T^{GT})$ and the training loss function can be formulated as the $L2$ norm of the error between the GT and predicted transformation parameters: $L = \left\|\Delta T^{GT} - \Delta T\right\|_2^2$

Network Inference: Algorithm 1 summarises the steps during network inference to detect a plane. The iterative approach gives rough estimates of the plane in the first few iterations and subsequently makes smaller and more accurate refinements. This coarse-to-fine adjustment improves accuracy and is less susceptible to different initialisations. To improve accuracy and convergence, we repeat Algorithm 1 with 5 random plane initialisations per volume and average their final transformations T_N after N iterations.

Transformation Representations: In ITN, plane transformation ΔT is rigid, comprising only translation and rotation. We explore the effect of using different transformation representations as the CNN regression outputs (Table 1) since there are few comparative studies that investigate this on deep networks. The first three representations explicitly separate translation and rotation in which rotation is represented by quaternions, Euler angles and rotation matrix respectively. α and β are weightings given to the translation and rotation losses. Specifically, anchor points [4] are defined as the coordinates of three fixed points on the plane (we use: centre, bottom-left and bottom-right corner). The points uniquely and jointly represent any translation and rotation in 3D space. During inference, the predicted values of certain representations need to be constrained to give valid rotation. For instance, quaternions need to be normalised to unit quaternions and rotation matrices need to be orthogonalised. Anchor points need to be converted to valid rotation matrices as described in [4].

Algorithm 2. Compute relative transformation ΔT

1: **procedure** COMPUTE TRANSFORM($\boldsymbol{t}, \boldsymbol{q}, \boldsymbol{P}, \boldsymbol{Q}$)

2: $\quad \boldsymbol{t}_{new} = \begin{pmatrix} \max\left(P_{c_1^+}, P_{c_1^-}\right) t_1 \\ \max\left(P_{c_2^+}, P_{c_2^-}\right) t_2 \\ \max\left(P_{c_3^+}, P_{c_3^-}\right) t_3 \end{pmatrix}$ $\qquad \triangleright$ Compute weighted translation

3: $\quad Q_{max} = \max\left(\boldsymbol{Q}\right)$ $\qquad\qquad\qquad\qquad \triangleright$ Compute weighted rotation

4: $\quad$ **if** $Q_{max} = Q_{k_x^+}$ **OR** $Q_{k_x^-}$ **then**

5: $\qquad$ Convert $\boldsymbol{q}$ to Euler angles $(\theta_x, \theta_y, \theta_z)$ using convention 'xyz'

6: $\qquad \boldsymbol{r}_{new} \leftarrow$ Rotation about x-axis with magnitude $Q_{max}\theta_x$

7: $\quad$ **else if** $Q_{max} = Q_{k_y^+}$ **OR** $Q_{k_y^-}$ **then**

8: $\qquad$ Convert $\boldsymbol{q}$ to Euler angles $(\theta_x, \theta_y, \theta_z)$ using convention 'yxz'

9: $\qquad \boldsymbol{r}_{new} \leftarrow$ Rotation about y-axis with magnitude $Q_{max}\theta_y$

10: $\quad$ **else if** $Q_{max} = Q_{k_z^+}$ **OR** $Q_{k_z^-}$ **then**

11: $\qquad$ Convert $\boldsymbol{q}$ to Euler angles $(\theta_x, \theta_y, \theta_z)$ using convention 'zxy'

12: $\qquad \boldsymbol{r}_{new} \leftarrow$ Rotation about z-axis with magnitude $Q_{max}\theta_z$

13: $\quad \Delta T \leftarrow (\boldsymbol{t}_{new}, \boldsymbol{r}_{new})$

14: $\quad$ **return** ΔT

Classification Probability as Confidence Measure: We further extend our ITN by incorporating classification probability as a confidence measure for the regressed values of translation and rotation. The method can be applied to any transformation representation but we use quaternions since it yields the best results. In addition to the regression outputs $\boldsymbol{t}$ and $\boldsymbol{q}$, the CNN also predicts two classification probability outputs $\boldsymbol{P}$ and $\boldsymbol{Q}$ for translation and rotation respectively. We divide translation into 6 discrete classification categories: positive and negative translation along each coordinate axis. Denoting c as the translation classification label, we have $c \in \{c_1^+, c_1^-, c_2^+, c_2^-, c_3^+, c_3^-\}$ where c_1^+ is the category representing translation along the positive x-axis. $\boldsymbol{P}$ is then a 6-element vector giving the probability of translation along each axis direction. Similarly, we divide rotation into 6 categories: clockwise and counter-clockwise rotation about each coordinate axis. Denoting k as the rotation classification label, we have $k \in \{k_1^+, k_1^-, k_2^+, k_2^-, k_3^+, k_3^-\}$ where k_1^+ is the category representing clockwise rotation about the x-axis. $\boldsymbol{Q}$ is then a 6-element vector giving the probability of rotation about each axis.

A training sample is represented by $(X, \boldsymbol{t}^{GT}, \boldsymbol{q}^{GT}, c^{GT}, k^{GT})$. c^{GT} gives the coordinate axis along which the current plane centre has the furthest absolute distance from the GT plane centre. Similarly, k^{GT} gives the coordinate axis about which the current plane will rotate the most to reach the GT plane. Appendix A derives the computations of c^{GT} and k^{GT} during training. The overall training loss function can then be written as:

$$L = \alpha \left\| \boldsymbol{t}^{GT} - \boldsymbol{t} \right\|_2^2 + \beta \left\| \boldsymbol{q}^{GT} - \frac{\boldsymbol{q}}{\|\boldsymbol{q}\|} \right\|_2^2 - \gamma \log P_{c^{GT}} - \delta \log Q_{k^{GT}} \qquad (1)$$

The first and second terms are the $L2$ losses for translation and rotation regression while the third and fourth terms are the cross-entropy losses for translation and rotation classification. α, β, γ and δ are weights given to the losses.

During inference, the CNN outputs t, q, P and Q are combined to compute the relative transformation ΔT (Algorithm 2). For translation, each component of the regressed translation t is weighted by the corresponding probabilities in the vector P. For rotation, we only rotate the plane about the most confident rotation axis as predicted by Q. In order to determine the magnitude of that rotation, the regressed quaternion q needs to be broken down into Euler angles using the appropriate convention in order to determine the rotation angle about that most confident rotation axis. An Euler angle representation using convention 'xyz' means a rotation about x-axis first followed by y-axis and finally z-axis. Hence, P and Q are used as confidence weighting for t and q, allowing the plane to translate and rotate to a greater extent along the more confident axis.

Network Architecture: ITN utilises a multi-task learning framework for predictions of multiple outputs. The architecture differs according to the number of outputs that the CNN predicts. All our networks comprise 5 convolution layers, each followed by a max-pooling layer. These layers contain shared features for all outputs. After the 5th pooling layer, the network branches into fully-connected layers to learn the specific features for each output. Details of all network architectures are described in Appendix B.

3   Experiments and Results

Data and Experiments: ITN is evaluated on 3D US volumes of fetal brain from 72 subjects. For each volume, TV and TC standard planes are manually selected by a clinical expert. 70% of the dataset is randomly selected for training and the rest 30% used for testing. All volumes are processed to be isotropic with mean dimensions of $324 \times 207 \times 279$ voxels. ITN is implemented using Tensorflow running on a machine with Intel Xeon CPU E5-1630 at $3.70\,\mathrm{GHz}$ and one NVIDIA Titan Xp 12GB GPU. We set plane size $s=225$, $N=10$ and $\alpha=\beta=\gamma=\delta=1$. During training, we use a batch size of 64. Weights are initialised randomly from a distribution with zero mean and 0.1 standard deviation. Optimisation is carried out for 100,000 iterations using the Adam algorithm with learning rate=0.001, $\beta_1=0.9$ and $\beta_2=0.999$. The predicted plane is evaluated against the GT using distance between the plane centres (δx) and rotation angle between the planes $(\delta\theta)$. Image similarity of the planes is also measured using peak signal-to-noise ratio (PSNR) and structural similarity (SSIM).

Results: Table 2 compares the plane detection results when different transformation representations are used by ITN. In general, there is little difference in the translation error. This is because all translation representations are the same, which use the three Cartesian axes except for anchor points which have slightly greater translation error. The rotation errors on TC plane suggest that quaternions are a good representation. Rotation matrices and anchor points

Table 2. Evaluation of ITN with different transformation representations for standard plane detection. Results presented as (Mean ± Standard Deviation).

CNN outputs	TV plane				TC plane			
	δx (mm)	$\delta\theta$ (°)	PSNR	SSIM	δx (mm)	$\delta\theta$ (°)	PSNR	SSIM
t, q	6.29±5.33	17.0±12.0	15.3±2.0	0.375±0.081	6.23±6.99	14.9±7.5	15.5±2.1	0.383±0.100
t, θ	5.69±5.85	17.0±8.5	15.2±1.7	0.372±0.084	7.13±9.00	16.0±5.9	14.6±2.4	0.357±0.119
t, R	5.79±6.10	17.7±11.6	15.8±1.9	0.389±0.091	6.39±7.39	17.3±15.4	15.5±2.4	0.385±0.118
A_1, A_2, A_3	6.64±8.66	17.0±10.4	15.9±2.4	0.399±0.099	7.88±10.0	16.3±12.6	15.0±2.7	0.351±0.124

over-parameterise rotation and can make network learning more difficult with greater degree of freedom. Since these parameters are not constrained, it is also harder to convert them back into valid rotations during inference. Quaternions have fewer parameters and slightly-off quaternion can still be easily normalised to give valid rotation. Compared to Euler angles, quaternions avoid the problem of gimbal lock. For TV plane, there is little difference in rotation error. This is because sonographers use the TV plane as a visual reference when acquiring 3D volumes. This causes the TV plane to lie roughly in the central plane of the volume with lower rotation variances, thus making the choice of rotation representation less important. Table 3 compares the performance of ITN with/without classification probability outputs. Given a baseline model (M1) that only has regression outputs t, q, the addition of classification probabilities P, Q improves the translation and rotation accuracy respectively (M2-M4). The classification probabilities act as confidence weights for the regression outputs to improve plane detection accuracy. Furthermore, the classification and regression outputs are trained in a multi-task learning fashion, which allows feature sharing and enables more generic features to be learned, thus preventing model overfitting. M1-M4 use one plane image as CNN input. We further improve our results by using three orthogonal plane images instead as this provides more information about the 3D volume (M4+). M4 and M4+ take 0.46 s and 1.35 s to predict one plane per volume. The supplementary material provides videos showing the update of a randomly initialised plane and its extracted image through 10 inference iterations.

Figure 2 shows a visual comparison between the GT planes and the planes predicted by M4. To evaluate the clinical relevance of the predicted planes, a

Table 3. Evaluation of ITN with/without confidence probability for standard plane detection. Results presented as (Mean ± Standard Deviation).

CNN outputs	TV plane				TC plane			
	δx (mm)	$\delta\theta$ (°)	PSNR	SSIM	δx (mm)	$\delta\theta$ (°)	PSNR	SSIM
M1: t, q	6.29±5.33	17.0±12.0	15.3±2.0	0.375±0.081	6.23±6.99	14.9±7.5	15.5±2.1	0.383±0.100
M2: t, q, P	5.14±5.37	16.8±9.9	16.0±2.1	0.408±0.092	5.12±5.50	13.9±7.1	15.8±2.2	0.393±0.115
M3: t, q, Q	6.07±6.32	14.0±8.1	15.7±2.5	0.399±0.108	7.66±7.14	12.7±6.0	15.5±3.0	0.386±0.123
M4: t, q, P, Q	3.83±2.10	12.7±7.7	16.4±1.9	**0.419±0.092**	3.80±1.85	12.6±6.1	16.5±2.1	0.407±0.110
M4+: t, q, P, Q	**3.49±1.81**	**10.7±5.7**	**16.6±1.8**	0.413±0.082	**3.39±2.13**	**11.4±6.3**	**16.8±2.1**	**0.437±0.110**

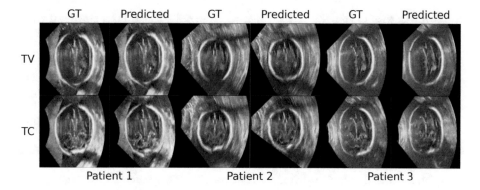

Fig. 2. Visualisation of GT planes and planes predicted by M4.

clinical expert manually measures the head circumference (HC) on both the predicted and GT planes and computes the standard deviation of the measurement error to be 1.05 mm (TV) and 1.25 mm (TC). This is similar to the intraobserver variability of 2.65 mm reported for HC measurements on TC plane [8]. Thus, accurate biometrics can be extracted from our predicted planes.

4   Conclusion

We presented ITN, a new approach for standard plane detection in 3D fetal US by using a CNN to regress rigid transformation iteratively. We compare the use of different transformation representations and show quaternions to be a good representation for iterative pose estimation. Additional classification probabilities are learned via multi-task learning which act as confidence weights for the regressed transformation parameters to improve plane detection accuracy. As future work, we are evaluating ITN on other plane detection tasks (*eg.* view plane selection in cardiac MRI). It is also worthwhile to explore new transformation representations and extend ITN to simultaneous detection of multiple planes.

Acknowledgments. Supported by the Wellcome Trust IEH Award [102431]. The authors thank Nvidia Corporation for the donation of a Titan Xp GPU.

References

1. Baumgartner, C.F., et al.: Sononet: real-time detection and localisation of fetal standard scan planes in freehand ultrasound. IEEE TMI **36**(11), 2204–2215 (2017)
2. Chen, H., et al.: Automatic fetal ultrasound standard plane detection using knowledge transferred recurrent neural networks. In: Navab, N., Hornegger, J., Wells, W.M., Frangi, A.F. (eds.) MICCAI 2015. LNCS, vol. 9349, pp. 507–514. Springer, Cham (2015). https://doi.org/10.1007/978-3-319-24553-9_62

3. Chen, H., Ni, D., Qin, J., Li, S., Yang, X., Wang, T., Heng, P.A.: Standard plane localization in fetal ultrasound via domain transferred deep neural networks. IEEE J. Biomed. Health Inf. **19**(5), 1627–1636 (2015)

4. Hou, B., et al.: Predicting slice-to-volume transformation in presence of arbitrary subject motion. In: Descoteaux, M., Maier-Hein, L., Franz, A., Jannin, P., Collins, D.L., Duchesne, S. (eds.) MICCAI 2017. LNCS, vol. 10434, pp. 296–304. Springer, Cham (2017). https://doi.org/10.1007/978-3-319-66185-8_34

5. Kendall, A., Grimes, M., Cipolla, R.: Posenet: a convolutional network for real-time 6-dof camera relocalization. In: ICCV 2015, pp. 2938–2946. IEEE (2015)

6. NHS: Fetal anomaly screening programme: programme handbook June 2015. Public Health England (2015)

7. Ryou, H., Yaqub, M., Cavallaro, A., Roseman, F., Papageorghiou, A., Noble, J.A.: Automated 3D ultrasound biometry planes extraction for first trimester fetal assessment. In: Wang, L., Adeli, E., Wang, Q., Shi, Y., Suk, H.-I. (eds.) MLMI 2016. LNCS, vol. 10019, pp. 196–204. Springer, Cham (2016). https://doi.org/10.1007/978-3-319-47157-0_24

8. Sarris, I., et al.: Intra-and interobserver variability in fetal ultrasound measurements. Ultrasound Obstet. Gynecol. **39**(3), 266–273 (2012)

Towards Radiotherapy Enhancement and Real Time Tumor Radiation Dosimetry Through 3D Imaging of Gold Nanoparticles Using XFCT

Caroline Vienne[1]([✉]), Adrien Stolidi[1], Hermine Lemaire[1], Daniel Maier[2],
Diana Renaud[2], Romain Grall[3], Sylvie Chevillard[3], Emilie Brun[4],
Cécile Sicard[4], and Olivier Limousin[2]

[1] CEA, LIST, DISC, 91191 Gif-sur-Yvette Cedex, France
caroline.vienne@cea.fr
[2] CEA/DRF/IRFU, CEA Saclay, 91191 Gif-sur-Yvette Cedex, France
[3] CEA/DRF/iRCM/LCE, CEA Fontenay, 92265 Fontenay-aux-Roses Cedex, France
[4] Université Paris Saclay, LCP, 91405 Orsay Cedex, France

Abstract. To enhance the efficiency of radiotherapy, a promising strategy consists in tumor exposure simultaneously to ionizing radiation (IR) and gold nanoparticles (GNPs). Indeed, when exposed to the radiation beam, these GNPs exhibit a photoelectric effect that generates reactive oxygen species (ROS) within the tumor and enhances the direct IR related deleterious effects. The measurement of this photoelectric effect thanks to an additional detector could give new insight for in vivo quantification and distribution of the GNPs in the tumor and more importantly for measuring the precise dose deposition. As a first step towards such a challenge, we present here materials and methods designed for detecting and measuring very low concentrations of GNPs in solution and for performing 3D reconstruction of small gold objects whose size is representative with respect to the considered application. A matrix image detector, whose sensitivity is first validated through the detection of few hundreds of micrograms of GNPs, is combined with a pinhole element and moved along a limited circular trajectory to acquire 2D fluorescence images of a motionless object. We implement a direct back-projection algorithm that provides a 3D image of these objects from this sparse set of data.

Keywords: X-ray fluorescence · Radiotherapy · Nanoparticles · CT

1 Introduction

The treatment of cancer is a major health challenge that mobilizes the scientific community from different fields. Due to the difficulty of eradicating resistant tumors, innovative approaches are proposed to enhance the efficiency of

© Springer Nature Switzerland AG 2018
A. F. Frangi et al. (Eds.): MICCAI 2018, LNCS 11070, pp. 401–409, 2018.
https://doi.org/10.1007/978-3-030-00928-1_46

radiotherapy. In the past decade, there has been a growing interest in using nanoparticles of high atomic number materials for dose enhancement and among them, gold nanoparticles (GNPs) offer several attractive features since they are generally considered chemically inert, biologically non-reactive and overall non toxic [1]. Depending on their size and on the route of administration, these nanoparticles can accumulate into the tumor, then during the radiotherapy, ionizing radiation (IR) will interact with the GNPs that will release free electrons. Once in contact with biological medium, those electrons will generate reactive oxygen species (ROS) and provoke an additional oxidative stress, compared to radiation alone, permitting to more effectively kill the tumor cells. In [2], Hainfeld et al. showed the beneficial effects of injecting GNPs to improve X-ray therapy. However, this promising idea faces a new challenge: up to now, there are no ways to know exactly how many GNPs reach the tumor and how long they are retained into it. All these data are crucial in order to estimate the applied radiative dose and to adjust GNPs delivery along the radiotherapy for optimizing the control of the tumor growth. To reach this goal, a promising idea consists in measuring the X-ray fluorescence of gold which follows the photoelectric effect [3,4]. By quantifying the intensity of Au-$K_{\alpha,\beta}$ fluorescence, it is possible to conclude on the concentration of GNPs in the tumor and on the IR dose. Fluorescence X-rays are commonly used for identifying the material composition of a given object but they can also be used when coupled with methods of tomography (XFCT), to determine the distribution of fluorescing elements. In this paper, we describe the considered setup based on the integration of a portable 16×16 pixels miniature imaging-spectrometer detector on a robotic arm. In Sect. 2, we present the materials and the performances of the proposed system for measuring GNPs in solution in view of biological aspects concerning the acceptable quantity of GNPs and dose that can be administered during radiotherapy. The second contribution of this paper concerns the validation of our XFCT strategy with this setup. A pinhole is added in front of the detector and the independent use of each pixel gives a 2D spectral image of a region of interest of a few centimeters. By moving the detector around this region of interest, a set of 2D images is acquired, post-processed and used as input of a back-projection algorithm for recovering the rough shape and dimension of small gold objects. XFCT results are detailed in Sect. 3. Due to the important drop of signal caused by the pinhole, the approach is here validated on pure gold objects but these first results pave the way for future optimizations.

2   Materials and Methods

An overall view of the proposed setup is displayed in Fig. 1. Both X-ray tube and detector are mounted on robotic arms, which facilitates the alignment of the setup and, above all, allows the acquisition of multiple views for XFCT approach. The detector is positioned at 90° of the X-ray beam in order to minimize the scattered radiation induced by ground.

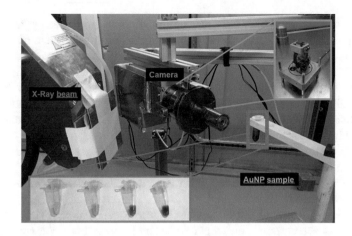

Fig. 1. View of the system. The X-ray beam is strongly filtered and collimated to create an incident pencil-beam with the desired spectral shape and the detector (camera) is also shielded by a collimator of 10 cm length and 1 cm diameter. In blue, the active surface of the detector without shielding is presented. In red, the different solutions of GNPs with increasing concentrations.

2.1   X-Ray Source Characteristics

A large majority of applications of XFCT are based on the use of a synchrotron source, which provides a bright monochromatic beam [5–7]. These beam characteristics are highly interesting for maximizing the efficiency of XFCT data acquisition since the incident energy can be selected according to the application. In particular, if a specific material is targeted, it is possible to choose the energy just above the absorption edge in order to obtain the best fluorescence signal. However, in practice, the use of synchrotrons is not realistic in laboratory or medical environments and polychromatic X-ray tubes have to be considered instead. The X-ray source used in this work is a Viscom XT 9225-D-ED microfocus tube used under 120 kV and at its maximum power (320 W). In order to limit the background noise during the measurement of the gold fluorescence, the X-ray tube is shielded with 1.4 mm of lead in addition to its native shielding and equipped with a 1 cm thick tungsten collimator, 3 mm in diameter. This collimator creates a circular illuminated region of 5 cm in diameter at the object position (30 cm from the source point).

2.2   Detector Performance and Calibration

The detector model is a CdTe imaging spectrometer namely Caliste-HD, which demonstrates high energy resolution over a large energy range [8]. This hybrid component is made of the assembly of one 16×16 pixel CdTe detector and eight analog front-end ASICs named IDeF-X HD equipped with 32 spectroscopic channels. Each pixel has a 625 μm pitch for a total size of the detector of $1\,cm^2$.

The main attractiveness to this design lies on the large energy range of the detector (1.5 keV to 1 MeV) and its good energy resolution down to 700 eV full width at half maximum (FWHM) at 60 keV. In the present configuration, the detector is installed into a light portable setup with limited cooling power. In addition to high count rates, the energy resolution degrades to 1.4 keV FWHM at 60 keV, still good enough for our demonstration. The energy resolution allows a good discrimination of the fluorescence X-rays lines for heavy metals such as gold. The whole detector chain is calibrated in energy thanks to a home-made plate covered with different element powders (Bismuth, Molybdenum, Tin, Gadolinium, Tungsten, Gold) that exhibit X-ray fluorescence lines at well-known energies. The plate is illuminated with the same X-ray source as used for the GNPs fluorescence.

When doing direct measurement of the fluorescence signal, the responses of the 256 pixels are summed up to generate the fluorescence spectrum. The performance of this detector for GNPs detection is validated using 1 mL of aqueous suspensions of GNPs at different concentrations. GNPs' size is 32 ± 6 nm. 20 min integration time is performed. The X-ray fluorescence of GNPs is clearly visible down to a mass of 144 μg of gold (see Fig. 2). A dose rate of 0.12 mGy/s at the location of the object is measured with a UNIDOS E dosemeter coupled with a TM 31013 PTW ionization chamber.

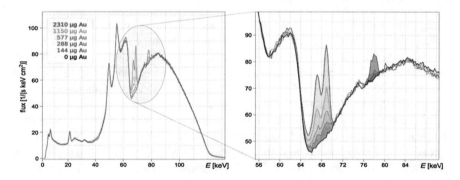

Fig. 2. Fluorescence spectrum obtained with different GNP concentrations in solution.

2.3   Pinhole X-Ray Fluorescence Imaging

For XFCT acquisition, a pinhole is added 10 cm in front of the image plane. This pinhole is made of 5 mm lead, attenuating all scattered or fluorescence signal, except for the aperture of 1 mm diameter. The distance between the pinhole and the object is 10 cm creating a magnification of 1 and allowing the inspection of a region of 1 cm^3. Contrarily to XFCT strategies based on a movable tightly collimated detector that inspects successively very small regions of the environment, the use of a pinhole coupled with a matrix image detector gives a direct 2D projection of the fluorescence distribution (see Fig. 3) and avoid additional translational movements of the detector. Pinhole use has been investigated couples of years ago in another emission imaging such as SPECT and PET [9,10] and more recently by Jung et al. in a simulation study [11].

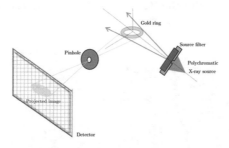

Fig. 3. Considered geometry for acquisition of XFCT data using a pinhole in front of the 2D detector.

3 XFCT Results

Due to the addition of the collimator and the use of the detector as an imaging spectrometer, which means that the signals from the 256 pixels are no longer summed up, the count of photons is greatly reduced in the XFCT configuration. For this reason, we chose here to validate the feasibility of our approach on pure gold objects with a representative size in a representative volume of interest (1 mm scale in a volume of few centimeters). Two small objects are considered in this case and described in Fig. 4.

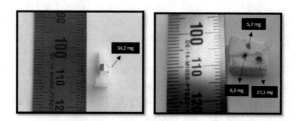

Fig. 4. Two gold samples used for XFCT: gold ring of 3 mm diameter and 1.2 mm height for 34.2 mg (left) and three pieces of gold of 1 to 2 mm size inserted in foam core with respective weight of 5.7 mg, 6.3 mg and 27.1 mg.

3.1 Acquisition Setup

The detector is now moved along a semi-circular trajectory around the sample in order to provide different views of the object. The acquisition plane crosses the X-ray beam perpendicularly in order to ensure that the detector is always put at 90° from the X-ray incident beam and 26 images are acquired with an angular step of 10°, corresponding to a maximal angular range of 250° (see Fig. 5). This angular limitation in the trajectory aims at taking into account the limited accessibility around the human body during radiotherapy.

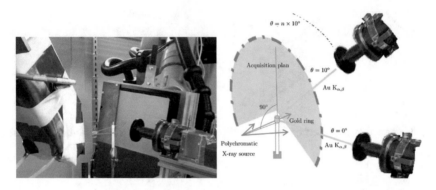

Fig. 5. Principle of XFCT data acquisition with the CdTe detector manipulated with the robotic arm.

3.2 Image Acquisition

For each pixel of the detector, the energy spectrum is recorded and 2D images are processed and used for the reconstruction. The 2D image of the gold ring corresponding to the first position of the detector along the trajectory ($\theta = 0°$) is displayed in Fig. 6. The left image corresponds to the complete spectrum. The second image corresponds to the hit-map of each pixel for all photons and the last one to the hit-map after selecting only photons whose energy is between 65 keV and 70 keV. Using the given spectrum, the energy resolution is about 1.9 keV FWHM at Au-K_{α_1}.

Figure 7 shows three different fluorescence images of the ring object (first row) and of the three pieces of gold (second row) acquired for three different positions of the detector ($-20°$, $100°$, $200°$). The projection of the objects is clearly visible with pixels red to yellow (counts), the scattered homogeneous signal of the environment creates a dark blue background signal and the corners of the image, shielded by the collimator, have a zero value (black color). The acquisition time for each projection is 2 min, resulting in a total acquisition time of 52 min and a deposited dose of almost 400 mGy.

3.3 Image Reconstruction

A 3D reconstruction of both objects is performed from the 26 projections. Contrarily to classical tomographic imaging methods where the inversion of the

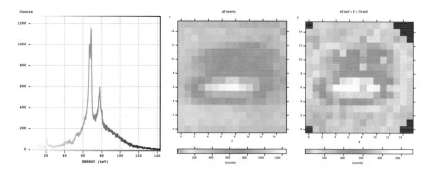

Fig. 6. Acquisition of a 2D image of gold fluorescence from the direct spectral signal measured in each pixel (left) to the corresponding hit-map created from all photons (center) and finally the hit-map for the photons whose energy is close to the energy range of the K_α fluorescence ray of gold (≈ 68 keV)(right).

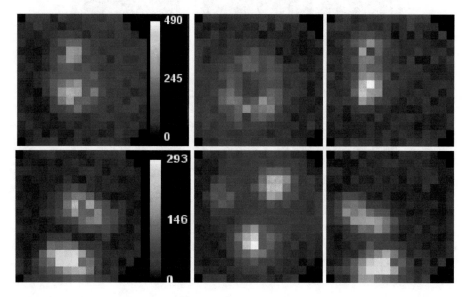

Fig. 7. Mutliple views of the gold objects provided by the 16×16 pixels detector.

Radon transform is based on Fourier back-projection methods, the reconstruction problem in XFCT involves iterative approaches that are better fitted for dealing with a sparse set of projections and a higher level of noise in the projections. Usually, maximum likelihood expectation maximization (MLEM) methods are chosen in this case. However, in our ideal conditions where the gold sample is put in an almost non attenuating foam, the object can be easily segmented from the background and we chose to apply a visual hull reconstruction approach [12] on the binarized images. The basic algorithm for visual hull extraction consists first in segmenting each input image in order to obtain the silhouette of the object. Then, using the parameters of the acquisition system (pinhole-detector distance and pixel size), the silhouette from each image is projected to 3D space thereby creating a visual cone. Finally the visual hull is obtained as the intersection of all the visual cones generated for different points of view. Reconstruction results are presented in Fig. 8. The 3D space is discretized in $100 \times 100 \times 100$ voxels of size 100 μm. An isosurface is applied to the reconstructed volume to display the global shape and dimension of the objects and give a first visual validation of the approach. In addition, a cross section of the reconstructed volumes (b, d) is displayed for each object. The gold ring appears slightly deformed with a diameter of about 3.2 mm, close to real value of 3 mm and the three tiny objects are well separated, which confirms that the spatial resolution is better than 1 mm.

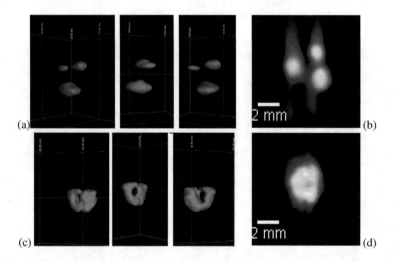

Fig. 8. Multiple views of the reconstructed objects (a, c) and cross section of the 3D images (b, d).

4   Conclusion

In this first step toward the validation of the feasability of measuring the dose deposited in the tumor during radiotherapy we focused on optimizing the system setup. A specific detector has been adapted and combined with a benchtop X-ray tube for this purpose. The sensitivity of the measurement has been validated on solutions with very low concentrations of GNPs. In addition, a first XFCT experiment has been successfully realized with small gold objects, representative in size of a tumor. The next two major steps of our developments consist in realizing XFCT of GNPs first in solution then in vivo.

References

1. Liu, A., Ye, B.: Application of gold nanoparticles in biomedical researches and diagnosis. Clin Lab. **8**(1–2), 23–36 (2013)
2. Hainfeld, J.F., Slatkin, D.N., Smilowitz, H.M.: The use of gold nanoparticles to enhance radiotherapy in mice. Phys. Med. Biol. **49**, 309–315 (2004)
3. Manohar, N., Reynoso, F.J., Diagaradjane, P., Krishnan, S., Cho, S.H.: Quantitative imaging of gold nanoparticle distribution in a tumor-bearing mouse using benchtop x-ray fluorescence computed tomography. Sci. Rep. **6**, 22079 (2016)
4. Le Loirec, C., Chambellan, D., Tisseur, D.: Image-guided treatment using an X-ray therapy unit and GNP: test of concept. Radiat. Prot. Dosim. **169**(1–4), 331–335 (2016)
5. Sunaguchi, N., Yuasa, T., Hyodo, K., Zeniya, T.: Fluorescent x-ray computed tomography using the pinhole effect for biomedical application. Opt. Commun. **297**, 210–214 (2013)
6. Sasaya, T., Sunaguchi, N., Lwin, T.T., Hyodo, K., Zeniya, T., Takeda, T., Yuasa, T.: Dual-energy fluorescent x-ray computed tomography system with a pinhole design: use of K-edge discontinuity for scatter correction. Sci. Rep. **7**, 44143 (2017)
7. Sasaya, T., Sunaguchi, N., Zeniya, T., Yuasa, T.: Multi-pinhole fluorescent x-ray computed tomography for molecular imaging. Sci. Rep. **7**, 5742 (2017)
8. Meuris A, et al.: Caliste HD: a new fine pitch Cd(Zn)Te imaging spectrometer from 2 keV up to 1 MeV. In: Nuclear Science Symposium Conference Record, pp. 4485–4488 (2011)
9. Jaszczak, R.J., et al.: Pinhole collimation for ultra-high-resolution, small-field-of-view SPECT. Phys. Med. Biol. **39**, 425–437 (1994)
10. Panin, V.Y., et al.: Fully 3-D PET reconstruction with system matrix derived from point source measurements. IEEE Trans. Med. Imaging **25**(7), 907–921 (2006)
11. Jung, S., Sung, W., Ye, S.J.: Pinhole X-ray fluorescence imaging of gadolinium and gold nanoparticles using polychromatic X-rays: a Monte Carlo study. Int. J. Nanomed. **12**, 5805–5817 (2017)
12. Laurentini, A.: The visual hull concept for silhouette based image understanding. IEEE Trans. Pattern Anal. Mach. Intell. **16**, 150–162 (1994)

Dual-Domain Cascaded Regression for Synthesizing 7T from 3T MRI

Yongqin Zhang[1,2], Jie-Zhi Cheng[3], Lei Xiang[1], Pew-Thian Yap[1],
and Dinggang Shen[1(✉)]

[1] Department of Radiology and BRIC, University of North Carolina at Chapel Hill,
Chapel Hill, NC 27599, USA
`dgshen@med.unc.edu`
[2] School of Information Science and Technology, Northwest University,
Xi'an 710127, China
[3] Shanghai United Imaging Intelligence Co., Ltd., Shanghai 201807, China

Abstract. Due to the high cost and low accessibility of 7T magnetic resonance imaging (MRI) scanners, we propose a novel dual-domain cascaded regression framework to synthesize 7T images from the routine 3T images. Our framework is composed of two parallel and interactive multi-stage regression streams, where one stream regresses on spatial domain and the other regresses on frequency domain. These two streams complement each other and enable the learning of complex mappings between 3T and 7T images. We evaluated the proposed framework on a set of 3T and 7T images by leave-one-out cross-validation. Experimental results demonstrate that the proposed framework generates realistic 7T images and achieves better results than state-of-the-art methods.

1 Introduction

Since early 2000s, 3T MRI has become the standard for research and clinical applications. In 2017, the first 7T MRI scanner was approved for clinical use by the United States Food and Drug Administration (FDA)[1]. Compared with 3T MRI, 7T MRI typically affords greater anatomical details and faster image reconstruction, which may benefit the diagnosis of diseases [1]. However, 7T MRI scanners are significantly more expensive and hence less common at hospitals and clinical institutions. To date, there are less than 100 7T MRI scanners worldwide [2]. Accordingly, this motivates the research on 7T image synthesis using the low-field images (e.g., 3T images). In this work, we show how the prediction of 7T MRI from 3T images can be improved by concurrently considering the spatial and frequency domains in a regression framework.

The basic goal of 7T image synthesis is to map low-resolution (LR) 3T images to high-resolution (HR) 7T images. But this is not a simple super-resolution

---

[1] https://www.fda.gov/NewsEvents/Newsroom/PressAnnouncements/ucm580154.htm.

The original version of this chapter was revised: A missing grant number has been added to the Acknowledgements section. The correction to this chapter is available at https://doi.org/10.1007/978-3-030-00928-1_100

A. F. Frangi et al. (Eds.): MICCAI 2018, LNCS 11070, pp. 410–417, 2018.
https://doi.org/10.1007/978-3-030-00928-1_47

problem because the appearance and contrast of 7T images can be different from those of 3T images. For this purpose, a number of machine learning methods have been proposed in recent years. Bhavsar et al. [3] introduced a group-sparse representation method for resolution enhancement of CT lung images. Roy et al. [4] presented an example-based super-resolution framework to synthesize HR MR images from multi-contrast atlases. To enhance the quality and resolution of neonatal images, Zhang et al. [5] proposed a super-resolution method with the guidance of longitudinal data. Bahrami et al. [6] proposed a hierarchical sparse representation method with multi-level canonical correlation analysis (M-CCA) for the reconstruction of 7T-like MR images from 3T MR images. A deep learning approach has appeared for resolution enhancement in [7]. Bahrami et al. [8] developed a CNN-based approach that takes into account appearance and anatomical features (CAAF) to predict 7T images from 3T images.

In this paper, we propose a dual-domain cascaded regression (DDCR) framework to synthesize realistic 7T from 3T images with two parallel and interactive multi-stage regression streams based on spatial and frequency domains. Our framework employs complementary cues on both domains to learn complex mappings from 3T to 7T modalities. Comparisons with the existing methods indicate that synthesized 7T images with higher quality can be obtained with DDCR.

2   Method

DDCR (Fig. 1) formulates the mapping between the 7T and 3T images as a regression problem. Specifically, DDCR regresses the local patches of 7T images from local patches of 3T images. DDCR uses intensity and spectral transformations to improve the quality of 7T image synthesis. DDCR consists of two steps: (1) image preprocessing and (2) multi-stage regression.

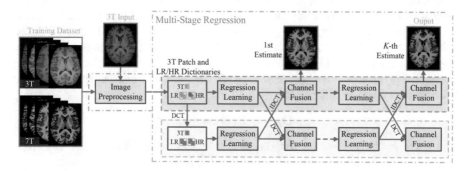

Fig. 1. Method overview. DCT and IDCT are the forward and inverse discrete cosine transforms, respectively.

2.1   Image Preprocessing

An input 3T image $\mathbf{Y}$ and pairs of 3T and 7T exemplar images $\{\mathbf{J}_{3T}, \mathbf{J}_{7T}\}$ are registered to MNI standard space [9] using FLIRT [10,11] to remove pose differences. Specifically, all 7T exemplar images are linearly registered to the MNI standard space with an individual template [9]. The 3T exemplar image is then rigidly aligned to its corresponding 7T image. After registration, bias correction [12] and skull stripping [13] are performed. The image intensity values are normalized using histogram matching and scaled to range of $[0, 1]$. Histogram matching is performed separately for 3T and 7T images. For 3T images, the histograms of all normalized 3T exemplar images are matched to the histogram of the normalized input 3T image. Following that, the normalized 7T exemplar image whose corresponding 3T exemplar image is nearest to the input 3T image in Euclidean distance is chosen as referenced 7T image for the histogram matching of all remaining 7T images.

2.2   Multi-stage Regression

To model the mapping from 3T (LR) to 7T (HR) modalities, a dual-domain multi-stage regression is developed. As shown in Fig. 1, the regression process is carried out on the two streams of spatial and frequency domains in multiple stages. In this study, the frequency domain is computed with the simple but efficient discrete cosine transform. For each stage of regression, the regression mapping from 3T to 7T modalities is performed separately. The regression results of spatial and frequency domains are then fused together as a new input for the later regression stage. It is worth noting that input image of the first stage regression is the normalized 3T image, whereas the input images of the remaining stages along each stream are the intermediate synthesized 7T images.

For the first stage, given an input 3T image $\mathbf{X} \in \mathcal{R}^{M \times N \times O}$ and Q pairs of 3T and 7T exemplar images $\mathbf{Z}_{3T}, \mathbf{Z}_{7T} \in \mathcal{R}^{M \times N \times O \times Q}$, we divide the input image into patches, denoted as $\mathbf{x}$, with size $p \times p \times p$ for patch regression. For each input patch, we collect L_1 most similar patches $\{\mathbf{z}_{3T,l} | l = 1, \cdots, L_1\}$ from the 3T exemplar images with block-matching method [14]. The 7T patches $\{\mathbf{z}_{7T,l} | l = 1, \cdots, L_1\}$ with the same locations of 3T exemplar patches are also collected from the corresponding 7T exemplar images. These 3T and 7T patch pairs are employed for the construction of the LR and HR dictionaries: $\mathbf{D}_{LR} = [\mathbf{z}_{3T,1}, \cdots, \mathbf{z}_{3T,L_1}]$ and $\mathbf{D}_{HR} = [\mathbf{z}_{7T,1}, \cdots, \mathbf{z}_{7T,L_1}]$ in the spatial domain, respectively. We propose a linear regression model to represent the mapping from the LR dictionary to the HR dictionary:

$$\mathbf{D}_{HR} = \mathbf{B}_s \mathbf{D}_{LR} + \varepsilon, \tag{1}$$

where $\mathbf{B}_s$ is the projection matrix, and ε is the error. We employ the ridge regression [15] to solve the inverse problem (1) in an optimization form:

$$\hat{\mathbf{B}}_s = \min_{\mathbf{B}_s} \|\mathbf{D}_{HR} - \mathbf{B}_s \mathbf{D}_{LR}\|_2^2 + \lambda \|\mathbf{B}_s\|_2^2, \tag{2}$$

where λ is a regularization parameter. By taking the first derivative of (2) with respect to the variable $\mathbf{B}_s$ and setting it to zero, the projection matrix can be expressed in a closed-form solution:

$$\hat{\mathbf{B}}_s = \mathbf{D}_{HR} \mathbf{D}'_{LR} \left(\mathbf{D}_{LR} \mathbf{D}'_{LR} + \lambda \mathbf{I} \right)^{-1}, \tag{3}$$

where $\mathbf{D}'_{LR}$ denotes the transpose of the matrix $\mathbf{D}_{LR}$, and $\mathbf{I}$ is an identity matrix. According to the inverse matrix identity [16], the estimated projection matrix $\hat{\mathbf{B}}_s$ in the spatial domain can be rewritten in another form with low computational complexity as follows:

$$\hat{\mathbf{B}}_s = \mathbf{D}_{HR}\left(\mathbf{D}'_{LR}\mathbf{D}_{LR} + \lambda\mathbf{I}\right)^{-1}\mathbf{D}'_{LR}. \tag{4}$$

By fixing $\hat{\mathbf{B}}_s$, the preliminary synthesized $\hat{\mathbf{y}}_{se}$ of the 7T MR patch $\mathbf{y}$ from the input 3T patch $\mathbf{x}$ becomes a simple matrix projection:

$$\hat{\mathbf{y}}_{se} = \hat{\mathbf{B}}_s\mathbf{x}. \tag{5}$$

On the other hand, we can also estimate a synthesized HR dictionary $\hat{\mathbf{D}}_{se}$ from the LR dictionary $\mathbf{D}_{LR}$ in the following form:

$$\hat{\mathbf{D}}_{se} = \hat{\mathbf{B}}_s\mathbf{D}_{LR}, \tag{6}$$

where $\hat{\mathbf{D}}_{se}$ is denoted as synthesized HR dictionary and can be referenced for the construction of LR dictionary for the next regression stage.

For the first stage of regression in the frequency domain, let α, $\mathbf{U}_{LR}$ and $\mathbf{U}_{HR}$ stand for the respective DCT coefficients of $\mathbf{x}$, $\mathbf{D}_{LR}$ and $\mathbf{D}_{HR}$, respectively. Similar to the regression in the spatial domain, the synthesized 7T component and the synthesized HR dictionary in the frequency domain can be separately computed as

$$\hat{\mathbf{v}}_{te} = \mathbf{U}_{HR}\left(\mathbf{U}'_{LR}\mathbf{U}_{LR} + \lambda\mathbf{I}\right)^{-1}\mathbf{U}'_{LR}\alpha, \tag{7}$$

and

$$\hat{\mathbf{U}}_{te} = \mathbf{U}_{HR}\left(\mathbf{U}'_{LR}\mathbf{U}_{LR} + \lambda\mathbf{I}\right)^{-1}\mathbf{U}'_{LR}\mathbf{U}_{LR}. \tag{8}$$

These temporary results can be referenced as the input and the construction of LR dictionary for the next stage.

After regression on both spatial and frequency domain, we further fuse the regression results of $\hat{\mathbf{y}}_{se}$, $\hat{\mathbf{D}}_{se}$, $\hat{\mathbf{v}}_{te}$ and $\hat{\mathbf{U}}_{te}$ in the spatial and frequency domains as follows:

$$\hat{\mathbf{y}} = \sqrt{(\hat{\mathbf{y}}_{se} \circ \hat{\mathbf{y}}_{se} + \mathrm{idct}\,(\hat{\mathbf{v}}_{te}) \circ \mathrm{idct}\,(\hat{\mathbf{v}}_{te}))\,/2}, \tag{9}$$

$$\hat{\mathbf{D}}_{HR} = \sqrt{\left(\hat{\mathbf{D}}_{se} \circ \hat{\mathbf{D}}_{se} + \mathrm{idct}(\hat{\mathbf{U}}_{te}) \circ \mathrm{idct}(\hat{\mathbf{U}}_{te})\right)/2}, \tag{10}$$

$$\hat{\mathbf{v}} = \sqrt{(\mathrm{dct}\,(\hat{\mathbf{y}}_{se}) \circ \mathrm{dct}\,(\hat{\mathbf{y}}_{se}) + \hat{\mathbf{v}}_{te} \circ \hat{\mathbf{v}}_{te})\,/2}, \tag{11}$$

$$\hat{\mathbf{U}}_{HR} = \sqrt{\left(\mathrm{idct}\left(\hat{\mathbf{D}}_{se}\right) \circ \mathrm{idct}\left(\hat{\mathbf{D}}_{se}\right) + \hat{\mathbf{U}}_{te} \circ \hat{\mathbf{U}}_{te}\right)/2}, \tag{12}$$

where $\mathrm{dct}\,(\cdot)$ and $\mathrm{idct}\,(\cdot)$ represent forward and inverse DCT functions, respectively, and the operator $\circ$ is the Hadamard product of two matrices.

With the computed $\hat{\mathbf{y}}$, $\hat{\mathbf{D}}_{HR}$, $\hat{\mathbf{v}}$ and $\hat{\mathbf{U}}_{HR}$, the cascaded stages of regression can be further carried out in the streams of respective domains. Specifically, for the cascaded regression in the spatial domain, the synthesized $\hat{\mathbf{y}}$ and dictionary $\hat{\mathbf{D}}_{HR}$ at the stage k are taken as the input $\mathbf{x}$ and the LR dictionary $\mathbf{D}_{LR}$ of the stage $k+1$, respectively. Similarly, in the frequency domain, the synthesized HR component $\hat{\mathbf{v}}$ and HR dictionary $\hat{\mathbf{U}}_{HR}$ at the stage k are treated as the input LR component α and the LR dictionary $\mathbf{U}_{LR}$ of the stage $k+1$. On the other hand, the HR dictionaries $\mathbf{D}_{HR}$ and $\mathbf{U}_{HR}$ from the stage k in the spatial and frequency domains are treated as the HR dictionaries of the stage $k+1$, respectively. With the setup of input, LR and HR dictionaries on both domains, we can perform the equations (5)–(8) to obtain regression results at the current stage. Then we can fuse the regression results with equations (9)–(12) again for the next stage. With K stages of regression, we further collect all synthesized 7T patches to construct the final result.

3   Experiments and Results

3.1   Dataset

With the local institutional review board (IRB), 15 adults were recruited for MR data acquisition in this study. The 3T and 7T brain images of all subjects were acquired with Siemens Magnetom Trio 3T and 7T MRI scanners, respectively. Specifically, for 3T images, T1 images of 224 coronal slices were obtained with the 3D magnetization-prepared rapid gradient-echo (MP-RAGE) sequence. The imaging parameters of 3D MP-RAGE sequence were as follows: repetition time (TR) = 1900 ms, echo time (TE) = 2.16 ms, inversion time (TI) = 900 ms, flip angle (FA) = $9°$, and voxel size = $1 \times 1 \times 1 \ mm^3$. For 7T images, T1 images of 191 sagittal slices were also obtained with the 3D MP2-RAGE sequence. The imaging parameters of 3D MP2-RAGE sequence were as follows: TR = 6000 ms, TE = 2.95 ms, TI = 800/2700 ms, FA = $4°/4°$, and voxel size = $0.65 \times 0.65 \times 0.65 \ mm^3$. As the gradient echo pulse sequences were used for image acquisition, there is only little distortion between the obtained 3T and 7T MR images, which ensures the imaging consistency across magnetic fields.

3.2   Experimental Setup

Extensive experiments were conducted to illustrate the effectiveness of the proposed method. In all experiments, we adopted leave-one-out cross-validation (LOOCV) for the evaluation. Specifically, in one fold of LOOCV, one 3T MR image was chosen for testing, whereas the remaining paired 3T and 7T MR images were treated as exemplars. The 7T image paired with the testing 3T image was treated as the ground truth image. For simplicity, we chose two stages for the implementation of the multi-stage strategy. The parameters of the proposed method were as follows: $p = 3$, $\lambda = 0.001$, $Q = 14$, $K = 2$, $L_1 = 25$ and $L_2 = 1$ in all experiments, where L_2 is the number of similar patches in the second stage regression. For the parameter settings, we manually tuned these parameters from the first stage to the last to ensure that the proposed method approximates its best performance.

3.3   Results

Several relevant methods like histogram matching (HMAT), M-CCA [6] and CAAF [8] were used as baseline methods for comparison. Meanwhile, to further illustrate the benefit of dual-domain strategy for the cascaded regression, DDCR was also compared with single spatial-domain cascaded regression, denoted as SDCR. For quantitative image quality assessment, we adopted two evaluation metrics: PSNR and Structural SIMilarity (SSIM) index [17]. All synthesized images from baseline methods and our method were compared with the real 7T images for the computation of PSNR and SSIM. Figure 2 shows the box-plots of PSNR and SSIM values of 15 synthesized 7T MR images. As can be observed, DDCR generally achieves higher PSNR and SSIM than the other baseline methods. Even though SDCR almost achieves the same PSNR values as DDCR, SDCR has distinctly lower SSIM values than DDCR. Figure 3 shows the axial, sagittal and coronal views of synthesized 7T MR images for one randomly selected subject. It can also be found from Fig. 3 that the synthesized 7T image by DDCR has better image quality and less distortion.

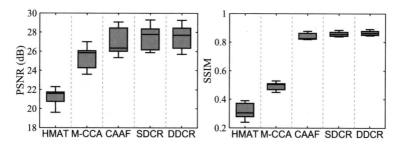

Fig. 2. Box-plots for PSNR and SSIM values. The middle line of each box is the median, the edges mark the 25th and 75th percentiles, and the whiskers extend to the minimum and the maximum. For all methods, the respective medians of PSNR and SSIM values are as follows: (a) HMAT (PSNR = 21.6 dB, SSIM = 0.30), (b) M-CCA (PSNR = 25.8 dB, SSIM = 0.50), (c) CAAF (PSNR = 26.3 dB, SSIM = 0.83), (d) SDCR (PSNR = 27.7 dB, SSIM = 0.85), and (e) DDCR (PSNR = 27.7 dB, SSIM = 0.86).

4   Discussion

Referring to Figs. 2 and 3, the proposed cascaded regression method can synthesize 7T images with better quality. Meanwhile, as can be found in Fig. 2, although the performance of DDCR w.r.t. the PSNR index is similar to that of SDCR, DDCR achieves higher SSIM values than SDCR. It is suggested that the synthesized 7T images by DDCR are more similar to real 7T images and thus validate the effectiveness of the dual-domain strategy.

We convert the image synthesis problem into a regression problem and solve it in a closed form. Multi-stage regression is also employed to further improve the quality of image synthesis. By introducing two complementary domains,

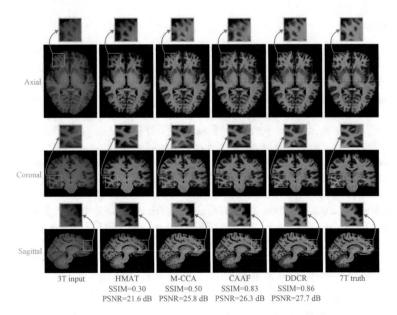

Fig. 3. Visual comparison of axial, sagittal and coronal views of synthesized 7T images with close-up views of specific regions for one subject.

two regression streams on respective spatial and frequency domains benefit each other in learning complex mappings between 3T and 7T images. The proposed method is simple and effective with low computational cost, which outperforms sparse representation based methods (e.g., M-CCA [6]) and can even compete with deep learning based methods (e.g., CAAF [8]). The proposed method is free of training process and does not require large amounts of training data. With limited 7T exemplar data, we can still achieve satisfactory 7T image synthesis. Therefore, the dependence of the proposed method on large training data, particularly less available 7T data, is not very strong.

5   Conclusion

In this paper, we have proposed a novel image synthesis method based on dual-domain cascaded regression. With the reference of pairs of 3T and 7T MR exemplar images, the proposed method can synthesize high-quality 7T images from 3T images. The experimental results suggest that the proposed method generally achieves better results than the state-of-the-art methods both qualitatively and quantitatively and thus corroborate the efficacy of the proposed method. For big training data, dual-domain convolutional neural network for image synthesis is left as our future research work.

Acknowledgements. This work was supported in part by NIH grants (EB006733, MH100217, MH108914, 1U01MH110274).

References

1. Zwaag, W., Schafer, A., Marques, J.P., Turner, R., Trampel, R.: Recent applications of UHF-MRI in the study of human brain function and structure: a review. NMR Biomed. **29**(9), 1274–1288 (2016)
2. Forstmann, B.U., Isaacs, B.R., Temel, Y.: Ultra high field MRI-guided deep brain stimulation. Trends Biotechnol. **35**(10), 904–907 (2017)
3. Bhavsar, A., Wu, G., Lian, J., Shen, D.: Resolution enhancement of lung 4D-CT via group-sparsity. Med. Phys. **40**(12), 121717 (2013)
4. Roy, S., Carass, A., Prince, J.L.: Magnetic resonance image example-based contrast synthesis. IEEE Trans. Med. Imaging **32**(12), 2348–2363 (2013)
5. Zhang, Y., Shi, F., Cheng, J., Wang, L., Yap, P. T., Shen, D.: Longitudinally guided super-resolution of neonatal brain magnetic resonance images. IEEE Trans. Cybern. (2018). https://doi.org/10.1109/TCYB.2017.2786161
6. Bahrami, K., Shi, F., Zong, X., Shin, H.W., An, H., Shen, D.: Reconstruction of 7T-like images from 3T MRI. IEEE Trans. Med. Imaging **35**(9), 2085–2097 (2016)
7. Dong, C., Loy, C.C., He, K., Tang, X.: Learning a deep convolutional network for image super-resolution. In: Fleet, D., Pajdla, T., Schiele, B., Tuytelaars, T. (eds.) ECCV 2014. LNCS, vol. 8692, pp. 184–199. Springer, Cham (2014). https://doi.org/10.1007/978-3-319-10593-2_13
8. Bahrami, K., Shi, F., Rekik, I., Shen, D.: Convolutional neural network for reconstruction of 7T-like images from 3T MRI using appearance and anatomical features. In: Carneiro, G., et al. (eds.) LABELS/DLMIA -2016. LNCS, vol. 10008, pp. 39–47. Springer, Cham (2016). https://doi.org/10.1007/978-3-319-46976-8_5
9. Holmes, C.J., Hoge, R., Collins, L., Woods, R., Toga, A.W., Evans, A.C.: Enhancement of MR images using registration for signal averaging. J. Comput. Assist. Tomogr. **22**(2), 324–333 (1998)
10. Jenkinson, M., Bannister, P., Brady, J.M., Smith, S.M.: Improved optimisation for the robust and accurate linear registration and motion correction of brain images. NeuroImage **17**(2), 825–841 (2002)
11. Jenkinson, M., Beckmann, C.F., Behrens, T.E., Woolrich, M.W., Smith, S.M.: FSL. NeuroImage **62**, 782–90 (2012)
12. Sled, J.G., Zijdenbos, A.P., Evans, A.C.: A nonparametric method for automatic correction of intensity nonuniformity in MRI data. IEEE Trans. Med. Imaging **17**(1), 87–97 (1998)
13. Shi, F., Fan, Y., Tang, S., Gilmore, J.H., Lin, W., Shen, D.: Neonatal brain image segmentation in longitudinal MRI studies. NeuroImage **49**(1), 391–400 (2010)
14. Brunig, M., Niehsen, W.: Fast full-search block matching. IEEE Trans. Circuits Syst. Video Technol. **11**(2), 241–247 (2001)
15. Zhang, Y., Liu, J., Yang, W., Guo, Z.: Image super-resolution based on structure-modulated sparse representation. IEEE Trans. Image Process. **24**(9), 2797–2810 (2015)
16. Petersen, K.B., Pedersen, M.S.: The Matrix Cookbook (2012)
17. Wang, Z., Bovik, A., Sheikh, H., Simoncelli, E.: Image quality assessment: from error visibility to structural similarity. IEEE Trans. Image Process. **13**(4), 600–612 (2004)

Machine Learning in Medical Imaging

Concurrent Spatial and Channel 'Squeeze & Excitation' in Fully Convolutional Networks

Abhijit Guha Roy[1,2]([⊠]), Nassir Navab[2,3], and Christian Wachinger[1]

[1] Artificial Intelligence in Medical Imaging (AI-Med),
KJP, LMU München, Munich, Germany
abhijit.guha-roy@tum.de
[2] Computer Aided Medical Procedures, Technische Universität München,
Munich, Germany
[3] Computer Aided Medical Procedures, Johns Hopkins University, Baltimore, USA

Abstract. Fully convolutional neural networks (F-CNNs) have set the state-of-the-art in image segmentation for a plethora of applications. Architectural innovations within F-CNNs have mainly focused on improving spatial encoding or network connectivity to aid gradient flow. In this paper, we explore an alternate direction of recalibrating the feature maps adaptively, to boost meaningful features, while suppressing weak ones. We draw inspiration from the recently proposed squeeze & excitation (SE) module for channel recalibration of feature maps for image classification. Towards this end, we introduce three variants of SE modules for image segmentation, (i) squeezing spatially and exciting channel-wise (cSE), (ii) squeezing channel-wise and exciting spatially (sSE) and (iii) concurrent spatial and channel squeeze & excitation (scSE). We effectively incorporate these SE modules within three different state-of-the-art F-CNNs (DenseNet, SD-Net, U-Net) and observe consistent improvement of performance across all architectures, while minimally effecting model complexity. Evaluations are performed on two challenging applications: whole brain segmentation on MRI scans and organ segmentation on whole body contrast enhanced CT scans.

1 Introduction

Deep learning, in particular, convolutional neural networks (CNN) have become the standard for image classification [1,2]. Fully convolutional neural networks (F-CNNs) have become the tool of choice for many image segmentation tasks in medical imaging [3–5] and computer vision [6–9]. The basic building block for all these architectures is the convolution layer, which learns filters capturing local spatial pattern along all the input channels and generates feature maps jointly encoding the spatial and channel information. While much effort is put into improving this joint encoding of spatial and channel information, encoding of the spatial and channel-wise patterns independently is less explored. Recent work attempted to address this issue by explicitly modeling the interdependencies

© Springer Nature Switzerland AG 2018
A. F. Frangi et al. (Eds.): MICCAI 2018, LNCS 11070, pp. 421–429, 2018.
https://doi.org/10.1007/978-3-030-00928-1_48

between the channels of feature maps. An architectural component called squeeze & excitation (SE) block [10] was introduced, which can be seamlessly integrated within any CNN model. The SE block factors out the spatial dependency by global average pooling to learn a channel specific descriptor, which is used to recalibrate the feature map to emphasize on useful channels. Its nomenclature is motivated by the fact that the SE block 'squeezes' along the spatial domain and 'excites' or reweights along the channels. A convolutional network with SE blocks won the first place in the ILSVRC 2017 classification competition on the ImageNet dataset, indicating its effectiveness [10].

In this work, we want to leverage the high performance of SE blocks for image classification to image segmentation with F-CNNs. We refer to the previously introduced SE block as channel SE (cSE), because it only excites channel-wise, which proved to be effective for classification. We hypothesize that for image segmentation, the pixel-wise spatial information is more informative. Hence, we introduce another SE block, which 'squeezes' along the channels and 'excites' spatially, termed *spatial* SE (sSE). Finally, we propose to have concurrent spatial and channel SE blocks (scSE) that recalibrate the feature maps separately along channel and space, and then combines the output. Encouraging feature maps to be more informative both spatially and channel-wise. To the best of our knowledge, this is the first time that spatial squeeze & excitation is proposed for neural networks and the first integration of squeeze & excitation in F-CNNs.

We integrate the proposed SE blocks (cSE, sSE and scSE) in three state-of-the-art F-CNN models for image segmentation to demonstrate that SE blocks are a generic network component to boost performance. We evaluate the segmentation performance in two important medical applications: whole-brain and whole-body segmentation. In whole-brain segmentation, we automatically identify 27 cortical and subcortical structures on magnetic resonance imaging (MRI) T1-weighted brain scans. In whole-body segmentation, we automatically label 10 visceral organs on contrast-enhanced CT scan of the abdomen.

Related Work: F-CNN architectures have successfully been used in a wide variety of medical image segmentation tasks to provide state-of-the-art performance. A seminal F-CNN model is U-Net [3], which has an encoder/decoder based architecture combined with skip connections between encoder and decoder blocks with similar spatial resolution. SkipDeconv-Net (SD-Net) [4] builds upon U-Net, using unpooling layers used in [7] for decoding, learnt by jointly optimizing logistic and Dice loss functions. A more recent architecture introduces dense connectivity within the encoder and decoder blocks, unlike U-Net and SD-Net which uses normal convolutions, termed fully convolutional DenseNet [9].

2   Methods

Let us assume an input feature map $\mathbf{X} \in \mathbb{R}^{H \times W \times C'}$ that passes through an encoder or decoder block $\mathbf{F}_{tr}(\cdot)$ to generate output feature map $\mathbf{U} \in \mathbb{R}^{H \times W \times C}$, $\mathbf{F}_{tr} : \mathbf{X} \to \mathbf{U}$. Here H and W are the spatial height and width, with C' and C being the input and output channels, respectively. The generated $\mathbf{U}$ combines the spatial and channel information of $\mathbf{X}$ through a series of convolutional layers and non-linearities defined by $\mathbf{F}_{tr}(\cdot)$. We place the SE blocks $\mathbf{F}_{SE}(\cdot)$ on $\mathbf{U}$ to recalibrate it to $\hat{\mathbf{U}}$. We propose three different variants of SE blocks, which are detailed next. The SE blocks can be seamlessly integrated within any F-CNN model by placing them after every encoder and decoder block, as illustrated in Fig. 1(a). $\hat{\mathbf{U}}$ is used in the subsequent pooling/upsampling layers.

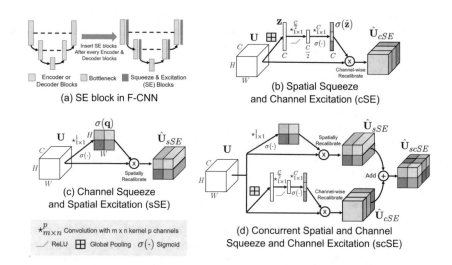

Fig. 1. Illustration of network architecture with squeeze & excitation (SE) blocks. (a) The proposed integration of SE blocks within F-CNN. (b–d) The architectural design of cSE, sSE and scSE blocks, respectively, for recalibrating feature map $\mathbf{U}$.

2.1 Spatial Squeeze and Channel Excitation Block (cSE)

We describe the spatial squeeze and channel excitation block, which was proposed in [10]. We consider the input feature map $\mathbf{U} = [\mathbf{u}_1, \mathbf{u}_2, \cdots, \mathbf{u}_C]$ as a combination of channels $\mathbf{u}_i \in \mathbb{R}^{H \times W}$. Spatial squeeze is performed by a global average pooling layer, producing vector $\mathbf{z} \in \mathbb{R}^{1 \times 1 \times C}$ with its kth element

$$z_k = \frac{1}{H \times W} \sum_i^H \sum_j^W \mathbf{u}_k(i,j). \tag{1}$$

This operation embeds the global spatial information in vector $\mathbf{z}$. This vector is transformed to $\hat{\mathbf{z}} = \mathbf{W}_1(\delta(\mathbf{W}_2\mathbf{z}))$, with $\mathbf{W}_1 \in \mathbb{R}^{C \times \frac{C}{2}}$, $\mathbf{W}_2 \in \mathbb{R}^{\frac{C}{2} \times C}$ being weights of two fully-connected layers and the ReLU operator $\delta(\cdot)$. This encodes the channel-wise dependencies. The dynamic range of the activations of $\hat{\mathbf{z}}$ are brought to the interval $[0, 1]$, passing it through a sigmoid layer $\sigma(\hat{\mathbf{z}})$. The resultant vector is used to recalibrate or excite $\mathbf{U}$ to

$$\hat{\mathbf{U}}_{cSE} = F_{cSE}(\mathbf{U}) = [\sigma(\hat{z}_1)\mathbf{u}_1, \sigma(\hat{z}_2)\mathbf{u}_2, \cdots, \sigma(\hat{z}_C)\mathbf{u}_C]. \tag{2}$$

The activation $\sigma(\hat{z}_i)$ indicates the importance of the ith channel, which are rescaled. As the network learns, these activations are adaptively tuned to ignore less important channels and emphasize the important ones. The architecture of the block is illustrated in Fig. 1(b).

2.2 Channel Squeeze and Spatial Excitation Block (sSE)

We introduce the channel squeeze and spatial excitation block that squeezes the feature map $\mathbf{U}$ along the channels and excites spatially, which we consider important for fine-grained image segmentation. Here, we consider an alternative slicing of the input tensor $\mathbf{U} = [\mathbf{u}^{1,1}, \mathbf{u}^{1,2}, \cdots, \mathbf{u}^{i,j}, \cdots, \mathbf{u}^{H,W}]$, where $\mathbf{u}^{i,j} \in \mathbb{R}^{1 \times 1 \times C}$ corresponding to the spatial location (i, j) with $i \in \{1, 2, \cdots, H\}$ and $j \in \{1, 2, \cdots, W\}$. The spatial squeeze operation is achieved through a convolution $\mathbf{q} = \mathbf{W}_{sq} \star \mathbf{U}$ with weight $\mathbf{W}_{sq} \in \mathbb{R}^{1 \times 1 \times C \times 1}$, generating a projection tensor $\mathbf{q} \in \mathbb{R}^{H \times W}$. Each $q_{i,j}$ of the projection represents the linearly combined representation for all channels C for a spatial location (i, j). This projection is passed through a sigmoid layer $\sigma(.)$ to rescale activations to $[0, 1]$, which is used to recalibrate or excite $\mathbf{U}$ spatially

$$\hat{\mathbf{U}}_{sSE} = F_{sSE}(\mathbf{U}) = [\sigma(q_{1,1})\mathbf{u}^{1,1}, \cdots, \sigma(q_{i,j})\mathbf{u}^{i,j}, \cdots, \sigma(q_{H,W})\mathbf{u}^{H,W}]. \quad (3)$$

Each value $\sigma(q_{i,j})$ corresponds to the relative importance of a spatial information (i, j) of a given feature map. This recalibration provides more importance to relevant spatial locations and ignores irrelevant ones. The architectural flow is shown in Fig. 1(c).

2.3 Spatial and Channel Squeeze & Excitation Block (scSE)

Finally, we introduce a combination of the above two SE blocks, which concurrently recalibrates the input $\mathbf{U}$ spatially and channel-wise. We obtain the concurrent spatial and channel SE, $\hat{\mathbf{U}}_{scSE}$, by element-wise addition of the channel and spatial excitation, $\hat{\mathbf{U}}_{scSE} = \hat{\mathbf{U}}_{cSE} + \hat{\mathbf{U}}_{sSE}$. A location (i, j, c) of the input feature map $\mathbf{U}$ is given higher activation when it gets high importance from both, channel re-scaling and spatial re-scaling. This recalibration encourages the network to learn more meaningful feature maps, that are relevant both spatially and channel-wise. The architecture of the combined scSE block is illustrated in Fig. 1(d).

Model Complexity: Let us consider an encoder/decoder block, with an output feature map of C channels. Addition of a cSE block introduces C^2 new weights, while a sSE block introduces C weights. So, the increase in model complexity of a F-CNN with h encoder/decoder blocks is $\sum_{i=1}^{h}(C_i^2 + C_i)$, where C_i is the number of output channels for the ith encoder/decoder block. To give a concrete example, the U-Net in our experiments has about 2.1×10^6 parameters. The scSE block adds 3.3×10^4 parameters, which is an approximate increase by 1.5%. Hence, SE blocks only increase overall network complexity by a very small fraction.

3   Experimental Results

In this section, we conducted extensive experiments to explore the impact of our proposed modules. We chose three state-of-the-art F-CNN architectures, U-Net [3], SD-Net [4] and Fully Convolutional DenseNet [9]. All of the networks have an encoder/decoder based architecture. The encoding and decoding paths consist of repeating blocks separated by down-sampling and up-sampling, respectively. We insert (i) channel-wise SE (cSE) blocks, (ii) spatial SE (sSE) blocks and (iii) concurrent spatial and channel-wise SE (scSE) blocks after every encoder and decoder block of the F-CNN architecture and compare against its vanilla version.

Datatsets: We use two datasets in our experiments. (i) Firstly, we tackle the task of segmenting MRI T1 brain scans into 27 cortical and sub-cortical structures. We use the Multi-Atlas Labelling Challenge (MALC) dataset [11], which is a part of OASIS [12], with 15 scans for training and 15 scans for testing consistent to the challenge instructions. The main challenge associated with the dataset are the limited training data with severe class imbalance between the target structures. Manual segmentations for MALC were provided by Neuromorphometrics, Inc.[1] (ii) Secondly, we tackle the task of segmenting 10 organs on whole-body contrast enhanced CT (ceCT) scans. We use data from the Visceral dataset [13]. We train on 65 scans from the silver corpus, and test on 20 scans with manual annotations from the gold corpus. The silver corpus was automatically labeled by fusing the results of multiple algorithms, yielding noisy labels. The main challenge associated with the whole-body segmentation is the highly variable shape of the visceral organs and the capability to generalize when trained with noisy labels. We use Dice score for performance evaluation.

Model Learning: In our experiments, all of the three F-CNN architectures had 4 encoder blocks, one bottleneck layer, 4 decoder blocks and a classification layer at the end. The logistic loss function was weighted with median frequency balancing [8] to compensate for the class imbalance. The learning rate was initially set to 0.01 and decreased by one order after every 10 epochs. The momentum was set to 0.95, weight decay constant to 10^{-4} and a mini batch size of 4. Optimization was performed using stochastic gradient descent. Training was continued till validation loss converged. All the experiments were conducted on an NVIDIA Titan Xp GPU with 12 GB RAM.

Quantitative Results: Table 1 lists the mean Dice score on test data for both datasets. Results of the standard networks together with the addition of cSE, sSE and scSE blocks are reported. Comparing along the columns, we observe that inclusion of any SE block consistently provides a statistically significant ($p \leq 0.001$, Wilcoxon signed-rank) increase in Dice score in comparison to the normal version for all networks, in both applications. We further observe that the spatial excitation yields a higher increase than the channel-wise excitation,

---

[1] http://Neuromorphometrics.com/.

Table 1. Mean and standard deviation of the global Dice scores for the different F-CNN models without and with cSE, sSE and scSE blocks on both datasets.

Networks	MALC dataset			
	No SE Block	+ cSE Block	+ sSE Block	+ scSE Block
DenseNets [9]	0.842 ± 0.058	0.865 ± 0.069	0.876 ± 0.061	**0.882 ± 0.063**
SD-Net [4]	0.771 ± 0.150	0.790 ± 0.120	0.860 ± 0.062	**0.862 ± 0.082**
U-Net [3]	0.763 ± 0.110	0.825 ± 0.063	0.837 ± 0.058	**0.843 ± 0.062**
Networks	Visceral dataset			
	No SE Block	+ cSE Block	+ sSE Block	+ scSE Block
DenseNets [9]	0.892 ± 0.068	0.903 ± 0.058	0.912 ± 0.056	**0.918 ± 0.051**
SD-Net [4]	0.871 ± 0.064	0.892 ± 0.065	0.901 ± 0.057	**0.907 ± 0.057**
U-Net [3]	0.857 ± 0.106	0.865 ± 0.086	0.872 ± 0.080	**0.881 ± 0.082**

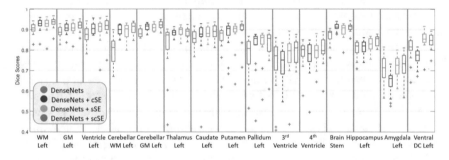

Fig. 2. Boxplot of Dice scores for all brain structures on the left hemisphere (due to space constraints), using DenseNets on MALC dataset, without and with proposed cSE, sSE, scSE blocks. Grey and white matter are abbreviated as GM and WM, respectively.

which confirms our hypothesis that spatial excitation is more important for segmentation. Spatial and channel-wise SE yields the overall highest performance, with an increase of 4–8% Dice for brain segmentation and 2–3% Dice for whole-body segmentation compared to the standard network. Particularly for brain, the performance increase is striking, given the limited increase in model complexity. Comparing the results across network architectures, DenseNets yield the best performance.

Figures 2 and 3 present structure-wise results for whole brain and whole body segmentation, respectively, for DenseNets. In Fig. 2, we observe that sSE and scSE outperform the normal model consistently for all the structures. The cSE model outperforms the normal model in most structures except some challenging structures like 3rd/4th ventricles, amygdala and ventral DC where its performance degrades. One possible explanation could be the small size of these structures, which might have got overlooked by only exciting the channels. The performance of sSE and scSE is very close. For whole body segmentation, in Fig. 3, we observe a similar pattern.

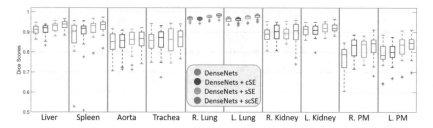

Fig. 3. Structure-wise Dice performance of DenseNets on Visceral dataset, without and with proposed cSE, sSE, scSE blocks. Left and right are indicated as L. and R. Psoas major muscle is abbreviated as PM.

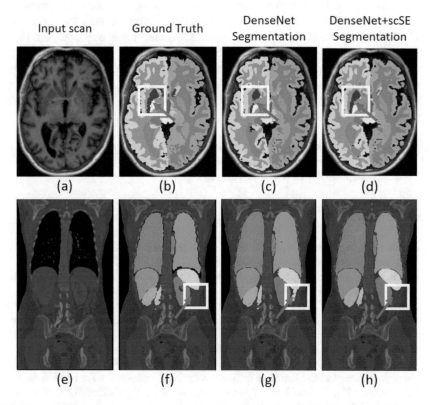

Fig. 4. Input scan, ground truth annotations, DenseNet segmentation and DenseNet+scSE segmentation for both whole-brain MRI T1 (a–d) and whole-body ceCT (e–h) are shown. ROIs are indicated by white box and red arrow highlighting regions where the scSE block improved the segmentation, for both applications.

Qualitative Results: Figure 4 presents segmentation results for MRI T1 brain scan in Fig. 4(a–d) and for Whole body ceCT scans in Fig. 4(e–h). We show the input scan, ground truth annotations, DenseNet segmentation along with our proposed DenseNet+scSE segmentation. We highlight ROIs with a white box and red arrow, to show regions where inclusion of scSE block improved the segmentation. For MRI brain scan segmentation, we indicate the structure left putamen, which is under segmented using DenseNet (Fig. 4(c)), but the segmentation improves with the inclusion of the scSE block (Fig. 4(d)). For whole body ceCT, we indicate the spleen, which is over segmented using DenseNet (Fig. 4(g)), and which is rectified with adding scSE block (Fig. 4(h)).

4   Conclusion

We proposed the integration of squeeze & excitation blocks within F-CNNs for image segmentation. Further, we introduced the *spatial* squeeze & excitation, which outperforms the previously proposed channel-wise squeeze & excitation. We demonstrated that SE blocks yield a consistent improvement for three different F-CNN architectures and for two different segmentation applications. Hence, recalibration with SE blocks seems to be a fairly generic concept to boost performance in CNNs. Strikingly, the substantial increase in segmentation accuracy comes with a negligible increase in model complexity. With the seamless integration, we believe that squeeze & excitation can be a crucial component for neural networks in many medical applications.

Acknowledgement. We thank the Bavarian State Ministry of Education, Science and the Arts in the framework of the Centre Digitisation.Bavaria (ZD.B) for funding and NVIDIA corporation for GPU donation.

References

1. Krizhevsky, A., Sutskever, I., Hinton, G.E.: Imagenet classification with deep convolutional neural networks. In: NIPS, pp. 1097–1105 (2012)
2. He, K., Zhang, X., Ren, S., Sun, J.: Deep residual learning for image recognition. In: CVPR, pp. 770–778. IEEE (2016)
3. Ronneberger, O., Fischer, P., Brox, T.: U-Net: convolutional networks for biomedical image segmentation. In: Navab, N., Hornegger, J., Wells, W.M., Frangi, A.F. (eds.) MICCAI 2015. LNCS, vol. 9351, pp. 234–241. Springer, Cham (2015). https://doi.org/10.1007/978-3-319-24574-4_28
4. Roy, A.G., Conjeti, S., Sheet, D., Katouzian, A., Navab, N., Wachinger, C.: Error corrective boosting for learning fully convolutional networks with limited data. In: Descoteaux, M., Maier-Hein, L., Franz, A., Jannin, P., Collins, D.L., Duchesne, S. (eds.) MICCAI 2017. LNCS, vol. 10435, pp. 231–239. Springer, Cham (2017). https://doi.org/10.1007/978-3-319-66179-7_27
5. Roy, A.G., Conjeti, S., Navab, N., Wachinger, C.: QuickNAT: segmenting MRI neuroanatomy in 20 seconds (2018). ArXiv:1801.04161
6. Long, J., Shelhamer, E., Darrell, T.: Fully convolutional networks for semantic segmentation. In: CVPR 2015, pp. 3431–40. IEEE (2015)
7. Noh, H., Hong, S., Han, B.: Learning deconvolution network for semantic segmentation. In: ICCV 2015, pp. 1520–28. IEEE (2015)
8. Badrinarayanan, V., Kendall, A., Cipolla, R.: Segnet: A deep convolutional encoder-decoder architecture for image segmentation. arXiv preprint arXiv:1511.00561 (2015)

9. Jégou, S., Drozdzal, M., Vazquez, D., Romero, A., Bengio, Y.: The one hundred layers tiramisu: fully convolutional densenets for semantic segmentation. In: CVPR Workshop, pp. 1175–1183. IEEE, July 2017
10. Hu, J., Shen, L., Sun, G.: Squeeze-and-excitation networks. In: CVPR 2018 (2018)
11. Landman, B., Warfield, S.: Miccai Workshop on Multiatlas Labeling. In: MICCAI Grand Challenge (2012)
12. Marcus, D.S., Fotenos, A.F., Csernansky, J.G., Morris, J.C., Buckner, R.L.: Open access series of imaging studies: longitudinal MRI data in nondemented and demented older adults. J. Cogn. Neurosci. **22**(12), 2677–2684 (2010)
13. Jimenez-del-Toro, O., et al.: Cloud-based evaluation of anatomical structure segmentation and landmark detection algorithms: VISCERAL anatomy benchmarks. IEEE TMI **35**(11), 2459–2475 (2016)

SPNet: Shape Prediction Using a Fully Convolutional Neural Network

S. M. Masudur Rahman Al Arif[1(✉)], Karen Knapp[2], and Greg Slabaugh[1]

[1] City, University of London, London, UK
S.Al-Arif@city.ac.uk
[2] University of Exeter, Exeter, UK

Abstract. Shape has widely been used in medical image segmentation algorithms to constrain a segmented region to a class of learned shapes. Recent methods for object segmentation mostly use deep learning algorithms. The state-of-the-art deep segmentation networks are trained with loss functions defined in a pixel-wise manner, which is not suitable for learning topological shape information and constraining segmentation results. In this paper, we propose a novel shape predictor network for object segmentation. The proposed deep fully convolutional neural network learns to predict shapes instead of learning pixel-wise classification. We apply the novel shape predictor network to X-ray images of cervical vertebra where shape is of utmost importance. The proposed network is trained with a novel loss function that computes the error in the shape domain. Experimental results demonstrate the effectiveness of the proposed method to achieve state-of-the-art segmentation, with correct topology and accurate fitting that matches expert segmentation.

1 Introduction

Shape is a fundamental topic in medical image computing and particularly important for segmentation of known objects in images. Shape has been widely used in segmentation methods, like the statistical shape model (SSM) [1] and level set methods [2], to constrain a segmentation result to a class of learned shapes. Recently proposed deep fully convolutional neural networks show excellent performance in segmentation tasks [3,4]. However, the neural networks are trained with a pixel-wise loss function, which fails to learn high-level topological shape information and often fails to constrain the object segmentation results to possible shapes (see Fig. 1a–c). Incorporating shape information in deep segmentation networks is a difficult challenge.

In [6], a deep Boltzmann machine (DBM) has been used to learn a shape prior from a training set. The trained DBM is then used in a variational framework to

---

Electronic supplementary material The online version of this chapter (https://doi.org/10.1007/978-3-030-00928-1_49) contains supplementary material, which is available to authorized users.

A. F. Frangi et al. (Eds.): MICCAI 2018, LNCS 11070, pp. 430–439, 2018.
https://doi.org/10.1007/978-3-030-00928-1_49

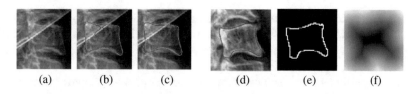

(a)   (b)   (c)   (d)   (e)   (f)

Fig. 1. (a–c) Advantage of shape prediction over pixel-wise classification (a) a noisy test image (b) segmentation result from a state-of-the-art deep network [5] (c) predicted shape from the proposed shape predictor network, SPNet. The green curve (−) represents the manually annotated vertebral boundary and the blue curve (−) represents the vertebral boundary of the predicted vertebra. The proposed SPNet can constrain the predicted shape to resemble a vertebra-like structure where the pixel-wise classification network failed in the presence of a strong image artifact. (d–f) Examples of a training vertebra (d) original image with manually annotated vertebral boundaries (e) pixels at the zero-level set (f) signed distance function. Darker tone represents negative values. (Color figure online)

perform object segmentation. A multi-network approach for incorporating shape information with the segmentation results was proposed in [7]. It uses a convolutional network to localize the segmentation object, an autoencoder to infer the shape of the object, and finally uses deformable models, a version of SSM, to achieve segmentation of the target object. Another method for localization of shapes using a deep network is proposed in [8] where the final segmentation is performed using SSM. All these methods consist of multiple components which are not trained in an end-to-end fashion and thus cannot fully utilize the excellent representation learning capability of neural networks for shape prediction. Recently, two methods were proposed which utilize a single network to achieve shape-aware segmentation. The method proposed in [9] uses a shallow convolutional network which is trained in two-stages. First, the network is trained in a supervised manner. Then the network is fine-tuned by using unlabelled data where the ground truth are generated with the help of a level set-based method. In contrast, the work presented in [5], proposed a shape-based loss term for training a deep segmentation network. However, both of these methods still use a cross-entropy loss function which is defined in a pixel-wise manner and thus not suitable to learn high-level topological shape information and constraints. In contrast to these methods, we propose a novel deep fully convolutional neural network, that is able to predict shapes instead of classifying each pixel separately. To the best of our knowledge, this is the first work that uses a fully convolutional deep neural network for shape prediction. We apply the proposed shape predictor network for segmentation of cervical vertebra in X-ray images where shape is of utmost importance and has constrained variation limits.

Most of the work in vertebra segmentation involves shape prediction [10,11]. Given the fact that a vertebra in an X-ray image mostly consists of homogeneous and noisy image regions separated by edges, active shape model and level set-based methods can be used to evolve a shape to achieve a segmentation [1,2,12].

While these methods work relatively well in many medical imaging modalities, inconsistent vertebral edges and lack of a difference in image intensities inside and outside the vertebra limits the performance of these methods in clinical X-ray image datasets.

Our proposed network is closely related to the state-of-the-art work on cervical vertebrae [5,13]. As mentioned earlier, [5] proposed a shape-based term in the loss function for training a segmentation network, UNet-S. The modified UNet [3] architecture produces a segmentation map for the input image patch which is defined over the same pixel space as the input. The UNet was further modified in [13], to achieve probabilistic spatial regression (PSR). Instead of classifying each pixel, the PSR network was trained to predict a spatially distributed probability map localizing vertebral corners.

In this work, we modify this UNet architecture to generate a signed distance function (SDF) from the input image. The predicted SDF is converted to shape parameters compactly represented in a shape space, in which the loss is computed. The contributions of this paper are two-fold: we propose (1) an innovative deep fully convolutional neural network that predicts shapes instead of segmentation maps and (2) a novel loss function that computes the error directly in the shape domain in contrast to the other deep networks where errors are computed in a pixel-wise manner. We demonstrate that the proposed approach outperforms the state-of-the-art method with topologically correct results, particularly on more challenging cases.

2 Dataset and Ground Truth Generation

This work utilizes the same dataset of lateral cervical X-ray images used in [5,13]. The dataset consists of 124 training images and 172 test images containing 586 and 797 cervical vertebrae, respectively. The dataset is collected from hospital emergency rooms and is full of challenging cases. The vertebra samples include low image intensity, high noise, occlusion, artifacts, clinical conditions such as osteophytes, degenerative change, and bone implants. The vertebral boundary of each vertebra in the dataset is manually annotated by expert radiologists (blue curve in Fig. 1d). The training vertebra patches were augmented using multiple scales and orientation angles. A total of 26,370 image patches are used for training the proposed deep network. The manual annotation for each of the training vertebrae is converted into a signed distance function (SDF). To convert the vertebral shapes into an SDF (Φ), the pixels lying on the manually annotated vertebral boundary curve have been assigned zero values. Then all other pixels are assigned values based on the infimum of the Euclidean distances between the corresponding pixel and the set of pixels with zero values. Mathematical details can be found in the supplementary materials. An example of the training vertebra with corresponding zero-level set pixels and SDF are illustrated in Fig. 1d–f. After converting all the training vertebral shapes to corresponding signed distance functions, principal component analysis (PCA) is applied. PCA allows each SDF (Φ) in the training data to be represented by a mean SDF ($\bar{\Phi}$), matrix of eigenvectors (W) and a vector of shape parameters, $\boldsymbol{b}$:

$$\phi = \bar{\phi} + W\boldsymbol{b}, \tag{1}$$

where ϕ and $\bar{\phi}$ are the vectorized form of Φ and $\bar{\Phi}$, respectively. For each training example, we can compute $\boldsymbol{b}$ as:

$$\boldsymbol{b} = W^T(\phi - \bar{\phi}) = W^T\phi_d, \tag{2}$$

where ϕ_d is the vectorized difference SDF, $\Phi_d = \Phi - \bar{\Phi}$. These parameters are used as the ground truth $(\boldsymbol{b}^{GT})$ for training the proposed network.

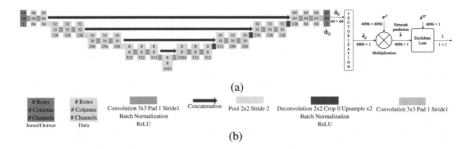

(a)

(b)

Fig. 2. SPNet: shape predictor network (a) network architecture (b) legend.

3   Methodology

To choose an appropriate network architecture for the application in hand, we follow the state-of-the-art work on cervical vertebrae [5,13]. We note that the choice can be altered based on the application, the complexity of the model and the available memory in the system for training. Our proposed shape predictor network, SPNet, takes a 64×64 vertebral image patch as input and produces its related difference SDF $(\hat{\Phi}_d)$ which is also defined over the same pixel space. We use the same network architecture as [13]. However, the final normalization layer has been removed. Instead, the last convolution layer outputs the difference signed distance function $(\hat{\Phi}_d)$ which is then sent to the final layer where it is converted to shape parameter vector $(\hat{\boldsymbol{b}})$ and compared with the ground truth $(\boldsymbol{b}^{GT})$. The network is illustrated in Fig. 2.

The forward pass through the final layer can be summarized below. First, the output of the last convolutional layer of the SPNet $(\hat{\Phi}_d)$ is vectorized as $\hat{\phi}_d$. Then the final prediction of network is computed as $\hat{\boldsymbol{b}}$:

$$\hat{\boldsymbol{b}} = W^T\hat{\phi}_d \text{ or in the element-wise form: } \hat{b}_i = \sum_{j=1}^{k} w_{ij}\hat{\phi}_{d_j}, i = 1, 2, \cdots, k; \tag{3}$$

where w_{ij} is the value at the i-th row and j-th column of the transposed eigen-vector matrix (W^T) and k is the number of shape parameters. Finally, the loss is defined as:

$$L = \sum_{i=1}^{k} L_i \text{ where } L_i = \frac{1}{2}(\hat{b}_i - b_i^{GT})^2. \tag{4}$$

The predicted shape parameter vector, $\hat{\boldsymbol{b}}$, has the same length as $\hat{\boldsymbol{\phi}}_d$ which is $64 \times 64 = 4096$. The initial version of the proposed network is designed to generate the full length shape parameter vector. However, the final version of the network is trained to generate fewer parameters which will be discussed in Sect. 5.

4 Experiments

The proposed network (SPNet) has been trained on a system with an NVIDIA Pascal Titan X GPU[1] for 30 epochs with a batch-size of 50 images. The network took approximately 22 h to train. We have also implemented a traditional convolutional neural network (CNN) where we predict the shape parameter vector $\boldsymbol{b}$ directly using a Euclidean loss function. The network consists of the contracting path of the proposed SPNet architecture, followed by two fully connected (FC) layers which regress the 4096 b-parameters at the output. This network will be mentioned as SP-FCNet in the following discussions. The SPNet has only 24,237,633 parameters where the SP-FCNet network has 110,123,968 trainable parameters. The FC layers cause a significant increase in the number of parameters. For comparison, we also show results of vertebral shape prediction based on the Chan-Vese level set segmentation method (LS-CV) [2,14]. Apart from these, we also compare our results with the segmentation networks described in [5]. Following their conventions, the shape-aware network will be referred to as UNet-S and the non-shape-aware version as UNet. The foreground predictions of these networks have been converted into shapes by tracking the boundary pixels. For the shape predictor networks, SPNet and SP-FCNet, the predicted b-parameters are converted into a signed distance function using Eq. 1. The final shape is then found by locating the zero-level set of this function. We compare the predicted shapes with the ground truth shapes using two error metrics: the average point to ground truth curve error (E_{p2c}) and the Hausdorff distance (d_H) between the prediction and ground truth shapes. Both metrics are reported in pixels.

5 Results

We first compare the three shape prediction methods in Table 1. We report the mean and standard deviation of the metrics over 797 test vertebrae. The Chan-Vese method (LS-CV) achieves an average E_{p2c} of 3.11 pixels, whereas the

[1] We gratefully acknowledge the support of NVIDIA Corporation with the donation of the Titan X Pascal GPU used for this research.

fully connected version of the shape predictor network (SP-FCNet) achieves 2.27 pixels and the proposed UNet-based shape predictor network (SPNet) achieves only 1.16 pixels. Hausdorff distance (d_H) shows more difference between the LS-CV and the deep networks. The comparison also illustrates how the proposed SPNet is superior to its traditional CNN-based counterpart, SP-FCNet. Both of these networks predict the shape parameter vector $(\boldsymbol{b})$ and the final loss is computed using Euclidean distance. It is the proposed SPNet's capabilities of generating the difference SDF $(\hat{\Phi}_d)$ and backpropagating the Euclidean loss on the SDF (Eq. 4) that make it perform better.

Table 1. Comparison of shape prediction methods.

Metrics	Average E_{p2c} (pixel)		Average d_H (pixel)	
Methods	Mean	Std	Mean	Std
LS-CV	3.11	1.13	10.94	3.68
SP-FCNet	2.27	0.83	6.74	3.25
SPNet (proposed)	**1.16**	**0.66**	**4.11**	**3.13**

Both of the deep networks have been trained to regress all 4096 shape parameters which are related to the corresponding eigenvectors. As the eigenvectors are ranked based on their eigenvalues, eigenvectors with small eigenvalues often result from noise and can be ignored. We evaluated the trained SPNet on a validation set at test time by varying the number of predicted parameters. The best performance was observed when only the first 18 b-parameters are kept which represents 98% of the total variation in the training dataset.

Table 2. Quantitative comparison of different methods.

Metrics	Average E_{p2c} (pixel)		Average d_H (pixel)		$nVmR$	Fit failure
Methods	Mean	Std	Mean	Std		(FF) %
LS-CV	3.107	1.13	10.94	3.68	0	85.45
SP-FCNet-18	2.082	0.78	6.48	3.32	0	43.54
UNet	1.114	1.29	5.06	6.11	57	8.53
UNet-S	0.999	0.67	4.37	4.02	45	6.02
SPNet-18	**0.996**	**0.55**	**4.17**	**3.06**	0	**4.14**

Based on this insight, we modified both versions of our deep networks to regress only 18 b-parameters and retrained the networks from randomly initialized weights. We report the performance of the retrained networks in Table 2. We also report the metrics for UNet and UNet-S networks from [5]. It can be seen that our proposed SPNet-18, outperforms all other networks quantitatively.

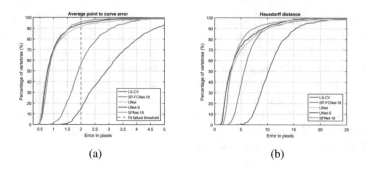

Fig. 3. Cumulative error curves (a) average E_{p2c} and (b) average d_H.

However, the improvement over UNet-S in terms of the E_{p2c} metric is small and not statistically significant according to the paired t-test at a 5% significance level. Quantitative improvements for SPNet-18 over all other cases pass the significance test.

The most important benefit of the proposed SPNet over the UNet and UNet-S is that the loss is computed in the shape domain, not in a pixel-wise manner. In the fifth column of the Table 2, we report the number of test vertebrae with multiple disjoint predicted regions $(nVmR)$. The pixel-wise loss function-based networks learn the vertebral shape implicitly, but this does not prevent multiple disjoint predictions for a single vertebra. The UNet and UNet-S produce 57 and 45 vertebrae, respectively with multiple predicted regions, whereas the proposed network does not have any such example indicating that the topological shape information has been learned based on the seen shapes. A few examples of these can be found in Fig. 4. We have also reported the fit failure (FF) for all the compared methods. Similar to [5], the FF is defined as the percentage of the test vertebrae having an E_{p2c} of greater than 2 pixels. The proposed SPNet-18 achieves the lowest FF. The cumulative error curves of the metrics are shown in Fig. 3. The performance of the proposed method is very close with the UNet and UNet-S in terms of the E_{p2c} metric. But in terms of the Hausdorff distance (d_H), the proposed method achieves noticeable improvement.

Moreover, the qualitative results in Fig. 4 distinctively demonstrate the benefit of using the proposed method. The UNet and UNet-S predict a binary mask and the predicted shape is located by tracking the boundary pixels. This is why the shapes are not smooth. In contrast, the proposed SPNet predicts b-parameters which are then converted to signed distance functions. The shape is then located based on the zero-level set of this function, resulting in smooth vertebral boundaries defined to the sub-pixel level which resembles the manually annotated vertebral boundary curves.

The worst performance is exhibited by the Chan-Vese method, LS-CV. The results of SP-FCNet-18 are better than the traditional Chan-Vese model, but underperform compared to the UNet-based methods. The reason can be attributed to the loss of spatial information because of the pooling operations.

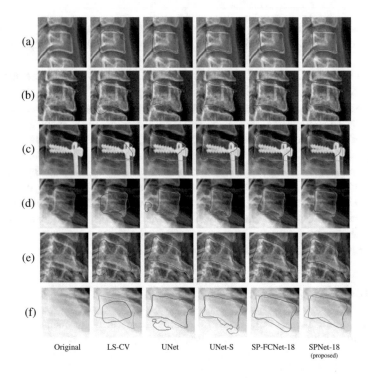

(a)

(b)

(c)

(d)

(e)

(f)

Original   LS-CV   UNet   UNet-S   SP-FCNet-18   SPNet-18
                                                                   (proposed)

Fig. 4. Qualitative results: predicted shape $(-)$ and ground truth $(-)$.

The UNet-based methods recover the spatial information in the expanding path by using concatenated data from the contracting path, thus perform much better than the fully connected version of the deep networks. Some relatively easy examples are shown in Fig. 4a and b. More challenging examples with bone implants (Fig. 4c), abrupt contrast change (Fig. 4d), clinical condition (Fig. 4e) and low contrast (Fig. 4f) are also reported. It can be seen even in these difficult situations, the SPNet-18 method predicts shapes which resembles a vertebra where the pixel-wise loss function-based UNet and UNet-S predict shapes with unnatural variations. More qualitative examples and further results with a fully automatic patch extraction process are illustrated in the supplementary material, demonstrating our method's capability of adjusting to variations in scale, orientation, and translation of the vertebral patch.

6   Conclusion

In this paper, we have proposed a novel method which exploits the excellent representation learning capability of the deep networks and the pixel-to-pixel mapping capability of the UNet-like encoder-decoder architectures to generate object shapes from the input images. Unlike the pixel-wise loss function-based segmentation networks, the loss for the shape predictor network is computed in the shape parameter space. This encourages better learning of high-level topological shape information and restricts the predicted shapes to a class of training shapes.

The proposed shape predictor network can also be adapted for segmentation of other organs in medical images where preservation of the shape is important. The network proposed in this paper is trained for segmentation of a single object in the input image. However, the level set method used for ground truth generation is inherently capable of representing object shapes that go through topological changes. Thus, given an appropriate object dataset, the same network can be used for segmentation of multiple and a variable number of objects in the input image. Similarly, the level set method can also be used to represent 3D object shapes. By replacing the UNet-like 2D deep network with a VNet-like [4] 3D network, our proposed method can be extended for 3D shape predictions. In future work, we plan to investigate the performance of our shape predictor network for segmentation of multiple and 3D objects.

References

1. Cootes, T.F., Taylor, C.J., Cooper, D.H., Graham, J.: Active shape models-their training and application. Comput. Vis. Image Underst. **61**, 38–59 (1995)
2. Tsai, A., et al.: A shape-based approach to the segmentation of medical imagery using level sets. IEEE Trans. Med. Imaging **22**(2), 137–154 (2003)
3. Ronneberger, O., Fischer, P., Brox, T.: U-Net: convolutional networks for biomedical image segmentation. In: Navab, N., Hornegger, J., Wells, W.M., Frangi, A.F. (eds.) MICCAI 2015. LNCS, vol. 9351, pp. 234–241. Springer, Cham (2015). https://doi.org/10.1007/978-3-319-24574-4_28
4. Milletari, F., Navab, N., Ahmadi, S.-A.: V-Net: fully convolutional neural networks for volumetric medical image segmentation. In: International Conference on 3D Vision (3DV), pp. 565–571. IEEE (2016)
5. Al Arif, S.M.M.R., Knapp, K., Slabaugh, G.: Shape-aware deep convolutional neural network for vertebrae segmentation. In: Glocker, B., Yao, J., Vrtovec, T., Frangi, A., Zheng, G. (eds.) MSKI 2017. LNCS, vol. 10734, pp. 12–24. Springer, Cham (2018). https://doi.org/10.1007/978-3-319-74113-0_2
6. Chen, F., Yu, H., Hu, R., Zeng, X.: Deep learning shape priors for object segmentation. In: Computer Vision and Pattern Recognition, pp. 1870–1877. IEEE (2013)
7. Avendi, M., Kheradvar, A., Jafarkhani, H.: A combined deep-learning and deformable-model approach to fully automatic segmentation of the left ventricle in cardiac MRI. Med. Image Anal. **30**, 108–119 (2016)
8. Mansoor, A., Cerrolaza, J.J., Idrees, R., Biggs, E., Alsharid, M.A., Avery, R.A., Linguraru, M.G.: Deep learning guided partitioned shape model for anterior visual pathway segmentation. IEEE Trans. Med. Imaging **35**, 1856–1865 (2016)
9. Tang, M., Valipour, S., Zhang, Z., Cobzas, D., Jagersand, M.: A deep level set method for image segmentation. In: Cardoso, M.J., et al. (eds.) DLMIA/ML-CDS - 2017. LNCS, vol. 10553, pp. 126–134. Springer, Cham (2017). https://doi.org/10.1007/978-3-319-67558-9_15

10. Roberts, M.G., Cootes, T.F., Adams, J.E.: Automatic location of vertebrae on DXA images using random forest regression. In: Ayache, N., Delingette, H., Golland, P., Mori, K. (eds.) MICCAI 2012. LNCS, vol. 7512, pp. 361–368. Springer, Heidelberg (2012). https://doi.org/10.1007/978-3-642-33454-2_45

11. Al Arif, S.M.M.R., Gundry, M., Knapp, K., Slabaugh, G.: Improving an active shape model with random classification forest for segmentation of cervical vertebrae. In: Yao, J., Vrtovec, T., Zheng, G., Frangi, A., Glocker, B., Li, S. (eds.) CSI 2016. LNCS, vol. 10182, pp. 3–15. Springer, Cham (2016). https://doi.org/10.1007/978-3-319-55050-3_1

12. Chen, T.F.: Medical image segmentation using level sets, Technical report. Canada, University of Waterloo, pp. 1–8 (2008)

13. Al-Arif, S.M.M.R., Knapp, K., Slabaugh, G.: Probabilistic spatial regression using a deep fully convolutional neural network. In: British Machine Vision Conference, BMVC 2017, London, 4–7 September 2017

14. Chan, T.F., Vese, L.A.: Active contours without edges. IEEE Trans. Image Process. **10**(2), 266–277 (2001)

Roto-Translation Covariant Convolutional Networks for Medical Image Analysis

Erik J. Bekkers[1(✉)], Maxime W. Lafarge[2(✉)], Mitko Veta[2],
Koen A. J. Eppenhof[2], Josien P. W. Pluim[2], and Remco Duits[1]

[1] Department of Mathematics and Computer Science,
Eindhoven University of Technology, Eindhoven, The Netherlands
`e.j.bekkers@tue.nl`
[2] Department of Biomedical Engineering, Eindhoven University of Technology,
Eindhoven, The Netherlands
`m.w.lafarge@tue.nl`

Abstract. We propose a framework for rotation and translation covariant deep learning using $SE(2)$ group convolutions. The group product of the special Euclidean motion group $SE(2)$ describes how a concatenation of two roto-translations results in a net roto-translation. We encode this geometric structure into convolutional neural networks (CNNs) via $SE(2)$ group convolutional layers, which fit into the standard 2D CNN framework, and which allow to generically deal with rotated input samples without the need for data augmentation.

We introduce three layers: a *lifting layer* which lifts a 2D (vector valued) image to an $SE(2)$-image, i.e., 3D (vector valued) data whose domain is $SE(2)$; a *group convolution layer* from and to an $SE(2)$-image; and a *projection layer* from an $SE(2)$-image to a 2D image. The lifting and group convolution layers are $SE(2)$ *covariant* (the output roto-translates with the input). The final projection layer, a maximum intensity projection over rotations, makes the full CNN rotation *invariant*.

We show with three different problems in histopathology, retinal imaging, and electron microscopy that with the proposed group CNNs, state-of-the-art performance can be achieved, without the need for data augmentation by rotation and with increased performance compared to standard CNNs that do rely on augmentation.

Keywords: Group convolutional network · Roto-translation group · Mitosis detection · Vessel segmentation · Cell boundary segmentation

1 Introduction

In this work we generalize $\mathbb{R}^2$ convolutional neural networks (CNNs) to $SE(2)$ group CNNs (G-CNNs) in which the data lives on position orientation space,

---

E.J. Bekkers and M.W. Lafarge—Joint main authors.

A. F. Frangi et al. (Eds.): MICCAI 2018, LNCS 11070, pp. 440–448, 2018.
https://doi.org/10.1007/978-3-030-00928-1_50

and in which the convolution layers are defined in terms of representations of the special Euclidean motion group $SE(2)$. In essence this means that we replace the convolutions (with translations of a kernel) by $SE(2)$ group convolutions (with roto-translations of a kernel). The advantage of the proposed approach compared to standard $\mathbb{R}^2$ CNNs is that rotation covariance is encoded in the network design and does not have to be learned by the convolution kernels. E.g., a feature that may appear in the data under several orientations does not have to be learned for each orientation, but only once. As a result, there is no need for data augmentation by rotation and the kernel weights (that no longer need to learn rotation covariance) become available to increase the CNNs expressive capacity. Moreover, the proposed group convolution layers are compatible with standard CNN modules, allowing for easy integration in popular CNN designs.

A main objective of medical image analysis is to develop models that are invariant to the shape and appearance variability of the structures of interest, including their arbitrary orientations. Rotation-invariance is a desired property, which our G-CNN framework generically deals with. We show state-of-the-art results with improvement over standard 2D CNNs on three different medical imaging tasks: mitosis detection in histopathology images, vessel segmentation in retinal images and cell boundary segmentation in electron microscopy (EM).

1.1 Related Work

In relation to other approaches that incorporate rotation invariance/covariance in the network design, such as harmonic networks [1], local transformation invariance learning [2], deep symmetry nets [3], scattering CNNs [4,5], and warped convolutions [6], the group convolution approaches [4,5,7–10] most naturally extend the standard CNNs by simply replacing the convolution operators.

In the work by Cohen and Welling [7] a comprehensive theoretical framework for G-CNNs is developed for discrete groups whose transformations stay on the pixel grid. In particular their focus was on the wall-paper groups p4 (group of translations + 90° rotations), for which a G-CNN approach was also developed by Dieleman et al. [8], and p4m (p4 + reflections). In their work it was convincingly demonstrated that including such symmetries, by replacing standard convolutions by group convolutions, substantially increases the network's performance without increasing the number of network variables. Although their theoretical G-CNN framework [7] holds for more general groups, their actual application scope was limited to discrete groups that stay on the pixel grid. In this paper, we are not restricted to such groups, but include efficient bi-linear interpolation that allows us to employ the full structure of the continuous roto-translation group $SE(2)$, which we can discretize to the sub-group $SE(2, N)$, with N rotations. Special cases of our framework are standard 2D CNNs when $N = 1$ and the p4 G-CNNs as proposed in [7,8] when $N = 4$.

In very recent work, Weiler et al. [9] describe a different approach to $SE(2)$ G-CNNs. Instead of relying on interpolation they used 2D complex-valued steerable kernels, which has the advantage that kernel rotations are exact. A disadvantage is, however, that these kernels are constrained to a specific combination of complex valued basis functions. With our interpolation approach, kernel rotation simply appears in the CNN architecture as a (sparse) matrix-vector multiplication, that maps a set of base weights to a full set of rotated kernels.

In work by Mallat, Oyallon, and Sifre [4,5] roto-translation invariant deep networks are formulated in the context of scattering theory. Their design involves a concatenation of separable group convolutions with hand-crafted (but well underpinned) filters, followed by the modulus as activation function. Learning takes place via support vector machines on the generated $SE(2)$ invariant descriptors. In our approach, the filters are learned without restrictions, the convolutions do not have to be separable, and we here use the common ReLU activation function.

In work by Bekkers et al. [10], an effective template matching method was proposed using group correlations in orientation scores, which are $SE(2)$ images obtained from a 2D image via lifting convolutions with a specific choice of kernel [11]. The $SE(2)$ templates were put in a B-spline basis (allowing for exact kernel rotations) and optimized via logistic regression. Their architecture fits within our framework as a single channel G-CNN of depth 2 with a fixed lifting kernel.

2 $SE(2)$ Convolutional Neural Networks

2.1   Group Theoretical Preliminaries

The Lie Group $SE(2)$: The group $SE(2) = \mathbb{R}^2 \rtimes SO(2)$ is the semi-direct product of the group of planar translations $\mathbb{R}^2$ and rotations $SO(2)$, and its group product is given by

$$g \cdot g' = (\mathbf{x}, \mathbf{R}_\theta) \cdot (\mathbf{x}', \mathbf{R}_{\theta'}) = (\mathbf{R}_\theta \mathbf{x}' + \mathbf{x}, \mathbf{R}_{\theta+\theta'}), \tag{1}$$

with group elements $g = (\mathbf{x}, \theta), g' = (\mathbf{x}', \theta') \in SE(2)$, with translations $\mathbf{x}, \mathbf{x}'$ and planar rotations by θ, θ'. The group acts on the space of positions and orientations $\mathbb{R}^2 \times S^1$ via $g \cdot (\mathbf{x}', \theta') = (\mathbf{R}_\theta \mathbf{x}' + \mathbf{x}, \theta + \theta')$. Since $(\mathbf{x}, \mathbf{R}_\theta) \cdot (\mathbf{0}, 0) = (\mathbf{x}, \theta)$, we can identify the group $SE(2)$ with the space of positions and orientations $\mathbb{R}^2 \times S^1$. As such we will often write $g = (\mathbf{x}, \theta)$, instead of $(\mathbf{x}, \mathbf{R}_\theta)$. Note that $g^{-1} = (-\mathbf{R}_\theta^{-1}\mathbf{x}, -\theta)$ since $g \cdot g^{-1} = g^{-1} \cdot g = (\mathbf{0}, 0)$.

Group Representations: The structure of the group can be mapped to other mathematical objects (such as 2D images) via representations. The left-regular $SE(2)$ representation on 2D images $f \in \mathbb{L}_2(\mathbb{R}^2)$ is given by

$$(\mathcal{U}_g f)(\mathbf{x}') = f(\mathbf{R}_\theta^{-1}(\mathbf{x}' - \mathbf{x})), \tag{2}$$

with $g = (\mathbf{x}, \theta) \in SE(2)$, $\mathbf{x}' \in \mathbb{R}^2$. It corresponds to a roto-translation of the image. The left-regular representation on functions $F \in \mathbb{L}_2(SE(2))$ on $SE(2)$, which we refer to as $SE(2)$-images, is given by

$$(\mathcal{L}_g F)(g') = F(g^{-1} \cdot g') = F(\mathbf{R}_\theta^{-1}(\mathbf{x}' - \mathbf{x}), \theta' - \theta), \tag{3}$$

with $g = (\mathbf{x}, \theta), g' = (\mathbf{x}', \theta') \in SE(2)$. It is a shift-twist (rotation + θ-shift) of F, see e.g. Figure 1. Next we define the G-CNN layers in terms of these representations.

2.2   The *SE(2)* Group Convolution Layers

In CNNs one can take a convolution or a cross-correlation viewpoint and since these operators simply relate via a kernel reflection, the terminology is often used interchangeably. We take the second viewpoint, our G-CNNs are implemented using cross-correlations. On $\mathbb{R}^2$ we define cross-correlation via inner products of translated kernels:

$$(k \star_{\mathbb{R}^2} f)(\mathbf{x}) := (\mathcal{T}_{\mathbf{x}}k, f)_{\mathrm{L}_2(\mathbb{R}^2)} := \int_{\mathbb{R}^2} k(\mathbf{x}' - \mathbf{x})f(\mathbf{x}')\mathrm{d}\mathbf{x}', \tag{4}$$

with $\mathcal{T}_{\mathbf{x}}$ the translation operator, the left-regular representation of the translation group $(\mathbb{R}^2, +)$. In the $SE(2)$ lifting layer we now simply replace translations of k by roto-translations via the $SE(2)$ representation $\mathcal{U}_g$ defined in Eq. (2).

The *SE(2)* Lifting Layer: Let $\underline{f}, \underline{k} : \mathbb{R}^2 \to \mathbb{R}^{N_c}$ be a vector valued 2D image and kernel (with N_c channels), with $\underline{f} = (f_1, \ldots, f_{N_c})$ and $\underline{k} = (k_1, \ldots, k_{N_c})$, then the group lifting correlations for vector valued images are defined by

$$(\underline{k} \tilde{\star} \underline{f})(g) := \sum_{c=1}^{N_c} (\mathcal{U}_g k_c, f_c)_{\mathrm{L}_2(\mathbb{R}^2)} = \sum_{c=1}^{N_c} \int_{\mathbb{R}^2} k_c(\mathbf{R}_\theta^{-1}(\mathbf{y} - \mathbf{x}))f_c(\mathbf{y})\mathrm{d}\mathbf{y}. \tag{5}$$

These correlations *lift* 2D image data to data that lives on the 3D position orientation space $\mathbb{R}^2 \times S^1 \equiv SE(2)$. The *lifting layer* that maps from a vector image $\underline{f}^{(l-1)} : \mathbb{R}^2 \to \mathbb{R}^{N_{l-1}}$, with N_{l-1} channels at layer $l-1$, to an $SE(2)$ vector image $\underline{F}^{(l)} : SE(2) \to \mathbb{R}^{N_l}$ using a set of N_l kernels $\mathbf{k}^{(l)} := (\underline{k}_1^{(l)}, \ldots, \underline{k}_{N_l}^{(l)})$, each with N_{l-1} channels, is then defined by

$$\underline{F}^{(l)} = \mathbf{k}^{(l)} \tilde{\star} \underline{f}^{(l-1)} := \left(\underline{k}_1^{(l)} \tilde{\star} \underline{f}^{(l-1)} , \quad \ldots \quad , \quad \underline{k}_{N_l}^{(l)} \tilde{\star} \underline{f}^{(l-1)} \right). \tag{6}$$

The *SE(2)* Group Convolution Layer: Let $\underline{F}, \underline{K} : SE(2) \to \mathbb{R}^{N_c}$ be a vector valued $SE(2)$ image and kernel, with $\underline{F} = (F_1, \ldots, F_{N_c})$ and $\underline{K} = (K_1, \ldots, K_{N_c})$, then the group correlations are defined as

$$(\underline{K} \star \underline{F})(g) := \sum_{c=1}^{N_c} (\mathcal{L}_g K_c, F_c)_{\mathrm{L}_2(SE(2))} = \sum_{c=1}^{N_c} \int_{SE(2)} K_c(g^{-1} \cdot h)F_c(h)\mathrm{d}h, \tag{7}$$

with $(K, F)_{\mathrm{L}_2(SE(2))} := \int_{SE(2)} K(h)F(h)\mathrm{d}h$, the inner product on $\mathrm{L}_2(SE(2))$. A set of $SE(2)$ kernels $\mathbf{K}^{(l)} := (\underline{K}_1^{(l)}, \ldots, \underline{K}_{N_l}^{(l)})$ defines a group convolution layer, mapping from $\underline{F}^{(l-1)}$ with $N_{(l-1)}$ channels to $\underline{F}^{(l)}$ with $N_{(l)}$ channels, via

$$\underline{F}^{(l)} = \mathbf{K}^{(l)} \star \underline{F}^{(l-1)} := \left(\underline{K}_1^{(l)} \star \underline{F}^{(l-1)} , \quad \ldots \quad , \quad \underline{K}_{N_l}^{(l)} \star \underline{F}^{(l-1)} \right). \tag{8}$$

The Projection Layer: Projects a multi-channel $SE(2)$ image back to $\mathbb{R}^2$ via

$$\underline{f}^{(l)}(\mathbf{x}) = \max_{\theta \in [0, 2\pi]} \underline{F}^{(l)}(\mathbf{x}, \theta). \tag{9}$$

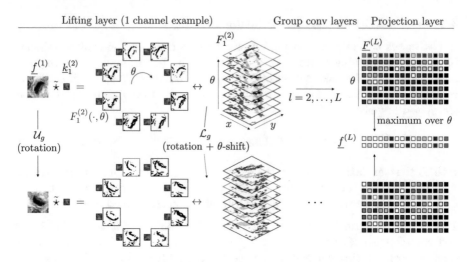

Fig. 1. Rotation co- and invariance. Top row: the activations after the lifting convolutions with a single kernel $\underline{k}_1^{(2)}$, stacked together it yields an $SE(2)$ image $F_1^{(2)}$ (cf. Eq. (6)). The projection layer at the end of the pipeline gives a rotation invariant feature vector. Bottom row: the same figures with a rotated input.

2.3 Discretization and Network Architecture

Discretization, Kernel Sizes and Rotation: Discretized 2D images are supported on a bounded subset of $\mathbb{Z}^2 \subset \mathbb{R}^2$ and the kernels live on a spatially rectangular grid of size $n \times n$ in $\mathbb{Z}^2$, with n the kernel size. We discretize the Lie group $SE(2,N) := \mathbb{Z}^2 \rtimes SO(2,N)$, with the space of 2D rotations in $SO(2)$ sampled with N rotation angles $\theta_i = \frac{2\pi}{N}i$, with $i = 0, \ldots, N-1$. The discrete lifting kernels $\mathbf{k}^{(l)}$ at layer l, mapping from a 2D image with N_{l-1} input channels to an $SE(2,N)$ image with N_l channels, thus have a shape of $n \times n \times N_{l-1} \times N_l$. The $SE(2,N)$ kernels $\mathbf{K}^{(l)}$ have a shape of $n \times n \times N \times N_{l-1} \times N_l$. A complete set of rotations of kernels $\mathbf{k}^{(l)}$ or $\mathbf{K}^{(l)}$ can be constructed with a single matrix multiplication from a vector that contains the shared kernel weights. This matrix is sparse and encodes bi-linear interpolation and kernel rotation.

3   Experiments and Results

We consider three different tasks in three different modalities. In each we consider the $SE(2,N)$ samplings with $N \in \{1, 2, 4, 8, 16\}$ to study the effect of the choice of N in the $SE(2,N)$ discretization. See Table 1 for the network settings. In each experiment the data is augmented at train and test time with transposed versions of the 2D input. For reference we also include transpose plus 90° rotation augmentation for the $N = 1$ experiment (as in [12,13]) in order to be able to show that these are not necessary in our $SE(2,N)$ networks for $N \geq 4$. Each experiment is repeated 3 times with random initialization and

Table 1. $SE(2, N)$ chain settings for different orientation samplings N.

N (Group)	1 ($\mathbb{Z}^2$)	2 ($\mathbb{Z}^2 \times p2$)	4 ($\mathbb{Z}^2 \times p4$)	8 ($SE(2,8)$)	16 ($SE(2,16)$)
Layer 1 - lifting with Eq. (6), $n = 5$					
N_1 ($\#_w$)	16 (1040)	13 (845)	10 (650)	8 (520)	6 (390)
Layer 2, 3, 4 - group conv. with Eq. (8), $n = 5$					
N_2 ($\#_w$)	16 (5408)	13 (7124)	10 (8420)	8 (10768)	6 (12108)
N_3 ($\#_w$)	16 (5408)	13 (7124)	10 (8420)	8 (10768)	6 (12108)
N_4 ($\#_w$)	64 (21632)	32 (17536)	16 (13472)	8 (10768)	4 (8072)
Layer 5 - group conv. with Eq. (8) + *projection with* Eq. (9), $n = 1$					
N_5 ($\#_w$)	16 (1056)	16 (1056)	16 (1056)	16 (1056)	16 (1056)
Layer 6 - standard conv. (output) layer, $n = 1$					
N_6 ($\#_w$)	1 (17)	1 (17)	1 (17)	1 (17)	1 (17)
Total $\#_w$	34561	33702	32035	33897	33751

sampling to get a rough estimate of the mean and variance on the performance. For a fair comparison for different N the overall number of weights is matched. For a fair comparison with the $\mathbb{R}^2$ approach, the number of "2D" activations ($N_l N$) in the last three layers is also matched. Each network optimizes a logistic loss using stochastic gradient descent with momentum using the same settings as in [12]. Our G-CNN implementations are available at https://github.com/tueimage/se2cnn. The results are given in Fig. 2, the tasks and metrics are summarized as follows.

Histopathology - Mitosis Detection: The task aims at detecting mitotic figures in hematoxylin-eosin stained slides. We used the public dataset AMIDA13 [14] that consists of high power field images from 23 breast cancer cases. Eight cases (458 mitoses) were used to train the networks with random batches of 68×68 image patches, balanced between mitotic and hard negative figures. This receptive field was obtained by means of max-pooling operations in the first three layers. Sets of candidate detections were generated as in [13] after selection of an operating point on four validation cases (92 mitoses). We assessed an F_1-score for each model based on the 11 test cases (533 mitoses) in the conditions of [14].

Retina - Vessel Segmentation: In this task the blood vessels in the retina are segmented. For validation we use the public DRIVE database [15], which consists of 40 retinal images with manual segmentations. The set is split in a training set (of which we use 16 for training, and 4 for validation) and a test set of also 20 images. The G-CNNs produce a probability for the vessel and background class. Training is done with 10000 patches (17×17) per class per image. The output probabilities can be thresholded to create a binary segmentation, which can be used to quantify performance in terms of sensitivity and specificity. The area under the receiver operator characteristic (ROC) curve, in short AUC, summarizes these performances into a single value.

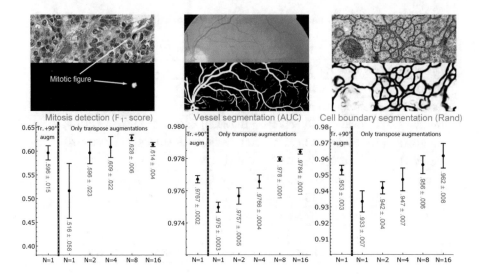

Fig. 2. Top row: Crop outs of images of the three tasks with the class probabilities generated by our method. Bottom row: Mean results (±1 std. dev.).

Electron Microscopy - Cell Boundary Segmentation: This task consists of segmenting the boundaries of cells that are imaged with EM. We use the data and evaluation system of the ISBI EM segmentation challenge [16]. The data consists of 2 volumes (1 train, 1 test), each containing 30 consecutive images from a serial section transmission EM. Both the segmentation and the evaluation is done by treating the volumes as sequences of 2D slices. To increase receptive field size we include max pooling in the first 2 layers. Training is done with 10000 patches (48 × 48) per class per image. The main evaluation criterion for the challenge is the Rand score, which measures the similarity between clusterings/connected components [17]. The reported Rand score is the maximum score (for several thresholds) computed for the connected components obtained after thinning of the binary cell boundary segmentation, see [16] for more details.

Results: In each experiment we see that the performance of the baseline with extra rotation augmentations is reached by the non-augmented G-CNNs for $N \geq 4$, and even is surpassed for $N \geq 8$. In the first two experiments we also observe that the variance on the output is reduced with increasing N. Our results on the public datasets match or improve upon the state of the art with the following scores: F_1-score $= 0.628 \pm 0.006$ for mitosis detection, AUC $= 0.9784 \pm 0.0001$ for vessel segmentation, Rand $= 0.962 \pm 0.008$ for cell boundary segmentation.

4   Discussion and Conclusions

We showed a consistent improvement of performances across three medical image analysis tasks when using G-CNNs compared to their corresponding CNN baselines. The reported results are in line with the benchmark of each dataset and the best performances were obtained for an orientation capacity $N \geq 4$, indicating the advantage of learning such rotation-invariant representations. We observed improved stability over the repeated experiments in mitosis detection and vessel segmentation for $N = 8$ and $N = 16$, suggesting a regularization effect due to the increased weight sharing with increasing N.

We conclude that it is beneficiary to include $SE(2)$ group convolution layers in CNN network design, as this avoids the need for rotation augmentation and it improves overall performance. In all three medical imaging problems we achieved state-of-the-art results with the same (basic) network design for each task. Based on these results we expect that our $SE(2)$ layers may lead to a further performance increase when embedded in more complex network designs, such as the popular UNets and ResNets.

Acknowledgements. The research leading to these results has received funding from the ERC council under the EC's 7th Framework Programme (FP7/2007–2013)/ERC grant agr. No. 335555.

References

1. Worrall, D.E., Garbin, S.J., Turmukhambetov, D., Brostow, G.J.: Harmonic networks: deep translation and rotation equivariance. In: CVPR, pp. 5028–5037 (2017)
2. Sohn, K., Lee, H.: Learning invariant representations with local transformations. In: CVPR, pp. 1339–1346. Omnipress (2012)
3. Gens, R., Domingos, P.M.: Deep symmetry networks. In: Advances in Neural Information Processing Systems, pp. 2537–2545 (2014)
4. Sifre, L., Mallat, S.: Rotation, scaling and deformation invariant scattering for texture discrimination. In: CVPR, pp. 1233–1240. IEEE (2013)
5. Oyallon, E., Mallat, S., Sifre, L.: Generic deep networks with wavelet scattering. arXiv preprint arXiv:1312.5940 (2013)
6. Henriques, J.F., Vedaldi, A.: Warped convolutions: efficient invariance to spatial transformations. In: International Conference on Machine Learning, pp. 1461–1469 (2017)
7. Cohen, T., Welling, M.: Group equivariant convolutional networks. In: International Conference on Machine Learning, pp. 2990–2999 (2016)
8. Dieleman, S., De Fauw, J., Kavukcuoglu, K.: Exploiting cyclic symmetry in convolutional neural networks. arXiv preprint arXiv:1602.02660 (2016)
9. Weiler, M., Hamprecht, F.A., Storath, M.: Learning steerable filters for rotation equivariant CNNs. arXiv preprint arXiv:1711.07289 (2017)
10. Bekkers, E.J., Loog, M., ter Haar Romeny, B.M., Duits, R.: Template matching via densities on the roto-translation group. IEEE tPAMI **40**(2), 452–466 (2018)
11. Duits, R., Felsberg, M., Granlund, G.H., ter Haar Romeny, B.M.: Image analysis and reconstruction using a wavelet transform constructed from a reducible representation of the Euclidean motion group. IJCV **72**(1), 79–102 (2007)
12. Lafarge, M.W., Pluim, J.P.W., Eppenhof, K.A.J., Moeskops, P., Veta, M.: Domain-adversarial neural networks to address the appearance variability of histopathology images. In: Cardoso, M.J., et al. (eds.) DLMIA/ML-CDS -2017. LNCS, vol. 10553, pp. 83–91. Springer, Cham (2017). https://doi.org/10.1007/978-3-319-67558-9_10

13. Cireşan, D.C., Giusti, A., Gambardella, L.M., Schmidhuber, J.: Mitosis detection in breast cancer histology images with deep neural networks. In: Mori, K., Sakuma, I., Sato, Y., Barillot, C., Navab, N. (eds.) MICCAI 2013. LNCS, vol. 8150, pp. 411–418. Springer, Heidelberg (2013). https://doi.org/10.1007/978-3-642-40763-5_51

14. Veta, M., et al.: Assessment of algorithms for mitosis detection in breast cancer histopathology images. MEDIA **20**(1), 237–248 (2015)

15. Staal, J., et al.: Ridge-based vessel segmentation in color images of the retina. IEEE TMI **23**(4), 501–509 (2004)

16. Arganda-Carreras, I., et al.: Crowdsourcing the creation of image segmentation algorithms for connectomics. Front. Neuroanat. **9**, 142 (2015)

17. Rand, W.M.: Objective criteria for the evaluation of clustering methods. J. Am. Stat. Assoc. **66**(336), 846–850 (1971)

Bimodal Network Architectures for Automatic Generation of Image Annotation from Text

Mehdi Moradi[✉], Ali Madani, Yaniv Gur, Yufan Guo, and Tanveer Syeda-Mahmood

IBM Research - Almaden Research Center, San Jose, USA
mmoradi@us.ibm.com

Abstract. Medical image analysis practitioners have embraced big data methodologies. This has created a need for large annotated datasets. The source of big data is typically large image collections and clinical reports recorded for these images. In many cases, however, building algorithms aimed at segmentation and detection of disease requires a training dataset with markings of the areas of interest on the image that match with the described anomalies. This process of annotation is expensive and needs the involvement of clinicians. In this work we propose two separate deep neural network architectures for automatic marking of a region of interest (ROI) on the image best representing a finding location, given a textual report or a set of keywords. One architecture consists of LSTM and CNN components and is trained end to end with images, matching text, and markings of ROIs for those images. The output layer estimates the coordinates of the vertices of a polygonal region. The second architecture uses a network pre-trained on a large dataset of the same image types for learning feature representations of the findings of interest. We show that for a variety of findings from chest X-ray images, both proposed architectures learn to estimate the ROI, as validated by clinical annotations. There is a clear advantage obtained from the architecture with pre-trained imaging network. The centroids of the ROIs marked by this network were on average at a distance equivalent to 5.1% of the image width from the centroids of the ground truth ROIs.

1 Introduction

Big data methods such as deep learning consume large quantities of labeled data. In medical imaging, such big data approaches have shown great impact in advancing segmentation and disease detection algorithms. To expedite the progress of this area of research, access to such datasets is vital. Much of the radiology data is recorded as paired image and radiology reports. While these are useful for training purposes and can be mined for labels, image level annotations are rarely recorded in clinical practice. Therefore, even though the diagnosis or finding is already described by a clinician in a report, clinical input is still required in marking the area depicting the finding back onto the image. In some

© Springer Nature Switzerland AG 2018
A. F. Frangi et al. (Eds.): MICCAI 2018, LNCS 11070, pp. 449–456, 2018.
https://doi.org/10.1007/978-3-030-00928-1_51

cases, such as mass or nodules of the lung in chest X-ray images, the finding could be limited to a small portion of a large organ.

In this work we propose to estimate the position of the region of interest (ROI) described in a text segment, written for a medical image, using a supervised neural network architecture. This area of work is fresh in medical image analysis. Attention networks have been proposed for highlighting an ROI in an image that contributes most to the output of a convolutional neural network (CNN). These have shown impressive outcomes in applications such as image captioning [12]. However, attention methods assume the availability of a detector and use only the image as the input, whereas our contribution is in facilitating the data curation step given the text reports. Other related work in data curation for medical image analysis include image to text mapping for automatic label generation for images [5]. This method does not mark ROIs on the image. There is also some work in crowd-sourcing of medical image annotations [4,8]. The automatic approach in the current paper can be used as a complement to crowd-sourcing where images can be annotated with some preliminary contours before being edited by human annotators.

The main contributions of this paper are bimodal (text+image) neural network architectures that estimate the ROIs coordinates, given an image and a text segment. We propose two bimodal architectures to facilitate two different common scenarios. **(I)** We train an end to end network that can process text using recurrent layers, and the images using convolutional layers, and merge the two to estimate the ROI coordinates. This integrated network is, however, difficult to train with limited annotated data. It is particularly difficult to sufficiently characterize the visual signature of relevant findings using limited data. **(II)** Since the main goal here is to limit the effort to annotate large quantities of images, we propose an alternative for situations when an organized collection of images, text and markings is scarce. This second approach separates the training of the image processing CNN, and the text processing network, from the network that maps the concatenated image and text features to the ROI coordinate space. The imaging network is trained on a very large public dataset to learn the features characterizing clinical findings in chest X-ray images.

To the best of our knowledge, the problem of generating image annotations for data curation purposes is among the less explored areas of medical image computing. Also, both architectures proposed here are novel combinations of network building blocks. One recent relevant work is the TieNet architecture proposed in [11]. TieNet addressed the disease classification problem using joint information from image and text features during training and using image only for prediction. Another relevant work is [9] which reports annotation from questions with an interactive process. We use reports both during training and prediction stages and the goal is mapping from text to image. Further, we model the anomaly localization as a regression problem on the polygonal bounding region coordinates. We have used these architectures on chest X-ray image annotation. We show that the availability of a large public dataset of X-ray images results in superior performance of the architecture with pre-trained image classifier.

2   Methodology

We describe two novel bimodal architectures for producing image level annotations. The ROI model selected here is a quadrilateral (a polygon with four edges). But the methodology can be generalized with more complex polygons. The outputs of both architectures are eight continuous values corresponding to the coordinates of vertices of the quadrilateral ROI. We describe the datasets used in this work, followed by the two architectures.

2.1   Datasets

DS1: Dataset 1 is a public dataset from Indiana University Hospital that includes chest X-ray images from approximately 3500 unique patients [1]. This collection is accompanied with corresponding reports. For a subset of this data, consisting of 494 images we performed image level annotations. We chose two groups of findings for image annotations. One was cardiomegaly which has a distinct signature showing an enlarged heart, and the second group was nodules, granuloma, and masses. These can appear in different areas of the lung and are more difficult to localize. Each of the 494 images paired with a text segment characterizing the anomaly, were presented to an experienced radiologist who marked a bounding quadrilateral around the finding. No limitation on size was enforced. The only limitation was to approximate the finding area with a four-corner convex shape.

DS2: Dataset 2 is the public collection of chest X-ray images released by National Institutes of Health (NIH). Known as the Chest-Ray14 dataset [10], this comprises of 112,120 frontal-view X-rays. 51,708 images have one or more finding labels of the following 14: atelectasis, cardiomegaly, consolidation, edema, effusion, emphysema, fibrosis, hernia, infiltration, mass, nodule, pleural thickening, pneumonia, and pneumothorax. The remaining 60,412 images do not contain any of the 14 findings and are labeled as "No Finding". Several groups have recently reported classifiers trained using this dataset [2]. The ground truth labels are mined from clinical records and are not validated. The use of this dataset in our current work is for building a rich and large network that can act as the source of features. We do not have image level annotations or reports for this dataset. Therefore, we could not use this in our end to end architecture.

2.2   Architecture 1: Integrated CNN+LSTM, Trained End to End

Figure 1 displays our proposed integrated architecture. The image is fed through a convolutional neural network which learns relevant visual features. In the reported version, there are four convolutional layers, and two fully-connected layers. Dropout, batch normalization, and ReLU activation functions are utilized in the CNN. The final layer of the CNN is a 256 node layer that represents the dimensionality reduced version of the image to be merged with the text network output layer.

On the text side, the findings and diagnoses in radiology reports have been manually coded with the standard Medical Subject Headings (MeSH) terms by domain experts [1]. MeSH is the medical vocabulary controlled by the US National Library of Medicine. The next step is embedding of each MeSH term into a quantitative vector. For this purpose, we used the GloVe (Global Vectors for Word Representation) algorithm [6]. Training of this embedding is performed on the term-term co-occurrence statistics from the 3500 reports in *DS1*. The next block within the text pipeline is a long short-term memory (LSTM) layer with 128 units. This is followed by a 256 node fully connected layer together listed as the LSTM block. While the mesh terms and embedding models are frozen, this LSTM encoder is trained along with the CNN network with the objective of estimating the ROI coordinates.

In the final component of the architecture, the textual features from LSTM output and image features are merged by concatenation and fed through a multi-layer perceptron (MLP). The MLP is a 3 layer fully-connected network. The output is a series of [x, y] coordinates for the polygon vertices. The loss is calculated as the mean squared error between the predicted coordinates and the actual coordinates.

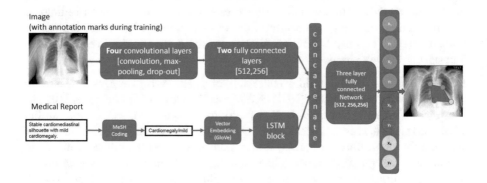

Fig. 1. Architecture 1: integrated text and imaging network.

2.3   Architecture 2: Trained DenseNet121 + Doc2Vec

Figure 2 demonstrates the components of the second architecture proposed in this paper. Given the limited size of the data with image level annotations, the CNN block of Architecture 1 is kept small and is still difficult to train. To solve this issue, we propose to learn the features characterizing the radiological findings within chest X-rays separately using *DS2*. To this end, we trained a DenseNet architecture [2] with 121 layers. This is inspired by [7]. However, in our architecture, the fully connected layer of DenseNet was replaced by a separate dense layer of dimension 1024 per finding class, followed by a sigmoid nonlinearity to create a 14-output network matching the 14 listed *DS2* labels. To train this network, we randomly divided *DS2* into a training set (80%) and a validation set (20%) and trained the network for 25 epochs with a batch size of 32, and with horizontal flip image augmentation. The performance was measured using the Area Under the Curve (AUC) by first generating the ROC curve per finding and averaging the AUC across all findings.

This pre-trained network was used as a source of features in Architecture 2. The image features were extracted from the output of the global average pooling (GAP) layer that operates on the last convolution layer of the CheXNet architecture. The GAP layer produced a feature vector of 1024 elements.

On the text side, we also replaced the embedding and trainable LSTM block with a pre-trained paragraph vector (PV) model that supplies a 128 dimensional feature vector given a text segment. We used the unsupervised method known as *PV-DBOW* to quantify text segments [3]. Unlike sequence learning through LSTM, PV-DBOW ignores context words in the input and predicts words randomly sampled from a text segment in the output. The model is capable of embedding input word sequences of variable length, and the learned representations are word-order independent, for which the encoding of a set of MeSH terms would be a good use case. We trained *PV-DBOW* using MeSH terms extracted from all 3500 reports available. Training was performed using stochastic gradient descent via backpropagation.

The two independently produced feature vectors for a text and image pair are then concatenated into a 1152 dimensional vector. After the input layer, there are three fully connected layers, with 1024, 512, and 128 neurons in each. Dropout is used throughout the network. The output layer feeds into the eight dimensional output representing the ROI coordinates. The network is trained using the mean squared error as measured by distance between estimated and annotated vertices. Backpropagation is used with Adam optimizer.

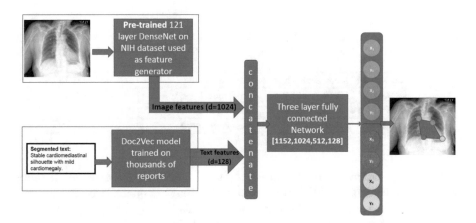

Fig. 2. Architecture 2: Image and text networks are trained separately. The resulting feature vectors are used to train a network that estimates ROI coordinates.

Experiments and Performance Metrics: All images were re-sized to 256×256. We included an additional 800 images from *DS1* that showed no clinically significant finding. For these images, the coordinates of the corresponding ROI were set to [0,0] for all four corners. These were used along with the 494 images with findings to train Architecture 1 and the final block of Architecture 2. One sanity check for the proposed solution is to not return a marking when there is no finding. For performance metrics, we report the centroid distance between the predicted and actual polygon normalized by image size. In experimenting with each of the two architectures, we performed 10 fold cross validation and report the average. All networks were trained on NVIDIA Titan X GPUs.

3 Results and Discussion

Architecture 1: The average distance between the centroids of the annotated and estimated quadrilaterals obtained from the Architecture 1 network was $7.2 \pm 5.1\%$ of the image size (measured only for the images with finding). The cardiomegaly cases were correctly annotated. The network also correctly returned values within 1% of [0,0] coordinates for all corners in all of the cases with a "no finding" label. For mass or nodules findings the estimated ROIs are close to ground truth, but not always overlapping.

Architecture 2: For Architecture 2, it is important to first understand the performance of the DenseNet feature generator on predicting labels for its classification task. The measured average AUC of the model over the 14 labels in *DS2* produced by our training process is 0.79. Table 1 lists the AUCs for the 14 labels. The result is comparable to the those reported in [2] and demonstrates that the feature learning process for the findings, including cardiomegaly and mass, is fairly successful.

Table 1. The area under ROC curves for the 14 labels present in the *DS2* dataset obtained from a 121 layer DenseNet trained as the feature generator of Architecture 2.

Atelectasis: **0.77**	Cardiomegaly: **0.89**	Effusion **0.86**	Infiltration: **0.70**
Nodule: **0.67**	Pneumonia: **0.73**	Pneumothorax: **0.81**	Consolidation: **0.80**
Emphysema: **0.84**	Fibrosis: **0.76**	Pleural thickening: **0.72**	Hernia: **0.78**
Edema: **0.90**	Mass: **0.79**	**Average: 0.79**	

The fully trained Architecture 2 network returned an average distance between the centroids of the annotated and estimated quadrilaterals that was equivalent to $5.1 \pm 4.0\%$ of the image width. This is a significant improvement compared to Architecture 1. Examples in Fig. 3 show that in this case, despite the over-estimations of ROI size in cases of mass and nodule, the results are generally accurate and the estimated ROI includes the ground truth. The cardiomegaly cases (right column of Fig. 3) show very accurate results. The overall

Dice coefficient was 61% compared to 46% for Architecture 2. Note that given the approximate nature of the markings, the Dice coefficient is not a good performance measure here. It was notable that 100% of the normal cases were mapped to the [0,0] corners and also all of the cardiomegaly cases were correctly mapped to the heart silhouette.

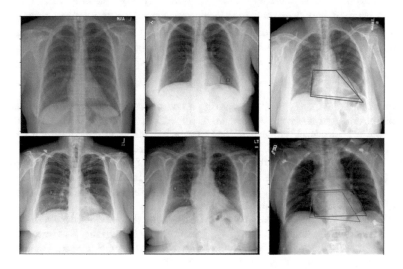

Fig. 3. Sample results from Architecture 2. Red is the estimated quadrilateral, blue is the one marked by a radiologist.

Comparison with an Image Only Network: In both of the reported architectures, one can cut off the text side of the network and produce the ROI coordinates using only images. While this image only scenario was not our target, it is fair to ask if text features contribute at all to the outcome. When we used only the imaging arm of Architecture 1, the average centroid distance went from $7.2 \pm 5.1\%$ to $21 \pm 10.9\%$ and the results also clearly deteriorated visually. For Architecture 2, the elimination of text features resulted in an average centroid distance of $7.8 \pm 7.7\%$ compared to $5.1 \pm 4.0\%$ in the bimodal network. In both architectures, removing text features also results in a complete collapse of the specificity with over 88% of normal images returning a non-zero ROI on Architecture 1, and 56% on Architecture 2. The text features clearly contribute to the accuracy of ROI estimation in both architectures.

4   Conclusion

We proposed two architectures for mapping findings from clinical reports onto the relevant region of the corresponding image. One design trains a CNN and an LSTM jointly. A second design relies on separate imaging and text networks trained on very large datasets as sources of features that are combined to predict the ROI coordinates. This second architecture provides more accurate results that can be used for building annotated datasets with minimal editing. We showed that the text arms of these bimodal networks clearly contribute to the accuracy of the generated annotations. We used a simple model of the ROI to ease the segmentation process. A more complex shape model can be adopted and estimated similarly. Furthermore, one can replace the final fully connected layers of each of the proposed architectures with a segmentation network and obtain a mask with no shape constraints. This can also accommodate the cases with multiple image findings which are not modeled in the current work.

References

1. Demner-Fushman, D., et al.: Preparing a collection of radiology examinations for distribution and retrieval. J. Am. Med. Inform. Assoc. **23**(2), 304–310 (2015)
2. Huang, G., Liu, Z., Weinberger, K.Q.: Densely connected convolutional networks. CoRR abs/1608.06993 (2016). http://arxiv.org/abs/1608.06993
3. Le, Q., Mikolov, T.: Distributed representations of sentences and documents. In: Xing, E.P., Jebara, T. (eds.) Proceedings of the 31st International Conference on Machine Learning. Proceedings of Machine Learning Research, vol. 32, pp. 1188–1196. PMLR, Bejing, China, 22–24 June 2014
4. Maier-Hein, L., et al.: Can masses of non-experts train highly accurate image classifiers? In: Golland, P., Hata, N., Barillot, C., Hornegger, J., Howe, R. (eds.) MICCAI 2014, Part II. LNCS, vol. 8674, pp. 438–445. Springer, Cham (2014). https://doi.org/10.1007/978-3-319-10470-6_55
5. Moradi, M., Guo, Y., Gur, Y., Negahdar, M., Syeda-Mahmood, T.: A cross-modality neural network transform for semi-automatic medical image annotation. In: Ourselin, S., Joskowicz, L., Sabuncu, M.R., Unal, G., Wells, W. (eds.) MICCAI 2016, Part II. LNCS, vol. 9901, pp. 300–307. Springer, Cham (2016). https://doi.org/10.1007/978-3-319-46723-8_35
6. Pennington, J., Socher, R., Manning, C.D.: Glove: Global vectors for word representation. In: Empirical Methods in Natural Language Processing (EMNLP), pp. 1532–1543 (2014). http://www.aclweb.org/anthology/D14-1162
7. Rajpurkar, P., et al.: Chexnet: Radiologist-level pneumonia detection on chest x-rays with deep learning. CoRR abs/1711.05225 (2017). http://arxiv.org/abs/1711.05225
8. Rodrguez, A.F., Muller, H.: Ground truth generation in medical imaging: a crowdsourcing-based iterative approach. In: Proceedings of the ACM Workshop on Crowdsourcing for Multimedia (2012)
9. Rupprecht, C., Peter, L., Navab, N.: Image segmentation in twenty questions. In: 2015 IEEE Conference on Computer Vision and Pattern Recognition (CVPR), pp. 3314–3322, June 2015
10. Wang, X., Peng, Y., Lu, L., Lu, Z., Bagheri, M., Summers, R.M.: Chestx-ray8: Hospital-scale chest x-ray database and benchmarks on weakly-supervised classification and localization of common thorax diseases. CoRR abs/1705.02315 (2017). http://arxiv.org/abs/1705.02315
11. Wang, X., Peng, Y., Lu, L., Lu, Z., Summers, R.M.: Tienet: Text-image embedding network for common thorax disease classification and reporting in chest x-rays. CoRR abs/1801.04334 (2018). http://arxiv.org/abs/1801.04334
12. Xu, K., et al.: Show, attend and tell: Neural image caption generation with visual attention. CoRR abs/1502.03044 (2015). http://arxiv.org/abs/1502.03044

Multimodal Recurrent Model with Attention for Automated Radiology Report Generation

Yuan Xue[1], Tao Xu[2], L. Rodney Long[3], Zhiyun Xue[3], Sameer Antani[3],
George R. Thoma[3], and Xiaolei Huang[1(✉)]

[1] College of Information Sciences and Technology,
Penn State University, University Park, PA, USA
sharon.x.huang@gmail.com
[2] Department of Computer Science and Engineering,
Lehigh University, Bethlehem, PA, USA
[3] National Library of Medicine, National Institutes of Health, Bethesda, MD, USA

Abstract. Radiologists routinely examine medical images such as X-Ray, CT, or MRI and write reports summarizing their descriptive findings and conclusive impressions. A computer-aided radiology report generation system can lighten the workload for radiologists considerably and assist them in decision making. Although the rapid development of deep learning technology makes the generation of a single conclusive sentence possible, results produced by existing methods are not sufficiently reliable due to the complexity of medical images. Furthermore, generating detailed paragraph descriptions for medical images remains a challenging problem. To tackle this problem, we propose a novel generative model which generates a complete radiology report automatically. The proposed model incorporates the Convolutional Neural Networks (CNNs) with the Long Short-Term Memory (LSTM) in a recurrent way. It is capable of not only generating high-level conclusive impressions, but also generating detailed descriptive findings sentence by sentence to support the conclusion. Furthermore, our multimodal model combines the encoding of the image and one generated sentence to construct an attention input to guide the generation of the next sentence, and henceforth maintains coherence among generated sentences. Experimental results on the publicly available Indiana U. Chest X-rays from the Open-i image collection show that our proposed recurrent attention model achieves significant improvements over baseline models according to multiple evaluation metrics.

1   Introduction

A radiologist completes a radiology report, by analyzing images from an examination, recognizing both normal and abnormal findings, and coming to a diagnosis. This process of medical image interpretation and reporting can be error-prone, however, even for experienced specialists. Where the discrepancies can

© Springer Nature Switzerland AG 2018
A. F. Frangi et al. (Eds.): MICCAI 2018, LNCS 11070, pp. 457–466, 2018.
https://doi.org/10.1007/978-3-030-00928-1_52

Input Image	Recurrent Attention	Ground Truth

Findings: The heart size and mediastinal contours appear within normal limits. No focal airspace consolidation , pleural effusion or pneumothorax. No acute bony abnormalities.
Impression: No acute cardiopulmonary finding.

Findings: The heart size and mediastinal silhouette are within normal limits for contour. The lungs are clear. No pneumothorax or pleural effusions. The XXXX are intact.
Impression: No acute cardiopulmonary abnormalities.

Findings: The heart size and mediastinal silhouette are within normal limits for contour. The lungs are clear. No focal airspace consolidation. No pleural effusion or pneumothorax. Normal cardiomediastinal silhouette. Heart size is normal.
Impression: Clear lungs. No acute cardiopulmonary abnormality.

Findings: Mediastinal contours are within normal limits. Heart size is within normal limits. No focal consolidation, pneumothorax or pleural effusion. No bony abnormality. Vague density in right mid lung, XXXX related to scapular tip and superimposed ribs. Not visualized on lateral exam.
Impression: Vague density in right XXXX, XXXX related to scapular tip and superimposed ribs. Consider oblique images to exclude true nodule. 2. No acute cardiopulmonary abnormality.

Fig. 1. Examples of original reports vs. reports generated by our recurrent attention model. Note that, Findings is a paragraph containing some descriptive sentences; Impression is a conclusive sentence. XXXXs are wrongly removed keywords due to de-identification.

come from the lack of knowledge or faulty reasoning by radiologists, staff shortage and excess workload also contribute to the errors in radiology reports [1]. To reduce workload and error occurrences, an automated or computer-aided reporting system can be helpful. An illustration of the automated report generation problem is shown in Fig. 1. The inputs are medical images of the same human subject from different views. In the resulting report, *Impression* is a single-sentence conclusion or diagnosis, and *Findings* is a paragraph containing multiple sentences that describe the radiologist's observations and findings regarding different regions in the images.

Most of the existing literature related to the report generation problem are based on deep learning technologies, following the encoder-decoder architecture originally used for machine translation [2]. While generation of the conclusive impression can be done by existing image captioning models that describe an image with a single sentence [15,19,20], Recurrent Neural Networks (RNNs) used by these existing models are known to be incapable of handling long sequences or paragraphs due to vanishing or exploding gradients [17]. Long Short-term Memory (LSTM) [8] alleviates this issue to some degree with a gating mechanism to learn long-term dependencies, but it still cannot completely prevent gradient from vanishing and thus is hard to model a very long sequence.

To generate a paragraph description, which is a very long sequence, some pioneering works have been done in the domain of natural image captioning, with hierarchical recurrent networks [12,13,21]. Mostly they use two levels of RNNs for paragraph generation: first, a paragraph-level RNN generates some topics, then a sentence-level RNN takes the topics as input and generates corresponding sentences. In [12,13], the authors utilize a pre-trained dense-captioning model [10] to detect semantic regions of the images. However, such pre-trained models are often not available for medical images. Toward the goal of medical image annotation, Shin *et al.* [18] proposed a deep learning framework to automatically annotate chest x-rays with Medical Subject Headings (MeSH) annotations for the first time. They use a CNN to classify the x-ray images with different disease labels. RNNs are then trained to describe the contexts of a detected disease with more details. Furthermore, a cascade model is applied to combine image and text contexts to improve annotation performance. Zhang et $al.$ [22] establish a direct multimodal mapping from medical images to diagnostic reports. They use an auxiliary attention sharpening (AAS) module to learn the image-language alignments more efficiently. However, their generated diagnostic reports are limited to describing five types of cell appearance features, which makes their problem less complex than general radiology report generation. Jing et $al.$ [9] adopt the hierarchical generation framework from [12] to generate detailed descriptions of medical images along with a co-attention model which can simultaneously attend to both visual and semantic features. Their work achieved impressive results on the IU chest x-ray dataset [4], although some repetitions can be found in their generated reports because their hierarchical model does not take contextual coherence into consideration.

In this paper, we focus on the generation of a findings paragraph. We break down the paragraph generation task into easier subtasks, where a subtask is concerned with generating one sentence at a time. To guarantee the intra-paragraph dependency and coherence among sentences, we develop a recurrent model, in which a first sentence is generated and then each succeeding sentence is generated by taking the encodings of both its preceding sentence and the image, as joint inputs. The main contributions of our work toward automated radiology report generation are: (1) we propose a novel recurrent generation model to generate the findings paragraph, sentence by sentence, whereby a succeeding sentence is conditioned upon multimodal inputs that include its preceding sentence and the original images, (2) we adopt an attention mechanism for our proposed multimodal model to improve performance. Extensive experiments on the Indiana U. Chest x-rays dataset demonstrate the effectiveness of our proposed methods.

2   Methodology

Assume we are generating a findings paragraph that contains L sentences. The probability of generating the i-th sentence with length T satisfies:

$$
\begin{aligned}
&\mathbb{P}(S_i = w_1, w_2, ..., w_T | V; \theta) \\
&= \mathbb{P}(S_1 | V) \prod_{j=2}^{i-1} \mathbb{P}(S_j | V, S_1, ...S_{j-1}) \mathbb{P}(w_1 | V, S_{i-1}) \prod_{t=2}^{T} \mathbb{P}(w_t | V, S_{i-1}, w_1, ...w_{t-1}),
\end{aligned}
\tag{1}
$$

where V is the given medical image, θ is the model parameter (we omit the θ in the right hand side), S_i represents the i-th sentence and w_t is the t-th token in the i-th sentence. Similar to the n-gram assumption in language models, we adopt the Markov assumption for sentence level generation with a "2-gram" model, which means the current sentence being generated depends only on its

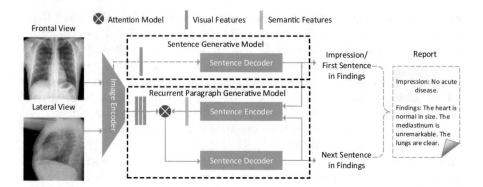

Fig. 2. The architecture of the proposed multimodal recurrent generation model with attention for radiology reports. Best viewed in color.

immediately preceding sentence and the image. This simplifies the estimated probability to be:

$$\hat{\mathbb{P}}(S_i = w_1, w_2, ... w_T | V; \theta) =$$

$$\underbrace{\mathbb{P}(S_1|V)}_{1} \underbrace{\prod_{j=2}^{i-1} \mathbb{P}(S_j|V, S_{j-1})}_{2} \underbrace{\mathbb{P}(w_1|V, S_{i-1}) \prod_{t=2}^{T} \mathbb{P}(w_t|V, S_{i-1}, w_1, ... w_{t-1})}_{3}. \tag{2}$$

Our goal is to find the optimal parameter for the Maximum Log-likelihood Estimate (MLE) as

$$\theta^* = \underset{\theta}{\operatorname{argmax}} \sum_{i=1}^{L} \log \hat{\mathbb{P}}(S_i = G_i | V; \theta), \tag{3}$$

where G_i is the ground truth for the i-th sentence in the findings paragraph.

As shown in Eq. 2, we separate that equation into 3 parts denoted by underbraces and introduce our model part by part. The overall architecture of our framework that takes medical images from multiple views as input and generates a radiology report with impression and findings is shown in Fig. 2. In order to generate the findings paragraph, we first use an encoder-decoder model which takes an image pair as input and generates the first sentence. Then the first sentence is fed into a sentence encoding network to output the semantic representation of that sentence. After that, both visual features of the image and semantic features of the preceding sentence are combined as the input to the multimodal recurrent generation network that generates the next sentence. This process is repeated until the model generates the last sentence in the paragraph. More details will be explained in the next subsections.

2.1   Image Encoder

In our model (Fig. 2), an image encoder is first applied to extract both global and regional visual features from the input images. The image encoder is a Convolutional Neural Network (CNN) that automatically extracts hierarchical visual features from images. More specifically, our image encoder is built upon the pre-trained resnet-152 [7]. We resize the input images to 224×224 to keep consistent with the pre-trained resnet-152 image encoder. Then, the local feature matrix $f \in \mathbb{R}^{1024 \times 196}$ (reshaped from $1024 \times 14 \times 14$) are extracted from the "res4b35" layer of resnet-152. Each column of f is one regional feature vector. Thus each image has 196 sub-regions. Meanwhile, we extract the global feature vector $f \in \mathbb{R}^{2048}$ from the last average pooling layer of resnet-152. For multiple input images from several views (e.g., frontal and lateral views as demonstrated in this paper), their regional and global features are concatenated accordingly before feeding into the following layers. For efficiency, all parameters in layers built from the resnet-152 are fixed during training.

2.2   Sentence Generative Model

In general, both the one-sentence impression and the first sentence in the findings paragraph contain some high level descriptions of the image. Thus, we develop a sentence generative model that takes the global visual features learned by the image encoder as input. Such a model can be trained to generate the impression. It can also be jointly trained with the recurrent generative model to generate the first sentence in the findings as an initialization of the recurrent model (formulated in part 1 of Eq. 2). In the sentence generative model, a single layer LSTM [8] is used for sentence decoding. The initial hidden states and cell states of the LSTM are set to be zero. The visual feature vector is used as the initial input of the LSTM to predict the first word of the sentence and then the whole sentence is produced word by word. Before being fed into the LSTM, a fully connected layer is utilized to transform the visual feature vector so that it has the same dimension as the word embedding. In all LSTM modules used in this paper, the dimensions of word embedding and the dimensions of hidden states are 512 and 1024, respectively.

2.3   Recurrent Paragraph Generative Model

As shown in Fig. 2, our recurrent paragraph generative model takes the sentence and regional image features as input and generates findings paragraph sentence by sentence. It has two main components: sentence encoder and attentional sentence decoder.

Sentence Encoder is used to extract semantic vectors from text descriptions. Two types of well-known text encoders are explored in this paper. The first one is a Bi-directional Long Short-Term Memory (Bi-LSTM) [6] which can encode better context information than the conventional one-directional LSTM. In the Bi-LSTM, each word corresponds to two hidden states, one for each direction. Inspired by [3], the 1D convolution neural network is also applied for sentence encoding. Our CNN model takes the 512 dimensional word embedding as input and has three convolution layers to learn hierarchical features. Each convolution layer has the kernel size 3, stride 1 and 1024 feature channels. The max-pooling operation is applied over feature maps extracted from each convolution layer, yielding a 1024 dimensional feature vector. The final sentence feature is the concatenation of feature vectors from different layers. We compare these two proposed encoder networks in Sect. 3.

Attentional Sentence Decoder takes regional visual features and the previously generated sentence as a multimodal input, and generates the next sentence. This solves both part 2 and part 3 of Eq. 2. The sentence decoder is a stacked 2-layer LSTM. The image pair V are converted as input to the 2-layer LSTM, then the learned encoding of the preceding sentence guides our model to generate the next sentence. We repeat this process until an empty sentence is generated, which indicates the end of the paragraph. In this way, the consistence of context in the paragraph is guaranteed.

To make different sentences focus on different image regions and capture the dependency between sentences, we propose a sentence based visual attention [15,20] mechanism for our recurrent generative model. Semantic features of the preceding sentence and regional visual representations are fed through a fully connected layer followed by a softmax layer to get the attention distribution over $k = 196$ image regions. First, we compute the attention weights over k regions as

$$a = W_{\mathrm{att}} \tanh(W_v v + W_s s 1^k), \tag{4}$$

where $v \in \mathbb{R}^{d_v \times k}$ are the regional visual features learned by the image encoder, $s \in \mathbb{R}^{d_s}$ represents the encoding of the preceding sentence. $W_{\mathrm{att}} \in \mathbb{R}^{1 \times k}$, $W_v \in \mathbb{R}^{k \times d_v}$ and $W_s \in \mathbb{R}^{k \times d_s}$ are parameters of the attention network. $1^k \in \mathbb{R}^{1 \times k}$ is a vector with all ones. $d_v = 1024$ is the dimension of the regional visual feature; d_s is the dimension of the sentence feature ($d_s = 2048$ for Bi-LSTM and $d_s = 3072$ for CNN sentence encoder). Next, we normalize it over all regions to get the attention distribution:

$$\alpha_i = \frac{\exp(a_i)}{\sum_i \exp(a_i)}, \tag{5}$$

where a_i is the i-th dimension in a. Finally, we compute the weighted visual representation as

$$v_{\mathrm{att}} = \sum_{i=1}^{k} \alpha_i v_i. \tag{6}$$

The input of the sentence decoder are now the weighted visual representation. When generating different sentences, the attention model focuses on different regions of the image based on the context of the preceding sentence. Features or regions which are not relevant to current sentence are filtered out and the model cannot see the sentence encoding directly so it is less likely to overfit to the semantic input. Performance comparison for the model with and without attention module can be found in Sect. 3.

All our proposed models are trained by the Adam optimizer [11]. The initial learning rate is set to be 1e−4 and learning rate decay is 0.9 for every 5 epochs.

The batch size is 460 for training. During the training, we adopt a teacher forcing policy, i.e., we always feed our decoder with ground truth word or sentence for the generation in the next timestep. During testing, greedy search is used for generating words and sentences in every timestep for efficiency. Previously generated words/sentences will be fed into the decoder as part of the input for the next word/sentence. The recurrent generative model will keep generating sentences until it generates an empty sentence. All modules are trained jointly in an end-to-end fashion by minimizing the cross entropy loss.

3   Experiments

We evaluate our model on the Indiana University Chest X-Ray collection [4]. The dataset contains 3,955 radiology reports from 2 large hospital systems within the Indiana Network for Patient Care database, and 7,470 associated chest x-rays from the hospitals' picture archiving systems. Each report is associated with a pair of images which are the frontal and lateral views, and contains comparison, indication, findings, and impression sections. All reports are fully anonymized for de-identification; however, 2.5% of findings/impression words are also removed during the de-identification, resulting in some keywords missing in the report. Since the original data are from multiple hospitals and are inconsistent, there are some images or findings missing in the original dataset. For our experiments, we filtered out reports without two complete image views or without complete sections of findings and impression, resulting in a smaller dataset with 2,775 reports associated with 5,550 images.

For data preparation, we tokenized all the words in the findings and impression in the dataset and obtained 2,218 unique words. Considering that the c size is already very small, we decided not to drop infrequent words with only once or twice appearances. We also added two special tokens, $\langle S \rangle$ and $\langle /S \rangle$, into the vocabulary to indicate the start and the end of a sentence. To evaluate our models, we randomly picked 250 reports to form the testing set. All evaluations are done on the testing set.

We use some common evaluation metrics for image captioning to provide a quantitative comparison. We report BLEU [16], METEOR [5] and ROUGE [14] scores of all proposed models and compare them with baseline models in Table 1. However, these evaluation metrics are not specially designed for medical report generation tasks. Hence we suggest another complementary metric. We construct a keyword dictionary from MTI annotations of the original dataset and some manual annotations. The dictionary contains 438 unique keywords, and we compute the keywords accuracy (KA) metric as the ratio of the number of keywords correctly generated by a model to the number of all keywords in the groundtruth findings. An example result can be found in Fig. 1.

For comparison, we reimplemented two baseline models [12,19] for radiology report generation. We use the same pre-trained resnet-152 image encoder for all models. Note that we do not have a pre-trained dense captioning model for medical images, thus we only use features learned by the image encoder directly for hierarchical generation [12]. Since Bi-LSTM encoding achieves better performance than convolution encoding in experiments, we adopt Bi-LSTM encoding for our final model. We also implemented a baseline model without attention module. In the recurrent generative model without attention, the sentence encoding learned by the sentence encoder are used as the initial hidden state and cell state of the sentence decoder. From Table 1, we can see that our final model with attention shows significant improvements over baseline models in all evaluation metrics. Moreover, although the hierarchical model [12] achieves reasonably high evaluation scores, the generated reports contain some repetitions and the paragraphs are not very coherent. In comparison, reports generated by our proposed model contain fewer repetitions and have more coherent context.

Table 1. Evaluation of generated reports on our testing set using BLEU, METEOR, ROUGE and KA metrics. We compare our models with two baseline models including a baseline implementation of the hierarchical generation model [12].

Methods	BLEU-1	BLEU-2	BLEU-3	BLEU-4	METEOR	ROUGE	KA
Vanilla CNN-RNN [19]	0.273	0.144	0.116	0.082	0.125	0.226	0.435
Hierarchical generation [12]	0.437	0.323	0.221	0.172	0.244	0.325	0.568
Ours-recurrent-conv	0.416	0.298	0.217	0.163	0.227	0.309	0.532
Ours-recurrent-BiLSTM	0.423	0.307	0.223	0.165	0.236	0.322	0.543
Ours-recurrent-attention	**0.464**	**0.358**	**0.270**	**0.195**	**0.274**	**0.366**	**0.596**

4   Discussions

In this paper, our main focus is on generating detailed findings for a report. For impression generation, a classification based method may be better at distinguishing abnormal cases and then giving the final conclusion. From the example results in Fig. 1 we can see that in the first row, both findings and impression are in accord with the groundtruth. However, in the second row of Fig. 1, both the generated findings and impression missed some abnormal descriptions. The main reason may be that we are training on a small training set, the training samples for abnormal cases are even fewer, and there are some inconsistency as well as noise in the original groundtruth reports. Moreover, our model does not create very well new sentences that have never appeared in the training set. This could be due to the difficulty in learning correct grammar from a small corpus since the objective function for training does not consider syntactic correctness. We expect that addressing the above limitations would require a larger and better annotated dataset, a new training strategy and a new evaluation metric which takes both keyword accuracy and grammar correctness into account.

5   Conclusions

In summary, we have proposed a multimodal recurrent model with attention for radiology report generation. A long and detailed paragraph can be generated recurrently sentence by sentence. Such a model can provide interpretable justifications as part of a computer-aided reporting system to assist clinicians in making decisions. We have shown that generating long and detailed paragraphs of findings is not only theoretical feasible but also practically useful. Experiments on a chest x-rays dataset demonstrate the effectiveness of our proposed method.

References

1. Brady, A., Laoide, R.Ó., McCarthy, P., McDermott, R.: Discrepancy and error in radiology: concepts, causes and consequences. Ulster Med. J. **81**(1), 3 (2012)
2. Cho, K., Van Merriënboer, B., Gulcehre, C., Bahdanau, D., Bougares, F., Schwenk, H., Bengio, Y.: Learning phrase representations using rnn encoder-decoder for statistical machine translation. arXiv preprint arXiv:1406.1078 (2014)
3. Conneau, A., Kiela, D., Schwenk, H., Barrault, L., Bordes, A.: Supervised learning of universal sentence representations from natural language inference data. arXiv preprint arXiv:1705.02364 (2017)
4. Demner-Fushman, D., Kohli, M.D., Rosenman, M.B., Shooshan, S.E., Rodriguez, L., Antani, S., Thoma, G.R., McDonald, C.J.: Preparing a collection of radiology examinations for distribution and retrieval. J. Am. Med. Inform. Assoc. **23**(2), 304–310 (2015)
5. Denkowski, M., Lavie, A.: METEOR universal: Language specific translation evaluation for any target language. In: Proceedings of the Ninth Workshop on Statistical Machine Translation, pp. 376–380 (2014)
6. Graves, A., Schmidhuber, J.: Framewise phoneme classification with bidirectional lstm and other neural network architectures. Neural Netw. **18**(5–6), 602–610 (2005)
7. He, K., Zhang, X., Ren, S., Sun, J.: Deep residual learning for image recognition. In: CVPR, pp. 770–778 (2016)
8. Hochreiter, S., Schmidhuber, J.: Long short-term memory. Neural Comput. **9**(8), 1735–1780 (1997)
9. Jing, B., Xie, P., Xing, E.: On the automatic generation of medical imaging reports. arXiv preprint arXiv:1711.08195 (2017)
10. Johnson, J., Karpathy, A., Fei-Fei, L.: Densecap: Fully convolutional localization networks for dense captioning. In: CVPR, pp. 4565–4574 (2016)
11. Kingma, D.P., Ba, J.: Adam: A method for stochastic optimization. arXiv preprint arXiv:1412.6980 (2014)
12. Krause, J., Johnson, J., Krishna, R., Fei-Fei, L.: A hierarchical approach for generating descriptive image paragraphs. In: CVPR, pp. 3337–3345 (2017)
13. Liang, X., Hu, Z., Zhang, H., Gan, C., Xing, E.P.: Recurrent topic-transition GAN for visual paragraph generation. CoRR, abs/1703.07022 2 (2017)
14. Lin, C.Y.: ROUGE: A package for automatic evaluation of summaries. Text Summarization Branches Out (2004)
15. Lu, J., Xiong, C., Parikh, D., Socher, R.: Knowing when to look: Adaptive attention via a visual sentinel for image captioning. In: CVPR, pp. 375–383 (2017)

16. Papineni, K., Roukos, S., Ward, T., Zhu, W.J.: BLEU: a method for automatic evaluation of machine translation. In: Proceedings of the 40th Annual Meeting on Association for Computational Linguistics, pp. 311–318. Association for Computational Linguistics (2002)
17. Pascanu, R., Mikolov, T., Bengio, Y.: On the difficulty of training recurrent neural networks. In: International Conference on Machine Learning, pp. 1310–1318 (2013)
18. Shin, H.C., Roberts, K., Lu, L., Demner-Fushman, D., Yao, J., Summers, R.M.: Learning to read chest x-rays: Recurrent neural cascade model for automated image annotation. In: CVPR, pp. 2497–2506 (2016)
19. Vinyals, O., Toshev, A., Bengio, S., Erhan, D.: Show and tell: A neural image caption generator. In: CVPR, pp. 3156–3164 (2015)
20. Xu, K., Ba, J., Kiros, R., Cho, K., Courville, A., Salakhudinov, R., Zemel, R., Bengio, Y.: Show, attend and tell: Neural image caption generation with visual attention. In: International Conference on Machine Learning, pp. 2048–2057 (2015)
21. Yu, H., Wang, J., Huang, Z., Yang, Y., Xu, W.: Video paragraph captioning using hierarchical recurrent neural networks. In: CVPR, pp. 4584–4593 (2016)
22. Zhang, Z., Xie, Y., Xing, F., McGough, M., Yang, L.: Mdnet: A semantically and visually interpretable medical image diagnosis network. In: CVPR, pp. 6428–6436 (2017)

Magnetic Resonance Spectroscopy Quantification Using Deep Learning

Nima Hatami[(✉)], Michaël Sdika, and Hélène Ratiney

Univ. Lyon, INSA-Lyon, Université Claude Bernard Lyon 1, UJM-Saint Etienne,
CNRS, Inserm, CREATIS UMR 5220, U1206, 69100 Lyon, France
hatami@creatis.insa-lyon.fr

Abstract. Magnetic resonance spectroscopy (MRS) is an important technique in biomedical research and it has the unique capability to give a non-invasive access to the biochemical content (metabolites) of scanned organs. In the literature, the quantification (the extraction of the potential biomarkers from the MRS signals) involves the resolution of an inverse problem based on a parametric model of the metabolite signal. However, poor signal-to-noise ratio (SNR), presence of the macro-molecule signal or high correlation between metabolite spectral patterns can cause high uncertainties for most of the metabolites, which is one of the main reasons that prevents use of MRS in clinical routine. In this paper, quantification of metabolites in MR Spectroscopic imaging using deep learning is proposed. A regression framework based on the Convolutional Neural Networks (CNN) is introduced for an accurate estimation of spectral parameters. The proposed model learns the spectral features from a large-scale simulated data set with different variations of human brain spectra and SNRs. Experimental results demonstrate the accuracy of the proposed method, compared to state of the art standard quantification method (QUEST), on concentration of 20 metabolites and the macromolecule.

Keywords: Convolutional Neural Networks · Short echo time
Magnetic Resonance Spectroscopy (MRS) · Deep learning
Metabolites · Time series regression · Parameter estimation

1 Introduction

Magnetic Resonance Spectroscopy Imaging (MRSI) allows detection and localization of spectra from several spatially distributed voxels. After each voxel signal quantification, it provides spatially resolved, non invasive and non-ionizing, metabolic information about the human body. The quantification process consists in analyzing the acquired spectra in order to estimate the metabolite concentrations, i.e. crucial biochemical information about the living cells and tissues.

© Springer Nature Switzerland AG 2018
A. F. Frangi et al. (Eds.): MICCAI 2018, LNCS 11070, pp. 467–475, 2018.
https://doi.org/10.1007/978-3-030-00928-1_53

1.1　MRS Quantification: Problematic and State of the Art

MRS signals are acquired in the time domain, but are usually inspected in the frequency domain as the metabolites are characterized by specific spectral patterns. A salient aspect of MRS is that the concentration of one molecule is directly proportional to the signal amplitude in the resulting signal. The signals acquired with short echo time, which is the focus of this paper, contain several (up to 20) metabolite contributions and also a macromolecular background. The MRS signal $y(t) = x(t) + b(t) + e$ can be described as parametric (metabolites' part $x(t)$) and non-parametric parts. $x(t)$ is defined as a linear combination of metabolite signals. $b(t)$ is called the background signal: originating from macromolecules, it is qualified as non-parametric because its model function is not known (partially at least). In addition, acquisition artifacts (such as eddy current effect or water residual) and Gaussian random noise e affect the acquired signal.

Up to now, all the proposed quantification methods solve an optimization problem attempting to minimize the difference between the data and a given parameterized model function. Most of the available methods employ local minimization and, in the case of short echo time, metabolite parameters are usually estimated by a non-linear least squares fit (in the time or the frequency domain) of the model (i.e. min $\|x - \hat{x}\|^2$) using a known basis set of the metabolite signals. Despite numerous proposed fitting methods (for example QUEST [1], LCModel [2], TARQUIN [3]), the robust, reliable and accurate quantification of brain metabolite concentration remains difficult. The major problems are: (1) strong metabolite spectral pattern overlapping (2) low signal to noise ratio, (3) unknown background and peak line shape. The problem is ill posed and current methods address it with different regularizations and constraint strategies (e.g. parameter bounds, penalizations), with possible large discrepancies in the results from one method to another [4].

Recently, as the application of machine learning expands into different domains, Das et. al [5] applied the Random Forest regressor for MRS quantification. It creates a set of decision trees from randomly selected subset of training set. This is the first and so far the only machine learning approach applied to this problem. In their work, a simplified problem with only three to five metabolites is addressed. We compare their approach to ours in the experiments section.

1.2　Contributions

The contributions of the current work can be summarized as follows: (i) addressing the MRS quantification problem using a deep learning approach for the first time. (ii) proposing a synthetic MRS signal generation framework for the quantification purpose. Such a framework can not only simulate the *in vivo* conditions, but also generate data free of cost and in a massive quantity. (iii) proposing an appropriate CNN model that outperforms the state-of-the art fitting methods. (iv) covering large number of metabolites (20) and the macromolecule. (v) studying the effect of different noise levels.

The remainder of this paper is organized as follows: the next section gives an overview on MRS imaging, its quantification and the state-of the art fitting methods. The Sect. 2 presents the proposed approach. The experiments, results and discussions are described in Sect. 3. Section 4 concludes the paper and suggests the possible future directions.

2   MRS Quantification: A Deep Learning Approach

The mathematical model for the parametric part is defined as follows:

$$x(t) = \sum_{m=1}^{M} a_m x_m(t) e^{\Delta\alpha_m t + 2i\pi \Delta f_m t} \tag{1}$$

where M is the number of metabolites, $x_m(t)$ is the known ideal pattern of the mth metabolite, and the parameters to be estimated are the amplitude (a_m), the damping factor $(\Delta\alpha_m)$ and the frequency shift (Δf_m). The amplitudes are directly proportional to the concentration of the metabolites. The quantification process aims to find the parameters (amplitude, damping factor and frequency shift) for each metabolite in a way that the result fits the input signal.

In this paper, a deep learning approach is presented as an alternative to the non-linear model fitting approaches of most methods in state of the art. Instead of finding the signal parameters as the solution of an inverse problem between the partial model given by Eq. 1 and the signal, our aim is to learn the inverse function once and for all on a training dataset. Once this function is learnt, it can be used on a new signal for the quantification of its parameters.

The MRS quantification problem is converted from an online regression problem (robustly extracting the parameters by solving an inverse problem) to an offline machine learning problem. The process can be decomposed in three parts described in the paragraphs below: one need to build the training dataset, to define a parametric representation of the inverse function and to setup a learning procedure to estimate the parameters of the inverse function.

2.1   Data Generation Framework

For any supervised learning technique to give satisfactory results, there should be enough training samples to be used in the learning process. Deep learning models in particular, require a relatively large amount of training data. A training dataset of *in vivo* MRS signal cannot be built as it requires costly acquisition on human subject. Moreover ground truth metabolite concentrations are not available for in vivo signals, even by using medical experts. This was the motivation to set up a synthetic data generation framework. The resulting dataset, if it succeeds to reproduce the distribution of realistic *in vivo* signals, has the advantage of being generated free of cost and on a massive scale.

The procedure to generate the dataset has been described in Fig. 1. Metabolite parameters a_m, (resp. $\Delta\alpha_m$), (resp. Δf_m) were randomly sampled

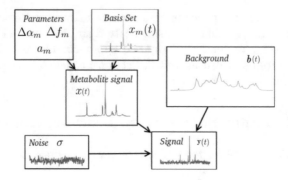

Fig. 1. The proposed synthetic MRS signal generation process.

with a distribution uniform in $[a_m^{\min}, a_m^{\max}]$, (resp. $[-\Delta\alpha^{\max}, \Delta\alpha^{\max}]$), (resp. $[-\Delta f^{\max}, \Delta f^{\max}]$). Knowing these parameters and the basis signals, the parametric signal x can be computed using the equation 1. Here, the background was considered as another metabolite: random scaling factor, damping and frequency shift was applied to the known background signal before it is added to x. Random complex Gaussian noise is finally added to get the final signal. To generate signal with a predefined SNR the standard deviation of the Gaussian distribution is set as the intensity of the first point of the noiseless signal divided by the SNR. This process can be repeated as many time as needed to create a large dataset of synthetic signals whose ground truth parameters are known.

2.2   Convolutional Neural Networks

There are two aspects of any CNN model that should be considered carefully: (i) designing an appropriate architecture, and (ii) choosing the right learning algorithm. Both architecture and learning rules should be chosen in a way that they are not only compatible with each other, but also fit the data and the application appropriately.

Architecture. CNN exploits spatially-local correlation by enforcing a local connectivity pattern between neurons of adjacent layers. Each layer is representing a different *feature-level* and consists of convolution (filter), activation function, and pooling (a.k.a. subsampling), respectively. The input and output of each layer are called *feature maps*. A filter layer convolves its input with a set of trainable kernels. The convolutional layer is the core building block of a CNN and exploits spatially local correlation by enforcing a local connectivity pattern between neurons of adjacent layers. The connections are local, but always extend along the entire depth of the input volume in order to produce the strongest response to a spatially local input pattern. Here we applied the recently proposed CReLU (Concatenated Rectified Linear Units) [6] because it demonstrated improvement in the recognition performance. It is based on an observation in CNN models that the filters in lower layers form pairs (i.e. filters with opposite phase). To avoid the model to learn redundant filters of both positive and negative phase information, CReLU is proposed as follows:

$$CRelu = Conc(r(x), -r(-x)) \tag{2}$$

where, $Conc$ is the concatenation operator and ReLU is defined as $r(x) = max(0, x)$.

Pooling reduces the resolution of input and makes it robust to small variations for previously learned features. It combines the outputs of i-1th layer into a single input in ith layer over a range of local neighborhood.

At the end of the feature extraction layers, the feature maps are flatten and fed into a fully connected (FC) layer for regression. FC layers connect every neuron in one layer to every neuron in another layer, which in principle are the same as the traditional multi-layer perceptron (MLP). The proposed pipeline for MRS quantification is shown in Fig. 2.

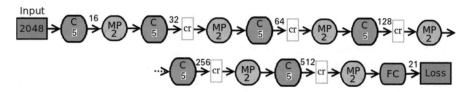

Fig. 2. The proposed CNN architecture for MRS quantification. The C, MP, cr, and FC represent convolution, max-pool, CReLu, and fully-connected layers, respectively.

Learning. Gradient-based optimization method (error back-propagation algorithm) is utilized to estimate parameters of the model. For faster convergence, the stochastic gradient descent (SGD) is used for updating the parameters. More details on CNN architecture and learning algorithm can be found in [7,8].

3   Experiments and Results

In the experiments, the metabolite basis set as well as the background signal provided by the ISMRM MRS Fitting Challenge 2016 were used. Although all parameters were used to generate the signal, only the amplitude, which are the main parameters of interest, were estimated by the neural network. Amplitudes were drawn in $[0, 1]$, Δa^{max} was set to $10\,\mathrm{Hz}$ as well as Δf^{max}.

Training datasets of up to 5×10^5 samples were generated. 80% of these samples are used to train the network and the rest is used as a validation dataset to evaluate the CNNs with different architectures, depths and solvers (optimization processes). Once the best CNN is chosen, it is applied and compared to state of the art quantification methods on a different unseen test set of 10,000 samples.

As shown in Fig. 2, a 7-layer CNN model is chosen with 2-channel (each real and imaginary part of the complex signal) input of size 2048 and the output layer with 21 neurons (20 metabolites amplitudes and a macromolecule scaling factor).

The Symmetric mean absolute percentage error (SMAPE) [9] over the whole test set is used to measure the accuracy of the models for each metabolite:

$$SMAPE = \frac{\sum_{n=1}^{N} |a - \hat{a}|}{\sum_{n=1}^{N} (a + \hat{a})} \tag{3}$$

where $\hat{a}$ and a are the estimated and ground truth amplitude values, respectively. SMAPE has been chosen as metric for its invariance to scale changes and its robustness to small values estimation.

Experiments were carried out using the Caffe framework [10] with the Adam solver and the maximum number of iterations set to 200,000. To initially move fast towards the local minimum, and move more slowly as approaching it, the "step" $(lr_0 \times \gamma^{floor(iter/step)})$ learning rate policy was chosen with $\gamma : 0.5$ and $lr_0 : 10^{-3}$.

The less deep architectures have less parameters to adjust. Therefore, they need less data to train. However, for learning more complex tasks, expanding the layers is one of the options, which consequently requires larger data size. In our case that the data can be generated in any desired size (except when there is time or computational restrictions), we should try deeper models, if it was beneficial. The goal is to find an optimal architecture that minimizes the bias and standard deviation of the estimator. Figure 3 shows the process of choosing the optimal data size for a given CNN model.

For the comparison and as a gold standard, quantitation based on semi-parametric quantum estimation (QUEST) [1] is used. This nonlinear least-squares algorithm ranked between the best methods in the ISMRM'16 MRS Fitting Challenge. We also compare our results with the only machine learning approach applied on MRS quantification i.e. random forest regression algorithm [5]. However, since the full details on the features used for the random forest is not given, we applied it on the raw data (no traditional hand-crafted feature extraction used).

Discussion: This work has tackled, through the proposed deep learning app-roach, the major bottleneck of MRS quantification which is the metabolite peak overlapping and macromolecular background contamination. One can also see that learning curves presented in Fig. 3 has the expected shape: this will allow to estimate the bias and generalization power of our CNN estimator. Remarkably, the SMAPE is high in QUEST for the metabolites that are known to have overlapped spectral pattern (and thus strong amplitude parameter correlation) such as GABA, Glu, Gln, but also Glc, Ins, sIns, while CNN CRelu and RF performance appear to be insensitive to spectral pattern overlapping. This results can be confirmed visually on the plot presented in Fig. 4. Results from Table 1 show that CNN quantification outperforms the two other methods both with

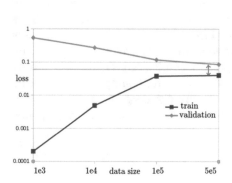

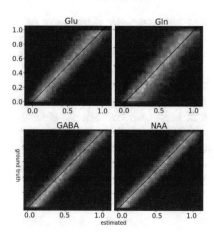

Fig. 3. Learning curves: training and validation loss as a function of the training set size. The green line and pink gap approximately represent the estimated bias and standard deviation, respectively.

Fig. 4. Ground truth vs. estimated metabolite concentrations using the CNN model for the test set (without noise).

Table 1. The SMAPE (%) of the QUEST and Random Forest ensemble (RF) vs. the deep CNN model on the short echo-time data with no noise (left) and 10 SNR (right).

Metabolite	Quest	RandForest	CNN CReLu	Metabolite	Quest	RandForest	CNN CReLu
Ala	6.64	22.05	**2.80**	Ala	31.21	24.39	21.03
Asc	6.44	22.13	**3.92**	Asc	28.80	24.24	**20.64**
Asp	8.81	24.12	**5.23**	Asp	41.98	**25.38**	25.87
Cr	**10.31**	20.70	12.28	Cr	26.30	22.92	**19.64**
GABA	15.48	16.86	**5.98**	GABA	37.63	25.14	**24.37**
GPC	5.53	14.96	**3.34**	GPC	25.06	19.33	**13.67**
GSH	7.94	21.52	**4.44**	GSH	26.81	23.70	**19.06**
Glc	10.89	22.00	**2.01**	Glc	33.42	24.07	**20.85**
Gln	18.11	23.60	**9.89**	Gln	36.09	24.94	**22.98**
Glu	15.97	23.07	**7.74**	Glu	34.88	24.82	**22.29**
Gly	12.44	23.57	**9.81**	Gly	29.78	24.18	**21.50**
Ins	11.84	20.89	**8.72**	Ins	28.03	23.73	**20.20**
Lac	6.34	20.46	**2.43**	Lac	28.80	24.32	**20.40**
NAA	9.26	20.87	**5.38**	NAA	26.69	22.93	**18.95**
NAAG	7.15	15.75	**3.76**	NAAG	23.58	21.85	**16.03**
PCho	6.13	16.10	**4.94**	PCho	21.44	19.60	**14.27**
PCr	**10.24**	20.67	11.19	PCr	26.40	22.77	**19.39**
PE	17.64	24.26	**10.96**	PE	43.29	24.84	**23.29**
Tau	14.81	23.25	**11.65**	Tau	36.82	24.20	**22.18**
sIns	6.80	16.91	**6.10**	sIns	23.02	17.72	**14.09**
Macromol.	1.32	5.06	**0.86**	Macromol.	14.45	17.59	**8.84**
# wins	2	0	**19**	# wins	0	1	**20**
Ave. Rank	2.47	2.52	**1.00**	Ave. Rank	2.95	2.00	**1.04**

and without noise. One can notice that without noise, the QUEST 's SMAPE were smaller than RF while it is not the case for noisy data. Note that the chosen noise level is really important here and most of the acquisitions are generally done with higher SNRs. The obtained results demonstrate the high noise robustness of machine learning approaches. Finally, these different methods were compared on data which metabolite relative concentrations/proportions do not mimic *in vivo* conditions. However, the present results demonstrate the ability of CNN to perform MRS quantification without being hampered by the usual limitations. The next step is to integrate more realistic signal in the data generation, for example by including phase variation due to eddy current, residual water or non ideal lineshapes.

4 Conclusions and Future Work

Quantification of metabolites in MRS imaging using deep learning is presented for the first time. A CNN model, as a class of deep, feed-forward artificial neural networks is used for accurate estimation of spectral parameters. Since efficient training of the CNN model requires large number of samples and such a data is not available *in vivo*, a new framework of generating a simulated human brain spectra is set up. Experiments are carried out on 20 metabolites and the macromolecule using different noise levels. The obtained results are compared to the Quest and the Random Forest regressor, highlighting the superiority of the proposed method. This study opens a new line of research to further investigate the application of deep learning techniques on MRS quantification problem.

Some future directions to extend the current work are (i) validation of the proposed CNN model on *in vivo* data, (ii) including the non-linear effects and artifacts (e.g. water residue and eddy current effect) in the synthetic data generation model for more realistic simulation of *in vivo* conditions, and (iii) investigating different deep learning models, architectures, and signal representations (e.g. image representation of spectral data [11]) for improving the accuracy.

Acknowledgement. This work is supported by the academic program of NVIDIA, the CNRS PEPS "APOCS" and the LABEX PRIMES (ANR-11-LABX-0063) of Université de Lyon, within the program "Investissements d'Avenir" (ANR-11-IDEX-0007). We also acknowledge the CC-IN2P3 for providing the computing resources.

References

1. Ratiney, H., Sdika, M., Coenradie, Y., Cavassila, S., van Ormondt, D., Graveron-Demilly, D.: Time-domain semi-parametric estimation based on a metabolite basis set. Nucl. Magn. Reson. Biomed. **18**, 1–13 (2005)
2. Provencher, S.W.: Estimation of metabolite concentrations from localized in vivo proton NMR spectra. Magn. Reson. Med. **30**(6), 672–679 (1993)
3. Wilson, M., Reynolds, G., Kauppinen, R., Arvanitis, T., Peet, A.: A constrained least-squares approach to the automated quantitation of in vivo 1h magnetic resonance spectroscopy data. Magn. Reson. Med. **65**(1), 1–12 (2011)

4. Bhogal, A., Schür, R., Houtepen, L., Bank, B., Boer, V., Marsman, A., et al.: 1H-MRS processing parameters affect metabolite quantification: the urgent need for uniform and transparent standardization. NMR Biomed. **30**(11), e3804 (2017)
5. Das, D., Coello, E., Schulte, R.F., Menze, B.H.: Quantification of metabolites in magnetic resonance spectroscopic imaging using machine learning. In: Descoteaux, M., Maier-Hein, L., Franz, A., Jannin, P., Collins, D.L., Duchesne, S. (eds.) MICCAI 2017. LNCS, vol. 10435, pp. 462–470. Springer, Cham (2017). https://doi.org/10.1007/978-3-319-66179-7_53
6. Shang, W., Sohn, K., Almeida, D., Lee, H.: Understanding and improving convolutional neural networks via concatenated rectified linear units. In: International Conference on Machine Learning, pp. 2217–2225 (2016)
7. LeCun, Y., Bottou, L., Orr, G.B., Müller, K.-R.: Efficient backprop. In: Orr, G.B., Müller, K.-R. (eds.) Neural Networks: Tricks of the Trade. LNCS, vol. 1524, pp. 9–50. Springer, Heidelberg (1998). https://doi.org/10.1007/3-540-49430-8_2
8. Bouvrie, J.: Notes on convolutional neural networks (2006)
9. Flores, B.E.: A pragmatic view of accuracy measurement in forecasting. Omega **14**, 93–98 (1986)
10. Jia, Y., et al.: Caffe: Convolutional architecture for fast feature embedding. arXiv preprint arXiv:1408.5093 (2014)
11. Hatami, N., Gavet, Y., Debayle, J.: Classification of time-series images using deep convolutional neural networks. In: ICMV (2017)

A Lifelong Learning Approach to Brain MR Segmentation Across Scanners and Protocols

Neerav Karani$^{(\boxtimes)}$, Krishna Chaitanya, Christian Baumgartner, and Ender Konukoglu

Computer Vision Lab, ETH Zurich, Zurich, Switzerland
`nkarani@vision.ee.ethz.ch`

Abstract. Convolutional neural networks (CNNs) have shown promising results on several segmentation tasks in magnetic resonance (MR) images. However, the accuracy of CNNs may degrade severely when segmenting images acquired with different scanners and/or protocols as compared to the training data, thus limiting their practical utility. We address this shortcoming in a lifelong multi-domain learning setting by treating images acquired with different scanners or protocols as samples from different, but related domains. Our solution is a single CNN with shared convolutional filters and domain-specific batch normalization layers, which can be tuned to new domains with only a few ($\approx$4) labelled images. Importantly, this is achieved while retaining performance on the older domains whose training data may no longer be available. We evaluate the method for brain structure segmentation in MR images. Results demonstrate that the proposed method largely closes the gap to the benchmark, which is training a dedicated CNN for each scanner.

1 Introduction

Segmentation of brain MR images is a critical step in many diagnostic and surgical applications. Accordingly, several approaches have been proposed for tackling this problem such as atlas-based segmentation [1], methods based on machine learning techniques such as CNNs [2], among many others as detailed in this recent survey [3]. One of the important challenges in many MRI analysis tasks, including segmentation, is robustness to differences in statistical characteristics of image intensities. These differences might arise due to using different scanners in which factors like drift in scanner SNR over time [4], gradient non-linearities [5] and others play an important role. Intensity variations may even arise when scanning protocol parameters (flip angle, echo or repetition time, etc.) are slightly changed on the same scanner. Figure 1(a, b) shows 2D slices from two T1-weighted MRI datasets from different scanners, along with their intensity histograms which show the aforementioned variations. Segmentation algorithms are often very sensitive to such changes. Furthermore, images acquired with different MR modalities, such as T1 and T2-weighted images, may have considerable high-level similarities in image content (see Fig. 1). While analyzing these

© Springer Nature Switzerland AG 2018
A. F. Frangi et al. (Eds.): MICCAI 2018, LNCS 11070, pp. 476–484, 2018.
https://doi.org/10.1007/978-3-030-00928-1_54

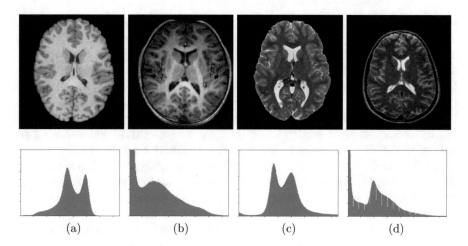

Fig. 1. Image slices (top) and corresponding histograms (bottom) of normalized T1w (a,b) and T2w (c,d) MRIs from different scanners. Despite high-level information similarity, there exists considerable intensity and contrast differences, which segmentation algorithms are often sensitive to.

images, humans can leverage such commonalities easily and it would be highly desirable if learning-based algorithms could mimic this trait.

In the parlance of transfer machine learning, images acquired from different scanners, protocols or similar MR modalities may be viewed as data points sampled from different domains, with the degree of domain shift potentially indicated by the differences in their intensity statistics. This perspective motivates us to employ ideas from the literature of domain adaptation [6], multi-domain learning [7] and lifelong learning [8] to the problem of brain segmentation across scanners/protocols. Domain adaptation/transfer learning refers to a situation where a learner trained on a source domain is able to perform well on a target domain, of which only a few labelled examples are available. However, in this case, the performance on the source domain may not be necessarily maintained after adaptation. Multi-domain learning aims to train a learner that can simultaneously perform well on multiple domains. Finally, in lifelong learning, a multi-domain learner is able to incorporate new domains with only few labelled examples, while preserving performance on previous domains.

Variants of image intensity standardization [9,10] and atlas intensity renormalization [11] have been proposed as pre-processing steps to insure conventional segmentation methods from inter-scanner differences. Among learning methods based on hand-crafted features, transfer learning approaches have been employed for multi-site segmentation [12] and classification [13]. While adaptive support vector machines used by [12] may be adapted for new scanners in a lifelong learning sense, they are likely to be limited by the quality of the hand-crafted features. Using CNNs, [14] propose to deal with inter-protocol differences by learning domain invariant representations. This approach may be limited to work with the least common denominator between the domains, while, as shown in [15], providing a few separate parameters for each domain allows for learning of domain specific nuances. Further, it is unclear how [14] can be extended to deal with new domains that may be encountered after the initial training. In the computer vision literature, several adaptations of batch normalization (BN) [16] have been suggested for domain adaptation [17,18] and multi-domain learning [15,19] for object recognition using CNNs. Broadly, these works employ BN for domain-specific scaling to account for domain shifts, while sharing the bulk of the CNN parameters to leverage the similarity between the domains.

In this work, we extend approaches based on adaptive BN layers for segmentation across scanning protocols in a lifelong learning setting. In particular, we train a CNN with common convolutional filters and specific BN parameters for each protocol/scanner. The network is initially trained with images from a few scanners to learn appropriate convolutional filters. It can then be adapted to new protocols/scanners by fine-tuning the BN parameters with only a few labelled images. Crucially, this is achieved without performance degradation on the older scanners, whose training data is not available after the initial training.

2   Method

Batch normalization (BN) was introduced in [16] to enable faster training of deep neural networks by preventing saturated gradients via normalization of inputs before each non-linear activation layer. In a BN layer, each batch x_B is normalized as shown in Eq. 1. During training, μ_B and σ_B^2 are the mean and variance of x_B, while at test time, they are the estimated population mean and variance as approximated by a moving average over training batches. γ, β are learnable parameters that allow the network to undo the normalization, if required. Inspired by [15], we propose to use separate batch normalization for each protocol/scanner.

$$BN(x_B) = \gamma \times \frac{x_B - \mu_B}{\sqrt{\sigma_B^2 + \epsilon}} + \beta \tag{1}$$

Notwithstanding variations in image statistics due to inter-scanner differences, a segmentation network would be confronted with images of the same organ, acquired with the same modality (MR). Hence, it is reasonable to postulate common characteristics between the domains and thus, shared support in an appropriate representation space. Following [15], we hypothesize that such a representation space can be found by using domain-agnostic convolutional filters and that the inter-domain differences can be handled by appropriate normalization via domain-specific BN modules. This approach is not only in line with the previous domain adaptation works [18], but also embodies the normalization idea of conventional proposals for dealing with inter-scanner variations [9–11]. Further, like [19], once suitable shared convolutional filters have been learned, we adapt the domain-specific BN layers to new related domains.

The training procedure in our framework is as follows. We use superscript bn to indicate a network with domain-specific BN layers. We initially train a network, $N_{12...d}^{bn}$ on d domains, with shared convolutional filters and separate BN parameters, bn_k, for each domain D_k. During training, each batch consists of only one domain, with all domains covered successively. In a training iteration when the batch consists of domain D_k, $bn_{k'}$ for k' $\neq$k are frozen. Now, consider a new domain D_{d+1}, with a few labelled images $I_{D_{d+1}}$. We split this small dataset into two halves, using one for training, $I_{D_{d+1}}^{tr}$ and the other for validation, $I_{D_{d+1}}^{vl}$. We evaluate the performance of $N_{12...d}^{bn}$ on $I_{D_{d+1}}^{tr}$, using each learned bn_k, $k = 1, 2, \cdots d$. If bn_{k*} leads to the best accuracy, we infer that among the already learned domains, D_{k*} is the closest to D_{d+1}. Then, keeping the convolutional filter weights fixed, an additional set of BN parameters bn_{d+1} is initialized with bn_{k*} and fine-tuned using $I_{D_{d+1}}^{tr}$ with standard stochastic gradient descent minimization. The optimization is stopped when the performance on $I_{D_{d+1}}^{vl}$ stops improving. Now, the network can segment all domains D_k, for $k = 1, 2, \ldots d, d + 1$ using their respective bn_k.

In the spirit of lifelong learning, this approach allows learning on new domains with only a few labelled examples. This is enabled by utilizing the knowledge obtained from learning on the old domains, in the form of the trained domain-agnostic parameters. The fact that the number of domain-specific parameters is small comes with two advantages. One, that they can be tuned for a new domain by training with a few labelled images quickly and with minimal risk of overfitting. Secondly, they can be saved for each domain without significant memory footprint. Finally, catastrophic forgetting [20] by performance degradation on previous domains does not arise in this approach by construction because of the explicit separate modeling of shared and private parameters.

3   Experiments and Results

Datasets: Brain MR datasets from several scanners, hospitals, or acquisition protocols are required to test the applicability of the proposed method for lifelong multi-domain learning. To the best of our knowledge, there are only a few publicly available brain MRI datasets with ground truth segmentation labels from human experts. Therefore, we use FreeSurfer [1] to generate pseudo ground truth annotations. While annotations from human experts would be ideal, we believe that FreeSurfer annotations can serve as a reasonable proxy to test our approach to lifelong multi-scanner learning.

We use images from 4 publicly available datasets: Human Connectome Project (HCP) [21], Alzheimer's Disease Neuroimaging Initiative (ADNI)[1], Autism Brain Imaging Data Exchange (ABIDE) [22] and Information eXtraction from Images (IXI)[2]. The datasets are split into different domains, as shown in Table 1. Domains D_1, D_2, D_3 are treated as initially available, and D_4, D_5 as

---

[1] adni.loni.usc.edu.

[2] brain-development.org/ixi-dataset/.

Table 1. Details of the datasets used for our experiments.

Domain	Dataset	Field	MR Modality	n_{train}	$n_{train}^{scratch}$	n_{test}
D_1	HCP	3T	T1w	30	30	20
D_2	HCP	3T	T2w	30	30	20
D_3	ADNI	1.5T	T1w	30	30	20
D_4	ABIDE, Caltech	3T	T1w	4	20	20
D_5	IXI	3T	T2w	4	20	20

new. The number of training and test images for each domain indicated in the table are explained later while describing the experiments.

Training Details: While the domain-specific BN layers can be incorporated in any standard CNN, we work with the widely used U-Net [2] architecture with minor alterations. Namely, our network has a reduced depth with three max-pooling layers and a reduced number of kernels: 32, 64, 128, 256 in the convolutional blocks on the contracting path and 128, 64, 32 on the upscaling path. Also, bilinear interpolation is preferred to deconvolutional layers for upscaling in view of potential checkerboard artifacts [23]. The network is trained to minimize the dice loss, as introduced in [24] to reduce sensitivity to imbalanced classes. Per image volume, the intensities are normalized by dividing by their 98th percentile. The initial network trains in about 6 h, while the domain-specific BN modules can be updated for a new domain in about 1 h, on a Nvidia Titan Xp GPU.

Experiments: We train three types of networks, as described below.

- Individual networks N_d: Trained for each domain d, with $n_{train}^{scratch}$ training images (see Table 1). For the known domains (D_1, D_2, D_3), the accuracy of N_d serves as a baseline that the other networks with shared parameters must preserve. For the new domains (D_4, D_5), the performance of N_d is the benchmark that we seek to achieve by training on much fewer training examples (n_{train}) and using the knowledge of the previously learned domains.
- A shared network N_{123}: Trained on D_1, D_2, D_3 with n_{train} images, with all parameters shared including the BN layers, bn_s. In contrast to the training regime of $N_{1,2,...d}^{bn}$ described in Sect. 2, while training N_{123} each batch randomly contains images from all domains to ensure that the shared BN parameters can be tuned for all domains. Histogram equalization [25] is applied to a new domain D_d before being tested N_{123}. For adapting N_{123} to D_d, all parameters are fine-tuned with n_{train} images of the new domain and the modified network is referred to as $N_{123 \rightarrow d}$.
- A lifelong multi-domain learning network N_{123}^{bn}: Trained on D_1, D_2, D_3, with shared convolutional layers and domain-specific BN layers. The updated network after extending N_{123}^{bn} for a new domain D_d according to the procedure described in Sec. 2 is called $N_{123,k^* \rightarrow d}$, where k^* is the closest domain to D_d.

Table 2. Segmentation dice scores for different domains for the three different types of networks, trained as explained in the experiments section.

Network	Test	BN	Thal	Hipp	Amyg	Ventr	Caud	Puta	Pall	Avg
N_1	D_1	bn_1	0.919	0.861	0.849	0.901	0.9	0.887	0.747	0.866
N_2	D_2	bn_2	0.912	0.84	0.836	0.891	0.889	0.876	0.736	0.854
N_3	D_3	bn_3	0.913	0.872	0.81	0.944	0.864	0.879	0.853	0.876
N_4	D_4	bn_4	0.924	0.879	0.853	0.933	0.912	0.9	0.851	0.893
N_5	D_5	bn_5	0.884	0.79	0.773	0.803	0.793	0.818	0.791	0.81
N_{123}	D_1	bn_s	0.909	0.846	0.824	0.891	0.878	0.877	0.745	0.853
N_{123}	D_2	bn_s	0.888	0.838	0.815	0.876	0.863	0.86	0.701	0.834
N_{123}	D_3	bn_s	0.905	0.851	0.792	0.938	0.863	0.873	0.828	0.864
N_{123}	D_4	bn_s	0.745	0.249	0.057	0.787	0.428	0.324	0.071	0.38
N_{123}	$D_{4,HistEq}$	bn_s	0.641	0.428	0.175	0.754	0.628	0.579	0.303	0.501
$N_{123 \to 4}$	D_4	bn_s	0.91	0.856	0.74	0.922	0.894	0.859	0.786	0.852
$N_{123 \to 4}$	D_1	bn_s	0.869	0.809	0.773	0.867	0.861	0.722	0.667	0.795
$N_{123 \to 4}$	D_2	bn_s	0.676	0.418	0.512	0.105	0.635	0.4	0.411	0.451
$N_{123 \to 4}$	D_3	bn_s	0.801	0.762	0.65	0.753	0.728	0.715	0.772	0.74
N_{123}	D_5	bn_s	0.418	0.178	0.182	0.438	0.268	0.197	0.025	0.244
N_{123}	$D_{5,HistEq}$	bn_s	0.294	0.143	0.16	0.437	0.261	0.293	0.01	0.228
$N_{123 \to 5}$	D_5	bn_s	0.861	0.777	0.761	0.799	0.76	0.796	0.741	0.785
$N_{123 \to 5}$	D_1	bn_s	0.267	0.022	0.173	0.004	0.05	0.002	0.004	0.075
$N_{123 \to 5}$	D_2	bn_s	0.574	0.574	0.564	0.739	0.657	0.521	0.526	0.594
$N_{123 \to 5}$	D_3	bn_s	0.147	0.029	0.16	0.006	0.114	0.039	0.003	0.071
N_{123}^{bn}	D_1	bn_1	0.916	0.852	0.84	0.894	0.893	0.884	0.729	0.858
N_{123}^{bn}	D_2	bn_2	0.91	0.853	0.843	0.887	0.882	0.873	0.749	0.857
N_{123}^{bn}	D_3	bn_3	0.911	0.868	0.818	0.944	0.867	0.879	0.846	0.876
N_{123}^{bn}	D_4	bn_1	0.621	0.288	0.218	0.173	0.676	0.576	0.457	0.43
N_{123}^{bn}	D_4	bn_2	0.162	0	0.001	0.001	0.04	0.017	0	0.032
N_{123}^{bn}	D_4	bn_3	0.721	0.271	0.305	0.549	0.569	0.515	0.297	0.461
$N_{123,3 \to 4}^{bn}$	D_4	bn_4	0.878	0.83	0.772	0.907	0.875	0.852	0.772	0.841
N_{123}^{bn}	D_5	bn_1	0.001	0.019	0.062	0.008	0.004	0	0	0.013
N_{123}^{bn}	D_5	bn_2	0.354	0.123	0.268	0.225	0.407	0.276	0.366	0.288
N_{123}^{bn}	D_5	bn_3	0	0.003	0.031	0.001	0	0	0	0.005
$N_{123,2 \to 5}^{bn}$	D_5	bn_5	0.774	0.687	0.687	0.761	0.669	0.714	0.713	0.715

Results: All networks are evaluated based on their mean Dice score for n_{test} images from the appropriate domain (see Table 1). Quantitative results of our experiments are shown in Table 2. The findings can be summarized as follows:

- N_{123} preserves the performance of N_1, N_2, N_3. Thus, a single network can learn to segment multiple domains, provided sufficient training data is available from all the domains at once. However, its performance severely degrades for unseen domains D_4 and D_5. Histogram equalization (denoted by $D_{d,HistEq}$) to the closest domain is unable to improve performance significantly, while fine-tuning the network for the new domains causes catastrophic forgetting [20], that is, degradation in performance on the old domains.
- N_{123}^{bn} also preserves the performance of N_1, N_2, N_3. For a new domain D_4, using the bn_3 parameters of the trained N_{123}^{bn} leads to the best performance. Thus, we infer that D_3 is the closest to D_4 among D_1, D_2, D_3. After fine-tuning the parameters of BN_3 to obtain those of BN_4, the dice scores for all the structures improve dramatically and are comparable to the performance of N_4. Crucially, as the original bn_k for k = 1, 2, 3 are saved, the performance on D_1, D_2, D_3 in the updated network $N_{123,3-4}^{bn}$ is exactly the same as in N_{123}^{bn}. Similar results can be seen for the other new domain, D_5. The improvement in the segmentations for new domains after fine-tuning the BN parameters can also be observed qualitatively in Fig. 2.

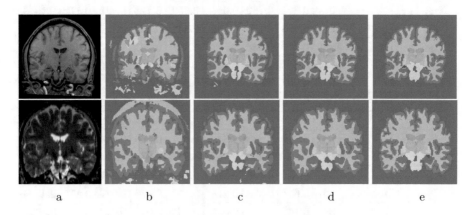

a   b   c   d   e

Fig. 2. Qualitative results: (a) images from domains D_d, segmentations predicted by (b) N_{123}^{bn}, bn_{k^*}, (c) $N_{123,k^*\to d}^{bn}$, bn_d, (d) N_d and (e) ground truth annotations, with $\{d, k^*\}$ as $\{4, 3\}$ (top) and $\{5, 2\}$ (bottom).

4   Conclusion

In this article, we presented a lifelong multi-domain learning approach to learn a segmentation CNN that can be used for related MR modalities and across scanners/protocols. Further, it can be adapted to new scanners or protocols with only a few labelled images and without degrading performance on the previous scanners. This was achieved by learning batch normalization parameters for each scanner, while sharing the convolutional filters between all scanners. In future work, we intend to investigate the possibility of extending this approach to MR modalities that were not present during the initial training.

To the best of our knowledge, this is the first work to tackle the lifelong machine learning problem for CNNs in the context of medical image analysis. We believe that this may set an important precedent for more research in this vein to handle data distribution changes which are ubiquitous in clinical data.

References

1. Fischl, B.: Freesurfer. Neuroimage **62**(2), 774–781 (2012)
2. Ronneberger, O., Fischer, P., Brox, T.: U-Net: convolutional networks for biomedical image segmentation. In: Navab, N., Hornegger, J., Wells, W.M., Frangi, A.F. (eds.) MICCAI 2015, Part III. LNCS, vol. 9351, pp. 234–241. Springer, Cham (2015). https://doi.org/10.1007/978-3-319-24574-4_28
3. Despotović, I., et al.: MRI segmentation of the human brain: challenges, methods, and applications. Comput. Math. Methods Med. **2015**, 23 (2015)
4. Preboske, G., et al.: Common MRI acquisition non-idealities significantly impact the output of the boundary shift integral method of measuring brain atrophy on serial MRI. Neuroimage **30**(4), 1196–1202 (2006)
5. Jovicich, J., et al.: Reliability in multi-site structural MRI studies: effects of gradient non-linearity correction on phantom and human data. Neuroimage **30**(2), 436–443 (2006)
6. Pan, S., et al.: A survey on transfer learning. IEEE Trans. Knowl. Data Eng. **22**(10), 1345–1359 (2010)
7. Dredze, M., et al.: Multi-domain learning by confidence-weighted parameter combination. Mach. Learn. **79**(1–2), 123–149 (2010)
8. Thrun, S.: Lifelong learning algorithms. In: Thrun, S., Pratt, L. (eds.) Learning to Learn, pp. 181–209. Springer, Boston (1998). https://doi.org/10.1007/978-1-4615-5529-2_8
9. Zhuge, Y., et al.: Intensity standardization simplifies brain MR image segmentation. Comput. Vis. Image Underst. **113**(10), 1095–1103 (2009)
10. Weisenfeld, N., et al.: Normalization of joint image-intensity statistics in MRI using the Kullback-Leibler divergence. In: IEEE International Symposium on Biomedical Imaging: Nano to Macro, vol. 2004, pp. 101–104. IEEE (2004)
11. Han, X., et al.: Atlas renormalization for improved brain MR image segmentation across scanner platforms. IEEE Trans. Med. Imaging **26**(4), 479–486 (2007)
12. Van Opbroek, A., Ikram, M.A., Vernooij, M., De Bruijne, M.: Transfer learning improves supervised image segmentation across imaging protocols. IEEE Trans. Med. Imaging **34**(5), 1018–1030 (2015)
13. Cheplygina, V., Pena, I.P., Pedersen, J.H., Lynch, D.A., Sørensen, L., de Bruijne, M.: Transfer learning for multi-center classification of chronic obstructive pulmonary disease. IEEE J. Biomed. Health Inform. **22**(5), 1486–1496 (2018)
14. Kamnitsas, K., et al.: Unsupervised domain adaptation in brain lesion segmentation with adversarial networks. In: Niethammer, M., et al. (eds.) IPMI 2017. LNCS, vol. 10265, pp. 597–609. Springer, Cham (2017). https://doi.org/10.1007/978-3-319-59050-9_47
15. Bilen, H., Vedaldi, A.: Universal representations: the missing link between faces, text, planktons, and cat breeds. arXiv preprint arXiv:1701.07275 (2017)

16. Ioffe, S., et al.: Batch normalization: accelerating deep network training by reducing internal covariate shift. In: International Conference on Machine Learning, pp. 448–456 (2015)
17. Li, Y., Wang, N., Shi, J., Liu, J., Hou, X.: Revisiting batch normalization for practical domain adaptation. arXiv preprint arXiv:1603.04779 (2016)
18. Carlucci, F., Porzi, L., Caputo, B., Ricci, E., Bulo, S.: Autodial: Automatic domain alignment layers. In: IEEE International Conference on Computer Vision (ICCV 2017), pp. 5077–5085. IEEE (2017)
19. Rebuffi, S., et al.: Learning multiple visual domains with residual adapters. In: Advances in Neural Information Processing Systems, pp. 506–516 (2017)
20. French, R.: Catastrophic forgetting in connectionist networks. Trends Cogn. Sci. **3**(4), 128–135 (1999)
21. Van Essen, D., et al.: The WU-Minn human connectome project: an overview. Neuroimage **80**, 62–79 (2013)
22. Di Martino, A., et al.: The autism brain imaging data exchange: towards a large-scale evaluation of the intrinsic brain architecture in autism. Mol. Psychiatry **19**(6), 659 (2014)
23. Odena, A., et al.: Deconvolution and checkerboard artifacts. Distill (2016)
24. Milletari, F., et al.: V-net: Fully convolutional neural networks for volumetric medical image segmentation. In: 2016 Fourth International Conference on 3D Vision (3DV), pp. 565–571. IEEE (2016)
25. Nyúl, L., et al.: New variants of a method of MRI scale standardization. IEEE Trans. Med. Imaging **19**(2), 143–150 (2000)

Respond-CAM: Analyzing Deep Models for 3D Imaging Data by Visualizations

Guannan Zhao[1], Bo Zhou[2], Kaiwen Wang[2], Rui Jiang[1], and Min Xu[2($\boxtimes$)]

[1] Department of Automation, Tsinghua University, Beijing, China
mxu1@cs.cmu.edu
[2] School of Computer Science, Carnegie Mellon University, Pittsburgh, PA, USA

Abstract. The convolutional neural network (CNN) has become a powerful tool for various biomedical image analysis tasks, but there is a lack of visual explanation for the machinery of CNNs. In this paper, we present a novel algorithm, Respond-weighted Class Activation Mapping (Respond-CAM), for making CNN-based models interpretable by visualizing input regions that are important for predictions, especially for biomedical 3D imaging data inputs. Our method uses the gradients of any target concept (e.g. the score of target class) that flow into a convolutional layer. The weighted feature maps are combined to produce a heatmap that highlights the important regions in the image for predicting the target concept. We prove a preferable sum-to-score property of the Respond-CAM and verify its significant improvement on 3D images from the current state-of-the-art approach. Our tests on Cellular Electron Cryo-Tomography 3D images show that Respond-CAM achieves superior performance on visualizing the CNNs with 3D biomedical image inputs, and is able to get reasonably good results on visualizing the CNNs with natural image inputs. The Respond-CAM is an efficient and reliable approach for visualizing the CNN machinery, and is applicable to a wide variety of CNN model families and image analysis tasks. Our code is available at: https://github.com/xulabs/projects/tree/master/respond_cam.

1 Introduction

3D imaging data is commonly used in biomedical research. Since biological structures are 3D in nature, 3D images capture substantially more information as compared to 2D images. Recently, convolutional neural network (CNN) has become one of the most powerful tools for analyzing 3D imaging data in biomedical research, especially for tasks like classification, object detection and segmentation [4]. However, there is lack of explanation for what exactly CNNs have learned, how they learn, and how to improve them. To make CNN models more interpretable and reliable, the visualization of deep models is desirable.

A number of methods have been proposed to visualize CNNs for understanding computer vision tasks in 2D natural images. Most of the state-of-the-art

---

G. Zhao and B. Zhou—Contributed equally.

© Springer Nature Switzerland AG 2018
A. F. Frangi et al. (Eds.): MICCAI 2018, LNCS 11070, pp. 485–492, 2018.
https://doi.org/10.1007/978-3-030-00928-1_55

works have been well summarized and integrated in [5]. Zeiler & Fergus proposed a method that mapped activations back to the input pixel space via Deconv-net, so that certain class-discriminative patterns in the input image were highlighted and visualized [8]. Class Activation Mapping (CAM) was proposed to highlight discriminative image regions for classification tasks [10]. However, it was only applicable to CNNs without fully-connected layers except the last layer. Selvaraju [6] generalized the CAM and proposed the Grad-CAM, which provided informative visualization for analyzing and diagnosing deep models for natural image classification and visual question answering. As to our knowledge, however, the visualization of CNN in biomedical applications, especially regarding 3D imaging data, has not been properly studied.

In this paper, we present a novel CNN visualization algorithm called Respond-CAM. The Respond-CAM is easy to implement, compatible with any CNN and is especially suited for CNNs using 3D biomedical images. We tested our Respond-CAM on the 3D images of macromolecular complex structures obtained from Cellular Electron Cryo-Tomography (CECT), an emerging imaging technique for visualizing these structures at their near-native state and at nanometer resolution. To show that our Respond-CAM is effective for a variety of inputs to the CNNs, we chose to use these macromolecular complexes for their large variations in shapes and sizes. This makes the CECT dataset ideal for testing the performance of the Respond-CAM. Previous studies have shown that CNN has important applications in CECT, including cellular structure segmentation, classification, etc. [2,7] We applied our visualization methods to two important CECT CNN models, denoted CNN-1 (taken from [7]) and CNN-2. We demonstrate that Respond-CAM achieves better visualization results than Grad-CAM, the current state-of-the-art method. Our theoretical analysis and experimental results both show that Respond-CAM has a preferable *sum-to-score* property, which makes the visualization results more consistent with CNN outputs than Grad-CAM [6]. These results indicate a significant improvement from Grad-CAM, especially in 3D biomedical images. In summary, our contributions are listed as follows:

- We propose a novel visualization approach (Respond-CAM) to analyze CNN models for 3D biomedical images, such as CECT;
- We prove the *sum-to-score* property of Respond-CAM and verify its significant improvement compared with current state-of-the-art approach.

2   Methods

Inspired by the work of [6], we propose the Respond-weighted Class Activation Mapping (Respond-CAM) to visualize and highlight the class-discriminative parts in a 3D image. The Respond-CAM can be easily extended to other tasks, such as segmentation and regression. Figure 1 gives an overview of our Respond-CAM architecture and its relationship to CNNs in various subtomogram analysis tasks. A *subtomogram* is a cubic subvolume of a CECT tomogram that is likely to contain only one macromolecule.

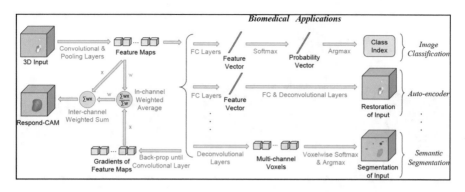

Fig. 1. Overview: for a trained CNN, we choose a differentiable scalar output of interest y (e.g. an entry of the feature vector) and calculate the gradient of y to the feature maps. Then we combine the feature maps and their gradients to get the Respond-CAM representing which areas in the input contribute the most to the output y.

For a class index c and an output A of a certain layer, we denote the corresponding Respond-CAM as $L_A^{(c)}$. Typically, we set A to be the last convolutional layer [6].

We first compute the gradients of $y^{(c)}$ (the *score* for class c before the softmax) with respect to all feature maps of the convolutional layer A. The gradients are denoted as $\frac{\partial y^{(c)}}{\partial A_{i,j,k}^{(l)}}$, where $A_{i,j,k}^{(l)}$ stands for the position (i,j,k) of the l-th feature map. For every feature map $A^{(l)}$, the forward activations are fairly smooth because of the spatial correlation of convolution operations. However, their gradients, fed backwards through fully-connected layers, can be quite noisy and scattered. In order to "smoothen" the gradients, we calculate the $\alpha_l^{(c)}$ which is the weighted-average of all the gradients in the feature map using Eq. 1:

$$\alpha_l^{(c)} = \frac{\sum_{i,j,k} A_{i,j,k}^{(l)} \frac{\partial y^{(c)}}{\partial A_{i,j,k}^{(l)}}}{\sum_{i,j,k} A_{i,j,k}^{(l)} + \epsilon} \tag{1}$$

where ϵ is a sufficiently small positive number for numerical stability and can be usually ignored. This $\alpha_l^{(c)}$ serves as an estimation of the "importance" of feature map $A^{(l)}$. The Respond-CAM $L_A^{(c)}$ has the same shape as every $A^{(l)}$, where l is the index of the feature map. We then take a linear combination of $A^{(l)}$ to compute the Respond-CAM:

$$L_A^{(c)} = \sum_l \alpha_l^{(c)} A^{(l)} \tag{2}$$

Although the result of Respond-CAM $L_A^{(c)}$ typically has a smaller shape than the input image does, we can resize it by interpolation in order to overlap it on the input image as a heatmap, as shown in the rightmost part of Fig. 2.

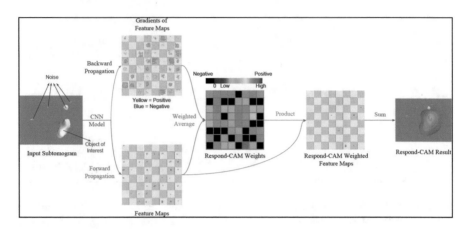

Fig. 2. Respond-CAM walk-through with an example. By applying the weighted average with each feature maps to their corresponding gradients, we get the Respond-CAM weights for each feature map. We calculate the Respond-CAM using Eq. 2 where the map with the largest weight (marked with red) contributes the most. As a result, the object-of-interest area gets highlighted.

The calculation process of Respond-CAM is demonstrated in Fig. 2. Our approach is named "Respond-CAM" because each of the weights $\alpha_l^{(c)}$ can be interpreted as the *responsiveness* of its corresponding feature map $A^{(l)}$: it shows how rapidly, and in which direction, the score of class c would change (i.e. *respond*) as the feature map $A^{(l)}$ changes.

We summarize three main advantages of Respond-CAM. (1) The algorithm is adaptive to any CNN architecture. (2) The calculation is efficient and simple to implement. (3) It approximately meets the *sum-to-scores* property better than the Grad-CAM.

The Sum-to-score Property of Respond-CAM. To demonstrate this property, we take CNNs with only one fully-connected layer as example. In such case, the gradients $\frac{\partial y^{(c)}}{\partial A_{i,j,k}^{(l)}}$ are exactly the weights of that fully-connected layer, which are constant once the CNN is trained. Therefore, it can be proved that the class score $y^{(c)}$ equals to the sum of Respond-CAM plus bias $b^{(c)}$ for the class (see Supplementary Section 1 of [9] for details), as shown in the following equation:

$$y^{(c)} = b^{(c)} + \sum_{i,j,k}(L_A^{(c)})_{i,j,k} \approx \sum_{i,j,k}(L_A^{(c)})_{i,j,k} \qquad (3)$$

The equation indicates that the Respond-CAM approximately sum to the class score. This is denoted as the *sum-to-score* property. Then, we examine CNNs which contain multiple fully-connected layers. Although the gradients $\frac{\partial y^{(c)}}{\partial A_{i,j,k}^{(l)}}$ are not constant for such CNNs, we find the approximation still reasonable. The detailed discussions about the approximation shown above can also be found in Supplementary Section 1 of [9].

3 Experiments and Results

3.1 Data Preparations

We simulated subtomograms in a similar way as previous works [1]. Each subtomogram consisted of 40^3 voxels. We set the tilt angle to $\pm 60°$, and the signal-to-noise ratio to $+\infty$ and 0.1 respectively. Two datasets, including *the noise-free* and *the noised* data, were collected. In each dataset, we acquired 23000 subtomograms of 23 structural classes. We separated the subtomograms into the training set and the test set with a ratio of 4:1. We train our CNN models using 80% subtomograms of the training set for fitting and the rest for validation. Only the data from test sets are used for visualizations in our experiments.

We adopt two CNN models for our experiments. One of them is the same model that achieved the best classification accuracy in [7] with simple architecture, which we denote as *CNN-1*. Another is a slightly modified version of CNN-1. It further increases the classification accuracy on our datasets to over 96% and is denoted as *CNN-2*. Their architectures are described in detail in Supplementary Section 2 of [9].

3.2 Experimental Results

Three representative examples that stress the difference between our Respond-CAM and Grad-CAM are shown in Fig. 3. The last convolution layer is used here. The subtomograms are classified correctly by both CNN-1 and CNN-2, so it is expected that the heatmaps highlight the object of interest with maximum positive values. However, as shown in Fig. 3, Grad-CAM sometimes gives noisy or even opposite results for the CECT volumetric data when noise is introduced, especially when applied to CNN-1, where the objects of interest are highlighted with negative values. In comparison, Respond-CAM produces significantly better heatmaps that indicate the locations of objects of interest with clean visualization result. One example of the visualization results for CNN-1 intermediate layers are also shown in Fig. 4.

The Respond-CAM and the Grad-CAM were also evaluated quantitatively by examining their *sum-to-score* property. Intuitively, the better the *sum-to-score* property is approximated, the more consistent the visualization results would be with the CNN outputs themselves. The L1 error and Kendall's Tau (KT) [3] were calculated over both trained models using all subtomograms in the test set. These two metrics were chosen to verify the *sum-to-score* property from different aspects. L1 error measures the *absolute difference* between the class score and the sum of Respond-CAM/Grad-CAM heatmap, while the KT checks their *relative consistency*, i.e. we expect that the top-n predictions are consistent whether the classes are sorted by the class scores or by the sums of heatmaps. For each subtomogram, the L1 error is defined using Eq. 4:

$$L_1 = \frac{1}{C} \sum_c \left| \sum_{i,j,k} L_A^{(c)} - y^{(c)} \right| \tag{4}$$

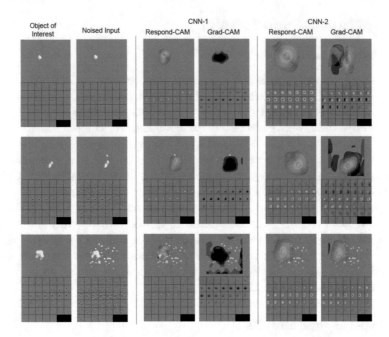

Fig. 3. Three cases in which Respond-CAM displays significant improvement. In each sub-figure, the same 3D image is presented in two ways. (1) Upper half: the parallel projection of subtomogram isosurface or Respond-CAM/Grad-CAM contours; (2) lower half: the corresponding 2D slices. Notice that heatmaps are resized so they can be overlaid on subtomograms.

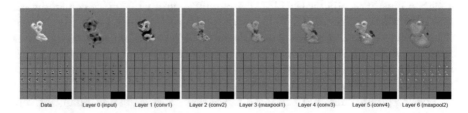

Fig. 4. The intermediate layer visualization of Respond-CAM using same classification network shown in Fig. 3. All layers before fully-connected layer are visualized.

where $\sum_{i,j,k} L_A^{(c)}$ is the sum of Grad-CAM/Respond-CAM for class c, $y^{(c)}$ is the corresponding score of class c, and C is the number of classes. The L_1 is ranged in $[0, +\infty]$ and reaches 0 for a perfect consistence.

The KT measures the similarity of two sequences of class indexes sorted by (a) scores and (b) the sum of Grad-CAM/Respond-CAM. It is defined in Eq. 5:

$$\tau = \frac{P - Q}{P + Q} \tag{5}$$

where P is the number of concordant pairs, and Q is the number of discordant pairs. The τ is ranged in $[-1, 1]$ and reaches 1 for a perfect consistence. The evaluation results are listed in Table 1. We can see that the L1 error of our Respond-CAM is significantly smaller than the L1 of Grad-CAM. The KT of our Respond-CAM is also much closer to 1 as compared to results from Grad-CAM. Thus, the Respond-CAM much more strongly exhibits the *sum-to-score* property than Grad-CAM on both CNN models in CECT data.

Table 1. Comparison between Grad-CAM and Respond-CAM on L1 error and Kendall's Tau (KT) on different CNNs and datasets.

Model	CNN-1	CNN-2	CNN-1	CNN-2
SNR	$+\infty$	$+\infty$	0.1	0.1
L1, Grad	15.344 ± 7.789	8.117 ± 3.854	21.142 ± 8.511	14.020 ± 5.232
L1, Respond	$\mathbf{0.601 \pm 0.187}$	$\mathbf{0.770 \pm 0.366}$	$\mathbf{1.006 \pm 0.721}$	$\mathbf{0.542 \pm 0.194}$
KT, Grad	0.273 ± 0.350	0.822 ± 0.097	-0.116 ± 0.341	0.458 ± 0.260
KT, Respond	$\mathbf{0.981 \pm 0.014}$	$\mathbf{0.976 \pm 0.018}$	$\mathbf{0.975 \pm 0.024}$	$\mathbf{0.984 \pm 0.013}$

4 Discussion and Conclusion

We presented a novel CNN visualization approach that can be applied to CNN models with 3D/2D image inputs. Specifically, we used CECT data as the example to test our approach. Both visualization examples and quantitative tests show that our Respond-CAM achieves significantly better CNN visualization results as compared to the current state-of-the-art approach (Grad-CAM) on the 3D imaging data. In the Grad-CAM, the weights are calculated by simply averaging the gradients of the feature maps, while ignoring the feature maps themselves. This information loss in Grad-CAM sometimes produces improper weights and leads to undesirable results, such as those shown in Fig. 3. Our experimental results also show that the Respond-CAM satisfies the *sum-to-score* property, which enables a more consistent and robust visualization of CNNs than Grad-CAM. Therefore, the Respond-CAM is a more reasonable visualization approach for CNNs, especially in the cases with 3D biomedical images, such as CECT. More details are available on [9].

In conclusion, our Respond-CAM achieved superior performance on visualizing the CNNs with biomedical 3D imaging data inputs. It is able to produce reasonably good results on visualizing the CNNs with 3D imaging data and can be applied to a wide variety of other imaging data. We believe the Respond-CAM is an efficient and reliable approach for visualizing the CNN machineries.

Acknowledgements. We thank Dr. Xiaodan Liang for suggestions. This work was supported in part by U.S. National Institutes of Health grant P41 GM103712. Min Xu acknowledges support from Samuel and Emma Winters Foundation. Rui Jiang is a RONG professor at the Institute for Data Science, Tsinghua University.

References

1. Beck, M., Malmström, J.A., Lange, V., Schmidt, A., Deutsch, E.W., Aebersold, R.: Visual proteomics of the human pathogen Leptospira interrogans. Nature Methods **6**(11), 817–823 (2009)
2. Chen, M., et al.: Convolutional neural networks for automated annotation of cellular cryo-electron tomograms. Nature Methods **14**(10), 983 (2017)
3. Kendall, M.G.: A new measure of rank correlation. Biometrika **30**(1/2), 81–93 (1938)
4. Litjens, G., et al.: A survey on deep learning in medical image analysis. Med. Image Anal. **42**, 60–88 (2017)
5. Olah, C., et al.: The building blocks of interpretability. Distill **3**(3), e10 (2018)
6. Selvaraju, R.R., Cogswell, M., Das, A., Vedantam, R., Parikh, D., Batra, D.: Grad-cam: Visual explanations from deep networks via gradient-based localization. https://arxiv.org/abs/1610.02391v3 (2016)
7. Xu, M., et al.: Deep learning based subdivision approach for large scale macromolecules structure recovery from electron cryo tomograms. arXiv preprint arXiv:1701.08404 (2017)
8. Zeiler, M.D., Fergus, R.: Visualizing and understanding convolutional networks. In: Fleet, D., Pajdla, T., Schiele, B., Tuytelaars, T. (eds.) ECCV 2014. LNCS, vol. 8689, pp. 818–833. Springer, Cham (2014). https://doi.org/10.1007/978-3-319-10590-1_53
9. Zhao,G., Zhou, B., Wang, K., Jiang, R., Min, X.: Respond-cam: Analyzing deep models for 3D imaging data by visualizations. arXiv preprint arXiv:1806.00102 (2018)
10. Zhou, B., Khosla, A., Lapedriza, A., Oliva, A., Torralba, A.: Learning deep features for discriminative localization. In: Proceedings of the IEEE Conference on Computer Vision and Pattern Recognition, pp. 2921–2929 (2016)

Generalizability *vs.* Robustness: Investigating Medical Imaging Networks Using Adversarial Examples

Magdalini Paschali[1](✉), Sailesh Conjeti[2], Fernando Navarro[1], and Nassir Navab[1,3]

[1] Computer Aided Medical Procedures, Technische Universität München, Munich, Germany
magda.paschali@tum.de
[2] German Center for Neurodegenerative Diseases (DZNE), Bonn, Germany
[3] Computer Aided Medical Procedures, Johns Hopkins University, Baltimore, MD, USA

Abstract. In this paper, for the first time, we propose an evaluation method for deep learning models that assesses the performance of a model not only in an unseen test scenario, but also in extreme cases of noise, outliers and ambiguous input data. To this end, we utilize adversarial examples, images that fool machine learning models, while looking imperceptibly different from original data, as a measure to evaluate the robustness of a variety of medical imaging models. Through extensive experiments on skin lesion classification and whole brain segmentation with state-of-the-art networks such as Inception and UNet, we show that models that achieve comparable performance regarding generalizability may have significant variations in their perception of the underlying data manifold, leading to an extensive performance gap in their robustness.

1 Introduction

Deep learning is being increasingly adopted within the medical imaging community for a plethora of tasks including classification, segmentation, detection *etc.* The classic approach towards the assessment of any machine learning model revolves around the evaluation of its *generalizability i.e.* its performance on unseen test scenarios. However, in case of *limited* training data, such as medical imaging datasets, using heavily over-parameterized deep learning models could lead to the "memorization" of the training data. Evaluating such models on an available non-overlapping test set is popular, yet significantly limited in its ability to explore the model's resilience to outliers and noisy data/labels (*i.e.* robustness). Additionally, the limited interpretability of deep learning models due to their "black-box" nature challenges their adoption into clinical practice.

Existing model evaluation routines look deeply into over-fitting but insufficiently into scenarios of model sensitivity to variations of the input. Robustness

© Springer Nature Switzerland AG 2018
A. F. Frangi et al. (Eds.): MICCAI 2018, LNCS 11070, pp. 493–501, 2018.
https://doi.org/10.1007/978-3-030-00928-1_56

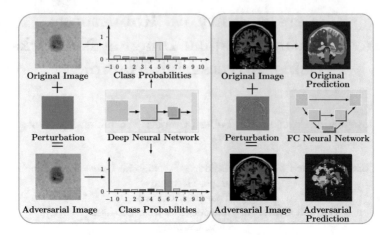

Fig. 1. Overview of Adversarial Crafting and its effect on network prediction. The difference between the generated adversarial image and the original image is imperceptible, yet deep neural networks are successfully fooled into anomalous predictions.

evaluation estimates potential failure probabilities when the model is *pushed* to its limits. In this paper, we approach evaluating a model by leveraging adversarial examples [1] that are crafted with the purpose of *fooling* a model and can uncover cases where its performance may degenerate. Our approach to using adversarial examples as benchmark is also significantly less laborious and expensive than constituting a sufficiently diverse test set with manual annotation.

Adversarial examples are images crafted to purposely fool machine learning models, while the added perturbations are imperceptible to human eyes [1], as shown in Fig. 1. Our work is among the first that explore adversarial examples in medical imaging and leverage them in a constructive fashion to benchmark model performance not only on clean and noisy but also on adversarially crafted data. Previously, Zhu et al. augmented their dataset with adversarial examples to control overfitting and improve their model's performance on mass segmentation [2]. Even though adversarial examples may not occur in naturally acquired data, utilizing them can present new opportunities for medical imaging researchers to investigate their models, with the ultimate goal of increasing robustness and optimizing the decision boundaries learned for different tasks.

Our contribution is two-fold: Firstly, we demonstrate on a variety of medical image computing tasks that widely adopted state-of-the art deep learning models are not immune to adversarial examples crafting. Secondly, we utilize adversarial examples to benchmark model robustness by comparing a variety of architectures, such as Inception [3] and UNet [4], for the tasks of skin lesion classification and whole brain segmentation.

2 Methodology

2.1 Adversarial Crafting

Given a trained model F, an original input image X with output label Y, we generate an adversarial example $\hat{X}$ by solving a box-constrained optimization problem $\min_{\hat{X}} \|\hat{X} - X\|$ subject to $F(X) = Y$, $F(\hat{X}) = \hat{Y}$, $\hat{Y} \neq Y$ and $\hat{X} \in [0,1]$. Such an optimization minimizes the added perturbation, say r (*i.e.* $\hat{X} = X + r$) while simultaneously *fooling* the model F [1]. By imposing an additional constraint such as $\|r\| \leq \epsilon$, we can restrict the perturbation to be small enough to be imperceptible to humans.

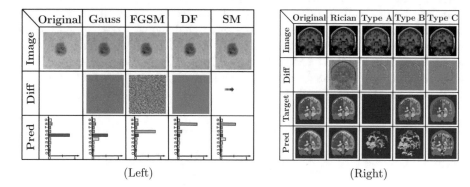

(Left)　　　　　　　　　　　　　(Right)

Fig. 2. Illustration of adversarial examples and their effect on model predictions. Left: Skin lesion classification and Right: Whole brain segmentation. The arrow in the case of the SM attack indicates the few pixels that were perturbed. Contrasting with prediction on original images, the crafted examples are able to successfully *fool* the models into either misclassification or generating incorrect segmentation maps.

Classification: Gradient-based adversarial example generation methods have been proposed with the objective of generating minimum amount of perturbation r that misclassifies $\hat{X}$. These include the Fast Gradient Sign Method (FGSM) [5], DeepFool (DF) [6], Saliency Map Attacks (SMA) [7] *etc.* Adversarial examples crafted with these methods are shown in Fig. 2. For a trained model F, FGSM performs a one-step pixel-level update along the sign of the gradient that maximizes the task loss J and the resultant perturbation is computed as $r = \epsilon \text{sign}(\nabla_X J(\theta, X, Y))$, where θ are the parameters of the model. The amount of perturbation is regulated by a hyper-parameter ϵ that is typically assigned a low value, so that $\hat{X}$ is visually imperceptible from X.

Differing from FGSM, DF follows an iterative greedy search process, where in each iteration the projections of the input sample to the decision boundaries of all the classes are computed and an r is calculated that will push X towards the closest decision boundary of a class, other than the correct one. In SMA, the impact of each pixel on the prediction of the model is estimated and the input is selectively perturbed to cause the most significant change to the output.

Segmentation: In [8], the authors introduced Dense Adversarial Generation (DAG) as a method for crafting adversarial examples for semantic segmentation, closely resembling per-pixel, targeted FGSM. Particularly, DAG utilizes an incorrect segmentation mask, given by the user, and a target set of non-background pixels. Its goal is to calculate a minimum perturbation r that will alter the prediction from the correct class to the incorrect target class.

We utilized DAG to craft adversarial examples, seen in Fig. 2, by creating targets with varying degrees of difficulty. Particularly, we set the target to be all background (Type A), randomly assign a small percentage of pixels to a randomly-selected adversarial class (Type B) and modify (dilate) only a particular target class while keeping all other classes intact (Type C). Of the aforementioned attack types, Type A is the most challenging, causing the largest amount of perturbation, while Type C is expected to distort the image the least, as can be seen in Fig. 2. The Mean Square Error (MSE) between the original and adversarial images remained extremely small, ranging from 0.004 for adversaries of Type A to 0.002 for B and C.

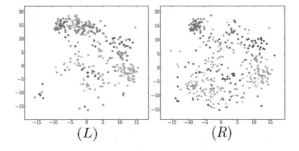

(L) (R)

Fig. 3. t-SNE representation of the embeddings of 3 classes (red, blue and green) from clean (•), noisy (○) and adversarial images (+). The noisy examples (○) are embedded closer to clean data (L), while adversarial ones are *pushed* to the model boundaries (R).

2.2   Model Evaluation with Adversarial Examples

The proposed pipeline for the evaluation of robustness involves benchmarking models against task-specific adversarial attacks and is similar across tasks. For classification, we crafted adversarial examples with FGSM, DF and SMA, while for segmentation we applied DAG with 3 different types of targets (Type A−C). Afterwards we attacked our models in a black-box fashion with examples generated by independently trained models, to maintain an unbiased attack scenario.

Contrasting with Noise: One could argue that applying noise on the test images before inference could replace the need for adversarial examples. However, that is not the case since hard ambiguous cases and outliers cannot be modeled by noise distributions. Adversarial examples, which are crafted with the purpose to force models to fail, are better suited for evaluating model behavior when subject to input extrema. To showcase that adversarial perturbations do not resemble noise distributions, we also crafted images distorted with modality-specific noise (Gaussian noise for dermatoscopic images and Rician noise for T1w MRI). For fairness, the Structural Similarity (SSIM) between the original and noisy images was the same as the one between the original and adversarial examples and ranged from 0.97 to 0.99.

We plot the t-Stochastic Neighbor Embedding representation (t-SNE) from IV3 for the clean, noisy and adversarial examples (FGSM) in Fig. 3 for the classification task to further illustrate this difference. Contrasting Fig. 3 (L) with Fig. 3 (R), we clearly observe that images distorted with noise are embedded close to the clean images, while adversarial examples are pushed further towards other classes. The anomalous nature of the adversarial examples clearly supports our hypothesis that their behavior is not akin to noise and can act as a harder benchmark for evaluating a model's robustness.

3   Experiments

To provide a proof-of-concept for the proposed robustness evaluation we chose the challenging tasks of fine-grained skin lesion classification and segmentation of the whole brain. The task-specific model learning is described as follows:

Classification: We fine-tune three state-of-the art deep learning architectures namely, InceptionV3 (IV3) [3], InceptionV4 (IV4) [3] and MobileNet (MN) [9] for this task. Both IV3 and IV4 are very-deep architectures (>100 layers), while MN is significantly compact. Comparing these architectures would help discover if any innate relationships exist between model complexity (in terms of depth and parameters) and their robustness. To keep the comparisons fair, all the models were initialized with their respective ImageNet parameters and fine-tuned with a weighted cross-entropy loss with affine data augmentation. Specifically, the models were trained with stochastic gradient descent with a decaying learning rate initialized at 0.01, momentum of 0.9 and dropout of 0.8 for regularization. We use the publicly-available Dermofit [10] image library consisting of 1300 high-quality dermatoscopic images, with histologically validated fine grained expert annotations (10 classes) for this task. The dataset was split at patient-level with non-overlapping folds (50% for training and rest for testing).

Segmentation: For this task we chose to evaluate three popular fully-convoluti-onal deep architectures, namely SegNet (SN) [11], UNet (UN) [4] and DenseNet (DN) [12]. Contrasting across these architectures, we evaluate the importance of skip connections with respect to robustness varying from no skip connections in SN to introducing long-range skips in UN and both long and short-range skip connections in DN. The model parameters (depth and layers) were chosen to maintain comparable model complexity, so as to exclusively factor out

Table 1. Comparative evaluation of the classification and segmentation models on clean, noisy and adversarial examples. We report the average accuracy and Dice overlap score along with the % drop in performance on adversarial examples with respect to performance on clean data.

			Noise	Adversarial	
		Clean	**Gaussian**	**Avg**	**% Drop**
Classification	**IV3** [3]	0.710	0.693	**0.641**	**6.897**
	IV4 [3]	**0.810**	**0.761**	0.633	17.72
	MN [9]	0.800	0.647	0.564	24.55
		Clean	**Rician**	**Avg**	**% Drop**
Segmentation	**SN** [11]	0.842	0.595	0.470	37.17
	UN [4]	**0.862**	0.759	0.453	40.92
	DN [12]	0.861	**0.848**	**0.667**	**19.53**

the impact of skip connections to robustness. The aforementioned models were trained with a composite loss of weighted-cross entropy and Dice loss [13] and model optimization was performed with ADAM optimizer with an initial learning rate of 0.001. We use 27 volumes from the publicly-available whole-brain segmentation benchmark (subset of Open Access Series of Imaging Studies (OASIS) dataset [14]) that was released as a part of the Multi-Atlas Labeling Challenge in MICCAI 2012 [15], with 80-20 patient-level splits for training and testing. The models for both tasks were trained until convergence using TensorFlow [16] and adversarial examples for DF and SMA attacks described in Sec. 2.2 were crafted using the FoolBox [17] library.

Following the model evaluation strategy presented in Sec. 2.2, adversarial examples were crafted for each of the trained models and their robustness is evaluated in terms of average classification accuracy and average Dice score. We report the overall performance of the models in Table 1, where we compare the performance of each model on clean and noisy images with their average score against all the attacks. Furthermore, in Table 2 we are reporting the performance of each model against all the black-box attacks separately.

4   Results and Discussion

4.1   Robustness Evaluation for Classification

Visual Evaluation: Fig. 2 (Left) illustrates adversarial examples crafted for an unseen test example (belonging to malignant melanoma class) for each of the classification related attacks (FGSM, DF and SMA) alongside an image perturbed with Gaussian noise for comparison. A scaled version of the difference image with respect to the original is also shown along with the posterior probabilities estimated using IV3 network. We observe that all the adversarial examples, regardless of the attack are consistently misclassified with very high confidence, while the addition of Gaussian noise only results in confidence reduction. Furthermore, FGSM induces perturbations dispersed across the whole image, while DF and SMA generate perturbations more localized to the lesion.

Attacks: From Table 1, we observe that IV4 and MN both achieve comparable performance on clean data (80–81%) superior to the one of IV3 (71%). By limiting model evaluation to generalizability (*i.e.* performance on clean data) one may prematurely conclude that IV3 demonstrates the worst comparative performance. However, upon comparing the robustness of these models with respect to average performance under all the attacks (Table 2), we observe a contrary trend. The performance drop for IV3 is significantly lower (7%) in comparison to IV4 (17%) and MN (25%). IV4 achieves higher accuracy on DF and SMA attacks, while IV3 is the most robust model against FGSM. Contrasting IV4 and MN, we observe that MN performs poorly not only on noisy samples but also on all of the attacks, as shown in Table 2. These contrasting observations clearly substantiate the core hypothesis within the paper that model evaluation should not be limited to generalizability and that performing robustness evaluation is equally important. Despite showing comparable performance in terms of generalizability, we can clearly conclude that IV4 is strongly preferred over MN.

Table 2. Comparative evaluation of model robustness using black-box attacks for the tasks of classification and segmentation. We report the average accuracy for classification and average Dice overlap score across structures for segmentation.

		FGSM			DF			SMA		
		IV3	IV4	**MN**	IV3	IV4	MN	IV3	IV4	MN
Classification	**IV3** [3]	**0.449**	**0.548**	**0.567**	0.729	0.707	0.664	**0.738**	0.701	0.669
	IV4 [3]	0.429	0.411	0.451	**0.743**	**0.768**	**0.697**	0.735	**0.778**	**0.683**
	MN [9]	0.335	0.275	0.213	0.726	0.731	0.672	0.732	0.735	0.661
		Type A			Type B			Type C		
		SN	UN	DN	SN	UN	DN	SN	UN	DN
Segmentation	**SN** [11]	0.277	0.272	0.309	0.397	0.473	0.428	0.669	0.702	0.705
	UN [4]	0.248	0.434	0.258	0.364	0.434	0.368	0.636	0.653	0.677
	DN [12]	**0.600**	**0.528**	**0.415**	**0.749**	**0.721**	**0.563**	**0.819**	**0.791**	**0.814**

4.2 Robustness Evaluation for Segmentation

Visual Evaluation: Fig. 2 (Right) illustrates how the prediction maps of the trained DN model transform when it is attacked. All the DAG attacks (Type A-C) successfully fool the model into producing an incorrect prediction map. However, the prediction on the image distorted with Rician noise is visually similar to the one of the original image and the ground truth. This clearly demonstrates that adding adversarial perturbation is not akin to adding random noise.

Attacks: From Table 1, we observe that DN (86.1%) and UN (86.2%) achieve almost identical performance on clean unseen test examples and fare better than SN (84.2%), highlighting the importance of skip connections. Furthermore, the fact that the performance drop caused by the addition of Rician noise remains low for UN and DN (10% and 1% respectively) reinforces the distinction between noise and adversarial perturbations. Regarding model performance with respect to adversarial attacks in Table 2, we observe that DN is not only resilient to noise but also significantly more robust than SN (by 18%) and UN (by 21%) to attacks crafted by any other model. Furthermore, SN and UN remain highly vulnerable to all the attacks with a significant 37–40% drop in their average Dice score. In consensus to the classification results discussed earlier, comparing the three segmentation models only in terms of generalizability would not have been sufficient to determine the best one. Both its resilience to samples distorted with Rician noise and its consistent resistance to adversarial attacks make DN the strongest model among its competitors for this task.

5   Conclusion

In this paper we explored adversarial examples in medical imaging for the tasks of classification and segmentation and proposed a strategy for model evaluation by leveraging task-specific adversarial attacks. We showed that for two models with comparable performance, their relative exploration of the underlying data manifold may have significant differences, hence resulting in varying robustness and model sensitivities. Specifically, we demonstrate that for segmentation tasks the use of dense blocks and skip connections contributes to both improved generalizability and robustness, while model depth seems to increase the resistance of classification models to adversarial examples.

References

1. Szegedy, C., et al.: Intriguing properties of neural networks. In: ICLR (2014)
2. Zhu, W., Xiang, X., Tran, T.D., Hager, G.D., Xie, X.: Adversarial deep structured nets for mass segmentation from mammograms. In: ISBI (2018)
3. Szegedy, C., Vanhoucke, V., Ioffe, S., Shlens, J., Wojna, Z.: Rethinking the inception architecture for computer vision. In: CVPR (2016)
4. Ronneberger, O., Fischer, P., Brox, T.: U-Net: convolutional networks for biomedical image segmentation. In: MICCAI (2015)
5. Goodfellow, I., Shlens, J., Szegedy, C.: Explaining and harnessing adversarial examples. In: ICLR (2015)
6. Moosavi-Dezfooli, S.M., Fawzi, A., Frossard, P.: DeepFool: a simple and accurate method to fool deep neural networks. In: CVPR (2016)
7. Papernot, N., McDaniel, P.D., Jha, S., Fredrikson, M., Berkay Celik, Z., Swami, A.: The limitations of deep learning in adversarial settings. In: EuroS&P (2016)

8. Xie, C., Wang, J., Zhang, Z., Zhou, Y., Xie, L., Yuille, A.L.: Adversarial examples for semantic segmentation and object detection. In: ICCV (2017)
9. Howard, A.G., et al.: MobileNets: efficient convolutional neural networks for mobile vision applications. CoRR abs/1704.04861 (2017)
10. Ballerini, L., Fisher, R.B., Aldridge, R.B., Rees, J.: A color and texture based hierarchical K-NN approach to the classification of non-melanoma skin lesions. In: Color Medical Image Analysis (2013)
11. Badrinarayanan, V., Kendall, A., Cipolla, R.: SegNet: a deep convolutional encoder-decoder architecture for image segmentation. IEEE Trans. Pattern Anal. Mach. Intell. **39**(12), 2481–2495 (2017)
12. Jégou, S., Drozdzal, M., Vázquez, D., Romero, A., Bengio, Y.: The one hundred layers tiramisu: fully convolutional DenseNets for semantic segmentation. CVPR Workshops (2017)
13. Roy, A.G., Conjeti, S., Sheet, D., Katouzian, A., Navab, N., Wachinger, C.: Error corrective boosting for learning fully convolutional networks with limited data. MICCAI (2017)
14. Marcus, D.S., Wang, T.H., Parker, J., Csernansky, J.G., Morris, J.C., Buckner, R.L.: Open Access Series of Imaging Studies (OASIS): Cross-sectional MRI data in young, middle aged, nondemented, and demented older adults. J. Cogn. Neurosc. **19**(9), 1498–1507 (2007)
15. Landman, B., Warfield, S.: MICCAI workshop on Multiatlas labeling. In: MICCAI Grand Challenge (2012)
16. Abadi, M., Agarwal, A., Barham, P., Brevdo, E., Chen, Z., Citro, C., et al.: TensorFlow: large-scale machine learning on heterogeneous distributed systems. CoRR abs/1603.04467 (2016)
17. Rauber, J., Brendel, W., Bethge, M.: Foolbox v0.8.0: A Python toolbox to benchmark the robustness of machine learning models. CoRR abs/1707.04131 (2017)

Subject2Vec: Generative-Discriminative Approach from a Set of Image Patches to a Vector

Sumedha Singla[1], Mingming Gong[2], Siamak Ravanbakhsh[3], Frank Sciurba[4], Barnabas Poczos[5], and Kayhan N. Batmanghelich[1,2,5(✉)]

[1] Computer Science Department, University of Pittsburgh, Pittsburgh, PA, USA
kayhan@pitt.edu
[2] Department of Biomedical Informatics, University of Pittsburgh, Pittsburgh, PA, USA
[3] Computer Science Department, University of British Columbia, Vancouver, Canada
[4] University of Pittsburgh School of Medicine, University of Pittsburgh, Pittsburgh, PA, USA
[5] Machine Learning Department, Carnegie Mellon University, Pittsburgh, PA, USA

Abstract. We propose an attention-based method that aggregates local image features to a subject-level representation for predicting disease severity. In contrast to classical deep learning that requires a fixed dimensional input, our method operates on a *set* of image patches; hence it can accommodate variable length input image without image resizing. The model learns a clinically interpretable subject-level representation that is reflective of the disease severity. Our model consists of three mutually dependent modules which regulate each other: (1) a *discriminative* network that learns a fixed-length representation from local features and maps them to disease severity; (2) an *attention* mechanism that provides interpretability by focusing on the areas of the anatomy that contribute the most to the prediction task; and (3) a *generative* network that encourages the diversity of the local latent features. The generative term ensures that the attention weights are non-degenerate while maintaining the relevance of the local regions to the disease severity. We train our model end-to-end in the context of a large-scale lung CT study of Chronic Obstructive Pulmonary Disease (COPD). Our model gives state-of-the art performance in predicting clinical measures of severity for COPD. The distribution of the attention provides the regional relevance of lung tissue to the clinical measurements.

1 Introduction

We propose a deep learning model that learns subject-level representation from a *set* of local features. Our model represents the image volume as a *bag* (or set) of local features (or patches) and can accommodate input images of variable sizes. We target diseases where the pathology is diffused and is not always located in the same anatomical region. The model learns by optimizing the objective

© Springer Nature Switzerland AG 2018
A. F. Frangi et al. (Eds.): MICCAI 2018, LNCS 11070, pp. 502–510, 2018.
https://doi.org/10.1007/978-3-030-00928-1_57

function that balances two goals: (1) to build a fixed length subject-level feature that is predictive of the disease severity, (2) to extract interpretable local features that identify regions of anatomy that contribute the most to the disease. Our motivation comes from the study of COPD, but the proposed model is applicable to a wide range of heterogeneous disorders.

Many diseases such as emphysema are highly heterogeneous [15] and show diffuse pattern in computed tomographic (CT) images of the lung. Having an objective way to characterize local patterns of the disease is important in diagnosis, risk prediction, and sub-typing [4,6,12,17]. Although various intensity and texture based feature descriptors are proposed to characterize the visual appearance of the disease [1,18,20], most image features are generic and are not necessarily optimized for the disease. Recent advances in deep learning enable researchers going directly from raw image to clinical outcome without specifying radiological features [3,5]. However, the classical deep learning methods, that operate on entire volume or slices [5], are challenging to interpret and they require resizing the input images to a fixed dimension. Reshaping voxels in a CT image without adjusting for the density, changes the interpretation of the intensity values.

In this paper, we view each subject as a *set* of image patches from the lung region. Previously, [1,16] viewed the subjects as sets and used handcrafted image features. In contrast, the *discriminative* part of our model uses deep learning approach and directly extracts features from the volumetric patches. Next, we use an attention mechanism [19] to adaptively weight local features and build the subject level representation, which is predictive of the disease severity. Our model is inspired by the Deep Set [21]. We extend it by adapting *generative* regularization, which prevents the redundancy of the hidden features. Furthermore, the *attention* mechanism provides interpretability by quantifying the relevance of a region to the disease. We evaluate the performance of our method on a simulated dataset and a COPD lung CT dataset where our method gives state-of-the-art performance in predicting the clinical measurements.

2   Method

We represent each subject as a set (bag) of volumetric image patches extracted from the lung region $\mathcal{X}_i = \{x_{ij}\}_{j=1}^{N_i}$, where N_i is the number of patches for subject i, which varies with subject. Our method maps x_{ij} to a low-dimensional latent space. It then aggregates the latent features to form a fix-length representation, by adaptively weighting the patches based on their contribution in prediction of disease severity (y_i). The general idea of our approach is shown in Fig. 1.

The method consists of three networks that are trained jointly: (1) a *discriminative* network, that aggregates the local information from patches in the set $\mathcal{X}_i$ to predict the disease severity y_i, (2) an *attention* mechanism, that helps discriminative network to selectively focus on patch-features by assigning weights to the patches in $\mathcal{X}_i$, and (3) a *generative* network, that regularizes the discriminative network to avoid redundant representation of patches in the latent space. The model is trained end to end, by minimizing the below objective function:

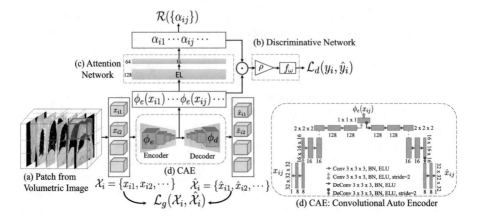

Fig. 1. (a) A subject is represented as a set of 3d image patches, (b) Discriminative Network: aggregates local features to form a fixed length representation for the subject and predicts the disease severity, (c) Attention Network: focuses attention on critical patches to provide interpretability, (d) Convolutional Auto Encoder (Generative Network): prevents redundancy of latent features.

$$\min_{\omega,\theta_e,\theta_d,\theta_a} \sum_i \mathcal{L}_d\left(y_i, \hat{y}_i(\mathcal{X}_i); \theta_e, \omega\right) + \lambda_1 \mathcal{L}_g\left(\mathcal{X}_i, \hat{\mathcal{X}}_i; \theta_e, \theta_d\right) + \lambda_2 \mathcal{R}\left(\mathcal{X}_i; \theta_e, \theta_a\right), \quad (1)$$

where $\mathcal{L}_d(\cdot, \cdot)$ and $\mathcal{L}_g(\cdot, \cdot)$ are the discriminative and generative loss functions respectively and $\mathcal{R}(\cdot)$ is a regularization over the attention. The θ_e, θ_d, θ_a and ω are the parameters of each term. λ_1, λ_2 controls the balance between the terms. The sum is over number of subjects. Next, we discuss each term in more detail.

2.1   Discriminative Network

The discriminative network transforms the input set of image patches and estimates the disease severity $\hat{y}_i(\mathcal{X}_i)$ as

$$\hat{y}_i(\mathcal{X}_i) = f\left(\rho\left(\phi_e\left(\mathcal{X}_i, \theta_e\right)\right), \omega\right). \quad (2)$$

The transformation is composed of three functions: (1) $\phi_e(\cdot; \theta_e)$ is an encoder function parameterized by θ_e. It extracts features from patches in the set $\mathcal{X}_i$ and outputs a set of features. (2) The $\rho(\cdot)$ function operates on the elements of the set and converts the variable length set $\phi_e(\mathcal{X}_i; \theta_e)$ into a fixed length vector. It is a permutation invariant function such as, maximum function $\rho(\cdot) = \max(\phi_e(x_{i,1}), \cdots, \phi_e(x_{i,N_i}))$ or mean function $\rho(\cdot) = \frac{1}{N_i}\sum_{j=1}^{N_i} \phi_e(x_{ij})$. This formulation ensures that, $\hat{y}_i(\mathcal{X}_i)$ is invariant to the order of patches in $\mathcal{X}_i$. We tried different ρ's and the mean function works well for our task. The mean function assumes all the instances within the set are contributing equally to the set-level feature vector. We extended it further to perform weighted mean, where weights are learned using the attention network in Sect. 2.2. (3) $f(\cdot; \omega)$ is a prediction function, parameterized by ω. It takes the set-level feature vector extracted by $\rho(\cdot)$ as input, and estimates the disease severity. Finally, $\mathcal{L}_d(y_i, \hat{y}_i(\mathcal{X}_i); \theta_e, \omega)$ is a ℓ_2 loss function between predicted and true value.

2.2 Attention Mechanism

The goal of our proposed model is twofold: first to provide a prediction of the disease severity and secondly, to provide a qualitative assessment of our prediction. Here, it is reasonable to assume that different regions in the lung contribute differently to the disease severity. We model this contribution by adaptively weighting the patches. The weight indicates the importance of a patch in predicting the overall disease severity of the lung. This idea is similar to attention mechanism in Computer Vision [19] and Natural Language Processing [9] communities.

We estimate the attention weights for the subject i ($\boldsymbol{\alpha}_i = \{\alpha_{i1}, \cdots, \alpha_{i,N_i}\}$) by the attention network as

$$\boldsymbol{\alpha}_i = A(\phi_e(\mathcal{X}_i; \theta_e); \theta_a). \tag{3}$$

Unlike the $\rho(\cdot)$ function, $A(\cdot; \theta_a)$ maps a set to another set. Permuting the order of elements in the set $\mathcal{X}_i$, should *equivariantly* permute the output set $\boldsymbol{\alpha}_i$. To ensure $A(\cdot)$ is a permutation equivariant function, we construct it as a neural network with equivariant layer (EL) [21]. Assuming $\mathbf{H}_i \in \mathbb{R}^{N_i,d}$ where k^{th} row is $\phi(x_{ik}; \theta_e) \in \mathbb{R}^d$, one possible way of modeling the equivariant layer is

$$[\mathbf{H}_i]_k = \mathbf{W}([\mathbf{H}_i]_k - \max(\mathbf{H}_i, 1)) + \mathbf{b}, \tag{4}$$

where $[\mathbf{H}_i]_k$ denotes k^{th} row of $\mathbf{H}_i$ and $\max(\mathbf{H}_i, 1)$ is the max over rows. $\mathbf{W} \in \mathbb{R}^{L \times d}$, $\boldsymbol{b} \in \mathbb{R}^L$ are the parameters of the EL. To ensure $A(\cdot; \theta_a)$ is permutation equivariant we construct it by composing few EL's. Also, we assume that the weights ($\boldsymbol{\alpha}_i$) are non-negative numbers that sums to 1. The output of the EL is passed to a softmax to obtain a distribution of weights over the patches. Finally, to ensure the weights are sparsely distributed, we added a regularization term $\mathcal{R}(\mathcal{X}_i; \theta_e, \theta_a) = \sum_{j=1}^{N_i} \log(\alpha_{ij} + \epsilon)$ to the loss function in Eq. 1.

2.3 Generative Network

The encoder function ϕ_e projects the raw patch x_{ij} to a d-dimensional latent representation $\left(i.e., \phi_e(x_{ij}; \theta_e) \in \mathbb{R}^d\right)$. Without extra regularization, the loss function focuses only on the prediction task, forcing ϕ_e to extract information that is only relevant to y. If y is low dimensional, ϕ_e learns a highly redundant latent space representation for each patch. Since α_{ij} is a function of $\phi_e(x_{ij}, \theta_e)$, redundant features result in uniform weights *i.e.*, ($\alpha_{ij} = \frac{1}{|\mathcal{X}_i|}$). This phenomenon makes interpretability difficult. We demonstrated this effect in our experiments.

To discourage loss of information, we added a convolutional auto-encoder (CAE) [11] to reconstruct patch as $\hat{x}_{ij} = \phi_d(\phi_e(x_{ij}; \theta_e); \theta_d)$. A generative loss $\mathcal{L}_g(\mathcal{X}_i, \hat{\mathcal{X}}_i; \theta_e, \theta_d) = \frac{1}{|\mathcal{X}_i|} \sum_{x_{ij} \in \mathcal{X}_i} ||x_{ij} - \hat{x}_{ij}||_2$ is added to the final loss function.

Table 1. Clinical measurement regression and GOLD stage classification accuracy by different methods on the COPDGene dataset.

Method	FEV1	FEV1/FVC	GOLD exact	GOLD one-off
Our method ($\lambda_1 = 0$)	**0.68**	**0.71**	**61.17 %**	**87.64 %**
Our method ($\lambda_1 = 10$)	**0.64**	0.70	**55.60 %**	**84.57%**
CNN [5]	0.53	—	51.1 %	74.9 %
Non-Parametric [16]	0.58	0.70	50.47 %	—
K-Means [16]	0.54	0.67	48.23 %	—
Baseline	0.52	0.69	49.06 %	—

2.4 Architecture Details

The $f(\cdot; \omega)$ is a linear function predicting the disease severity y_i. The architecture of generative network is elaborated in Fig. 1. The convolutional layer employs batch-normalization for regularization, followed by an exponential linear unit (ELU) [2] for non-linearity. The attention network $A(\cdot; \theta_a)$ has 2 equivalence layers with sigmoid activation function, followed by a softmax layer. The model is trained using Adam optimizer [7] with a fixed learning rate of 0.001.

3 Experiments

We evaluate the prediction and interpretation of our method on synthetic and real datasets. To evaluate the interpretability of our method quantitatively, we synthesize a dataset where the set-level target (y) are simulated from a subset of instances. Hence by viewing the attention weights as a detector of the relevant instances, we are able to evaluate the interpretability of our approach.

3.1 Synthetic Data

In this experiment, we build 10,000 training and 8,000 testing sets. The instances in the set are randomly drawn images from MNIST [8] dataset. The size of the sets varies between 20 to 100 instances. Each image is a 28×28 pixel monochrome image of a handwritten digit between $0 - 9$. The set-label (y) is the sum of prime numbers $(2, 3, 5, 7)$ in that set. Our method predicts the set-label with a high accuracy ($R^2 = 0.99$ on held-out data). We view the attention weights as detectors of prime numbers. Note that no instance level supervision is used. We make an ROC (Receiver Operating Characteristic) curve per set, and compute one average ROC curve across the held-out dataset. Figure 2(a) shows the average and error bar for all the sets. The figure compares our method (blue) with equal weights (red) (*i.e.*, $\alpha_{ij} = 1/|\mathcal{X}_i|$) and uniform random weights (green). Our method can detect correct instances in the set, with only weak supervision over the set (*i.e.*, set-level label y). Here we used $\lambda_1 = 100$ and $\lambda_2 = 0.01$.

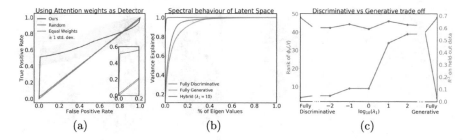

Fig. 2. (a) ROC curve of detecting true relevant instances on synthetic dataset using attention weights, (b) Spectral properties of patch-level features for different values of λ_1. (c) The trade-off between rank of latent space (red, y-axis on left) and predictive power (blue, y-axis on right) for different values of λ_1. Left represents fully discriminative and right represents fully generative models.

3.2   COPD

We evaluate our model on 6,400 subjects with different degrees of severity of the COPD from the COPDGene dataset [13]. As clinical measures, we use the Forced Expiratory Volume in one second (FEV1), the ratio of FEV1 and Forced Vital Capacity (FVC), and discrete score (between 0–4) called the Global Initiative for Chronic Obstructive Lung Disease (GOLD). We first segment the lung area on the inspiratory images using CIP library [14]. Each subject is represented as a bag of equal size 3D patches, with some overlap. Large patch size and percentage overlap leads to GPU memory issues. We experimented with different values and finally used patch-size of $32 \times 32 \times 32$ with 40% overlap in our experiments.

We perform three experiments: (1) *Prediction:* we compare the performance of our method against the sate-of-art for predicting the clinical measurements, (2) *Generative regularizer (λ_1):* we study the effect of the generative regularizer (*i.e.,* λ_1) in terms of prediction accuracy and information preserved in latent space, (3) *Visualization:* we visualize the interpretation of the model on the subject and population level. Unlike λ_1, the choice of λ_2 don't have any significant effect on the prediction accuracy. The value of λ_2 influences the sparsity and diversity of the attention weights. In the experiments, we fixed λ_2 to 0.0001.

Prediction: We compare to several baselines: (a) **Baseline**: Two threshold-based features measuring the percentage of voxels with intensity less than -950 Hounsfield Unit (HU) for the inspiratory and -856 HU for expiratory images. These measurements reflect the clinical measure to quantify emphysema and the degree of gas trapping. (b) **Non-parametric**: Schabdach et al. [16] view each subject as a set of hand-crafted histogram and texture features from supervoxels. They represent each subject in an embedding space using a non-parametric distance between sets. (c) **CNN**: Gonzalez et al. [5] use deep features learned from a composite image of four canonical views of a CT scan to quantify FEV1 and stage COPD. (d) **BOW**: It extracts features similar to [16] from supervoxels, but applies k−means to extract the subject-level representation. We perform

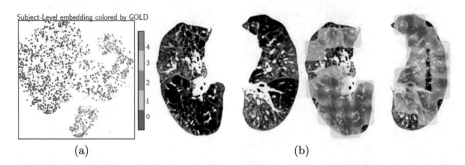

Fig. 3. (a) Embedding the subjects in 2D using tSNE. The dots represents one subject colored by the GOLD score. (b) An axial view of the attention map on a subject. Red color indicate higher relevance to the disease severity.

10-fold cross-validation and report R^2 for the continuous measurements (*i.e.*, FEV1 and FEV/FVC) and accuracy for the GOLD score. For GOLD score we also report the percentage of cases whose classification lays within one class of the true value (*one-off*). The Table 1 summarizes the results of the experiments. Our method outperforms the state-of-the-art on predicting FEV1 and GOLD score. Adding the generative regularization ($\lambda_1 = 10$) reduces the accuracy but provides better interpretability. In the following, we study the effect of λ_1.

Generative regularizer (λ_1): The Fig. 2(b) reports the spectral behaviors of the latent features (*i.e.*, $\phi_e(\mathcal{X}_i)$) for varying λ_1. For small λ_1 the loss function doesn't optimize for the generative loss. Hence, the latent space representation becomes highly redundant, and all the attention weights α_{ij} converges to $\frac{1}{|\mathcal{X}_i|}$. The Fig. 2(c) shows the trade-off between effective rank of the latent feature and R^2 for predicting FEV1. Although, the R^2 drops a little, the rank, which represents the diversity of the latent features, improves drastically. The gap between accuracies of $\lambda_1 = 0$ and $\lambda_1 > 0$ is the price we pay for the interpretability. Fully generative model ($\lambda_1 \rightarrow \infty$) does not produce good prediction.

Visualization: We use tSNE [10] to visualize subject-level features in two dimension. In Fig. 3(a), each dot represents a subject colored by the GOLD score. Even in two dimension, subjects with GOLD score of (0,1) and (3,4) are quite separable and 2's are in between. The bimodal distribution of GOLD stages 3 and 4, is sensitive to t-SNE parameterization and requires further investigation. 3(b) visualizes the attention weights on one subject. The dark area on the left lung, which is severely damaged, received hight attention.

4   Conclusion

We developed a novel attention-based model that achieves high prediction while maintaining interpretability. The method outperforms state-of-art and detects correct instances on the simulated data. Our current model does not account for spatial locations of the patches. As a future direction, we plan to extend the model to accommodate relationship between patches.

Acknowledgement. This work is partially supported by NIH Award Number 1R01HL141813-01. We gratefully thank NVIDIA Corporation for their donation of the Titan X Pascal GPU. We thank Competitive Medical Research Fund (CMRF) grant for their funding.

References

1. Cheplygina, V., Peña, I.P., Pedersen, J.H., Lynch, D.A., Sørensen, L., de Bruijne, M.: Transfer learning for multi-center classification of chronic obstructive pulmonary disease, January 2017
2. Clevert, D.A., Unterthiner, T., Hochreiter, S.: Fast and Accurate Deep Network Learning by Exponential Linear Units (ELUs), November 2015
3. Dubost, F., et al.: GP-Unet: lesion detection from weak labels with a 3D regression network. In: Descoteaux, M., Maier-Hein, L., Franz, A., Jannin, P., Collins, D.L., Duchesne, S. (eds.) MICCAI 2017. LNCS, vol. 10435, pp. 214–221. Springer, Cham (2017). https://doi.org/10.1007/978-3-319-66179-7_25
4. Estépar, R.S.J., Kinney, G.L.: Computed tomographic measures of pulmonary vascular morphology in smokers and their clinical implications. AJRCCM **188**(2), 231–239 (2013)
5. González, G., Ash, S.Y., Vegas-Sánchez-Ferrero, G.: Disease staging and prognosis in smokers using deep learning in chest computed tomography. AJRCCM **197**(2), 193–203 (2017)
6. Hayhurst, M.D., MacNee, W., Flenley, D.C.: Diagnosis of pulmonary emphysema by computerised tomography. Lancet **2**(8398), 320–322 (1984)
7. Kingma, D.P., Ba, J.: Adam: A Method for Stochastic Optimization, December 2014
8. LeCun, Y., Cortes, C.: MNIST handwritten digit database. AT&T Labs (2010)
9. Luong, M.T., Pham, H., Manning, C.D.: Effective Approaches to Attention-based Neural Machine Translation, August 2015
10. van der Maaten, L., Hinton, G., Visualizing Data using t-SNE: Visualizing Data using t-SNE. J. Mach. Learn. Res. **9**, 2579–2605 (2008)
11. Masci, J., Meier, U., Cireşan, D., Schmidhuber, J.: Stacked convolutional auto-encoders for hierarchical feature extraction. In: Honkela, T., Duch, W., Girolami, M., Kaski, S. (eds.) ICANN 2011. LNCS, vol. 6791, pp. 52–59. Springer, Heidelberg (2011). https://doi.org/10.1007/978-3-642-21735-7_7
12. Müller, N.L., Staples, C.A., Miller, R.R., Abboud, R.T.: Density mask: an objective method to quantitate emphysema using computed tomography. Chest **94**, 782–787 (1988)
13. Regan, E.A., et al.: Genetic epidemiology of COPD (COPDGene) study design. J. COPD **7**(1), 32–43 (2010)
14. San Jose Estepar, R., Ross, J.C., Harmouche, R., Onieva, J., Diaz, A.A., Washko, G.R.: CIP: an open-source library and workstation for quantitative chest imaging. Am. J. Respir. Crit. Care Med. **191**, A4975 (2015)
15. Satoh, K., Kobayashi, T., Murota, M.: CT assessment of subtypes in pulmonary emphysema in smokers. JJCR **46**(1), 98–102 (2001)

16. Schabdach, J., Wells, W.M., Cho, M., Batmanghelich, K.N.: A likelihood-free approach for characterizing heterogeneous diseases in large-scale studies. In: Niethammer, M., et al. (eds.) IPMI 2017. LNCS, vol. 10265, pp. 170–183. Springer, Cham (2017). https://doi.org/10.1007/978-3-319-59050-9_14
17. Shapiro, S.D.: Evolving concepts in the pathogenesis of chronic obstructive pulmonary disease. Clin. Chest Med. **21**(4), 621–632 (2000)
18. Sorensen, L., Nielsen, M., Lo, P., Ashraf, H., Pedersen, J.H., de Bruijne, M.: Texture-based analysis of COPD: a data-driven approach. IEEE Trans. Med. Imaging **31**(1), 70–78 (2012)
19. Xu, K., et al.: Show, attend and tell: neural image caption generation with visual attention. In: International Conference on Machine Learning, February 2015
20. Yang, J., et al.: Unsupervised discovery of spatially-informed lung texture patterns for pulmonary emphysema: the MESA COPD study. In: Descoteaux, M., Maier-Hein, L., Franz, A., Jannin, P., Collins, D.L., Duchesne, S. (eds.) MICCAI 2017. LNCS, vol. 10433, pp. 116–124. Springer, Cham (2017). https://doi.org/10.1007/978-3-319-66182-7_14
21. Zaheer, M., Kottur, S., Ravanbakhsh, S., Poczos, B., Salakhutdinov, R., Smola, A.: Deep sets. In: Advances in Neural Information Processing Systems, pp. 3391–3401, March 2017

3D Context Enhanced Region-Based Convolutional Neural Network for End-to-End Lesion Detection

Ke Yan[1], Mohammadhadi Bagheri[2], and Ronald M. Summers[1(✉)]

[1] Imaging Biomarkers and Computer-Aided Diagnosis Laboratory,
Bethesda, MD, USA
[2] Clinical Image Processing Service, Department of Radiology and Imaging Sciences,
National Institutes of Health Clinical Center, Bethesda, MD 20892-1182, USA
{ke.yan,mohammad.bagheri,rms}@nih.gov

Abstract. Detecting lesions from computed tomography (CT) scans is an important but difficult problem because non-lesions and true lesions can appear similar. 3D context is known to be helpful in this differentiation task. However, existing end-to-end detection frameworks of convolutional neural networks (CNNs) are mostly designed for 2D images. In this paper, we propose 3D context enhanced region-based CNN (3DCE) to incorporate 3D context information efficiently by aggregating feature maps of 2D images. 3DCE is easy to train and end-to-end in training and inference. A universal lesion detector is developed to detect all kinds of lesions in one algorithm using the DeepLesion dataset. Experimental results on this challenging task prove the effectiveness of 3DCE.

1 Introduction

Automated lesion detection in computed tomography (CT) scans plays an important role in computer-aided disease screening and tracking. To differentiate lesions from non-lesions, 3D context is crucial [4–6,9]. However, existing detection frameworks using convolutional neural networks (CNNs) [2,8] are typically designed for 2D images. Therefore, algorithms that can take 3D context information into consideration are in need.

As a direct solution, Liao et al. [6] extended the region proposal network (RPN) [8] to 3D RPN to process volumetric CT data. However, 3D CNNs are very memory-consuming so that sometimes it is hard to fit a single sample into the memory of a mainstream GPU [6]. To solve this problem, [6] used small 3D patches as the input of the network. Besides, 3D bounding-boxes are generally more difficult to annotate than 2D ones, which leads to sparse training data for 3D RPNs. Hence, data augmentation was used in [6] to combat over-fitting. In [4], 2D networks were first applied to generate lesion candidates, then 3D CNN classifiers were trained for false positive reduction (FPR). Some researchers trained classifiers on the aggregation of multiple 2D slices (e.g. three orthogonal

A. F. Frangi et al. (Eds.): MICCAI 2018, LNCS 11070, pp. 511–519, 2018.
https://doi.org/10.1007/978-3-030-00928-1_58

views (2.5D) or random views of the candidate lesion) for FPR [9]. FPR-based approaches have two stages and are not end-to-end.

In this paper, we propose 3D context enhanced region-based CNNs (3DCE) to incorporate 3D context into 2D regional CNNs. Multiple neighboring slices are sent into a 2D detection network to generate feature maps separately, which are then aggregated for final prediction. We improve the region-based fully convolutional network (R-FCN) [2] for this task. 3DCE has many advantages: (1) Compared with the 2-stage candidate generation + FPR approaches, 3DCE is more efficient and end-to-end in both training and inference. (2) It can leverage popular 2D CNN backbones and pretrained weights such as VGG-16 [11]. The weights are learned from millions of images [3] and are known to be beneficial for transfer learning [10]. On the contrary, 3D CNNs lack such pretrained models and have to be trained from scratch. (3) 3DCE only requires 2D bounding-box annotations to train. Compared with 3D methods, it can obtain large-scale training data more easily, e.g., from radiologists' routine lesion measurements [12].

Previous studies on lesion detection generally focused on specific types of lesions, such as lung nodules and liver lesions. While some common types receive much attention, many infrequent but still clinically significant types have been ignored. In this paper, we apply the proposed algorithm on DeepLesion [12], a large-scale and diverse lesion dataset. It contains over 32 K 2D annotations of lesions with a variety of types. Using this dataset, we develop a universal lesion detection algorithm that finds all types of lesions with one unified framework. After incorporating 3D contexts with 3DCE, the sensitivity of lesion detection with 4 false positives per image is improved from 80.32% to 84.37% on the test set of the challenging dataset, proving the effectiveness of 3DCE.

2   Method

Our goal is to consider 3D context in lesion detection, meanwhile leveraging pretrained 2D CNN weights for transfer learning [10]. A simple solution [4] is to input multiple neighboring slices into object detection frameworks with pretrained backbones. Since current detectors are mostly designed for natural images with three channels (RGB), it is necessary to extend the filters in the first layer and pad it with zeros for the extra input channels. Thus, the new network can start from using the three channels with non-zero weights, and gradually learn the new weights in the first layer to fit the extra input channels. The drawback of this data-level fusion strategy is that the pretrained weights may need to change greatly to adapt to 3D textures. Our idea is to fuse information in the feature map level. We first group slices to 3-channel images and extract good feature maps for each image, then aggregate the feature maps of neighboring images to collect 3D information, and finally build lesion classifiers on top of the fused features. Therefore, the backbone network structure for 2D images can be kept, whereas its representation capability is enhanced for 3D by feature aggregation.

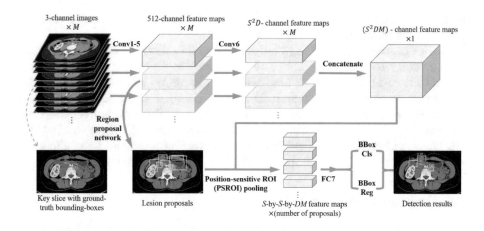

Fig. 1. The framework of 3DCE for lesion detection.

2.1   3DCE

The framework of the proposed 3D context enhanced region-based CNN (3DCE) is presented in Fig. 1. We adopt the R-FCN [2] for this task, which we find is faster, and more accurate and memory-efficient than the widely-used faster region-based CNN (faster RCNN) [4,8]. Different from faster RCNN, R-FCN constructs a set of position-sensitive score maps, each encoding the object class or position information in a relative spatial position of the object. After that, a position-sensitive region of interest (PSROI) pooling layer summarizes these score maps on each lesion proposal. The object classification and bounding-box regression results are finally obtained by another pooling operation [2].

We first improve R-FCN by adding 3 new layers after PSROI pooling: a 2048D fully-connected (FC) layer, a ReLU layer, and two FC layers for classification and bounding-box regression, respectively. A performance boost (0.7%) was observed with these additional layers, whereas the speed is comparable to the original R-FCN because we have made the feature maps before FC7 thinner. The last two pooling layers (pool4 and pool5) in VGG-16 are removed to enhance the resolution of the feature map, since lesions are often small and sparse. In 3DCE, $3M$ slices are grouped to M 3-channel images, as shown in Fig. 1. During training, the central slice contains the ground-truth bounding-box and the other slices provide the 3D context. We combine the M images to be a sample to input into the convolutional blocks (Conv1–5 of VGG-16) to produce M feature maps. Only the feature map derived from the central image is sent to the region proposal network (RPN) to generate lesion proposals. All feature maps undergo another convolutional layer (Conv6). They are then concatenated to aggregate the 3D information, forming an S^2DM-channel feature map, where $S = 7$ is the size of the pooled feature map for each proposal. D controls the number of 2D feature maps of 3DCE. We empirically set $D = 10$ in this paper. M determines the amount of 3D context to be incorporated. Larger M brings more information and more memory cost and risk of over-fitting. We found $M = 3 \sim 9$ ($18 \sim 54$ mm) a reasonable range in our lesion detection task.

In 3DCE, the weights of Conv1–6 are shared for different images in a sample. This strategy reduces the number of parameters to be learned compared with the 3D filters in 3D CNNs. Thus, 3DCE is less prone to overfitting. The 2D feature extractor (Conv1–6) and 3D feature classifier (FC7–end) are trained simultaneously, so Conv1–6 can learn useful features for both lesions and their contexts. This strategy can also be viewed as factorizing 3D filters to 2D + 1D [7]. There are four loss terms in 3DCE: lesion classification loss and bounding-box regression loss in RPN and improved R-FCN. They are optimized jointly.

2.2 Implementation Details

The algorithms were implemented using MXNet [1] and run on an NVIDIA Titan X Pascal GPU. We initialized the weights in Conv1–Conv5 with an ImageNet [3] pretrained VGG-16 model. All other layers were randomly initialized. Five anchor scales (16, 24, 32, 48, 96) and three anchor ratios (1:2, 1:1, 2:1) were used in RPN. The loss weight of bounding-box regression in improved R-FCN was set to be 10. In training, each mini-batch had 2 samples (each sample had M 3-channel images) when $M < 7$ and 1 sample when $M \geq 7$. We adopted the stochastic gradient descent (SGD) optimizer and set the base learning rate to 0.001, then reduced it by a factor of 10 after the 4th and 5th epochs.

3 Experiments

3.1 DeepLesion Dataset

The DeepLesion dataset [12] was mined from a hospital's picture archiving and communication system (PACS) based on bookmarks, which are markers annotated by radiologists during their daily work to highlight significant image findings. It is a large-scale dataset with 32,735 lesions on 32,120 axial slices from 10,594 CT studies of 4,427 unique patients. Different from existing datasets that typically focus on one type of lesion, DeepLesion contains a variety of lesions including those in lungs, livers, kidneys, etc., and enlarged lymph nodes in the chest, abdomen, and pelvis (see examples in Fig. 3). Their diameters range from 0.21 to 342.5 mm. The great diversity in type and size makes lesion detection in this dataset a challenging task. We rescaled the 12-bit CT intensity range to floating-point numbers in [0,255] using a single windowing (-1024–3071 HU) that covers the intensity ranges of the lung, soft tissue, and bone. Every image slice was resized so that each pixel corresponds to 0.8 mm. The slice intervals of most CT scans in the dataset are either 1 mm or 5 mm. We interpolated in the z-axis to make the intervals of all volumes 2 mm. The black borders in images were clipped for computation efficiency. We divided DeepLesion into training (70%), validation (15%), and test (15%) sets by randomly splitting the dataset at the patient level. No data augmentation was performed.

3.2   Results and Discussion

A predicted box was regarded as correct if its intersection over union (IoU) with a ground-truth box is larger than 0.5. The free-response receiver operating characteristic (FROC) curves of several methods are shown in Fig. 2.

- Improved R-FCN, 1 slice: Only the key slice with the lesion annotation was used for training and inference, thus no 3D context information was exploited. Its inferior accuracy indicates the importance of 3D context.
- Faster RCNN, 3 slice: The baseline method. Images composed of 3 neighboring slices were input to faster RCNN [8] with VGG-16 backbone. Pool4 and pool5 were removed similar to the improved R-FCN.
- Improved R-FCN, 3 slices: See Sec. 2.1. It outperformed faster RCNN using the same 3-slice 3D context.
- Data-level fusion, 11 slices: In this method, multiple slices are input into improved R-FCN. We found that 11 slices achieved the best performance, but it is still lower than 3DCE with 9 input slices, proving that the feature fusion strategy of 3DCE can better leverage the 3D context information.
- 3DCE: We tested applying 9, 15, 21, 27 slices ($M = 3, 5, 7, 9$). They achieved the best accuracy among all methods compared on the dataset.

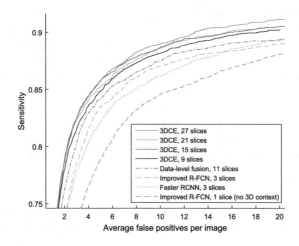

Fig. 2. FROC curves of various methods on the test set of DeepLesion (4802 images).

To analyze the detection accuracy on different lesions and images, we split the test set according to three criteria and display the results in Table 1. Eight lesion types are provided in DeepLesion. It is found that lung, mediastinum, and liver lesions have high sensitivity, probably because their intensity and appearance is relatively distinctive from the background. The sensitivity of all types were improved by 3DCE. Bone, soft tissue, pelvis, and abdomen lesions were improved the most. The complex and cluttered appearance of abdominal structures makes

Table 1. Sensitivity (%) at 4 false positives (FPs) per image on the test set of DeepLesion. The baseline is the faster RCNN algorithm. Lesions were sorted according to their types, sizes, and the slice intervals of the CT scans. The abbreviations of lesion types stand for lung, mediastinum, liver, soft tissue, pelvis, abdomen, kidney, and bone, respectively [12]. The mediastinum type mainly consists of lymph nodes in the chest. Abdomen lesions are miscellaneous ones that are not in liver or kidney. The soft tissue type contains lesions in the muscle, skin, and fat.

	Lesion type								Lesion diameter (mm)			Slice interval (mm)	
	LU	ME	LV	ST	PV	AB	KD	BN	<10	10~30	>30	<2.5	>2.5
Baseline	88	84	80	76	76	75	72	55	72	83	80	80	80
3DCE	91	88	84	82	81	80	76	63	78	86	84	85	83

3D context more important in the area. It is interesting to find that lesions with lower performance in the baseline method were generally improved more by 3DCE. As for lesion size, smaller lesions ($< 10\,\mathrm{mm}$) are harder to detect and benefited more by 3D context. 3DCE works better on CT scans with finer slice intervals because more precise information can be provided by the intermediate slices, compared with the interpolated slices in scans with bigger intervals.

During experiments, we noticed that sometimes the detector identified smaller parts of a large or scattered lesion with a big ground-truth bounding-box. Although the IoU is less than 0.5 in such cases, the detection may still be viewed as a true positive (TP) and it can also help the radiologists. To overcome this evaluation bias, we utilized the intersection over the detected bounding-box area ratio (IoBB) as another criterion. Besides, there are missing lesion annotations in the test set, because DeepLesion is based on radiologists' bookmarks, who typically mark only representative lesions in their daily work. Thus, an FP prediction may actually be a TP. We invited two experienced radiologists to re-annotate all lesions on 300 random slices in the test set of DeepLesion. The number of ground-truth lesions in the 300 slices grew from 305 to 768. We also assessed the algorithms on this all-lesion test set. The results are shown in Table 2.

Table 2. Sensitivity (%) at 4 FPs per image of different methods. Both the original test set and the all-lesion test set are investigated using two overlap computation criteria.

	Original test set		All-lesion test set		Inference
	IoU	IoBB	IoU	IoBB	time (ms)
No 3D context	76.51	80.16	66.90	72.47	**19**
Faster RCNN, 3 slices	80.32	85.34	71.60	80.31	32
Improved R-FCN, 3 slices	81.53	85.89	74.39	81.88	**19**
Data-level fusion, 11 slices	82.94	86.52	74.56	80.49	28
3DCE, 9 slices	83.57	87.81	**76.31**	**82.75**	56
3DCE, 27 slices	**84.37**	**87.85**	75.09	**82.75**	114

In Table 2, 3DCE still has the best accuracy despite the test sets and evaluation criteria. The performance computed using IoBB is better than IoU. The sensitivity at 4 FPs on the all-lesion test set actually became lower than the original test set of DeepLesion. DeepLesion consists of only representative lesions that radiologists think are measurable in their daily work, which are often subjective choices. Meanwhile, the all-lesion set was intensively labeled to include every abnormality. Some lesions in the all-lesion set are not measurable or too small, thus do not exist in the training set, which affects the algorithms' performance. In other words, both the number of FPs and the sensitivity are decreased by the new annotations. The inference time is also shown in Table 2. The improved R-FCN spent significantly less time than the baseline faster RCNN (since faster RCNN needs to run 4 FC layers on a thick feature map) while still got better accuracy. 3DCE's time complexity is roughly linearly proportional to the number of input slices, since it generates feature maps for multiple images. However, if tested on volumetric data, this extra time cost can be largely reduced because the feature maps of neighboring slices can be cached and reused.

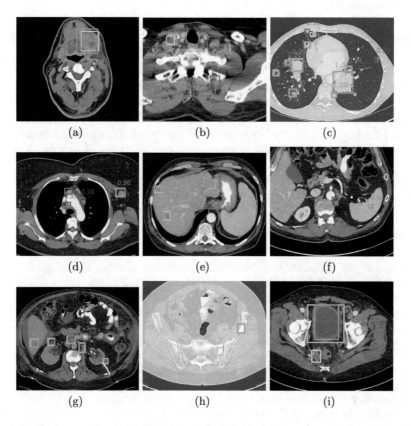

Fig. 3. Detection results of 3DCE with scores >0.9 on the test set of DeepLesion. Yellow, orange, green, and red boxes correspond to ground-truths in the test set, additional ground-truths in the all-lesion test set, predicted true positives, and false positives.

2D candidate generation + 3D/2.5D false positive reduction (FPR) methods were also tested. The accuracy of the FPR classifiers on this dataset is not promising, which is possibly due to the small inter-class variance (lesions and non-lesions look very similar) and large intra-class variance (many lesion types) of the candidates. We also designed a 3D CNN that receives 27-slice inputs (same as 3DCE), extracts features using 3D filters, and predicts 2D boxes on the key slice. It was adapted from improved R-FCN and trained from scratch. Its sensitivity at 4 FPs per image is 79.7% compared with 3DCE's 84.4%, proving that 3DCE with pretrained weights and factorized filters is superior.

Sample detection results are shown in Fig. 3. There are a large variety of lesions in DeepLesion. In (c), 14 lung nodules/masses were annotated and 10 were detected (the two FPs are actually TPs with bigger boxes). In (d), an axillary enlarged lymph node was detected but three small mediastinum ones were incorrectly spotted. The detector sometimes cannot distinguish enlarged and normal lymph nodes due to its scale robustness.

4   Conclusion

In this paper, we presented 3D context enhanced region-based CNN (3DCE) to leverage the 3D context when detecting lesions in volumetric data. 3DCE is memory-friendly, end-to-end, and simple to implement and train. It consistently improved the detection accuracy on the DeepLesion dataset. We expect it to be applicable in various detection problems where 3D context is helpful. We also developed a detector that can help radiologists find all types of lesions with one unified framework. It may serve as an initial screening tool and send its detection results to other specialist systems trained on certain types of lesions.

Acknowledgments. This research was supported by the Intramural Research Program of the NIH Clinical Center. We thank NVIDIA for the GPU card donation.

References

1. Chen, T., et al.: MXNet: A Flexible and Efficient Machine Learning Library for Heterogeneous Distributed Systems (2015). arXiv:1512.01274
2. Dai, J., Li, Y., He, K., Sun, J.: R-FCN: object detection via region-based fully convolutional networks. In: NIPS, pp. 379–387 (2016)
3. Deng, J., Dong, W., Socher, R., Li, L.J., Li, K., Fei-Fei, L.: ImageNet: a large-scale hierarchical image database. In: IEEE CVPR, pp. 248–255 (2009)
4. Ding, J., et al.: Accurate pulmonary nodule detection in computed tomography images using deep convolutional neural networks. In: MICCAI (2017)
5. Dou, Q., et al.: Multilevel contextual 3-D CNNs for false positive reduction in pulmonary nodule detection. IEEE Trans. Biomed. Eng. **64**(7), 1558–1567 (2017)
6. Liao, F., Liang, M., Li, Z., Hu, X., Song, S.: Evaluate the malignancy of pulmonary nodules using the 3D deep leaky noisy-or network (2017). arXiv:1711.08324
7. Qiu, Z., Yao, T., Mei, T.: Learning spatio-temporal representation with pseudo-3D residual networks. In: ICCV, pp. 5534–5542 (2017)

8. Ren, S., He, K., Girshick, R., Sun, J.: Faster R-CNN: towards real-time object detection with region proposal networks. In: NIPS, pp. 91–99 (2015)
9. Roth, H.R., et al.: Improving computer-aided detection using convolutional neural networks and random view aggregation. IEEE Trans. Med. Imaging **35**(5), 1170–1181 (2016)
10. Shin, H.C., et al.: Deep convolutional neural networks for computer-aided detection: CNN architectures, dataset characteristics and transfer learning. IEEE Trans. Med. Imaging **35**(5), 1285–1298 (2016)
11. Simonyan, K., Zisserman, A.: Very deep convolutional networks for large-scale image recognition. In: ICLR, pp. 1–14 (2015)
12. Yan, K., et al.: Deep lesion graphs in the wild: relationship learning and organization of significant radiology image findings in a diverse large-scale lesion database. In: IEEE CVPR (2018)

Keep and Learn: Continual Learning by Constraining the Latent Space for Knowledge Preservation in Neural Networks

Hyo-Eun Kim[(✉)], Seungwook Kim, and Jaehwan Lee

Lunit Inc., Seoul, South Korea
{hekim,swkim,jhlee}@lunit.io

Abstract. Data is one of the most important factors in machine learning. However, even if we have high-quality data, there is a situation in which access to the data is restricted. For example, access to the medical data from outside is strictly limited due to the privacy issues. In this case, we have to learn a model sequentially only with the data accessible in the corresponding stage. In this work, we propose a new method for preserving learned knowledge by modeling the high-level feature space and the output space to be mutually informative, and constraining feature vectors to lie in the modeled space during training. The proposed method is easy to implement as it can be applied by simply adding a reconstruction loss to an objective function. We evaluate the proposed method on CIFAR-10/100 and a chest X-ray dataset, and show benefits in terms of knowledge preservation compared to previous approaches.

1 Introduction

In a restricted multi-center learning environment where each chunk of data is only available at the corresponding center, we should learn a model incrementally without previous data chunks. Consider the scenario in which privacy-sensitive medical data are spread across multiple hospitals such that a machine learning model has to be learned sequentially. If all data are available to be used concurrently, learning just with state-of-the-art deep learning models such as ResNet for image recognition [5] or GNMT for machine translation [15] can be a good solution. However, if a data chunk from one stage is not available anymore in the following learning stages, it is hard to preserve the knowledge learned from the old data chunk because of the phenomenon known as catastrophic forgetting [4]. This becomes more problematic especially in neural networks optimized with gradient descent [12].

Overcoming catastrophic forgetting is one of the key research topics in deep learning. One naive approach is to fine-tune (FT) the model with the data accessible at each stage by learning from the up-to-date model parameters [2]. Learning without Forgetting (LwF) is a representative method for overcoming

© Springer Nature Switzerland AG 2018
A. F. Frangi et al. (Eds.): MICCAI 2018, LNCS 11070, pp. 520–528, 2018.
https://doi.org/10.1007/978-3-030-00928-1_59

catastrophic forgetting in neural networks [11]. Before starting training in the current stage, output logits (LwF-logits) of the current training examples are calculated first, so that each example is paired with its true label and also the pre-calculated LwF-logit. The LwF-logits are used as pseudo labels for preserving old knowledge. Elastic Weight Consolidation (EWC) maintains old knowledge by constraining important weights (i.e. model parameters) not to vary too much [8]. The relative importance between weights is defined based on Fisher information matrix. Deep Generative Replay (GR) [13] uses a generative adversarial network [3]. GR learns a generative model and a task solving model at the same time, and the learned generator is used for sampling old data during current learning stage. The concept of GR is interesting, but samples from generative models are not suitable for use in certain applications such as medical imaging where pixel-level details include important radiographic features for diagnosis.

LwF and EWC are representative approaches for preventing catastrophic forgetting in neural networks based on two distinctive philosophies: controlling the output activation (LwF) or the model parameters (EWC). In this work, we preserve knowledge by modeling the feature space directly.[1] Based on the assumption that there exists better feature space for knowledge preservation, we model the high-level feature space and the output (logit) space to be mutually informative each other, and constrain the feature space to be in the modeled space during training. With experimental validation, we show that the proposed method preserves more knowledge than previous approaches.

2   Baseline Models

LwF and EWC are originally proposed for preventing catastrophic forgetting in *multi-task learning* where each task has its own data and the data used in previous tasks are not available when solving the current task. We call this as multi-center multi-task learning. We focus on *multi-center single-task learning* where the model is learned with different data-chunk of the same task and access to each data-chunk is restricted. In this section, we define several baseline models for the multi-center single-task learning environment.

Fine-tuning (FT) trains a model incrementally based on the model parameters learned in the previous stage. Figure 1(a) shows the model architecture for FT. X_n, Z, and Y_n are random variables for the input, latent, and output spaces, respectively. Target loss function $L_n(\theta)$ (e.g., negative-log-likelihood for classification) optimizes the model parameters θ which consist of θ_s (shared) and θ_n (new). In the first stage, θ is randomly initialized. In the following stages, θ is restored from the model learned in the previous stage.

Learning without Forgetting (LwF) trains a model using both ground-truth labels and pseudo labels (pre-calculated LwF-logits). Figure 1(b) demonstrates

---

[1] We denote *feature space* to be the space of feature vectors, usually from the layer before the output layer. [11] showed that using the LwF-vectors of the second last hidden layer instead of the LwF-logits of the output layer had no benefit.

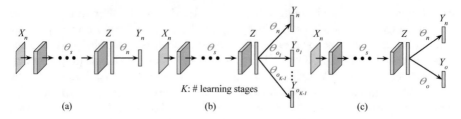

Fig. 1. Model architectures: (a) FT/EWC, (b) LwF, and (c) modified LwF (LwF+).

the K-th learning stage. Y_n and Y_{o_i} are the model's output for the current and the i-th stages for i in $\{1, ..., K-1\}$. The loss function is described as,

$$L(\theta) = L_n(\theta) + L_{LwF}(\theta), \qquad L_{LwF}(\theta) = \sum_i \lambda_{LwF} L_{o_i}(\theta), \qquad (1)$$

where $L_n(\theta)$ is the loss between the model output $y_n \in Y_n$ and its ground-truth label. $L_{o_i}(\theta)$ is the loss between the model output $y_{o_i} \in Y_{o_i}$ and its LwF-logit, and λ_{LwF} is a weighting constant. θ_s and θ_n are initialized randomly in the first stage and restored from the previous stage in the following stages. In the K-th stage, $\theta_{o_{K-1}}$ is initialized with θ_n of the $(K-1)$-th stage and fine-tuned until the final stage. In the third stage, for example, θ_{o_1} and θ_{o_2} are restored from θ_{o_1} and θ_n of the second stage, respectively. For classification tasks, $L_n(\theta)$ and $L_{o_i}(\theta)$ are typically the cross-entropy loss.

In the multi-center multi-task learning environment, LwF preserves old knowledge by constraining the outputs of the old task-specific layers with corresponding pseudo labels. But, finding out the optimal feature space in terms of all the tasks becomes hard as the number of tasks (i.e. output branches) increases.

Modified LwF (LwF+): LwF can be modified for the multi-center single-task learning. All the previous task-specific layers are merged into a single knowledge-preserving layer as shown in Fig. 1(c). So the loss function becomes,

$$L(\theta) = L_n(\theta) + L_{LwF+}(\theta), \qquad L_{LwF+}(\theta) = \lambda_{LwF+} L_o(\theta), \qquad (2)$$

where $L_o(\theta)$ is the loss between $y_o \in Y_o$ and its pseudo label (LwF-logit). θ_s and θ_n are initialized randomly in the first stage and restored from the previous model in the following stages. θ_o is initialized with θ_n from the first stage and fine-tuned until the end of the learning stages.

Elastic Weight Consolidation (EWC) constrains the model parameters by defining the importance of weights. Each parameter has its own weight-decay constant; the more important a parameter is, the larger the weight-decay constant. Based on the model in Fig. 1(a), the loss function is,

$$L(\theta) = L_n(\theta) + L_{EWC}(\theta), \qquad L_{EWC}(\theta) = \sum_j \frac{\lambda_{EWC}}{2} F_j(\theta_j - \theta^*_{p,j})^2, \qquad (3)$$

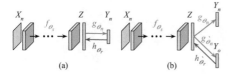 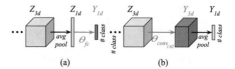

Fig. 2. Proposed model architecture: (a) the first learning stage and (b) the following learning stages.

Fig. 3. Top layers of ResNet: based on (a) fc layer or (b) $conv_{1\times1}$ layer. Both are functionally equivalent.

where $\theta_{p,j}^*$ is the j-th model parameter learned in the previous stage and F_j is the j-th element of the diagonal of the Fisher matrix F for weighting the j-th model parameter θ_j. λ_{EWC} is a weighting constant. θ_s, θ_n are randomly initialized in the first stage and restored from the previous model for the following stages.

EWCLwF (EWCLwF+) is the combined model of EWC and LwF (LwF+). Since both methods keep old knowledge based on two distinctive approaches, they can be used complementarily. Based on the model architecture described in Fig. 1(b) with the loss function in Eq. (1), $L_{EWC}(\theta)$ in Eq. (3) is merged so the loss function becomes $L(\theta) = L_n(\theta) + L_{LwF}(\theta) + L_{EWC}(\theta)$. EWCLwF+ is similar to EWCLwF. Based on the model LwF+ in Fig. 1(c) with the loss in Eq. (2), target loss becomes $L(\theta) = L_n(\theta) + L_{LwF+}(\theta) + L_{EWC}(\theta)$.

All the presented models are originated from the two representative methods for knowledge preservation in neural networks. Details of the experimental set-up for the baseline models will be explained in Sect. 4.

3 Proposed Methodology

In a general neural network model as in Fig. 1(a), the output Y_n of the input data X_n is compared with its true label, and the error is propagated backward from top to bottom, which encourages the latent variable Z to be task-specific. To keep the previously learned knowledge, the latent space Z should be informative enough to include the information of the input X_n.

During learning the feature extractor f of θ_s and the classifier g of θ_n, inverse function h of g ($h = g^{-1}$) can be approximately modeled by minimizing the L2 distance between the latent vector $z \in Z$ and its reconstruction $h(g(z))$ like Fig. 2(a). Without any constraints, minimizing the reconstruction loss easily makes the latent space Z to be trivial in terms of the information that Z can represent such that $\mathbf{H}(Z)$ which is an entropy of Z is low. Since Z should be informative enough to minimize the task solving loss $L_n(\theta)$, joint learning with both the reconstruction and task solving losses prevents Z from being trivial. It is known that minimizing the conditional entropy $\mathbf{H}(Z|Y_n)$ can be done by minimizing the reconstruction error of Z under the auto-encoder framework [14]. And minimizing the task solving loss $L_n(\theta)$ keeps $\mathbf{H}(Z)$ not to reduce too much.

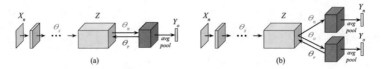

Fig. 4. Proposed model described in Fig. 2 based on the modified ResNet in Fig. 3.

As a result, Z and Y_n are being mutually informative from the joint learning with the two losses.[2]

Figure 2 shows the proposed model architecture. In the first stage, f, g, and h (respectively parameterized by θ_s, θ_n, and θ_r; initialized randomly in the first stage) are learned by minimizing the task solving and reconstruction losses concurrently. In the next stage, the parameters θ_o and θ_r of the functions g' and h' are restored from the θ_n and θ_r of the first stage and fixed during the rest of the learning stages.[3] Y_n and Y_o are the outputs for solving the task with current data and preserving previously-learned knowledge, respectively. Based on the loss function for LwF+ in Eq.(2), target Z space modeled in the first stage can be kept in the following stages by fixing θ_o of g' and θ_r of h' and guiding the output Y_o with LwF-logits. The loss function is shown below,

$$L(\theta) = L_n(\theta) + L_{LwF+}(\theta) + L_{rec}(\theta), \qquad L_{rec}(\theta) = \lambda_{rec} L2(\theta), \qquad (4)$$

where λ_{rec} is a weighting constant for the reconstruction loss. LwF-logits for Y_o are calculated in the same manner as in LwF+. θ_s and θ_n in the second stage are initialized with the parameters learned from the first stage and fine-tuned using the data in the corresponding stages until the end of the learning process.

Since we bound the Z space with the space modeled in the first stage and fix the θ_o, θ_r and Y_o (with LwF-logits), f tries to pull the new data examples into the modeled space which is remembering the previous data examples.

4   Experiments

We compare the proposed method with the baseline models in several image classification tasks. Base network is ResNet [5] which consists of multiple residual blocks and average-pooling (*avgpool*) followed by a fully-connected (*fc*) layer as shown in Fig. 3(a). The 3-D feature map Z_{3d} extracted from the top-most residual block is pooled into a 1-D feature vector Z_{1d} via *avgpool*, and the output vector Y_{1d} is obtained from Z_{1d} through the final *fc*. Given $z_{3d} \in Z_{3d}$ of an input example, $y_{1d} \in Y_{1d}$ is given by $g_{\theta_{fc}}(avgpool(z_{3d}))$, where g is the *fc* layer parameterized by θ_{fc}. g and *avgpool* are commutative because *avgpool* is a linear operation. Based on the modified model in Fig. 3(b), the output y_{1d} can be described as $y_{1d} = avgpool(g_{\theta_{conv_{1\times1}}}(z_{3d}))$, where g is now an 1×1 convolution

---

[2] Note that the mutual information between Z and Y_n is $\mathbf{I}(Z; Y_n) = \mathbf{H}(Z) - \mathbf{H}(Z|Y_n)$.
[3] θ_o, θ_r are used to restore the modeled space, so they do not need to be fine-tuned.

Table 1. Layer components. N, C, R are # of residual blocks, a conv layer, a residual block, respectively; e.g., R_1 of ResNet-110 has 18 # of two consecutive 3×3 conv layers with filter width 64. Downsampling with stride 2 is performed by R_2 and R_3.

	N	C_{init}	R_1	R_2	R_3	$C_{1 \times 1}$
ResNet-56	9	$3 \times 3, 16$	$[3 \times 3, 16] \times 2$	$[3 \times 3, 32] \times 2$	$[3 \times 3, 64] \times 2$	$1 \times 1, 10$
ResNet-110	18	$3 \times 3, 16$	$[3 \times 3, 64] \times 2$	$[3 \times 3, 128] \times 2$	$[3 \times 3, 256] \times 2$	$1 \times 1, 100$
ResNet-21	3	$3 \times 3, 32$	$[3 \times 3, 32] \times 2$	$[3 \times 3, 64] \times 2$	$[3 \times 3, 128] \times 2$	$1 \times 1, 2$

layer ($conv_{1 \times 1}$) parameterized by $\theta_{conv_{1 \times 1}}$. We used the modified ResNet in order to model the approximate inverse function h accurately before $avgpool$. Both are equivalent in terms of their function, but the modified model requires more computation than the original ResNet. The proposed network architecture is shown in Fig. 4. θ_n and θ_o are the model parameters of $conv_{1 \times 1}$ layers which are the replacement of fc layers in the original ResNet.

Three datasets are used for experimental validation; CIFAR-10/100 [9] and chest X-rays (CXRs) for natural image and medical image classification. ResNet-56, 110, 21 are the base models for CIFAR-10, CIFAR-100, and CXRs, respectively. Each network consists of an initial convolution layer, three sets of N consecutive residual blocks, and a final $conv_{1 \times 1}$ layer. In ResNet-21, an additional convolution layer (kernel 3×3, filter width 32, stride 2) with maxpooling (kernel 2×2, stride 2) is added as conv-bn-relu-maxpool (bn: batch normalization [7], relu: rectified linear unit [10]) before the initial convolution to expand receptive field for large-size CXRs. Table 1 summarizes the layer components. The top layer of ResNet-21 is modified from its original architecture and this will be explained in Sect. 4.2. Approximate inverse function h (of g) parameterized by θ_r in Fig. 4 consists of multiple consecutive convolutions. h in ResNet-56, 110, 21 for CIFAR-10, 100, CXRs includes four, three, three consecutive 3×3 (stride 1) convolution layers with filter widths (64, 128, 128, 64), (256, 256, 256), (32, 64, 128) followed by a single bn-relu, respectively.

For CIFAR-10/100, the initial learning rate of 0.1 is decayed by $\frac{1}{10}$ every 40 epochs until the 120-th epoch. For CXRs, the initial learning rate of 0.01 is decayed by $\frac{1}{10}$ every 20 epochs until the 80-th epoch. Weight decay constant of 0.0001 and stochastic gradient descent with momentum 0.9 are used. For CIFAR-10/100, 32×32 image is randomly cropped from 40×40 zero-padded image (4 pixels on each side of the original 32×32 image) during training [5]. Each CXR is resized to 500×500 and randomly cropped 448×448 image is used for training. λ_{EWC} for CIFAR-10, CIFAR-100, and CXRs are 0.1, 10.0, and 1.0, respectively. They are selected from the set $\{0.1, 1.0, 10.0\}$ by cross validation. λ_{LwF} in Eq. (1) is $\frac{0.1}{K-1}$, where K is the number of learning stages including the current one. λ_{LwF+} and λ_{rec} are 0.1 and 1.0. All experiments are done with tensorflow [1].

Table 2. CIFAR-10/100: test set (10k images) error rates - mean (std) of five trials.

	CIFAR-10				CIFAR-100			
	stage-1	stage-2	stage-3	stage-4	stage-1	stage-2	stage-3	stage-4
FT	20.21(.151)	16.76(.419)	15.40(.174)	15.02(.174)	50.13(1.25)	42.79(.692)	40.53(.467)	38.96(.354)
EWC	19.87(.421)	16.70(.178)	15.42(.258)	14.77(.331)	49.93(.937)	42.52(.299)	40.72(.231)	38.94(.504)
LwF	20.28(.532)	16.62(.453)	15.46(.220)	14.68(.304)	50.41(.422)	42.70(.334)	39.50(.417)	37.51(.319)
LwF+	19.88(.574)	16.57(.194)	15.02(.238)	14.05(.115)	50.69(.760)	42.64(.887)	39.31(.490)	37.30(.558)
EWCLwF	**19.79(.122)**	16.62(.041)	15.45(.413)	14.49(.183)	50.15(.552)	42.22(.481)	39.62(.338)	37.44(.526)
EWCLwF+	20.26(.474)	16.99(.410)	15.34(.440)	14.25(.239)	50.10(.439)	42.49(.335)	39.32(.288)	37.21(.377)
Proposed	20.11(.431)	**16.12(.253)**	**14.54(.175)**	**13.74(.195)**	49.87(.461)	**42.00(.479)**	**38.81(.438)**	**36.42(.373)**

4.1   CIFAR-10/100

CIFAR-10/100 have 10/100 classes with 32×32 50k/10k training/test images, respectively. In our experiment, 10k training images are used for validation and the model which performs the best on the validation set is selected for evaluation on the test set. The remaining 40k training images are splitted into four sets (10k/set). Each model is trained continually in the multi-center single-task learning set-up, where each center has 10k training images and the task is 10/100-class classification. Table 2 shows the error rates on the test set with mean (std) of five trials. LwF+, EWCLwF+ mostly perform better than LwF, EWCLwF; i.e. LwF+, EWCLwF+ are more appropriate for the multi-center single-task learning. The proposed method performs the best as shown in this table.

After stage-1, training data of the stage-1 (st-1-trn) is not used in the following stages anymore. So, we evaluate the final model with st-1-trn to see how much of st-1-trn has been forgotten after the final stage. For CIFAR-10, 85.75%, 85.97%, 88.64%, 88.22%, 89.40% of st-1-trn are still preserved as correct at stage-4 for FT, EWC, LwF+, EWCLwF+, Proposed, respectively. For CIFAR-100, 58.67%, 58.85%, 65.57%, 66.91%, 69.34% of st-1-trn are preserved correctly at the final stage (with the same ordering).

4.2   Chest X-Rays for Tuberculosis

We experiment with a real-field medical dataset in order to verify the proposed method is also valid in a practical set-up. A total of 10,508 de-identified CXRs (from the Korean Institute of Tuberculosis [6]) are used. It consists of 3,556 abnormal (tuberculosis; TB) and 6,952 normal cases. CXRs are commonly used for screening TB. The cases which require a follow-up test are recalled by radiologists. Among the 3,556 abnormal cases, 1,438 cases were diagnosed as active TB (TB-A) at the screening stage. The status of the remaining 2,118 cases which needed a follow-up sputum test could not be specified radiologically at the screening stage (TB-U). 80% of the data are randomly selected for training and divided into four sets; 288(TB-A), 424(TB-U), 1390(Normal) per each set. The remaining 20% are splitted evenly for validation and test; 143(TB-A), 211(TB-U), 696(Normal) for each set.

We modified the output layer of the model in order to exploit the status information of abnormality. Two output $conv_{1 \times 1}$ layers are used for 2-class (TB

Table 3. CXRs for TB: test set AUC - mean (std) of five trials.

	stage-1	stage-2	stage-3	stage-4
FT	0.811(.025)	0.842(.019)	0.882(.011)	0.892(.015)
EWC	0.812(.016)	0.832(.025)	0.865(.012)	0.887(.008)
LwF	0.814(.020)	0.853(.026)	0.882(.020)	0.891(.019)
LwF+	0.806(.010)	0.844(.022)	0.881(.018)	0.898(.014)
EWCLwF	**0.821(.019)**	0.841(.021)	0.869(.018)	0.890(.023)
EWCLwF+	0.817(.012)	0.852(.018)	0.871(.019)	0.884(.017)
Proposed	0.813(.035)	**0.869(.021)**	**0.896(.017)**	**0.909(.013)**

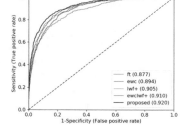

Fig. 5. ROC curves at stage-4 with stage-1 training data.

vs normal) and 3-class (TB-A, TB-U, and normal) classification, respectively. The 3-class $conv_{1\times1}$ is used for knowledge preservation. The 2-class $conv_{1\times1}$ is just for the performance measurement (AUC; area under ROC curve).

Table 3 summarizes AUC of each model with mean (std) of five trials. Except for the first stage, the proposed method is always better than the others. The proposed method also performs the best in terms of the ensemble performance of the five trials; 0.9257, 0.9205, 0.9217, 0.9271, 0.9228, 0.9172, 0.9363 for FT, EWC, LwF, LwF+, EWCLwF, EWCLwF+, Proposed, respectively. Figure 5 is the ROC curves of the st-1-trn at stage-4 (similar to CIFAR-10/100), which implicitly shows that the proposed method is helpful to preserve old knowledge.

5 Conclusion

In this work, we raise the problem of catastrophic forgetting in multi-center single-task learning environment and propose a new way to preserve old knowledge in neural networks. By modeling the high-level feature space to be appropriate for knowledge preservation in the first stage and constraining the feature space to be in the modeled space during training in the following stages, we can preserve the knowledge learned in preceding stages. The proposed method is shown to be beneficial in terms of keeping the old knowledge in classification tasks. We need more experimental analysis beyond the classification such as lesion detection or segmentation, and we leave this for future work.

References

1. Abadi, M., Agarwal, A., et al.: TensorFlow: large-scale machine learning on heterogeneous systems (2015). http://tensorflow.org/
2. Girshick, R., Donahue, J., et al.: Rich feature hierarchies for accurate object detection and semantic segmentation. In: CVPR (2014)
3. Goodfellow, I., Pouget-Abadie, J., et al.: Generative adversarial nets. In: NIPS (2014)
4. Goodfellow, I.J., Mirza, M., et al.: An empirical investigation of catastrophic forgetting in gradient-based neural networks. In: ICLR (2014)

5. He, K., Zhang, X., et al.: Deep residual learning for image recognition. In: CVPR (2016)

6. Hwang, S., Kim, H.E., et al.: A novel approach for tuberculosis screening based on deep convolutional neural networks. In: SPIE Medical Imaging (2016)

7. Ioffe, S., Szegedy, C.: Batch normalization: accelerating deep network training by reducing internal covariate shift. In: ICML (2015)

8. Kirkpatrick, J., Pascanu, R., et al.: Overcoming catastrophic forgetting in neural networks. In: PNAS (2017)

9. Krizhevsky, A., Hinton, G.: Learning multiple layers of features from tiny images. In: Technical report, University of Toronto (2009)

10. Krizhevsky, A., Sutskever, I., Hinton, G.E.: Imagenet classification with deep convolutional neural networks. In: NIPS (2012)

11. Li, Z., Hoiem, D.: Learning without forgetting. In: ECCV (2016)

12. McCloskey, M., Cohen, N.J.: Catastrophic interference in connectionist networks: the sequential learning problem. Psychol. Learn. Motiv. **24**, 109–165 (1989)

13. Shin, H., Lee, J.K., et al.: Continual learning with deep generative replay (2017). arXiv:1705.08690

14. Vincent, P., Larochelle, H.: Stacked denoising autoencoders: learning useful representations in a deep network with a local denoising criterion. JMLR **11**, 3371–3408 (2010)

15. Wu, Y., Schuster, M., et al.: Google's neural machine translation system: Bridging the gap between human and machine translation (2016)

Distribution Matching Losses Can Hallucinate Features in Medical Image Translation

Joseph Paul Cohen$^{(\boxtimes)}$, Margaux Luck, and Sina Honari

Montreal Institute for Learning Algorithms, University of Montreal,
Montreal, Canada
{cohenjos,luckmarg,honaris}@iro.umontreal.ca

Abstract. This paper discusses how distribution matching losses, such as those used in CycleGAN, when used to synthesize medical images can lead to mis-diagnosis of medical conditions. It seems appealing to use these new image synthesis methods for translating images from a source to a target domain because they can produce high quality images and some even do not require paired data. However, the basis of how these image translation models work is through matching the translation output to the distribution of the target domain. This can cause an issue when the data provided in the target domain has an over or under representation of some classes (e.g. healthy or sick). When the output of an algorithm is a transformed image there are uncertainties whether all known and unknown class labels have been preserved or changed. Therefore, we recommend that these translated images should not be used for direct interpretation (e.g. by doctors) because they may lead to misdiagnosis of patients based on hallucinated image features by an algorithm that matches a distribution. However there are many recent papers that seem as though this is the goal.

Keywords: Distribution matching · Image synthesis
Domain adaptation

1 Introduction

The introduction of adversarial losses [1] made it possible to train new kinds of models based on implicit distribution matching. Recently, adversarial approaches such as CycleGAN [2], pix2pix [3], UNIT [4], Adversarially Learned Inference (ALI) [5], and GibbsNet [6] have been proposed for un-paired and paired image translation between two domains. These approaches have been used recently in medical imaging research for translating images between domains such as MRI and CT. However, there is a bias when the output of these models are used for interpretation. When translating images from a source domain to a target domain, these models are trained to match the target domain distribution, where they may hallucinate images by adding or removing image features. This

© Springer Nature Switzerland AG 2018
A. F. Frangi et al. (Eds.): MICCAI 2018, LNCS 11070, pp. 529–536, 2018.
https://doi.org/10.1007/978-3-030-00928-1_60

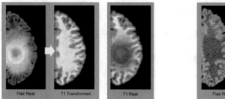 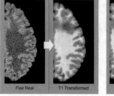

(a) A translation removing tumors   (b) A translation adding tumors

Fig. 1. Examples of two CycleGANs trained to transform MRI images from Flair to T1 types. We show healthy images in green and tumor images in red. In (a) the model was trained with a bias to remove tumors because the target distribution did not have any tumor examples so the transformation was forced to remove tumors in order to match the target distribution. Conversely in (b) the tumors were added to the image to match the distribution which was composed of only tumor examples during training.

can cause a problem when the target distribution during training has over or under representation of known or unknown labels compared to the test time distribution. Due to such a bias, we recommend until better solutions are proposed that maintain the vital information, such translated images should not be used for medical diagnosis, since they can lead to mis-diagnosis of medical conditions. This issue should be discussed because recently several papers have been published performing image translation using distribution matching. The main motivation for many of these approaches was to translate images from a source domain to a target domain such that they could be later used for interpretation (e.g. by doctors). Applications include MR to CT [7,8], CS-MRI [9,10], CT to PET [11], and automatic H&E staining [12].

We demonstrate the problem with a caricature example in Fig. 1 where we *cure cancer* (in images) and *cause cancer* (in images) using a CycleGAN that translates between Flair and T1 MRI samples. In Fig. 1(a) the model has been trained only on healthy T1 samples which causes it to remove cancer from the image. This model has learned to match the target distribution regardless of maintaining features that are present in the image. In the following sections, we demonstrate how these methods introduce a bias in image translation due to matching the target distribution.

We draw attention to this issue in the specific use case where the images are presented for interpretation. However, we do not aim to discourage work using these losses for data augmentation to improve the performance of a classification, segmentation, or other model.

2   Problem Statement

Our argument is that the composition of the source and target domains can bias the image transformation to cause an unwanted feature hallucination. We systematically review the objective functions used for image translation in Table 1 and discuss how they each exhibit this bias.

Let's first consider a standard GAN model [1] where the generator is a transformation function $f_{a,b}(a)$ which maps samples from the source domain D_a to samples from the target domain D_b. The discriminator is trained given samples from D_b through which the transformation function can match the distribution of D_b.

$$\text{GAN Disc: } \max_{b \sim D_b} \mathbb{E}\, [logD(b)] + \mathbb{E}_{a \sim D_a}\, [log(1 - D(f_{a,b}(a)))]$$

In order to minimize this objective the transformation function will need to produce images that match real images from the distribution D_b. Here there are no constraints to force a correct mapping between D_a and D_b, so for a non-finite D_a we can consider it to be equal to a Gaussian noise $\mathcal{N}$ typically used in a GAN.

In order to better enforce the mapping between the domains CycleGAN [2] extends the generator loss to include cycle consistency terms:

$$\text{Cycle Consistency: } |f_{b,a}(f_{a,b}(a)) - a|$$

Here the function $f_{a,b}$ is composed of the inverse transformation $f_{b,a}$ to create a reconstruction loss that will regularize both transformations to not ignore the source image. However, this process does not provide a guarantee that a correct mapping will be made. In order to match the target distribution, image features can be hallucinated and information to reconstruct an image in the other domain can be encoded [13]. Moreover, due to having un-paired source and target data, the target distribution that the generator is trained on may be even distinct from the target distribution that corresponds to the data in the source domain (e.g. having only tumor targets while the source is all healthy). This makes the models such as CycleGAN even more prone to hallucinate features due to the way the data in the target domain is gathered.

Another approach to solve this problem is using a conditional discriminator [3,14]. The intuition here is that giving the discriminator the source image a as well as the transformed image $f_{a,b}(a)$, we can model the joint distribution. This approach requires paired examples in order to provide real source and target pairs to the discriminator. The dataset D_b still plays a role in determining what the discriminator learns and therefore how the transformation function operates. The discriminator is trained by:

$$\max_{(a,b) \sim (D_a, D_b)} \mathbb{E}\, [logD(b, a)] + \mathbb{E}_{a \sim D_a}\, [log(1 - D(f_{a,b}(a), a))]$$

Even in the case of CondGAN that the source and target domain distributions correspond to each other due to having paired data, the discriminator can assign more/less capacity to a feature (e.g. tumors), due to having over/under representation of those features in the target distribution. This can be a source of bias in how those features are translated.

Table 1. Loss formulations divided into two phases of training. On the left the discriminator loss is shown (when applicable) and on the right the transformation/generator loss is shown. Note that for GAN losses the generator matches the target distribution indirectly through gradients it receives from the discriminator.

	Discriminator Loss (max)	Domain Transformer/Generator Loss (min)
GAN	$\underset{b\sim D_b}{\mathbb{E}}[logD(b)] + \underset{a\sim D_a}{\mathbb{E}}[log(1 - D(f_{a,b}(a)))]$	$\underset{a\sim D_a}{\mathbb{E}}[-log(D(f_{a,b}(a)))]$
CycleGAN	$\underset{b\sim D_b}{\mathbb{E}}[logD(b)] + \underset{a\sim D_a}{\mathbb{E}}[log(1 - D(f_{a,b}(a)))]$	$\underset{a\sim D_a}{\mathbb{E}}[-log(D(f_{a,b}(a))) + |f_{b,a}(f_{a,b}(a)) - a|]$
CondGAN	$\underset{(a,b)\sim(D_a,D_b)}{\mathbb{E}}[logD(b,a)] + \underset{a\sim D_a}{\mathbb{E}}[log(1 - D(f_{a,b}(a),a))]$	$\underset{a\sim D_a}{\mathbb{E}}[-log(D(f_{a,b}(a),a))]$
L1	-	$\underset{(a,b)\sim(D_a,D_b)}{\mathbb{E}}||f_{a,b}(a) - b||_1$

Finally, we look at how to train a transformation using only a L1 loss without any adversarial distribution matching term. With this classic approach we consider transformations based on minimizing the pixel wise error:

$$\underset{(a,b)\sim(D_a,D_b)}{\mathbb{E}}||f_{a,b}(a) - b||_1$$

Unlike GAN models that match the target distribution over the entire image, L1 predicts each pixel locally given its receptive field without the need to account for global consistency. As long as some pixels present the category of interest in the image (e.g. tumor), L1 can learn a mapping. However, L1 still can suffer from a bias when the train and test distributions are different, e.g. when no tumor pixels are provided during training, which can be caused by having new known or unknown labels at test time.

With all these approaches to domain translation we find there is the potential for bias in the training data (specifically D_b for our experiments below).

3   Bias Impact

We use the BRATS2013 [15] synthetic MRI dataset because we can visually inspect the presence of a tumor, it is freely available to the public, and we have paired data to inspect results. Our task for analysis is to transform Flair MRI images (source domain) into T1-weighted images (target domain). We start with 1700 image slices where 50% are healthy and 50% have tumors. We use 1400 to construct training sets for the models and 300 as a holdout test set used to test if the transformation added or removed tumors.

In this section, we construct two training scenarios: unpaired and paired. For the CycleGAN we use an unpaired training scenario which keeps the distribution fixed in the source domain (with 50% healthy and 50% tumor samples)

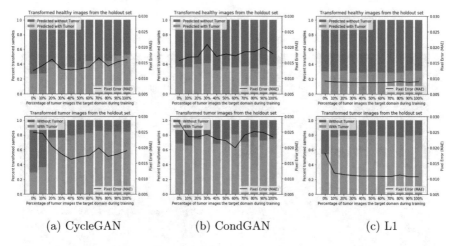

(a) CycleGAN   (b) CondGAN   (c) L1

Fig. 2. We plot the classifier's prediction on 300 (53% tumor) unseen samples (holdout test set) as we vary the distribution of tumor samples in the target domain from 0% to 100% of three models (CycleGAN, CondGAN, L1). This corresponds to 33 trained models. We split the source domain samples of the holdout test set into healthy (top row) and tumor (bottom row) and apply a classifier on the translated images. Green represents translated samples predicted by the classifier as healthy and red represents samples predicted with tumors. If the translation was without bias the percentage of healthy to tumor images should not change across the 11 models trained for each loss. For CycleGAN, we observe that the percentage of the images diagnosed with tumors increases as the percentage of tumor images in the target distribution increases. The black line represents the mean absolute pixel error between translated and ground truth target samples. While CondGAN seems to have a more stable classification results compared to CycleGAN, the pixel error indicates how much the translated images are away from ground truth samples and subject to change for different percentage of tumor composition in the target domain. L1 loss seem to suffer the least from target distribution matching and produces high error only when the target distribution has 0% of tumors (during training) and is asked to translate tumor samples. This case corresponds to 0% L1 on the bottom row.

and changes the ratio of healthy to cancer samples in the target domain D_b to simulate how the distribution matching works when the target distribution is irrelevant to the source distribution. For the CondGAN and L1 models we use a paired training scenario where both the source and target domains have the same proportion of healthy to tumor examples because they have to be presented as pairs to the model.

We train 3 models under 11 different percentages of tumor examples in the target distribution, which vary from 0% to 100% with tumors. In place of a doctor to classify the transformed samples we use an impartial CNN classifier (4 convolutional layers with ReLU and Stride-2 convolutions, 1 fully connected layer with no non-linearity, and a two-way softmax output layer) which obtains 80% accuracy on the test set. The results of using this classifier on the generated

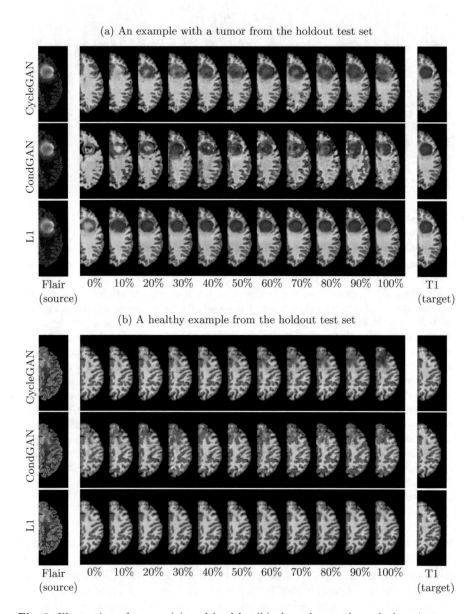

Fig. 3. Illustration of tumor (a) and healthy (b) class change through domain translation while changing the ratio of the healthy to tumor samples in the target domain D_b for all three models (CycleGAN, CondGAN, L1). We vary the distribution of D_b from 0% tumor to 100% examples to train 33 different models. We show images of the source domain (Flair) on the left and the corresponding ground truth image in the target domain (T1) on the right. We can observe visually the magnitude of the changes introduced.

T1 samples with different target domain composition is shown in Fig. 2. As we change the composition of the target domain we can observe the bias impact on the class of the transformed examples from the holdout test set. If there was no bias in matching the target distribution due to the composition of the samples in the target domain, there would be no difference in the percentage of the images diagnosed with a tumor as we change the target domain composition in Fig. 2. We also compute the mean absolute pixel reconstruction error between the ground truth image in the target domain and the translated image. If a large feature is added or removed it should produce a large pixel error. If the translation was doing a perfect job, the pixel error should have been 0 for all cases.

We draw the readers attention to CycleGAN which produces the most dramatic change in class labels, since the model learns to map a balanced (tumor to healthy) source domain to an unbalanced composition in the target domain, which encourages the model to add or remove features. This indicates such models are subject to even more bias due to the composition of the features in the target domain that can be different from the ones in the source domain.

For CondGAN, the pixel error changes across as the composition of tumor/healthy changes, indicating there is a bias due to the training data composition. Perceptually the L1 loss appears the most consistent producing the least bias. However, it has error when it is trained on 0% tumor and the model is asked to translate tumor samples at test time (0% for L1 in Fig. 2 bottom row and Fig. 3(a)), which is due to a mis-match between train and test distributions. It indicates that if at test time images with new known or unknown labels (e.g. a new disease) are presented to the model, it cannot transform them properly. In Fig. 3 we show examples of the translated images between the models. Note how for GAN based models the cancer tumor gradually appears and gets bigger from left to right. L1 mostly suffers in Fig. 3(a) for 0%. Interestingly, in the case of 100% tumor it can translate healthy images even though it was not trained with healthy images. We believe this is due to having both healthy and tumor regions in each image which allows the network to see healthy sub-regions and learn to translate both categories.

4   Conclusion

In this work we discussed concerns about how distribution matching losses, such as those used in CycleGAN, can lead to mis-diagnosis of medical conditions. We have presented experimental evidence that when the output of an algorithm matches a distribution, for unpaired or paired data translation, all known and unknown class labels might not be preserved. Therefore, these translated images should not be used for interpretation (e.g. by doctors) without proper tools to verify the translation process. We illustrate this problem using dramatic examples of tumors being added and removed from MRI images. We hope that future methods will take steps to ensure that this bias does not influence the outcome of a medical diagnosis.

Acknowledgements. We thank Adriana Romero Soriano, Michal Drozdzal, and Mohammad Havaei for their valuable input and assistance on the project. This work is partially funded by a grant from the U.S. National Science Foundation Graduate Research Fellowship Program (grant number: DGE-1356104) and the Institut de valorisation des donnees (IVADO). This work utilized the supercomputing facilities managed by the Montreal Institute for Learning Algorithms, NSERC, Compute Canada, and Calcul Quebec.

References

1. Goodfellow, I.J., et al.: Generative adversarial networks. In: Neural Information Processing Systems (2014)
2. Zhu, J.Y., Park, T., Isola, P., Efros, A.A.: Unpaired image-to-image translation using cycle-consistent adversarial networks. In: International Conference on Computer Vision (2017)
3. Isola, P., Zhu, J.Y., Zhou, T., Efros, A.A.: Image-to-image translation with conditional adversarial networks. In: Computer Vision and Pattern Recognition (2017)
4. Liu, M.Y., Breuel, T., Kautz, J.: Unsupervised image-to-image translation networks. In: Neural Information Processing Systems (2017)
5. Dumoulin, V., et al.: Adversarially learned inference. In: International Conference on Learning Representations (2017)
6. Lamb, A., Hjelm, D., Ganin, Y., Cohen, J.P., Courville, A., Bengio, Y.: GibbsNet: Iterative adversarial inference for deep graphical models. In: Neural Information Processing Systems (2017)
7. Wolterink, J.M., Dinkla, A.M., Savenije, M.H., Seevinck, P.R., van den Berg, C.A., Išgum, I.: Deep MR to CT synthesis using unpaired data. In: Workshop on Simulation and Synthesis in Medical Imaging (2017)
8. Nie, D., Trullo, R., Petitjean, C., Ruan, S., Shen, D.: Medical image synthesis with context-aware generative adversarial networks. In: Medical Image Computing and Computer-Assisted Intervention (2016)
9. Quan, T.M., Nguyen-Duc, T., Jeong, W.K.: Compressed sensing MRI reconstruction using a generative adversarial network with a cyclic loss. IEEE Trans. Med. Imaging **37**(6), 1488–1497 (2018)
10. Yang, G., et al.: DAGAN: Deep De-Aliasing generative adversarial networks for fast compressed sensing MRI reconstruction. IEEE Trans. Med. Imaging **37**(6), 1310–1321 (2018)
11. Ben-Cohen, A., Klang, E., Raskin, S.P., Amitai, M.M., Greenspan, H.: Virtual PET images from CT data using deep convolutional networks: initial results. In: Tsaftaris, S.A., Gooya, A., Frangi, A.F., Prince, J.L. (eds.) SASHIMI 2017. LNCS, vol. 10557, pp. 49–57. Springer, Cham (2017). https://doi.org/10.1007/978-3-319-68127-6_6
12. Bayramolu, N., Kaakinen, M., Eklund, L.: Towards virtual H&E staining of Hyperspectral lung histology images using conditional generative adversarial networks. In: International Conference on Computer Vision (2017)
13. Chu, C., Zhmoginov, A., Sandler, M.: CycleGAN, a master of Steganography. In: Neural Information Processing Systems Workshop on Machine Deception (2017)
14. Mirza, M., Osindero, S.: Conditional Generative Adversarial Nets (2014). arXiv 1411.1784
15. Menze, B.H., Jakab, A., Bauer, S.: The Multimodal Brain Tumor Image Segmentation Benchmark (BRATS). IEEE Transactions on Medical Imaging **34**(10), 1993–2024 (2015)

Generative Invertible Networks (GIN): Pathophysiology-Interpretable Feature Mapping and Virtual Patient Generation

Jialei Chen[1,2]([✉]), Yujia Xie[3], Kan Wang[1,2], Zih Huei Wang[4], Geet Lahoti[1,2], Chuck Zhang[1,2], Mani A. Vannan[5], Ben Wang[1,2,6], and Zhen Qian[5]([✉])

[1] Georgia Tech Manufacturing Institute, Georgia Institute of Technology, Atlanta, Georgia
jialei.chen@gatech.edu
[2] H. Milton Stewart School of Industrial and Systems Engineering, Georgia Tech, Atlanta, Georgia
[3] School of Computational Science and Engineering, Georgia Tech, Atlanta, Georgia
[4] Department of Industrial Engineering and Engineering Management, National Tsing Hua University, Hsinchu, Taiwan
[5] Marcus Heart Valve Center, Piedmont Heart Institute, Atlanta, Georgia
Zhen.Qian@piedmont.org
[6] School of Materials Science and Engineering, Georgia Tech, Atlanta, Georgia

Abstract. Machine learning methods play increasingly important roles in pre-procedural planning for complex surgeries and interventions. Very often, however, researchers find the historical records of emerging surgical techniques, such as the transcatheter aortic valve replacement (TAVR), are highly scarce in quantity. In this paper, we address this challenge by proposing novel generative invertible networks (GIN) to select features and generate high-quality *virtual patients* that may potentially serve as an additional data source for machine learning. Combining a convolutional neural network (CNN) and generative adversarial networks (GAN), GIN discovers the pathophysiologic meaning of the feature space. Moreover, a test of predicting the surgical outcome directly using the selected features results in a high accuracy of 81.55%, which suggests little pathophysiologic information has been lost while conducting the feature selection. This demonstrates GIN can generate virtual patients not only visually authentic but also pathophysiologically interpretable.

Keywords: Virtual patients · Generative Neural Networks

1 Introduction

For pre-surgical planning of complex surgeries and interventions, it remains difficult to build a comprehensive pathophysiology-based model incorporating the dynamic interactions between the human body and the medical device. Developing machine learning models from historical surgical data to help predict and

© Springer Nature Switzerland AG 2018
A. F. Frangi et al. (Eds.): MICCAI 2018, LNCS 11070, pp. 537–545, 2018.
https://doi.org/10.1007/978-3-030-00928-1_61

optimize the surgical outcome has become a promising alternative. In literature, machine learning methods (e.g., random forests [1], logistic regression [2]) have been used for various prediction purposes based on pre-selected features, while recently, deep learning methods (e.g., convolutional neural networks [3]) have emerged for feature selection and outcome prediction directly based on the input images. However, the key challenge to most surgery-related machine learning problems is that, while existing machine learning methods typically require large amounts of data, the dataset available consists of data from only a limited number of patients, which is usually too small for training considering the high dimensional input data (usually a fusion of medical images and clinical records). Furthermore, the highly unbalanced prediction input (e.g., age, blood pressure) and output (e.g., surgical outcome) add another layer of difficulty. In short, machine learning methods based on existing surgical records have limitations, and an enhancement of data size is imperative.

One immediate method to enlarge the data size is data augmentation [4], including image translation, rotation, changing in brightness and tune, etc. Nevertheless, most image augmentation methods used in natural images may impose alterations with pathophysiologic significance to medical images. For example, in CT scans, image intensity corresponds to specific substances of human tissue, alterations of which may change the tissue type and lead to a different surgical outcome. This difference limits the effectiveness of image augmentation in medical images. Meanwhile, a bypass method that is also widely adopted is transfer learning technique [5]. Researchers try to adapt the pre-trained model from natural images and modify a small amount of the model parameters for medical applications with less training data [3]. Yet a strong assumption of transfer learning is that the image features learnt from natural images would work similarly in medical images. For the prediction of surgical outcomes, the rationality of that is not clear, because a surgery involves a complex and dynamic interaction between the human anatomy and the surgical device, and the visual cues extracted from the medical images may not be sufficient for such a prediction. In one of our recent work, the predictive performance for transcatheter aortic valve replacement (TAVR) outcome using transfer learning is inferior to a CNN learnt from scratch [6]. This urges us to explore other possibilities.

Another way of data size enhancement is to generate *virtual patients*. Different from some literature, here it refers to the digital models that mimic the patient organ but are not exactly the same as any real patients [7]. The virtual patients can be 3D printed for a bench-top surgical simulation to assess surgical outcomes just like in the real patients as an enhancement to the dataset [8]. While medical image simulation based on a 4D extended cardiac-torso (XCAT) phantom is widely investigated [9], a complete *generative* model from scratch is lacking in medical literature. Some models from the machine learning community have the potential for virtual patient generation, including restrict Boltzmann machine (RBM) and variational auto-encoder (VAE) [5]. Yet these methods usually lead to sever blurriness in generated images. Recently, a deep learning framework, generative adversarial networks (GAN) was proposed to generate high-quality images, based on the distribution of the training images (see Sect. 2.2), which can be authentic enough to fool human eyes [10]. A straightforward idea is to adapt GAN for virtual patient generation. However, all of the generative methods above result in generating virtual patients that *visually* look like real patients, but with unclear pathophysiologic meanings.

In this work, we proposed a novel, deep learning framework - generative invertible networks (GIN) to extract the features from the real patients and generate virtual patients, which were both visually and pathophysiologically plausible, using the features (see Sect. 2). Specifically, GIN tries to find the feature mapping from the high-dimensional human issue/organ space (represented by CT images) to a low-dimensional feature space and, more importantly, its reverse (see Fig. 1). In contrast, GAN only finds the one-direction mapping from the feature space to the image space (i.e. generating), which makes it difficult to build the connection between the input images and the physical meaning of the feature space. In Sect. 3, we performed a case study using GIN to find the bidirectional feature mapping for the patients who underwent TAVR with the pre-surgical CT images as the input. Using the reverse mapping CNN, important clinical markers for the prediction of TAVR outcomes, such as the annular calcification, have been captured by the low-dimensional feature space (see Fig. 2). Moreover, a test of predicting the surgical outcome directly using the selected features results in a high accuracy (see Fig. 4). This shows GIN preserves the pathophysiologically meaningful features while conducting the dimension reduction and can generate virtual patients with different possible surgical outcomes.

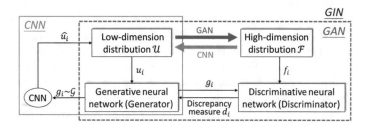

Fig. 1. The overall architecture of GIN. It contains a GAN and a CNN.

2 Methodology

2.1 Preparing TAVR Dataset with Augmentation

Aortic stenosis (AS) is one of the most common yet severe valvular heart diseases. Transcatheter aortic valve replacement (TAVR) is a less-invasive treatment option for AS patients who have a high risk of open-heart surgery [11]. The deployment of the TAVR prosthesis involves a complex interaction between the prosthesis, the native aortic root, and the blood flow, which are not fully understood and may affect the procedural outcome, such as the degree of paravalvular leakage (PVL) and the risk of thrombosis/stroke [11]. We studied the pre-procedural CT images of 168 AS patient (with an average age of 78) who received TAVR using a self-expandable prosthetic valve (CoreValve, Medtronic) from 2013 to 2016. All of the patients had pre-TAVR contrast-enhanced CT scans, which were performed on a 320-detector row CT scanner (Aquilion ONE, Toshiba). CT images were reconstructed with 10% increments throughout the cardiac cycle, and the cardiac phase of the peak aortic valve opening was used. Each CT dataset contained a 3D volume of the cardiothoracic region. For computational purpose, we chose only one slide at the aortic annulus (selected by a clinician) for this study. The method itself can be easily generalized to the 3D image volume. Post-TAVR PVL was set to be the major endpoint and was dichotomized to two groups: group 1 included none or low (trace to mild) PVL, while group 2 included high (moderate to severe) PVL.

We preformed routine data augmentation by slightly rotating the annular plane to add more samples. The regions of interest were rotated in 3D by four rotation angles in the annulus plane and one rotation angle in the longitudinal X-Z plane, from the original orientation. This led to an augmentation of 10 times the training set size. The augmented dataset was used to train the GIN.

2.2   Starting from GAN

The architecture of the GAN is shown in the blue dash box of Fig. 1 [5]. The key idea of the image generation by GAN is regarding the training set images as realizations of a distribution $\mathcal{F}$, which has extremely high-dimensional support (i.e. number of pixels of images). The distribution $\mathcal{F}$ can be physically interpreted as the group of images we are interested in (e.g., the aortic annulus). GAN can actually find a transformation from an easy-to-generate distribution $\mathcal{U}$ (usually, multi-uniform) to a distribution $\mathcal{G}$, which eventually is close enough to the target $\mathcal{F}$. In particular, GAN contains 2 neural networks (NN, see blue dash box of Fig. 1). In each training step of stochastic gradient descent (SGD), the realizations u_i of $\mathcal{U}$ is fed into the *generator* to generate g_i following $\mathcal{G}^{(i)}$. Generated image g_i is fed into the *discriminator* to be compared with the training set data f_i and find the discrepancy d_i, which is served as the loss function for the generator. The two NN's are trained by alternative optimization, until we think the generated distribution $\mathcal{G}$ is close enough to the true distribution $\mathcal{F}$.

GIN contains a GAN part for generation (blue dash box of Fig. 1). Moreover, in our framework, the support of distribution $\mathcal{U}$ is regarded as the feature space (it does not yet have any physical meaning) and realizations of the distribution $\mathcal{U}$ are the hidden features of the corresponding valves. This means given a feature vector (a realization of distribution $\mathcal{U}$), the GAN part in GIN can generate a virtual valve based on that feature vector.

2.3   Adding a CNN for Reverse Mapping

As mentioned, the generation using only GAN lacks pathophysiologic interpretation. The reason is that it only gives one-direction mapping from the feature space $\mathcal{U}$ to the real valve distribution $\mathcal{F}$ (assuming the final $\mathcal{G}$ is close enough to the true distribution $\mathcal{F}$, see Sect. 2.2). Thus, the feature space itself is difficult to interpret, and we are generating virtual patients without meaningful guidance. One way to introduce the pathophysiologic meaning to the feature space is to find corresponding locations of the real patients in that space, since the real patients have surgical records, such as the post-TAVR PVL level, which can be used to label the space and conduct classification. In other words, we need to find the backward mapping from the real valve distribution $\mathcal{F}$ to the feature space $\mathcal{U}$. Therefore, besides GAN, we add a CNN to the framework regarding the generated images g_i from $\mathcal{G}$ as input and the feature $u_i \sim \mathcal{U}$ as the output (see red box of Fig. 1). After the CNN is trained, we may feed the model with real patients data $f_i \sim \mathcal{F}$ and find its corresponding feature in the feature space.

In most literature, CNN is used for classification [3], which means the supervised value for each data set is discrete. Here, we use the CNN for regression, which means the label $u_i \sim \mathcal{U}$ (features) is a continuous vector with a non-zero measure. This is much more difficult for training when the dimension of $\mathcal{U}$ is high. But the advantage is that we are using the realization of distribution $\mathcal{G}$ (instead of $\mathcal{F}$) as the training set, in which, theoretically speaking, the available data size is infinitely large. In reality, we restrict the dimension of $\mathcal{U}$ to be less than 20 (10 in the case study) to gain a stable training result from CNN.

2.4 GIN Framework

Putting everything together, GIN contains three NN's, two of them first form a GAN (one generator and one discriminator) to find the transformation from the feature space to the CT images space, then the other NN finds the reverse mapping from the CT images space to the feature space (see Fig. 1). Finally, we have the bidirectional mapping between features and CT images. Furthermore, the feature space selected by GIN captures the pathophysiologic information hidden in CT images, which can be used to predict surgical complications (PVL). This allows us to conduct arithmetic operations in the feature space and make sure any generated virtual patients have physical and pathophysiologic meanings (e.g., we can generate a virtual patient knowing it may lead to high PVL or not).

It is important to note that our method is essentially different from adversarially learned inference (ALI) or bidirectional GAN (BiGAN) [12] in the literature. In order to invest the feature space with pathophysiologic meanings, we need a *hard* inverse, i.e. CNN=Generator^{-1} for every input sample. Thus, GIN has a sequential order of GAN and CNN to make sure the sample-to-sample inverse is explicitly trained and thus has better expressibility (see reconstruction test in Sect. 3.1). In contrast, BiGAN or ALI uses one discriminator to supervise both generator and encoder, the generator and encoder would be inverse to each other, as claimed, yet only in distribution level, which is not rigorous enough for medical image applications. Moreover, it uses coupling training of 3 NNs. This complicated architecture requires more fine tuning and therefore less suitable for our sparse dataset (see Sect. 2.1).

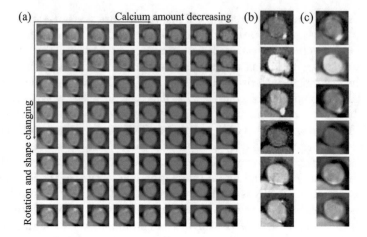

Fig. 2. The training results of GIN. (a) the characteristic valve CT images in the feature space, (b) The real patients valve CT image, (c) reconstruction test of the real valves in (b).

3 Results

In this test, the dimension of the feature space $\mathcal{U}$ is chosen to be 10, the results can be sharper if the feature dimension is increased to 20. But the training cost will also increase dramatically. The two NN's of the GAN part adapt 2-layer vanilla neural networks with 512 hidden nodes in each hidden layer and ReLu activations. CNN has approximately the same complexity with leaky ReLu activation and batch normalization in each layer (see [10] for more details).

3.1 Pathophysiology-Interpretable Feature Mapping

After training the GIN, a 2D cross-section in the feature space of the valves are shown in Fig. 2(a). The small figures at different locations mean the corresponding characteristic valve CT images in the specific locations of the feature space. We may find some physical meaning for the two features. In every column, from top to bottom, the valve rotates clockwise and the shape of the valve wall is gradually changed. In every row, from left to right, the amount of calcification (which is the brightest region in the CT images) decreases. According to clinical observations, high amounts of annular calcification could be an important risk factor of post-TAVR PVL. Thus, we may speculate that the left region in the feature space, which has visually more calcium, may be associated with higher rates of surgical complications.

Since the bidirectional mapping between the feature space and the valve space (see Sect. 2.4) is found by GIN, We may conduct the following reconstruction test to visualize the information loss by the framework. The features of the real patients' CT images were first extracted by the CNN part, and then the extracted features were used to generate virtual CT images by the GAN part. Ideally, if there is no information loss in both feature extraction (CNN) and generation (GAN), the reconstructed images should be identical to the real ones. The test results of some representative real CT images (Fig. 2(b)) are shown in Fig. 2(c). In the test, the reconstructed images look similar to their real counterparts, especially the overall shape and orientation of the valve. Meanwhile, some of the important details like calcification are also captured. This shows that the GIN captures pathophysiologically meaningful features. Yet some of the details are missing and also the reconstructed images are not as sharp as the real ones. This may be because the training set data is too small even with the augmentation to generate high fidelity images and the feature space is set to be too low to capture higher order features. Comparing our reconstruction test and the ones in the BiGAN paper [12], we would conclude that GIN is better in extracting the features and finding a sample-to-sample hard inverse.

3.2   Post-TAVR PVL Prediction

In order to assess the pathophysiologic mean-ing of the feature space, we look for the rela-tionship between the selected features and PVL. The first 2 Isomap [13] features are shown in Fig. 3, where the red squares rep-resent the patients with high PVL and the blue crosses represent the patients with low PVL. The two groups of different PVL lev-els follow different, visually distinguishable dis-tribution, even projecting to a 2D feature plane.

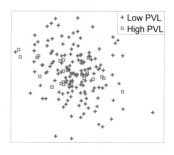

Fig. 3. The feature mapping of the real patients in the feature space with different PVL levels.

A more rigorous approach is to quantify the pathophysiologic significance by predicting the post-TAVR PVL level using the features selected. A simple random forest classifier (total 500 deci-sion trees) was used to classify the two groups, namely high PVL and low PVL. A 4-fold cross validation (75% of data as a training set and 25% as a validation set) was adopted to check the prediction performance as shown in Fig. 4. The average of the test accuracy, sensitivity, and specificity were 81.55%, 70.76%, and 82.42% respectively. The receiver-operating characteris-tic (ROC) curves are shown in Fig. 4 of each val-idation and the AUC values are 0.77, 0.84, 0.82, and 0.88 respectively. All of these turned out to be statistically significant ($p < 0.001$). This promising result shows that the features selected

K-fold CV	Accuracy	Sensitivity	Specificity
1	80.95%	75.00%	81.58%
2	76.19%	66.67%	76.92%
3	78.57%	71.43%	79.49%
4	90.48%	83.33%	91.67%
Average	81.55%	70.76%	82.42%

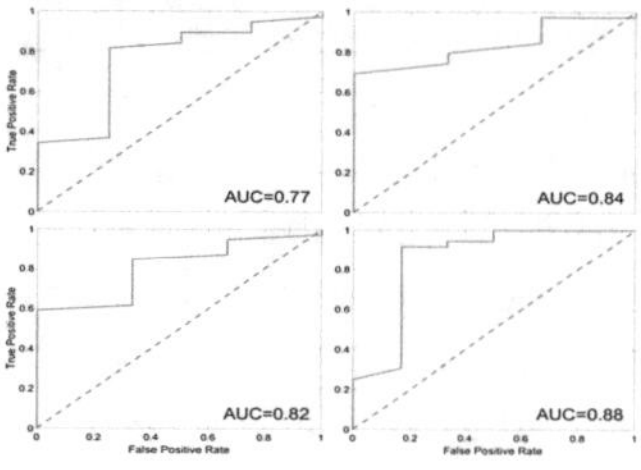

Fig. 4. The accuracy measure-ments (upper) and ROC curves (bottom) of the random forest model in predicting PVL.

by GIN is pathophysiologically interpretable and the information related to PVL outcomes in CT image is well-preserved.

3.3   CT Image Generation

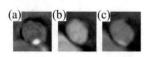

Fig. 5. Virtual patient generation with possibly different PVL levels.

More importantly, the pathophysiologically interpretable features captured by GIN can be used for virtual patient generation. Recall that the GAN can only generate the virtual patients that look like real patients. However, GIN can generate virtual patients with specific pathophysiologic appearances. The random forests classifier (see Sect. 3.2) actually segments the feature space to two parts according to its predicted PVL level. Thus, we may generate a virtual patient with a high probability of resulting in a high PVL by selecting a feature vector in the high PVL part of the space. As shown in Fig. 5(a), the generated CT image visually contains a large calcified nodule, which may lead to a high level post-TAVR PVL. We can also generate a virtual patient that is most likely with a low or none PVL as shown in Fig. 5(b). Also, we may generate a virtual patient with the features near the decision boundary as shown in Fig. 5(c). Despite the high prediction accuracy shown in Fig. 4, the sensitivity is relatively low. Thus, we may generate more virtual patients with a high PVL (Fig. 5(a)) to reduce the imbalance outcome of the dataset. Also, generating virtual patients with the features near decision boundary (Fig. 5(c)) can be extremely helpful to improve the prediction ability of the future predictive model. The generated virtual patients can then be 3D printed and go through virtual surgeries to obtain the PVL label in vitro (see [7] for more experimental details) as future work.

4   Conclusion

We proposed a new generative framework – GIN – to generate visually authentic virtual patients by finding the bidirectional feature mapping between the features and the real CT images (see Fig. 2). Moreover, a test of predicting the surgical outcome directly using the selected features resulted in a high accuracy, which suggests that features contain pathophysiologic meaning (see Fig. 4). This means GIN can generate virtual patients with different surgical outcomes for later 3D printing and in-vitro experiments (see Fig. 5). These virtual patients can be crucial in enhancing the model prediction power as an additional data source and more importantly, understanding the nature of the disease and performing optimal pre-surgical planning. In general, applying GIN to generate physically interpretable virtual samples has great potential for image related machine learning methods with limited and unbalanced datasets.

References

1. Statnikov, A., Wang, L., Aliferis, C.F.: A comprehensive comparison of random forests and support vector machines for microarray-based cancer classification. BMC Bioinform. **9**(1), 319 (2008)
2. Kim, H.-J., Fay, M.P., Feuer, E.J., Midthune, D.N.: Permutation tests for joinpoint regression with applications to cancer rates. Stat. Med. **19**(3), 335–351 (2000)
3. Shin, H.-C., et al.: Deep convolutional neural networks for computer-aided detection: CNN architectures, dataset characteristics and transfer learning. IEEE Trans. Med. Imaging **35**(5), 1285–1298 (2016)
4. Greenland, S., Christensen, R.: Data augmentation priors for Bayesian and semi-Bayes analyses of conditional-logistic and proportional-hazards regression. Stat. Med. **20**(16), 2421–2428 (2001)
5. Goodfellow, I., Bengio, Y., Courville, A., Bengio, Y.: Deep Learning, vol. 1. MIT Press, Cambridge (2016)
6. Wang, Z.H., et al.: Prediction of paravalvular leak post transcatheter aortic valve replacement using a convolutional neural network. In: 2018 IEEE 15th International Symposium on Biomedical Imaging (ISBI 2018), pp. 1088–1091, April 2018
7. Qian, Z., et al.: Quantitative prediction of paravalvular leak in transcatheter aortic valve replacement based on tissue-mimicking 3D printing. JACC Cardiovasc. Imaging **10**(7), 719–731 (2017)
8. Wang, K., Chang, Y.-H., Chen, Y., Zhang, C., Wang, B.: Designable dualmaterial auxetic metamaterials using three-dimensional printing. Mater. Des. **67**, 159–164 (2015)
9. Segars, W., Sturgeon, G., Mendonca, S., Grimes, J., Tsui, B.M.: 4D XCAT phantom for multimodality imaging research. Med. Phys. **37**(9), 4902–4915 (2010)
10. Arjovsky, M., Chintala, S., Bottou, L.: Wasserstein GAN. arXiv preprint arXiv:1701.07875 (2017)
11. Conti, C.A., et al.: Biomechanical implications of the congenital bicuspid aortic valve: a finite element study of aortic root function from in vivo data. J. Thorac. Cardiovasc. Surg. **140**(4), 890–896 (2010)
12. Donahue, J., Krahenbuhl, P., Darrell, T.: Adversarial feature learning. arXiv preprint arXiv:1605.09782 (2016)
13. Tenenbaum, J.B., De Silva, V., Langford, J.C.: A global geometric framework for nonlinear dimensionality reduction. Science **290**(5500), 2319–2323 (2000)

Training Medical Image Analysis Systems like Radiologists

Gabriel Maicas[1]([✉]), Andrew P. Bradley[2], Jacinto C. Nascimento[3], Ian Reid[1], and Gustavo Carneiro[1]

[1] Australian Institute for Machine Learning, School of Computer Science,
The University of Adelaide, Adelaide, Australia
gabriel.maicas@adelaide.edu.au
[2] Science and Engineering Faculty, Queensland University of Technology,
Brisbane, Australia
[3] Institute for Systems and Robotics, Instituto Superior Tecnico, Lisbon, Portugal

Abstract. The training of medical image analysis systems using machine learning approaches follows a common script: collect and annotate a large dataset, train the classifier on the training set, and test it on a hold-out test set. This process bears no direct resemblance with radiologist training, which is based on solving a series of tasks of increasing difficulty, where each task involves the use of significantly smaller datasets than those used in machine learning. In this paper, we propose a novel training approach inspired by how radiologists are trained. In particular, we explore the use of meta-training that models a classifier based on a series of tasks. Tasks are selected using teacher-student curriculum learning, where each task consists of simple classification problems containing small training sets. We hypothesize that our proposed meta-training approach can be used to pre-train medical image analysis models. This hypothesis is tested on the automatic breast screening classification from DCE-MRI trained with weakly labeled datasets. The classification performance achieved by our approach is shown to be the best in the field for that application, compared to state of art baseline approaches: DenseNet, multiple instance learning and multi-task learning.

Keywords: Meta-learning · Curriculum learning · Multi-task training Breast image analysis · Breast screening · Magnetic resonance imaging

1 Introduction

Radiologists are exceptionally trained specialists who play a crucial role interpreting and assisting other doctors and specialists in diagnosing and treating diseases. Their training program typically requires the trainee to solve tasks

Supported by Australian Research Council through grants DP180103232, CE140100016 and FL130100102.

of increasing difficulty [1], where each task contains a relatively small number of "training images". Such a program bears little resemblance to the training of medical image analysis systems based on machine learning that are modeled to solve narrowly defined, but complex classification problems [2], requiring large training sets. Once trained, these models cannot be easily adapted to new problems – they must be re-trained with new large training sets. The use of pre-trained models [3] as a way of initializing a model is the first step towards a more similar approach to the training program of radiologists. However, pre-training does not train a model to be able to learn new tasks – instead it is a "trick" to improve convergence and generalization. Meanwhile, machine learning researchers have developed more effective *learning to learn* approaches [4] – such approaches are motivated by the ability of humans to learn new tasks quickly and with limited "training sets". The optimization in such approaches penalizes classification loss and inefficient learning on new tasks (i.e., classification problems) by using a training scheme that continuously samples new tasks, mimicking the human training process. Our hypothesis is that medical machine learning methods could benefit from such an radiologist's style training process.

In this paper, we introduce an improved model agnostic meta-learning [4] (MAML) as a way of pre-training a classifier. The training process maximizes the ability of the classifier to adapt to new tasks using relatively small training sets. We also propose a technical innovation for MAML [4], by replacing the random task selection with teacher-student curriculum learning as an improved way for selecting tasks [5]. This task selection process is based on the model's performance on the tasks, trying to mimic radiologists' training. Our improved MAML is tested on weakly-supervised breast screening from DCE-MRI, where samples are globally annotated with classes (i.e. volume-level labels): *no findings*, *benign lesions* and *malignant lesions*, but these samples do not have lesion delineations. Note that the use of weakly-labeled datasets is becoming increasingly important for medical image analysis as this is the data available in clinical practice [2].

We test our proposed approach on a dataset of dynamic contrast enhanced MRI for the breast screening classification. Results show that our proposed approach improves the area under the ROC curve (AUC), outperforming baselines such as DenseNet [6], which holds the state-of-the-art (SOTA) for many classification problems; multiple-instance learning [7], which holds SOTA for breast screening in mammography; and multi-task learning [8]. Our learning approach produces an AUC of 0.90, which is better than the best result from the baseline methods that achieves an AUC of 0.85.

2   Literature Review

Breast screening from DCE-MRI aims at early detection of breast cancer in women at high-risk [9]. Currently, this screening process is mostly done manually, where its success depends on the radiologist's abilities [10]. An automated breast screening system working as a second reader can help radiologists reduce variability and increase the sensitivity and specificity of their readings. Traditionally, such systems rely on classifiers trained with large-scale strongly labeled datasets (i.e., containing lesion delineation and global classification) [11–15]. The non-scalability of this process (due to costs related to the annotation process) motivated the development of learning methods that can use weakly-labeled training sets [7] (i.e., samples contain only global classification). However, these methods still follow traditional machine learning approaches, which means that they still need large-scale training sets, even when the model has been pre-trained from other classification problems [3].

Contrasting with traditional machine learning algorithms, humans excel at learning new skills and new "classification" problems, where new learning tasks often require fewer training samples than the ones before. This *learning to learn* ability has inspired the development of a new generation of machine learning algorithms. For example, multi-task learning uses an optimization function that is trained to simultaneously minimize the loss of several different, but related classification problems [8], helping the regularization of the training procedure. Nevertheless, multi-task learning does not address the issue of making a model effective at learning new classification problems with small datasets. This issue is addressed by *meta-learning* [4], which has been designed to solve the *few-shot* learning problem, where the classifier is trained to train for new classification problems with previously unseen classes containing a small number of images. In meta-learning for few-shot classification, the model is *meta-trained* to solve classification problems for many randomly sampled tasks (i.e., the tasks are not fixed as in multi-task learning). Then the model is *meta-tested* by classifying unseen classes after being able to adapt using *few* training images of such unseen classes.

We explore the potential to improve the meta-learning process using a more useful (i.e., non random) task sampling procedure. For example, formulating the task sampling as a multi-armed bandit problem has been shown to produce faster convergence and better generalization [16]. Similarly, Matiisen *et al.* [5] proposed a new form of curriculum learning [17] that selects new tasks based not on their performance but on their performance improvement. However, these task sampling approaches have been applied in traditional machine learning problems, such as supervised and reinforcement learning problems, which means that our proposed application of curriculum learning for task selection in meta-learning is novel, to the best of our knowledge[1].

3   Methodology

Our methodology consists of three stages (see Fig. 1). We first **meta-train** the model using different tasks (each containing relatively small training sets) to find

---

[1] While writing the final draft of this paper, we noticed a recent approach by Sharma et al. [18]. However, they sample tasks for the problem of multi-task learning. In addition, sampling tasks is not based on the improvement of performance, but tasks where the performance is worse.

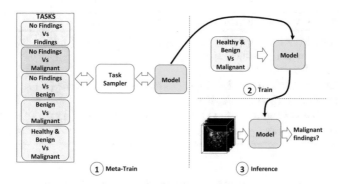

Fig. 1. The model is first meta-trained using several tasks containing relatively small training sets. The meta-trained model is then used to initialize the usual training process for breast screening (i.e., healthy and benign versus malignant). The probability of malignancy is estimated from a forward pass during the inference process.

a good initialization that is then used to **train** the model for the breast screening task (i.e., the healthy and benign versus malignant task). The **inference** is performed using previously unseen test data. Below, we define the dataset and describe each stage.

3.1 Dataset

Let the dataset be represented by $\mathcal{D} = \{(\mathbf{v}_i, \mathbf{t}_i, b_i, d_i, y_i)\}_{i=1}^{|\mathcal{D}|}$ where $\mathbf{v} : \Omega \to \mathbb{R}$ is the first subtraction DCE-MRI volume (Ω denotes the volume lattice), $\mathbf{t} : \Omega \to \mathbb{R}$ is the T1-weighted volume, $b \in \{\text{left}, \text{right}\}$ indicates if this is the left or right breast of the patient, $d_i \in \mathbb{N}$ denotes patient identification, and $y \in \mathcal{Y} = \{0, 1, 2\}$ is the volume label ($y_i = 2$: breast contains a malignant lesion, $y_i = 1$: breast contains at least one benign and no malignant findings, and $y_i = 0$: no findings). We divide $\mathcal{D}$ using the patient identification into the training set $\mathcal{T}$, validation set $\mathcal{V}$ and testing set $\mathcal{S}$, with no overlap between these sets.

For the meta-training phase, we use the meta-training set defined by $\{\mathcal{D}_j\}_{j=1}^{5}$ where each meta-set $\mathcal{D}_j \subseteq \mathcal{T}$ contains the relevant volumes for the classification task K_j, defined as follows: (1) K_1 classifies volumes that contain any findings (benign or malignant); (2) K_2 discriminates between volumes with no findings and malignant findings; (3) K_3 discriminates between volumes with no findings and benign findings; (4) K_4 discriminates volumes with benign findings against malignant findings; and (5) K_5 addresses breast screening, i.e. finding volumes that contain malignant findings.

3.2 Model

We **meta-train** a model across a number of tasks so that it can be quickly trained to new unseen tasks from few images, or fine-tuned to become more effective at one of the tasks used in the meta-training phase. See algorithm 1 for an overview of the methodology.

Algorithm 1 Overview of the meta-training procedure

1: **procedure** META-TRAIN($\{K_1 \ldots K_5\}$, $\{\mathcal{D}_1 \ldots \mathcal{D}_5\}$, model f_θ)
2:     Initialise model parameters θ
3:     **for** $m = 1$ *to* M **do**   ▷ Meta-update Loop
4:         **Create** meta-batch $\mathcal{K}_m$ by sampling $|\mathcal{K}_m|$ tasks from $\{K_1 \ldots K_5\}$
5:         **for** each task $K_j \in \mathcal{K}_m$ **do**
6:             **Adapt** model with (1) using samples from $\mathcal{D}_j$ ▷ Adaptation
7:         **Update** model parameters with (2)   ▷ Meta-update

---

Let f_θ be the model parameterized by θ. For each meta update, the model adapts to the multiple tasks using the meta-batch set $\mathcal{K}_m$. The tasks included in $\mathcal{K}_m$ are sampled according to one of the methods described below in Sect. 3.3. For each task $K_j \in \mathcal{K}_m$, we sample from $\mathcal{D}_j$ a training set $\mathcal{D}_j^{tr}$ and a validation set $\mathcal{D}_j^{val}$ with N^{tr} and N^{val} volumes, respectively. The model parameter θ **adaptation** is performed with the following gradient descent at time step t:

$$\theta_j'^{(t)} = \theta^{(t)} - \alpha \frac{\partial \mathcal{L}_{K_j}\left(f_{\theta^{(t)}}\left(\mathcal{D}_j^{tr}\right)\right)}{\partial \theta}, \tag{1}$$

where α denotes the adaptation learning rate, and $\mathcal{L}_{K_j}\left(f_\theta\left(\mathcal{D}_j^{tr}\right)\right)$ is the cross-entropy loss to train for the classification task K_j. Finally, given the adapted models $f_{\theta_j'^{(t)}}$ for each task $K_j \in \mathcal{K}_m$, the model parameter θ is **meta-updated** from the error on the validation volumes $\mathcal{D}_j^{val}$ of the task w.r.t. the initial parameters $\theta^{(t)}$:

$$\theta^{(t+1)} = \theta^{(t)} - \beta \sum_{K_j \in \mathcal{K}_m} \frac{\partial \mathcal{L}_{K_j}\left(f_{\theta_j'^{(t)}}\left(\mathcal{D}_j^{val}\right)\right)}{\partial \theta}, \tag{2}$$

where β denotes the meta-learning rate. In summary, the **meta-training** phase consists of updating the parameters of the model based on the error in validation images after being *adapted* to a task using few images. This is equivalent to the following optimization:

$$\min_\theta \sum_{K_j \in \mathcal{K}_m} \mathcal{L}_{K_j} f_{\theta_j'^{(t)}}(\mathcal{D}_j^{val}) = \min_\theta \sum_{K_j \in \mathcal{K}_m} \mathcal{L}_{K_j}\left(f_{\theta^{(t)} - \alpha \frac{\partial \mathcal{L}_{K_j}\left(f_{\theta^{(t)}}\left(\mathcal{D}_j^{tr}\right)\right)}{\partial \theta}}(\mathcal{D}_j^{val})\right) \tag{3}$$

The resulting model f_θ obtained after the completion of the meta-training process is then fine-tuned using the cross entropy loss for the breast screening binary classification problem. This process consists of the **training phase**, where we use the training set $\mathcal{T}$ for training and validation set $\mathcal{V}$ for model selection. The final model is tested during the **inference phase** by feeding testing volumes from $\mathcal{S}$ through the network to estimate their probability of malignancy.

3.3   Task Sampling

The sampling process to select $|\mathcal{K}|$ tasks from $\bigcup_{j=1}^{5} K_j$ (step 4 of Algoritjm 1) is currently based on random sampling [4]. However, we consider this to be a crucial step in that algorithm, and therefore propose four sampling methods for step 4 of Algorithm 1. In particular, we study the following sampling methods: (1) **Random:** randomly sample all tasks with replacement [4]; (2) **All-task:** sample all $|\mathcal{K}| = 5$ tasks exactly once; (3) **Teacher-Student Curriculum Learning (CL)** [5]: sample tasks that can achieve a higher improvement on their performance. This is formalized by a partially observable Markov decision process (POMDP) parametrized by the *state*, which is the current parameter vector $\theta^{(t)}$; the next *action* to perform, which is the task K_j to train on; the *observation* O_{K_j}, consisting of the AUC improvement after adapting the parameters from $\theta^{(t)}$ to $\theta'^{(t)}$ for task K_j; and the *reward* R_{K_j}, which is computed from the AUC improvement of the current observation O_{K_j} minus the AUC improvement obtained from the last time the task K_j was sampled. The goal of the sampling algorithm is to maximize the score of all tasks, which is solved based on reinforcement learning using Thompson sampling. More specifically, a buffer $\mathcal{B}_j$ stores the last B rewards for task K_j, and at sampling time, a *recent reward* is randomly chosen from each of the buffers $\mathcal{B}_j$. The next task for the meta-training is the one associated with the buffer that produced the highest absolute valued *recent reward*. This procedure chooses to lean a task until its improvement stabilizes, and then different tasks will be sampled and so on. Note that by sampling according to the absolute value, tasks where the performance is decreasing will tend to be sampled again; and (4) **Multi-armed bandit (MAB)** [16]: sample in the same way as the CL approach above, but the observation O_{K_j} is stored in the buffer instead of the reward R_{K_j}. Also, the next task is selected based on the highest valued *recent observation* (not its absolute value).

4   Experiments and Results

We assess our methodology on a breast DCE-MRI dataset containing 117 patients, divided into a training set with 45 patients, a validation with 13 and a test set with 59 patients [15, 19]. Each sample for each patient in this dataset contains T1-weighted and dynamically-contrast enhanced MRI volumes. Given the current interest in decreasing the number of scans [12, 15], only the first subtraction volume is used. Although all patients contain at least one lesion (benign or malignant, confirmed by biopsy), not all breasts contain lesions. The T1-weighted volume is only used to automatically segment and extract the left and right breasts into volumes of size $100 \times 100 \times 50$ [15] and assign separate labels to them, where the label of a breast can be "no-finding", "malignant" (if it contains at least one malignant lesion), or "benign" (if all lesions are benign). All evaluations below are based on the area under the ROC curve (AUC).

The model f_θ, implemented in 3D, is based on the DenseNet [6], which currently holds the best classification performance in several computer vision applications. The model architecture and hyper-parameters are selected based on the

Table 1. Baseline AUC for classifiers trained on breast screening.

Baseline	AUC
DenseNet [6]	0.83
MIL [7]	0.85
Multi-task [8]	0.85

Table 2. AUC for our proposed models depending on the meta-batch size and task sampling methods and trained for breast screening.

Model	$|\mathcal{K}|$	AUC per sampling method			
		Random	All-task	MAB	CL
BSML	3	0.86	N/A	0.88	**0.90**
BSML	5	0.85	0.89	0.89	**0.90**
BSML-NS	4	0.85	0.88	0.87	0.89

highest AUC for the breast screening problem in the validation set. The architecture is composed of five dense blocks of two dense layers each and is trained with a learning rate of 0.01 and a batch size of 2 volumes. For our proposed methodology (labeled as BSML), the number of meta-updates is $M = 3000$, the meta-learning rate $\beta = 0.001$, the number of training and validation volumes selected for task K_j from the meta-set $\mathcal{D}_j$ is $N^{tr} = N^{val} = 4$, the number of gradient descent updates is 5, and the adaptation learning rate $\alpha = 0.1$. We check the influence of the meta-batch size $|\mathcal{K}| \in \{3, 5\}$. Also, we evaluate the influence of all task sampling approaches listed in Sect. 3.3. Finally, we also run experiments to check the performance of our model when the task of breast screening is not used for meta-training (BSML-NS). This means that the training process has to learn an unseen task starting from the initialization achieved in the meta-training step. In this case, we use $|\mathcal{K}| = 4$ and test the influence of the different task sampling approaches.

Our proposed model is compared against the following baselines: (1) a *DenseNet* trained for the breast screening binary task; (2) the pre-trained DenseNet (1) fine-tuned using a multiple-instance learning framework *(MIL)* [7] – this approach holds the SOTA for the breast screening problem in mammography; and (3) a DenseNet trained with a *multi-task* loss [8] using the 5 tasks defined in Sect 3.1.

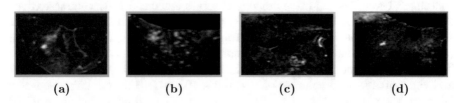

(a)   (b)   (c)   (d)

Fig. 2. Classification examples. Image (2a) shows a correct negative classification of a volume containing a benign lesion, images (2b) and (2c) show a correct positive classification of a volume containing a malignant lesion, and image (2d) shows an false negative classification of a volume containing a small malignant lesion.

Tables 1 and 2 contain the AUC for baselines and experiments detailed above. Figure 2 shows examples of the classification produced by our methodology.

5 Discussion and Conclusion

We presented a methodology to train medical image analysis systems that tries to mimic the process of training a radiologist. This is achieved by meta-training the model with several tasks containing small meta-training sets, followed by a subsequent training to solve the particular problem of interest. We established a new SOTA for the weakly supervised breast screening problem when compared to several baselines such as DenseNet [6], a multi-task trained DenseNet [8] and a DenseNet fine-tunned in a MIL framework [7]. Note that the MIL setup does not achieve a large improvement as reported in the original paper [7]. We believe that this is due to the use of DenseNet, which tends to show better classification results than Alexnet [7]. Also, it is worth mentioning that our proposed method has not shown any false positive classification in the test set.

As reflected in the experiments, the sampling of the tasks to meta-train is an important step of our proposed methodology. In particular, the CL sampling showed more accurate classification than random sampling, which yields similar results to the baselines. The MAB sampling improved over random selection, but it is still not as competitive as curriculum learning. We conjecture that sampling according to the best performance (i.e., MAB) keeps selecting more often the tasks that produce the highest reward, while CL samples tasks with a larger margin for improvement because they can achieve a larger slope in the learning curve. Consequently, CL aims at improving the reward for ALL tasks. Also, the meta-batch size does not appear to have much influence in the results. Furthermore, the BLML-NS results in Table 2 show that our proposed methodology can be successfully trained for breast screening even when this task is not included in the meta-training phase. In particular, notice that the AUC is competitive, being 1 point smaller than our best result (that includes breast screening in meta-training), but between 4 and 6 points better than the baselines.

References

1. The Royal Australian and New Zealand College of Radiologists: Training in Clinical Radiology (2009)
2. Wang, X., Peng, Y., et al.: Chestx-ray8: hospital-scale chest x-ray database and benchmarks on weakly-supervised classification and localization of common thorax diseases. In: CVPR (2017)
3. Bar, Y., Diamant, I., et al.: Deep learning with non-medical training used for chest pathology identification. In: Medical Imaging: Computer-Aided Diagnosis (2015)
4. Finn, C., Abbeel, P., Levine, S.: Model-agnostic meta-learning for fast adaptation of deep networks. In: ICML (2017)
5. Matiisen, T., Oliver, A., Cohen, T., Schulman, J.: Teacher-student curriculum learning. arXiv preprint arXiv:1707.00183 (2017)

6. Huang, G., Liu, Z.: Densely connected convolutional networks. In: CVPR (2017)
7. Zhu, W., Lou, Q., Vang, Y.S., Xie, X.: Deep multi-instance networks with sparse label assignment for whole mammogram classification. In: Descoteaux, M., Maier-Hein, L., Franz, A., Jannin, P., Collins, D.L., Duchesne, S. (eds.) MICCAI 2017. LNCS, vol. 10435, pp. 603–611. Springer, Cham (2017). https://doi.org/10.1007/978-3-319-66179-7_69
8. Xue, W., Brahm, G.: Full left ventricle quantification via deep multitask relationships learning. Med. Image Anal. **43**, 54–65 (2018)
9. Smith, R.A., Andrews, K.S.: Cancer screening in the United States, 2017: a review of current American cancer society guidelines and current issues in cancer screening. CA Cancer J. Clin. **67**, 100–121 (2017)
10. Vreemann, S., Gubern-Merida, A.: The frequency of missed breast cancers in women participating in a high-risk MRI screening program. Breast Cancer Res. Treat. **169**, 323–331 (2018)
11. Gubern-Mérida, A., Martí, R.: Automated localization of breast cancer in DCE-MRI. Med. Image Anal. **20**, 265–274 (2015)
12. Dalmış, M.U., Vreemann, S.: Fully automated detection of breast cancer in screening MRI using convolutional neural networks. J. Med. Imaging **5**, 014502 (2018)
13. Amit, G., et al.: Hybrid mass detection in breast MRI combining unsupervised saliency analysis and deep learning. In: Descoteaux, M., Maier-Hein, L., Franz, A., Jannin, P., Collins, D.L., Duchesne, S. (eds.) MICCAI 2017. LNCS, vol. 10435, pp. 594–602. Springer, Cham (2017). https://doi.org/10.1007/978-3-319-66179-7_68
14. Jäger, P.F., et al.: Revealing hidden potentials of the q-Space signal in breast cancer. In: Descoteaux, M., et al. (eds.) MICCAI 2017. LNCS, vol. 10433, pp. 664–671. Springer, Cham (2017). https://doi.org/10.1007/978-3-319-66182-7_76
15. Maicas, G., Carneiro, G., Bradley, A.P., Nascimento, J.C., Reid, I.: Deep reinforcement learning for active breast lesion detection from DCE-MRI. In: Descoteaux, M., Maier-Hein, L., Franz, A., Jannin, P., Collins, D.L., Duchesne, S. (eds.) MICCAI 2017. LNCS, vol. 10435, pp. 665–673. Springer, Cham (2017). https://doi.org/10.1007/978-3-319-66179-7_76
16. Gutiérrez, B., Peter, L., Klein, T., Wachinger, C.: A multi-armed bandit to smartly select a training set from big medical data. In: Descoteaux, M., Maier-Hein, L., Franz, A., Jannin, P., Collins, D.L., Duchesne, S. (eds.) MICCAI 2017. LNCS, vol. 10435, pp. 38–45. Springer, Cham (2017). https://doi.org/10.1007/978-3-319-66179-7_5
17. Bengio, Y., Louradour, J., et al.: Curriculum learning. In: ICML (2009)
18. Sharma, S., Jha, A.K., Hedge, P., Ravindran, B.: Learning to multi-task by active sampling. In: ICLR (2018)
19. McClymont, D., Mehnert, A., et al.: Fully automatic lesion segmentation in breast MRI using mean-shift and graph-cuts on a region adjacency graph. In: JMRI (2014)

Joint High-Order Multi-Task Feature Learning to Predict the Progression of Alzheimer's Disease

Lodewijk Brand[1], Hua Wang[1(✉)], Heng Huang[2], Shannon Risacher[3],
Andrew Saykin[3], and Li Shen[3,4]
for the ADNI

[1] Department of Computer Science, Colorado School of Mines, Golden, CO, USA
lbrand@mines.edu, huawangcs@gmail.com
[2] Department of Electrical and Computer Engineering,
University of Pittsburgh, Pittsburgh, PA, USA
heng.huang@pitt.edu
[3] Department of Radiology and Imaging Sciences, Department of BioHealth
Informatics, Indiana University, Indianapolis, IN, USA
{srisache,asaykin}@iupui.edu
[4] Department of Biostatistics, Epidemiology and Informatics,
University of Pennsylvania, Philadelphia, PA, USA
Li.Shen@pennmedicine.upenn.edu

Abstract. Alzheimer's disease (AD) is a degenerative brain disease that
affects millions of people around the world. As populations in the United
States and worldwide age, the prevalence of Alzheimer's disease will only
increase. In turn, the social and financial costs of AD will create a difficult environment for many families and caregivers across the globe.
By combining genetic information, brain scans, and clinical data, gathered over time through the Alzheimer's Disease Neuroimaging Initiative
(ADNI), we propose a new *Joint High-Order Multi-Modal Multi-Task
Feature Learning* method to predict the cognitive performance and diagnosis of patients with and without AD.

Keywords: Alzheimer's disease · Multi-modal · Longitudinal · Tensor

1 Introduction

Alzheimer's disease (AD) is a neurodegenerative condition characterized by the
progressive loss of memory and cognitive functions. The *Alzheimer's Association*

H. Wang—To whom all correspondence should be addressed.

ADNI—Data used in preparation of this article were obtained from the Alzheimers
Disease Neuroimaging Initiative (ADNI) database (ad-ni.loni.usc.edu). As such, the
investigators within the ADNI contributed to the design and implementation of
ADNI and/or provided data but did not participate in analysis or writing of this
report. A complete listing of ADNI investigators can be found at: https://adni.loni.
usc.edu/wp-content/uploads/how_to_apply/ADNI_Acknowledgement_List.pdf

© Springer Nature Switzerland AG 2018
A. F. Frangi et al. (Eds.): MICCAI 2018, LNCS 11070, pp. 555–562, 2018.
https://doi.org/10.1007/978-3-030-00928-1_63

recently released a report [1] in which they described various societal costs of AD in the United States. They found that in 2017 the total spending of caring for individuals with AD surpassed \$259 billion. In addition, they report that 1 in 10 people aged 65 or older suffer from some form of Alzheimer's dementia. Given the widespread effects of AD on patients, their families, and caregivers, it is important that the scientific community investigates methods that can accurately predict the progression of AD.

Following the body of work done through the Alzheimer's Disease Neuroimaging Initiative (ADNI), we present a new joint regression and classification model, inspired by our previous works [13,14], that has shown great performance in the identification of relevant genetic and phenotypic biomarkers in patients with AD. Our newly proposed method consists of three major components as follows. First, we use the $\ell_{2,1}$-norm regularization [5] to effectively associate input features over-time and generate a sparse solution. Second, we utilize a new group ℓ_1-norm regularization proposed in our previous works [10–12,14] to globally associate the weights of the input imaging and genetic modalities, where a *modality* indicates a single data grouping (*e.g.* brain imaging data, genetic data, diagnostic data, *etc.*). The group ℓ_1-norm regularization is able to determine which input modality is most effective at predicting a particular output. Third, we incorporate the trace norm regularization [2,4,15,16] to determine relationships that occur within modalities.

2 Joint Multi-modal Regression and Classification for Longitudinal Feature Learning

Joint multi-task learning (*e.g.* performing regression and classification at the same time) can help discover more robust patterns than those discovered when the tasks are performed using separate objectives [13,14]. These robust patterns can arise when the learned parameters for the regression task become outliers for the classification task.

In the ADNI data set, a collection of input modalities (*e.g.* VBM, FreeSurfer, SNP) have been collected from patients in every six months. The input imaging features are represented by a set of matrices $\mathcal{X} = \{X_1, X_2, \ldots, X_T\} \in \mathbb{R}^{D \times n \times T}$. The stacked matrices in $\mathcal{X}$ correspond to measurements recorded at T consecutive time points. Each matrix $X_t \in \mathbb{R}^{D \times n}$ is composed of k input modalities where $X_t = [X_{11}, X_{12}, \ldots, X_{1k}]$. Each input modality X_{tj} consists of d_j features such that $D = \sum_{j=1}^{k} d_j$. $\mathcal{X}$ is a tensor with D imaging features, n samples, and T time points.

In addition to the input modalities, the ADNI also collected cognitive information from each patient. The output of our model, a prediction of cognitive diagnoses and scores, is represented by the tensor $\mathcal{Y} = \{Y_1, Y_2, \ldots, Y_T\} \in \mathbb{R}^{n \times c \times T}$ where at each time point t from $(1 \leq t \leq T)$ a matrix $Y_t = [Y_{tr} \ Y_{tc}]$ represents the horizontal concatenation of the clinical diagnoses (classification tasks) and cognitive scores (regression tasks) of each patient who participated in the ADNI study.

In order to associate the longitudinal imaging markers and the genetic markers to predict cognitive scores and diagnoses over time, we introduce a tensor implementation of the widely used $\ell_{2,1}$-norm:

$$\left\|\mathcal{W}_{(1)}\right\|_{2,1} = \sum_{i=1}^{d} \sqrt{\sum_{t=1}^{T} \left\|\mathbf{w}_t^i\right\|_2^2}, \tag{1}$$

where $\mathbf{w}_t^i$ denotes the i-th row of the coefficient matrix W_t at time t. Here we define $\mathcal{W}_{(n)}$ as the unfolding operation of $\mathcal{W}$ along the n-th mode. Given this definition, it follows that $\mathcal{W}_{(1)} = [W_1 \ W_2 \ \ldots \ W_T] \in \mathbb{R}^{d \times (c \times T)}$. The $\ell_{2,1}$-norm regularization in Eq. (1) will ensure that each feature will either have small, or large values, over the longitudinal dimension.

In heterogeneous feature fusion, the features of a specific input modality can be more discriminative than others for a given task. For example, the features associated with the brain imaging modality may be more useful in determining cognitive scores than the corresponding genetic modality. Conversely, the genetic modality may be more discriminative in predicting a disease diagnosis. To incorporate this global relationship between modalities we use the group ℓ_1-norm (G_1-norm) proposed in our previous works [10,11,14]:

$$\left\|\mathcal{W}_{(1)}\right\|_{G_1} = \sum_{i=1}^{c} \sum_{j=1}^{k} \left\|\mathbf{w}_j^i\right\|_2, \tag{2}$$

where k is the number of input modalities.

The regularizations defined above in Eqs. (1–2) couple the learning tasks over time and learn the relative significance of each input modality for a given task. We know, as AD develops, that many cognitive measures are related to one another. This kind of correlation, when combined with a multivariate regression model and the hinge loss from a support vector machine (SVM) classifier, can be modeled by minimizing the rank of the unfolded coefficient matrix $\mathcal{W}$ in the following objective:

$$\min_{\mathcal{W}} J_2 = \sum_{t=1}^{T} \left\|X_t^T W_{tr} - Y_{tr}\right\|_F^2 + \sum_{t=1}^{T} h(X_t, Y_{tc})$$
$$+ \gamma_1 \left\|\mathcal{W}_{(1)}\right\|_{2,1} + \gamma_2 \left\|\mathcal{W}_{(1)}\right\|_{G_1} + \gamma_3 \left\|\mathcal{W}_{(1)}\right\|_*, \tag{3}$$

where $\|M\|_* = Tr(MM^T)^{1/2}$ denotes the trace norm of the matrix $M \in \mathbb{R}^{n \times m}$, which has been shown as the best convex approximation of the rank-norm [2]. The rank minimization will develop joint correlations across each of the learning tasks at different time points. We call J_2 in Eq. (3) the *Joint High-Order Multi-Modal Multi-Task Feature Learning* model. We will use this newly proposed model to effectively predict the cognitive scores and diagnoses of AD patients.

The algorithm to solve the proposed objective in Eq. (3) is summarized in Algorithm 1. Due to the space limit, the derivation of this algorithm and the rigorous proof of its global convergence will be supplied in an extended journal version of this paper.

Algorithm 1: A new algorithm to minimize J_2 in Equation (3)

Data: $\mathcal{X} = \{X_1, X_2, ..., X_T\} \in \mathbb{R}^{D \times n \times T}$, $\mathcal{Y} = [\mathcal{Y}_r, \mathcal{Y}_c] = \{Y_1, Y_2, ..., Y_T\} \in \mathbb{R}^{n \times c \times T}$.

1. Initialize $\mathcal{W}^{(0)} = [\mathcal{W}_r^{(0)}, \mathcal{W}_c^{(0)}] \in \mathbb{R}^{D \times c \times T}$ where $\mathcal{W}_r^{(0)} \in \mathbb{R}^{D \times c_r \times T}$ is generated using the regression results (Y_{tr}) at each individual time point and $\mathcal{W}_c^{(0)} \in \mathbb{R}^{D \times c_c \times T}$ is derived from T multi-class SVMs fit to Y_{tc}.

while *not converges* **do**

> **2.** Calculate the diagonal matrices D_r and D_c where the k-th diagonal element is computed as $D_j(i,i) = \dfrac{1}{2\sqrt{\sum_{t=1}^{T} \|\mathbf{w}_j^k\|_2^2}}$;
>
> **3.** Calculate the block-diagonal matrices $\bar{D}_r^i (1 \leq i \leq c_r)$ and $\bar{D}_c^i (1 \leq i \leq c_c)$ where the k-th diagonal block of D_j^i is $\dfrac{1}{2\|(\mathbf{w}_j)_i^k\|_2} I_k$;
>
> **4.** Calculate the diagonal matrices $\hat{D}_r$ and $\hat{D}_c$ where $\hat{D}_j = \frac{1}{2}\left(\mathcal{W}_{j(0)}(\mathcal{W}_{j(0)})^T\right)$;
>
> **5.** Update each W_{tr} by $W_{tr} = (X_t X_t^T + \gamma_1 D_r + \gamma_2 \bar{D}_r^i + \gamma_3 \hat{D}_r)^{-1} X_t Y_{tr}$;
>
> **6.** For each $\mathbf{w}_i (1 \leq i \leq c_c)$ in each W_{tc}, calculate $(\mathbf{w}_{t+1})_i = \tilde{D}_c^{-\frac{1}{2}}(\tilde{\mathbf{w}}_t)_i$, where $\tilde{\mathbf{w}}_i = arg\min_{\tilde{\mathbf{w}}_i} f_i(\tilde{\mathbf{w}}_i, b_i; \tilde{X}) + \tilde{\mathbf{w}}_i^T \tilde{\mathbf{w}}_i, \tilde{X} = \tilde{D}_c^{-\frac{1}{2}} X$ and $\tilde{D}_c = \gamma_1 D_c + \gamma_2 \bar{D}_c^i + \gamma_3 \hat{D}_c$;
>
> **7.** Update each W_t by $W_t = [W_r, W_c]$;
>
> **8.** $t = t + 1$.

Result: $\mathcal{W} = \{W_1, W_2, ..., W_T\} \in \mathbb{R}^{D \times c \times T}$.

---

3   Experiments

In this section, we will evaluate the proposed method on the data set provided by the ADNI. The goal of our experiments is to determine the relationships between the brain imaging data (FreeSurfer and VBM), genotypes encoded by SNPs, and the corresponding cognitive scores and AD diagnoses.

We downloaded 1.5 T MRI scans, SNP genotypes, and demographic information for 821 ADNI-1 participants. We performed voxel-based morphometry (VBM) and FreeSurfer automated parcellation on the MRI data by following [6], and extracted mean modulated gray matter (GM) measures for 90 target regions of interest (ROIs). We followed the SNP quality control steps discussed in [8]. We also downloaded the longitudinal scores of the participants' Rey Auditory Verbal Learning Test (RAVLT) and their clinical diagnoses in three categories: healthy control (HC), mild cognitive impairment (MCI), and AD. The details of these cognitive assessments can be found in the ADNI procedure manuals. The time points examined in this study for both imaging markers and cognitive assessments included baseline (BL), Month 6 (M6), Month 12 (M12) and Month 24 (M24). All the participants with no missing BL/M6/M12/M24 MRI measurements, SNP genotypes, and cognitive measures were included in this study; this resulted in a set of 412 subjects with 155 HC, 110 MCI, and 147 AD.

3.1 Joint Regression and Classification Performance

In order to evaluate the effectiveness of our new *Joint High-Order Multi-Modal Multi-Task Feature Learning* method, we tested its regression and classification performance against an array of popular machine learning models. In each experiment, we fine tune the parameters of our model (γ_1, γ_2 and γ_3) by searching a grid of powers of 10 between 10^{-5} to 10^5. The experiments are performed using a classical 5-fold cross-validation strategy for each of the chosen algorithms.

Table 1. Regression: Root mean squared error (RMSE) results of the proposed algorithm compared to linear regression, ridge regression, Lasso regression, K-nearest neighbors (KNN), and a multi-layer perceptron (MLP) classifier. **Classification:** F_1 scores of classifying HC, MCI, and AD patients of the proposed algorithm compared to logistic regression, random forest, support vector machine (SVM) (with *RBF* kernel), K-nearest-neighbors (KNN), and a multi-layer perceptron (MLP) regressor.

Regression Performance (RAVLT)			
	Linear	**Ridge**	**Lasso**
RMSE	1.41e+13±1.19e+12	0.333±0.016	0.333±0.016
	KNN	**MLP**	**Ours**
RMSE	0.344±0.009	0.318±0.026	**0.284±0.011**

Classification Performance (Diagnosis)			
	Logistic	**RandomForest**	**SVM**
F_1 *(HC)*	0.472±0.054	0.434±0.048	0.310±0.073
F_1 *(MCI)*	0.420±0.065	0.448±0.045	0.460±0.071
F_1 *(AD)*	0.456±0.044	0.494±0.098	0.450±0.088
	KNN	**MLP**	**Ours**
F_1 *(HC)*	0.340±0.069	0.424±0.089	**0.560±0.034**
F_1 *(MCI)*	0.396±0.054	0.386±0.092	**0.508±0.039**
F_1 *(AD)*	0.354±0.093	0.444±0.039	**0.644±0.120**

Results. In Table 1 we can see that our proposed algorithm performs significantly better than a collection of "out-of-the-box" machine learning methods. The significant performance improvements in both regression and classification are due to the fact that our algorithm is the only one capable of incorporating the important longitudinal information into its prediction. The various regularizations ($\ell_{2,1}$-, group ℓ_1- and trace norms) that we apply to the unfolded matrix $\mathcal{W}$ ensure that our proposed algorithm is able to incorporate the longitudinal patterns that are intrinsic to many clinical studies (including the ADNI).

3.2 Identification of Longitudinal Imaging Biomarkers

FreeSurfer. The coefficients associated with the FreeSurfer modality in $\mathcal{X}$ are extracted from $\mathcal{W}$ at each time point (BL, M6, M12, M24). Each corresponding coefficient is mapped onto Automated Anatomical Labeling (AAL) [9] regions of the brain (Fig. 1). When we look at the FreeSurfer brain heatmap we can draw a few interesting conclusions. First, the images show the same sparse image representation over time. This observation shows us that that the $\ell_{2,1}$-norm is working as expected and is successfully associating features across time, which illustrates the longitudinal predictive potential (a clinically important distinction) of our method. Second, we see that multiple parts of the brain related to the frontal gyrus have high weights compared to other parts of the brain not connected to AD, which is nicely consistent with existing clinical findings [3].

Voxel-Based Morphometry. The coefficients associated with the VBM modality in $\mathcal{X}$ are extracted from the coefficient matrix $\mathcal{W}$ at each time point. Each coefficient weight is mapped onto AAL regions of the brain (Fig. 2). The images associated with the VBM modality share the same longitudinal sparsity that we observed in the FreeSurfer coefficient matrix. Although, in this case, a completely different set of brain imaging features was discovered: features associated with the hippocampus. Here we see the remarkable effect of the G_1-norm regularization combined with the trace norm. Hippocampus atrophy has been shown to be highly predictive of AD.

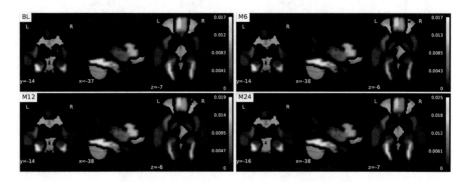

Fig. 1. Visualization of the FreeSurfer modality coefficients derived from $\mathcal{W}$ at various times (BL/M6/M12/M24). The top ten AAL regions are as follows (largest to smallest): *Fusiform_L, Fusiform_R, Frontal_Med_Orb_L, Frontal_Inf_Tri_L, Frontal_Med_Orb_R, Frontal_Inf_Tri_R, ParaHippocampal_L, Insula_L, Pallidum_R,* and *Pallidum_L.*

Single Nucleotide Polymorphism. The coefficients associated with the SNP modality in $\mathcal{X}$ are extracted from the coefficient matrix $\mathcal{W}$. Similar to two previous modalities, there was little difference between the coefficient matrices at each time point. The only orange bar in Fig. 3 is the coefficient that is associated with the *rs429358* SNP: the apolipoprotein E (ApoE) gene. *Schuff et al.* [7] and many others have discovered that the ApoE gene is related to increased rates of hippocampus atrophy. It is surprising that no other SNPs show up given that SNPs on the same gene are frequently associated with one another. One reason for this could be that the tuning coefficient on the $\ell_{2,1}$-norm is too large.

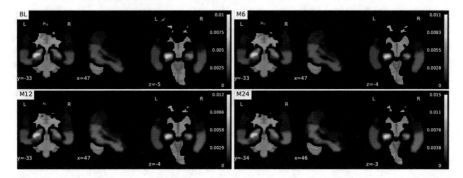

Fig. 2. Visualization of the voxel-based morphometry modality coefficients derived from $\mathcal{W}$ at various times (BL/M6/M12/M24). The top ten AAL regions are as follows (largest to smallest): *Hippocampus_L, Amygdala_L, Hippocampus_R Temporal_Inf_R Temporal_Mid_R, Temporal_Inf_L, ParaHippocampal_L, Amygdala_R, Temporal_Mid_L, ParaHippocampal_R, Angular_R,* and *Temporal_Pole_Sup_L.*

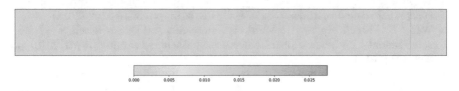

Fig. 3. Heatmap visualization of the SNPs along the x-axis against the corresponding coefficients derived from $\mathcal{W}$. The single orange line on the right-hand side is the weight associated with *rs429358*.

4   Conclusion

Learning effective mappings between different input and output modalities is an important research task in AD research. In the proposed *Joint High-Order Multi-Modal Multi-Task Feature Learning* model, we use various regularizations to learn the relationships between modalities over time. Our proposed method shows superior performance compared to traditional machine learning models.

Acknowledgement. This research was partially supported by NSF-IIS 1423591 and NSF-IIS 1652943; NSF-IIS 1302675, NSF-IIS 1344152, NSF-DBI 1356628, NSF-IIS 1619308, NSF-IIS 1633753, and NIH R01 AG049371; NIH R01 EB022574, NIH R01 LM011360, NIH R01 AG19771, NIH U19 AG024904, and NIH P30 AG10133.

References

1. Alzheimer, Association, Sciencestaff, Alzorg: 2017 Alzheimer's disease facts and figures (2017). https://doi.org/10.1016/j.jalz.2017.02.001
2. Candès, E.J., Recht, B.: Exact matrix completion via convex optimization. Found. Comput. Math. **9**(6), 717 (2009). https://doi.org/10.1007/s10208-009-9045-5

3. Galton, C.J., et al.: Differing patterns of temporal atrophy in Alzheimer's disease and semantic dementia. Neurology **57**(2), 216–225 (2001)
4. Lu, L., Wang, H., Yao, X., Risacher, S., Saykin, A., Shen, L.: Predicting progressions of cognitive outcomes via high-order multi-modal multi-task feature learning. In: IEEE ISBI 2018, pp. 545–548 (2018)
5. Nie, F., Huang, H., Cai, X., Ding, C.H.: Efficient and robust feature selection via joint $\ell_{2,1}$-norms minimization. In: NIPS 2010, pp. 1813–1821 (2010)
6. Risacher, S.L., et al.: Longitudinal MRI atrophy biomarkers: relationship to conversion in the ADNI cohort. Neurobiol. Aging **31**(8), 1401–1418 (2010)
7. Schuff, N., et al.: MRI of hippocampal volume loss in early Alzheimers disease in relation to ApoE genotype and biomarkers. Brain **132**(4), 1067–1077 (2009)
8. Shen, L.: Whole genome association study of brain-wide imaging phenotypes for identifying quantitative trait loci in MCI and AD: a study of the ADNI cohort. NeuroImage **53**(3), 1051–1063 (2010). imaging Genetics
9. Tzourio-Mazoyer, N., et al.: Automated anatomical labeling of activations in SPM using a macroscopic anatomical parcellation of the MNI MRI single-subject brain. NeuroImage **15**(1), 273–289 (2002)
10. Wang, H., Nie, F., Huang, H., Ding, C.: Heterogeneous visual features fusion via sparse multimodal machine. In: IEEE CVPR 2013, pp. 3097–3102 (2013)
11. Wang, H., Nie, F., Huang, H.: Multi-view clustering and feature learning via structured sparsity. In: International Conference on Machine Learning (ICML 2013), pp. 352–360 (2013)
12. Wang, H.: Identifying quantitative trait loci via group-sparse multitask regression and feature selection: an imaging genetics study of the ADNI cohort. Bioinformatics **28**(2), 229–237 (2011)
13. Wang, H., et al.: Identifying AD-sensitive and cognition-relevant imaging biomarkers via joint classification and regression. In: Fichtinger, G., Martel, A., Peters, T. (eds.) MICCAI 2011. LNCS, vol. 6893, pp. 115–123. Springer, Heidelberg (2011). https://doi.org/10.1007/978-3-642-23626-6_15
14. Wang, H., et al.: Identifying disease sensitive and quantitative trait-relevant biomarkers from multidimensional heterogeneous imaging genetics data via sparse multimodal multitask learning. Bioinformatics **28**(12), i127–i136 (2012)
15. Wang, H., et al.: From phenotype to genotype: an association study of longitudinal phenotypic markers to alzheimer's disease relevant SNPs. Bioinformatics **28**(18), i619–i625 (2012)
16. Wang, H., et al.: High-order multi-task feature learning to identify longitudinal phenotypic markers for alzheimer's disease progression prediction. In: NIPS 2012, pp. 1277–1285 (2012)

Fast Multiple Landmark Localisation Using a Patch-Based Iterative Network

Yuanwei Li[1]($\boxtimes$), Amir Alansary[1], Juan J. Cerrolaza[1], Bishesh Khanal[2],
Matthew Sinclair[1], Jacqueline Matthew[2], Chandni Gupta[2], Caroline Knight[2],
Bernhard Kainz[1], and Daniel Rueckert[1]

[1] Biomedical Image Analysis Group, Imperial College London, London, UK
yuanwei.li09@imperial.ac.uk
[2] School of Biomedical Engineering and Imaging Sciences,
King's College London, London, UK

Abstract. We propose a new Patch-based Iterative Network (PIN) for fast and accurate landmark localisation in 3D medical volumes. PIN utilises a Convolutional Neural Network (CNN) to learn the spatial relationship between an image patch and anatomical landmark positions. During inference, patches are repeatedly passed to the CNN until the estimated landmark position converges to the true landmark location. PIN is computationally efficient since the inference stage only selectively samples a small number of patches in an iterative fashion rather than a dense sampling at every location in the volume. Our approach adopts a multi-task learning framework that combines regression and classification to improve localisation accuracy. We extend PIN to localise multiple landmarks by using principal component analysis, which models the global anatomical relationships between landmarks. We have evaluated PIN using 72 3D ultrasound images from fetal screening examinations. PIN achieves quantitatively an average landmark localisation error of 5.59 mm and a runtime of 0.44 s to predict 10 landmarks per volume. Qualitatively, anatomical 2D standard scan planes derived from the predicted landmark locations are visually similar to the clinical ground truth.

1 Introduction

Anatomical landmark localisation is a key challenge for many medical image analysis tasks. Accurate landmark identification can be used for (a) extracting biometric measurements of anatomical structures, (b) landmark-based registration of 3D volumes, (c) extracting 2D clinical standard planes from 3D volumes and (d) initialisation of tasks such as image segmentation. However, manual landmark detection is time-consuming and suffers from high observer variability. Thus, there is a need to develop automatic methods for fast and accurate

Electronic supplementary material The online version of this chapter (https:// doi.org/10.1007/978-3-030-00928-1_64) contains supplementary material, which is available to authorized users.

A. F. Frangi et al. (Eds.): MICCAI 2018, LNCS 11070, pp. 563–571, 2018.
https://doi.org/10.1007/978-3-030-00928-1_64

landmark localisation. Recently, deep learning approaches have been proposed for this purpose [1,3,5–8] but there remain major challenges: (a) typically only a limited amount of annotated medical images is available, (b) model training and inference for 3D medical images is computationally intensive, making real-time applications challenging and (c) when multiple landmarks are detected jointly, their spatial relationships should be taken into account.

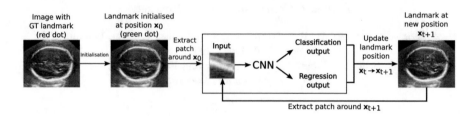

Fig. 1. Overall framework of PIN for single landmark localisation.

Related Work: Deep learning methods for landmark localisation can be divided into two categories: The first category adopts an end-to-end learning strategy where the entire image is taken as input to a convolutional neural network (CNN) while the output is a map from which the landmark coordinates can be inferred directly. Payer *et al.* [5] and Laina *et al.* [3] output a heatmap in which Gaussians are located at the landmark positions. Xu *et al.* [6] train a supervised action classifier (SAC) that outputs an action map whose classification labels denote the direction towards the true landmark location. However, end-to-end learning methods are typically applied to 2D images since 3D volumetric networks require large receptive fields for landmark tasks. Such 3D networks are computationally intensive, which inhibits real-time performance, and require a large amount of memory during training, which is beyond current hardware's capabilities.

The second category uses image patches as training samples to learn a classification or regression model. Zheng *et al.* [8] extract a patch around each voxel in the image and use a neural network to classify if a landmark is present at the patch centre. Zhang *et al.* [7] and Aubert *et al.* [1] use a CNN-based regression model that learns the association between an image patch and its 3D displacement to the true landmark. Ghesu *et al.* [2] propose a deep reinforcement learning (DRL) approach that also operates on patches. Most patch-based methods require dense sampling of many image patches during prediction which is computationally intensive. Furthermore, most methods require the training of separate models to detect each landmark. This is time-consuming and neglects the spatial relationships among multiple landmarks.

Contribution: In this paper, we propose a novel landmark localisation approach that uses a patch-based CNN to predict multiple landmarks efficiently in an iterative manner. We term this approach Patch-based Iterative Network (PIN). PIN has distinct advantages that address the key challenges of landmark localisation in 3D medical images: **(1)** During inference, PIN guides the patch towards the true landmark location using iterative sparse sampling. This approach reduces the computational cost by avoiding dense sampling at every voxel of the volume. **(2)** PIN uses a 2.5D representation to approximate the 3D patch as network input. This accelerates computation as only 2D convolutions are required. **(3)** PIN treats landmark localisation as a combined regression and classification problem for which a joint network is learned via multi-task learning. This prevents model overfitting, improves generalisation ability of the learned features and increases localisation accuracy. **(4)** PIN detects multiple landmarks jointly using a single model and takes the global anatomical spatial relationships among landmarks into account. We evaluate the landmark localisation accuracy of PIN using 3D ultrasound images of the fetal brain. In addition, clinically useful scan planes can be extracted from the predicted landmarks which visually resemble the anatomical standard planes as defined by fetal screening standards, *e.g.,* [4].

2   Method

Overall Framework: Figure 1 illustrates the overall PIN framework for single landmark localisation. We show the 2D case for clarity but the method works similarly in 3D. Given an image, the goal is to predict the true landmark coordinates (red dot in Fig. 1). A position x_0 is first initialised at instant $t = 0$ and a patch centred around x_0 is extracted (solid green box in Fig. 1). The CNN takes the patch as input and predicts regression and classification outputs that are used to compute a new position x_{t+1} from the previous position x_t, bringing the patch closer to the true landmark location. The patch at x_{t+1} (dashed green box in Fig. 1) is then given as input to the CNN and the process is repeated until the patch reaches the true landmark position.

Network Input: For 3D data, the CNN input can be a 3D volume patch. However, 3D convolution operations on volume patches are computationally expensive. To this end, we use a 2.5D representation to approximate the full 3D patch. Specifically, given a particular position $x = (x, y, z)^T$ in a volume V, we extract three 2D image patches centred around x at the three orthogonal planes (Fig. 2a). The patch extraction function is denoted as $I(V, x, s)$ where s is the length of the square patch. The three 2D patches are then concatenated together as a 3-channel 2D patch which is passed as input to the CNN. Such a representation is computationally efficient since it requires only 2D convolutions and still provides a good approximation of the full 3D volume patch.

Joint Regression and Classification: PIN jointly predicts the magnitude and direction of movement of a current point towards the true landmark by combining a regression and a classification task together in a multi-task learning framework. This joint framework shares model parameters in the convolutional layers and is experimentally shown to learn more generalisable features, which improves overall performance.

The regression task estimates how much the point at the current position should move to get to the true landmark location. The regression output $d =$

$(d_1, d_2, \ldots, d_{n_o})^T$ is a displacement vector that predicts the relative distance between the current and true landmark positions. In single landmark localisation, d has $n_o = 3$ elements which give the displacement along each coordinate axis.

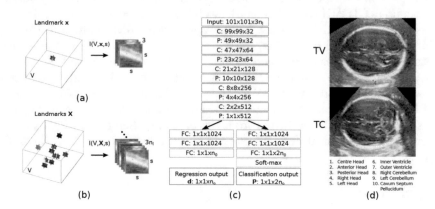

Fig. 2. (a) Patch extraction of a single landmark. (b) Patch extraction of multiple landmarks. (c) CNN architecture combining regression and classification. Output size of each layer is represented as width × height × (# feature maps). (d) Landmarks defined on the TV and TC plane for fetal sonographic examination.

The classification task estimates the direction of current point movement towards the true landmark by dividing direction into 6 discrete classification categories: positive and negative direction along each coordinate axes [6]. Denoting c as the classification label, we have $c \in \{c_1^+, c_1^-, c_2^+, c_2^-, c_3^+, c_3^-\}$. For instance, c_1^+ is the category representing movement along the direction of positive x-axis. The classification output $\boldsymbol{P}$ is then a vector with $2n_o = 6$ elements, each representing the probability/confidence of movement in that direction. Mathematically, $\boldsymbol{P} = (P_{c_1^+}, P_{c_1^-}, \ldots, P_{c_{n_o}^+}, P_{c_{n_o}^-})^T$ where $P_{c_1^+} = \text{Prob}(c = c_1^+)$.

Given a volume V and its ground truth landmark point $\boldsymbol{x}^{GT}$, a training sample is represented by $(I(V, \boldsymbol{x}, s), \boldsymbol{d}^{GT}, \boldsymbol{P}^{GT})$ where $\boldsymbol{x}$ is a point randomly sampled from V and $I(V, \boldsymbol{x}, s)$ is its associated patch. The ground truth displacement vector is given by $\boldsymbol{d}^{GT} = \boldsymbol{x}^{GT} - \boldsymbol{x}$. To obtain $\boldsymbol{P}^{GT}$, we first determine the ground truth classification label c^{GT} by selecting the component of $\boldsymbol{d}^{GT}$ with the maximum absolute value and taking into account its sign,

$$c^{GT} = \begin{cases} c_i^+, & \text{if } d_i^{GT} > 0 \\ c_i^-, & \text{otherwise.} \end{cases} \tag{1}$$

where $i = \text{argmax}(\text{abs}(\boldsymbol{d}^{GT}))$. For a vector $\boldsymbol{a}$, $\text{argmax}(\boldsymbol{a})$ returns the index of the vector component with maximum value. During training, a hard classification label is used. As such, the probability vector $\boldsymbol{P}^{GT}$ is obtained as a one-hot vector where component $P_{c^{GT}}$ is set to 1 and all others set to 0. The CNN is trained by minimising the following combined loss function:

$$L = (1 - \alpha)\frac{1}{n_0 n_{batch}} \sum_{n=1}^{n_{batch}} \left\| \boldsymbol{d}_n^{GT} - \boldsymbol{d}_n \right\|_2^2 - \alpha\frac{1}{n_{batch}} \sum_{n=1}^{n_{batch}} \log\left(P_{c^{GT},n}\right) \qquad (2)$$

The first term is the Euclidean loss of the regression task and the second term is the cross-entropy loss of the classification task. α is the weighting between the two losses. n_{batch} is the number of training samples in a mini-batch. $\boldsymbol{d}_n$ and $P_{c^{GT},n}$ denote respectively the regression and classification outputs predicted by the CNN on the nth sample.

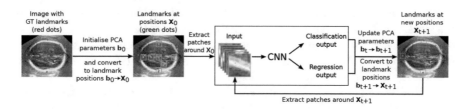

Fig. 3. Overall framework of PIN for multiple landmarks localisation.

CNN Architecture: Figure 2c shows the PIN CNN architecture combining the classification and regression tasks. The network comprises five convolution (C) layers, each followed by a max-pooling (P) layer. These layers are shared by both tasks. After the 5th pooling layer, each task has three separate fully-connected (FC) layers to learn the task-specific features. All convolution layers use 3x3 kernels with stride $=1$ and all pooling layers use 2x2 kernels with stride $=2$. ReLU activation is applied after all convolution and FC layers except for the last FC layer of each task. Drop-out is added after each FC layer.

PIN Inference: Given an unseen 3D volume, we initialise 19 points in the volume (one at the volume centre and 18 others at fixed distance of one-quarter image size around it). The patch extracted from each point is forward passed into the CNN and the point is moved to its new position based on the CNN outputs ($\boldsymbol{d}$ and $\boldsymbol{P}$) and a chosen update rule. This process is repeated for T iterations until there is no significant change in the displacement of the point. The final positions of the 19 points at iteration T is averaged and taken to be the final landmark prediction. Multiple initialisations average out errors and improve the overall localisation accuracy.

PIN Update Rules: We proposed three update rules (A–C). Let $\boldsymbol{x}_t$ be the position of a point at iteration t and $\boldsymbol{x}_{t+1}$ be the new updated position. Rule A is based only on the classification output $\boldsymbol{P}$. It updates the current landmark position by moving it one pixel in the direction category which has the highest probability as predicted by $\boldsymbol{P}$. Rule B is based only on the regression output $\boldsymbol{d}$ and is given by: $\boldsymbol{x}_{t+1} = \boldsymbol{x}_t + \boldsymbol{d}$. Rule C uses both the classification and regression outputs for the update and is given by:

$x_{t+1} = x_t + P_{max} \odot d$ where $\odot$ is the element-wise multiplication operator and $P_{max} = (\max(P_{c_1^+}, P_{c_1^-}), \max(P_{c_2^+}, P_{c_2^-}), \ldots, \max(P_{c_{n_o}^+}, P_{c_{n_o}^-}))^T$. Intuitively, Rule C moves the point to its new position by an amount specified by the regression output weighted by a confidence probability specified by the classification output. This ensures smaller movement in the less confident direction and vice versa.

Multiple Landmarks Localisation: The above approach for single landmark localisation has two drawbacks: **(1)** Separate CNN models are required for each landmark which increase the parametrisation significantly and thus computational cost for training and inference. **(2)** Individual landmark prediction ignores the anatomical relationships between the different landmarks. To overcome these problems, we extend our approach to localise multiple landmarks simultaneously using only one CNN model which also accounts for inter-landmark relationships by working in a reduced dimensional space.

Let $X = (x_1, y_1, z_1, \ldots, x_{n_l}, y_{n_l}, z_{n_l})^T$ be the 3D coordinates of all n_l landmarks of one volume. Given a training set of X, we use PCA to transform X into a lower dimensional space. The transformations between the original and reduced dimensional spaces are given by,

$$X = \bar{X} + Wb \tag{3}$$

$$b = W^T(X - \bar{X}), \tag{4}$$

where $\bar{X}$ is the mean of the training set, b is a n_b-element vector where $n_b < 3n_l$ and the columns of matrix W are the n_b eigenvectors. In our case, $n_l = 10$ and we set $n_b = 15$ to explain 99.5% of the total variations in the training set.

We can directly apply our PIN approach to the reduced dimensional space by replacing all occurrences of x by b. Figure 3 illustrates the PIN approach for multiple landmarks. Specifically, 3 orthogonal patches are extracted for every landmark and concatenated together so that a $s \times s \times 3n_l$ block is passed as CNN input (Fig. 2b). d becomes the displacement vector in the reduced dimensional space with $n_o = n_b$ elements. The number of classification categories becomes $2n_b$ which include positive and negative directions along each dimension of the reduced space. Hence, P is a $2n_b$-element vector. Training can be carried out similar to Eq. 2 with the only difference being $d^{GT} = b^{GT} - b$ where b^{GT} is transformed from x^{GT} using Eq. 4 and b is randomly sampled. During inference, we update b iteratively using $b_{t+1} = b_t + P_{max} \odot d$ (Rule C) and use Eq. 3 to convert b_{t+1} back to X_{t+1} for patch extraction in the next iteration. We use multiple initialisations of b_0 (one initialisation with $b_0 = 0$ and five random initialisations) and take their mean results as the final landmarks prediction.

3   Experiments and Results

Data: PIN is evaluated on 3D ultrasound volumes of the fetal head from 72 subjects. Each volume is annotated by a clinical expert with 10 anatomical landmarks that lie on two standard planes (transventricular (TV) and transcerebellar

(TC)) commonly used for fetal sonographic examination as defined in the UK FASP handbook [4] (Fig. 2d). 70% of the dataset is randomly selected for training and the remaining 30% is used for testing. All volumes are processed to be isotropic and resized to $324 \times 207 \times 279$ voxels with voxel size $0.5 \times 0.5 \times 0.5 \, \mathrm{mm}^3$.

Experiment Setup: PIN is implemented using Tensorflow running on a machine with Intel Xeon CPU E5-1630 at 3.70 GHz and one NVIDIA Titan Xp 12 GB GPU. Patch size s is set to 101. During training, we set $n_{batch} = 64$. Weights are initialised randomly from a distribution with zero mean and 0.1 standard deviation. Optimisation is carried out for 100,000 iterations using the Adam algorithm with learning rate $= 0.001$, $\beta_1 = 0.9$ and $\beta_2 = 0.999$. We choose $\alpha = 0.5$ empirically unless otherwise stated. During inference, $T = 350$ for Rule A and $T = 10$ for Rule B and C.

Results: Table 1 compares the landmark localisation errors of a single landmark, cavum septum pellucidum (CSP), using several PIN variants which differ in the CNN model training and the inference update rule. Given the same inference rules, the model trained using both classification and regression losses ($\alpha = 0.5$) achieves lower error than the models trained using either loss alone ($\alpha = 1$ or 0) (PIN1 vs PIN3, PIN2 vs PIN4). This illustrates the benefits of multi-task learning. Using the model trained with joint losses, we then compare the effect of different inference rules. PIN3 uses only the classification output which can result in landmarks getting stuck and oscillating between two opposing classification categories during iterative testing (*e.g.*, c_1^+ and c_1^-). PIN3 also takes longer during inference since the patch moves by one pixel at each test iteration and requires more iterations to converge. PIN4 uses only the regression output, which improves the localisation accuracy and runtime as the patch 'jumps' towards the true landmark position at each iteration. This requires much fewer iterations to converge. PIN5 achieves the best localisation accuracy by combining the classification and regression outputs where the regression output gives the magnitude of movement weighted by the classification output giving the probability of movement in each direction. Our proposed PIN approach also outperforms a recent state-of-the-art landmark localisation approach using DRL [2].

Table 2 shows the localisation errors for all ten landmarks. PIN-Single trains a separate model for each landmark while PIN-Multiple trains one joint model that predicts all the landmarks simultaneously. Since PIN-Multiple accounts for

Table 1. Localisation error (mm) and runtime (s) of different approaches for single landmark (CSP) localisation. C and R denote classification and regression training loss respectively. Results presented as (Mean ± Standard Deviation).

	PIN1	PIN2	PIN3	PIN4	PIN5	DRL [2]
Training loss	C	R	C+R	C+R	C+R	-
Inference rule	Rule A	Rule B	Rule A	Rule B	Rule C	-
Localisation error	7.53 ± 6.48	6.45 ± 3.96	6.34 ± 3.62	6.08 ± 3.90	$\mathbf{5.47 \pm 4.23}$	7.37 ± 5.86
Running time (s)	3.56	0.09	3.50	0.09	**0.09**	6.58

Table 2. Localisation error (mm) of PIN for single and multiple landmark localisation. Results presented as (Mean ± Standard Deviation).

Landmarks	1	2	3	4	5	6
PIN-Single	5.62 ± 2.85	11.30 ± 7.24	8.13 ± 3.90	7.23 ± 3.73	7.11 ± 4.73	4.39 ± 2.07
PIN-Multiple	4.34 ± 2.21	8.80 ± 4.27	6.28 ± 2.77	6.31 ± 3.32	5.56 ± 2.71	4.68 ± 2.27
	7	8	9	10	Overall	
	5.45 ± 2.73	4.04 ± 2.22	5.50 ± 3.64	5.47 ± 4.23	6.42 ± 4.49	
	5.15 ± 2.90	4.70 ± 2.33	4.57 ± 1.92	5.50 ± 2.79	**5.59 ± 3.09**	

Patient 1 TV   Patient 1 TC   Patient 2 TV   Patient 2 TC   Patient 3 TV   Patient 3 TC

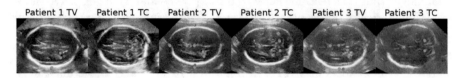

Fig. 4. Visualisation of landmarks predicted by PIN-Multiple (green dots) vs. ground truth landmarks (red dots).

anatomical relationships among the landmarks, it has a lower overall localisation error than PIN-Single. PIN-Single needs a total of 0.94 s to predict all ten landmarks in sequence while PIN-Multiple needs 0.44 s to predict all ten landmarks simultaneously. Figure 4 shows the TV and TC planes containing the ground truth landmarks as red dots. The landmarks predicted by PIN-Multiple are projected onto these standard planes as green dots. The supplementary materials provide visual comparison of standard planes obtained from ground truth and predicted landmarks as well as videos showing several initialisations converging towards the true landmark positions (and standard planes) after ten inference updates.

4 Conclusion

We have presented PIN, a new approach for anatomical landmark localisation. Its patch-based and iterative nature enables training on limited data and fast prediction on large 3D volumes. A joint regression and classification model is trained by multi-task learning to improve localisation accuracy. PIN is capable of multiple landmark localisation and uses PCA to impose anatomical constraints among landmarks. PIN is generic to landmark localisation and as future work, we are extending PIN to other medical applications. It is also worthwhile to replace PCA with an autoencoder to model non-linear correlations among landmarks.

Acknowledgments. Supported by the Wellcome Trust IEH Award [102431]. The authors thank Nvidia Corporation for the donation of a Titan Xp GPU.

References

1. Aubert, B., Vazquez, C., Cresson, T., Parent, S., Guise, J.D.: Automatic spine and pelvis detection in frontal X-rays using deep neural networks for patch displacement learning. In: ISBI 2016, pp. 1426–1429 (2016)
2. Ghesu, F.C., Georgescu, B., Mansi, T., Neumann, D., Hornegger, J., Comaniciu, D.: An artificial agent for anatomical landmark detection in medical images. In: Ourselin, S., Joskowicz, L., Sabuncu, M.R., Unal, G., Wells, W. (eds.) MICCAI 2016. LNCS, vol. 9902, pp. 229–237. Springer, Cham (2016). https://doi.org/10.1007/978-3-319-46726-9_27
3. Laina, I., et al.: Concurrent segmentation and localization for tracking of surgical instruments. In: Descoteaux, M., Maier-Hein, L., Franz, A., Jannin, P., Collins, D.L., Duchesne, S. (eds.) MICCAI 2017. LNCS, vol. 10434, pp. 664–672. Springer, Cham (2017). https://doi.org/10.1007/978-3-319-66185-8_75
4. NHS: Fetal anomaly screening programme: programme handbook June 2015. Public Health England (2015)
5. Payer, C., Štern, D., Bischof, H., Urschler, M.: Regressing heatmaps for multiple landmark localization using CNNs. In: Ourselin, S., Joskowicz, L., Sabuncu, M.R., Unal, G., Wells, W. (eds.) MICCAI 2016. LNCS, vol. 9901, pp. 230–238. Springer, Cham (2016). https://doi.org/10.1007/978-3-319-46723-8_27
6. Xu, Z., et al.: Supervised action classifier: approaching landmark detection as image partitioning. In: Descoteaux, M., Maier-Hein, L., Franz, A., Jannin, P., Collins, D.L., Duchesne, S. (eds.) MICCAI 2017. LNCS, vol. 10435, pp. 338–346. Springer, Cham (2017). https://doi.org/10.1007/978-3-319-66179-7_39
7. Zhang, J., Liu, M., Shen, D.: Detecting anatomical landmarks from limited medical imaging data using two-stage task-oriented deep neural networks. IEEE Trans. Image Process. **26**(10), 4753–4764 (2017)
8. Zheng, Y., Liu, D., Georgescu, B., Nguyen, H., Comaniciu, D.: 3D deep learning for efficient and robust landmark detection in volumetric data. In: Navab, N., Hornegger, J., Wells, W.M., Frangi, A.F. (eds.) MICCAI 2015. LNCS, vol. 9349, pp. 565–572. Springer, Cham (2015). https://doi.org/10.1007/978-3-319-24553-9_69

Omni-Supervised Learning: Scaling Up to Large Unlabelled Medical Datasets

Ruobing Huang[(✉)], J. Alison Noble, and Ana I. L. Namburete

Institute of Biomedical Engineering, Department of Engineering Science,
University of Oxford, Oxford, UK
ruobing.huang@eng.ox.ac.uk

Abstract. Two major bottlenecks in increasing algorithmic performance in the field of medical imaging analysis are the typically limited size of datasets and the shortage of expert labels for large datasets. This paper investigates approaches to overcome the latter via *omni-supervised learning*: a special case of semi-supervised learning. Our approach seeks to exploit a small annotated dataset and iteratively increase model performance by scaling up to refine the model using a large set of unlabelled data. By fusing predictions of perturbed inputs, the method generates new training annotations without human intervention. We demonstrate the effectiveness of the proposed framework to localize multiple structures in a 3D US dataset of 4044 fetal brain volumes with an initial expert annotation of just 200 volumes (5% in total) in training. Results show that structure localization error was reduced from 2.07 ± 1.65 mm to 1.76 ± 1.35 mm on the hold-out validation set.

1 Introduction

Recent years have witnessed machine learning revolutionize the field of computer science. This data-driven technology is capable of processing large-scale datasets and in fact, is nourished by increasing availability of data. Many applications, such as natural language processing and image recognition, have since benefited from this feature as a vast amount of data and annotations are obtainable online via crowd-sourcing. This mechanism is not easily reproduced in the medical field, for two principal reasons. Firstly, there are the relatively limited size of medical datasets; collecting medical data is relatively difficult, costly, and may depend on the morbidity. Sharing/transferring medical datasets is usually restricted due to ethical and/or privacy concerns. Secondly, the shortage of expert annotations for large datasets. In most scenarios, human labelling is tedious and time-consuming. Furthermore, the labelling of medical data can require specialized knowledge and skills. As a result, comprehensive labelling for many medical datasets is infeasible owing to the scarcity and costliness of expert resources.

This paper seeks to overcome the latter by proposing a family of algorithms that scale up from a small annotated dataset to potentially infinite unlabelled data, requiring no additional human intervention. We tackle this omni-supervised

A. F. Frangi et al. (Eds.): MICCAI 2018, LNCS 11070, pp. 572–580, 2018.
https://doi.org/10.1007/978-3-030-00928-1_65

learning problem by an iterative training/prediction paradigm that distils knowledge from different models and available data. The accuracy of the framework is lower-bounded by that of a model solely trained on the small annotated set and can be continuously boosted by automatically generated labels.

We demonstrate this general framework for a localization task on a large 3D US dataset of 4044 fetal brain volumes. Starting from a small labelled subset of 200 volumes (5% of the whole dataset), the framework gradually incorporates unlabelled data and generates labels for the **full** dataset.

2   Related Work

Semi-supervised learning is a class of machine learning techniques that falls between unsupervised and supervised learning. It attempts to use unlabelled data to improve the performance of the model trained with a smaller annotated dataset. Self-training is one type of semi-supervised method in which model prediction is used as ground truth to train a new model. However, a naïve implementation of self-training is meaningless as it provides no information gain. A number of methods have been proposed to address this problem. One of the most intuitive approaches is active learning, where predictions are screened and adjusted by human experts before model retraining [1]. This can greatly reduce the amount of data to be annotated but requires expert resource along the process.

Radosavovic et al. proposed *data distillation* to tackle self-training [2]. It generates annotations for unlabelled data by aggregating predictions of perturbed versions of one example using one trained model. These generated labels are then used to train new models and the process is iterated. It is intuitive, as perturbing data (augmentation) can generate useful information that is known to help training (avoid over-fitting). Meanwhile, it is accepted that averaging predictions from different models outperforms the results produced by a single model [3]. This idea is extended to transfer knowledge from trained models (teacher models) to a new model (i.e. student model) which is termed as *model distillation* [4]. It is typically accomplished by first combining predictions of an ensemble of teacher models as soft targets to train new models. It can enhance model performance which suggests model distillation can also extract useful signal to help self-training.

This paper, for the first time, combines model distillation and data distillation to build and evaluate an integrated semi-supervised framework. The framework is applied to tackle a real-world medical imaging problem, addressing the challenges of limited annotated data. This work does not emphasize building a specific, sophisticated base model, but rather on exploring a general method that is readily extended to different applications.

3   Methods

The proposed framework can be summarized as follows: (1) Building a group of teacher/base models and training them with the manually labelled dataset respectively; (2) Perturbing unlabelled data (i.e. via geometric transformations) to generate multiple copies of each image; (3) Applying the trained models on these transformed images; (4) Ensembling predictions from different models and different transformations via weighting or averaging; (5) Training a student model using the mixture of generated and manual labels (see Fig. 1).

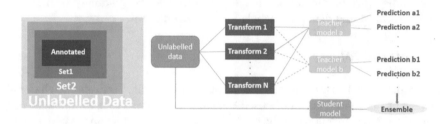

Fig. 1. Schematic of the proposed framework. The figure on the left shows the framework starts from a small annotated subset, to train the base models, and gradually expands to the full unlabelled set. The flow-chart shows unlabelled data are transformed to generate multiple of copies, and are sent to different base models for evaluation. The predictions are aggregated to generate new labels to train student models.

One of the key parts of our framework is model distillation. The general principle is that 'soft targets' (predicted class probability: $0 \leq p \leq 1$) provide richer information than the 'hard targets' (e.g. 0/1 binary score). The predicted probability includes additional information of similarity between inputs and targets thus it is more informative in training new models. Moreover, an ensemble of models is usually superior in classification accuracy than any single component. It suggests different models might be complementary to each other and combining their predictions can be advantageous in self-training. Note that the base models (also referred to as teacher models) can be more complicated, while the student models usually have a compact size to ensure fast inference.

Another contribution of our framework is the incorporation of data distillation. Perturbations of inputs can produce a useful signal for self-training. It does not modify network structures and is simple to implement. Here we also highlight the importance of selecting suitable types of transformations, especially for medical datasets. Later experiments show that certain transformations can be more informative than others in a specific application.

After automatic annotations are generated for the unlabelled data, the results are merged with the initial annotated dataset as the new training set. This new training set can be used to fine-tune the base models or train new student models from scratch. In practice, fine-tuning the model usually encourages faster convergence, but it might be limited when the base model converges to a poor local extrema. We investigate this point further in Sect. 4.

4   Experiments on Structure Localization

Clinical Task Definition. We evaluate the proposed method on structure detection in 3D fetal brain neurosonography: a complex task in a challenging imaging modality. A standard fetal 3D neurosonography examination requires identification and evaluation of several key brain anatomies; namely, the lateral ventricles (LV), cavum septi pellucidi (CSP), thalami (Tha), cerebellum (CE), brain stem (BS) and eye (Eye) (Fig. 2). Identifying these structures in ultrasound (US) is non-trivial as: (1) image quality is greatly affected by speckle, skull calcification and the position of the US probe with respect to the brain; (2) developing brain structures change continuously over gestation, both in size and appearance; (3) the position and orientation of the fetal head are highly variable, and commonly observed in reverse positions (see Fig. 3). As a result, interpreting a 3D fetal US volume is time-consuming and requires a high-level of expertise. An automatic method to localize brain structures across a large gestational age (GA) range is desirable to lessen the clinical burden of interpreting 3D scans and assist routine evaluation.

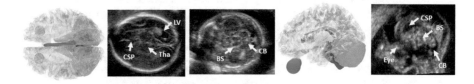

Fig. 2. Key brain structures. Schematics of CSP (blue), LV (green), TH (yellow), CB (red) and BS (grey), Eye (purple) are shown in axial and sagittal views. Examples of the structures shown in an US volume are displayed accordingly.

Datasets. 4044 3D US fetal brain volumes were acquired to a standard clinical 3D acquisition protocol and gestational age ranged between 20 and 30 weeks. As the fan-shaped US beam is bordered by a large black region, each volume was cropped at the centre of size 160 × 160 × 160 (with isotropic voxels of 0.6 × 0.6 × 0.6 mm^3) and to homogenize the data dimensions. 388 volumes were annotated and separated into a set of 200 to train the initial teacher model, and 188 were held out for validation. The remaining unlabelled 3656 volumes were divided into sets of 403, 811, 2242 respectively for self-training. In total, annotating the 388 volumes took approximately **120** hours of expert time. Manual annotation of the full dataset would require **1251** hours (over 30 weeks of work, given a 40 h/week work schedule) which is not feasible.

Base Model Design. One of the most popular current methods in object detection is the R-CNN [5] and its variants [6], which consists of a region proposal part (RPP) and a region classification part. The state-of-the-art RPP uses a sliding-window scheme [6] which is not well-suited for fetal neurosonography as scans are taken from different angles. Our task seeks orientation-sensitive predictions instead of axis-aligned boxes. Moreover, as we work with a 3D modality, an exhaustive search for RPP in full 3D space is excessively computationally expensive.

Alternatively, we found the task could be framed as a segmentation problem which can be solved using the well-known 3D U-Net [7], which provides a more straight-forward and unified approach than a two-step framework [5]. As a 3D U-Net supports volumetric input, it is able to incorporate global information that might be hard to obtain in an individual region. Moreover, it provides a denser supervision that enables model distillation. One major obstacle in transfer learning knowledge for localization is that it is usually defined as a regression problem (to the desired coordinates). A single value of the predicted coordinate does not carry inheritable probability information, which is indispensable in model distillation. Our approach transforms the task into a voxel-wise classification problem that naturally produces probability heat-maps (output voxel values $\in [0, 1]$) for each class. These maps are the soft targets that carry rich information that can be passed on to new models. For simplicity, we consider two base models, namely $\mathcal{M}_{CE}$ and $\mathcal{M}_{Dice}$, that have identical network architecture but were trained using different loss functions: binary cross-entropy (CE) and dice similarity loss (Dice), respectively.

Multi-transform Inference. Many types of geometric transformation can be used in data distillation, such as cropping, flipping, and rotation. Radosavovic et al. used scaling and horizontal flipping [2] to improve the model. Here we investigate the influence of geometric transformation type in more detail. Specifically, we retrain the model on labels generated using two different groups of transformation: $\mathcal{T}_t$: flipping and translation. Input volumes were flipped horizontally and vertically. To generate realistic input, each raw volume was translated by $t = \{-10, 0, 10\}$ in each orthogonal direction. In total, this resulted in 7 perturbed versions of an input. $\mathcal{T}_r$: flipping and rotation. Here, input volumes were rotated in the axial and the coronal views by $\pm 10°$. This group also had 7 perturbed versions of each input. For simplicity, predictions were aggregated via averaging across different perturbations and different models for all the experiments.

Implementation Details. Each 3D U-Net model contained four convolutional (CONV) and down-sampling layers and four CONV and up-sampling layers. The kernel numbers for the first two CONV layers are 16, 32, and 64 for all remaining CONV layers. Kernel size is $3 \times 3 \times 3$ voxels. The feature maps were fed into six sigmoid layers to yield the bounding box masks for each target. Model training was done end-to-end simultaneously via the Adam optimizer with an initial learning rate of 10^{-3} (decayed by a factor of 0.1 every 15 epochs). Batch-normalization, ReLU, and max-pooling were used after each linear CONV layer. On average, a 3D volume was processed in 1.3 s on an 11 GB RAM workstation with one NVIDIA GTX 1080 TI.

5   Results and Conclusion

Base Models. The two base models: $\mathcal{M}_{CE}$, $\mathcal{M}_{Dice}$ were trained from scratch using 200 manually annotated volumes. The first two rows of Table 1 report their accuracy on the held-out validation set. The two models performed similarly in finding the centre of targets. $\mathcal{M}_{Dice}$ outperformed $\mathcal{M}_{CE}$ in IoU metric but scored inferiorly in estimating size. This can be explained as the CE loss identifies the class of each voxel (local evaluation): more voxels are correctly labelled, which leads to more accurate volume estimation. While the Dice loss evaluates the gross overlap (global evaluation), the IoU metric quantifies this property. Given the complexity of fetal brain anatomy, an ideal model should utilize information on both local appearance and global information. Thus the combination of their predictions should assist training new models.

Transformation Type. To evaluate the influence of the geometric transformation in data distillation, we compared prediction accuracy of the two student models, $\mathcal{T}_t$, $\mathcal{T}_r$, which were learned from labels generated using transform groups $\mathcal{T}_t$ and $\mathcal{T}_r$, respectively (as defined in Sect. 4). In each case, the training set consisted of 200 manually labelled volumes and 403 automatically annotated volumes. Comparing the performance of $\mathcal{T}_t$, $\mathcal{T}_r$ with $\mathcal{M}_{Dice}$, Table 1 shows localization accuracy was enhanced in both cases for all evaluated metrics. Moreover, $\mathcal{T}_r$ outperformed $\mathcal{T}_t$. This is as expected as the targets in fetal neurosonography have large orientation variations. Perturbing data rotationally may produce informative signals for the data distillation. This highlights the importance of selecting a data-specific transformation to distil knowledge from unlabelled medical data. We opt for transformation $\mathcal{T}_r$ for all following experiments.

Table 1. Model performance. The predictions and annotations were compared by evaluating the distance between their centre (Cen Err), the average volume difference (Vol Err) and the 3D Intersection over Union (IoU).

Model	Loss	Training size	Cen Err (mm)	Vol Err (%)	3D IoU (%)
$\mathcal{M}_{CE}$	CE	200	2.07 ± 1.65	22.8 ± 19.6	57.9 ± 15.2
$\mathcal{M}_{Dice}$	Dice	200	2.00 ± 1.57	24.3 ± 17.4	59.5 ± 13.6
$\mathcal{T}_t$	Dice	603	1.96 ± 1.60	17.6 ± 14.4	60.6 ± 15.1
$\mathcal{T}_r$	Dice	603	1.94 ± 1.56	17.1 ± 13.7	60.9 ± 14.9
Fine tuned	Dice	603	1.96 ± 1.74	17.3 ± 14.1	60.9 ± 15.2
Our method	Dice	603	$\mathbf{1.90 \pm 1.54}$	$\mathbf{16.2 \pm 14.5}$	$\mathbf{61.8 \pm 15.1}$

Model Re-Training. To compare fine-tuning with training from scratch, we fine-tuned a model based on $\mathcal{M}_{Dice}$. The weights of the first two layers were fixed and the initial learning rate was set to be 0.5×10^{-4}. To compare with a

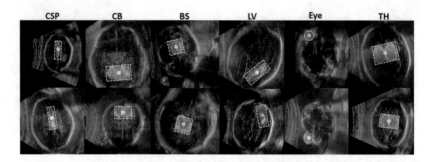

Fig. 3. Target structures viewed on US slices from random subjects (ground truth - yellow box, prediction - transparent overlay). The centre of each structure is plotted as a white dot. The image contrast, fetal head size, and orientation, vary dramatically. Speckle and acoustic shadows also influence structure visibility.

model trained from scratch ($\mathcal{T}_r$), the **Fine tuned** model was trained using the same dataset as $\mathcal{T}_r$ for consistency. Table 1 (row 4, 5) suggests that retraining from scratch resulted in slightly better performance. This shows local optimum trapping might have larger effects on model learning, which agrees with the findings reported in [2]. All other experiments are conducted by fully retraining.

Full Framework. Next, we report the result of the full framework (last row in Table 1), that combines model distillation (using $\mathcal{M}_{CE}$ and $\mathcal{M}_{Dice}$), and data distillation (using $\mathcal{T}_r$). The final model is the best at localizing the six targeted structures. Furthermore, the full framework outperformed the model only using data distillation (row 4, $\mathcal{T}_r$). This shows that information learned by different models can be effectively combined for self-training.

Table 2. Model performance with increasing training set size. The predictions and annotations were evaluated in the same manner as Table 1.

Model	Training size	Cen Err (mm)	Vol Err (%)	3D IoU (%)
$\mathcal{M}_{Dice}1$	200	2.07 ± 1.65	22.8 ± 19.6	57.9 ± 15.2
$\mathcal{M}_{Dice}2$	603	1.90 ± 1.54	16.2 ± 14.5	61.8 ± 15.1
$\mathcal{M}_{Dice}3$	1414	1.78 ± 1.48	15.8 ± 15.0	62.8 ± 13.6
$\mathcal{M}_{Dice}4$	3856	$\mathbf{1.76 \pm 1.35}$	$\mathbf{15.6 \pm 14.0}$	$\mathbf{62.8 \pm 13.0}$

Scaling Up to the Full Dataset. In a *supervised* setting, deep learning surpasses other machine learning techniques as it can be continuously improved given more training data. Here we show similar results using our *semi-supervised* framework. Visual results refer to Fig. 3. Table 2 shows that model performance scaled with training set size. In Table 2, $\mathcal{M}_{Dice}4$ used all the available unlabelled data, and achieved the best accuracy. Compare to $\mathcal{M}_{Dice}1$, it successfully boosted the model performance by nearly 7% in predicting volume size, 5% in 3D IoU, and is 0.7 mm more accurate in centre-point localization on average. It shows that the proposed framework can exploit unlabelled data to benefit subsequent retraining. $\mathcal{M}_{Dice}3$ and $\mathcal{M}_{Dice}4$ had similar mean accuracy while the latter had smaller variance. This suggests the framework performance might saturate given a limited number of base models and data transformation types. While a direct comparison is not possible (dataset is not publicly available), our results are comparable with fully-supervised approaches [8]. Furthermore, our best model $\mathcal{M}_{Dice}4$ outperformed the results reported in the recently published [9], thus adding credibility to our baseline model.

To visually evaluate model performance on the 3856 unlabelled data, we used Procrustes analysis to align the centre of the detected structures thereby registering their US volumes accordingly (see Fig. 4). After alignment, the mean volume corresponds better with the anatomical diagram (all shown in coronal view). It suggests the final model can be extended to build a rigid registration tool and create a brain atlas for further analysis and processing.

To conclude, this paper has presented an original semi-supervised framework that can efficiently scale up to a large medical dataset given a small annotated subset. Validation experiments were carried out on a large 3D US dataset, containing 4044 fetal brain volumes, for a multi-stream localization task. The method has potential to be applied to other tasks to greatly reduce the expert resource required for labelling large-scale medical datasets.

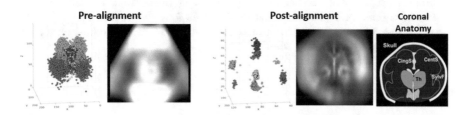

Fig. 4. Rigid registration of all unlabelled volumes using predicted structure locations. Each color in the point clouds represents a structure: blue-CSP, red-TH, yellow-BS, green-CB, cyan-LV, purple-Eye. The mean volumes of the unlabelled volumes before and after alignment are shown accordingly. The figure on the right is a schematic of the fetal brain in the coronal view.

Acknowledgement. We acknowledge the *Intergrowth*-21st study [10] for the image datasets. This work was supported by the National Institutes of Health (NIH) through National Institute on Alcohol Abuse and Alcoholism (NIAAA) (2 U01 AA014809-14), the Royal Academy of Engineering under the Engineering for Development Research Fellowship Scheme, and the EPSRC Programme Grant Seebibyte (EP/M013774/1).

References

1. Gur, Y., Moradi, M., Bulu, H., Guo, Y., Compas, C., Syeda-Mahmood, T.: Towards an efficient way of building annotated medical image collections for big data studies. In: Cardoso, M.J., et al. (eds.) LABELS/CVII/STENT -2017. LNCS, vol. 10552, pp. 87–95. Springer, Cham (2017). https://doi.org/10.1007/978-3-319-67534-3_10
2. Radosavovic, I., Dollár, P., Girshick, R., Gkioxari, G., He, K.: Data distillation: Towards omni-supervised learning. arXiv preprint arXiv:1712.04440 (2017)
3. Hinton, G., Vinyals, O., Dean, J.: Distilling the knowledge in a neural network. arXiv preprint arXiv:1503.02531 (2015)
4. Bucila, C., Caruana, R., Niculescu-Mizil, A.: Model compression: making big, slow models practical. In: Proceedings of the 12th International Conference on Knowledge Discovery and Data Mining (KDD 2006) (2006)
5. Girshick, R., Donahue, J., Darrell, T., Malik, J.: Rich feature hierarchies for accurate object detection and semantic segmentation. In: CVPR (2014)
6. He, K., Gkioxari, G., Dollár, P., Girshick, R.: Mask R-CNN. In: 2017 IEEE International Conference on Computer Vision (ICCV), pp. 2980–2988. IEEE (2017)
7. Çiçek, Ö., Abdulkadir, A., Lienkamp, S.S., Brox, T., Ronneberger, O.: 3D U-Net: Learning dense volumetric segmentation from sparse annotation. In: Ourselin, S., Joskowicz, L., Sabuncu, M.R., Unal, G., Wells, W. (eds.) MICCAI 2016. LNCS, vol. 9901, pp. 424–432. Springer, Cham (2016). https://doi.org/10.1007/978-3-319-46723-8_49
8. Sofka, M., Zhang, J., Good, S., Zhou, S.K., Comaniciu, D.: Automatic detection and measurement of structures in fetal head ultrasound volumes using sequential estimation and integrated detection network (IDN). IEEE TMI 33(5), 1054–1070 (2014)
9. Huang, R., Xie, W., Noble, J.A.: VP-Nets: efficient automatic localization of key brain structures in 3D fetal neurosonography. Med. Image Anal. 47, 127–139 (2018)
10. Papageorghiou, A.T.: International standards for fetal growth based on serial ultrasound measurements: the fetal growth longitudinal study of the intergrowth-21st project. Lancet 384(9946), 869–879 (2014)

Recurrent Neural Networks for Classifying Human Embryonic Stem Cell-Derived Cardiomyocytes

Carolina Pacheco$^{(\boxtimes)}$ and René Vidal

Center for Imaging Science, Mathematical Institute for Data Science,
Department of Biomedical Engineering, Johns Hopkins University,
Baltimore, USA
cpachec2@jhu.edu

Abstract. Classification of human embryonic stem cell-derived cardiomyocytes (hESC-CMs) is important for many applications in cardiac regenerative medicine. However, a key challenge is the lack of ground truth labels for hESC-CMs: Whereas adult phenotypes are well-characterized in terms of their action potentials (APs), the understanding of how the shape of the AP of immature CMs relates to that of adult CMs remains limited. Recently, a new metamorphosis distance has been proposed to determine if a query immature AP is closer to a particular adult AP phenotype. However, the metamorphosis distance is difficult to compute making it unsuitable for classifying a large number of CMs. In this paper we propose a semi-supervised learning framework for the classification of hESC-CM APs. The proposed framework is based on a recurrent neural network with LSTM units whose parameters are learned by minimizing a loss consisting of two parts. The supervised part uses labeled data obtained from computational models of adult CMs, while the unsupervised part uses the metamorphosis distance in an efficient way. Experiments confirm the benefit of integrating information from both adult and stem cell-derived domains in the learning scheme, and also show that the proposed method generates results similar to the state-of-the-art (94.73%) with clear computational advantages when applied to new samples.

Keywords: Semi-supervised learning · LSTM
Embryonic cardiomyocytes

1 Introduction

The unquestioned cardiomyogenic potential of human embryonic stem cells [1] and the well-established protocols for their isolation and maintenance [2] make them one of the most promising sources of cardiomyocytes (CMs) for applications such as cell-based cardiac repair [3] and drug screening [4]. However, their use is still hampered by the current limited understanding of the phenotypic traits of

© Springer Nature Switzerland AG 2018
A. F. Frangi et al. (Eds.): MICCAI 2018, LNCS 11070, pp. 581–589, 2018.
https://doi.org/10.1007/978-3-030-00928-1_66

human stem cell-derived cardiomyocytes (hESC-CMs) and their relationship to the phenotypes of adult CMs [3]. To characterize the phenotype of hESC-CMs, prior work [5] studies the expression of specific genes and ion channel-encoding subunits. Alternatively, [6,7] apply thresholding to simple features extracted from the cell's action potential (AP). However, simple classification methods based on handcrafted features and subjective criteria not only discard most of the information contained in the AP, but also are hardly transferable.

Recently, automatic methods have been proposed to analyze the heterogeneity of hESC-CMs APs using the whole AP as an input. For instance, the existence of different clusters was studied via a spectral grouping-based algorithm in [8], and the metamorphosis distance proposed in [9] was adapted in [10] to classify embryonic APs by computing their distances to adult APs with known phenotype. While this new method shows better interpolation and clustering results [11], it is too computationally intensive to be applicable to large-scale datasets.

In this paper we propose a new method for classifying hESC-CMs APs based on recurrent neural networks (RNNs) with long short term memory (LSTM) units [12]. LSTMs have recently re-gained popularity for time series classification because of their great performance in applications to speech recognition [13] and activity recognition [14]. However, while LSTMs have also been successfully applied to the analysis of physiological signals [15,16], standard LSTMs are not directly applicable to the classification of hESC-CMs because of the lack of labels for embryonic APs. In this context, the contribution of this paper is to propose a semi-supervised approach that exploits the abundance of labels for adult APs, which can be obtained via simulation of electrophysiological models for the typical adult phenotypes (atrial, ventricular, etc.). The proposed semi-supervised approach uses a novel loss function to train an LSTM that combines a classification loss for adult APs (supervised part) and a contrastive loss for embryonic APs (unsupervised part). For the supervised part we use synthetic APs obtained from computational models of adult atrial [17] and ventricular [18] CMs, while for the unsupervised part we compute similarities between APs, making efficient use of Euclidean and metamorphosis distances.

Experiments on a dataset of 6940 hESC-CMs APs show that our semi-supervised approach provides smooth clustering results that are comparable to those presented in [11] in terms of Davies-Bouldin Index (DBI), and also confirm the benefit of integrating information from both adult and embryonic APs. Furthermore, the semi-supervised approach is able to use the Euclidean metric more effectively than previous methods, considerably outperforming the 1-nearest neighbor scheme (87.88% vs 62.90% of agreement with the best result published in [11]). When the metamorphosis distance is used, our method achieves 94.73% of agreement with the best results published in [11], but it is significantly less computationally expensive when applied to new data.

2   Methods

Let the sequence $\mathbf{x}_j^e = \{x_j^e(k) \in \mathbb{R}\}_{k=1}^T$, where T is the total number of samples in one cycle length, represent the jth embryonic AP. Let $\mathbf{x}_i^a$ be the ith adult AP and let $y_i^a \in \{0,1\}$ be its ground truth label, where $y_i^a = 0$ denotes atrial and $y_i^a = 1$ denotes ventricular. We consider the problem of assigning a label $\hat{y}_j^e$ to each $\mathbf{x}_j^e$, where $\hat{y}_j^e = 0$ denotes atrial-like and $\hat{y}_j^e = 1$ denotes ventricular-like.

A simple approach is to use a 1 nearest-neighbor (1NN) classifier with the Euclidean distance $d_E(\mathbf{x}_j^e, \mathbf{x}_i^a) = \frac{1}{\sigma_M}\sqrt{\sum_{k=1}^{T}\left(x_j^e(k) - x_i^a(k)\right)^2}$, where σ_M is a normalization parameter. However, the Euclidean distance can be affected by nuisance factors such as changes in AP shape induced by the maturation process.

An alternative approach is to use 1NN classification with the metamorphosis distance, which generates an interpolation path $x(k, s)$ between an embryonic AP, $x(k, 0) = x_j^e(k)$, and an adult AP, $x(k, S) = x_i^a(k)$, that minimizes the amount of deformation between the two, which depends on a certain velocity $\mathbf{v}$:

$$d_M^2(\mathbf{x}_j^e, \mathbf{x}_i^a) = \min_{\mathbf{x},\mathbf{v}} \sum_{s=0}^{S-1} \|v(k,s)\|_V^2 + \tfrac{1}{\sigma_M^2}\|x(k + v(k,s), s+1) - x(k,s)\|_2^2, \quad (1)$$

where $\|\cdot\|_V^2$ is a Sobolev norm and σ_M^2 is a balancing parameter (see [10,11]). However, the metamorphosis distance is computationally intensive to evaluate.

2.1   Classifier Architecture

Long Short-Term Memory (LSTM) units [12] are recurrent blocks whose key elements are input gates $i(k)$, forget gates $f(k)$ and output gates $o(k)$ that modulate the evolution of the state $c(k)$ and its output $h(k)$ at time k as follows

$$
\begin{aligned}
i(k) &= \sigma\left(W_i x(k) + U_i h(k-1) + b_i\right) \in \mathbb{R}^p \\
f(k) &= \sigma\left(W_f x(k) + U_f h(k-1) + b_f\right) \in \mathbb{R}^p \\
o(k) &= \sigma\left(W_o x(k) + U_o h(k-1) + b_o\right) \in \mathbb{R}^p \\
c(k) &= f(k) \circ c(k-1) + i(k) \circ \tanh\left(W_c x(k) + U_c h(k-1) + b_c\right) \in \mathbb{R}^p \\
h(k) &= o(k) \circ \tanh\left(c(k)\right) \in \mathbb{R}^p
\end{aligned}
\quad (2)
$$

where p denotes the layer dimension, $\sigma(z) = \frac{1}{1+e^{-z}}$ is the sigmoidal function, $x(k)$ is the input sequence at time k and $\circ$ denotes the Hadamard product.

The proposed architecture for the classifier is depicted in Fig. 1: an RNN with one hidden LSTM layer of dimension $p = 3$, and one sigmoid unit as the output layer (64 parameters in total). This sigmoid unit operates only in the last value of the cell output $h(T)$, once all the sequence $x(k)$ has been processed by the LSTM layer.

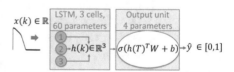

Fig. 1. Network architecture: one hidden LSTM layer $(p = 3)$ and a sigmoid unit.

2.2   Semi-supervised Objective Function

We use the binary crossentropy loss $\ell(y, \hat{y}) = -y \log(\hat{y}) - (1 - y)\log(1 - \hat{y})$ to quantify how close the LSTM prediction $\hat{y} = \sigma(h(T)^T W + b)$ is to label y. More specifically, given N_a adult APs $\{\mathbf{x}_i^a\}$ and their labels $\{y_i^a\}$, our supervised loss is

$$\frac{1}{N_a} \sum_{i=1}^{N_a} \{-y_i^a \log(\hat{y}_i^a) - (1 - y_i^a) \log(1 - \hat{y}_i^a)\}. \tag{3}$$

Now, while we do not have labels for the embryonic APs $\{\mathbf{x}_j^e\}$, we can still use $\ell(\hat{y}_j^e, \hat{y}_{j'}^e)$ to compare the predicted labels for two different embryonic APs. Intuitively, we would like similar APs to have the same labels, and dissimilar APs to have different labels. Therefore, given N_e APs, we use a contrastive loss

$$\frac{1}{N_e (N_e - 1)} \sum_{j=1}^{N_e} \sum_{j' \neq j} s_{(j,j')} \cdot \ell\left(\hat{y}_j^e, \hat{y}_{j'}^e\right) + \left(1 - s_{(j,j')}\right) \cdot \ell\left((1 - \hat{y}_j^e), \hat{y}_{j'}^e\right), \tag{4}$$

where $s_{(j,j')}$ represents the similarity between AP $\mathbf{x}_j^e$ and AP $\mathbf{x}_{j'}^e$. We define the similary between two APs based on their distance $d\left(\mathbf{x}_j^e, \mathbf{x}_{j'}^e\right)$ (Euclidean or metamorphosis) as $s_{(j,j')} = \exp\left(-\frac{d^4\left(\mathbf{x}_j, \mathbf{x}_{j'}\right)}{\sigma_s^4}\right)$, where σ_s is chosen as $\sigma_s^4 = \overline{d^4}$, where d is the distance variable and the top bar denotes average operator.

After combining the supervised and unsupervised terms of the loss, we obtain

$$\frac{1 - \lambda}{N_a} \left(\sum_{j=1}^{N_a} \ell\left(y_j^a, \hat{y}_j^a\right)\right) + \frac{\lambda}{N_e - 1} \sum_{j=2}^{N_e} s_{(j,j-1)} \cdot \ell\left(\hat{y}_j^e, \hat{y}_{j-1}^e\right)$$
$$+ \left(1 - s_{(j,j-1)}\right) \cdot \ell\left((1 - \hat{y}_j^e), \hat{y}_{j-1}^e\right), \tag{5}$$

where λ is a balancing parameter between supervised and unsupervised parts. Instead of making pairwise comparisons between all APs, we propose to compare an AP $\mathbf{x}_j^e$ with the previous one $\mathbf{x}_{j-1}^e$, so fewer distance computations are needed.

2.3   Clustering Quality Index

Since no ground truth labels are available for embryonic APs, the Davies-Bouldin Index (DBI) [19] is considered as a measure of clustering quality. Let $\Omega_0 = \{\mathbf{x}_j^e \mid \hat{y}_j^e < 0.5\}$ and $\Omega_1 = \{\mathbf{x}_j^e \mid \hat{y}_j^e \geq 0.5\}$ be the sets containing the different clusters, let S_y be the mean distance from elements of class y to the average signal of the same class, $\mu_y(k) = \frac{1}{|\Omega_y|} \sum_{\mathbf{x}_j^e \in \Omega_y} x_j^e(k)$, and let M_{01} be the distance between the averages $\mu_0(k)$ and $\mu_1(k)$. The DBI is defined as the ratio between the intra-cluster dispersion and the distance between clusters

$$DBI\left(\Omega_0, \Omega_1\right) = \frac{S_0 + S_1}{M_{01}}, \tag{6}$$

and should be as small as possible. For computational reasons, and since the Euclidean distance d_E is a good approximation of the metamorphosis distance d_M for small distances, the intra-cluster dispersions S_0 and S_1 are computed using d_E, whereas the distance between clusters M_{01} is computed using d_M.

3 Experiments

3.1 Adult CMs APs Data

A population of 2000 synthetic adult APs was generated by using computational models. The O'hara-Rudy model (ORd) [18] and the Nygren model [17] were paced at 1.5 Hz with 1000 random sets of parameters each (varying between 80% and 120% of their nominal values) to generate ventricular and atrial mature CMs APs, respectively. The parameters varied were the maximum conductances and permeabilities of ion channels (g_{Na}, g_{NaL}, g_{t_0}, g_{Kr}, g_{Ks}, g_{K1}, g_{NC_X}, g_{Kb}, g_{pCa}, P_{Ca}, P_{NaK}, P_{Nab}, P_{Cab} in ORd model, and g_{CaL}, g_{Ks}, g_{Kr}, g_{K1}, g_{Nab} and g_{Cab} in Nygren model). Normalization was applied to each AP so that its maximum voltage and resting membrane potential are 1 and 0, respectively. The Sparse Modeling for Representatives Selection (SMRS) method [20] was then applied to select a subset of $N_a = 300$ templates shown in Fig. 2a.

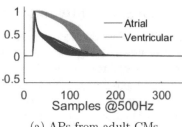

(a) APs from adult CMs

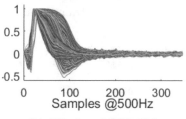

(b) APs from hESC-CMs

Fig. 2. Action potentials: (a) 300 adult CMs, (b) 6940 hESC-CMs.

3.2 hESC-CMs Data

A population of $N_e = 6940$ hESC-CMs APs obtained from 9 cell aggregates paced at 1.5 Hz and optically mapped at a sampling rate of 500 Hz was obtained in [21]. The APs were averaged over beating cycles, a 5×5 boxcar spatial filter was applied for denoising, and then they were normalized (see Fig. 2b). Only 1600 APs (fixed and coming from 2 cell aggregates) were used for training, but labels were predicted for the whole dataset.

3.3 Implementation Details

The classifier architecture was implemented in Keras [22] with TensorFlow backend and trained using the RMSProp optimizer (learning rate 0.003) using batches of 19 APs (3 adult and 16 embryonic). 90 batches were used for training and 10 batches for validation, completing $N_a = 300$ adult APs and $N_e = 1600$ embryonic APs in total. The metamorphosis parameter was set as $\sigma_M = 0.3$.

Three cases are studied: Supervised learning $\lambda = 0$ (Sup-LSTM), Semi-supervised learning $\lambda = 0.1$ with Euclidean distances (Semi-LSTM-E), and Semi-supervised learning $\lambda = 0.1$ with metamorphosis distances (Semi-LSTM-M). In

each case the network was trained 5 times (100 epochs for the Sup-LSTM case
and 200 epochs for the Semi-LSTM cases), and the average of the classification
results at the last epoch is analyzed.

3.4   Experimental Results

The average classification results generated by the RNN LSTM in the studied
cases are shown in Fig. 3 for the 9 cell aggregates. In all cases the proposed classifier generates smooth classification regions and suggests heterogeneity in most
of the cell aggregates, which coincides with previous findings [11,21]. Observe
that the classification result produced by semi-supervised learning is significantly
different from the one produced by supervised learning, with the former being
significantly better in terms of DBI. This emphasizes that adult and embryonic
APs intrinsically belong to different domains, and therefore classifying embryonic
APs with a network trained only with adult APs is not adequate.

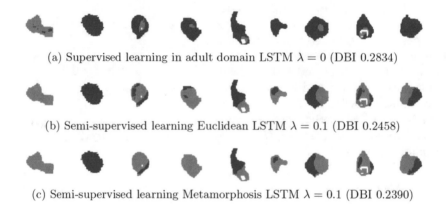

(a) Supervised learning in adult domain LSTM $\lambda = 0$ (DBI 0.2834)

(b) Semi-supervised learning Euclidean LSTM $\lambda = 0.1$ (DBI 0.2458)

(c) Semi-supervised learning Metamorphosis LSTM $\lambda = 0.1$ (DBI 0.2390)

Fig. 3. LSTM classification results (each pixel corresponds to one hESC-CM AP). Blue
indicates atrial-like phenotype and red indicates ventricular-like phenotype.

Table 1 compares our results to those of the method presented in [11] (1NN
classifier with $N_a = 20$ synthetic adult AP templates). Observe that supervised
learning shows significantly higher DBI than the rest, which is expected since
it does not consider hESC-CMs data during training. On the other hand, the
semi-supervised learning scheme outperforms the 1NN scheme when Euclidean
distances are used (DBI 0.2458 vs 0.2558). 1NN with Euclidean distances was
replicated with the same 300 adult AP templates used to train the network (see
Table 1), confirming that the improvement in clustering quality observed in the
semi-supervised scheme is not attributable to the number of templates used, but
to the method itself: Euclidean metric is a good approximation of metamorphosis for small distances, so it performs better when distances within hESC-CMs
domain are computed (proposed semi-supervised framework) than when distances between hESC-CMs and adult CMs domains are computed (1NN).

Table 1. Comparing the results of the proposed method (LSTM) with the results presented in [11]. Accuracy* is computed assuming 1NN classification with metamorphosis distance as ground truth (E: Euclidean, M: Metamorphosis).

Method	1NN	1NN	1NN	Sup-LSTM	Semi-LSTM	Semi-LSTM
Templates	20 [11]	20 [11]	300 SMRS	300 SMRS	300 SMRS	300 SMRS
Metric	M	E	E		E	M
DBI	0.2297	0.2558	0.2566	0.2834	0.2458	0.2390
Accuracy*	1	0.6488	0.6290	0.4723	0.8788	0.9473

1NN metamorphosis results presented in [11] show the best clustering quality (DBI 0.2297), followed by the Semi-LSTM-M (DBI 0.2390). The classification accuracy assuming 1NN metamorphosis as the ground truth was computed and plotted vs the DBI in Fig. 4. The use of metamorphosis distance in semi-supervised learning not only produces lower DBI but also consistently generates bet-

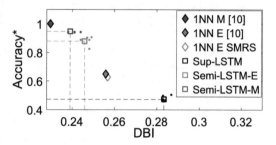

Fig. 4. Accuracy* vs DBI. 1NN M as ground truth (E: Euclidean, M: Metamorphosis).

ter classification accuracy than when the Euclidean distance is used (small dots in Fig. 4 represent single trials results, and squares represent the average classification per case). An improvement of 24.98% in the classification accuracy is observed between 1NN and the semi-supervised learning scheme when 300 templates and only Euclidean distances are used, achieving 87.88% accuracy without any metamorphosis distance computation.

4   Conclusion

The proposed method not only successfully integrates labeled data from a different domain to solve the task, but also proves to be a powerful framework to improve the performance of Euclidean-based methods in the classification of hESC-CMs APs. Moreover, it reaches 94.73% of agreement with the state-of-the-art, trading off accuracy with computational complexity: whereas the classification of a new sample in state-of-the-art method requires to solve 20 computationally intensive optimization problems (6.74 sec/sample in 2 8-core computer nodes with 8 2.3 GHz CPUs per node [11]), in the proposed method it just needs to be processed by a small RNN with fixed weights (less than 6 sec for the whole 6940 APs dataset in one 2.2 GHz CPU with 2 cores, 4 threads).

Acknowlegement. The authors thank Dr. Giann Gorospe for insightful discussions, and Dr. Renjun Zhu and Prof. Leslie Tung for providing the hESC-CMs dataset. CP is supported by CONICYT BECAS CHILE 73170418.

References

1. Kehat, I., et al.: Human embryonic stem cells can differentiate into myocytes with structural and functional properties of cardiomyocytes. J. Clin. Investig. **108**(3), 407–414 (2001)
2. Turksen, K.: Human embryonic stem cell protocols. vol. 331. Springer (2006)
3. Zhu, W.Z., Hauch, K.D., Xu, C., Laflamme, M.A.: Human embryonic stem cells and cardiac repair. Transp. Rev. **23**(1), 53–68 (2009)
4. Braam, S.R.: Prediction of drug-induced cardiotoxicity using human embryonic stem cell-derived cardiomyocytes. Stem Cell Res. **4**(2), 107–116 (2010)
5. Sartiani, L.: Developmental changes in cardiomyocytes differentiated from human embryonic stem cells: a molecular and electrophysiological approach. Stem Cells **25**(5), 1136–1144 (2007)
6. Peng, S., Lacerda, A., Kirsch, G., Brown, A., Bruening-Wright, A.: The action potential and comparative pharmacology of stem cell-derived human cardiomyocytes. J. Pharmacol. Toxicol. Methods **61**(3), 277–286 (2010)
7. He, J.Q., Ma, Y., Lee, Y., Thomson, J.A., Kamp, T.J.: Human embryonic stem cells develop into multiple types of cardiac myocytes: action potential characterization. Circul. Res. **93**(1), 32–39 (2003)
8. Gorospe, G., Zhu, R., Millrod, M., Zambidis, E., Tung, L., Vidal, R.: Automated grouping of action potentials of human embryonic stem cell-derived cardiomyocytes. IEEE Trans. Biomed. Eng. **61**(9), 2389–2395 (2014)
9. Trouvé, A., Younes, L.: Metamorphoses through Lie group action. Found. Comput. Math. **5**(2), 173–198 (2005)
10. Gorospe, G., Younes, L., Tung, L., Vidal, R.: A metamorphosis distance for embryonic cardiac action potential interpolation and classification. In: Mori, K., Sakuma, I., Sato, Y., Barillot, C., Navab, N. (eds.) MICCAI 2013. LNCS, vol. 8149, pp. 469–476. Springer, Heidelberg (2013). https://doi.org/10.1007/978-3-642-40811-3_59
11. Gorospe, G., et al.: Efficient metamorphosis computation for classifying embryonic cardiac action potentials. In: 5th Workshop on Mathematical Foundations of Computational Anatomy (2015)
12. Hochreiter, S., Schmidhuber, J.: Long short-term memory. Neural Comput. **9**(8), 1735–1780 (1997)
13. Graves, A., Jaitly, N.: Towards end-to-end speech recognition with recurrent neural networks. In: International Conference on Machine Learning, pp. 1764–1772 (2014)
14. Donahue, J., et al.: Long-term recurrent convolutional networks for visual recognition and description. In: IEEE Conference on Computer Vision and Pattern Recognition, pp. 2625–2634 (2015)
15. Lipton, Z.C., Kale, D.C., Elkan, C., Wetzel, R.: Learning to diagnose with LSTM recurrent neural networks. arXiv:1511.03677 (2015)
16. Zihlmann, M., Perekrestenko, D., Tschannen, M.: Convolutional recurrent neural networks for electrocardiogram classification. arXiv:1710.06122 (2017)
17. Nygren, A., et al.: Mathematical model of an adult human atrial cell: the role of k+ currents in repolarization. Circul. Res. **82**(1), 63–81 (1998)

18. O'Hara, T., Virág, L., Varró, A., Rudy, Y.: Simulation of the undiseased human cardiac ventricular action potential: model formulation and experimental validation. PLoS Comput. Biol. **7**(5), e1002061 (2011)
19. Davies, D.L., Bouldin, D.W.: A cluster separation measure. IEEE Trans. Pattern Anal. Mach. Intell. **2**, 224–227 (1979)
20. Elhamifar, E., Sapiro, G., Vidal, R.: See all by looking at a few: Sparse modeling for finding representative objects. In: IEEE Conference on Computer Vision and Pattern Recognition, pp. 1600–1607 (2012)
21. Zhu, R., Millrod, M.A., Zambidis, E.T., Tung, L.: Variability of action potentials within and among cardiac cell clusters derived from human embryonic stem cells. Sci. Rep. **6**, 18544 (2016)
22. Chollet, F., et al.: Keras (2015). https://keras.io

Group-Driven Reinforcement Learning for Personalized mHealth Intervention

Feiyun Zhu[1], Jun Guo[2], Zheng Xu[1], Peng Liao[2], Liu Yang[4],
and Junzhou Huang[1,3(✉)]

[1] Department of CSE, University of Texas at Arlington, Arlington, TX 76013, USA
[2] Department of Statistics, Univeristy of Michigan, Ann Arbor, MI 48109, USA
[3] Tencent AI Lab, Shenzhen 518057, China
jzhuang@uta.edu
[4] School of Software, Central South University, Changsha 410075, Hunan, China

Abstract. Due to the popularity of smartphones and wearable devices nowadays, mobile health (mHealth) technologies are promising to bring positive and wide impacts on people's health. State-of-the-art decision-making methods for mHealth rely on some ideal assumptions. Those methods either assume that the users are completely homogenous or completely heterogeneous. However, in reality, a user might be similar with some, but not all, users. In this paper, we propose a novel group-driven reinforcement learning method for the mHealth. We aim to understand how to share information among similar users to better convert the limited user information into sharper learned RL policies. Specifically, we employ the K-means clustering method to group users based on their trajectory information similarity and learn a shared RL policy for each group. Extensive experiment results have shown that our method can achieve clear gains over the state-of-the-art RL methods for mHealth.

1 Introduction

In the wake of the vast population of smart devices (smartphones and wearable devices such as the Fitbit Fuelband and Jawbone etc.) users worldwide, mobile health (mHealth) technologies become increasingly popular among the scientist communities. The goal of mHealth is to use smart devices as great platforms to collect and analyze raw data (weather, location, social activity, stress, etc.). Based on that, the aim is to provide in-time interventions to device users according to their ongoing status and changing needs, helping users to lead healthier lives, such as reducing the alcohol abuse [4] and the obesity management [11].

Formally, the tailoring of mHealth intervention is modeled as a sequential decision making (SDM) problem. It aims to learn the optimal decision rule to decide when, where and how to deliver interventions [7,10,13,17] to best serve

---

This work was partially supported by NSF IIS-1423056, CMMI-1434401, CNS-1405985, IIS-1718853 and the NSF CAREER grant IIS-1553687.

A. F. Frangi et al. (Eds.): MICCAI 2018, LNCS 11070, pp. 590–598, 2018.
https://doi.org/10.1007/978-3-030-00928-1_67

users. This is a brand-new research topic. Currently, there are two types of reinforcement learning (RL) methods for mHealth with distinct assumptions: (a) the off-policy, batch RL [16,17] assumes that all users in the mHealth are completely homogenous: they share all information and learn an identical RL for all the users; (b) the on-policy, online RL [7,17] assumes that all users are completely different: they share no information and run a separate RL for each user. The above assumptions are good as a start for the mHealth study. However, when mHealth are applied to more practical situations, they have the following drawbacks: (a) the off-policy, batch RL method ignore the fact that the behavior of all users may be too complicated to be modeled with an identical RL, which leads to potentially large biases in the learned policy; (b) for the on-policy, online RL method, an individual user's trajectory data is hardly enough to support a separate RL learning, which is likely to result in unstable policies that contain lots of variances [14].

A more realistic assumption lies between the above two extremes: a user may be similar to some, but not all, users and similar users tend to have similar behaviors. In this paper, we propose a novel group driven RL for the mHealth. It is in an actor-critic setting [3]. The core idea is to find the similarity (cohesion) network for the users. Specifically, we employ the clustering method to mine the group information. Taking the group information into consideration, we learn K (i.e., the number of groups) shared RLs for K groups of users respectively; each RL learning procedure makes use of all the data in that group. Such implementation balances the conflicting goals of reducing the complexity of data while enriching the number of samples for each RL learning process.

2   Preliminaries

The Markov Decision Process (MDP) provides a mathematical tool to model the dynamic system [2,3]. It is defined as a 5-tuple $\{\mathcal{S}, \mathcal{A}, P, R, \gamma\}$, where $\mathcal{S}$ is the state space and $\mathcal{A}$ is the action space. The state transition model $\mathcal{P} : \mathcal{S} \times \mathcal{A} \times \mathcal{S} \mapsto [0, 1]$ indicates the probability of transiting from one state s to another s' under a given action a. $\mathcal{R} : \mathcal{S} \times \mathcal{A} \mapsto \mathbb{R}$ is the corresponding reward, which is assumed to be bounded over the state and action spaces. $\gamma \in [0, 1)$ is a discount factor that reduces the influence of future rewards. The stochastic policy $\pi (\cdot \mid s)$ determines how the agent acts with the system by providing each state s with a probability over all the possible actions. We consider the parameterized stochastic policy, i.e., $\pi_\theta (a \mid s)$, where θ is the unknown coefficients.

Formally, the quality of a policy π_θ is evaluated by a value function $Q^{\pi_\theta} (s, a) \in \mathbb{R}^{|\mathcal{S}| \times |\mathcal{A}|}$ [12]. It specifies the total amount of rewards an agent can achieve when starting from state s, first choosing action a and then following the policy π_θ. It is defined as follows [3]:

$$Q^{\pi_\theta} (s, a) = \mathbb{E}_{a_i \sim \pi_\theta, s_i \sim \mathcal{P}} \left\{ \sum_{t=0}^{\infty} \gamma^t \mathcal{R} (s_t, a_t) \mid s_0 = s, a_0 = a \right\}. \tag{1}$$

The goal of various RL methods is to learn an optimal policy π_{θ^*} that maximizes the Q-value for all the state-action pairs [2]. The objective is $\pi_{\theta^*} = \arg\max_\theta \widehat{J}(\theta)$ (such procedure is called the actor updating [3]), where

$$\widehat{J}(\theta) = \sum_{s\in\mathcal{S}} d_{\mathrm{ref}}(s) \sum_{a\in\mathcal{A}} \pi_\theta(a \mid s) Q^{\pi_\theta}(s,a), \tag{2}$$

where $d_{\mathrm{ref}}(s)$ is a reference distribution over states; $Q^{\pi_\theta}(s,a)$ is the value for the parameterized policy π_θ. It is obvious that we need the estimation of $Q^{\pi_\theta}(s,a)$ (i.e. the critic updating) to determine the objective function (2).

3   Cohesion Discovery for the RL Learning

Suppose we are given a set of N users; each user is with a trajectory of T points. Thus in total, we have $NT = N \times T$ tuples summarized in $\mathcal{D} = \{\mathcal{D}_n \mid n = 1, \cdots, N\}$ for all the N users, where $\mathcal{D}_n = \{\mathcal{U}_i \mid i = 1, \cdots, T\}$ summarizes all the T tuples for the n-th user and $\mathcal{U}_i = (s_i, a_i, r_i, s_i')$ is the i-th tuple in $\mathcal{D}_n$.

3.1   The Pooled-RL and Separate RL (Separ-RL)

The first RL method (i.e. Pooled-RL) assumes that all the N users are completely homogenous and following the same MDP; they share all information and learn an identical RL for all the users [16]. In this setting, the critic updating (with an aim of seeking for solutions to satisfy the Linear Bellman equation [2,3]) is

$$\mathbf{w} = f(\mathbf{w}) = \arg\min_{\mathbf{h}} \frac{1}{|\mathcal{D}|} \sum_{\mathcal{U}_i\in\mathcal{D}} \left\| \mathbf{x}(s_i, a_i)^\mathsf{T}\mathbf{h} - \left[r_i + \gamma\mathbf{y}(s_i';\theta)^\mathsf{T}\mathbf{w}\right] \right\|_2^2 + \zeta_c \|\mathbf{h}\|_2^2, \tag{3}$$

where $\mathbf{w} = f(\mathbf{w})$ is a fixed point problem; $|\mathcal{D}|$ represents the number of tuples in $\mathcal{D}$; $\mathbf{x}_i = \mathbf{x}(s_i, a_i)^\mathsf{T}$ is the value feature at the time point i; $\mathbf{y}_i = \mathbf{y}(s_i';\theta) = \sum_{a\in\mathcal{A}}\mathbf{x}(s_i', a)\pi_\theta(a \mid s_i')$ is the feature at the next time point; ζ_c is a tuning parameter. The least-square temporal difference for Q-value (LSTDQ) [5,6] provides a closed-form solver for (3) as follows

$$\widehat{\mathbf{w}} = \left(\zeta_c\mathbf{I} + \frac{1}{|\mathcal{D}|} \sum_{\mathcal{U}_i\in\mathcal{D}} \mathbf{x}_i(\mathbf{x}_i - \gamma\mathbf{y}_i)^\mathsf{T} \right)^{-1} \left(\frac{1}{|\mathcal{D}|} \sum_{\mathcal{U}_i\in\mathcal{D}} \mathbf{x}_i r_i \right). \tag{4}$$

As $d_{\mathrm{ref}}(s)$ is generally unavailable, the T-trial objective for (2) is defined as

$$\hat{\theta} = \arg\max_\theta \frac{1}{|\mathcal{D}|} \sum_{\mathcal{U}_i\in\mathcal{D}} \sum_{a\in\mathcal{A}} Q(s_i, a; \widehat{\mathbf{w}})\pi_\theta(a|s_i) - \frac{\zeta_a}{2}\|\theta\|_2^2, \tag{5}$$

where $Q(s_i, a; \widehat{\mathbf{w}}) = \mathbf{x}(s_i, a)^\mathsf{T}\widehat{\mathbf{w}}$ is the newly defined Q-value which is based on the critic updating result in (4); ζ_a is the tuning parameter to prevent overfitting.

In case of large feature spaces, one can iteratively update $\widehat{\mathbf{w}}$ via (4) and $\widehat{\theta}$ in (5) to reduce the computational cost.

The Pooled-RL works well when all the N users are very similar. However, there are great behavior discrepancies among users in the mHealth study because they have different ages, races, incomes, religions, education levels etc. Such case makes the current Pooled-RL too simple to simultaneously fit all the N different users' behaviors. It easily results in lots of biases in the learned value and policy.

The second RL method (Separ-RL), such as Lei's online contextual bandit for mHealth [7,15], assumes that all users are completely heterogeneous. They share no information and run a separate online RL for each user. The objective functions are very similar with (3), (4), (5). This method should be great when the data for each user is very large in size. However, it generally costs a lot of time and other resources to collect enough data for the Separ-RL learning. Taking the HeartSteps for example, it takes 42 days to do the trial, which only collects 210 tuples per user. What is worse, there are missing and noises in the data, which will surely reduce the effective sample size. The problem of small sample size will easily lead to some unstable policies that contain lots of variances.

3.2 Group driven RL learning (Gr-RL)

We observe that users in mHealth are generally similar with some (but not all) users in the sense that they may have some similar features, such as age, gender, race, religion, education level, income and other socioeconomic status [8]. To this end, we propose a group based RL for mHealth to understand how to share information across similar users to improve the performance. Specifically, the users are assumed to be grouped together and likely to share information with others in the same group. The main idea is to divide the N users into K groups, and learn a separate RL model for each group. The samples of users in a group are pooled together, which not only ensures the simplicity of the data for each RL learning compared with that of the Pooled-RL, but also greatly enriches the samples for the RL learning compared with that of the Separ-RL, with an average increase of $(N/K - 1) \times 100\%$ on sample size (cf. Sect. 3.1).

To cluster the N users, we employ one of the most benchmark clustering method, i.e., K-means. The behavior information (i.e. states and rewards) in the trajectory is processed as the feature. Specifically, the T tuples of a user are stacked together $\mathbf{z}_n = [s_1, r_1, \cdots, s_T, r_T]^{\mathsf{T}}$. With this new feature, we have the objective for clustering as $J = \sum_{n=1}^{N} \sum_{k=1}^{K} r_{nk} \|\mathbf{z}_n - \boldsymbol{\mu}_k\|^2$, where $\boldsymbol{\mu}_k$ is the k-th cluster center and $r_{nk} \in \{0,1\}$ is the binary indicator variable that describes which of the K clusters the data $\mathbf{z}_n$ belongs to. After the clustering step, we have the group information $\{\mathcal{G}_k \mid k = 1, \cdots, K\}$, each of which includes a set of similar users. With the clustering results, we have the new objective for the critic updating as $\mathbf{w}_k = f(\mathbf{w}_k) = \mathbf{h}_k^*$ for $k = 1, \cdots K$, where $\mathbf{h}_k^*$ is estimated as

$$\min_{\{\mathbf{h}_k | k=1, \cdots, K\}} \sum_{k=1}^{K} \left\{ \frac{1}{|\mathcal{G}_k|} \sum_{\mathcal{U}_i \in \mathcal{G}_k} \|\mathbf{x}_i^{\mathsf{T}} \mathbf{h}_k - (r_i + \gamma \mathbf{y}_i^{\mathsf{T}} \mathbf{w}_k)\|_2^2 + \zeta_c \|\mathbf{h}_k\|_2^2 \right\}, \quad (6)$$

which could be solved via the LSTDQ. The objective for the actor updating is

$$\max_{\{\theta_k | k=1,\cdots,K\}} \sum_{k=1}^{K} \left\{ \frac{1}{|\mathcal{G}_k|} \sum_{\mathcal{U}_i \in \mathcal{G}_k} \sum_{a \in \mathcal{A}} Q\left(s_i, a; \widehat{\mathbf{w}}_k\right) \pi_{\theta_k}\left(a | s_i\right) - \frac{\zeta_a}{2} \|\theta_k\|_2^2 \right\}. \tag{7}$$

The objectives (6) and (7) could be solved independently for each cluster. By properly setting the value of K, we could balance the conflicting goal of reducing the discrepancy between connected users while increasing the number of samples for each RL learning: (a) a small K is suited for the case where T is small and the users are generally similar; (b) while a large K is adapted to the case where T is large and users are generally different from others. Besides, we find that the proposed method is a generalization of the conventional Pooled-RL and Separ-RL: (a) when $K = 1$, the proposed method is equivalent to the Pooled-RL; (b) when $K = N$, our method is equivalent to the Separ-RL.

4   Experiments

There are three RL methods for comparison: (a) the Pooled-RL that pools the data across all users and learn an identical policy [16,17] for all the users; (b) the Separ-RL, which learns a separate RL policy for each user by only using his or her data [7]; (c) The group driven RL (Gr-RL) is the proposed method.

The HeartSteps dataset is used in the experiment. It is a 42-days trial study where there are 50 participants. For each participant, 210 decision points are collected—five decisions per participant per day. At each time point, the set of intervention actions can be the intervention type, as well as whether or not to send interventions. The intervention is sent via smartphones, or via wearable devices like a wristband [1]. In our study, there are two choices for a policy $\{0,1\}$: $a = 1$ indicates sending the positive intervention, while $a = 0$ means no intervention [16,17]. Specifically, the parameterized stochastic policy is assumed to be in the form $\pi_\theta\left(a \mid s\right) = \frac{\exp[-\theta^\mathsf{T}\phi(s,a)]}{\sum_{a'}\exp[-\theta^\mathsf{T}\phi(s,a)]}$, where $\theta \in \mathbb{R}^q$ is the unknown variance and $\phi\left(\cdot, \cdot\right)$ is the feature processing method for the policy, i.e., $\phi\left(s, a\right) = [as^\mathsf{T}, a]^\mathsf{T} \in \mathbb{R}^m$, which is different from the feature for the value function $\mathbf{x}\left(s, a\right)$.

4.1   Experiments Settings

For the nth user, a trajectory of T tuples $\mathcal{D}_n = \{(s_i, a_i, r_i)\}_{i=1}^{T}$ are collected via the micro-randomized trial [7,10]. The initial state is sampled from the Gaussian distribution $S_0 \sim \mathcal{N}_p\{0, \Sigma\}$, where Σ is the $p \times p$ covariance matrix with predefined elements. The policy of selecting action $a_t = 1$ is drawn from the random policy with a probability of 0.5 to provide interventions, i.e. $\mu\left(1 \mid s_t\right) = 0.5$ for all states s_t. For $t \geq 1$, the state and immediate reward are generated as follows

$$\begin{aligned}
S_{t,1} &= \beta_1 S_{t-1,1} + \xi_{t,1}, \\
S_{t,2} &= \beta_2 S_{t-1,2} + \beta_3 A_{t-1} + \xi_{t,2}, \\
S_{t,3} &= \beta_4 S_{t-1,3} + \beta_5 S_{t-1,3} A_{t-1} + \beta_6 A_{t-1} + \xi_{t,3}, \\
S_{t,j} &= \beta_7 S_{t-1,j} + \xi_{t,j}, \qquad \text{for } j = 4, \ldots, p
\end{aligned} \tag{8}$$

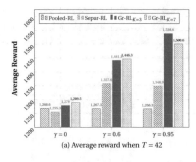 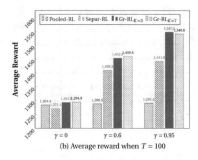

Fig. 1. Average reward of 3 RL methods: (a) Pooled-RL, (b) Separ-RL, (c) Gr-RL$_{K=3}$ and Gr-RL$_{K=7}$. The left sub-figure shows the results when the trajectory is short, i.e. $T = 42$; the right one shows the results when $T = 100$. A larger value is better.

$$R_t = \beta_{14} \times [\beta_8 + A_t \times (\beta_9 + \beta_{10} S_{t,1} + \beta_{11} S_{t,2}) + \beta_{12} S_{t,1} - \beta_{13} S_{t,3} + \varrho_t], \quad (9)$$

where $\boldsymbol{\beta} = \{\beta_i\}_{i=1}^{14}$ are the main parameters for the MDP; $\{\xi_{t,i}\}_{i=1}^{p} \sim \mathcal{N}\left(0, \sigma_s^2\right)$ is the noise in the state (9) and $\varrho_t \sim \mathcal{N}\left(0, \sigma_r^2\right)$ is the noise in the reward model (9). To mimic N users that are similar but not identical, we need N different $\boldsymbol{\beta}$s, each of which is similar with a set of others. Formally, there are two steps to obtain $\boldsymbol{\beta}$ for the i-th user: (a) select the m-th basic $\boldsymbol{\beta}$, i.e. $\boldsymbol{\beta}_m^{\text{basic}}$; it determines which group the i-th user belongs to; (b) add the noise $\boldsymbol{\beta}_i = \boldsymbol{\beta}_m^{\text{basic}} + \boldsymbol{\delta}_i$, for $i \in \{1, 2, \cdots, N_m\}$ to make each user different from others, where N_m indicates the number of users in the m-th group, $\boldsymbol{\delta}_i \sim \mathcal{N}\left(0, \sigma_b \mathbf{I}_{14}\right)$ is the noise and $\mathbf{I}_{14} \in \mathbb{R}^{14 \times 14}$ is an identity matrix. The value of σ_b specifies how different the users are. Specially in our experiment, we set $M = 5$ groups (each group has $N_m = 10$ people, leading to $N = 50$ users involved in the experiment). The basic $\boldsymbol{\beta}$s for the M groups are set as follows

$$\boldsymbol{\beta}_1^{\text{basic}} = [0.40, 0.25, 0.35, 0.65, 0.10, 0.50, 0.22, 2.00, 0.15, 0.20, 0.32, 0.10, 0.45, 800]$$
$$\boldsymbol{\beta}_2^{\text{basic}} = [0.45, 0.35, 0.40, 0.70, 0.15, 0.55, 0.30, 2.20, 0.25, 0.25, 0.40, 0.12, 0.55, 700]$$
$$\boldsymbol{\beta}_3^{\text{basic}} = [0.35, 0.30, 0.30, 0.60, 0.05, 0.65, 0.28, 2.60, 0.35, 0.45, 0.45, 0.15, 0.50, 650]$$
$$\boldsymbol{\beta}_4^{\text{basic}} = [0.55, 0.40, 0.25, 0.55, 0.08, 0.70, 0.26, 3.10, 0.25, 0.35, 0.30, 0.17, 0.60, 500]$$
$$\boldsymbol{\beta}_5^{\text{basic}} = [0.20, 0.50, 0.20, 0.62, 0.06, 0.52, 0.27, 3.00, 0.15, 0.15, 0.50, 0.16, 0.70, 450],$$

Besides, the noises are set $\sigma_s = \sigma_r = 1$ and $\sigma_\beta = 0.01$. Other variances are $p = 3$, $q = 4$, $\zeta_a = \zeta_c = 0.01$. The feature processing for the value estimation $Q^{\pi_\theta}(s, a)$ is $\mathbf{x}(s, a) = [1, s^\mathsf{T}, a, s^\mathsf{T} a]^\mathsf{T} \in \mathbb{R}^{2p+2}$ for all the compared methods.

4.2 Evaluation Metric and Results

In the experiments, the expectation of long run average reward (ElrAR) $\mathbb{E}\left[\eta^{\pi_{\hat{\theta}}}\right]$ is proposed to evaluate the quality of a learned policy $\pi_{\hat{\theta}}$ [9,10]. Intuitively in

Table 1. The average reward of three RL methods when the discount factor γ changes from 0 to 0.95: (a) Pooled-RL, (b) Separ-RL, (c) Gr-RL$_{K=3}$ and Gr-RL$_{K=7}$. A larger value is better. The **bold value** is the best and the *blue italic value* is the 2nd best.

γ	Average reward ($T = 42$)			
	Pooled-RL	Separ-RL	Gr-RL$_K = 3$	Gr-RL$_K = 7$
0	1268.6 ± 68.2	1255.3 ± 62.3	*1279.0 ± 66.6*	**1289.5 ± 64.5**
0:2	1268.1 ± 68.3	1287.6 ± 76.8	*1318.3 ± 62.5*	**1337.3 ± 56.7**
0:4	1267.6 ± 68.4	1347.0 ± 54.1	*1368.8 ± 57.6*	**1389.7 ± 50.7**
0:6	1267.3 ± 68.5	1357.6 ± 57.9	*1441.3 ± 48.2*	**1446.3 ± 46.7**
0:8	1266.8 ± 68.7	1369.4 ± 51.6	**1513.9 ± 38.8**	*1484.0 ± 44.5*
0:95	1266.3 ± 68.7	1348.9 ± 53.4	**1538.6 ± 34.3**	*1500.6 ± 42.8*
Avg	1267.4	1327.6	**1410.0**	*1407.9*
γ	*Average reward ($T = 100$)*			
0	1284.4 ± 64.1	1271.1 ± 70.7	*1293.5 ± 62.1*	**1294.9 ± 63.7**
0:2	1285.8 ± 63.9	1301.2 ± 65.6	*1329.6 ± 58.5*	**1332.9 ± 58.7**
0:4	1287.1 ± 63.8	1370.1 ± 49.1	*1385.5 ± 52.1*	**1393.0 ± 49.2**
0:6	1288.5 ± 63.6	1409.3 ± 42.2	*1452.9 ± 44.3*	**1459.6 ± 40.9**
0:8	1289.9 ± 63.4	1435.0 ± 37.6	**1519.0 ± 39.5**	*1518.0 ± 38.5*
0:95	1291.2 ± 63.2	1441.9 ± 35.9	**1547.2 ± 37.2**	*1540.6 ± 38.1*
Avg	1287.8	1371.4	*1421.3*	**1423.2**

The value of γ specifies different RL methods: (a) $\gamma = 0$ means the contextual bandit [7],(b) $0 < \gamma < 1$ indicates the discounted reward RL.

the HeartSteps application, ElrAR measures the average step a user could take each day when he or she is provided by the intervention via the learned policy $\pi_{\hat{\theta}}$. Specifically, there are two steps to achieve the ElrAR [10]: (a) get the $\eta^{\pi_{\hat{\theta}}}$ for each user by averaging the rewards over the last $4,000$ elements in the long run trajectory with a total number of $5,000$ tuples; (b) ElrAR $\mathbb{E}[\eta^{\pi_{\hat{\theta}}}]$ is achieved by averaging over the $\eta^{\pi_{\hat{\theta}}}$'s of all users.

The experiment results are summarized in Table 1 and Fig. 1, where there are three RL methods: (a) Pooled-RL, (b) Separ-RL, (c) Gr-RL$_{K=3}$ and Gr-RL$_{K=7}$. $K = 3, 7$ is the number of cluster centers in our algorithm, which is set different from the true number of groups $M = 5$. Such setting is to show that Gr-RL does not require the true value of M. There are two sub-tables in Table 1. The top sub-table summarizes the experiment results of three RL methods under six γ settings (i.e. the discount reward) when the trajectory is short, i.e. $T = 42$. While the bottom one displays the results when the trajectory is long, i.e. $T = 100$. Each row shows the results under one discount factor, $\gamma = 0, \cdots, 0.95$; the last row shows the average performance over all the six γ settings.

As we shall see, Gr-RL$_{K=3}$ and Gr-RL$_{K=7}$ generally perform similarly and are always among the best. Such results demonstrate that our method doesn't require the true value of groups and is robust to the value of K. In average, the proposed method improves the ElrAR by 82.4 and 80.3 steps when $T = 42$ as well as 49.8 and 51.7 steps when $T = 100$, compared with the best result of the state-of-the-art methods, i.e. Separ-RL. There are two interesting observations: (1) the improvement of our method decreases as the trajectory length T increases; (2) when the trajectory is short, i.e. $T = 42$, it is better to set small Ks, which emphasizes the enriching of dataset; while the trajectory is long, i.e. $T = 100$, it is better to set large Ks to simplify the data for each RL learning.

5   Conclusions and Discussion

In this paper, we propose a novel group driven RL method for the mHealth. Compared with the state-of-the-art RL methods for mHealth, it is based on a more practical assumption that admits the discrepancies between users and assumes that a user should be similar with some (but not all) users. The proposed method is able to balance the conflicting goal of reducing the discrepancy between pooled users while increasing the number of samples for each RL learning. Extensive experiment results verify that our method gains obvious advantages over the state-of-the-art RL methods in the mHealth.

References

1. Dempsey, W., Liao, P., Klasnja, P., Nahum-Shani, I., Murphy, S.A.: Randomised trials for the fitbit generation. Significance **12**(6), 20–23 (2016)
2. Geist, M., Pietquin, O.: Algorithmic survey of parametric value function approximation. IEEE TNNLS **24**(6), 845–867 (2013)
3. Grondman, I., Busoniu, L., Lopes, G.A.D., Babuska, R.: A survey of actor-critic reinforcement learning: standard and natural policy gradients. IEEE Trans. Syst. Man Cybern. **42**(6), 1291–1307 (2012)
4. Gustafson, D.: A smartphone application to support recovery from alcoholism: a randomized clinical trial. JAMA Psychiatry **71**(5), 566–572 (2014)
5. Kolter, J.Z., Ng, A.Y.: Regularization and feature selection in least-squares temporal difference learning. In: International Conference on Machine Learning, pp. 521–528 (2009)
6. Lagoudakis, M.G., Parr, R.: Least-squares policy iteration. J. Mach. Learn. Res. **4**, 1107–1149 (2003)
7. Lei, H., Tewari, A., Murphy, S.: An actor-critic contextual bandit algorithm for personalized interventions using mobile devices. In: NIPS 2014 Workshop: Personalization: Methods and Applications, pp. 1–9 (2014)
8. Li, T., Levina, E., Zhu, J.: Prediction models for network-linked data. CoRR abs/1602.01192, February 2016
9. Liao, P., Tewari, A., Murphy, S.: Constructing just-in-time adaptive interventions. Ph.D. Section Proposal, pp. 1–49 (2015)
10. Murphy, S.A., Deng, Y., Laber, E.B., Maei, H.R., Sutton, R.S., Witkiewitz, K.: A batch, off-policy, actor-critic algorithm for optimizing the average reward. CoRR abs/1607.05047 (2016)
11. Patrick, K., Raab, F., Adams, M., Dillon, L., Zabinski, M., Rock, C., Griswold, W., Norman, G.: A text message-based intervention for weight loss: randomized controlled trial. J. Med. Internet Res. **11**(1), e1 (2009)

12. Sutton, R.S., Barto, A.G.: Reinforcement Learning: An Introduction, 2nd edn. MIT Press, Cambridge (2012)
13. Xu, Z., Li, Y., Axel, L., Huang, J.: Efficient preconditioning in joint total variation regularized parallel MRI reconstruction. In: Navab, N., Hornegger, J., Wells, W.M., Frangi, A.F. (eds.) MICCAI 2015, Part II. LNCS, vol. 9350, pp. 563–570. Springer, Cham (2015). https://doi.org/10.1007/978-3-319-24571-3_67
14. Xu, Z., Wang, S., Zhu, F., Huang, J.: Seq2seq fingerprint: An unsupervised deep molecular embedding for drug discovery. In: ACM Conference on Bioinformatics, Computational Biology, and Health Informatics (2017)
15. Zhu, F., Guo, J., Li, R., Huang, J.: Robust actor-critic contextual bandit for mobile health (mhealth) interventions. arXiv preprint arXiv:1802.09714 (2018)
16. Zhu, F., Liao, P.: Effective warm start for the online actor-critic reinforcement learning based mhealth intervention. In: The Multi-disciplinary Conference on Reinforcement Learning and Decision Making, pp. 6–10 (2017)
17. Zhu, F., Liao, P., Zhu, X., Yao, Y., Huang, J.: Cohesion-driven online actor-critic reinforcement learning for mhealth intervention. arXiv:1703.10039 (2017)

Joint Correlational and Discriminative Ensemble Classifier Learning for Dementia Stratification Using Shallow Brain Multiplexes

Rory Raeper[1], Anna Lisowska[2], Islem Rekik[1(✉)],
and The Alzheimer's Disease Neuroimaging Initiative

[1] BASIRA lab, CVIP group, School of Science and Engineering, Computing,
University of Dundee, Dundee, UK
irekik@dundee.ac.uk
[2] Department of Computer Science, The University of Warwick, Coventry, UK
http://www.basira-lab.com

Abstract. The demented brain wiring undergoes several changes with dementia progression. However, in early dementia stages, particularly early mild cognitive impairment (eMCI), these remain challenging to spot. Hence, developing accurate diagnostic techniques for eMCI identification is critical for early intervention to prevent the onset of Alzheimer's Disease (AD). There is a large body of machine-learning based research developed for classifying different brain states (e.g., AD vs MCI). These works can be fundamentally grouped into two categories. The first uses *correlational* methods, such as canonical correlation analysis (CCA) and its variants, with the aim to identify most correlated features for diagnosis. The second includes *discriminative* methods, such as feature selection methods and linear discriminative analysis (LDA) and its variants to identify brain features that distinguish between two brain states. However, existing methods examine these correlational and discriminative brain data *independently*, which overlooks the complementary information provided by both techniques, which could prove to be useful in the classification of patients with dementia. On the other hand, how early dementia affects cortical brain *connections in morphology* remains largely unexplored. To address these limitations, we propose a joint correlational and discriminative ensemble learning framework for eMCI diagnosis that leverages a novel brain network representation, derived from the cortex. Specifically, we devise 'the shallow convolutional brain multiplex' (SCBM), which not only measures the similarity in morphology between pairs of brain regions, but also encodes the relationship between two morphological brain networks. Then, we represent each individual brain using a set of SCBMs, which are used to train joint ensemble CCA-SVM and LDA-based classifier. Our framework outperformed several state-of-the-art methods by 3-7% including independent correlational and discriminative methods.

© Springer Nature Switzerland AG 2018
A. F. Frangi et al. (Eds.): MICCAI 2018, LNCS 11070, pp. 599–607, 2018.
https://doi.org/10.1007/978-3-030-00928-1_68

1   Introduction

Early mild cognitive impairment (eMCI) is an early stage of dementia, that affects brain function and cognition in subtle ways that remain challenging to spot when mapping brain connections using Magnetic Resonance Imaging (MRI) in the disordered brain. Undoubtedly, understanding how early dementia alters specific brain connections across different patients might help better diagnose and stratify early stages of brain dementia, treat patients effectively, and eventually slow down worsening of symptoms and conversion to Alzheimer's Disease (AD). Within this scope, several machine learning approaches leveraged multimodal (MRI) data including resting-state functional MRI (rsfMRI) and diffusion MRI (dMRI) to distinguish between patients with MCI and healthy controls [1]. However, the very early brain states of dementia including eMCI remain least investigated in dementia literature, compared with AD and MCI states.

Recent machine-learning methods were devised for MCI identification using connectomic brain data [2,3]. However, existing works mainly used functional networks (derived from rsfMRI) and structural networks (derived from dMRI). These exclude the recent landmark works [4–6], which devised morphological brain networks (MBN) for mapping morphological 'connections' in the cortex. Basically, an MBN is generated by measuring the difference in morphology between two cortical regions based on a specific cortical attribute (e.g., sulcal depth). More importantly, [4,6] proposed to embed multiple brain networks into a multiplex network structure composed of intra-layer and inter-layer networks. Each intra-layer network in the multiplex represents an MBN derived from a specific cortical attribute, whereas an inter-layer network is a network-to-network similarity slid between two consecutive intra-layers. The integrated inter-layer network is able to capture high-order brain alterations at the morphological level. While [6] used correlational inter-layers in the brain multiplex structure for late dementia diagnosis, [4] proposed convolutional inter-layers produced by convolving two consecutive MBNs (intra-layers) in the multiplex for early dementia stratification. Notably, both multiplex architectures outperformed conventional single-layer and multi-layer brain network representations. Furthermore, while [6] used a machine learning method that identifies discriminative connectional features for dementia classification, [4] proposed a correlation-based ensemble learning framework, which identifies highly correlated multiplex features. Such approaches disentangle correlational from discriminative approaches, which might limit our understanding of disordered connectional changes in the diseased brain.

Broadly, existing classification approaches can be categorized into two groups: (1) methods that aim to identify highly correlated features such as Canonical Correlation Analysis (CCA) [4,7,8], and (2) methods that seek to identify the most discriminative features using feature selection methods such as [9] or discriminative analysis [10]. The first group includes all related CCA works and their variants such as sparse CCA (sCCA) [11] and non-linear kernel CCA (kCCA) [12]. Typically, CCA maps input features into a shared space where their correlation is maximized, and the mapped features can then be fused. The second group comprises discriminative machine learning approaches, such as Linear Discriminant Analysis (LDA), where the input features are projected onto a space where their disparity and discriminability are maximized [10]. Other methods integrate a discriminative feature selection method such as mutual information (MutInf-FS) [9] and Infinite Feature Selection (Inf-FS) [6,13]. However, a fundamental limitation of the above methods and works reviewed in [14] consists in either identifying correlational features or discriminative features for stratifying dementia states. This overlooks the complementary information that can be integrated from both correlational and discriminative approaches to further the eMCI/NC classification accuracy.

To fill this gap, we propose a joint correlational and discriminative ensemble learning framework, which first pairs multi-source brain multiplex data generated from a set of MBNs. Next, each pair is communicated to two different blocks of our framework: the first block including a set of discriminative classifiers and the second block including a set of correlational classifiers. Ultimately, we aggregate labels predicted by both blocks using majority voting to output the final label for a target testing subject. In addition to this landmark contribution, we propose a novel multi-layer brain network architecture, the shallow convolutional brain multiplex (SCBM), which unlike the deep CBM proposed in [4], is generated using only two MBNs. This avoids creating redundant features when pairing multiplexes prior to passing them forward to classifiers.

2 Ensemble LDA and CCA-SVM Paired Classifier Learning using Shallow Convolutional Brain Multiplexes

In this section, we introduce the concept of a shallow convolutional brain multiplex and present our novel joint correlational and discriminative ensemble learning framework. Fig. 1 shows the different steps for (A) shallow convolutional brain multiplex construction from cortical surface, and (B) multi-source SCBM data pairing for training the correlational block comprising a set of CCA-based SVM classifiers and the discriminative block including a set of LDA classifiers. Below we detail the different steps of our eMCI/NC classification framework.

Single-View Morphological Brain Network (MBN) Construction. For each cortical attribute (e.g., cortical thickness), we construct a single-view network for each subject. Such network comprises a set of nodes (anatomical brain regions) and a collection of edges interconnecting the nodes (representing the difference between the two brain regions in *morphology*). The average value of a cortical attribute was calculated for each anatomical region of interest (ROI). For each cortical attribute, the strength of each network edge connecting two ROIs is then computed as the absolute difference between their average values, thereby quantifying their dissimilarity (Fig. 1). The same procedure was followed to obtain the connectivity matrices from different cortical attributes (e.g., sulcal depth, curvature) [4,6].

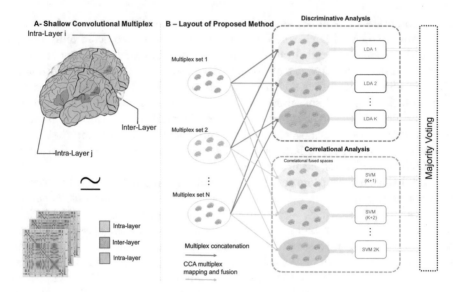

Fig. 1. *Pipeline of the proposed joint correlational and discriminative ensemble learning using shallow convolutional brain multiplexes.* (A) shows the construction of a single multiplex where the inter-layers are created between two intra-layers (two MBNs derived from the cortical surface). (B) We first represent each subject using N multiplexes, produced using different combinations of morphological brain networks. Next, for all possible combinations of multiplex pairs, each pair of multiplexes is passed into the ensemble framework, consisting of a correlational learning block (where they are mapped by CCA and classified by SVM) and a discriminative block (where they are mapped and separated into two classes by LDA). The two blocks produce predicted class labels for the test subjects based on analysis of subsequent pairs of multiplexes. The final class label is assigned through majority voting on labels assigned by the two blocks.

Convolutional Brain Multiplex Construction. In a generic way, we define a brain multiplex $\mathcal{M}$ using a set of M intra-layers (or MBNs) $\{\mathbf{V}_1, \ldots, \mathbf{V}_M\}$, each representing a single view of the brain morphology (i.e., cortical attribute), where between two consecutive intra-layers $\mathbf{V}_i$ and $\mathbf{V}_j$ we slide an inter-layer $\mathbf{C}_{i,j}$, which is defined by convolving two consecutive intra-layers. Convolution captures the signal within a subgraph (a small patch in the connectivity matrix) extracted from a first layer (whole matrix) as an expression of other subgraphs extracted from a second layer. One can think of the inter-layer network as a 'blending' of both intra-layers, expressing the amount of overlap of first intra-layer as it is shifted over the second intra-layer.

Each element in row a and column b within the convolutional inter-layer matrix $\mathbf{C}_{i,j}$ between views $\mathbf{V}_i$ and $\mathbf{V}_j$ is defined as: $\mathbf{C}_{i,j}(a,b) = \sum_p \sum_q \mathbf{V}_i(p,q)\mathbf{V}_j(a-p+1,b-q+1)$. The multiplex architecture allows not only to explore how different brain views get altered by a specific disorder, but how their relationship might get affected. Since the morphological brain connectivity matrices are symmetric (**Fig.** 1–A), we extract features from each MBN by directly concatenating the off-diagonal weights of all connectivities in each upper triangular matrix. For each network of size $n \times n$, we extract a feature vector of size $(n \times (n-1)/2)$. Previously, in [4], the generalized multiplex architecture was proposed: $\mathcal{M} = \{\mathbf{V}_1, C_{1,2}, \mathbf{V}_2, \ldots, \mathbf{V}_j, \mathbf{C}_{i,j}, \mathbf{V}_j, \ldots, \mathbf{V}_M\}$. Next, to capture the inter-relationship between all possible combinations of intra-layers in a multiplex, a set of N multiplexes were generated for each subject through reordering the intra-layer networks, thereby generating an *ensemble of brain multiplexes* $\mathbb{M} = \{\mathcal{M}_1, \ldots, \mathcal{M}_N\}$. However, this approach resulted in many highly correlated features used for the ensemble learning, which may somewhat mislead classifier learning. To minimize the correlation between different multiplexes when pairing them for ensemble classifier training, we propose a shallow (i.e., 2-layer) convolutional brain multiplex structure. We define a *shallow* multiplex $\mathcal{M} = \{\mathbf{V}_i, \mathbf{C}_{i,j}, \mathbf{V}_j\}$ using 2 intra-layers $\mathbf{V}_i$ and $\mathbf{V}_j$ and an inter-layer $\mathbf{C}_{i,j}$ encoding the relationship between $\mathbf{V}_i$ and $\mathbf{V}_j$, slid in between them (Fig. 1–A). We note that each subject-specific brain multiplex $\mathcal{M}$ in $\mathbb{M}$ captures unique similarities between two different morphological brain network views (e.g., sulcal depth network and cortical thickness network) that are not present in a different shallow multiplex.

Proposed Joint Canonical Correlational and Discriminative Mappings of SCBM Sets. Since each multiplex $\mathcal{M}_k \in \mathbb{M}$ captures a unique and complex relationship between different brain network views, one needs to examine all morphological brain multiplexes in the ensemble $\mathbb{M}$. This will provide us with a more holistic understanding of how explicit morphological brain connections can be altered by dementia onset as well as how their implicit high-order (a connection of connections) relationship can be affected. To make use of all the information available from different multiplexes, in the *correlational learning block* of our framework (outlined in green Fig. 1–B), we use CCA [7,8] to map pairs of multiplex features extracted from different sets into a shared subspace that depicts highly-correlated relevant features. We then concatenate the CCA-mapped multiplex features from the first and second sets. This correlational block allows to minimize the multiplex set-specific noise and reduces multiplex data dimensionality. Next, we use each CCA-mapped pair of multiplex features $\tilde{\mathbf{M}}_{k,l}^c$ to train a linear support vector machine (SVM) classifier (Fig. 1–B). Noting that for each training subject we have N multiplexes estimated, we perform C_N^2 mappings of each SCBM pair in $\mathbb{M}$.

Simultaneously, we train *the paralleled discriminative block* (outlined in red Fig. 1–B) aggregating sets of regularized LDA classifiers using the paired SCBM features from different sets in a *supervised* manner. Specifically, each LDA classifier attempts to maximize the difference between multiplex features so that there are distinct groups based on the given class labels. All training multiplex features are mapped into a discriminative space guided by the labels, where discriminative paired multiplex features are generated $\tilde{\mathbf{M}}_{k,l}^d$. In the testing stage, we use the learned correlational and discriminative transformations to respectively map each pair of testing multiplex feature vector onto their corresponding

CCA space where they are communicated to an SVM classifier and LDA space, respectively. Finally, to identify the label of the testing subject, we use majority voting by selecting the highly frequent predicted label outputted by classifiers in both blocks. We note that LDA performs both feature dimensionality reduction and classification, while CCA only maps the features, thus requires to be combined with a classifier such as SVM.

3   Results and Discussion

Data. We used leave-one-out cross validation to evaluate the proposed classification framework on 82 subjects (42 eMCI and 42 NC) from ADNI GO public dataset[1], each with structural T1-w MR image. We used FreeSurfer [15] to reconstruct both right and left cortical surfaces for each subject from T1-w MRI. Then we parcellated each cortical hemisphere into 35 cortical regions using Desikan-Killiany Atlas. For the deep CBM, we defined $N = 6$ multiplexes, each using $M = 4$ MBNs, anchored at $\mathbf{V}_1$. For each cortical attribute (signal on the cortical surface), we compute the strength of the morphological network connection linking i^{th} ROI to the jth ROI as the absolute difference between the averaged attribute values in both ROIs. Multiplex $\mathcal{M}_1$ includes cortical attribute views $\{\mathbf{V}_1, \mathbf{V}_2, \mathbf{V}_3, \mathbf{V}_4\}$, $\mathcal{M}_2$ includes $\{\mathbf{V}_1, \mathbf{V}_2, \mathbf{V}_4, \mathbf{V}_3\}$, $\mathcal{M}_3$ includes $\{\mathbf{V}_1, \mathbf{V}_3, \mathbf{V}_4, \mathbf{V}_2\}$, $\mathcal{M}_4$ includes $\{\mathbf{V}_1, \mathbf{V}_3, \mathbf{V}_2, \mathbf{V}_4\}$, $\mathcal{M}_5$ includes $\{\mathbf{V}_1, \mathbf{V}_4, \mathbf{V}_2, \mathbf{V}_3\}$, and $\mathcal{M}_6$ includes $\{\mathbf{V}_1, \mathbf{V}_4, \mathbf{V}_3, \mathbf{V}_2\}$. For each cortical region, $\mathbf{V}_1$ denotes the maximum principal curvature brain view, $\mathbf{V}_2$ denotes the mean cortical thickness brain view, $\mathbf{V}_3$ denotes the mean sulcal depth brain view, and $\mathbf{V}_4$ denotes the mean average curvature brain view. As for the proposed SCBM, we define $N = C_4^2 = 6$ shallow multiplexes by considering all possible pairings of 2 views out of 4. For our experiments, we created 4 representations of MBN data: (1) 'Views' by concatenating all MBNs, (2) 'Correlational multiplexes' with inter-layer computed using Pearson correlation, (3) 'Convolutional multiplexes' composed of 4 intra-layers with inter-layers generated using 2D convolution, and (4) 'Shallow convolutional multiplexes' composed of 2 intra-layers with inter-layers generated using 2D convolution.

Comparison Methods and Evaluation. To demonstrate the effectiveness of integrating correlational and discriminative methods into a single framework, we benchmarked our method against several discriminative methods including: Eigenvector Centrality (ECFS) [16], Mutual Information (MutInf-FS) [17], and Infinite Feature Selection (Inf-FS) [13]. We also benchmarked our method against the CCA-based eMCI/NC classification framework in [4]. We also evaluated the performance of each of the aforementioned discriminative methods when combined with CCA using our proposed framework using MBNs derived from the right hemisphere since significantly greater cortical atrophy is observed in the right hemisphere of MCI patients compared with the left hemisphere [18]. A leave-one-out (LOO) cross-validation (CV) scheme was used to test all these

---

[1] http://adni.loni.usc.edu.

Table 1. Average eMCI/NC classification accuracy using our method and different comparison methods.

Method	Dataset	Accuracy	Sensitivity(%)	Specificity(%)
Ensemble SVM Paired Classifiers using CCA[4]	Views	67.86	61.9	73.81
	Correlational	58.33	64.29	52.38
	Convolutional	71.43	73.81	69.05
	Shallow Conv	73.81	76.19	71.43
Ensemble SVM Paired Classifiers using ECFS[14]	Views	73.81	64.29	**83.33**
	Correlational	73.81	73.81	73.81
	Convolutional	76.19	73.81	78.57
	Shallow Conv	66.67	66.67	66.67
Ensemble SVM Paired Classifiers using CCA[6]+ ECFS[14]	Views	69.05	64.29	73.81
	Correlational	57.14	61.9	52.38
	Convolutional	70.24	73.81	66.67
	Shallow Conv	78.57	78.57	78.57
Ensemble SVM Paired Classifiers using MutInf-FS[15]	Views	72.62	66.67	78.57
	Correlational	63.1	61.9	64.29
	Convolutional	64.29	64.29	64.29
	Shallow Conv	76.19	78.57	73.81
Ensemble SVM Paired Classifiers Using CCA[6]+ MutInf-FS[15]	Views	66.67	61.9	71.43
	Correlational	54.76	57.14	52.38
	Convolutional	71.43	71.43	71.43
	Shallow Conv	77.38	78.57	76.19
Ensemble LDA Paired Classifiers[9]	Views	70.24	61.9	78.57
	Correlational	71.43	71.43	71.43
	Convolutional	77.38	78.57	76.19
	Shallow Conv	73.81	73.81	73.81
Ensemble LDA[9] and CCA-SVM[6] Paired Classifiers (**Ours**)	Views	70.24	69.05	71.43
	Correlational	70.24	66.67	73.81
	Convolutional	79.76	**78.57**	80.95
	Shallow Conv	80.95	**83.33**	**78.57**

methods, with a 5-fold nested CV to optimize the number of selected features for discriminative methods. Furthermore, each of these methods was evaluated using the 4 representations of MBN data.

Best performance. Table 1 displays the results for our proposed framework and all comparison methods. Overall, merging discriminative and correlational methods in an ensemble learning framework consistently outperformed the base methods when used independently. Furthermore, our method, combining CCA and LDA, achieved the best classification accuracy 80.95% using shallow convolutional brain multiplexes. Compared with other correlational-discriminative frameworks (e.g., CCA + ECFS) and the recent work [4], our method increased the classification accuracy by ~3-7%.

Shallow vs. deep convolutional brain multiplexes. The proposed SCBM consistently outperformed concatenated MBN views and correlation brain multiplexes across all methods –except for independent ECFS. Since different deep multiplexes contain overlapping sets of features, resulting in highly-correlated input data, it might result in a suboptimal ensemble performance. Hence, the new shallow multiplex structure solved this problem by reducing the correlation between individual classifiers in the ensemble and overall produced a better ensemble classifier performance compared to the ensemble classifier using deep convolutional multiplex structure [4].

4   Conclusion

Diagnosing early brain symptoms of dementia such as early Mild Cognitive Impairment (eMCI) is vital to prevent worsening of symptoms. To assist this diagnosis, we proposed a joint correlational and discriminative ensemble learning framework using shallow convolution brain multiplexes. Our method attained a large increase in accuracy when using both the shallow and deep convolutional data against several benchmark methods including [4], and numerous discriminative methods. A reported increase of over 7% was attained for the shallow data which supports our theory that utilizing both correlational and discriminative analysis methods yields an increase in overall performance. Another conclusion drawn from these results is the similar accuracy between the shallow and deep convolutional data with the shallow having a higher prediction accuracy frequently. This shows that investigating the similarity between two brain networks can be convenient when analyzing the multi-level effects dementia has on brain connections. Future work may integrate genomic, functional and structural networks as well as explore a wider variety of discriminative feature selection methods together with a broad array of correlational methods (such as Sparse CCA or Kernel CCA) to explore.

References

1. Brown, C.J., Hamarneh, G.: Machine learning on human connectome data from MRI. arXiv preprint arXiv:1611.08699 (2016)
2. Chen, X., Zhang, H., Gao, Y., Wee, C.Y., Li, G., Shen, D.: High-order resting-state functional connectivity network for MCI classification. Human brain mapping **37**, 3282–3296 (2016)
3. Wee, C.Y., Yang, S., Yap, P.T., Shen, D., Initiative, A.D.N., et al.: Sparse temporally dynamic resting-state functional connectivity networks for early MCI identification. Brain imaging and behavior **10**, 342–356 (2016)
4. Lisowska, A., Rekik, I., Initiative, A.D.N., et al.: Pairing-based ensemble classifier learning using convolutional brain multiplexes and multi-view brain networks for early dementia diagnosis, Springer (2017) 42–50

5. Soussia, M., Rekik, I.: High-order connectomic manifold learning for autistic brain state identification. International Workshop on Connectomics in Neuroimaging (2017) 51–59
6. Mahjoub, I., Mahjoub, M.A., Rekik, I.: Brain multiplexes reveal morphological connectional biomarkers fingerprinting late brain dementia states. Scientific reports **8**, 4103 (2018)
7. Zhu, X., Suk, H.I., Lee, S.W., Shen, D.: Canonical feature selection for joint regression and multi-class identification in alzheimer's disease diagnosis. Brain imaging and behavior **10**, 818–828 (2016)
8. Hardoon, D.R., Szedmak, S., Shawe-Taylor, J.: Canonical correlation analysis: An overview with application to learning methods. Neural computation **16**, 2639–2664 (2004)
9. Peng, H., Long, F., Ding, C.: Feature selection based on mutual information criteria of max-dependency, max-relevance, and min-redundancy. IEEE Transactions on pattern analysis and machine intelligence **27**, 1226–1238 (2005)
10. Mika, S., Ratsch, G., Weston, J., Scholkopf, B., Mullers, K.R.: Fisher discriminant analysis with kernels. Neural networks for signal processing IX, 1999. Proceedings of the 1999 IEEE signal processing society workshop. (1999) 41–48
11. Hardoon, D.R., Shawe-Taylor, J.: Sparse canonical correlation analysis. Machine Learning **83**, 331–353 (2011)
12. Akaho, S.: A kernel method for canonical correlation analysis. arXiv preprint cs/0609071 (2006)
13. Roffo, G., Melzi, S., Cristani, M.: Infinite feature selection. Proceedings of the IEEE International Conference on Computer Vision (2015) 4202–4210
14. Rathore, S., Habes, M., Iftikhar, M.A., Shacklett, A., Davatzikos, C.: A review on neuroimaging-based classification studies and associated feature extraction methods for Alzheimer's disease and its prodromal stages. NeuroImage **155**, 530–548 (2017)
15. Fischl, B.: Freesurfer. Neuroimage **62**, 774–781 (2012)
16. Roffo, G., Melzi, S.: Features selection via eigenvector centrality. Proceedings of New Frontiers in Mining Complex Patterns (NFMCP 2016)(Oct 2016) (2016)
17. Bennasar, M., Hicks, Y., Setchi, R.: Feature selection using joint mutual information maximisation. Expert Systems with Applications **42**, 8520–8532 (2015)
18. Apostolova, L.G., Steiner, C.A., Akopyan, G.G., Dutton, R.A., Hayashi, K.M., Toga, A.W., Cummings, J.L., Thompson, P.M.: Three-dimensional gray matter atrophy mapping in mild cognitive impairment and mild Alzheimer disease. Archives of neurology **64**, 1489–1495 (2007)

Statistical Analysis for Medical Imaging

FDR-HS: An Empirical Bayesian Identification of Heterogenous Features in Neuroimage Analysis

Xinwei Sun[1,6], Lingjing Hu[2(✉)], Fandong Zhang[3,6], Yuan Yao[4(✉)], and Yizhou Wang[5,6]

[1] School of Mathematical Science, Peking University, Beijing 100871, China
[2] Yanjing Medical College, Capital Medical University, Beijing 101300, China
hulj@ccmu.edu.cn
[3] Key Laboratory of Machine Perception (Ministry of Education),
Department of Machine Intelligence, School of Electronics Engineering
and Computer Science, Peking University, Beijing 100871, China
[4] Hong Kong University of Science and Technology and Peking University,
Hong Kong, China
yuany@ust.hk
[5] National Engineering Laboratory for Video Technology,
Key Laboratory of Machine Perception, School of EECS, Peking University,
Beijing 100871, China
[6] Deepwise Inc., Beijing 100085, China

Abstract. Recent studies found that in voxel-based neuroimage analysis, detecting and differentiating "procedural bias" that are introduced during the preprocessing steps from lesion features, not only can help boost accuracy but also can improve interpretability. To the best of our knowledge, GSplit LBI is the first model proposed in the literature to simultaneously capture both procedural bias and lesion features. Despite the fact that it can improve prediction power by leveraging the procedural bias, it may select spurious features due to the multicollinearity in high dimensional space. Moreover, it does not take into account the heterogeneity of these two types of features. In fact, the procedural bias and lesion features differ in terms of volumetric change and spatial correlation pattern. To address these issues, we propose a "two-groups" Empirical-Bayes method called "FDR-HS" (False-Discovery-Rate Heterogenous Smoothing). Such method is able to not only avoid multicollinearity, but also exploit the heterogenous spatial patterns of features. In addition, it enjoys the simplicity in implementation by introducing hidden variables, which turns the problem into a convex optimization scheme and can be solved efficiently by the expectation-maximum (EM) algorithm. Empirical experiments have been evaluated on the Alzheimer's

Dedicated to Professor Bradley Efron on the occasion of his 80th birthday.

Electronic supplementary material The online version of this chapter (https://doi.org/10.1007/978-3-030-00928-1_69) contains supplementary material, which is available to authorized users.

© Springer Nature Switzerland AG 2018
A. F. Frangi et al. (Eds.): MICCAI 2018, LNCS 11070, pp. 611–619, 2018.
https://doi.org/10.1007/978-3-030-00928-1_69

Disease Neuroimage Initiative (ADNI) database. The advantage of the proposed model is verified by improved interpretability and prediction power using selected features by FDR-HS.

Keywords: Voxel-based Structural Magnetic Resonance Imaging False Discovery Rate Heterogenous Smoothing · Procedural Bias Lesion voxel

1   Introduction

In recent years, the issue of model interpretability attracts an increasing attention in voxel-based neuroimage analysis of disease prediction, e.g. [5,9]. Examples include, but not limited to, the preprocessed features on structural Magnetic Resonance Imaging (sMRI) images that usually contain the following voxel-wise features: (1) lesion features that are contributed to the disease (2) procedural bias introduced during the preprocessing steps and shown to be helpful in classification [3,12] (3) irrelevant or null features which are uncorrelated with disease label. Our goal is to stably select non-null features, i.e. lesion features and procedural bias with high power/recall and low false discovery rate (FDR).

The lesion features have been the main focus in disease prediction. In dementia disease such as Alzheimer's Disease (AD), such features are thought to be geometrically clustered in atrophied regions (hippocampus and medial temporal lobe etc.), as shown by the red voxels in Fig. 1(A). To explore such spatial patterns, multivariate models with Total Variation [10] regularization can be applied by enforcing smoothness on the voxels in neighbor, e.g. the n^2GFL [15] can stably identify the early damaged regions in AD by harnessing the lesions.

Recently, another type of features called procedural bias, which are introduced during the preprocessing steps, are found to be helpful for disease prediction [12]. Again, taking AD as an example, the procedural bias refer to the mistakenly enlarged Gray Matter (GM) voxels surrounding locations with cerebral spinal fluid (CSF) spaces enlarged, e.g. lateral ventricle, as shown in Fig. 1(A). This type of features has been ignored in the literature until recently, when the GSplit LBI [12] was targeted on capturing both types of features via a split of tasks of TV regularization (for lesions) and disease prediction with general linear model (with procedural bias). By leveraging such bias, it can outperform models which only focus on lesions in terms of prediction power and interpretability.

However, GSplit LBI may suffer from inaccurate feature selection due to the following limitations in high dimensional feature space:[1] (1) multicollinearity: high correlation among features in multivariate models [14]; (2) "heterogenous features": the procedural bias and lesion features differ in terms of volumetric change (enlarged v.s. atrophied) and particularly spatial pattern (surroundingly distributed v.s. spatially cohesive). Specifically, the multicollinearity could select spurious null features which are inter-correlated with non-nulls. Moreover, GSplit

---

[1] Please refer supplementary material for detailed and theoretical discussion.

LBI fails to take into account the heterogeneity since it enforces correlation on features without differentiation. Such problems altogether may result in inaccurate selection of non-nulls, especially procedural bias. As shown in Fig. 1(B) and Table 2, the procedural bias selected by GSplit LBI are unstably scattered on regions that are less informative than ventricle. Moreover, the collinearity among features tends to select a subset of features among correlated ones, as discussed in [16]. Such a limitation leads to the ignorance of many meaningful regions (such as medial temporal lobe, thalamus etc.) of GSplit LBI in selecting lesion features, as identified by the purple frames of FDR-HS in Fig. 1(B). Moreover, the two problems above may get worse as dimensionality grows. In our experiments with a fine resolution ($4 \times 4 \times 4$ of 20,091 features), the prediction accuracy of GSplit LBI deteriorates to 89.77% (as shown in Table 3), lower than 90.91% reported in [12] with a coarse resolution ($8 \times 8 \times 8$ of 2,527 features).

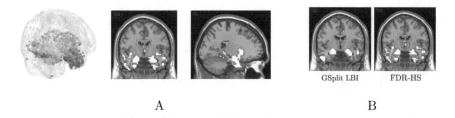

GSplit LBI   FDR-HS

A   B

Fig. 1. A: the features selected by FDR-HS (green denotes procedural bias; red denotes lesion features which are geometrically clustered) B: comparison with GSplit LBI

To resolve the problems above, we propose a "two-groups" empirical Bayes method to identify heterogenous features, called FDR-HS standing for "FDR Heterogenous smoothing" in this paper. As a univariate FDR control method, it avoids the collinearity problem by proceeding voxel-by-voxel, as discussed in [7]. Moreover, it can deal with heterogeneity by regularizing on features with different levels of spatial coherence in different feature groups, which remedies the problem of losing spatial patterns that most conventional mass-univariate models suffer from, such as two sample T-test, BH_q [4] and LocalFDR [7]. By introducing a binary latent variable, our problem turns into a convex optimization and can be solved efficiently via EM algorithm like [13]. The method is applied to a voxel-based sMRI analysis for AD with a fine resolution ($4 \times 4 \times 4$ of 20,091 features). As a result, our proposed method exhibits a much stabler feature extraction than GSplit LBI, and achieves much better classification accuracy at 91.48%.

2   Method

Our dataset consists of p voxels and N samples $\{x_i, y_i\}_1^N$ where x_{ij} denotes the intensity value of the jth voxel of the ith sample and $y_i = \{\pm 1\}$ indicates the disease status (-1 denotes AD). The FDR-HS method is proposed to select non-null features. Such method is the combination of "two-groups" model and heterogenous regularization, which is illustrated in Fig. 2 and discussed below.

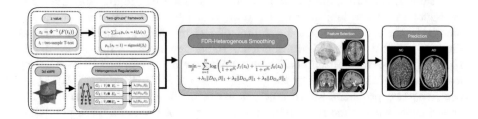

Fig. 2. Illustration of FDR-HS model.

Model Formulation. Assuming for each voxel $i \in \{1, ..., p\}$, the statistic z_i is sampled from the following mixture:

$$z_i \sim \sum_{k=0}^{1} \mathrm{p}(s_i = k)\mathrm{p}(z_i|s_i = k) = c_i f_1(z_i) + (1 - c_i) f_0(z_i), \qquad (2.1)$$

where s_i is a latent variable indicating if the voxel i belongs to the group of null features ($s_i = 0$) or the group of non-null ones ($s_i = 1$), $c_i = \mathrm{p}(s_i = 1) = \mathrm{sigmoid}(\beta_i) = e^{\beta_i}/\left(1 + e^{\beta_i}\right)$ and $z_i = \Phi^{-1}\left(F_{N-2}(t_i)\right)$ with t_i computed by two-sample t-test. Correspondingly, $f_0(\cdot)$ is density function of nulls, i.e. uncorrelated with AD and $f_1(\cdot)$ is that of non-nulls, i.e. procedural bias and lesions. The loss function can thus be defined as negative log-likelihood of z_i:

$$\ell(\beta) = - \sum_{i=1}^{N} \log \left(\frac{e^{\beta_i}}{1 + e^{\beta_i}} f_1(z_i) + \frac{1}{1 + e^{\beta_i}} f_0(z_i) \right) \qquad (2.2)$$

which can be viewed as logistic regression (when f_0 and f_1 are replaced with binaries, as (2.6)) with identity design matrix since (2.1) proceeds voxel-by-voxel. Hence, it does not have the problem of multicollinearity.

Selecting Features. To select features, we compute the posterior distribution of s_i conditioned on z_i and $\widehat{\beta}_i$ (estimated β_i) and features with

$$\mathrm{p}(s_i = 0|z_i, \widehat{\beta}_i) = \frac{(1 - \widehat{c}_i) f_0(z_i)}{\widehat{c}_i f_1(z_i) + (1 - \widehat{c}_i) f_0(z_i)} < \gamma \ \left(\widehat{c}_i = e^{\widehat{\beta}_i}/\left(1 + e^{\widehat{\beta}_i}\right)\right) \quad (2.3)$$

are selected. The $\gamma \in (0, 1)$ is pre-setting threshold parameter.

Heterogenous Spatial Smoothing. However, (2.1) may lose spatial structure of non-nulls, especially lesion features. Besides, note that the procedural bias and lesion features are heterogenous in terms of volumetric change and level of spatial coherence. Hence, to capture the spatial structure of heterogenous features, we split the graph of voxels which denotes as G^2 into three subgraphs, i.e. $G = G_1 \cup G_2 \cup G_3$ with:

$$G_1 = (V_1, E_1), \ V_1 = \{i : z_i \leq 0\}, \ E_1 = \{(i,j) \in E : z_i \leq 0, z_j \leq 0\} \quad (2.4a)$$
$$G_2 = (V_2, E_2), \ V_2 = \{i : z_i > 0\}, \ E_2 = \{(i,j) \in E : z_i > 0, z_j > 0\} \quad (2.4b)$$
$$G_3 = (V_3, E_3), \ V_3 = V_1 \cup V_2, \ E_3 = \{(i,j) \in E : z_i > 0, z_j \leq 0\} \quad (2.4c)$$

where G_1 denotes the subgraph restricted on enlarged voxels (procedural bias since -1 denotes AD); G_2 denotes the subgraph restricted on degenerate voxels (lesion features); G_3 denotes the bipartite graph with the edges connecting enlarged and degenerate voxels. The optimization function can be redefined as:

$$g(\beta) = \ell(\beta) + \lambda_{pro}\|D_{G_1}\beta\|_1 + \lambda_{les}\|D_{G_2}\beta\|_1 + \lambda_{pro\text{-}les}\|D_{G_3}\beta\|_1 \quad (2.5)$$

where $D_{G_k}\beta = \sum_{(i,j)\in E_k} \beta_i - \beta_j$ for $k \in \{1,2,3\}$ denote graph difference operator on $G_{k=1,2,3}$. By setting the group of regularization hyper-parameters $\{\lambda_{pro}, \lambda_{les}, \lambda_{pro\text{-}les}\}$ with different values, we can enforce spatial smoothness on three subgraphs at different level in a contrast to the traditional homogeneous regularization in [13]. The choice of each hyper-parameter, similar to [13], it is a trade-off between over-fitting and over-smoothing. Too small value tends to select features more than needed, while too large value will oversmooth hence the features are less clustered. Note that lesion features are more spatially coherent than procedural bias and they are located in different regions, the reasonable choice of regularization hyper-parameters tend to have $\lambda_{les} \leq \lambda_{pro} \leq \lambda_{pro\text{-}les}$.

Optimization. Note that the function (2.5) is not convex. Hence we adopted the same idea in [13] that introduced the latent variables s_i and $= 1$ if $z_i \sim f_1(z)$ and 0 if $z_i \sim f_0(z)$. The $\ell(\beta)$ and $g(\beta)$ are modified as:

$$\ell(\beta, s) = \sum_{i=1}^{N} \left\{ \log\left(1 + e^{\beta_i}\right) - s_i\beta_i \right\} \quad (2.6)$$

$$g(\beta, s) = \ell(\beta, s) + \lambda_{pro}\|D_{G_1}\beta\|_1 + \lambda_{les}\|D_{G_2}\beta\|_1 + \lambda_{pro\text{-}les}\|D_{G_3}\beta\|_1 \quad (2.7)$$

To solve (2.7), we can implement Expectation-Maximization (EM) algorithm to alternatively solve β and s. Suppose currently we are in the $(k+1)^{th}$ iteration. *In the E-step,* we can estimate s_i by expectation value conditional on (β^k, z_i):
$\tilde{s}_i = \mathrm{E}(s_i|\beta^k, z_i) = \frac{c_i^k f_1(z_i)}{c_i^k f_1(z_i)+(1-c_i^k)f_0(z_i)}$.
In the M-step, we plug $\tilde{s}_i$ into (2.7), denote $\widetilde{D}_G = \left[D_{G_1^T}, \frac{\lambda_{les}}{\lambda_{pro}}D_{G_2^T}, \frac{\lambda_{pro\text{-}les}}{\lambda_{pro}}\right.$

$\left. D_{G_3^T}\right]^T$ and expand $\ell(\beta|\tilde{s}^k)$ using a second-order Taylor approximation at the β^k. Then the M-step turns into a generalized lasso problem with square loss:

$$\min_{\beta} \frac{1}{2}\|\tilde{y} - \widetilde{X}\beta\|_2^2 + \lambda_{pro}\|\widetilde{D}_G\beta\|_1 \quad (2.8)$$

---

[2] Here $G = (V, E)$, where V is the node set of voxels, E is the edge set of voxel pairs in neighbor (e.g. 3-by-3-by-3).

where $\widetilde{X} = diag\{\sqrt{w_1}, ..., \sqrt{w_p}\}$ and $\tilde{y}_i = \sqrt{w_i}\left(\beta_i^k - \nabla_\beta \ell(\beta|\tilde{s}_i^k)_{|_{\beta^k}}/w_i\right)$ with $w_i = \nabla_\beta^2 \ell(\beta|\tilde{s}_i)_{|_{\beta^k}}$. Note that X and $\widetilde{D}_G$ are sparse matrices, hence (2.8) can be efficiently solved by Alternating Direction Method of Multipliers (ADMM) [6] which has a complexity of $O(p \log p)$.

Estimation of f_0 and f_1. Before the iteration, we need to estimate $f_0(z)$ and $f_1(z)$. The marginal distribution of z can be regarded as mixture models with p components: $z \sim \frac{1}{p}\sum_{i=1}^{p} g_i(z)$, $g_i(z) = p(s_i)p(z|s_i) = c_i f_1(z) + (1 - c_i)f_0(z)$ Hence, the marginal distribution of z is $f(z) = \bar{c}f_1(z) + (1 - \bar{c})f_0(z)$, which is equivalent to LocalFDR [7]. We can therefore implement the CM (Central Matching) [7] method to estimate $\{f_0(z), \bar{c}\}$ and kernel density to estimate $f(z)$. The $f_1(z)$ can thus be given as $(f(z) - f_0(z)\bar{c})/(1 - \bar{c})$.

3 Experimental Results

In this section, we evaluate the proposed method by applying it on the ADNI database http://adni.loni.ucla.edu. The database is split into 1.5 T and 3.0T (namely 15 and 30) MRI scanner magnetic field strength datasets. The 15 dataset contains 64 AD, 110 MCI (Mild Cognitive Impairment) and 90 NC, while the 30 dataset contains 66 AD and 110 NC. After applying DARTEL VBM [2] preprocessing pipeline on the data with scale of $4 \times 4 \times 4$ mm^3 voxel size, there are in total 20,091 voxels with average values in GM population on template greater than 0.1 and they are served as input features. We designed experiments on 1.5T AD/NC, 1.5T MCI/NC and 3.0T AD/NC tasks, namely 15ADNC, 15MCINC and 30ADNC, respectively.

3.1 Prediction Results

To test the efficacy of selected features by FDR-HS and compare it with other univariate models (as listed in Table 1), we feed them into elastic net classifier, which has been one of the state-of-the-arts in the prediction of neuroimage data [11]. The hyper-parameters are determined by grid-search. In details, the threshold hyper-parameter of p-value in T-test and q-value in BH$_q$ are optimized through $\{0.001, 0.01, 0.02, 0.05, 0.1\}$; the threshold hyper-parameter for choosing non-nulls, i.e. γ for FDR-HS (2.3) and the counterpart of LocalFDR [7], are chosen from $\{0.1, 0.2, ..., 0.5\}$. Besides, the regularization parameters λ_{pro}, λ_{les} and $\lambda_{pro\text{-}les}$ of FDR-HS are ranged in $\{0.1, 0.2, ..., 2\}$. For elastic net, the regularization parameter is chosen from $\{0.1, 0.2, ..., 2, 5, 10\}$; the mixture parameter α is from $\{0, 0.01, ..., 1\}$. Moreover, we compare our model to GSplit LBI and elastic net, adopting the same optimized strategy for hyper-parameters in [12] (the top 300 negative voxels are identified as procedural bias [12]) and those of elastic net following after the univariate models, as mentioned above.

A 10-fold cross-validation strategy is applied and the classification results for all tasks are summarized in Table 1. As shown, our method yields better results than others in all cases, that includes: (1) FDR-HS can select features with more prediction power than other univariate models due to the ability to capture heterogenous spatial patterns; (2) FDR-HS can achieve better classification results than multivariate methods in high dimensional settings, in which the non-nulls may be represented by other nulls that are highly correlated with them.

Table 1. Comparison between FDR-HS and others on 10-fold classification result

	Univariate + ElasticNet				Multivariate	
	T-test	BH$_q$ [4]	LocalFDR [7]	FDR-HS	GSplit LBI [12]	Elastic Net [16]
15ADNC	89.61%	89.61%	87.01%	**90.26%**	85.06%	87.01%
15MCINC	70.50%	71.00%	73.50%	**75.00%**	72.50%	72.00%
30ADNC	88.64%	89.77%	89.77%	**91.48%**	89.77%	88.07%

3.2 Feature Selection Analysis

We used 2-d images of 30ADNC to visualize the features of all methods under the hyper-parameters that give the best accuracy. As shown in Fig. 3, the lesion features selected by FDR-HS are located clustered in early damaged regions; while procedural bias are surrounding around lateral ventricle. Besides, such a result is given by $\lambda_{les} < \lambda_{pro} < \lambda_{pro\text{-}les}$, which agrees with that the larger value results in features with lower level of spatial coherence. In contrast, the lesions selected by T-test and BH$_q$ are scattered and redundant; some procedural bias around lateral ventricle are missed by BH$_q$ and LocalFDR. Moreover, GSplit LBI selected procedural bias on regions with CSF space less enlarged than lateral ventricle; besides, it ignored lesions located in medial temporal lobe, Thalamus and Fusiform etc., which are believed to be the early damaged regions [1,8].

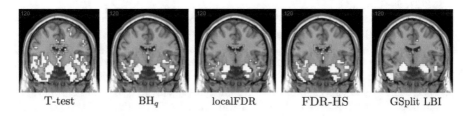

| T-test | BH$_q$ | localFDR | FDR-HS | GSplit LBI |

Fig. 3. The comparison of FDR-HS between others in terms of feature selection (30ADNC). Red denotes lesions; blue denotes procedural bias.

Besides, we also evaluated the stability of selected features using multi-set Dice Coefficient (mDC) measurement defined in [15]. Larger mDC implies more stable feature selection. As shown in Table 2, our model can obtain more stable results than GSplit LBI which suffer the "collinearity" problem.

Table 2. Comparison between FDR-HS and others on stability (measured by mDC)

	T-test	BH$_q$	LocalFDR	FDR-HS	GSplit LBI
mDC$^{(+)}$ (Lesion features)	0.6705	0.6248	0.6698	**0.6842**	0.4598
mDC$^{(-)}$ (Procedural Bias)	0.6267	0.5541	0.5127	**0.6540**	0.3033

4 Conclusions

In this paper, a "two-groups" Empirical-Bayes model is proposed to stably and efficiently select interpretable heterogenous features in voxel-based neuroimage analysis. By modeling prior probability voxel-by-voxel and using a heterogenous regularization, the model can avoid multicollinearity and exploit spatial patterns of features. With experiments on ADNI database, the features selected by our models have better interpretability and prediction power than others.

Acknowledgements.. This work was supported in part by 973-2015CB351800, NSFC-61625201, 61527804, National Basic Research Program of China (Nos. 2015CB85600, 2012CB825501), NNSF of China (Nos. 61370004, 11421110001), HKRGC grant 16303817, Scientific Research Common Program of Beijing Municipal Commission of Education (No. KM201610025013) and grants from Tencent AI Lab, Si Family Foundation, Baidu BDI and Microsoft Research-Asia.

References

1. Aggleton, J.P., Pralus, A., Nelson, A.J., Hornberger, M.: Thalamic pathology and memory loss in early alzheimer's disease: moving the focus from the medial temporal lobe to papez circuit. Brain **139**(7), 1877–1890 (2016)
2. Ashburner, J.: A fast diffeomorphic image registration algorithm. Neuroimage **38**(1), 95–113 (2007)
3. Ashburner, J., Friston, K.J.: Why voxel-based morphometry should be used. Neuroimage **14**(6), 1238–1243 (2001)
4. Benjamini, Y., Hochberg, Y.: Controlling the false discovery rate: a practical and powerful approach to multiple testing. J. R. Stat. Soc.. Ser. B (Methodol.), pp. 289–300 (1995)
5. Bießmann, F., et al.: On the interpretability of linear multivariate neuroimaging analyses: filters, patterns and their relationship. In: Proceedings of the 2nd NIPS Workshop on Machine Learning and Interpretation in Neuroimaging. Lake Tahoe: Harrahs and Harveys, (2012). Citeseer
6. Boyd, S., Parikh, N., Chu, E., Peleato, B., Eckstein, J.: Distributed optimization and statistical learning via the alternating direction method of multipliers. foundations and Trends®. Mach. Learn. **3**(1), 1–122 (2011)
7. Efron, B., Hastie, T.: Computer age statistical inference: algorithms. evidence and data science. In: Institute of Mathematical Statistics Monographs (2016)
8. Galton, C.J., et al.: Differing patterns of temporal atrophy in alzheimer's disease and semantic dementia. Neurology **57**(2), 216–225 (2001)

9. Haufe, S., Meinecke, F., Görgen, K., Dähne, S., Haynes, J.D., Blankertz, B., Bießmann, F.: On the interpretation of weight vectors of linear models in multivariate neuroimaging. Neuroimage **87**, 96–110 (2014)

10. Rudin, L.I., Osher, S., Fatemi, E.: Nonlinear total variation based noise removal algorithms. Phys. D: Nonlinear Phenom. **60**(1–4), 259–268 (1992)

11. Shen, L., et al.: Identifying neuroimaging and proteomic biomarkers for MCI and AD via the elastic net. In: Liu, T., Shen, D., Ibanez, L., Tao, X. (eds.) MBIA 2011. LNCS, vol. 7012, pp. 27–34. Springer, Heidelberg (2011). https://doi.org/10.1007/978-3-642-24446-9_4

12. Sun, X., Hu, L., Yao, Y., Wang, Y.: GSplit LBI: taming the procedural bias in neuroimaging for disease prediction. In: Descoteaux, M., Maier-Hein, L., Franz, A., Jannin, P., Collins, D.L., Duchesne, S. (eds.) MICCAI 2017. LNCS, vol. 10435, pp. 107–115. Springer, Cham (2017). https://doi.org/10.1007/978-3-319-66179-7_13

13. Tansey, W., Koyejo, O., Poldrack, R.A., Scott, J.G.: False discovery rate smoothing. J. Am. Stat. Assoc (2017). (just-accepted)

14. Tu, Y.K., Kellett, M., Clerehugh, V., Gilthorpe, M.S.: Problems of correlations between explanatory variables in multiple regression analyses in the dental literature. Br. Dent. J. **199**(7), 457 (2005)

15. Xin, B., Hu, L., Wang, Y., Gao, W.: Stable feature selection from brain sMRI. In: AAAI, pp. 1910–1916 (2014)

16. Zou, H., Hastie, T.: Regularization and variable selection via the elastic net. J. R. Stat. Soc.: Ser. B (Stat. Methodol.) **67**(2), 301–320 (2005)

Order-Sensitive Deep Hashing for Multimorbidity Medical Image Retrieval

Zhixiang Chen[1,2,3], Ruojin Cai[1], Jiwen Lu[1,2,3(✉)], Jianjiang Feng[1,2,3], and Jie Zhou[1,2,3]

[1] Department of Automation, Tsinghua University, Beijing, China
lujiwen@tsinghua.edu.cn
[2] State Key Lab of Intelligent Technologies and Systems, Tsinghua University, Beijing, China
[3] Beijing National Research Center for Information Science and Technology, Beijing, China

Abstract. In this paper, we propose an order-sensitive deep hashing for scalable medical image retrieval in the scenario of coexistence of multiple medical conditions. The pairwise similarity preservation in existing hashing methods is not suitable for this multimorbidity medical image retrieval problem. To capture the multilevel semantic similarity, we formulate it as a multi-label hashing learning problem. We design a deep hash model for powerful feature extraction and preserve the ranking list with a triplet based ranking loss for better assessment assistance. We further introduce the cross-entropy based multi-label classification loss to exploit multi-label information. We solve the optimization problem by continuation to reduce the quantization loss. We conduct extensive experiments on a large database constructed on the NIH Chest X-ray database to validate the efficacy of the proposed algorithm. Experimental results demonstrate that our order sensitive deep hashing leads to superior performance compared with several state-of-the-art hashing methods.

1 Introduction

The pictures of internal body structures produced by CT and MRI scans are important for the diagnosis and assessment of disease. The interpretation of the imaging results is objective and with high inter-observer variability due to the requirement of expertise accumulation and practical experience. To circumvent the discrepancy between expert interpretations, prior cases with similar manifestations could be presented to form a reference based assessment by content based image retrieval. For better assistance in assessment, such retrieval system should be with plenty cases of various disease manifestations, which in turn requires the similar retrieval algorithm to be both scalable and accurate.

Z. Chen and R. Cai—Co-first authors.

© Springer Nature Switzerland AG 2018
A. F. Frangi et al. (Eds.): MICCAI 2018, LNCS 11070, pp. 620–628, 2018.
https://doi.org/10.1007/978-3-030-00928-1_70

Learning based hashing methods arise to be a promising solution for such retrieval system by encoding images as compact binary codes with similarity preservation in the Hamming space [1].

Learning based hashing methods leverage the statistical properties of data samples to learn the mapping functions to generate compact binary codes. They can be broadly categorized into shallow learning based hashing methods and deep learning based hashing methods. The former takes handcrafted features like SIFT and GIST as input and learns hashing functions to transform them into compact binary codes. Representative works in this class includes Spectral Hashing (SH) [2] that solves eigenvectors of the graph Laplacian with bit balance and bit independent constraints, Iterative Quantization (ITQ) [3] that further improves the results by reducing the quantization loss through feature rotation, Semi-supervised Hashing (SSH) [4] that exploits both the unlabelled and labelled data. They learn the hashing functions in a two stage manner to optimize transformations with feature fixed, which may lead to suboptimal performance. In contrast, deep learning based hashing methods are able to tailor features for hashing through end-to-end learning on the images directly and further enhance the performance with powerful convolutional neural network. The seminal work includes Deep Hashing (DH) [5] that utilizes multi-layer neural network to capture the nonlinear neighborhood relationship between samples, Deep Supervised Hashing (DSH) [6] that introduces a regularizer to encourage outputs of neural networks to be close to binary values, HashNet [7] that continuously approximates the sign activation with smooth activations. This motivates us to leverage the deep learning framework for hashing function learning.

For similarity preservation, the objective function of hash learning, both shallow and deep learning based hashing methods, is designed to align the distances or similarities computed from the input space and the Hamming space. The alignment is usually measured over a pair of samples with discrepancy minimization [8], such as the similarity-distance production minimization in spectral hashing. The pairwise distance in the Hamming space is desired to be smaller if the pairwise similarity in the input space is larger. Such similarity preservation is also used to develop the application specific hashing methods in the community of medical image computing, such as Deep Multiple Instance Hashing for tumor assessment [9], binary code tagging and Deep Residual Hashing for chest X-ray images [10,11], etc. Note that such similarity preservation is suitable for samples with single class label. However, in the scenario of medical image, multiple symptoms or diseases may be observed from one medical image. Multilevel semantic structural similarity exists between samples, which the above pairwise alignment cannot capture. To this end, it is important to design objective function with multilevel similarity preservation in parallel to these existing methods.

In this work, we propose an order sensitive deep hashing (termed as OSDH) method for scalable medical image retrieval with multimorbidity awareness, as shown in Fig. 1. We formulate this multimorbidity aware retrieval as a multi-label hash learning problem and leverage the convolutional neural network for feature extraction. We propose to solve it by optimizing the objective of triplet based ranking similarity preservation over binary codes. We further narrow the semantic gap between learned binary codes and the associated concepts with classification supervision. We apply the proposed OSDH algorithm to clinical chest X-ray database to validate the efficacy and demonstrate superior performance over several state-of-the-art hashing methods.

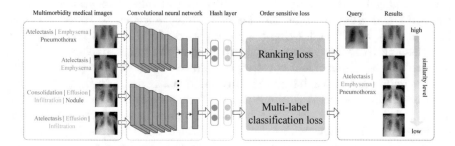

Fig. 1. Overview of the OSDH method. We learn to hash on multimorbidity medical images with order preserving by deep learning model. The retrieval results with learned binary codes are expected to preserve the multilevel similarity

2   Methodology

Mathematically, given a set of training samples $X = \{x_1, \ldots, x_N\}$ and corresponding class labels $L = \{1, \ldots, C\}$, where each sample x_i is associated with a subset of labels $Y_i \subseteq L$, our goal is to learn the hash functions to generate binary codes $B = \{b_1, \ldots, b_N\} \in \{-1, 1\}^k$ such that the multilevel semantic structural similarity of samples is preserved by the binary codes. For scalable retrieval, the length of binary code k is much smaller than the dimension of input sample.

2.1   Deep Hash Model

As shown in Fig. 1, we develop a deep hash model to jointly learn visual feature extraction and the subsequent mapping to compact binary codes. The learning procedure is applied on raw pixels of input images by using convolutional neural network for feature extraction. Such hierarchical non-linear function exhibits powerful learning capacity and encourages the learned feature to capture the multilevel semantic information. The convolutional neural network could be an off-the-shelf architecture, such as AlexNet [12] or an application specific network. On top of the network, the output of the last fully connected layer h_i is fed into the succeeding hash layer for dimensional reduction and binarization. We leverage a fully connected layer to map h_i to a k-dimension feature vector $\hat{h}_i^k$. $\hat{h}_i^k$ is then quantized to $[-1, 1]$ to produce the binary code b_i. To reduce the quantization loss, $\hat{h}_i^k$ is usually passed through an activation layer to scale the magnitude within $[-1, 1]$ before applying the binarization. While most existing works use the hyperbolic tangent function $\tanh(\hat{\boldsymbol{h}}_i^k)$ in the activation layer, we design a parameterized hyperbolic tangent function $\tanh(\alpha\hat{\boldsymbol{h}}_i^k)$ to approximate the sgn$(\cdot)$ function, as will be detailed in Sect. 2.3. By denoting the mapping from raw pixels of image $\boldsymbol{x}_i$ to the output of activation $\tanh(\alpha\hat{\boldsymbol{h}}_i^k)$ as $\boldsymbol{g}(\cdot)$ and its parameters as Θ, we can formulate the derivation of binary code as

$$\boldsymbol{b}_i = \text{sgn}\left(\boldsymbol{g}\left(\boldsymbol{x}_i, \Theta\right)\right) \tag{1}$$

2.2 Order Sensitive Supervision

To facilitate efficient multimorbidity aware retrieval, the learned binary codes are expected to preserve the multilevel semantic similarity between samples. In the context of multiple labels, the similarity between samples can be measured by the ranking order of neighbors. For each query sample $\boldsymbol{x}_q$, its semantic similarity level r with respect to a sample $\boldsymbol{x}_i$ in the database can be computed by the number of common labels shared by both $|\boldsymbol{Y}_q \cap \boldsymbol{Y}_i|$. By assigning a similarity level for each sample in the database, a ground truth ranking list for $\boldsymbol{x}_q$ can be formed by sorting samples in the decreasing order of similarity level. For each query $\boldsymbol{x}_q$ and its corresponding ranking list $\{\boldsymbol{x}_i\}_{i=1}^M$, we can define a triplet based ranking loss over binary codes,

$$\mathcal{L}_R(\boldsymbol{x}_q) = \sum_{i=1}^M \sum_{j:r_j<r_i} \frac{2^{r_i} - 2^{r_j}}{Z} max(0, D(\boldsymbol{b}_q, \boldsymbol{b}_i) - D(\boldsymbol{b}_q, \boldsymbol{b}_j) + \rho) \tag{2}$$

$D(\boldsymbol{b}_1, \boldsymbol{b}_2)$ measures the Hamming distance between the binary codes $\boldsymbol{b}_1$ and $\boldsymbol{b}_2$. ρ is introduced to control the minimum margin between the Hamming distances of the two pairs. r_i and r_j are the ground truth similarity levels of samples $\boldsymbol{x}_i$ and $\boldsymbol{x}_j$ with respect to query $\boldsymbol{x}_q$. Z is a constant related to the length of ranking list, which will be explained in Sect. 3. The coefficient $\frac{2^{r_i}-2^{r_j}}{Z}$ assigns larger weight for pair $(\boldsymbol{x}_i, \boldsymbol{x}_j)$ when $\boldsymbol{x}_i$ is more relevant to $\boldsymbol{x}_q$ than $\boldsymbol{x}_j$. By summing over all the samples $\boldsymbol{x}_i$ in the ranking list and its pair $(\boldsymbol{x}_i, \boldsymbol{x}_j)$, the minimization of (2) is able to encourage the preservation of the ranking list in the Hamming space for query $\boldsymbol{x}_q$. To preserve the semantic multilevel similarity structure, we can choose to optimize the summation of (2) over all training samples, $\sum_{\boldsymbol{x}_q \in \boldsymbol{X}} \mathcal{L}_R(\boldsymbol{x}_q)$.

While the loss in (2) is related to the relative similarity level, the label information is not fully exploited to learn hash functions. Previous works on single label data further take advantage of the label information by directly applying it to train the network [13,14]. The training procedure is performed either in the framework of two-stream multi-task learning including classification and hash or by classification over the binary codes directly. The basic assumption of such algorithm is that the binary codes should be ideal for classification. In order to further exploit the multi-label information, we choose to expect the activation output $\boldsymbol{g}(\boldsymbol{x}_i, \Theta)$ optimal for classification and jointly learn both the network and the classifier. Specifically, we design the loss of multi-label classification in the form of cross entropy,

$$\mathcal{L}_C(\boldsymbol{y}_i, \hat{\boldsymbol{y}}_i) = -\sum_{c=1}^{C} (\boldsymbol{y}_{ic} \ln \hat{\boldsymbol{y}}_{ic} + (1 - \boldsymbol{y}_{ic}) \ln (1 - \hat{\boldsymbol{y}}_{ic}))) \tag{3}$$

The ground truth label $\boldsymbol{y}_{ic} \in \{0, 1\}$ indicates whether sample $\boldsymbol{x}_i$ is with the c-th label. For sample $\boldsymbol{x}_i$, the probability belonging to the c-th class inferred by a linear classifier. By accumulating the cross-entropy loss of each class, (3) presents the multi-label classification loss for sample $\boldsymbol{x}_i$. The summation of this loss over all training samples $\sum_{i=1}^{N} \mathcal{L}_C(\boldsymbol{y}_i, \hat{\boldsymbol{y}}_i)$ could be used for optimization.

2.3   Optimization with Continuation

With the ranking preserving loss in (2) and the semantic classification loss in (3), we derive the overall objective for hash learning as

$$\arg \min_{\Theta} \mathcal{L} = \lambda_R \sum_{\boldsymbol{x}_q \in X} \mathcal{L}_R(\boldsymbol{x}_q) + \lambda_C \sum_{i=1}^{N} \mathcal{L}_C(\boldsymbol{y}_i, \hat{\boldsymbol{y}}_i) + \lambda_p \mathcal{L}_p \tag{4}$$

where λ_R, λ_C and λ_p are hyper-parameters to balance the effects of the three terms. The third term is the regularizer term over parameters of the mapping $\boldsymbol{g}$. This objective is non-differentiable due to the binary constraint of $\boldsymbol{b}_i \in \{-1, 1\}$ in (2), which makes the standard back-propagation method infeasible to train the deep model. With the activation of $\tanh(\cdot)$ being within $[-1, 1]$, most existing works circumvent the non-smooth problem with the error-prone relaxation to approximate sgn function with tanh function. In contrast, we leverage the continuation method [7] to gradually smoothing the objective with parameterized hyperbolic tangent functions with enlarging scale parameter α. The sgn function can be regarded as the parameterized tanh function with infinity scale parameter

$$\lim_{\alpha \to \infty} \tanh(\alpha \hat{\boldsymbol{h}}_i^k) = \text{sgn}\left(\hat{\boldsymbol{h}}_i^k\right) \tag{5}$$

Thus, we train the network with the initial value of scale parameter α_0 as 1 and increase it according to the predefined sequence. For each scale parameter α_i, after the network converges, we use the converged network parameters to initialize the training over next scale parameter α_{i+1}.

3   Experiments and Results

Database: Our database builds on the NIH Chest X-ray database [15], which is currently the largest public chest X-ray database. The NIH Chest X-ray database comprises of 112,120 frontal-view X-ray images from 30,805 unique patients. Each image is with multiple labels, attached with one or more of fourteen common thoracic pathologies mined from the associated radiological reports. To build our database, we selected 13,000 images of 13 most frequent pathologies, which are Atelectasis, Consolidation, Infiltration, Pneumothorax, Edema,

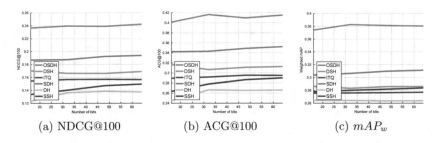

(a) NDCG@100   (b) ACG@100   (c) mAP_w

Fig. 2. Comparison of ranking performance of OSDH and other hashing methods

Emphysema, Fibrosis, Effusion, Pneumonia, Pleural_thickening, Cardiomegaly, Nodule and Mass. We constitute the training (80%) and testing (20%) sets with both patient and pathology-level non-overlapping splits to avoid positive bias.

Evaluation Settings: We compare our method with shallow learning based method: ITQ [3] and SSH [4], and deep learning based method: DH [5], SDH [5] and DSH [6]. We report their results by running the source codes provided by their respective authors to train the models by ourselves. We directly use the raw pixels as input for the convolutional neural network and 1024-D GIST feature otherwise.

In our implementation, we utilize the AlexNet network structure [12] and implement it in the Caffe [16] framework. We train the network from scratch by setting the batch size as 256, momentum as 0.9, and weight decay as 0.005. The learning rate is set to an initial value of 10^{-4} with 40% decrease every 10,000 iterations. We set the length of the ranking list M as 3 to include the samples those share all, at least one and none of the labels with the query sample. For parameter tuning, we evenly split the training set into ten parts to cross validate the parameters. We set ρ as 5, α as a sequence of 10 values from 1 to infinity, λ_R as 10^{-1}, λ_C as 1 and λ_p as 10^{-4}.

We evaluate the retrieval performance of generated binary codes with three main metrics: Normalized Discounted Cumulative Gain (NDCG) [17], Average Cumulative Gain (ACG) [17] and weighted mean Average Precision (mAP$_w$). NDCG for the truncated ranking list with p results is computed as $NDCG@p = \frac{1}{Z} \sum_{i=1}^{p} \frac{2^{r_i}-1}{\log(1+i)}$ where Z is a constant related to p to ensure the NDCG score for the correct order as 1. ACG is computed by $ACG@p = \frac{1}{p} \sum_{i=1}^{p} r_i$. And mAP$_w$ is computed by $mAP_w = \frac{1}{Q} \sum_{q=1}^{Q} \frac{\sum_{p=1}^{M} \delta(r_p>0)ACG@p}{M_{r>0}}$ with indicator function $\delta(\cdot) \in \{0,1\}$ and $M_{r>0}$ being the number of relevant samples. We evaluate the performance over binary codes with lengths of 16, 32, 48, and 64 bits.

Table 1. Performance in terms of NDCG@100 of different hashing methods

Methods	16 bits	32 bits	48 bits	64 bits
DH	0.1233	0.1364	0.1384	0.1374
ITQ	0.1545	0.1568	0.1569	0.1565
SSH	0.1337	0.1403	0.1472	0.1495
SDH	0.1868	0.1874	0.1923	0.1937
DSH	0.1701	0.1645	0.1624	0.1670
OSDH	**0.2366**	**0.2396**	**0.2390**	**0.2422**

Table 2. Performance in terms of NDCG@100, ACG@100 and mAP$_w$ for variants of the proposed OSDH method with the length of binary code as 32 bits

Methods	NDCG	ACG	mAP$_w$
OSDH-R	0.2145	0.3937	0.3645
OSDH-C	0.2091	0.3709	0.3313
OSDH	0.2396	0.4163	0.3826

Results and Analysis: Table 1 demonstrates the retrieval performance of different hashing methods in terms of NDCG@100 for different lengths of binary codes. We can observe that OSDH consistently outperforms both deep learning based hashing methods and shallow hashing methods by 5%–11%. While the deep learning based hashing methods present higher performance than the shallow ones, our OSDH further improves the results by order sensitive loss and continuation optimization. The ranking performances of all evaluated metrics are shown in Fig. 2.

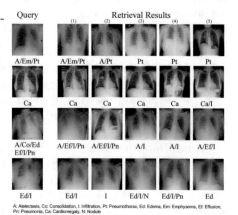

Fig. 3. Qualitative results for OSDH

Significant gaps between our OSDH and state-of-the-art methods are observed for all ranking metrics over various lengths of binary codes. The effects of ranking preservation and multi-label classification are validated. In Fig. 3, we show some retrieved results for our OSDH. Images sharing more pathologies with the query image are preferred to be ranked at top. This indicates our OSDH is able to preserve the multilevel similarity and return images with high similarity level for better assessment assistance.

To study the effects of different terms in the objective, we perform ablative testing by setting λ_R as 0 (OSDH-R) or λ_C as 0 (OSDH-C). The performance results are listed in Table 2 for 32-bit binary codes. From the table, we can find that the multi-label classification term contributes more to the performance improvement compared against the ranking list preservation. Note that the performances of both OSDH-R and OSDH-C are higher than the performances of state-of-the-art hashing methods as reported in Table 1. Combining these two loss terms, the performance is higher than individual baselines. This implies the label information is not fully exploit by the triplet based ranking loss and the ranking list information is important to capture the multilevel similarity.

4   Conclusion

In this paper, we have proposed a learning-based hashing method for scalable multimorbidity medical image retrieval for better assessment assistance. By formulating the retrieval problem as a multi-label hash learning problem, we develop an order sensitive deep hashing method to capture the multilevel semantic similarity by both ranking list preservation and multi-label classification. We propose to optimize the learning problem with continuation to reduce the quantization loss. We conduct extensive experiments to validate the superiority of the proposed OSDH in comparison with several state-of-the-art hashing methods.

Acknowledgment. This work was supported in part by the National Key Research and Development Program of China under Grant 2017YFA0700802, the National Natural Science Foundation of China under Grants 61672306, U1713214, 61572271, and 61527808, the National 1000 Young Talents Plan Program, the National Postdoctoral Program for Innovative Talents under Grant BX201700137, China Postdoctoral Science Foundation under Grant 2018M630159, Tsinghua University Initiative Scientific Research Program.

References

1. Zhang, X., Liu, W., Dundar, M., Badve, S., Zhang, S.: Towards large-scale histopathological image analysis: Hashing-based image retrieval. TMI **34**(2), 496–506 (2015)
2. Weiss, Y., Torralba, A., Fergus, R.: Spectral hashing. In: NIPS, pp. 1753–1760 (2008)
3. Gong, Y., Lazebnik, S., Gordo, A., Perronnin, F.: Iterative quantization: a procrustean approach to learning binary codes for large-scale image retrieval. TPAMI **35**(12), 2916–2929 (2013)
4. Wang, J., Kumar, S., Chang, S.: Semi-supervised hashing for large-scale search. TPAMI **34**(12), 2393–2406 (2012)
5. Liong, V.E., Lu, J., Wang, G., Moulin, P., Zhou, J.: Deep hashing for compact binary codes learning. In: CVPR, pp. 2475–2483 (2015)
6. Liu, H., Wang, R., Shan, S., Chen, X.: Deep supervised hashing for fast image retrieval. In: CVPR, pp. 2064–2072 (2016)
7. Cao, Z., Long, M., Wang, J., Yu, P.S.: Hashnet: deep learning to hash by continuation. In: ICCV, pp. 5608–5617 (2017)
8. Wang, J., Zhang, T., Song, J., Sebe, N., Shen, H.T.: A survey on learning to hash. CoRR abs/1606.00185 (2016)
9. Conjeti, S., Paschali, M., Katouzian, A., Navab, N.: Deep multiple instance hashing for scalable medical image retrieval. In: MICCAI, pp. 550–558 (2017)
10. Sze-To, A., Tizhoosh, H.R., Wong, A.K.C.: Binary codes for tagging x-ray images via deep de-noising autoencoders. In: IJCNN, pp. 2864–2871 (2016)
11. Conjeti, S., Roy, A.G., Katouzian, A., Navab, N.: Hashing with residual networks for image retrieval. In: MICCAI, pp. 541–549 (2017)
12. Krizhevsky, A., Sutskever, I., Hinton, G.E.: Imagenet classification with deep convolutional neural networks. In: NIPS, pp. 1106–1114 (2012)

13. Li, Q., Sun, Z., He, R., Tan, T.: Deep supervised discrete hashing. In: NIPS, pp. 2479–2488 (2017)
14. Yang, H., Lin, K., Chen, C.: Supervised learning of semantics-preserving hash via deep convolutional neural networks. TPAMI **40**(2), 437–451 (2018)
15. Wang, X., Peng, Y., Lu, L., Lu, Z., Bagheri, M., Summers, R.M.: Chestx-ray8: hospital-scale chest x-ray database and benchmarks on weakly-supervised classification and localization of common thorax diseases. In: CVPR, pp. 3462–3471 (2017)
16. Jia, Y., et al.: Caffe: convolutional architecture for fast feature embedding. In: ACM MM, pp. 675–678 (2014)
17. Järvelin, K., Kekäläinen, J.: IR evaluation methods for retrieving highly relevant documents. In: SIGIR, pp. 41–48 (2000)

Exact Combinatorial Inference
for Brain Images

Moo K. Chung[1(✉)], Zhan Luo[1], Alex D. Leow[2], Andrew L. Alexander[1],
Richard J. Davidson[1], and H. Hill Goldsmith[1]

[1] University of Wisconsin, Madison, USA
mkchung@wisc.edu
[2] University of Illinois, Chicago, USA

Abstract. The permutation test is known as the exact test procedure in statistics. However, often it is not exact in practice and only an approximate method since only a small fraction of every possible permutation is generated. Even for a small sample size, it often requires to generate tens of thousands permutations, which can be a serious computational bottleneck. In this paper, we propose a novel combinatorial inference procedure that enumerates all possible permutations combinatorially without any resampling. The proposed method is validated against the standard permutation test in simulation studies with the ground truth. The method is further applied in twin DTI study in determining the genetic contribution of the minimum spanning tree of the structural brain connectivity.

1 Introduction

The permutation test is perhaps the most widely used nonparametric test procedure in sciences [1,7,10]. It is known as the exact test in statistics since the distribution of the test statistic under the null hypothesis can be exactly computed if we can calculate all possible values of the test statistic under every possible permutation. Unfortunately, generating every possible permutation for whole images is still extremely time consuming even for modest sample size.

When the total number of permutations are too large, various resampling techniques have been proposed to speed up the computation in the past. In the resampling methods, only a small fraction of possible permutations are generated and the statistical significance is computed *approximately*. This approximate permutation test is the most widely used version of the permutation test. In most of brain imaging studies, 5000–1000000 permutations are often used, which puts the total number of generated permutations usually less than 1% of all possible permutations. In [10], 5000 permutations are out of possible $\binom{27}{12} = 17383860$ permutations (2.9%) were used. In [7], for instance, 1 million permutations out of $\binom{40}{20}$ possible permutations (0.07%) were generated using a super computer.

In this paper, we propose a novel *combinatorial inference* procedure that enumerates all possible permutations combinatorially and simply avoids resampling that is slow and approximate. Unlike the permutation test that takes few

© Springer Nature Switzerland AG 2018
A. F. Frangi et al. (Eds.): MICCAI 2018, LNCS 11070, pp. 629–637, 2018.
https://doi.org/10.1007/978-3-030-00928-1_71

hours to few days in a desktop, our exact procedure takes few seconds. Recently combinatorial approaches for statistical inference are emerging as an powerful alternative to existing statistical methods [1,5]. Neykov et al. proposed a combinatorial technique for graphical models. However, their approach still relies on bootstrapping, which is another resampling technique and still approximate [5]. Chung et al. proposed another combinatorial approach for brain networks but their method is limited to integer-valued graph features [1]. Our main contributions of this paper are as follows.

(1) A new combinational approach for the permutation test that does not require resampling. While the permutation tests require exponential run time and approximate [1], our combinatorial approach requires $\mathcal{O}(n^2)$ run time and exact. (2) Showing that the proposed method is a more sensitive and powerful alternative to the existing permutation test through extensive simulation studies. (3) A new formulation for testing the brain network

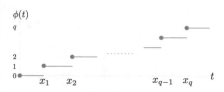

Fig. 1. Monotone sequence $x_1 < x_2 < \cdots < x_q$ is mapped to integers between 1 and q *without* any gap via $\phi(t)$.

differences by using the minimum spanning tree differences. The proposed framework is applied to a twin DTI study in determining the heritability of the structural brain network.

2   Exact Combinatorial Inference

The method in this paper extends our previous *exact topological inference* [1], which is limited to integer-valued monotone functions from graphs. Through Theorem 1, we extend the method to any arbitrary monotone function.

Definition 1. *For any sets G_1 and G_2 satisfying $G_1 \subset G_2$, function f is strictly monotone if it satisfies $f(G_1) < f(G_2)$. $\subset$ denotes the strict subset relation.*

Theorem 1. *Let f be a monotone function on the nested set $G_1 \subset G_2 \subset \cdots \subset G_q$. Then there exists a nondecreasing function ϕ such that $\phi \circ f(G_j) = j$.*

Proof. We prove the statement by actually constructing such a function. Function ϕ is constructed as follows. Let $x_j = f(G_j)$. Then obviously $x_1 < x_2 < \cdots < x_q$. Define an increasing step function ϕ such that

$$\phi(t) = 0 \text{ if } t < x_1, \quad \phi(t) = j \text{ if } x_j \leq t < x_{j+1}, \quad \phi(t) = q \text{ if } x_q \leq t.$$

The step function ϕ is illustrated in Fig. 1. Then it is straightforward to see that $\phi \circ f(G_j) = j$ for all $1 \leq j \leq q$. Further ϕ is nondecreasing. □

Consider two nested sets $F_1 \subset F_2 \subset \cdots \subset F_q$ and $G_1 \subset G_2 \subset \cdots \subset G_q$. We are interested in testing the null hypothesis H_0 of the equivalence of two monotone functions defined on the nested sets:

$$f(F_1) < f(F_2) < \cdots < f(F_q) \quad \text{vs.} \quad g(G_1) < g(G_2) < \cdots < g(G_q).$$

We have nondecreasing functions ϕ and ψ on $f(F_j)$ and $g(G_j)$ respectively that satisfies the condition Theorem 1. We use pseudo-metric

$$D_q = \max_t |\phi(t) - \psi(t)|$$

as a test statistic that measures the similarity between two monotone functions. The use of maximum removes the problem of multiple comparisons. The distribution of D_q can be determined by combinatorially.

Theorem 2. $P(D_q \geq d) = 1 - \frac{A_{q,q}}{\binom{2q}{q}}$, where $A_{u,v}$ satisfies $A_{u,v} = A_{u-1,v} + A_{u,v-1}$ with the boundary condition $A_{0,v} = A_{u,0} = 1$ within band $|u - v| < d$ and initial condition $A_{0,0} = 0$ for $u, v \geq 1$.

Proof. Let $x_j = \phi \circ f(F_j)$ and $y_j = \phi \circ g(G_j)$. From Theorem 1, the sequences $x_1, \cdots, x_q$ and $y_1, \cdots, y_q$ are monotone and integer-valued between 1 and q *without* any gap. Perform the permutation test on the sorted sequences. If we identify each x_j as moving one grid to right and y_j as moving one grid to up, each permutation is mapped to a walk from $(0,0)$ to (q, q). There are total $\binom{2q}{q}$ number of such paths and each permutation can be mapped to a walk uniquely.

Note $\max_{1 \leq j \leq q} |x_j - y_j| < d$ if and only if $|x_j - y_j| < d$ for all $1 \leq j \leq q$. Let $A_{q,q}$ be the total number of paths within $|x - y| < d$ (Fig. 2 for an illustration). Then it follows that $A_{q,q}$ is iteratively given as $A_{u,v} = A_{u-1,v} + A_{u,v-1}$ with $A_{0,0} = 0$, $A_{0,v} = A_{u,0} = 1$, within $|u - v| < d$. Thus $P(D_q < d) = \frac{A_{q,q}}{\binom{2q}{q}}$. □

For example, $P(D_3 \geq 2)$ is computed sequentially as follows (Fig. 2). We start with the bottom left corner $A_{0,0} = 0$ and move right or up toward the upper corner. $A_{1,0} = 1$, $A_{0,1} = 1 \rightarrow A_{1,1} = A_{1,0} + A_{0,1} \rightarrow \cdots \rightarrow A_{3,3} = A_{3,2} + A_{2,3} = 8$. The probability is then $P(D_3 \geq 2) = 1 - 8/\binom{6}{3} = 0.6$. The computational complexity of the combinatorial inference is $\mathcal{O}(q^2)$ for computing $A_{q,q}$ in the grid while the permutation test is exponential.

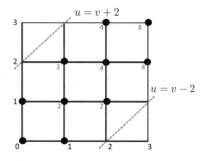

Fig. 2. In this example, $A_{u,v}$ is computed within the boundary (dotted red line) from $(0,0)$ to $(3,3)$.

3   Inference on Minimum Spanning Trees

As a specific example of how to apply the method, we show how to test for shape differences in minimum spanning trees (MST) of graphs. MST are often used in speeding up computation and simplifying complex graphs as simpler trees [9]. We et al. used MST in edge-based segmentation of lesion in brain MRI [9]. Stam et al. used MST as an unbiased skeleton representation of complex brain networks [6]. Existing statistical inference methods on MST rely on using graph theory features on MST such as the average path length. Since the probability distribution of such features are often not well known, the permutation test is frequently used, which is not necessarily exact or effective. Here, we apply the proposed combinatorial inference for testing the shape differences of MST.

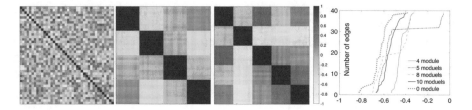

Fig. 3. Randomly simulated correlation matrices with 0, 4 and 5 modules. The plot shows the number of nodes over the largest edge weights added into MST construction during Kruskal's algorithm for 4, 5, 8, 10 and 0 modules.

For a graph with p nodes, MST is often constructed using Kruskal's algorithm, which is a greedy algorithm with runtime $\mathcal{O}(p \log p)$. The algorithm starts with an edge with the smallest weight. Then add an edge with the next smallest weight. This sequential process continues while avoiding a loop and generates a spanning tree with the smallest total edge weights. Thus, the edge weights in MST correspond to the order, in which the edges are added in the construction of MST. Let M_1 and M_2 be the MST corresponding to $p \times p$ connectivity matrices C_1 and C_2. We are interested in testing hypotheses

$$H_0 : M_1 = M_2 \quad \text{vs.} \quad H_1 : M_1 \neq M_2.$$

The statistic for testing H_0 vs. H_1 is as follows. Since there are p nodes, there are $p-1$ edge weights in MST. Let $w_1^1 < w_2^1 < \cdots < w_{p-1}^1$ and $w_1^2 < w_2^2 < \cdots < w_{p-1}^2$ be the sorted edge weights in M_1 and M_2 respectively. These correspond to the order MST are constructed in Kruskal's algorithm. w_j^1 and w_j^2 are edge weights obtained in the j-th iteration of Kruskal's algorithm. Let ϕ and ψ be monotone step functions that map the the edge weights obtained in the j-th iteration to integer j, i.e., $\phi(w_j^1) = j$, $\psi(w_j^2) = j$. ϕ and ψ can be interpreted as the number of nodes added into MST in the j-th iteration.

4   Validation and Comparisons

For validation and comparisons, we simulated the random graphs with the ground truth. We used $p = 40$ nodes and $n = 10$ images, which makes possible permutations to be exactly $\binom{10+10}{10} = 184756$ making the permutation test manageable. The data matrix $X_{n \times p} = (x_{ij}) = (\mathbf{x}_1, \mathbf{x}_2, \cdots, \mathbf{x}_p)$ is simulated as standard normal in each component, i.e., $x_{ij} \sim N(0,1)$. or equivalently each column is multivariate normal $\mathbf{x}_j \sim N(0,I)$ with identity matrix as the covariance.

Table 1. Simulation results given in terms of p-values. In the case of no network differences (0 vs. 0 and 4 vs. 4), higher p-values are better. In the case of network differences (4 vs. 5, 4 vs. 8 and 5 vs. 10), smaller p-values are better.

	Combinatorial	Permute 0.1%	Permute 0.5%	Permute 1%
0 vs. 0	0.831 ± 0.187	0.746 ± 0.196	0.745 ± 0.195	0.744 ± 0.196
4 vs. 4	0.456 ± 0.321	0.958 ± 0.075	0.958 ± 0.073	0.958 ± 0.073
4 vs. 5	0.038 ± 0.126	0.381 ± 0.311	0.377 ± 0.311	0.378 ± 0.311
4 vs. 8	0.053 ± 0.138	0.410 ± 0.309	0.411 ± 0.306	0.411 ± 0.306
5 vs. 10	0.060 ± 0.126	0.391 ± 0.283	0.395 ± 0.284	0.395 ± 0.283

Let $Y = (y_{ij}) = (\mathbf{y}_1, \cdots, \mathbf{y}_p) = X$. So far, there is no statistical dependency between nodes in Y. We add the following block modular structure to Y. We assume there are $k = 4, 5, 8, 10, 40$ modules and each module consists of $c = p/k = 10, 8, 5, 4, 1$ number of nodes. Then for the i-th node in the j-th module, we simulate

$$\mathbf{y}_{c(j-1)+i} = \mathbf{x}_{c(j-1)+1} + N(0, \sigma I) \quad \text{for } 1 \le i \le c, 1 \le j \le k \tag{1}$$

with $\sigma = 0.1$. Subsequently, the connectivity matrix $C = (c_{ij})$ is given by $c_{ij} = corr(\mathbf{y}_i, \mathbf{y}_j)$. This introduces the block modular structure in the correlation network (Fig. 3). For 40 modules, each module consists of just 1 node, which is basically a network with 0 module.

Using (1), we simulated random networks with 4, 5, 8, 10 and 0 modules. For each network, we obtained MST and computed the distance D between networks. We computed the p-value using the combinatorial method. In comparison, we performed the permutation tests by permuting the group labels and generating 0.1, 0.5 and 1% of every possible permutation. The procedures are repeated 100 times and the average results are reported in Table 1.

In the case of no network differences (0 vs. 0 and 4 vs. 4), higher p-values are better. The combinatorial method and the permutation tests all performed well for no network difference. In the case of network differences (4 vs. 5, 4 vs. 8 and 5 vs. 10), smaller p-values are better. The combinatorial method performed far superior to the permutation tests. None of the permutation tests detected modular structure differences. The proposed combinatorial approach on MST seems to be far more sensitive in detecting modular structures. The performance of the permutation test does not improve even when we sample 10% of all possible permutations. The permutation test doesn't converge rapidly with increased samples. The codes for performing exact combinatorial inference as well as simulations can be obtained from http://www.stat.wisc.edu/~mchung/twins.

5   Application to Twin DTI Study

Subjects. The method is applied to 111 twin pairs of diffusion weighted images (DWI). Participants were part of the Wisconsin Twin Project [2]. 58 monozy-

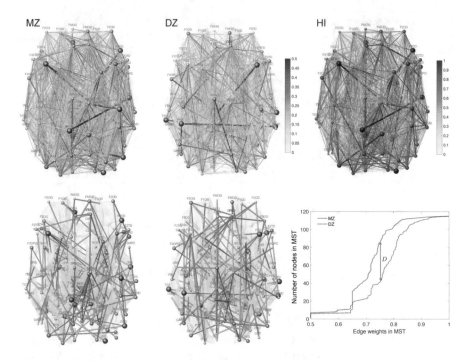

Fig. 4. Top: Correlation network of MZ- and DZ-twins and heritability index (HI). Bottom: Minimum spanning trees (MST) constructed using Kruskal's algorithm on 1-correlation. Plot: The number of added nodes is plotted over the largest edge weights of MST for MZ- (solid red) and DZ-twins (dotted black) during the MST construction. The pseudo-metric D is 46 at edge weight 0.75 (corresponding to correlation 0.25).

gotic (MZ) and 53 same-sex dizygotic (DZ) twins were used in the analysis. We are interested in knowing the extent of the genetic influence on the structural brain network of these participants and determining its statistical significance between MZ- and DZ-twins. Twins were scanned in a 3.0 Tesla GE Discovery MR750 scanner with a 32-channel receive-only head coil. Diffusion tensor imaging (DTI) was performed using a three-shell diffusion-weighted, spin-echo, echo-planar imaging sequence. A total of 6 non-DWI (b = 0 s·mm2) and 63 DWI with non-collinear diffusion encoding directions were collected at b = 500, 800, 2000 (9, 18, 36 directions). Other parameters were TR/TE = 8575/76.6 ms; parallel imaging; flip angle = 90°; isotropic 2 mm resolution (128 × 128 matrix with 256 mm field-of-view).

Image Processing. FSL were used to correct for eddy current related distortions, head motion and field inhomogeneity. Estimation of the diffusion tensors at each voxel was performed using non-linear tensor estimation in CAMINO. DTI-TK was used for constructing the study-specific template [3]. Spatial normalization was performed for tensor-based white matter alignment using a non-parametric diffeomorphic registration method [11]. Each subject's tractography was constructed in the study template space using the streamline method, and tracts

were terminated at FA-value less than 0.2 and deflection angle greater than 60°
[4]. Anatomical Automatic Labeling (AAL) with $p = 116$ parcellations were used
to construct $p \times p$ structural connectivity matrix that counts the number of white
matter fiber tracts between the parcellations [8].

Exact Combinatorial Inference. From the individual structural connectivity
matrices, we computed pairwise twin correlations in each group using Spearman's correlation. The resulting twin correlations matrices C_{MZ} and C_{DZ} (edge
weights in Fig. 4) were used to compute the heritability index (HI) through
Falconer's formula, which determines the amount of variation due to genetic
influence in a population: HI $= 2(C_{MZ} - C_{DZ})$ [1]. Although HI provides quantitative measure of heritability, it is not clear if it is statistically significant. We
tested the significance of HI by testing the equality of C_{MZ} and C_{DZ}. We used
$1 - C_{MZ}$ and $1 - C_{DZ}$ as edge weights in finding MST using Kruskal's algorithm. This is equivalent to using C_{MZ} and C_{DZ} as edge weights in finding the
maximum spanning trees. Figure 4 plot shows how the number of nodes increase
as the edges are added into the MST construction. At the same edge weights,
MZ-twins are more connected than DZ-twins in MST. This implies MZ-twins are
connected less in lower correlations and connected more in higher correlations.

Results. At edge weight 0.75, which is the maximum gap and corresponding
to correlation 0.25, the observed distance D was 46. The corresponding p-
value was computed as $P(D \geq 46) = 1.57 \times 10^{-8}$. The localized regions of
brain that genetically contribute the most can also be identified by identifying the nodes of connections around edge weight 0.75 (0.75 ± 0.2). The following AAL regions are identified as the region of statistically significant MST
differences: Frontal-Mid-L, Frontal-Mid-R, Frontal-Inf-Oper-R, Rolandic-Oper-
R, Olfactory-L, Frontal-Sup-Medial-L, Frontal-Sup-Medial-R, Occipital-Inf-L,
SupraMarginal-R, Precuneus-R, Caudate-L, Putamen-L, Temporal-Pole-Sup-L,
Temporal-Pole-Sup-R, Temporal-Pole-Mid-R, Cerebelum-Crus2-R, Cerebelum-
8-R, Vermis-8 (Fig. 5). The identified frontal and temporal regions are overlapping with the previous MRI-based twin study [7].

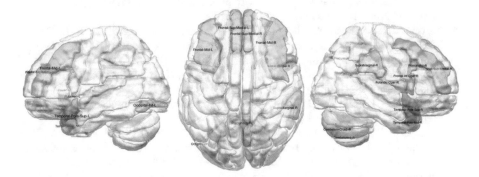

Fig. 5. Regions corresponding to the maximum difference between MST of MZ- and
DZ-twins.

6   Conclusion and Discussion

We presented the novel exact combinatorial inference method that outperforms the traditional permutation test. The main innovation of the method is that it works for any monotone features. Given any two sets of measurements, all it requires is to sort them and we can apply the method. Thus, the method can be applied to wide variety of applications. For this study, we have shown how to apply the method in testing the shape differences in MST of the structural brain networks. The method was further utilized in localizing brain regions influencing such differences.

In graphs, there are many monotone functions including the number of connected components, total node degrees and the sorted eigenvalues of graph Laplacians. These monotone functions can all be used in the proposed combinatorial inference. The proposed method is also equally applicable to wide variety of monotonically decreasing graph features such as the largest connected components [1]. If $\phi \circ f$ is monotonically decreasing, $-\phi \circ f$ is monotonically increasing, thus the same method is applicable to decreasing functions. The applications of other features are left for future studies.

Acknowledgements. This work was supported by NIH grants R01 EB022856, R01 MH101504, P30 HD003352, U54 HD09025, UL1 TR002373. We thank Nagesh Adluru, Yuan Wang, Andrey Gritsenko (University of Wisconsin-Madison), Hyekyoung Lee (Seoul National University), Zachery Morrissey (University of Illinois-Chicago) and Sourabh Palande, Bei Wang (University of Utah) for valuable supports.

References

1. Chung, M.K., Villalta-Gil, V., Lee, H., Rathouz, P.J., Lahey, B.B., Zald, D.H.: Exact topological inference for paired brain networks *via* persistent homology. In: Niethammer, M. (ed.) IPMI 2017. LNCS, vol. 10265, pp. 299–310. Springer, Cham (2017). https://doi.org/10.1007/978-3-319-59050-9_24
2. Goldsmith, H.H., Lemery-Chalfant, K., Schmidt, N.L., Arneson, C.L., Schmidt, C.K.: Longitudinal analyses of affect, temperament, and childhood psychopathology. Twin Res. Hum. Genet. **10**, 118–126 (2007)
3. Hanson, J.L., Adluru, N., Chung, M.K., Alexander, A.L., Davidson, R.J., Pollak, S.D.: Early neglect is associated with alterations in white matter integrity and cognitive functioning. Child Develop. **84**, 1566–1578 (2013)
4. Lazar, M., et al.: White matter tractography using tensor deflection. Hum. Brain Mapp. **18**, 306–321 (2003)
5. Neykov, M., Lu, J., Liu, H.: Combinatorial inference for graphical models. arXiv preprint arXiv:1608.03045 (2016)
6. Stam, C.J., Tewarie, P., Van Dellan, E., van Straaten, E.C.W., Hillebrand, A., Van Mieghem, P.: The trees and the forest: Characterization of complex brain networks with minimum spanning trees. Int. J. Psychophysiol. **92**, 129–138 (2014)
7. Thompson, P.M., et al.: Genetic influences on brain structure. Nat. Neurosci. **4**, 1253–1258 (2001)

8. Tzourio-Mazoyer, N., et al.: Automated anatomical labeling of activations in spm using a macroscopic anatomical parcellation of the MNI MRI single-subject brain. NeuroImage **15**, 273–289 (2002)

9. Wu, Z., Leahy, R.: An optimal graph theoretic approach to data clustering: theory and its application to image segmentation. IEEE Trans. Pattern Anal. Mach. Intell. **15**, 1101–1113 (1993)

10. Zalesky, A., et al.: Whole-brain anatomical networks: does the choice of nodes matter? NeuroImage **50**, 970–983 (2010)

11. Zhang, H., Yushkevich, P.A., Alexander, D.C., Gee, J.C.: Deformable registration of diffusion tensor MR images with explicit orientation optimization. Med. Image Anal. **10**, 764–785 (2006)

Statistical Inference with Ensemble of Clustered Desparsified Lasso

Jérôme-Alexis Chevalier[1,2]([✉]), Joseph Salmon[2], and Bertrand Thirion[1]

[1] Parietal Team, Inria, CEA, Paris-Saclay University, Paris, France
{jerome-alexis.chevalier,thirion}@inria.fr
[2] Telecom ParisTech, Paris, France
joseph.salmon@telecom.paristech.fr

Abstract. Medical imaging involves high-dimensional data, yet their acquisition is obtained for limited samples. Multivariate predictive models have become popular in the last decades to fit some external variables from imaging data, and standard algorithms yield point estimates of the model parameters. It is however challenging to attribute confidence to these parameter estimates, which makes solutions hardly trustworthy. In this paper we present a new algorithm that assesses parameters statistical significance and that can scale even when the number of predictors $p \geq 10^5$ is much higher than the number of samples $n \leq 10^3$, by leveraging structure among features. Our algorithm combines three main ingredients: a powerful inference procedure for linear models –the so-called Desparsified Lasso– feature clustering and an ensembling step. We first establish that Desparsified Lasso alone cannot handle $n \ll p$ regimes; then we demonstrate that the combination of clustering and ensembling provides an accurate solution, whose specificity is controlled. We also demonstrate stability improvements on two neuroimaging datasets.

1 Introduction

Prediction problems in medical imaging are typically high-dimensional small-sample problems. Training such models can be seen as an inference procedure. As in all research fields, this inference has to come with probabilistic guarantees in order to assess its reliability and to clarify further interpretation. In such settings, linear models have raised a strong interest. In particular the Lasso, introduced in [9], has been thoroughly investigated in [5]. Specifically, for settings in which the number of features p is greater than the number of samples n –though commensurate– numerous inference solutions have been proposed: see among others [2,3,8,11,12]. However, when $n \ll p$, these inference solutions are not scalable. In practice they fail to be informative, as we will show in our first simulation (cf. Sec. 3.1). Indeed, in these regimes, due to the curse of dimensionality, localizing statistical effects becomes much harder and an informative inference seems hopeless without dimensionality reduction. However, in high dimension, datasets often exhibit a particular data structure and inter-predictors correlation. This makes dimension reduction possible by the means of

© Springer Nature Switzerland AG 2018
A. F. Frangi et al. (Eds.): MICCAI 2018, LNCS 11070, pp. 638–646, 2018.
https://doi.org/10.1007/978-3-030-00928-1_72

clustering algorithms which should respect data structure as described in [10]. The issue with clustering-based solutions is that clustering is almost surely suboptimal and unstable; it carries some arbitrariness related to initialization or estimators heuristics. A solution to mitigate this confounding factor is to embed it in a bagging strategy, as done e.g. in [10].

Our contribution is an algorithm for statistical inference in high-dimensional scenarios, combining the Desparsified Lasso procedure, first introduced in [12], with clustering and bagging steps: the Ensemble of Clustered Desparsified Lasso. We describe it in detail and provide experiments on simulated and real data to assess its potential on multivariate linear models for medical imaging.

2   Theoretical and Algorithmic Framework

Notations. For clarity, scalars are denoted with normal font, vectors with bold lowercase, and matrices with bold uppercase letters. For $p \in \mathbb{N}$, $[p] = \{1, \ldots, p\}$.

Inference on Linear Models. Our aim is to give confidence bounds on the coefficients of the parameter vector denoted $\mathbf{w}^*$ in the following linear model:

$$\mathbf{y} = \mathbf{X}\mathbf{w}^* + \sigma_* \boldsymbol{\varepsilon} \;, \tag{1}$$

where $\mathbf{y} \in \mathbb{R}^n, \mathbf{X} \in \mathbb{R}^{n \times p}, \mathbf{w}^* \in \mathbb{R}^p$, $\boldsymbol{\varepsilon} \sim \mathcal{N}(\mathbf{0}, \mathbf{I}_n)$ and $\sigma_* > 0$. The matrix $\mathbf{X}$ is the design matrix, its columns are called the predictors, $\mathbf{y}$ is called the response vector, $\boldsymbol{\varepsilon}$ is the noise (or the error vector) of the model and σ_* is the (unknown) noise standard deviation. The signal to noise ratio (SNR), defined by $\mathrm{SNR}_y = \|\mathbf{X}\mathbf{w}^*\|_2 / (\sigma_* \|\boldsymbol{\epsilon}\|_2)$, is a measure that describes the noise regime in any given experiment. The true support is defined as $S_* = \{j \in [p]; w_j^* \neq 0\}$ and its size is $s_* = |S_*|$. It is noteworthy that our problem is not a prediction problem, we are not aiming at finding $\hat{\mathbf{w}}$ minimizing $\|\mathbf{X}\hat{\mathbf{w}} - \mathbf{X}\mathbf{w}^*\|_2$, but an estimation problem, in which we want to control $\|\hat{\mathbf{w}} - \mathbf{w}^*\|_\infty$ statistically.

Desparsified Lasso for High-Dimensional Inference. The Desparsified Lasso (DL) estimator denoted $\hat{\mathbf{w}}^{\mathrm{DL}}$, introduced in [12], can be seen as a generalization of the Ordinary Least Squares (OLS) estimator for inference in $n < p$ settings. Under some assumptions (notably the sparsity of $\mathbf{w}^*$) that are made explicit in [3], $\hat{\mathbf{w}}^{\mathrm{DL}}$ has the following property:

$$\forall j \in [p], \quad \sigma_*^{-1} (\Omega_{jj})^{-1/2} (\hat{w}_j^{\mathrm{DL}} - w_j^*) \sim \mathcal{N}(0, 1) \;, \tag{2}$$

where the diagonal of $\boldsymbol{\Omega}$ (estimated precision matrix; inverse of $\mathbf{X}^\top \mathbf{X}/n$) is computed concurrently with $\hat{\mathbf{w}}^{\mathrm{DL}}$, as described in [12]. From (2) we can compute confidence intervals and p-values of the coefficients of the weight vector.

In [3], several high-dimensional inference solutions are discussed and compared. DL displays an interesting trade-off between good control of the family-wise error rate (FWER) and strong power. The FWER is defined as FWER = $\mathrm{Prob}(\mathrm{FP} \geq 1)$ where FP is the number of false positives.

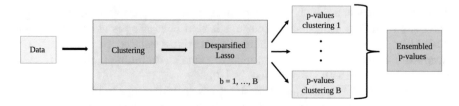

Fig. 1. To leverage Desparsified Lasso inference procedure on medical images, our algorithm relies on feature clustering and an ensembling step on randomized solutions.

Clustering to Handle Structured High-Dimensional Data. In high-dimensional inference, variables are often highly correlated. Specifically, a medical image has a 3D representation and a given voxel is highly correlated with its neighbors; $\mathbf{w}$ obviously carries the same structure. In addition $n \ll p$ and $n < s_*$ make the statistical inference challenging without data structure assumptions as shown in [3]. To leverage data structure, we introduce a clustering step that reduces data dimensionality before applying our inference procedure. Here, we consider a spatially-constrained hierarchical clustering algorithm described in [10] that uses Ward criterion while respecting the image geometrical structure. The combination of this clustering algorithm and the DL inference procedure will be referred to as the Clustered Desparsified Lasso (CDL) algorithm.

Bagging to Alleviate Dependency on Clustering. It is preferable not to rely on a particular clustering as small perturbations on it have a dramatic impact on the final solution. We followed the approach presented in [10] that argues in favor of the randomization over a spatially-constrained clustering method: to build B clusterings of the predictors, they use the same clustering method but with B different random subsamples of size $\lfloor 0.7n \rfloor$ from the full sample.

Inference with Ensemble of Clustered Desparsified Lasso. We now have all the elements to present our Ensemble of Clustered Desparsified Lasso (ECDL) algorithm which is summarized in Fig. 1. ECDL consists in B repetitions of the CDL algorithm (using random subsamples of size $\lfloor 0.7n \rfloor$ for the clustering and the full sample for the DL procedure) and an ensembling step analogous to the bagging method introduced by [1]. Once the CDL algorithm has been run B times, we have B partitions into C clusters, each cluster being associated with a p-value. We denote by $P^{(b,c)}$ the p-value for the cth cluster in the bth fold. The p-value $P_j^{(b)}$ of the coefficient $j \in [p]$ in the bth repetition is $P^{(b,c)}$ whenever j belongs to cluster c, i.e. we attribute the same p-value to all the predictors in a given cluster. This yields B p-values for each coefficient. Finally, to ensemble the p-values one has to use specific techniques which ensure that the resulting p-value is meaningful as a frequentist hypothesis test. Thus, to derive the p-value P_j of the jth coefficient, we have considered the ensembling solution presented in [8] that has the required properties and consists in taking the median of $\{P_j^{(b)} \text{ for } b \in [B]\}$ multiplied by 2.

3   Simulation and Experimental Results

3.1   First Simulation: The Importance of Dimension Reduction

Simulation. This simulation has a 1D structure and we set $n = 100$ and $p = 2000$. We construct the design matrix $\mathbf{X}$ such that predictors are normally distributed and two consecutive predictors have a fixed correlation $\rho = 0.95$. The weight $\mathbf{w}^*$ is such that $w_j^* = 1$ for $1 \leq j \leq 50$ and $w_j^* = 0$ otherwise, then $s_* = 50$. We also set $\sigma_* = 10$ such that $\mathrm{SNR}_y = 3$ (cf. Sec. 3.3).

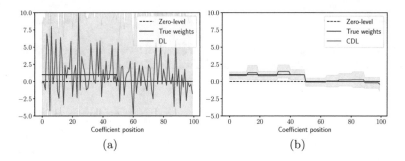

(a)   (b)

Fig. 2. (a) 95% coefficient intervals given by the raw Desparsified Lasso (DL) fail to retrieve the true support. (b) 95% coefficient intervals given by the Clustered Desparsified Lasso (CDL) are much narrower, and yield a good support accurately.

Results. We compare the DL procedure applied to the uncompressed data, displayed in Fig. 2-(a), and the CDL algorithm in Fig. 2-(b). The number of clusters, whose impact will be discussed in Sec. 4, has been set to $C = 200$, allowing to reduce the dimension from $p = 2000$ to $C = 200$ before performing the inference. This reduction tames the estimator variance and yields useful confidence intervals that could not be reached by DL only.

3.2   Second Simulation: Improvement by Bootstrap and Aggregation

Simulation. Here, we consider a simulation with a 3D structure, that aims at approximating the statistics of the Oasis experiment (cf. Sec. 3.3). The volume considered is a 3D-cube with edge length $H = 50$, with $n = 400$ samples and $p = H^3 = 125\,000$ predictors (voxels). To construct $\mathbf{w}^*$, we define a 3D weight vector $\tilde{\mathbf{w}}^*$ with five regions of interest (ROIs) represented in Fig. 3-(a) and then make a bijective transformation of $\tilde{\mathbf{w}}^*$ in a vector of size p. Each ROI is a cube of width $h = 6$, leading to a size of support $s_* = 5h^3 = 1080$. Four ROIs are situated in corners of the cubic map and the last ROI is situated in the center of the cube. To construct $\mathbf{X}$, we first define the 3D design matrix $\tilde{\mathbf{X}}$ from p random normal vectors of size n smoothed with 3D Gaussian filter with bandwidth σ_{smth} (smoothing is performed across all predictors for each sample), then we use the same transformation as before and derive the $n \times p$ design matrix. The choice $\sigma_{\mathrm{smth}} = 2$ is made to achieve similar correlations as for the Oasis experiment. We also set $\sigma_* = 8$, i.e. $\mathrm{SNR}_y = 3$ (cf. Sec. 3.3).

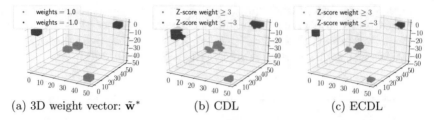

(a) 3D weight vector: $\tilde{\mathbf{w}}^*$ (b) CDL   (c) ECDL

Fig. 3. In this simulation, comparing the original 3D weight vector with CDL and ECDL solutions, we observe that the ECDL solution is much more accurate.

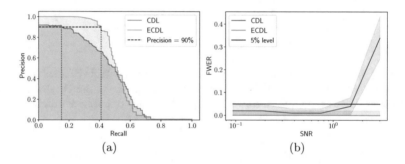

(a)   (b)

Fig. 4. (a) The precision-recall curve for the recovery of $\mathbf{w}$ is much better adding an ensembling step over CDL. (b) FWER (nominal rate 5%) is well controlled by the ECDL algorithm while for high level of SNR it is not controlled by the CDL algorithm.

Results. To derive the ECDL solutions we aggregated $B = 25$ different CDL solutions during the ensembling step. To obtain the results presented in Fig. 4, we ran 100 simulations. In Fig. 4-(a), we display the precision-recall curve (cf. Scikit-learn `precision_recall_curve` function) of the solutions obtained by each algorithm with $C = 500$ clusters. ECDL very strongly outperforms CDL: for precision of at least 90%, the ECDL recall is 42% while the CDL recall is only 16%.

In order to check the FWER control, we define a neutral region that separates ROIs from the non-active region. Indeed, since the predictors are highly correlated, the detection of a null predictor in the vicinity of an active one is not a mistake. Thus, neutral regions enfold ROIs with a margin of 5 voxels. We compare different values of σ_* from 2^3 to 2^8 giving SNR_y lying between .1 and 3. In Fig. 4-(b), one can observe that the FWER is always well controlled using ECDL; the later is even conservative since the empirical FWER stays at 0% for a 5% nominal level. On the opposite, the FWER is not well controlled by

CDL: its empirical value goes far above the 5% rate for high SNR. This is due to the shape of the discovered regions that do not always correspond to the exact shape and location of ROIs. This effect is also observable watching thresholded Z-score maps yielded by CDL and ECDL in Fig. 3. By increasing the number of clusters, we would obtain discovered regions more similar to the true ROIs, yet their statistical significance would drop and the power would collapse.

3.3   Experiments on MRI Datasets

Haxby Dataset. Haxby is a functional MRI dataset that maps the brain responses of subjects watching images of different objects (see [6]). In our study we only consider the responses related to images of faces and houses for the first subject, to identify brain regions that discriminate between these two stimuli, assuming that this problem can be modeled as a regression problem. Here $n = 200$, $p = 24k$, (estimated) $SNR_y = 1.0$ and we used $C = 500$ and $B = 25$.

Oasis Dataset. The Oasis MRI dataset (see [7]) provides anatomical brain images of several subjects together with their age. The SPM voxel-based morphometry pipeline was used to obtain individual gray matter density maps. We aim at identifying which regions are informative to predict the age of a given subject. Here $n = 400$, $p = 125k$ and (estimated) $SNR_y = 3.0$; we also took $C = 500$ and $B = 25$ as in Sec. 3.2.

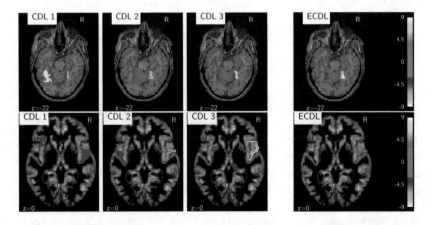

Fig. 5. Results of the CDL and ECDL algorithms on Haxby (top) and Oasis (bottom) experiments. CDL algorithm outcomes are highly dependent on the clustering, which creates a jitter in the solution. Drawing consensus among many CDL results, ECDL removes the arbitrariness related to the clustering scheme.

Results. The results of these experiments are displayed in Fig. 5 with Z-transform of the p-values. For clarity, we thresholded the Z-score maps at 3 (and -3) keeping only the regions that have a high probability of being discriminative. The solutions given by the CDL algorithm with three different choices of clustering look noisy and unstable while the ECDL solution defines a synthesis of the CDL results and exhibits a nice symmetry in the case of Haxby. Thus, these results clearly illustrate that the ensembling step removes the arbitrariness due to the clustering.

Stability of Bagging Estimator. This last experiment quantifies the gain in stability when adding the ensembling step. From the two previous experiments, we derive 25 ECDL solution maps (with $B = 25$) and 25 CDL solution maps and measure the variability of the results. Correlation between the full maps and Jaccard index of the detected areas (here, voxels with an absolute Z-score greater than 3) show that ECDL is substantially more stable than CDL (Fig. 6).

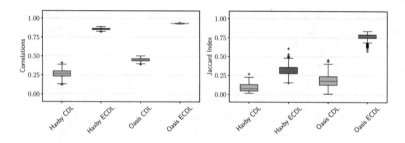

Fig. 6. Correlation (left) and Jaccard Index (right) are much higher with the ECDL algorithm than with CDL across 25 replications of the analysis of the imaging datasets.

4   Discussion

Recapitulation. We have introduced ECDL, an algorithm for high-dimensional inference on structured data which scales even when the number of predictors $p \geq 10^5$ is much higher than the number of samples $n \leq 10^3$. It can be summarized as follows: i) perform B repetitions of the CDL algorithm, that runs Desparsified Lasso (DL) inference on a model compressed by clustering, yielding several p-values for each predictor; ii) use an ensemble method aggregating all p-values to derive a single p-value per predictor. In Sec. 3.1, we have shown that the clustering step, justified by specific data structures and locally high inter-predictor correlation, was necessary to yield an informative inference solution when $n \ll p$. Then, we have demonstrated, in Sec. 3.2, that randomizing and bagging the CDL solution improves the control of the FWER and the precision-recall curve. While the ensembling step obviously removes the arbitrariness of the clustering choice, in Sec. 3.3 we showed it also increases stability.

ECDL Parameter Setting. The number of clusters C is the main free parameter, and an optimal value depends on characteristics of the data (inter-predictor correlation, SNR). In our simulations, we observe a bias/variance trade-off: a small number of clusters reduces variance and enhances statistical power, while a greater number yields refined solutions. The ensembling step helps improving shape accuracy without loss in sensitivity, as the combination of multiple CDL solutions recovers finer spatial information.

Computational Cost of ECDL. The most expensive step is the DL inference, which includes the resolution of $\mathcal{O}(C)$ Lasso problems with n samples and C features. This is repeated B times in ECDL, making it embarrassingly parallel; we could run the ECDL algorithm on standard desktop stations with $n = 400$, $C = 500$ and $B = 25$ in less than 10 min.

Additional Work Related to ECDL. In Haxby experiment (cf. 3.3) we approximated the problem as a regression one. Thus, an interesting extension would be to adapt ECDL to classification settings. Another matter is the comparison with bootstrap and permutation-based approaches e.g. [4], that we leave for future work. Note however that, in [3], a study of bootstrap approaches points out some unwanted properties and they do not outperform DL.

Usefulness for Medical Imaging. For structured high-dimensional data, our algorithm is relevant to assess the statistical significance of a set of predictors when fitting a target variable. Our experimental results show that ECDL is very promising for inference problems in medical imaging.

Acknowledgements. This research was supported by Labex DigiCosme (project ANR-11-LABEX-0045-DIGICOSME) operated by ANR as part of the program "Investissement d'Avenir" Idex Paris Saclay (ANR-11-IDEX-0003-02). This work is also funded by the FAST-BIG project (ANR-17-CE23-0011).

References

1. Breiman, L.: Bagging predictors. Mach. Learn. **24**(2), 123–140 (1996)
2. Bühlmann, P.: Statistical significance in high-dimensional linear models. Bernoulli **19**(4), 1212–1242 (2013)
3. Dezeure, R., Bühlmann, P., Meier, L., Meinshausen, N.: High-dimensional inference: confidence intervals, p-values and R-software hdi. Stat. Sci. **30**(4), 533–558 (2015)
4. Gaonkar, B., Davatzikos, C.: Deriving statistical significance maps for SVM based image classification and group comparisons. In: Ayache, N., Delingette, H., Golland, P., Mori, K. (eds.) MICCAI 2012. LNCS, vol. 7510, pp. 723–730. Springer, Heidelberg (2012). https://doi.org/10.1007/978-3-642-33415-3_89
5. Hastie, T.J., Tibshirani, R., Wainwright, M.: Statistical Learning with Sparsity: The Lasso and Generalizations. CRC Press, Boca Raton (2015)
6. Haxby, J., Gobbini, I., Furey, M., Ishai, A., Schouten, J., Pietrini, P.: Distributed and overlapping representations of faces and objects in ventral temporal cortex. Science **293**(5539), 2425–2430 (2001)
7. Marcus, D., Wang, T., Parker, J., Csernansky, J., Morris, J., Buckner, R.: Open access series of imaging studies (OASIS): cross-sectional MRI data in young, middle aged, nondemented, and demented older adults. J. Cognit. Neurosci. **19**(9), 1498–1507 (2007)

8. Meinshausen, N., Meier, L., Bühlmann, P.: P-values for high-dimensional regression. J. Am. Stat. Assoc. **104**(488), 1671–1681 (2009)
9. Tibshirani, R.: Regression shrinkage and selection via the lasso. J. R. Stat. Soc. Ser. B Stat. Methodol. **58**, 267–288 (1994)
10. Varoquaux, G., Gramfort, A., Thirion, B.: Small-sample brain mapping: sparse recovery on spatially correlated designs with randomization and clustering (2012)
11. Wasserman, L., Roeder, K.: High-dimensional variable selection. Ann. Stat. **37**(5A), 2178–2201 (2009)
12. Zhang, C.-H., Zhang, S.S.: Confidence intervals for low dimensional parameters in high dimensional linear models. J. R. Stat. Soc. Ser. B Stat. Methodol. **76**(1), 217–242 (2014)

Low-Rank Representation
for Multi-center Autism Spectrum
Disorder Identification

Mingliang Wang[1], Daoqiang Zhang[1(✉)], Jiashuang Huang[1],
Dinggang Shen[2(✉)], and Mingxia Liu[2(✉)]

[1] College of Computer Science and Technology, Nanjing University of Aeronautics
and Astronautics, Nanjing, China
dqzhang@nuaa.edu.cn
[2] Department of Radiology and BRIC, University of North Carolina at Chapel Hill,
Chapel Hill, NC, USA
dgshen@med.unc.edu, mxliu@unc.edu

Abstract. Effective utilization of multi-center data for autism spectrum
disorder (ASD) diagnosis recently has attracted increasing attention,
since a large number of subjects from multiple centers are beneficial
for investigating the pathological changes of ASD. To better utilize the
multi-center data, various machine learning methods have been proposed.
However, most previous studies do not consider the problem of data
heterogeneity (*e.g.*, caused by different scanning parameters and subject populations) among multi-center datasets, which may degrade the
diagnosis performance based on multi-center data. To address this issue,
we propose a multi-center low-rank representation learning (MCLRR)
method for ASD diagnosis, to seek a good representation of subjects
from different centers. Specifically, we first choose one center as the target domain and the remaining centers as source domains. We then learn
a domain-specific projection for each source domain to transform them
into an intermediate representation space. To further suppress the heterogeneity among multiple centers, we disassemble the learned projection
matrices into a shared part and a sparse unique part. With the shared
matrix, we can project target domain to the common latent space, and
linearly represent the source domain datasets using data in the transformed target domain. Based on the learned low-rank representation,
we employ the k-nearest neighbor (KNN) algorithm to perform disease
classification. Our method has been evaluated on the ABIDE database,
and the superior classification results demonstrate the effectiveness of
our proposed method as compared to other methods.

1 Introduction

Autism spectrum disorder (ASD) is associated with a range of phenotypes,
such as poor social communication abilities, repetitive patterns of behavior, and

This study was supported by National Natural Science Foundation of China under
Grant 61876082, 61861130366, 61703301, and 61473149.

A. F. Frangi et al. (Eds.): MICCAI 2018, LNCS 11070, pp. 647–654, 2018.
https://doi.org/10.1007/978-3-030-00928-1_73

restricted interest. It was reported that there were 62.2 million ASD cases in the world in 2015 [1]. However, the pathological mechanism of ASD is unclear, and conventional diagnosis of ASD is usually based on symptoms [2], and thus the precise diagnosis is the main challenge in the research literature of ASD.

Neuroimaging is a powerful tool for characterizing neural patterns of functional connectivity using resting-state functional magnetic resonance imaging (rs-fMRI) data, and has been widely applied to ASD diagnosis. Recently, multi-center rs-fMRI datasets are available for studying of ASD disease and many researchers have devoted their efforts to take advantage of increasing amounts of multi-center data. Existing methods [3–5] either try to diagnose ASD using data from each imaging center separately, or straightforwardly combine multi-center datasets for disease analysis. However, these methods do not consider the facts that there is usually a limited number of imaging data at each center and datasets from different centers often have heterogeneous characteristics. Recently, low-rank representation (LRR) [6] has been successfully applied to neuroimage-based brain disease analysis, which helps uncover the underlying structure of data by suppressing noisy features. For example, Adeli et $al.$ [7] developed a joint feature-sample selection method to diagnose Parkinson's disease with a low-rank constraint. Vounou et $al.$ [8] proposed a sparse reduced-rank regression model to identify potential genetic data associated with Alzheimer's disease. However, these studies generally ignore the problem of data heterogeneity ($e.g.$, caused by different scanning parameters and subject populations) among different centers, thus leading to sub-optimal performance.

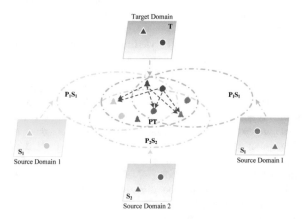

Fig. 1. Illustration of our multi-center low-rank representation learning method. There are I source domains and a target domain. Each source domain (denoted as $\mathbf{S}_i$) and the target domain (denoted as $\mathbf{T}$) contain two samples (marked as triangles and circles) belonging to two categories. Our method transforms each source domain $\mathbf{S}_i$ into an intermediate representation $\mathbf{P}_i\mathbf{S}_i$, and each transformed sample can be linearly represented by the target samples with a common latent projection ($i.e.$, $\mathbf{PT}$).

Accordingly, in this paper, we propose a novel unsupervised multi-center low-rank representation (MCLRR) learning method to learn the latent representation of multi-center data for ASD disease diagnosis. The framework of our proposed method is described in Fig. 1. As illustrated in Fig. 1, we treat the center that needs to be analyzed as target domain and the remaining centers as source domains. In addition, we also assume that no label information is available for samples in the target domain, while samples in source domains are well labeled. Then we transform each source domain into an intermediate latent representation space, such that each transformed sample can be linearly represented by samples in the target domain. As a result, the heterogeneity across different centers can be partly alleviated. To further reduce the heterogeneity of different centers, we disassemble each learned projection matrix of source domains into a shared projection matrix and a space unique matrix. And the target domain can be transformed into the latent space using the learned shared projection. With the transformed target domain dataset, we can well represent the source domain datasets. Finally, we employ the k-nearest neighbor (KNN) algorithm on the latent space by using the labeled source domain datasets to arrive a final classification decision of the target domain.

2   Method

Data and Pre-processing: In this study, we use rs-fMRI data from the Autism Imaging Data Exchange (ABIDE) database[1], a large multi-center autism dataset. It contains a total of 871 quality rs-fMRI data from 17 different centers. Due to the limited number of participates in several centers, we select 468 subjects from 5 different centers (with the number of subjects >50), including *Leuven, NYU, UCLA, UM* and *USM*. Specifically, there are 250 ASD patients and 218 normal controls (NCs), and the numbers of patients and NCs in each center are comparable.

We download the pre-processed rs-fMRI data with the Configurable Pipeline for the Analysis of Connectomes (C-PAC) from the Preprocessed Connectome Project[2]. The image pre-possessing steps include slice timing corrected, motion correction, and normalization of the intensity. Subsequently, the signal fluctuations induced by head motion, respiration, cardiac pulsation, and scanner drift were removed by conducting the nuisance regression. Afterward, the anatomical automatic labeling (AAL) atlas with 116 pre-defined regions-of-interest (ROIs) was aligned onto each image, followed by extracting ROI-based mean time series for each subject. Finally, based on the pairwise Pearson correlation coefficients, a functional connectivity matrix was conducted, where each edge weight is the correlation between a pair of ROIs. For simplicity, the upper triangle (symmetric with lower triangle) and the diagonal values (*i.e.*, correlation of an ROI to itself) of the matrix were removed, and the remaining triangles were converted

---

[1] http://fcon_1000.projects.nitrc.org/indi/abide/.

[2] http://preprocessed-connectomes-project.org.

to a vector as the features. Thus, we obtained a 6,670 dimensional feature vector for representing each subject.

Multi-center Low-Rank Representation: In this study, we formulate the multi-center ASD diagnosis as a low-rank representation based classification problem, where one center is chosen as the target domain and the remaining centers as source domains. Suppose there are I source domains, each source domain is composed of a set of N_i subjects $\mathbf{S}_i = [\mathbf{s}_1, \ldots, \mathbf{s}_{N_i}] \in \mathbb{R}^{d \times N_i}$, and a set of N_T subjects $\mathbf{T} = [\mathbf{t}_1, \ldots, \mathbf{t}_{N_T}] \in \mathbb{R}^{d \times N_T}$ in the target domain, where d is the dimension of the feature vector. Our aim is to find an intermediate latent space, via the low-rank transformation matrix $\mathbf{P}_i$ to represent source domains using the target domain. The proposed objective function is defined as:

$$\min_{\mathbf{P}_i, \mathbf{Z}_i, \mathbf{E}_i^Z} \sum_{i=1}^{I} \left(rank(\mathbf{Z}_i) + \alpha \|\mathbf{E}_i^Z\|_1 \right)$$

$$\text{s.t. } \mathbf{P}_i \mathbf{S}_i = \mathbf{T}\mathbf{Z}_i + \mathbf{E}_i^Z, i = 1, \cdots, I \tag{1}$$

where $rank(\mathbf{Z}_i)$ is the rank of matrix $\mathbf{Z}_i$, $\|\mathbf{E}_i^Z\|_1 = \sum_{j=1}^{N_i} \sum_{i=1}^{d} | \mathbf{E}_{i,j}^Z |$ is ℓ_1-norm, and α is a parameter to balance the contributions of low-rank constraint and sparse regularization. Although it is difficult to solve the rank minimization in Eq. (1) directly, *nuclear norm* provides a good surrogate for addressing it. Therefore, the Eq. (1) can be rewritten as:

$$\min_{\mathbf{P}_i, \mathbf{Z}_i, \mathbf{E}_i^Z} \sum_{i=1}^{I} \left(\|\mathbf{Z}_i\|_* + \alpha \|\mathbf{E}_i^Z\|_1 \right)$$

$$\text{s.t. } \mathbf{P}_i \mathbf{S}_i = \mathbf{T}\mathbf{Z}_i + \mathbf{E}_i^Z, i = 1, \cdots, I \tag{2}$$

where $\| \cdot \|_*$ denotes the nuclear norm of a matrix, which can be calculated by the sum of singular values of the matrix.

It is worth noting that it could be sub-optimal to reconstruct data from source domain in the original target domain, since data acquired from different centers are usually heterogeneous. Since the underlying pathology of ASD disease among multiple centers is the same, it is intuitive to assume that multiple centers share an intrinsic latent representation space. Accordingly, we can disassemble the transformation matrix $\mathbf{P}_i$ into a shared latent space via both a low-rank matrix $\mathbf{P}$ and a unique sparse matrix $\mathbf{E}_i^P$ for the i-th source domain. By transforming the target domain to the latent space with the matrix $\mathbf{P}$, our multi-center low-rank representation (MCLRR) learning method can be described as:

$$\min_{\mathbf{P}, \mathbf{P}_i, \mathbf{Z}_i, \mathbf{E}_i^Z, \mathbf{E}_i^P} \|\mathbf{P}\|_* + \sum_{i=1}^{I} \left(\|\mathbf{Z}_i\|_* + \alpha \|\mathbf{E}_i^Z\|_1 + \beta \|\mathbf{E}_i^P\|_1 \right)$$

$$\text{s.t. } \mathbf{P}_i \mathbf{S}_i = \mathbf{P}\mathbf{T}\mathbf{Z}_i + \mathbf{E}_i^Z, \tag{3}$$

$$\mathbf{P}_i = \mathbf{P} + \mathbf{E}_i^P, i = 1, \cdots, I$$

$$\mathbf{P}\mathbf{P}^T = \mathbf{I}$$

where β is the balanced parameter between shared and variance part, and the orthogonal constraint $\mathbf{PP}^T = \mathbf{I}$ is imposed to avoid trivial solutions of matrix $\mathbf{P}$. In Eq. (3), the common low-rank matrix $\mathbf{P}$ can uncover most of the shared information amongst multi-center ASD datasets. The rank of matrix $\mathbf{E}_i^Z$ tends to find a representation coefficient on the transformed target domain space. The minimization of $\|\mathbf{E}_i^Z\|_1$ and $\|\mathbf{E}_i^P\|_1$ encourages the error of reconstruction matrix and variance matrix to be sparse.

Optimization: The problem in Eq. (3) is a typical mixed nuclear norm and ℓ_1-norm minimization optimization. In this paper, we adopt the Augmented Lagrange Multiplier (ALM) to solve the objective function. We first transform Eq. (3) into the following equivalent formulation:

$$\min_{\mathbf{J},\mathbf{P},\mathbf{P}_i,\mathbf{Z}_i,\mathbf{E}_i^Z,\mathbf{E}_i^P,\mathbf{F}_i} \|\mathbf{J}\|_* + \sum_{i=1}^I \left(\|\mathbf{F}_i\|_* + \alpha\|\mathbf{E}_i^Z\|_1 + \beta\|\mathbf{E}_i^P\|_1\right)$$

$$\text{s.t. } \mathbf{P}_i\mathbf{S}_i = \mathbf{PTZ}_i + \mathbf{E}_i^Z, \qquad (4)$$

$$\mathbf{P}_i = \mathbf{P} + \mathbf{E}_i^P, i = 1, \cdots, I$$

$$\mathbf{PP}^T = \mathbf{I}, \mathbf{P} = \mathbf{J}, \mathbf{Z}_i = \mathbf{F}_i$$

Then the augmented Lagrange function can be defined as follows:

$$\min_{\substack{\mathbf{J},\mathbf{P},\mathbf{P}_i,\mathbf{Z}_i,\mathbf{E}_i^Z,\mathbf{E}_i^P, \\ \mathbf{F}_i,\mathbf{Y}_{1,i},\mathbf{Y}_{2,i},\mathbf{Y}_{3,i},\mathbf{Y}_4}} \|\mathbf{J}\|_* + \sum_{i=1}^I (\|\mathbf{F}_i\|_* + \alpha\|\mathbf{E}_i^Z\|_1 + \beta\|\mathbf{E}_i^P\|_1 + \frac{\mu}{2}\|\mathbf{P}_i\mathbf{S}_i -$$

$$\mathbf{PTZ}_i - \mathbf{E}_i^Z\|_F^2 + \frac{\mu}{2}\|\mathbf{P}_i - \mathbf{P} - \mathbf{E}_i^P\|_F^2 + \frac{\mu}{2}\|\mathbf{Z}_i - \mathbf{F}_i\|_F^2 +$$

$$\langle\mathbf{Y}_{1,i},\mathbf{P}_i\mathbf{S}_i - \mathbf{PTZ}_i - \mathbf{E}_i^Z\rangle + \langle\mathbf{Y}_{2,i},\mathbf{P}_i - \mathbf{P} - \mathbf{E}_i^P\rangle +$$

$$\langle\mathbf{Y}_{3,i},\mathbf{Z}_i - \mathbf{F}_i\rangle) + \langle\mathbf{Y}_4,\mathbf{P} - \mathbf{J}\rangle + \frac{\mu}{2}\|\mathbf{P} - \mathbf{J}\|_F^2$$

$$(5)$$

where $\langle\cdot,\cdot\rangle$ denotes the inner product of two matrices, $i.e.$, $\langle\mathbf{A},\mathbf{B}\rangle = tr(\mathbf{A}^T\mathbf{B})$. $\mathbf{Y}_1,\mathbf{Y}_2,\mathbf{Y}_3$ and $\mathbf{Y}_4$ are Lagrange multipliers and $\mu > 0$ is a penalty parameter.

While it is difficult to jointly update the variables in Eq. (5), we can still optimize each of them in the leave-one-out fashion. Hence, we alternately optimize each variable iteratively with fixed values of the others and resort to ALM to solve the objective function. Once we obtain the representation of transformed target domain ($i.e.$, $\mathbf{PT}$) and source domains ($i.e.$, $\mathbf{PTZ}_i$), we can use the KNN algorithm to estimate the final label of a test sample.

3   Experiments

Experimental Settings: We evaluated the proposed MCLRR method in ASD vs. NC classification based on multi-center data from the ABIDE database.

The performance was measured via four criteria, *i.e.*, classification accuracy (ACC), sensitivity (SEN), specificity (SPE) and area under the ROC curve (AUC).

We first compared our MCLRR method with 3 baseline methods, including KNN, support vector machine (SVM), and classical low-rank representation (LRR) method [6]. To investigate the influence of our learned latent representation, we further compare MCLRR with its variant (denoted as MCLRR-1) without mapping data of target domain to the latent space. That is, MCLRR-1 directly employ data in the original target domain to represent data in source domains (without learning the shared transform matrix), while MCLRR transforms the target domain to a shared space for representing multiple source domains. Different from KNN and SVM methods that use the original rs-fMRI features for classification, LRR and our methods (*i.e.*, MCLRR-1 and MCLRR) first learn new representations of data and then feed the new features into a 5-nearest neighbor classifier for disease classification. Besides, we compare MCLRR with 3 state-of-the-art methods for ASD diagnosis, including a graph-based convolutional network [3] with hinge loss (denoted as sGCN-1) and global loss (denoted as sGCN-2), functional connectivity association analysis with leave-one-out classifier (FCA) [4], and a denoising autoencoder (DAE) [5] with two autoencoders.

In the experiments, we select one from multiple centers in turn as the target domain and regard the remaining ones as source domains. A 5-fold cross-validation (CV) strategy was used for performance evaluation. Specifically, the subjects of each domain are randomly partitioned into 5 subsets, and the subjects within one subset are selected as the test data each time, while all other subjects in the remaining subsets are used to train the models. To obtain the optimal parameters in different methods, we further performed a 5-fold inner CV using training data. The parameters in MCLRR-1 (*i.e.*, α) and MCLRR (*i.e.*, α and β) are chosen from $\{1e^{-3}, \cdots, 1e^3\}$, respectively. The parameter λ in LRR was also set to $\{1e^{-3}, \cdots, 1e^3\}$ to balance the low-rank constraint and the outliers detection. For SVM method, we use the linear SVM classifier with parameters (*i.e.*, C) selected from the range of $\{2^{-5}, \cdots, 2^5\}$. The parameter k for the KNN method was chosen from $\{3, 5, 7, 9, 11, 15\}$.

Results: We report the experimental results achieved by our method and those baseline methods in Fig. 2. As can be seen from Fig. 2, we can derive several interesting observations. *First*, low-rank-based methods (*i.e.*, LRR, MCLRR-1, and MCLRR) generally achieve better performance in most cases. For example, the average ACC values (*i.e.*, across multiple centers) achieved by low-rank-based methods are 63.92%, 63.60% and 68.74% respectively, which are noticeably higher than those of KNN and SVM methods (*i.e.*, 58.71% and 61.02%). This demonstrates that low-rank-based representation is useful in dealing with the problem of data heterogeneity by discovering the underlying data structure among different imaging centers. *In addition*, our proposed MCLRR method consistently outperforms MCLRR-1 in terms of ACC, SEN and AUC on

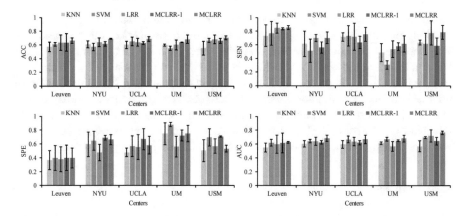

Fig. 2. Performance of proposed MCLRR method and three baseline methods in ASD vs. NC classification using multiple centers data.

multiple centers datasets. These results validate the efficacy of our proposed strategy that projects multi-center data into an intermediate latent representation space.

We further report the comparison between our method and state-of-the-art methods for ASD identification on the *NYU* center in Table 1. It can be seen from Table 1 that our MCLRR method achieves higher accuracy (*i.e.*, 69.10%), specificity (*i.e.*, 66.43%) and AUC (*i.e.*, 68.33%) than 4 competing methods, even though sGCN and DAE are two deep-learning methods.

Table 1. Comparison with state-of-the-art methods for ASD identification using rs-fMRI ABIDE data. FNC: Functional Network Connectivity; KNN: k-nearest neighbor algorithm.

Methods	Feature type	Classifier	ACC (%)	SEN (%)	SPE (%)	AUC (%)
sGCN-1 [3]	FNC	KNN	60.50	–	–	57.00
sGCN-2 [3]	FNC	KNN	63.50	–	–	61.00
FCA [4]	FNC	*t*-test	63.00	72.00	58.00	–
DAE [5]	FNC	Softmax regression	66.00	66.00	65.00	–
MCLRR (ours)	FNC	KNN	**69.10**	70.24	**66.43**	**68.33**

4 Conclusion

We present a novel low-rank representation method using multi-center data for ASD diagnosis. Specifically, to alleviate the heterogeneities of multi-center datasets, we first learn the projection matrices to transform the source domains into a latent representation space. Also, we disassemble the learned projection matrix into a shared matrix and a sparse matrix. Then, we transform the target domain into the latent space with the shared projection matrix, and linearly represent the source domain datasets using data in the transformed target domain. A k-nearest neighbor method is employed to arrive at a final classification decision. Results on the ABIDE database demonstrate the effectiveness of our method in ASD diagnosis using rs-fMRI data acquired from multiple centers. In the future, we will perform data-driven feature extraction for rs-fMRI data via deep learning [9–11] rather than using current hand-crafted (*i.e.*, ROI) features, which is expected to further improve the diagnostic performance.

References

1. Catal-Lpez, F., et al.: Risk of mortality among children, adolescents, and adults with autism spectrum disorder or attention deficit hyperactivity disorder and their first-degree relatives: a protocol for a systematic review and meta-analysis of observational studies. Syst. Rev. **6**(1), 189 (2017)
2. Wang, J., et al.: Multi-task diagnosis for autism spectrum disorders using multimodality features: a multi-center study. Hum. Brain Mapp. **38**(6), 3081–3097 (2017)
3. Ktena, S.I., et al.: Metric learning with spectral graph convolutions on brain connectivity networks. Neuroimage **169**, 431–442 (2017)
4. Nielsen, J.A., et al.: Multisite functional connectivity MRI classification of autism: ABIDE results. Front. Hum. Neurosci. **7**(599), 1–12 (2013)
5. Heinsfeld, A.S., Franco, A.R., Craddock, R.C., Buchweitz, A., Meneguzzi, F.: Identification of autism spectrum disorder using deep learning and the ABIDE dataset. Neuroimage Clin. **17**, 16–23 (2017)
6. Liu, G., Lin, Z., Yu, Y.: Robust subspace segmentation by low-rank representation. In: Proceedings of the 27th International Conference on Machine Learning, ICML 2010, Haifa, pp. 663–670 (2010)
7. Adeli, E., et al.: Joint feature-sample selection and robust diagnosis of Parkinson's disease from MRI data. Neuroimage **141**, 206–219 (2016)
8. Vounou, M., et al.: Sparse reduced-rank regression detects genetic associations with voxel-wise longitudinal phenotypes in Alzheimer's disease. Neuroimage **60**(1), 700–16 (2012)
9. Liu, M., Zhang, J., Adeli, E., Shen, D.: Landmark-based deep multi-instance learning for brain disease diagnosis. Med. Image Anal. **43**, 157–168 (2018)
10. Lian, C., et al.: Multi-channel multi-scale fully convolutional network for 3D perivascular spaces segmentation in 7T MR images. Med. Image Anal. **46**, 106–117 (2018)
11. Zhang, J., Liu, M., Shen, D.: Detecting anatomical landmarks from limited medical imaging data using two-stage task-oriented deep neural networks. IEEE Trans. Image Process. **26**(10), 4753–4764 (2017)

Exploring Uncertainty Measures in Deep Networks for Multiple Sclerosis Lesion Detection and Segmentation

Tanya Nair[1(✉)], Doina Precup[2], Douglas L. Arnold[3,4], and Tal Arbel[1]

[1] Centre for Intelligent Machines, McGill University, Montreal, Canada
tnair@cim.mcgill.ca
[2] School of Computer Science, McGill University, Montreal, Canada
[3] Montreal Neurological Institute, McGill University, Montreal, Canada
[4] NeuroRx Research, Montreal, Canada

Abstract. Deep learning (DL) networks have recently been shown to outperform other segmentation methods on various public, medical-image challenge datasets [3,11,16], especially for large pathologies. However, in the context of diseases such as Multiple Sclerosis (MS), monitoring all the focal lesions visible on MRI sequences, even very small ones, is essential for disease staging, prognosis, and evaluating treatment efficacy. Moreover, producing deterministic outputs hinders DL adoption into clinical routines. Uncertainty estimates for the predictions would permit subsequent revision by clinicians. We present the first exploration of multiple uncertainty estimates based on Monte Carlo (MC) dropout [4] in the context of deep networks for lesion detection and segmentation in medical images. Specifically, we develop a 3D MS lesion segmentation CNN, augmented to provide four different voxel-based uncertainty measures based on MC dropout. We train the network on a proprietary, large-scale, multi-site, multi-scanner, clinical MS dataset, and compute lesion-wise uncertainties by accumulating evidence from voxel-wise uncertainties within detected lesions. We analyze the performance of voxel-based segmentation and lesion-level detection by choosing operating points based on the uncertainty. Empirical evidence suggests that uncertainty measures consistently allow us to choose superior operating points compared only using the network's sigmoid output as a probability.

Keywords: Uncertainty · Segmentation · Detection
Multiple Sclerosis

1 Introduction

Deep learning (DL) has become ubiquitous in computer vision and other applications [7,13], yet its adoption in medical imaging has been comparatively slow, due, in part, to the shortage of large-scale annotated datasets. Recently, DL frameworks have been shown to outperform other segmentation methods on a

© Springer Nature Switzerland AG 2018
A. F. Frangi et al. (Eds.): MICCAI 2018, LNCS 11070, pp. 655–663, 2018.
https://doi.org/10.1007/978-3-030-00928-1_74

variety of public challenge datasets [3,11,16], particularly on metrics focused on large pathologies. For neurological diseases such as Multiple Sclerosis (MS), lesions can be very small (e.g. 3–5 voxels) and the detection and segmentation of lesions of *all sizes* on MRI sequences is a key component for clinical assessment of disease stage and prognosis, as well as for evaluating the efficacy of treatments during clinical trials. Early DL approaches have shown success in the segmentation of large lesions [2], and recent work has shown how using a tissue-prior or lesion-prior can improve detection for medium and small lesions on small, private datasets [6]. However, current DL methods have not yet been shown to outperform other machine learning methods in the detection of small lesions, leading to potential errors in patient lesion counts, which may have serious consequences in clinical trials. Moreover, DL methods typically produce predictors with deterministic outcomes. In contrast, traditional Bayesian machine learning provides not only a prediction, but also an uncertainty about it, through a probability density over outcomes. While mathematically principled, traditional Bayesian approaches to DL have not been widely used in applications due to implementation challenges and excessive training times. Recently, Gal and Ghahramani [4] presented a simpler approach to uncertainty estimation for DL, by training a dropout network and taking Monte Carlo (MC) samples of the prediction using dropout at test time. This approach produces an approximation of the posterior of the network's weights. In computer vision, modeling uncertainty improves the performance of a standard scene understanding network with no additional parameterization [9]. In the first application to medical image analysis, [12] leverage MC sample variance in a two-stage lung nodule detection system where they rely on uncertainty at nodule contours, and an initial prediction into the second stage, without an analysis of the usefulness of the uncertainty measure. In [10], the authors perform an evaluation of the MC sample variance for image-based diabetic retinopathy diagnosis. They show that the sample variance is useful for referring cases to experts in this context.

We present the first qualitative and quantitative comparison of the effectiveness of *several different uncertainty measures* derived from MC dropout in the context of DL for lesion segmentation and detection in medical images. We develop a 3D MS lesion segmentation CNN, augmented to provide four voxel-based uncertainty measures based on MC dropout: predictive variance, MC sample variance, predictive entropy, and mutual information. The network is trained on a large proprietary, multi-scanner, multi-center, clinical trial dataset of patients with Relapsing-Remitting MS (RRMS). Voxel-wise uncertainties are combined to estimate lesion-level uncertainties. The resulting voxel-based segmentation and lesion-level detection performance are examined when choosing operating points on ROC curves (TPR vs. FDR) based on thresholded uncertainty levels. Our results indicate that while bigger lesions have large voxel-based uncertainties primarily along the border, the smallest lesions have the highest lesion-level detection errors, along with the highest uncertainty. Selecting operating points based on dropout uncertainty measures proves to be a more robust and principled approach than typical thresholding based on the network's sigmoid output.

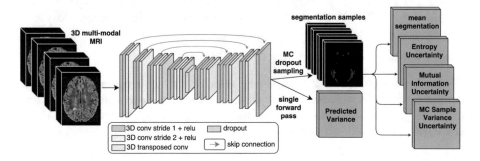

Fig. 1. Network architecture. All convolutional operations are 3D and we use additive skip connections instead of concatenating ones to reduce the number of parameters

2   Proposed Method

We develop a 3D fully convolutional neural network (CNN) with dropout to segment lesions from MRI sequences, by providing binary labels (lesion/non-lesion) to all voxels. The network is simultaneously trained to estimate uncertainty, as we will describe in detail below. Figure 1 contains the flowchart of our method. During testing, we pass an unseen multi-modal MR volume, x^*, through the network T times to obtain MC samples and estimate the uncertainty. The mean of the sample segmentations is used to obtain a single prediction.

2.1   Dropout as a Bayesian Approximation

During training, pairs of multi-sequence 3D MRIs, $\mathbf{X}$, and their associated binary ground truth T2 lesion labels, $\mathbf{Y}$, are used to learn the weights, W, of the 3D CNN. To capture uncertainty in the model, a prior distribution is placed over W, and an estimate of the posterior $p(W|\mathbf{X}, \mathbf{Y})$ is computed. Although computing this posterior analytically is intractable, variational methods can approximate it with a parameterized distribution $q(W)$ which minimizes the Kullback-Leibler (KL) divergence [1]:

$$q^*(W) = \underset{q(W)}{\arg\min}\, KL(q(W) \;||\; p(W|\mathbf{X}, \mathbf{Y})). \tag{1}$$

In [4], the authors show that minimizing the cross-entropy loss of a network with dropout applied after each layer of weights is equivalent to the minimization of the KL-divergence in Eq. (1), where the approximating distribution, $q(W)$, is a mixture of two Gaussians: $\mathcal{N}(0, \epsilon\mathbf{I})$ and $\mathcal{N}(M, \epsilon\mathbf{I})$ with small variances ϵ, mixing coefficients p and $1-p$ respectively, and where M are the variational parameters for weights W. Their derivation treats sampling from the mixture of Gaussians as sampling from a Bernoulli random variable returning either 0 or M, and links this to the application of dropout in a deep network. This is a key result, and means that we can sample from a dropout network's outputs to approximate the posterior $p(\hat{Y}|X^*, W)$ over the lesion label prediction $\hat{Y}$ for an input MRI X^*.

2.2   Measures of Uncertainty in DL Networks

We now describe the four uncertainty measures we will compute: prediction variance, which is learned directly from the training data and was discussed in [4], and three stochastic sampling-based measure based on dropout: variance of MC samples, predictive entropy, and mutual information.

Prediction Variance. During training, in addition the labels, the weights of the network are also trained to produce the prediction variance $\hat{V}$ at the output (Fig. 1). DL networks for classification typically pass network outputs, F_W, through a sigmoid or softmax function to obtain predictions $\hat{Y} \in [0, 1]$, which are then used in a loss function that compares them against ground truth labels Y. In our model, we follow the approach of [8], and assume the network outputs are corrupted by Gaussian noise with mean 0, and variance V at every voxel. The network is trained to output an estimate, $\hat{V}_W$, of the noise variance by reformulating prediction $\hat{Y}_W$ as:

$$\hat{Y}_W = sigmoid(F_W + \mathcal{N}(0, \mathbf{I}\hat{V}_W)). \tag{2}$$

During training, the Gaussian distribution is integrated out by taking T MC samples of $\hat{Y}_W$ and $\hat{V}_W$. We then use the standard weighted, binary cross-entropy function, averaging across the MC samples. Because the prediction variance is used to compute segmentations $\hat{Y}$, and subsequently the cross-entropy loss, the weight updates to the network during backpropagation push the network to learn the variance estimates without having explicit labels for them.

MC Sample Variance. As in previous work applying MC dropout methods [9, 10, 12], the MC sample variance is a measure of uncertainty derived from the variance of the T MC samples of the predicted segmentation, $var(\hat{Y}_1, ..., \hat{Y}_T)$.

Predictive Entropy. The predictive entropy is a measure of how much information is in the model predictive density function at each voxel i. We approximate the entropy for an input voxel x_i^* across T MC samples and C classes with the following biased estimator [5]:

$$H[\hat{y}_i|x_i^*, \mathbf{X}, \mathbf{Y}] \approx -\sum_{c=1}^{C} \frac{1}{T} \sum_{t=1}^{T} p(\hat{y}_i = c|x_i^*, W_t) log(\frac{1}{T} \sum_{t=1}^{T} p(\hat{y}_i = c|x_i^*, W_t)). \tag{3}$$

Mutual Information. Finally, the mutual information between the model posterior density function and the prediction density function is approximated at each voxel i as the difference between the entropy of the expected prediction, and the expectation of the model prediction entropies across samples [5]:

$$MI[\hat{y}_i, W | x_i^*, \mathbf{X}, \mathbf{Y}] \approx H[\hat{y}_i | x_i^*, \mathbf{X}, \mathbf{Y}] - E[H[\hat{y}_i | x_i^*, W]]. \tag{4}$$

2.3 Uncertainty-Based Filtering in Lesion Segmentation/Detection

The network outputs $\hat{y}_i$ computed as in Eq. (2) as well as the four defined measures of uncertainty $U_m(i), i = 1 \ldots 4$ at every voxel x_i^*. The standard approach to generate a classification would be to compute the indicator function $\mathbf{1}_{\hat{y}_i \geq \theta}$ where the threshold θ is specified (e.g. 0.9). When we use the uncertainty measure, we will additionally require that $U_m(i)$ is below another chosen threshold η in order to produce the prediction. If the predictions that are incorrect are uncertain, this filtering should increase the performance on remaining predictions.

In the context of neurological diseases such as MS, it important to perform lesion-level detection because changes in the a patient's lesion count are indicative of disease activity and progression. This requires a strategy to merge voxel-level uncertainty measures into lesion-level uncertainty, which is then used to perform lesion-wise filtering. Suppose we can generate a large set of candidate lesions. For a candidate l, composed of voxels $p, ..., q$, we will compute the lesion-uncertainty $U_m(l)$ from the voxel-wise uncertainties as: $U_m(l) = \sum_{i=p}^{q} log(U_m(i))$. Taking the log-sum of the voxel-level uncertainties reflects the simplifying assumption that neighbouring voxels are conditionally independent, given that they are part of l. To make the uncertainties comparable through a single threshold value, we rescale the values $U_m(l)$ to $[0, 1]$ by subtracting by the minimum lesion uncertainty and dividing by the range; we do this separately for each measure m. Detection is then performed using the uncertainty threshold and outputs in the same case as for the voxel-level. Further implementation details can be found in the supplementary material and code is available at https://github.com/tanyanair/segmentation_uncertainty.

3 Experiments and Results

The method was evaluated on a proprietary, multi-site, multi-scanner, clinical trial dataset of 1064 Relapsing-Remitting MS (RRMS) patients, scanned annually over a 24-month period. T1, T2, FLAIR, and PDW MRI sequences were acquired at a 1 mm × 1 mm × 3 mm resolution and pre-processed with brain extraction [15], N3 bias field inhomogeneity correction [14], Nyul image intensity normalization, and registration to the MNI-space. Ground truth T2 lesion segmentation masks were provided with the data. These were obtained using a proprietary approach where the result of an automated segmentation method was manually corrected by expert human annotators. The network was trained on 80% of the subjects, with 10% held out for validation and 10% for testing (2182/251/251 scans for training/validation/testing respectively). We take 10 MC samples during training and testing for the evaluation of the uncertainties.

To see if the uncertainty measures are useful and describe different information, we plot the voxel-level True Positive Rate ($TPR = \frac{TP}{TP+FN}$), and False Detection Rate ($FDR = 1 - \frac{TP}{TP+FP}$) Receiver Operating Characteristic (ROC) curves for the retained voxels at different uncertainty thresholds, and them compare against a baseline ROC in which no uncertainty thresholding is performed (Fig. 2a). At operating points of interest ($FDR < 0.3$), different measures lead to different percentage levels of voxel retention. The notably high TPR of the predicted variance curve can be attributed to the significantly lower voxel-level retention.

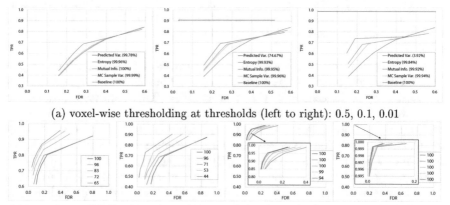

(a) voxel-wise thresholding at thresholds (left to right): 0.5, 0.1, 0.01

(b) lesion-wise thresholding across (left to right): all, small, medium, and large lesions

Fig. 2. FDR vs. TPR of retained predictions when (a) voxel-wise thresholding with each uncertainty measure and (b) lesion-wise thresholding with the entropy measure. In (a) the % of voxels retained is provided with each uncertainty measure in the legend. In (b), the % of lesions retained for each curve's uncertainty threshold is provided in the color coded legend for that plot. The uncertainty threshold used to generate a given color's curve in a plot is the same across these plots. Points along a curve correspond to different sigmoid thresholds used to binarize the model's segmentation output. Each plot contains a reference curve (100%) corresponding to the model's baseline performance when no uncertainty thresholding is performed.

To obtain lesion-level statistics from voxel segmentations, ground truth lesions smaller than 3 voxels were removed, as per clinical protocol. We performed voxel-level classification and candidate lesions are then obtained from lesion voxels by considering a surrounding, 18-connected neighbourhood in order to mitigate the impact of under-segmented ground truth in this dataset. A true positive (TP) lesion is detected when the segmentation, including its 18-connected neighbourhood, overlaps with at least three, or more than 50%, of the

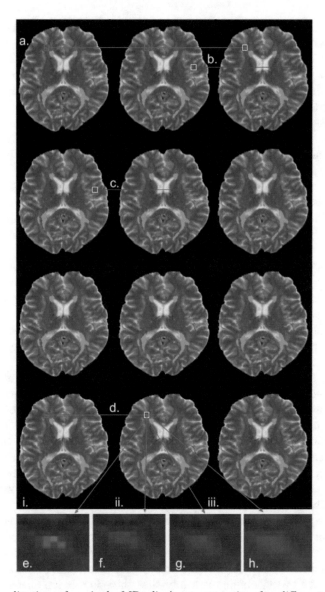

Fig. 3. Visualization of a single MR slice's segmentation for different uncertainty thresholds. From top to bottom we use the following uncertainty measures: entropy, mutual information, MC sample variance, and predicted variance. From left to right we show **i.** Baseline (no uncertainty thresholding) lesion segmentation. **ii.**, **iii.** Segmentation at two different thresholds for the uncertainty corresponding to that row (i.e. more lesions are excluded in iii.). Lesions are coloured with the following scheme: TP: green, FP:red, FN: blue, and True Negative (TN): white. Lesions **a, d** show the uncertainty corresponding to a FP in the baseline segmentation turned into a TN as the uncertainty threshold is increased. **b, c** show a TP (from another slice) becoming a FN. **d** shows a FP (from another slice) becoming a TN. The lesion uncertainties at **d** are shown for **e** entropy, **f** mutual information, **g** MC sample variance, and **h** predicted variance. Note that the threshold to turn lesions into TN's or FN's is different for different uncertainty measures. All MRI are courtesy of Neurorx Research.

ground truth lesion voxels. Insufficient overlap results in a false negative (FN), and candidate lesions of 3 or more voxels that do not overlap with a ground truth lesion are counted as false positives (FP). Lesion-level TPR, and FDR ROC curves for retained predictions at different entropy thresholds are shown in Fig. 2b. Results for the other measures can be found in the supplementary material, as they were extremely similar to one another. At all operating points, across all measures, using uncertainty to exclude uncertain predictions improves performance on remaining predictions, even when excluding just 2% of the most uncertain lesions, due to the resulting reduction in the number of both FP and FN assertions. In an analysis across small (3–10 vox), medium (11–50 vox), and large (51+) lesion bin sizes (Fig. 2b), we find that using uncertainty to exclude predictions is helpful for small lesions regardless of the exact uncertainty measure used. This is because the model does not perform as well for small lesions, which constitute 40% of lesions in the dataset, so removing the uncertain FP and FN segmentations improves the overall performance. However, for medium and large lesions, performance reduces slightly compared to non-thresholded segmentations because the DL model has very few FP's and FN's for medium and large lesions. Filtering out these sized lesions reduces TP's, reducing the performance for those sizes.

Figure 3(e–h) provides an example of uncertainties themselves. In general, measures computed from stochastic dropout samples are more uncertain around lesion contours. Relative to other work [12], the MC sample variance is very small, even around lesion contours, but mutual information and predictive entropy reflect the boundary-uncertainty more intensely. The learned, predictive variance reflects data uncertainty throughout contours in the entire MRI (e.g. boundaries between white matter and grey matter). Despite these voxelwise differences, when accumulating evidence to the lesion-level, the different measures tend to rank lesions is the same order of certainty, albeit on different scales, which leads to filtering out the same lesions, at different thresholds (i.e. Fig. 3c, d)). One interpretation is that between taking MC dropout samples, and computing the uncertainty measures, no new information is added. We also note that small lesions are relatively more uncertain than medium and large lesions. This is a consequence of computing lesion uncertainty from the log sum of all the uncertainty values in a detected lesion area. Although large lesions have larger, more uncertain contours, the accumulation of lesion-evidence within the boundary provides an overwhelming certainty that there is a lesion there. This is not the case for small lesions (less evidence).

4   Conclusion

We developed a 3D MS lesion segmentation CNN, augmented to provide four voxel-based uncertainties, and showed how these can be accumulated to estimate lesion-level uncertainties. Our results indicate that filtering based on uncertainty greatly improves lesion detection accuracy for small lesions, which make up 40% of the dataset, indicating that high uncertainty does indeed reflect incorrect predictions. Moreover, uncertainty measures in the results of an automatic, DL detection or segmentation method provide clinicians or radiologists with information permitting them to quickly assess whether to accept or reject lesions of high uncertainty, for example, or further analyze uncertain lesion boundaries. This could facilitate the wider adoption of DL methods into clinical work-flows.

Acknowledgements. This work was supported by the Canadian NSERC Discovery and CREATE grants, and an award from the International Progressive MS Alliance (PA-1603-08175).

References

1. Blei, D.M., et al.: Variational inference. ASA **112**(518), 859–877 (2017)
2. Brosch, T., et al.: Deep 3D convolutional encoder networks with shortcuts for multiscale feature integration applied to multiple sclerosis lesion segmentation. TMI **35**(5), 1229–1239 (2016)
3. Carass, A., et al.: Longitudinal multiple sclerosis lesion segmentation: resource and challenge. NeuroImage **148**, 77–102 (2017)
4. Gal, Y., Ghahramani, Z.: Dropout as a bayesian approximation: representing model uncertainty in deep learning. In: ICML, pp. 1050–1059 (2016)
5. Gal, Y., et al.: Deep Bayesian active learning with image data. In: ICML (2017)
6. Ghafoorian, M., et al.: Non-uniform patch sampling with deep convolutional neural networks for white matter hyperintensity segmentation. In: ISBI, pp. 1414–1417 (2016)
7. Hernandez, C., et al.: Team delft's robot winner of the amazon picking challenge 2016. In: Behnke, S., Sheh, R., Sariel, S., Lee, D.D. (eds.) RoboCup 2016. LNCS (LNAI), vol. 9776, pp. 613–624. Springer, Cham (2017). https://doi.org/10.1007/978-3-319-68792-6_51
8. Kendall, A., Gal, Y.: What uncertainties do we need in Bayesian deep learning for computer vision? In: NIPS, pp. 5580–5590 (2017)
9. Kendall, A., et al.: Bayesian SegNet: model uncertainty in deep convolutional encoder-decoder architectures for scene understanding. In: BMVC (2017)
10. Leibig, C., et al.: Leveraging uncertainty information from deep neural networks for disease detection. Nature **7**(1) (2017). https://doi.org/10.1038/s41598-017-17876-z
11. Menze, B.H., et al.: The multimodal brain tumor image segmentation benchmark (BRATS). TMI **34**(10), 1993–2024 (2015)
12. Ozdemir, O., et al.: Propagating uncertainty in multi-stage Bayesian convolutional neural networks with application to pulmonary nodule detection. In: NIPS (2017)
13. Russakovsky, O., et al.: Imagenet large scale visual recognition challenge. IJCV **115**(3), 211–252 (2015)
14. Sled, J.G., Zijdenbos, A.P., Evans, A.C.: A nonparametric method for automatic correction of intensity nonuniformity in MRI data. TMI **17**(1), 87–97 (1998)
15. Smith, S.M.: Fast robust automated brain extraction. HBM **17**(3), 143–155 (2002)
16. Styner, M., et al.: 3D segmentation in the clinic: a grand challenge II: MS lesion segmentation. MIDAS **2008**, 1–6 (2008)

Inherent Brain Segmentation Quality Control from Fully ConvNet Monte Carlo Sampling

Abhijit Guha Roy[1,2]([⊠]), Sailesh Conjeti[3], Nassir Navab[2,4],
and Christian Wachinger[1]

[1] Artificial Intelligence in Medical Imaging (AI-Med), KJP, LMU München,
Munich, Germany
abhijit.guha-roy@tum.de

[2] Computer Aided Medical Procedures, Technische Universität München,
Munich, Germany

[3] German Center for Neurodegenerative Diseases (DZNE), Bonn, Germany

[4] Computer Aided Medical Procedures, Johns Hopkins University, Baltimore, USA

Abstract. We introduce inherent measures for effective quality control of brain segmentation based on a Bayesian fully convolutional neural network, using model uncertainty. Monte Carlo samples from the posterior distribution are efficiently generated using dropout at test time. Based on these samples, we introduce next to a voxel-wise uncertainty map also three metrics for structure-wise uncertainty. We then incorporate these structure-wise uncertainty in group analyses as a measure of confidence in the observation. Our results show that the metrics are highly correlated to segmentation accuracy and therefore present an inherent measure of segmentation quality. Furthermore, group analysis with uncertainty results in effect sizes closer to that of manual annotations. The introduced uncertainty metrics can not only be very useful in translation to clinical practice but also provide automated quality control and group analyses in processing large data repositories.

1 Introduction

Magnetic resonance imaging (MRI) delivers high-quality, *in-vivo* information about the brain. Whole-brain segmentation [1,2] provides imaging biomarkers of neuroanatomy, which form the basis for tracking structural brain changes associated with aging and disease. Despite efforts to deliver robust segmentation results across scans from different age groups, diseases, field strengths, and manufacturers, inaccuracies in the segmentation outcome are inevitable [3]. A manual quality assessment is therefore recommended before continuing with the analysis. However, the manual assessment is not only time consuming, but also subject to inter- and intra-rater variability.

The underlying problem is that most segmentation algorithms provide results without a measure of confidence or quality. Bayesian approaches are an alterna-

© Springer Nature Switzerland AG 2018
A. F. Frangi et al. (Eds.): MICCAI 2018, LNCS 11070, pp. 664–672, 2018.
https://doi.org/10.1007/978-3-030-00928-1_75

tive, because they do not only provide the mode (i.e., the most likely segmentation) but also the posterior distribution. However, most Bayesian approaches use point estimates in the inference, whereas marginalization over parameters has only been proposed in combination with Markov Chain Monte Carlo sampling [4] or the Laplace approximation [5]. While sampling-based approaches incorporate fewer assumptions, they are computationally intense and have so far only been used for the segmentation of substructures but not the whole-brain [4].

Recent advances in Bayesian deep learning enabled approximating the posterior distribution by dropping out neurons at test time [6]. This does not require any additional parameters and is achieved by sampling from the Bernoulli distribution across the network weights. In addition, this approach enables to represent uncertainty in deep learning without sacrificing accuracy or computational complexity, allowing for fast Monte Carlo sampling. This concept of uncertainty was later extended for semantic segmentation within fully convolutional neural networks (F-CNN) [7] providing a pixel-wise uncertainty estimation. At the same time, F-CNNs started to achieve state-of-the-art performance for whole-brain segmentation, while requiring only seconds for a 3D volume [8,9].

In this work, we propose inherent measures of segmentation quality based on a Bayesian F-CNN for whole-brain segmentation. To this end, we extend the F-CNN architecture [8] with dropout layers, which allows for highly efficient Monte Carlo sampling. From the samples, we compute the voxel-wise segmentation uncertainty and introduce three metrics for quantifying uncertainty per brain structure. We show that these metrics are highly correlated with the segmentation accuracy and can therefore be used to predict segmentation accuracy in absence of ground truth. Finally, we propose to effectively use the uncertainty estimates as quality control measures in large-scale group analysis to estimate reliable effect sizes. We believe that uncertainty measures are not only essential for the translation of quantitative measures to clinical practice but also provide automated quality control and group analyses in large data repositories.

Prior Art: Evaluating segmentation performance without ground truth has been studied in medical imaging before. In early work, the common agreement strategy (STAPLE) was used to evaluate classifier performance for segmenting brain scans into WM, GM and CSF [10]. In another approach, features corresponding to a segmentation map were used to learn a separate regressor for predicting the Dice score [11]. Recently, the reverse classification accuracy was proposed, which involves training a separate classifier on the segmentation outcome of the method to evaluate, serving as pseudo ground truth [12]. In contrast to these previous approaches, we provide a quality measure that is *inherently* computed within the segmentation framework, derived from model uncertainty and does therefore not require training a second, independent classifier for evaluation, which itself may be subject to prediction errors.

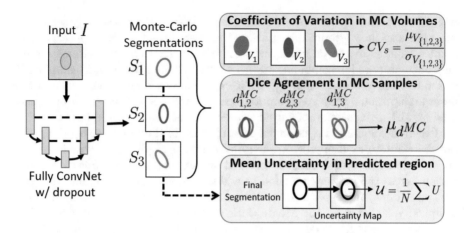

Fig. 1. A single input scan results in different Monte Carlo (MC) segmentations (S_1, S_2, S_3) based on different dropouts in the fully ConvNet. The samples are used to estimate three variants of structure-wise uncertainty. The final segmentation is the average of the MC samples, used in the third variant.

2   Method

Bayesian Inference: We employ dropout [13] to create a probabilistic encoder-decoder network, which approximates probabilistic neuron connectivity similar to a Bayesian neural network (BNN) [6]. Dropout is commonly used in training and then turned-off at testing time. By using dropout also at testing, we can sample from the posterior distribution of the model. We modify the architecture in [8] by *inserting dropout layers after every encoder and decoder block* with a dropout rate of q.

A given input I is feed-forwarded N times with different dropped out neurons, generating N different Monte Carlo (MC) samples of segmentation $\{S_1, \cdots S_N\}$. This inference strategy is similar to variational inference in BNNs, assuming a Bernoulli distribution over the weights [6]. The final probability map is given by computing the average over MC probability maps. We set the dropout rate to $q = 0.2$ and produce $N = 15$ MC samples (<2 min), after which performance saturates. We pre-train the network on 581 volumes of the IXI dataset[1] with FreeSurfer [2] segmentations and subsequently fine-tune on 15 of the 30 manually annotated volumes from the Multi-Atlas Labelling Challenge (MALC) dataset [14]. This trained model is used for all our experiments. In this work, we segment 33 cortical and sub-cortical structures.

---

[1] http://brain-development.org/ixi-dataset/.

2.1 Uncertainty Measures

1. Voxel-wise Uncertainty: The model uncertainty U_s for a given voxel $\mathbf{x}$, for a specific structure s is estimated as entropy over all N MC probability maps p_s

$$U_s(\mathbf{x}) = -\sum_{i=1}^{N} p_s^i(\mathbf{x}) \log(p_s^i(\mathbf{x})). \tag{1}$$

The voxel-wise uncertainty is the sum over all structures, $U = \sum_s U_s$. Voxels where uncertainty is low (i.e. entropy is low) receive the same predictions, in spite of different neurons being dropped out.

2. Structure-wise Uncertainty: For many applications, it is helpful to have an uncertainty measure per brain structure. We propose three different strategies for computing structure-wise uncertainty from MC segmentations, illustrated in Fig. 1 for $N = 3$ MC samples.

Type-1: We measure the variation of the volume across the MC samples. We compute the coefficient of variation $CV_s = \frac{\sigma_s}{\mu_s}$ for a structure s, with mean μ_s and standard deviation σ_s of MC volume estimates. Note that this estimate is agnostic to the size of the structure.

Type-2: We use the overlap between samples as a measure of uncertainty. To this end, we compute the average Dice score over all pairs of MC samples

$$d_s^{MC} = E\left[\{Dice((S_i == s), (S_j == s))\}_{i \neq j}\right]. \tag{2}$$

Type-3: We define the uncertainty for a structure s as mean voxel-wise uncertainty over the voxels which were labeled as s, $\mathcal{U}_s = E\left[\{U(\mathbf{x})\}_{\mathbf{x} \in \{S==s\}}\right]$.

Note that d_s^{MC} is directly related to segmentation accuracy, while $\mathcal{U}_s$ and CV_s are inversely related to accuracy.

2.2 Segmentation Uncertainty in Group Analysis

We propose to integrate the structure-wise uncertainty in group analysis. To this end, we solve a weighted linear regression model with weight w_i for subject i

$$\hat{\boldsymbol{\beta}} = \arg\min \sum_i \omega_i (V_i - \mathbf{X}_i \boldsymbol{\beta}^\top)^2 \tag{3}$$

with design matrix $\mathbf{X}$, vector of coefficients $\boldsymbol{\beta}$, and brain structure volume V_i. We use the first two types of structure-wise uncertainty and set the weight ω_i to $\frac{1}{CV_s}$ or $\frac{1}{1-d_s^{MC}}$. Including weights in linear regression increases its robustness as scans with reliable segmentation are emphasized. Setting all weights to a constant results in standard regression. In our experiments, we set

$$\mathbf{X}_i = [1, A_i, S_i, D_i] \qquad \boldsymbol{\beta} = [\beta_0, \beta_A, \beta_S, \beta_D] \tag{4}$$

with age A_i, sex S_i and diagnosis D_i for subject i. Of particular interest is the regression coefficient β_D, which estimates the effect of diagnosis on the volume of a brain structure V.

3   Experimental Results

Datasets: We test on the 15 volumes of the **MALC** dataset [14] that were not used for training. Further, we deployed the model on un-seen scans across 3 different datasets not used for training: (i) **ADNI-29**: The dataset consists of 29 scans from ADNI dataset [15], with a balanced distribution of Alzheimer's Disease (AD) and control subjects, and scans acquired with 1.5T and 3T scanners. The objective is to observe uncertainty changes due to variability in scanner and pathologies. (ii) **CANDI-13**: The dataset consists of 13 brain scans of children (age 5–15) with psychiatric disorders, part of the CANDI dataset [16]. The objective is to observe changes in uncertainty for data with age range not included in training. (iii) **IBSR-18**: The dataset consist of 18 scans publicly available at https://www.nitrc.org/projects/ibsr. The objective is to see the sensitivity of uncertainty with low resolution and poor contrast scans. Note that the training set (MALC) did not contain scans with AD or scans from children. Manual segmentations for MALC, ADNI-29, and CANDI-13 were provided by Neuromorphometrics, Inc.[2]

Table 1. Results on 4 different datasets with global Dice scores and correlation of Dice scores with 3 types of uncertainty.

Datasets	Mean dice score (DS)	Mean	Corr($\cdot$, DS)		
		CV_s	$\mathcal{U}_s$	CV_s	d_s^{MC}
MALC-15	$\mathbf{0.88} \pm 0.02$	0.38	-0.85	-0.81	$\mathbf{0.86}$
ADNI-29	0.83 ± 0.02	0.46	-0.72	-0.71	$\mathbf{0.78}$
CANDI-13	0.81 ± 0.03	0.54	-0.84	-0.86	$\mathbf{0.90}$
IBSR-18	0.81 ± 0.02	0.57	-0.76	-0.76	$\mathbf{0.80}$

Quantitative Analysis: To quantify the performance of the uncertainty in predicting the segmentation accuracy, we compute the correlation coefficient between the Dice scores and the three types of structure-wise uncertainty. Table 1 reports the correlations for all 4 test datasets, together with the Dice score of the inferred segmentation. Firstly, we observe that the segmentation accuracy is highest on MALC and that the accuracy drops (5–7%) for other datasets (ADNI, CANDI, IBSR). This decrease in performance is to be expected when transferring the model to other datasets and is also reflected in the uncertainty estimate (Mean CV_s). Secondly, for the three measures of structure-wise uncertainty, the Dice agreement in MC samples d_s^{MC} shows highest correlations across all datasets. The overall high correlation for d_s^{MC} indicates that it is a suitable proxy for measuring segmentation accuracy without the presence of ground truth annotations. Figure 2 shows scatter plots for the three uncertainty variants with respect to actual Dice score on CANDI-13.

---

[2] http://Neuromorphometrics.com/.

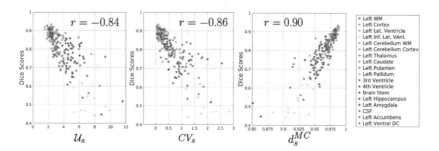

Fig. 2. Scatter plot of three types of uncertainty and Dice scores on CANDI-13 dataset (one dot per scan and structure), with their corresponding correlation coefficient (r). For clarity, structures only on the left hemisphere are shown.

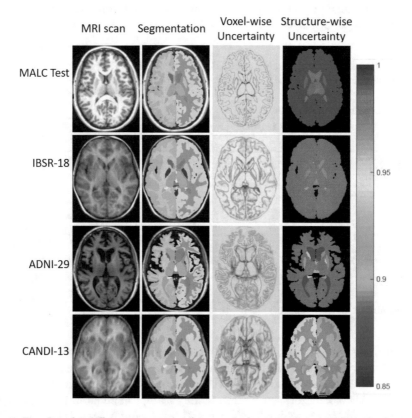

Fig. 3. Results of 4 different cases, one from each dataset, corresponding to the worst Dice score. The MRI scan, segmentation, voxel-wise uncertainty and structure-wise uncertainty (d_s^{MC}) are presented. Red in the heat map indicates high reliability in segmentation, while blue indicates poor segmentation.

Qualitative Analysis: Figure 3 illustrates qualitative results with MRI scan, segmentation, voxel-wise uncertainty map and structure-wise uncertainty (d_{MC}) heat map. In the heat map, red indicates higher reliability in segmentation. The first row shows results on a test sample from the MALC dataset, where segmentation is good with high reliability in prediction. The second row presents the scan with worst performance on IBSR-18 dataset, consisting of poor contrast with prominent ringing artifacts. Its voxel-wise and structure-wise uncertainty maps shows less reliability in comparison to MALC. The third row presents the scan with worst performance in ADNI-29, a subject of age 95 with severe AD. Prominent atrophy in cortex along with enlarged ventricles are visible in the MRI scan, with ringing artifacts at the top. Its d_s^{MC} heat maps shows higher uncertainty in some subcortical structures with brighter shades. The last row presents the MRI scan with the worst performance on CANDI-13 dataset, a subject of age 5 with high motion artifact together with poor contrast. Its voxel-wise uncertainty is higher in comparison to others, with dark patches prominent in subcortical regions. The heat map shows the lowest confidence for this scan, in comparison to other results.

Table 2. Results of group analyses on ADNI-29 and ABIDE datasets with pathologies (Alzheimer's and autism), with and without using uncertainty.

AD biomarkers	ADNI-29							
	Ground truth		Normal regression		CV_s		d_s^{MC}	
	β_D	p_D	β_D	p_D	β_D	p_D	β_D	p_D
Hippocampus	1.16	0.0010	1.26	0.0002	1.21	0.0002	1.25	0.0002
Lat. Ventricle	−0.15	0.6658	−0.19	0.5826	−0.15	0.6650	−0.16	0.6342
Autism biomarkers	ABIDE							
	Normal regression		Robust regression		CV_s		d_s^{MC}	
	β_D	p_D	β_D	p_D	β_D	p_D	β_D	p_D
Amygdala	−0.14	0.0140	−0.07	0.0499	−0.32	0.0001	−0.27	0.0001
Lat. Ventricles	−0.01	0.8110	−0.05	0.1294	−0.38	0.0089	−0.19	0.0843
Pallidum	−0.07	0.2480	−0.01	0.8727	−0.40	0.0051	−0.28	0.0165
Putamen	−0.07	0.2186	−0.01	0.8125	−0.43	0.0035	−0.39	0.0057
Accumbens	−0.08	0.1494	−0.03	0.4386	−0.21	0.0013	−0.17	0.0031

Uncertainty for Group Analysis: In this section, we evaluate the integration of structure-wise uncertainty in group analyses. First, we perform group analysis on ADNI-29 with 15 control and 14 AD subjects. We focus our analysis on most prominent AD biomarkers, the volume of hippocampus and lateral ventricles [17]. Table 2 reports the regression coefficient and p-value for diagnosis (β_D, p_D). The coefficient is computed by solving Eq. 3, where we use two types of uncertainty (CV_s, d_s^{MC}) and compare to normal regression. Although the dataset is small, it comes with ground truth annotations and therefore allows for estimating the actual β_D. Comparing, we observe that both versions of weighted regression results in β_D closer to the actual effect in comparison to normal regression. Also, we note that CV_s provides a better weighting than $(1 - d_s^{MC})$. Next, we perform group analysis on the ABIDE-I dataset [18] consisting of $1,112$ scans, with 573 normal subjects and 539 subjects with autism. The dataset is collected from 20 different sites with a high variability in scan quality. To factor out changes due to site, we added site as a covariate in Eq. 3. We report β_D with corresponding p-values for the volume of brain structures that have recently been associated to autism in a large ENIGMA study [19]. We compare uncertainty weighted regression to normal regression, and include robust regression with Huber norm. CV_s provides the highest effect sizes, followed by $(1 - d_s^{MC})$. Strikingly, uncertainty weighted regression results in significant associations to autism, identical to [19], whereas normal regression is only significant for amygdala.

4   Conclusion

We introduced a Bayesian F-CNN model for whole-brain segmentation that produces MC samples by using dropout at test time. Based on the samples, we introduced metrics for quantifying structure-wise uncertainty. We show a high correlation with segmentation accuracy of these metrics on 4 out-of-sample datasets, thus providing segmentation quality. In addition, we proposed to integrate the confidence in the observation into group analysis, yielding improved effect sizes.

Acknowledgement. We thank SAP SE and the Bavarian State Ministry of Education, Science and the Arts in the framework of the Centre Digitisation.Bavaria (ZD.B) for funding and the NVIDIA corporation for GPU donation.

References

1. Jenkinson, M., Beckmann, C.F., Behrens, T.E., Woolrich, M.W., Smith, S.M.: FSL. Neuroimage **62**(2), 782–790 (2012)
2. Fischl, B., Salat, D.H., Busa, E., Albert, M., et al.: Whole brain segmentation: automated labeling of neuroanatomical structures in the human brain. Neuron **33**(3), 341–355 (2002)
3. Keshavan, A.: Mindcontrol: a web application for brain segmentation quality control. NeuroImage **170**, 365–372 (2018)
4. Iglesias, J.E., Sabuncu, M.R., Van Leemput, K.: Improved inference in Bayesian segmentation using Monte Carlo sampling: application to hippocampal subfield volumetry. Med. Image Anal. **17**(7), 766–778 (2013)
5. Wachinger, C., Fritscher, K., Sharp, G., Golland, P.: Contour-driven atlas-based segmentation. IEEE TMI **34**(12), 2492–2505 (2015)
6. Gal, Y., Ghahramani, Z.: Dropout as a Bayesian approximation: representing model uncertainty in deep learning. In: Proceedings of ICML, pp. 1050–1059 (2016)
7. Kendall, A., Badrinarayanan, V., Cipolla, R.: Bayesian segnet: model uncertainty in deep convolutional encoder-decoder architectures for scene understanding. In: Proceedings of BMVC (2017)
8. Roy, A.G., Conjeti, S., Navab, N., Wachinger, C.: . QuickNAT: Segmenting MRI Neuroanatomy in 20 seconds (2018). ArXiv:1801.04161

9. Roy, A.G., Conjeti, S., Sheet, D., Katouzian, A., Navab, N., Wachinger, C.: Error corrective boosting for learning fully convolutional networks with limited data. In: Descoteaux, M., Maier-Hein, L., Franz, A., Jannin, P., Collins, D.L., Duchesne, S. (eds.) MICCAI 2017. LNCS, vol. 10435, pp. 231–239. Springer, Cham (2017). https://doi.org/10.1007/978-3-319-66179-7_27

10. Bouix, S., et al.: On evaluating brain tissue classifiers without a ground truth. Neuroimage **36**(4), 1207–1224 (2007)

11. Kohlberger, T., Singh, V., Alvino, C., Bahlmann, C., Grady, L.: Evaluating segmentation error without ground truth. In: Ayache, N., Delingette, H., Golland, P., Mori, K. (eds.) MICCAI 2012. LNCS, vol. 7510, pp. 528–536. Springer, Heidelberg (2012). https://doi.org/10.1007/978-3-642-33415-3_65

12. Valindria, V., et al.: Reverse classification accuracy: predicting segmentation performance in the absence of ground truth. TMI **36**(8), 1597–1606 (2017)

13. Srivastava, N., Hinton, G., Krizhevsky, A., Sutskever, I., Salakhutdinov, R.: Dropout: a simple way to prevent neural networks from overfitting. J. Mach. Learn. Res. **15**(1), 1929–1958 (2014)

14. Landman, B, Warfield, S.: Miccai workshop on multiatlas labeling. In: MICCAI Grand Challenge (2012)

15. Jack, C.R., Bernstein, M.A., Fox, N.C., Thompson, P., et al.: The Alzheimer's disease neuroimaging initiative (ADNI): MRI methods. JMRI **27**(4), 685–691 (2008)

16. Kennedy, D.N., Haselgrove, C., Hodge, S.M., Rane, P.S., Makris, N., Frazier, J.A.: CANDIShare: a resource for pediatric neuroimaging data (2012)

17. Thompson, P.M., Hayashi, K.M., et al.: Mapping hippocampal and ventricular change in Alzheimer disease. Neuroimage **22**(4), 1754–1766 (2004)

18. Di Martino, A., Yan, C.G., Li, Q., Denio, E.: The autism brain imaging data exchange: towards a large-scale evaluation of the intrinsic brain architecture in autism. Mol. Psychiatry **19**(6), 659 (2014)

19. Van Rooij, D., Anagnostou, E., Arango, C., Auzias, G., et al.: Cortical and subcortical brain morphometry differences between patients with autism spectrum disorder and healthy individuals across the lifespan: results from the ENIGMA ASD working group. Am. J. Psychiatry **175**(4), 359–369 (2018)

Perfect MCMC Sampling in Bayesian MRFs for Uncertainty Estimation in Segmentation

Saurabh Garg and Suyash P. Awate$^{(\boxtimes)}$

Computer Science and Engineering Department,
Indian Institute of Technology (IIT) Bombay, Mumbai, India
suyash@cse.iitb.ac.in

Abstract. Typical segmentation methods produce a single optimal solution and fail to inform about (i) the confidence/*uncertainty* in the object boundaries or (ii) alternate close-to-optimal solutions. To estimate uncertainty, some methods intend to sample segmentations from an associated posterior model using Markov chain Monte Carlo (MCMC) sampling or perturbation models. However, they cannot guarantee sampling from the true posterior, deviating significantly in practice. We propose a novel method that guarantees *exact MCMC sampling*, in finite time, of multi-label segmentations from *generic Bayesian Markov random field* (MRF) models. For exact sampling, we propose Fill's strategy and *extend it to generic MRF models* via a novel *bounding chain* algorithm. Results on simulated data and clinical brain images from 4 classic problems show that our uncertainty estimates gain accuracy over the state of the art.

Keywords: Segmentation · Uncertainty · Hidden MRF · Bayesian
EM · MCMC · Perfect/exact sampling · Brain · Multiatlas · Tumor
Tissue · Lesion

1 Introduction and Related Work

Accounting for *uncertainty* in automated segmentation results can improve risk analysis in clinical procedures (e.g., neurosurgery [1], radiotherapy [8]) and reliability in clinical diagnosis and studies. Segmentation methods, e.g., using expectation maximization (EM) and hidden Markov random fields (MRFs) or graph cuts, typically produce a single optimal solution, failing to inform about object-boundary uncertainty or alternate close-to-optimal solutions.

For a small class of MRF models that allow segmentation inference via graph cuts, efficient methods exist to exactly estimate label uncertainty [6]. For general MRFs, typical uncertainty estimation methods approximate modeling or sampling. While [3] uses (non-exact) Markov chain Monte Carlo (MCMC) to sample

---

The authors are grateful for funding from IIT Bombay Seed Grant 14IRCCSG010.

A. F. Frangi et al. (Eds.): MICCAI 2018, LNCS 11070, pp. 673–681, 2018.
https://doi.org/10.1007/978-3-030-00928-1_76

nonparametric curves, [8] uses a Gaussian-process approximation for label distributions. In tumor segmentation, [1] approximates the Gumbel perturbation models in [9] to sample from the underlying Bayesian MRF. For multiatlas segmentation, [2] uses bootstrap resampling to learn nonparametric regression models and error-convergence rates indicating voxelwise uncertainty for a *population* of images (not a specific image). In contrast, we propose the *perfect/exact MCMC* paradigm and a novel perfect-MCMC sampler for *generic Bayesian MRFs*, to estimate uncertainty in multilabel and multiatlas segmentation.

For uncertainty estimation in image registration, while some methods [7] use bootstrap data resampling to approximate the data distribution (unlike the posterior), others use MCMC sampling. Unlike typical MCMC [3] that is only asymptotically exact and can suffer from insufficient burn-in (fixing one very large burn-in for *all* tasks makes computational costs exorbitant), we guarantee exact MCMC in *finite time* and eliminate adhoc heuristics to determine burn-in.

We introduce a new framework for uncertainty estimation in segmentation by relying on *perfect MCMC sampling*, in finite time, from *generic Bayesian MRF* models. We propose to perfect-sample label images: (i) by combining coupling-from-the-past (CFTP) [10] with the bounding-chain (BC) [5] scheme, called CFTP-BC, and, more importantly, (ii) by extending Fill's algorithm (FA) [4] using the BC scheme, called FA-BC. Results on clinical brain images from 4 applications (segmenting tissues, subcortical structures, tumor, lobes) show that our uncertainty estimates gain accuracy over the state of the art.

2   Methods

We describe our frameworks for perfect MCMC sampling to estimate uncertainty.

MCMC Sampling. Let observed image y, with V voxels, be generated from (i) a hidden label image x that is modeled by MRF X with prior probability mass function (PMF) $P(X)$ and (ii) a likelihood model $P(Y|X)$. MRF X has a neighborhood system $\mathcal{N} := \{\mathcal{N}_v\}_{v=1}^V$, where $\mathcal{N}_v$ is the set of voxels neighboring voxel v. To sample from the posterior $Q(X) := P(X|y)$, MCMC methods construct a Markov chain $\mathcal{M}$ as the MRF sequence $X^1, X^2, \cdots, X^t, \cdots$, an associated *transition kernel* $K(\cdot, \cdot)$ with $P(X^{t+1}|X^t) := K(X^t, \cdot)$, and *stationary* PMF $Q(X)$. Typically, $\mathcal{M}$ is positive, recurrent, and aperiodic (such a chain is called *ergodic*), thereby having a unique stationary PMF and that PMF being $Q(X)$. $\mathcal{M}$ also typically satisfies *detailed balance*, or *reversibility*, which implies that kernel $K(\cdot, \cdot)$ also applies to the time-reversed chain. The Gibbs sampler is a Metropolis-Hastings MCMC sampler (with an ergodic reversible Markov chain); it iteratively selects a random voxel and draws from its local conditional PMF.

Coupling from the Past (CFTP) for Perfect MCMC Sampling. Gibbs sampler, and typical Metropolis samplers, need to run infinitely long to guarantee draws from the associated stationary PMF $Q(X)$. CFTP [10] theoretically guarantees the sampled state to be from the desired PMF $Q(X)$ by ensuring that any long-running Markov chain, irrespective of its initial state, would have reached the chosen sampled state, using a specific sequence of interstate-transition maps. CFTP tracks *coupled* parallel chains, one chain started in each possible state of the state space, until all of them *coalesce* to a single state.

Theorem 1. *Propp-Wilson [10]: The CFTP algorithm terminates in finite time and returns a draw from the stationary distribution of the Markov chain.*

Interpretation: Markov chain ergodicity implies, $\forall$ states x, a non-zero probability $> \epsilon > 0$ of reaching x, from any state x' in a finite number of transitions N_x. For a given instance of a sequence of interstate-transition maps (or, equivalently, random numbers) in the Markov chain, coalescence to some state must occur for some finite number of transitions $M \geq \max_x N_x$. Indeed, the probability of coalescence failing to occur $\to 0$ as $M \to \infty$. M is almost-surely *finite* because the probability of coalescence in any finite number of transitions is positive. Assume that coalescence occurred when the chain ran from time $t = -M$ to $t = 0$, using a specific sequence of transition maps. A chain running from $-\infty$ to 0 that uses this sequence of transition maps within $[-M, 0]$ reaches the same state at $t = 0$. Because the state reached by a chain running infinitely long is a draw from the stationary PMF $Q(X)$, the coalesced state at $t = 0$ is a draw from $Q(X)$.

For some PMFs $Q(X)$, the Gibbs sampler is *monotonic* [10] where transitions of coupled chains preserve a partial order on the states, and this allows CFTP to simplify parallel-chain tracking to tracking only two chains, each started from one of the extremal states (minimum and maximum) under the partial order. While monotonicity holds for the special case of the ferromagnetic Ising model, it fails to apply to many popular binary-MRF/ Potts models. For general cases, perfect sampling can use the *bounding chain* principle [5] as we propose next.

CFTP with Bounding Chain (CFTP-BC). For Gibbs sampling, CFTP-BC uses the following modified sampler $\mathcal{G}$ to draw label X_v, at each voxel v, from the conditional PMF $P(X_v|x_{-v})$ conditioned on all other label values x_{-v}.

1. Draw label l uniformly from the label set $\mathcal{L} := \{1, \cdots, L\}$. Draw $u \sim U(0, 1)$.
2. If $u < P(X_v = l|x_{-v})$, set $X_v := l$ and terminate; otherwise, iterate.

Provably, $\forall l$, the probability of $\mathcal{G}$ terminating with $X_v = l$ is $P(X_v = l|x_{-v})$.

For the Gibbs sampler relying on $\mathcal{G}$, the bounding chain algorithm [5] efficiently tracks the states of coupled parallel chains (monotone or not). CFTP-BC uses this tracking strategy to detect coalescence. Consider a new kind of a Markov chain $\mathring{\mathcal{M}}$ with state space $(2^{\mathcal{L}})^V$, where $2^{\mathcal{L}}$ is the set of subsets of $\mathcal{L}$. For $\mathring{\mathcal{M}}$, each state, say, $\mathring{X}$, contains a set of states $X \in \mathcal{L}^V$. $\mathring{\mathcal{M}}$ is associated with a state sequence $\mathring{X}^1, \mathring{X}^2, \cdots$ where the transition kernel $\mathring{K}(\cdot, \cdot)$ on $\mathring{X}$ is defined in terms of the transition kernel $K(\cdot, \cdot)$ acting on each state $X \in \mathring{X}$.

Definition 1. *Huber [5]: $\mathring{\mathcal{M}}$ is a bounding chain for $\mathcal{M}$ if there exists a coupling between $\mathring{\mathcal{M}}$ and $\mathcal{M}$ such that $X_v^t \in \mathring{X}_v^t, \forall v, \implies X_v^{t+1} \in \mathring{X}_v^{t+1}, \forall v$.*

Consider all coupled parallel chains $\mathcal{M}$ running $\mathcal{G}$ and visiting voxel v at time t. The bounding chain $\mathring{\mathcal{M}}$ keeps track of the set $\mathring{X}_v \subseteq \mathcal{L}$ of possible labels, at each v, across all chains $\mathcal{M}$ at any given time; it initializes $\mathring{X}_v := \mathcal{L}$ and detects coalescence when $|\mathring{X}_v| = 1, \forall v$. Each chain $\mathcal{M}$ has its conditional PMFs $P(X_v|x_{-v})$, dependent on MRF-neighborhood configurations $x_{\mathcal{N}_v}$. For each label l, let the minimum and maximum of conditional probabilities $P(X_v = l|x_{-v})$, over all chains $\mathcal{M}$, be $P^{\min}(X_v = l|x_{-v})$ and $P^{\max}(X_v = l|x_{-v})$, computed over all possible neighborhood label configurations in the cross-product space $\mathring{X}_{w_1} \times \mathring{X}_{w_2} \times \cdots$ over all $w_i \in \mathcal{N}_v$. Partition the set of all chains $\mathcal{M}$ into equivalence classes, based on possible MRF-neighborhood label values $x_{\mathcal{N}_v}$, within which Gibbs samplers $\mathcal{G}$ behave identically at voxel v. Now do the following at voxel v:

1. In the bounding chain $\mathring{\mathcal{M}}$, initialize the set of possible labels $\mathring{X}_v := \emptyset$.
2. Draw l uniformly from the label set $\mathcal{L}$. Draw $u \sim U(0, 1)$.
3. If $u > P^{\max}(X_v = l|x_{-v})$, then *no* chain $\mathcal{M}$ has changed state. So, do nothing.
4. If $u \in [P^{\min}(X_v = l|x_{-v}), P^{\max}(X_v = l|x_{-v})]$, then some of the equivalence classes of chains $\mathcal{M}$ have set $X_v \leftarrow l$. So, insert label l into set $\mathring{X}_v$.
5. If $u < P^{\min}(X_v = l|x_{-v})$, then all chains $\mathcal{M}$ set $X_v \leftarrow l$, indicating "local" coalescence that is a sufficient condition for every chain $\mathcal{M}$ to have undergone *at least one* transition where sampler $\mathcal{G}$ terminated. So, insert l into $\mathring{X}_v$. Exit. $\mathring{\mathcal{M}}$ avoids explicitly tracking a possibly exponential number of equivalence classes, but allows a possibly looser bound (larger $|\mathring{X}_v|$) resulting from some chains $\mathcal{M}$ running $\mathcal{G}$ multiple times and including *all* sampled labels in $\mathring{X}_v$.
6. Repeat from Step 2.

When, $\forall v$, set $\mathring{X}_v$ is a singleton, say, $\{\widehat{x}_v\}$, then all Markov chains $\mathcal{M}$ have coalesced to label image $\widehat{x}$ that is guaranteed to be a draw from the stationary PMF $Q(X)$. Ergodicity of $\mathcal{M}$ ensures coalescence almost-surely in finite time.

Fill's Algorithm (FA) for Perfect MCMC Sampling. A limitation of the CFTP strategy proposed in [10], including monotone-chain CFTP [10] and CFTP-BC [5], is that the CFTP running time M and the sampled state $\widehat{X}$ are *dependent* variables. M is unbounded whose order of magnitude is typically unknown a priori. So, some states x require a very long run from $-M$ to 0, with large unpredictable M. Impatient users who abort CFTP when M starts becoming large, add bias to the sampled states' PMF. In contrast, FA [4] makes the sampled state independent of the running time; it relies on acceptance-rejection (AR) sampling. The FA in [4] works only for monotone $\mathcal{M}$, as below.

1. Choose a random time $T > 0$ and a random label image $X^T := z$.
2. Run a Markov chain $\mathcal{M}$ from $T \to 0$, with initial $X^T := z$, reaching $X^0 := x$.
3. Let $S^T(x, z)$ be the event that a Markov chain starting at x ran for time T to reach z; this occurs for some set of pseudo-random number sequences $\mathcal{U}^{x \to z}$. Let $C^T(z)$ be the event that coupled parallel chains ran for time T and coalesced in z; this occurs for some set of pseudo-random number sequences $\mathcal{U}' \subseteq \mathcal{U}^{x \to z}$. With probability $P(C^T(z)|S^T(x, z))$, accept x as a draw from the stationary PMF $Q(X)$ and terminate; otherwise iterate from Step (1).

$P(C^T(z)|S^T(x, z))$ is computationally intractable, but AR decisions can be made by (i) simulating a $\sqcap^{x \to z} \in \mathcal{U}^{x \to z}$ to ensure $S^T(x, z)$ occurs and (ii) tracking coupled parallel chains, transitioning as per $\sqcap^{x \to z}$, to detect if $C^T(z)$ occurs.

Theorem 2. *Fill [4]: Fill's algorithm, with constrained monotone chains, guarantees that the sampled state is from the stationary PMF $Q(X)$.*

This is true because the underlying AR sampler generates a proposal x from the T-step transition kernel $K^T(z, \cdot)$ and, knowing that $M_z K^T(z, \cdot)$ is an upper bound for the stationary PMF $Q(\cdot)$ for $M_z := Q(z)/P(C^T(z))$, accepts the proposed x with probability $Q(x)/(M_z K^T(z, x))$ that equals $P(C^T(z)|S^T(x, z))$.

Fill's Algorithm with Bounding Chain (FA-BC). Previous works limit Fill's algorithm to monotone chains that apply to a very small class of PMFs $Q(X)$; for monotone chains, detecting $C^T(z)$ constrained on $S^T(x, z)$ needs the tracking of only two extremal states. We generalize Fill's algorithm to generic Bayesian MRFs by efficiently tracking constrained parallel *arbitrary* chains using a *novel constrained bounding chain* algorithm, as follows.

At time t and voxel v, for each label l, let $P^{\min}(X_v^t = l|x_{-v}^t)$ and $P^{\max}(X_v^t = l|x_{-v}^t)$ be defined as before. Let l^* be the label at voxel v for time $t+1$ along the Markov chain path $x \to z$. At time t, let $P^*(X_v^t = l^*|x_{-v}^t)$ be the label probability conditioned on neighboring labels for the path $x \to z$. Clearly, $P^{\min}(X_v^t = l|x_{-v}^t) \leq P^*(X_v^t = l^*|x_{-v}^t) \leq P^{\max}(X_v^t = l|x_{-v}^t)$. Initialize $t := 0$, $x^0 := x$.

1. At time t, do the following at each voxel v:
   (a) In the bounding chain $\mathcal{M}$, initialize the set of possible labels $\mathring{X}_v := \emptyset$.
   (b) Draw l uniformly from the label set $\mathcal{L}$.
   (c) If $l \neq l*$, draw $u \sim U(P^*(X_v^t = l^*|x_{-v}^t), 1)$; otherwise draw $u \sim U(0, 1)$. This sampling strategy simulates $\sqcap^{x \to z} \sim \mathcal{U}^{x \to z}$, ensuring that x^t transitions to x^{t+1} on the path $x \to z$, thereby leading to $S^T(x, z)$. The next steps track parallel coupled chains to detect if $C^T(z)$ occurs for $\sqcap^{x \to z}$.
   (d) If $u > P^{\max}(X_v^t = l|x_{-v}^t)$, then *no* chain $\mathcal{M}$ changes state. Go to Step 1b.
   (e) If $u \in [P^{\min}(X_v^t = l|x_{-v}^t), P^{\max}(X_v^t = l|x_{-v}^t)]$, then some chains $\mathcal{M}$ accept label l. Insert l into $\mathring{X}_v$. Go to Step 1b.
   (f) If $u < P^{\min}(X_v^t = l|x_{-v}^t)$, then all chains $\mathcal{M}$ set $X_v = l$. Insert l into $\mathring{X}_v$. Go to Step 1a to process a new voxel.
2. Increment t by 1. If $t < T$, repeat Step 1. If $t = T$ and coalescence has occurred, i.e., $|\mathring{X}_v| = 1, \forall v$, then accept the initial x as a draw from $Q(X)$.

Theorem 3. *Our modification of the Fill's algorithm, with constrained bounding chain, guarantees that the sampled state is from the stationary PMF $Q(X)$.*

Proof. We show that our random number generation scheme in Step 1c ensures $S^T(x, z)$ by simulating a $\sqcap^{x \to z} \in \mathcal{U}^{x \to z}$. At time t and voxel v, let E^* be the event that, for the chain going from $x \to z$, the label at voxel v at time $t+1$ is l^*. Let the $x \to z$ chain's *unconstrained* modified Gibbs sampler be $\mathcal{G}^*$ and the label probabilities be $P^*(X_v^t = l|x_{-v}^t)$. For E^* to occur, $\mathcal{G}^*$ accepted label l^* in some iteration i. In any iteration, $\mathcal{G}^*$ picked some l and some random u. Given E^*: if $\mathcal{G}^*$ picked an $l \neq l^*$, then u must have been within $[P^*(X_v^t = l|x_{-v}^t), 1]$; otherwise u could have been anywhere within $[0, 1]$. Now consider *parallel coupled* chains, one starting at each possible state, running sampler $\mathcal{G}$ for T transition steps. At iteration i, if $\mathcal{G}$ picks $l \neq l^*$, then $\mathcal{G}$ must pick u within $[P^*(X_v^t = l|x_{-v}^t), 1]$

because, otherwise, the chain started at x can incorrectly accept $l \neq l^*$ and E^* can fail to occur. At iteration i, if $\mathcal{G}$ picks $l = l^*$, then $\mathcal{G}$ can pick u within $[0, 1]$, leading to a non-zero probability for the chain started at x accepting l^* and leading to E^*. Steps 1d–1f track all chains, as in CFTP-BC, to detect $C^T(z)$ for the chosen $\sqcap^{x \to z}$. The result then follows from Theorem 2.   □

Exact Sampling to Estimate Uncertainty in Segmentation. We apply our FA-BC perfect-MCMC sampler to estimate uncertainty in Bayesian segmentation that models the *label image* prior as a *hidden MRF X* with the Potts model. We use FA-BC (i) during parameter estimation via EM, in the E step for Monte Carlo sampling label image X from its posterior, and (ii) after parameter estimation, to estimate uncertainty by sampling label maps from the posterior, given optimal parameters, and measuring their variability per voxel. We apply to 4 classic segmentation problems, in brain magnetic resonance imaging (MRI), with different likelihood models: (i) EM segmentation of tissues with mild lesions, with a Gaussian mixture model (GMM) for the intensities. (ii) EM segmentation of tumor, with a 2-component GMM for the tumor and non-tumor intensity patches on multimodal MRI, (iii) multiatlas segmentation of subcortical structures, and (iv) multiatlas segmentation of 4 lobes. Both (iii) and (iv) use a basic voxelwise nonparametric label-likelihood model for proof-of-concept, as follows. Let the multiatlas database $\mathcal{D} := \{z^j, s^j\}_{j=1}^J$ have template MRI images z^j paired with label images s^j. At voxel i, the observed-image patch $y_{\mathcal{N}_i}$ has likelihood $P(y_{\mathcal{N}_i}|X_i = l, \mathcal{D}) := \sum_{j=1}^J \mathbf{1}_l(s_i^j) G(\breve{y}_{\mathcal{N}_i}; \breve{z}_{\mathcal{N}_i}^j, \sigma^2 \mathbf{I}) / \sum_{j=1}^J \mathbf{1}_l(s_i^j)$ where $\mathbf{1}_l(a) = 1$ if $l = a$ (0 otherwise), $\mathbf{I}$ is the identity matrix, σ^2 the Gaussian kernel variance, and $\breve{y}_{\mathcal{N}_i}$ and $\breve{s}_{\mathcal{N}_i}^j$ are normalized patches with mean 0 and variance 1.

3   Results and Discussion

We show results on simulated data and on 4 classic brain-MRI analyses for 3 methods: (i) ours, (ii) approximate Gumbel perturbation model (aGPM) [1], (iii) Gibbs sampler with limited burn-in. For posterior-sampled label images (sample size 10^3), we compute mean and standard deviation (SD) per voxel (for the multi-category case, we generalize SD by square-root of unalikeability).

Validation on Simulated Data. The aGPM approximation of the true sampling PMF (in [9], which is intractable) can be severe (Fig. 1(a)–(c)), leading to a strong bias in the empirical mean estimate near edges (Fig. 1(d)). Our empirical mean estimate (Fig. 1(d)) is much closer to ground truth.

Results on Clinical Brain MRI. For many segmentation tasks, typical maximum-a-posteriori (MAP) segmentations can be very misleading by failing to expose regions with high uncertainty, e.g., (i) in subcortical structures, the hippocampus tail region (Fig. 2), (ii) in tumor, the edema regions (Fig. 3), (iii) in tissues, regions with mild lesions in white matter (Fig. 4). In these cases, the empirical means and SDs resulting from posterior-sampled label images are far more informative than the MAP estimate. However, in *all* these cases, unlike

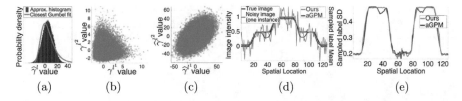

Fig. 1. Validation on Simulated Data: 128-voxel 1D image, 2 labels. Differences between *ideal* Gumbel perturbations γ in [9] (intractable for label-image sampling) and their tractable *approximations* $\widehat{\gamma}$ in aGPM [1]: (**a**) For a label image l, empirical histogram for $\widehat{\gamma}^l := \sum_{i=1}^{128} \gamma_i^{l_i}$, as per aGPM's notation, is almost Gaussian (central limit theorem), deviating significantly from Gumbel. (**b**)–(**c**) For label images l^1 and l^2, scatter between aGPM draws $\widehat{\gamma}^{l^1}$ and $\widehat{\gamma}^{l^2}$ (both using *same* sample for $\gamma_i^{\bullet}$) deviates from that between Gumbel draws γ^{l^1} and γ^{l^2}. (**d**)–(**e**) Sample mean and SD (voxelwise) of label images drawn from hidden-MRF posterior for aGPM [1] and our FA-BC sampler, averaged over multiple simulated image instances with different noise instances.

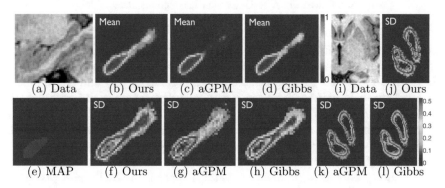

Fig. 2. Clinical brain MRI: Multiatlas segmentation, subcortical structures

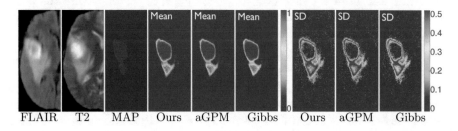

Fig. 3. Clinical multimodal brain MRI: Tumor segmentation.

our approach, both aGPM and Gibbs significantly underestimate the label SDs. Our FA-BC clearly improves over CFTP-BC [5] (Fig. 4) when, unlike our FA-BC, for large values of the smoothness parameter (say, β) in the Potts-MRF model, CFTP-BC takes far too many transition steps T and computation times, or virtually fails to terminate (for $\beta > 0.66$). For multiatlas hippocampus

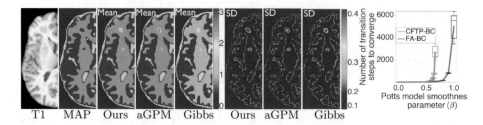

T1   MAP   Ours   aGPM   Gibbs   Ours   aGPM   Gibbs

Fig. 4. Clinical brain MRI, simulated mild lesion: Tissue segmentation.

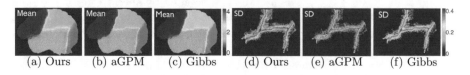

(a) Ours   (b) aGPM   (c) Gibbs   (d) Ours   (e) aGPM   (f) Gibbs

Fig. 5. Clinical brain MRI: Multiatlas segmentation of lobes.

segmentation (Fig. 2(b)–(d)), compared to our method, aGPM and Gibbs severely underestimate the label means as well. For tissue segmentation (Fig. 4), within the mild lesion with intensities between those of gray and white matter, our label mean is halfway between the label values of gray and white matter and indicates a greater uncertainty. In contrast, aGPM (or Gibbs) labels the lesion more confidently as gray (or white) matter, which is undesirable. For multiatlas multimodal-MRI tumor segmentation (Fig. 3), tissue segmentation with mild lesions (Fig. 4), and lobe segmentation (Fig. 5), aGPM and Gibbs severely underestimate label SDs, unlike our method that theoretically and practically guarantees sampled label images from the true posterior.

Computation Times: Gibbs's convergence time varies severely with the MRF model and the data, making it very difficult to predict burn-in. With a safe-side burn-in of 5000, as per the plot in Fig. 4, our FA-BC is 10–20× faster.

Conclusion. We introduced a new framework for uncertainty estimation in segmentation relying on *perfect MCMC sampling* of label images from their posteriors, defined using a *generic MRF model*. Our FA-BC extended Fill's algorithm to use a bounding-chain scheme, *improving theoretically and practically* over the state of the arts for (i) uncertainty estimation, e.g., aGPM and naive Gibbs, and (ii) perfect sampling, e.g., CFTP-BC, for analyzing simulated data and clinical brain MRI (segmenting tissues, subcortical structures, tumor, lobes).

References

1. Alberts, E., et al.: Uncertainty quantification in brain tumor segmentation using CRFs and random perturbation models. In: IEEE International Symposium on Biomedical Imaging, pp. 428–431 (2016)
2. Awate, S., Whitaker, R.: Multiatlas segmentation as nonparametric regression. IEEE Trans. Med. Imaging **33**(9), 1803–17 (2014)
3. Fan, A.C., Fisher, J.W., Wells, W.M., Levitt, J.J., Willsky, A.S.: MCMC curve sampling for image segmentation. In: Ayache, N., Ourselin, S., Maeder, A. (eds.) MICCAI 2007. LNCS, vol. 4792, pp. 477–485. Springer, Heidelberg (2007). https:// doi.org/10.1007/978-3-540-75759-7_58
4. Fill, J.: An interruptible algorithm for perfect sampling via Markov chains. Ann. Appl. Prob. **8**(1), 131–62 (1998)
5. Huber, M.: Perfect sampling using bounding chains. Ann. Appl. Prob. **14**(2), 734–753 (2004)
6. Kohli, P., Torr, P.: Measuring uncertainty in graph cut solutions. Comp. Vis. Image Underst. **112**, 30–8 (2008)
7. Kybic, J.: Bootstrap resampling for image registration uncertainty estimation without ground truth. IEEE Trans. Image Process. **19**(1), 64–73 (2010)
8. Le, M., Unkelbach, J., Ayache, N., Delingette, H.: Sampling image segmentations for uncertainty quantification. Med. Image Anal. **34**, 42–51 (2016)
9. Papandreou, G., Yuille, A.: Perturb-and-MAP random fields: using discrete optimization to learn and sample from energy models. In: International Conference on Computer Vision (2011)
10. Propp, J., Wilson, D.: Exact sampling with coupled Markov chains and applications to statistical mechanics. Random Struct. Algorithms **9**(1), 223–52 (1996)

On the Effect of Inter-observer Variability for a Reliable Estimation of Uncertainty of Medical Image Segmentation

Alain Jungo[1]($\boxtimes$), Raphael Meier[2], Ekin Ermis[3], Marcela Blatti-Moreno[3], Evelyn Herrmann[3], Roland Wiest[2], and Mauricio Reyes[1]

[1] Institute for Surgical Technologies and Biomechanics, University of Bern, Bern, Switzerland
alain.jungo@istb.unibe.ch
[2] SCAN, Institute for Diagnostic and Interventional Neuroradiology, Inselspital, Bern University Hospital, University of Bern, Bern, Switzerland
[3] University Clinic for Radio-oncology, Inselspital, Bern University Hospital, University of Bern, Bern, Switzerland

Abstract. Uncertainty estimation methods are expected to improve the understanding and quality of computer-assisted methods used in medical applications (e.g., neurosurgical interventions, radiotherapy planning), where automated medical image segmentation is crucial. In supervised machine learning, a common practice to generate ground truth label data is to merge observer annotations. However, as many medical image tasks show a high inter-observer variability resulting from factors such as image quality, different levels of user expertise and domain knowledge, little is known as to how inter-observer variability and commonly used fusion methods affect the estimation of uncertainty of automated image segmentation. In this paper we analyze the effect of common image label fusion techniques on uncertainty estimation, and propose to learn the uncertainty among observers. The results highlight the negative effect of fusion methods applied in deep learning, to obtain reliable estimates of segmentation uncertainty. Additionally, we show that the learned observers' uncertainty can be combined with current standard Monte Carlo dropout Bayesian neural networks to characterize uncertainty of model's parameters.

Keywords: Inter-observer variability · Uncertainty estimation Semantic segmentation

1 Introduction

The performance of medical image segmentation has increased with the advances in supervised machine learning and is reported to achieve close to human performance for specific tasks [6]. Despite the success of deep learning and its merit

© Springer Nature Switzerland AG 2018
A. F. Frangi et al. (Eds.): MICCAI 2018, LNCS 11070, pp. 682–690, 2018.
https://doi.org/10.1007/978-3-030-00928-1_77

in recent state-of-the-art methods [9], modern systems still lack in robustness and yield unexpected errors which hinders the adoption of such systems in medical applications. Uncertainty estimates of computer's results can help to foster understanding and trustworthiness of the underlying deep learning models. Various works have been proposed to produce uncertainty estimates in neural networks [1,2]. The Bayesian approach through Monte Carlo dropout proposed by Gal and Ghahramani [2] is probably the most popular due to its simple realization. Most methods built on Bayesian approaches stem from computer vision applications whereon ground truth definition has low inter-observer variability. However, calculation of segmentation uncertainty in medical images is particularly difficult, as the image content and quality can vary (e.g., image resolution, patient motion, partial volume effect), and often times medical images only partially describe the anatomy or (patho)physiology of interest. This can lead to a large inter-observer variability that is exacerbated by clinical domain-knowledge required to manually segment medical images. To deal with inter-observer variability in medical image segmentation, supervised learning approaches are typically trained using ground truth generated by common fusion techniques (e.g., majority voting, STAPLE [10]). However, as inter-observer variability reflects the disagreement among experts, we postulate that a supervised learning approach needs to likewise reflect experts disagreement when providing uncertainty estimates on new unseen cases. Little is known as to how inter-observer variability and commonly used fusion methods affect the estimation of image segmentation uncertainty. We hypothesize that inter-observer variability needs to be taken into account when learning models aiming at producing reliable estimations of segmentation uncertainty.

To this end, in this paper we analyze the effect of common image label fusion techniques on uncertainty estimation, and propose to learn the uncertainty among observers. Additionally, we show that the learned observers' uncertainty can be combined with current standard Monte Carlo dropout Bayesian neural networks to characterize uncertainty of model's parameters. Due to the absence of a real ground truth in medical images we first analyze the effect on a synthetic dataset that simulates inter-observer variability. In a final experiment, we analyze the behavior on a clinical post-operative brain tumor cavity dataset with multiple observer annotations.

2   Uncertainty Estimation in Deep Learning

This section introduces two types of uncertainty considered below: uncertainty linked to inter-observer variability, and the intrinsic model's uncertainty linked to the difficulty of a given model to make a prediction.

2.1   Uncertainty Linked to Inter-observer Variability

We analyze uncertainty linked to inter-observer variability through simulated scenarios including inter-observer variability and two different levels of image entropy. These are: (i) inter-observer variability and low entropy of the input image (i.e. crisp or sharp image edges), and (ii) inter-observer variability and high entropy of the input image (i.e. diffuse image edges). While case (ii) better reflects the reality in medical applications, case (i) was created to test whether the image content (in terms of difficulty of the segmentation task) affects the estimation of uncertainty. Following the initial postulate, we are interested to analyze the model's capability to learn the inter-observer variability into the estimation of segmentation uncertainty regardless of the image content. Figure 1 illustrates these configurations.

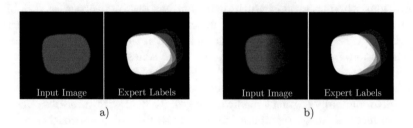

Fig. 1. Synthetic analysis using two simulated image-label scenarios. (a) low entropy of the input image and inter-observer variability, (b) high entropy of the input image and inter-observer variability.

2.2   Uncertainty Linked to Model's Parameters

Parameter uncertainty can be modeled by Bayesian neural networks [5,7] with distributions for the model weights. As presented by Gal and Ghahramani [2], dropout regularization can be interpreted as an approximation for Bayesian inference over the weights of the network. If applied at test time, dropout produces randomly sampled networks, which can be viewed as Monte Carlo samples over the posterior distribution of the model weights. Be I an input image that leads to a predicted class $y_i \in C$ at pixel i, where C is the set of classes. Then the approximative class probability resulting from T Monte Carlo samples is $p(y_i = c \mid I) \approx \frac{1}{T}\sum_{t=1}^{T} p(y_{i,t} = c \mid I, W^t)$ with sampled weights W^t. The uncertainty can be computed by the predictive entropy $H \approx -\sum_{c \in C} p(y_i = c \mid I) \log p(y_i = c \mid I)$. With increasing dataset size the model's parameter uncertainty decreases [3]. This makes it well-suited for the use in medical images, where training datasets are typically small. Since computing uncertainty estimations via Monte Carlo dropout does not pose any restrictions on the learning procedure, the uncertainty linked to the inter-observer variability can be combined with the model's parameter uncertainty.

3   Experimental Setup

3.1   Deep Learning Architecture

For both experiments, we used a U-net-based [8] architecture. We chose this architecture because of its popularity and its vast use in the medical imaging domain. We modify the standard architecture by adding a dropout layer ($p =$ 0.2) after each convolution layer [3]. For all experiments we use $T = 20$ Monte Carlo samples.

3.2   Experiment 1: Synthetic

In this experiment, we aim at examining the impact of the fusion method (or absence of) on the uncertainty estimation. We analyzed the following approaches: (a) no fusion (i.e. all labels used during training), (b) majority vote, (c) STAPLE [10], (d) intersection (to simulate a strict expert agreement) and (e) union of all observers (all experts' results are merged).

We produced a synthetic dataset to circumvent the absence of a multi-observer dataset with known underlying ground truth. The dataset aims at mimicking the situations described in Sect. 2.1 without introducing additional complexity. A synthetic sample of the dataset is created in four steps, as follows:

Ground Truth Generation: Eight perimeter points, initially equidistantly lying on a circle, are randomly perturbed with respect to the circle's center (angles: $\pm 15°$, distance factor: $[0.75, 1.5]$) and interpolated with a B-spline model.

Low-Entropy (i.e. unperturbed) Images: Input images I were derived from the ground truth by: (a) varying the maximum value (initially 255) randomly $[30, 255]$, (b) adding a Gaussian blur with random sigma $[2, 8]$, (c) adding Gaussian noise (factor: $0.15(\max(I) - \min(I))$. See input image of Fig. 1(a).

Observer Annotations: Perturbations to the simulated expert annotations were conducted by randomly perturbing the three rightmost perimeter points of the ground truth (angles: $\pm 10°$, distance: $\pm 0.4 \cdot d$ with d the distance to the center).

High-Entropy (i.e. perturbed) Image: Observer annotations are first summed up to the ground truth with random intensities $[50, 255]$, followed by an intensity normalization. Afterwards, maximum intensities are randomized ($[30, 255]$); an intensity gradient is added (random exponential decay $[0.5, 6.5]$ towards the right part of the image, and Gaussian blur (random sigma $[2, 8]$) and noise (factor: $0.15(\max(I) - \min(I))$ are introduced. See input image of Fig. 1(b).

The dataset of synthetic images consists of 100 samples, each containing a ground truth, five observer annotations, and perturbed and unperturbed grayscale images.

Implementation Details. Due to the low complexity of the task for the synthetic data, the U-net model consists only of two pooling/upsampling steps with an initial filter size of 16. For all fusion methods (and the absence of fusion) a network was trained for 100 epochs, with the last model being selected. In the absence of fusion, the observer annotations are sampled randomly. Adam [4] optimizer with a learning rate of 10^{-3} was used.

3.3   Experiment 2: Brain Tumor Cavity

In this experiment, we aim at validating the findings of the synthetic experiment on clinical data. We compared the uncertainty obtained by training without fusion and chose majority vote as fusion method yielding best segmentation performance. Since the underlying ground truth is unknown, a qualitative evaluation of the segmentation was performed.

MRI Patient Data. The clinical dataset consists of 30 post-operative brain tumor magnetic resonance images, with isotropic voxel size $(1 \times 1 \times 1\,\text{mm})$ acquired in the four standard sequences (T1-weighted (T1), T1-weighted post-contrast (T1c), T2-weighted (T2) and Fluid-attenuated inversion-recovery (FLAIR)), which are used to evaluate post-operative status of glioblastoma patients. The binary label maps delineate the cavity after tumor resection, and it is used for radiotherapy planning. The dataset contains annotations of three clinical radiation oncology experts with different levels of expertise (two years, four years, and over six years of clinical experience). This dataset is particularly interesting as post-operative resection cavities are ill-defined due to the presence of blood products producing pseudo-image gradients, CSF infiltration and air pockets.

Implementation Details. To adapt to the much more complex task of segmenting post-operative brain tumor resection cavities, we chose five pooling/upsampling steps and a initial filter size to 48. We used a two-dimensional input of the network and applied it on the axial slices of the brain volumes. The networks were trained for 35 epochs with selection of the last model. The optimizer is Adam with learning rate 10^{-3}. Due to the small dataset size, a six-fold cross-validation was performed.

3.4   Evaluation Metrics

As postulated, we seek reliable estimations of uncertainty that reflect expert disagreement as a result of the complexity of the task and different levels of expertise. As part of the Asimolar set of principles in A.I, this is known as *capability caution* on the upper limits of performance for systems learning from experts. To assess this, we assessed how fusion methods (or absence of) affect uncertainty in regions where expert disagreement is observed. We quantify this via $WME = \frac{1}{N}\sum_{i=1}^{N} \hat{H}_i \cdot H_i$, which is the weighted mean of the predictive entropy H over N pixels, and with $\hat{H}$ corresponding to the entropies of the expert disagreement. In order to capture the overall uncertainty produced by a model, we also evaluated the mean predictive entropy. This allows us to detect models yielding a high uncertainty but not reflecting the disagreement among the experts. Additionally, the Dice coefficient was used to assess segmentation performance.

4   Results and Discussion

4.1   Experiment 1: Synthetic

The weighted mean entropy (WME), the mean entropy (ME), and the Dice coefficient were computed in relation to the known ground truth. Quantitative results are shown in Table 1 and Fig. 4(a). The results particularly highlight the simultaneous increase of WME and ME for the model trained without any label fusion, as compared to the other models. This suggests that the uncertainty derived by a model trained with all labels (i.e. no fusion) better describes expert disagreement. On the contrary, training with intersection or union of labels reduces the reliability of the estimated uncertainty. In terms of segmentation performance, it is observed that training with all labeled information (i.e. no fusion) performs as well as those trained with either majority voting or STAPLE. This result suggests that a more reliable uncertainty does not come with a reduced segmentation accuracy, as it could have been expected when training models with non-fused label data.

Figure 2 presents qualitative results, showing that models trained with fused labels tend to underestimate the uncertainty with respect to the reference expert variability (second column of Fig. 2). Conversely, the model trained without any fusion better resembles the reference expert variability. Results on the unperturbed images (top row of Fig. 2) show that despite of the clear edge information of the input image, the uncertainty estimates reflect the underlying expert disagreement. This result verifies our postulate that a model can learn inter-observer variability regardless of the image content.

Table 1. Quantitative results of the synthetic experiment. The fusion methods are compared on weighted mean entropy (WME), mean entropy (ME) and Dice coefficient. U and P stand for *unperturbed* and *perturbed* and describe the state of the input image.

		No fusion	Majority	STAPLE	Union	Intersection
WME	U	**.68** $\pm$ .08	.54 $\pm$ .10	.59 $\pm$ .09	.29 $\pm$ .13	.30 $\pm$ .12
	P	**.67** $\pm$ .07	.47 $\pm$ .09	.56 $\pm$ .08	.30 $\pm$ .08	.20 $\pm$ .08
ME	U	**.12** $\pm$ .03	.09 $\pm$ .02	.10 $\pm$ .02	.08 $\pm$ .02	.08 $\pm$ .02
	P	**.12** $\pm$ .03	.08 $\pm$ .02	.09 $\pm$ .02	.08 $\pm$ .02	.09 $\pm$ .03
Dice	U	.99 $\pm$ .01	**.99** $\pm$ .01	.98 $\pm$ .01	.90 $\pm$ .02	.89 $\pm$ .03
	P	.96 $\pm$ .02	**.96** $\pm$ .02	**.96** $\pm$ .02	.92 $\pm$ .03	.88 $\pm$ .04

4.2   Experiment 2: Brain Tumor Cavity

Figure 4(b) illustrates the obtained variability of WME on the 30 cross-validated cavity images. Results were divided by segmentation performance in two groups, separated by the median Dice. For underperforming segmentation results (below

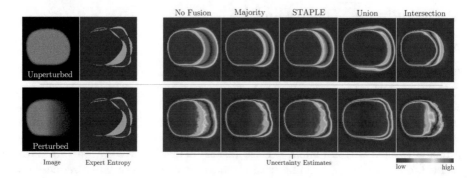

Fig. 2. Uncertainty estimations obtain from models trained on differently fused labels on the synthetic dataset. Top and bottom row correspond to training with unperturbed and perturbed input images, respectively. Columns correspond to the fusion method used.

median), results show no benefit in employing all label data for training and estimating uncertainty. Conversely, for segmentation results where the Dice was equal or larger than the median Dice, a benefit on using all label data was observed. This result suggests the existence of a link between segmentation performance and reliability of uncertainty estimation.

Figure 3 presents a qualitative result. It shows that the model trained on all labels is able to produce reliable uncertainty in regions of highest expert disagreement (right cavity side).

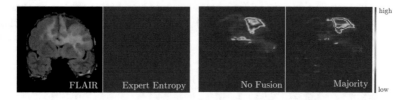

Fig. 3. Exemplary uncertainty estimations on the cavity dataset in comparison to the expert entropy.

The experiments on the synthetic and clinical dataset reveal that uncertainty estimations is linked to inter-observer variability, and that reliable uncertainty (i.e. reflecting expert disagreement) may be learned by avoiding label fusion in the training data. This is of high relevance in systems where for example, uncertainty estimations are used by experts to monitor and correct computer-generated results. In addition, we observed a link between segmentation performance and reliability of segmentation uncertainty estimates.

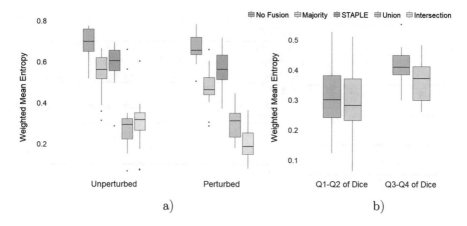

Fig. 4. Quantitative results of the weighted mean entropy (WME) metric. (a) results obtained for fusion methods on perturbed and unperturbed images of the synthetic dataset, (b) cavity dataset results separated by Dice performance (Q1-Q2: below median, Q3-Q4: above median).

5   Conclusion

In this paper, we analyzed the impact of fusion methods on the uncertainty estimation. Experiments were performed on a synthetic multi-observer dataset and a clinical dataset. First evidence verifies the link between uncertainty estimations from trained deep learning models and inter-observer variability, which is inherent of medical image applications. We conclude that the benefit of using fusion methods for reliable segmentation uncertainty estimations is conditioned to the performance of the underlying segmentation accuracy, and hence it needs to be assessed when considering fusion methods for ground truth generation.

Acknowledgments. This work was supported by the Swiss National Foundation by grant number 169607.

References

1. Blundell, C., Cornebise, J., Kavukcuoglu, K., Wierstra, D.: Weight uncertainty in neural network. In: ICML, pp. 1613–1622 (2015)
2. Gal, Y., Ghahramani, Z.: Bayesian convolutional neural networks with Bernoulli approximate variational inference. In: ICLR Workshop Track (2016)
3. Kendall, A., Gal, Y.: What uncertainties do we need in Bayesian deep learning for computer vision? In: NIPS, pp. 5580–5590 (2017)
4. Kingma, D., Ba, J.: Adam: a method for stochastic optimization. In: ICLR (2015)
5. MacKay, D.J.C.: A practical Bayesian framework for backpropagation networks. Neural Comput. **4**(3), 448–472 (1992)
6. Meier, R., et al.: Clinical evaluation of a fully-automatic segmentation method for longitudinal brain tumor volumetry. Sci. Rep. **6**, (2016). https://doi.org/10.1038/srep23376

7. Neal, R.M.: Bayesian Learning for Neural Networks, vol. 118. Springer, New York (2012). https://doi.org/10.1007/978-1-4612-0745-0
8. Ronneberger, O., Fischer, P., Brox, T.: U-Net: convolutional networks for biomedical image segmentation. In: Navab, N., Hornegger, J., Wells, W.M., Frangi, A.F. (eds.) MICCAI 2015. LNCS, vol. 9351, pp. 234–241. Springer, Cham (2015). https://doi.org/10.1007/978-3-319-24574-4_28
9. Shen, D., Wu, G., Suk, H.I.: Deep learning in medical image analysis. Annu. Rev. Biomed. Eng. **19**, 221–248 (2017)
10. Warfield, S.K., Zou, K.H., Wells, W.M.: Validation of image segmentation and expert quality with an expectation-maximization algorithm. In: Dohi, T., Kikinis, R. (eds.) MICCAI 2002. LNCS, vol. 2488, pp. 298–306. Springer, Heidelberg (2002). https://doi.org/10.1007/3-540-45786-0_37

Towards Safe Deep Learning: Accurately Quantifying Biomarker Uncertainty in Neural Network Predictions

Zach Eaton-Rosen[1(✉)], Felix Bragman[1], Sotirios Bisdas[2,3],
Sébastien Ourselin[4], and M. Jorge Cardoso[1,4]

[1] Centre for Medical Image Computing, University College London, London, UK
z.eaton-rosen@ucl.ac.uk
[2] Department of Neuroradiology, The National Hospital for Neurology
and Neurosurgery, University College London NHS Foundation Trust, London, UK
[3] Department of Brain Repair and Rehabilitation, Institute of Neurology,
University College London, London, UK
[4] Biomedical Engineering and Imaging Sciences, Kings College London, London, UK

Abstract. Automated medical image segmentation, specifically using deep learning, has shown outstanding performance in semantic segmentation tasks. However, these methods rarely quantify their uncertainty, which may lead to errors in downstream analysis. In this work we propose to use Bayesian neural networks to quantify uncertainty within the domain of semantic segmentation. We also propose a method to convert voxel-wise segmentation uncertainty into volumetric uncertainty, and calibrate the accuracy and reliability of confidence intervals of derived measurements. When applied to a tumour volume estimation application, we demonstrate that by using such modelling of uncertainty, deep learning systems can be made to report volume estimates with well-calibrated error-bars, making them safer for clinical use. We also show that the uncertainty estimates extrapolate to unseen data, and that the confidence intervals are robust in the presence of artificial noise. This could be used to provide a form of quality control and quality assurance, and may permit further adoption of deep learning tools in the clinic.

1 Introduction

Deep convolutional neural nets (CNNs) are becoming the dominant method for medical image semantic segmentation, markedly improving on previous techniques in a variety of tasks. Standard deep learning models produce a point-estimate of the 'probability' that a voxel belongs to each segmentation class—but these estimates typically lack any quantification of error. In medical applications safety is paramount: misreporting a biomarker or outright missing a pathological finding may endanger patients. If uncertainty estimates are not propagated through a clinical pipeline, or if errors are not properly quantified and calibrated, this can result in false conclusions downstream, e.g. when comparing volume estimates longitudinally. Models that can quantify uncertainty in their predictions may thus be useful in making safer and more actionable analysis pipelines.

© Springer Nature Switzerland AG 2018
A. F. Frangi et al. (Eds.): MICCAI 2018, LNCS 11070, pp. 691–699, 2018.
https://doi.org/10.1007/978-3-030-00928-1_78

While it remains uncommon to calculate estimates of uncertainty in probabilistic segmentation – indeed, many methods preclude it entirely – Bayesian models of segmentation incorporate estimates of model parameter variance explicitly, and even downstream errors such as volume estimates [1]. These methods have however seen limited adoption: they are computationally expensive, especially compared with modern CNNs, and have worse accuracy. In addition, the formulation in [1] relies on having a probabilistic atlas to use as a prior term, which may not be amenable to highly variable pathological tissues such as tumours or Multiple Sclerosis lesions. Bayesian neural networks can be used to approximate model uncertainty even without probabilistic atlases. One method of approximating a Bayesian neural network is to use 'dropout', which was originally proposed as a regularising technique [2]. In dropout, a randomly-determined subset of neurons in the network are 'dropped' randomly (have zero output) at each iteration. With modern neural networks having upwards of millions of parameters, this means that the same dropout mask is unlikely to ever be chosen twice for the network. At each iteration, one essentially uses a specific, thinned, version of the network. The stochastic nature of these networks can be used to approximate a Bayesian neural network [3]. From a practical point of view, predictive uncertainty is estimated by calculating the sample variance of predictions made from different forward passes from the network.

Bayesian modeling of uncertainties in CNNs is still not commonplace. To the best of our knowledge, no prior work has made use of these uncertainties to estimate the impact and reliability of downstream biomarker uncertainty (e.g. volume estimated from a segmentation), nor to describe how uncertainty estimates are related to data quality. In this work, we utilise a Bayesian deep learning model to measure the uncertainty of image segmentation. We fit network architectures with differing levels of stochasticity. We then measure the effects of uncertainty on volume estimation and propose to use these stochastic network outputs to build 'contours' of increasing segmentation volume that better approximate the unknown volume uncertainties. Because these techniques can be applied to any neural networks trained with dropout, our proposed method can be employed to give calibrated estimates for volume measurements at little additional cost.

2   Methods

In the Brain Tumour Segmentation (BraTS) challenge [4,5], CNNs have been used to produce winning submissions in recent years and have been established as the dominant fully-automated method for the task. We use data from the BraTS 2017 training dataset which contains 285 subjects with high- or low-grade gliomas. Each subject has $T_1$1-weighted, T_1-weighted with Gd contrast (T_1ce), T_2-weighted and FLAIR MRI scans. One expert segmentation is given for each subject, with 3 foreground labels: (1) Gd-enhancing tumour, (2) edema, and (3) the necrotic/non-enhancing tumour. These are combined to get binary hierarchical segmentations of 'active' (1), 'core' (1 + 3) and 'whole' (1 + 2 + 3), which we use henceforth.

This work concentrates on introducing a generalisable technique for quantifying uncertainty in a network's outputs rather than on designing a new neural network architecture. To that end, we used multiple variants of 'High-Res Net' [6], a residual network that uses dilated convolutions to increase the effective receptive field and the context of the representation. The proposed architectures are designed to test the effects of different levels of uncertainty throughout the network. The dropout rate p is kept constant at 0.5 except if applied in the input layer, in which case it is set to 0.05 (a low value is chosen to allow low-level image features into the network). The value of 0.5 maximises the variance of the layer outputs, which can be seen as maximising the effect of dropout. The number of kernels is larger than in [6] to allow the network to cope with the reduced capacity caused by dropout. We also train a non-stochastic (no dropout) network with the same number of parameters as a baseline.

In total, we trained four variants of the High-Res Net architecture: all networks use filter sizes of {24, 24, 48, 96, 96} for the first convolutional layer, the three convolutional blocks, and the next convolutional layer respectively. We define: HR_{default}: a non-stochastic network (no dropout); HR_{drop_last}: a stochastic network with dropout in the last layer; HR_{drop_all}: a stochastic network with dropout after each residual block, and a stochastic network with a heteroscedastic noise model HR_{hetero}. The heteroscedastic model uses the same network architecture as a trunk that branches into (a): a convolution with kernel of dimension $3 \times 3 \times 3$ and 120 filters before the softmax layer (for segmentation) and (b): a convolutional layer of dimension $3 \times 3 \times 3$ and 80 filters that connects to a softplus layer to output the estimate of the standard deviation.

'Predictive variance' denotes variance obtained by running these models several times and calculating variance over multiple trials. The heteroscedastic variant, HR_{hetero}, also adds an additive 'aleatoric' variance, which quantifies uncertainty over the data itself.

All optimisation is performed with the Adam optimiser with learning rate 0.001. All results are reported on withheld 'test' data with a 70:20:10 train: validation: test split. Training is halted when the validation loss does not improve for over 5 epochs. The work is implemented using NiftyNet [7], and code will be made publicly available.

2.1 Bayesian Deep Learning

In Bayesian neural networks, model weights $\mathbf{W}$ are assumed to have a distribution, rather than being point estimates. We aim to approximate the posterior $p(\mathbf{W}|\mathbf{X},\mathbf{Y})$ over the weights $\mathbf{W}$ given training data $\{\mathbf{X},\mathbf{Y}\}$. Dropout samples from the space of sub-models of a network architecture, where sampling is parameterised by a randomly-sampled Bernoulli dropout mask, to ultimately estimate model parameters and their uncertainties. Using this formulation, the neural network approximates a Gaussian Process [3].

In the proposed networks, we predict probabilities for a voxel to belong to each segmentation class. At test-time, we output the model T times, with T different dropout masks, and use these predictions to estimate the uncertainty.

Here, y is the prediction of the network and $\hat{y}$ is the result of one stochastic approximation. This variance can then be given explicitly by $\mathrm{Var}_{epi}(y) \approx \frac{1}{T}\sum_{t=1}^{T}\hat{y}^2 - \left(\frac{1}{T}\sum_{t=1}^{T}\hat{y}\right)^2$, i.e. estimated by measuring the variance of the forward passes. For networks except HR_{hetero}, we use a cross-entropy loss function.

This variance takes into account the uncertainty in the model itself by using different dropout masks for differing predictions. However, other sources of variance can also be measured. As in [8], an additional term can be introduced to model the uncertainty that is intrinsic to the problem—known as *aleatoric* uncertainty. With this new term, the variance can now be expressed as: $\mathrm{Var}(y) \approx \mathrm{Var}_{epistemic}(y) + \frac{1}{T}\sum_{t=1}^{T}\sigma_t^2$. While this aleatoric uncertainty can be approximated in many ways, for numerical stability, we follow [8] in assuming that the error has a normal distribution in logit space (un-normalised probabilities), and add the aleatoric noise to the logits directly in the network: $\hat{x}_{i,t} = f_i^W + \sigma_i^W \epsilon_t, \epsilon_t \sim \mathcal{N}(0,1)$. This noise model can then be used in an heteroscedastic setup through the following loss function $\mathcal{L}_x = \frac{1}{N}\sum_i^N \log \frac{1}{T}\sum_t \exp(\hat{x}_{i,t,c} - \log\sum_{c'}\exp\hat{x}_{i,t,c'})$. Note that this loss requires multiple passes over several noise realisations, and that increasing the noise in a voxel will reduce the logit differences and, correspondingly, the certainty of the predictions.

2.2 From Stochastic Segmentation Samples to Calibrated Volumetric Uncertainty

The uncertainty in these models can be visualised directly in the segmentation space, but it is harder to propagate this uncertainty from pixel-wise segmentation to volume estimation.

For a given subject i, the foreground volume $V = \sum_{i=1}^{n} p(x_i)$. Combining errors from the i voxels, we get: $Var(V) = \sum_{i=1}^{n}\sum_{j=1}^{n} cov(x_i, x_j)$. Although the covariance terms could be measured empirically, we instead decided to explicitly spatially regularise the data. We did this by predicting the probability of being in the foreground class repeatedly. We then take quantiles of this measurement at each voxel to build a cumulative distribution. In terms of 'combining errors', this is the equivalent of maximising the correlation between all voxels.

Maximising this correlation between voxels' predictions is not guaranteed to *calibrate* the volumetric estimates. To do this, we introduce a step to fit the error bars for the validation data. Practically, this is achieved by using the validation to fit an affine transformation on the percentiles of the volumetric CDF to a uniform distribution—equivalent to a 1-D histogram equalization. This mapping enforces the correct proportion of ground truths to appear in a given confidence interval. For final results, the parameters of the scaling for the 'test' set are fitted on all the 'validation' data. In the 'validation' data, to avoid test-train contamination, the parameters of the fit are determined through a 3-fold paradigm.

3   Results

We first compute and visualise the predictive uncertainties and segmentations over 20 samples of the model. In Fig. 1, we display the mean predicted segmentation, and the standard deviation of these outputs. Regions of high predictive variance are common at the borders of segmentation classes. From left to right, with the models becoming more complicated, we see that predicted variance becomes more localised and concentrated around the class boundaries. Empirically, we have found that the model with dropout in every layer produced the most stable variance estimates, whilst being computationally simple to implement. The mean Dice score, for the 'whole' label was HR_{drop_all}: 0.86, HR_{hetero}: 0.84, HR_{drop_last}: 0.83 and $HR_{default}$: 0.79. These numbers are average for this task (although the point of this paper is not to win the challenge). For HR_{hetero}, the scale of the aleatoric variance was orders of magnitude lower than the predictive uncertainty and it made no measurable contribution to the overall uncertainty (while being a more expensive model). Because HR_{drop_all} had the highest Dice scores on average and the aleatoric uncertainty was negligible, we used HR_{drop_all} for all further results.

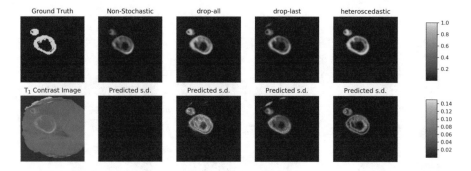

Fig. 1. Top row: mean confidences (over 20 forward passes) for the given model to belong to the 'Active' class. Bottom row: $\sigma_{predicted}$, the standard deviation across predictions. Different methods display similar predictions, but the level of uncertainty varies depending on the network used.

In Fig. 2 we plot the value of the probabilistic estimate in the 5th and 95th percentile, produced using the technique in Sect. 2.2. The volumes form a cumulative distribution function (CDF) over the percentiles. This image provides intuition for our choice to spatially correlate the voxels. The confidence intervals here encompass the ground truth.

After fitting the networks, we compare their results in Fig. 3. In Fig. 3a, we plot the predicted volume against the true volume for each of the test subjects. While volumes perform well, with observations clustered around equality there is a pronounced lack of variation in the predictions (it is actually impossible to see that 20 points are plotted per subject). This is true for all fitted networks.

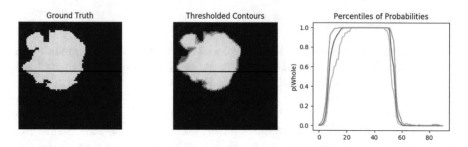

Fig. 2. Left: ground truth 'Whole' segmentation. Middle: 5th percentile volumetric measurement (yellow), contained within the 50th percentile (dark green) and outside that, the 95th percentile (cyan). Right: the probability of a voxel along the black line belonging to the 'Whole Tumour' class, as given by different percentiles in the volume space. These percentiles are not yet calibrated, but do contain the ground truth.

It is immediately apparent that the multiple predictions from any presented model are highly correlated, and do not end up producing samples with enough variation to include the true value (dashed black line). The range of estimates is not large enough to act as a confidence interval.

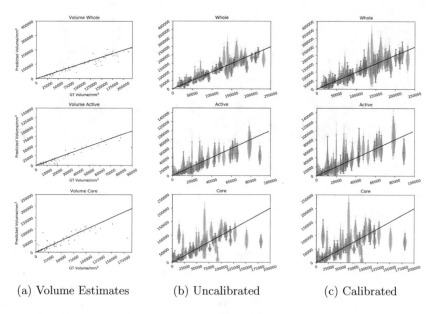

(a) Volume Estimates   (b) Uncalibrated   (c) Calibrated

Fig. 3. In Fig. 3a, we plot point estimates for 20 estimates of the volume from HR_{drop_all}. Despite 20 estimates being plotted, there is almost no variation that can be seen in the plots. This lack of variation is present in all methods (unshown). In Fig. 3b, we see the uncalibrated estimates of uncertainty, and in Fig. 3c we plot the calibrated estimates. Subjects in the 'validation' set are blue and 'test' orange.

We thus proceed to forming our volumetric CDF. We plot the distribution of each percentile from this distribution in Fig. 3b, with the mean and 95% confidence interval being plotted marked with horizontal lines. This data is inferred from 200 predicted volumes per subject. While the estimated volumes remain the same in expectation, the spread of the predictions is more commensurate with the known ground truth, although it may remain too small. In Fig. 3c we present the volume confidence intervals after applying our calibration step. The confidence intervals, especially in the 'Core' segmentation, have longer tails and thus overlap with the line of equality more of the time. That the affine scaling enlarges the confidence intervals can be seen empirically correcting the distribution for unmodelled sources of uncertainty.

As a sanity check, we test volume estimation and uncertainty maps on a subject with varying levels of Gaussian noise added to the data in Fig. 4. As noise increases, we see the segmentation error increase: also, we see the estimated volume reducing with added noise: crucially the confidence intervals still contain the ground truth value. One reason that the volume estimate may decrease with added noise is that in regions of uncertainty, cross-entropy loss functions tend to produce the most likely class (in this case, background)—we did not use weighted cross-entropy. The interaction of this stochastic framework with other loss functions would be an interesting avenue for exploration. While the performance under noise would require more extensive validation, it does raise the possibility of using predicted uncertainty as a proxy for image quality.

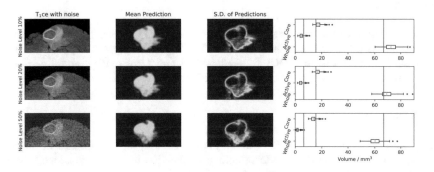

Fig. 4. Left column: T_1ce image with varying Gaussian noise added, with the σ parameter being the labelled percentage of mean foreground intensity. Centre-left: average for 'Whole' class for 200 estimates. Centre-right: the predictive uncertainty. Right: volume-level uncertainty, with ground-truth marked blue.

4   Discussion

In this work, we have investigated the suitability of single-model estimates of uncertainty in CNNs for producing calibrated confidence intervals of downstream biomarkers. Firstly, we showed these techniques may be applied in medical image segmentation to produce estimates of predictive uncertainty. We also illustrated how measuring volume from different forward passes of the stochastic network was wholly inadequate for producing a range of volumetric estimates that included the ground truth. We then proposed and implemented a solution to calibrate the uncertainty on estimating the volume.

Limitations: The main limitation of the proposed work is that while we take into account uncertainty in the model parameters and (with HR_{hetero}) the data itself, this is not an exhaustive quantification of the error. Factors such as the choice of neural network architecture could also be marginalised over in a Bayesian setting, as alluded to in [9]. The empirical nature of calibrating the probabilities is another limitation—in some settings, there may not be enough withheld data to properly perform the calibration. The calibration step is also, like many machine learning techniques, sensitive to domain shift and relies on continuing statistical similarity between images in the training set and the images for which the application will be used.

Further work will focus on validating this approach with other medical imaging data. We will investigate extending the proposed methodology for other biomarkers: for instance, uncertainty in shape parameters, or estimates of counts (e.g. for MS lesions). We will also focus on explicitly modeling the effect of network parameter choices on measured uncertainty (for example, by employing a diverse ensemble of architectures).

In conclusion, we have shown how to produce calibrated confidence intervals for volumetric analysis, with a non-disruptive extension to a typical deep-learning pipeline.

Acknowledgements. ZER is supported by the EPSRC Doctoral Prize. FB and MJC are supported by CRUK Accelerator Grant A21993. SB is supported by the National Institute for Health Research UCL Biomedical Research Centre. We gratefully acknowledge NVIDIA Corporation for the donation of hardware.

References

1. Iglesias, J.E., Sabuncu, M.R., Van Leemput, K.: Improved inference in bayesian segmentation using monte carlo sampling: application to hippocampal subfield volumetry. Med. Image Anal. **17**(7), 766–778 (2013)
2. Srivastava, N.: Dropout: a simple way to prevent neural networks from overfitting. J. Mach. Learn. Res. **15**(1), 1929–1958 (2014)
3. Gal, Y., Ghahramani, Z.: Dropout as a bayesian approximation: representing model uncertainty in deep learning. In: International Conference on Machine Learning, pp. 1050–1059 (2016)
4. Menze, B.: The multimodal brain tumor image segmentation benchmark (brats). IEEE Trans. Med. Imaging **34**(10), 1993–2024 (2015)
5. Bakas, S., et al.: Advancing the cancer genome atlas glioma mri collections with expert segmentation labels and radiomic features. Sci. Data **4**, 170117 (2017)
6. Li, W., Wang, G., Fidon, L., Ourselin, S., Cardoso, M.J., Vercauteren, T.: On the compactness, efficiency, and representation of 3D convolutional networks: brain parcellation as a pretext task. In: Niethammer, M. (ed.) IPMI 2017. LNCS, vol. 10265, pp. 348–360. Springer, Cham (2017). https://doi.org/10.1007/978-3-319-59050-9_28

7. Gibson, E.: Niftynet: a deep-learning platform for medical imaging. Comput. Methods Programs Biomed. **158**, 113–122 (2018)
8. Kendall, A., Gal, Y.: What uncertainties do we need in Bayesian deep learning for computer vision? In: Advances in Neural Information Processing Systems, pp. 5580–5590 (2017)
9. Kamnitsas, K., et al.: Ensembles of multiple models and architectures for robust brain tumour segmentation. arXiv preprint arXiv:1711.01468 (2017)

Image Registration Methods

Registration-Based Patient-Specific Musculoskeletal Modeling Using High Fidelity Cadaveric Template Model

Yoshito Otake[1(✉)], Masaki Takao[2], Norio Fukuda[1], Shu Takagi[3],
Naoto Yamamura[3], Nobuhiko Sugano[3], and Yoshinobu Sato[1]

[1] Graduate School of Information Science,
Nara Institute of Science and Technology, Ikoma, Japan
otake@is.naist.jp
[2] Graduate School of Medicine, Osaka University, Osaka, Japan
[3] Department of Mechanical Engineering, The University of Tokyo, Tokyo, Japan

Abstract. We propose a method to construct patient-specific musculoskeletal model using a template obtained from a high fidelity cadaver images. Musculoskeletal simulation has been traditionally performed using a *string-type* muscle model that represent the line-of-forces of a muscle with strings, while recent studies found that a more detailed model that represents muscle's 3D shape and internal fiber arrangement would provide better simulation accuracy when sufficient computational resources are available. Thus, we aim at reconstructing patient-specific muscle fiber arrangement from clinically available modalities such as CT or (non-diffusion) MRI. Our approach follows a conventional biomedical modeling approach which first constructs a highly accurate generic *template* model which is then registered using the patient-specific measurement. Our template is created from a high-resolution cryosectioned volume and newly proposed registration method aligns the surface of bones and muscles as well as the local orientation inside the muscle (i.e., muscle fiber direction). The evaluation was performed using cryosectioned volumes of two cadavers, one of which accompanies images obtained from clinical CT and MRI. Quantitative evaluation demonstrated that the mean fiber distance error between the one estimated from CT and the ground truth was 4.16, 3.76, and 2.45 mm for the gluteus maximus, medius, and minimus muscles, respectively. The qualitative visual assessment on 20 clinical CT images suggested plausible fiber arrangements that would be able to be translated to biomechanical simulation.

Keywords: Muscle fiber modeling · Fiber arrangement · Clinical CT

1 Introduction

We aim at a patient-specific modeling of musculoskeletal structures for biomechanical simulation in pre-operative surgical planning and postoperative rehabilitation. While *string-type* muscle model simplifying each muscle as a few string

© Springer Nature Switzerland AG 2018
A. F. Frangi et al. (Eds.): MICCAI 2018, LNCS 11070, pp. 703–710, 2018.
https://doi.org/10.1007/978-3-030-00928-1_79

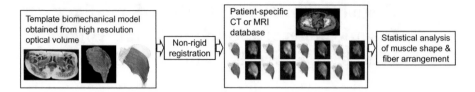

Fig. 1. Workflow of the proposed method. The shape and fiber arrangement of the target muscle (gluteus maximus in this figure) is obtained from a high-resolution optical volume of a cadaver specimen. The template is then registered to each subjects CT or MRI using the proposed non-rigid registration algorithm, from which the statistical model is created.

elements has been most commonly used in biomechanical simulations (such as in [12], etc.) by virtue of low computational cost and ease of modeling, 3D volumetric muscle models containing the muscle fiber architecture [3,14] have been investigated to improve accuracy of musculoskeletal simulation when sufficient computational resource is available. The modeling of muscle fiber arrangement has been attempted using medical imaging modalities such as ultrasound [15], diffusion tensor MRI [8], and micro CT [7], the limited field-of-view and long scan time precludes its use in clinical routine. On the other hand, the biomechanics community has proposed several method for modeling muscle fibers to achieve an accurate biomechanical simulation, one of which employs computational fluid dynamics [6] to obtain a physically plausible non-intersecting streamlines that connect origin and insertion areas. But the downside is its fidelity to patient-specific fiber arrangement.

Otake et al. [10] proposed a compromise solution in which a simple 3D geometric pattern representing fiber arrangement (e.g., a cluster of lines in a unit cube connecting top and bottom face) is spatially mapped to the muscle considering local orientation inside the muscle derived from the texture of patient's CT. Although it successfully modeled patient-specific and physically plausible fiber arrangement with a high-resolution optical volume, its robustness was limited especially for muscles with complicated fiber arrangement such as the gluteus medius in CT, and the authors demonstrated improved accuracy by addition of manually traced fiber lines, which should be highly operator dependent. Automated segmentation of musculoskeletal structures has been widely studied [1,11]. Especially, since the emergence of deep neural networks, it is approaching a viable option in clinical routine. Therefore, in this study, we assumed the segmentation label of the target bones and muscles are sou available. We propose a method to model patient-specific muscle fiber arrangement robustly from patient's medical images such as CT or (non-diffusion) MRI. Our approach follows a conventional biomedical modeling approach which first constructs a highly accurate generic *template* model, and then the template is non-rigidly registered to a noisy patient-specific image. Our template is created from a high-resolution cryosectioned volume [5] using the previously proposed method [10]. The contribution of this paper is twofold: (1) Introduction of a new cost function containing two

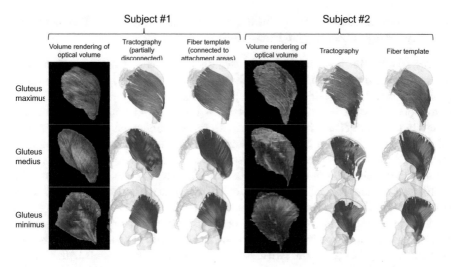

Fig. 2. High fidelity fiber arrangement templates obtained from optical image volume of two cadaver specimens in Visible Korean Human data set that were used as the ground truth in this study. A previously proposed algorithm [10] that fits a fiber template to the structure tensor field is employed. Tractography is also computed from the structure tensor field for comparison. The fitted fiber template correctly provided fiber lines that connect the origin and insertion areas, while tractography is partially disconnected due to noise in the tensor field. The color in the fiber rendering corresponds to the orientation at each line segment. X, Y, and Z components of the orientation vector were assigned to R, G, and B components.

data fitting terms, the surface fitness term and local orientation fitness term, and (2) evaluation with high-resolution optically acquired cryosection image volumes of two cadaver specimens. Quantitative evaluation of fiber arrangement is challenging also in brain tractography since obtaining the ground truth is difficult. We accomplished a validation with a highly reliable ground truth by using two series of cryosection images one of them accompanies CT and MR images.

2 Method

2.1 Overview of the Proposed Method

As illustrated in Fig. 1, the proposed method first construct a high fidelity template biomechanical model from a high resolution cryosection volume, then it is adapted to each patient using the information from patient-specific images. Since a large-scale image database is available for routinely used modalities such as CT and MR, the method allows statistical analysis of population-specific biomechanical parameters.

2.2　Construction of High Fidelity Fiber Arrangement Template and Preprocessing of Patient-Specific Images

Figure 2 shows the high fidelity fiber arrangement templates that we created from two optical cryosection image volumes (0.1 mm^3/voxel) using the method previously reported in [10]. As for the patient-specific image, CT or MRI, first, the regions of target bone and muscles are segmented. Although we used labels manually traced in 20 clinical CTs in this study, we confirmed with a larger scale CT database that automation of the segmentation using these 20 training data sets is viable with a deep neural network approach. The muscle attachment area was obtained using the method proposed by Fukuda et al. in [4]. Then, similar to [10], we obtain the local orientation within a neighborhood at each voxel by computing the eigenvector corresponding to the smallest eigenvalue of the gradient-based structure tensor [2]. A Gaussian filter (with standard deviation of σ_1) was applied to the image before computing gradient to suppress noise and after computing the gradient (with std. of σ_2) to smooth the tensor field. $\sigma_1 = 0.5$ mm and $\sigma_2 = 2$ mm were experimentally found to be effective in this method and used in the experiment below.

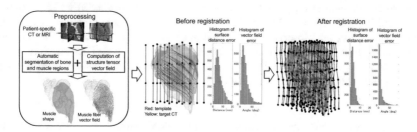

Fig. 3. The proposed non-rigid registration method with a cost function consisting of surface distance error and structure tensor vector field error.

2.3　Non-rigid Registration Using Shape and Local Orientation Cost

The proposed non-rigid registration and a representative registration result were illustrated in Fig. 3. The cost function consists of three terms, namely surface distance term (C_1), vector field difference term (C_2), and smoothness penalty term (g).

$$\hat{\Theta} = \arg\min_{\Theta}(1 - \alpha)C_1(\Theta) + \alpha C_2(\Theta) + \lambda g(\Theta) \tag{1}$$

The parameter α changes the balance between the two data fitness terms and λ is the regularization weight. Each term is as follows.

$$C_1(\Theta) = \frac{1}{N_m}\sum_{i \in S_m}\min_{j \in S_f}\|p_{m,i}(\Theta) - p_{f,j}\| + \frac{1}{N_f}\sum_{j \in S_f}\min_{i \in S_m}\|p_{m,i}(\Theta) - p_{f,j}\|$$

where S_m, N_m and S_f, S_m represents the surface and the number of vertices of moving and fixed surfaces, respectively. In this study, the moving and fixed surfaces contain three objects, the pelvis, femur, and the target muscle. $p_{m,i}$ and $p_{f,i}$ represents ith vertex in S_m and S_f, respectively. This term represents the symmetric surface distance.

$$C_2(\boldsymbol{\Theta}) = -Dice(\Omega_f, \Omega_m)\frac{1}{N}\sum_{i,j,k\in\Omega_f\cap\Omega_m} G(\theta_{i,j,k}(\boldsymbol{\Theta})); \sigma_{cost})$$

where Ω_f and Ω_m represent the regions covered by the moving and fixed surface, and $\theta_{i,j,k}$ represents the angular difference between vectors in the two vector fields at the voxed indexed by (i, j, k). $G(A; \sigma)$ is a Gaussian function with a standard deviation of σ. $g(\boldsymbol{\Theta})$ is a commonly used smoothness penalty term [13] represented as follows.

$$g(\boldsymbol{\Theta}) = \sum_{i=1}^{x}\sum_{j=1}^{y}\sum_{k=1}^{z}$$
$$\left[\left(\frac{\partial^2 T}{\partial x^2}\right)^2 + \left(\frac{\partial^2 T}{\partial y^2}\right)^2 + \left(\frac{\partial^2 T}{\partial z^2}\right)^2 + 2\left(\frac{\partial^2 T}{\partial xy}\right)^2 + 2\left(\frac{\partial^2 T}{\partial yz}\right)^2 + 2\left(\frac{\partial^2 T}{\partial xz}\right)^2\right]$$

2.4   Evaluation Method

The cadaveric data set that we used in this study [5] includes optical image volumes of two specimens, and one of the specimen (denoted as *subject*1 in the figures) accompanies images obtained by clinical CT and MRI (voxel size: 1.0 mm^3). Thus, as shown in Fig. 4, we constructed a high fidelity template from the optical image of *subject*2 and registered to CT and MRI of *subject*1 and evaluated the result using a ground truth obtained from the optical image of *subject*1. As for the error metric, we employed the fiber distance error which is defined as the mean distance between pairs of corresponding points on the nearest fiber [9], which is one of the metrics used in evaluation of white matter fibers in brain tractography.

3   Results

Figures 5 and 6 show the results of fiber arrangement of the gluteus maximus, medius, and minimus muscles computed from CT and MRI using the proposed non-rigid registration. Figure 5 shows quantitative evaluation in *subject*1 where the accurate ground truth obtained from the optical image was available. The proposed method was compared also with two previous methods that 1) used the grid fitting to the CT [10] (denoted as *Previous method 2* in the figure) and 2) used computational fluid dynamics [6] that computes fiber arrangement from its surface shape (denoted as *Previous method 2* in the figure). Fiber distance error for the gluteus medius muscle (Fig. 5a) for the estimation from CT, MRI, previous method 1, and 2, were 3.76 ± 1.24 mm, 3.26 ± 0.85 mm, 4.15 ± 2.29 mm, 8.72 ± 4.40 mm, respectively. The *previous method 1* had larger number

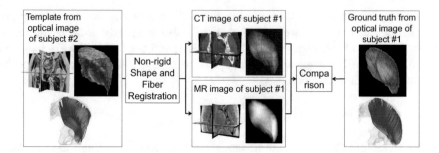

Fig. 4. Illustration of the evaluation scheme used in this study. Two cadaveric specimens are used. A high fidelity muscle fiber template obtained from an optical volume of one subject (subject 2) was registered to CT and MR images of the other subject (subject 1). The registration accuracy was evaluated by fiber distance error metric using the ground truth obtained from the optical volume of subject 1.

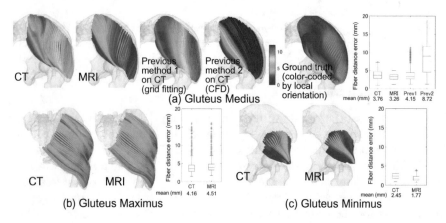

Fig. 5. Results of quantitative evaluation using the ground truth obtained from high resolution optical volume. The fiber arrangements estimated from CT and MRI in gluteus (a) medius, (b) maximus, and (c) minimus muscles were illustrated by the colormap corresponding to the fiber distance error from the ground truth.

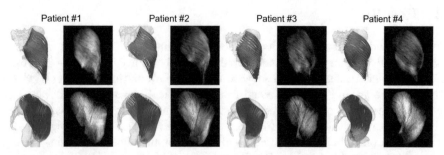

Fig. 6. Results of muscle fiber arrangement modeling of the gluteus maximus, and medius muscles of four representative patients (out of 20 patients analyzed in the study). The color corresponds to the local orientation (see the caption of Fig. 2)

of outliers in the anterior region (right side in the figure). We found that in this region of this subject, the amount of fat tissue was relatively low and there was almost no texture, resulting in a highly noisy structure tensor vectors. The proposed method was robust in this region owing to the cost function containing the fitness of the bone surface, where the attachment areas lay on, in addition to the vector field fitness. The *previous method 2* showed larger error overall, suggesting that the information from internal texture contributed significantly. The fiber distance errors for CT and MRI were 4.16 ± 2.34 mm, and 4.51 ± 2.38 mm, for the gluteus maximus and 2.45 ± 0.76 mm, and 1.77 ± 0.70 mm, for the gluteus minimus, respectively. Since the fiber distance error computes the average distance with the nearest fiber, the shorter fibers tend to show smaller error. Since fiber length is different between the muscles, direct comparison is difficult, but estimation from MRI shows smaller error in the gluteus medius, and minimus, and almost the same for the gluteus maximus. The results in Fig. 6 was obtained from clinical CTs, where no ground truth is available. Qualitative visual evaluation on the clinical CTs shown in Fig. 6 suggested a reasonable reconstruction for the three muscles.

4   Discussion and Conclusion

We proposed a non-rigid registration method with a cost function containing both surface distance error and the vector field angle error, and quantitatively evaluated its accuracy and demonstrated applications in patient-specific biomechanical modeling using a database of 20 clinical CTs. Compared to the previously proposed grid fitting method [10] that takes account for only the vector field, the proposed method was found to be more robust in the area with higher noise in the structure tensor field. Using the robust registration method, we proposed an approach to patient-specific biomechanical modeling using the high fidelity generic template model constructed from cadaveric images. One of the limitations in current study is that the evaluation used only two specimens only one of which has clinical CT and MRI. Enlarging the template database as well as introducing a new method to obtain the ground truth from clinical CTs are our ongoing work. Another potential future work is the statistical analysis using a large-scale CT database. The robustness of the proposed registration method even in the presence of noise in clinical CT would become a strong advantage in the large-scale cohort analysis of biomechanical parameters, since CT is the most common modality especially in the orthopedic surgery where the biomechanical simulation is most profitable.

Acknowledgment. This research was supported by MEXT/JSPS KAKENHI 26108004, JST PRESTO 20407, AMED/ETH the strategic Japanese-Swiss cooperative research program. The authors extend their appreciation to Professor Min Suk Chung (Ajou University School of Medicine) for providing us the Visible Korean Human dataset.

References

1. Andrews, S., Hamarneh, G.: The generalized log-ratio transformation: learning shape and adjacency priors for simultaneous thigh muscle segmentation. IEEE Trans. Med. Imaging **34**(9), 1773–1787 (2015)
2. Bigun, J.: Optimal orientation detection of linear symmetry. In: Proceedings of the IEEE First International Conference on Computer Vision, pp. 433–438 (1987)
3. Blemker, S.S., Delp, S.L.: Three-dimensional representation of complex muscle architectures and geometries. Ann. Biomed. Eng. **33**(5), 661–73 (2005)
4. Fukuda, N.: Estimation of attachment regions of hip muscles in CT image using muscle attachment probabilistic atlas constructed from measurements in eight cadavers. Int. J. Comput. Assist. Radiol. Surg. **12**(5), 733–742 (2017)
5. Jin, S.: Visible korean human: Improved serially sectioned images of the entire body. IEEE Trans. Med. Imaging **24**(3), 352–360 (2005)
6. Joshua, I., et al.: Fiber tractography for finite-element modeling of transversely isotropic biological tissues of arbitrary shape using computational fluid dynamics. In: Proceedings of the Conference on Summer Computer Simulation, pp. 1–6 (2015)
7. Kupczik, K.: Reconstruction of muscle fascicle architecture from iodine-enhanced microct images: a combined texture mapping and streamline approach. J. Theor. Biol. **382**, 34–43 (2015)
8. Levin, D.I.W.: Extracting skeletal muscle fiber fields from noisy diffusion tensor data. Med. Image Anal. **15**(3), 340–353 (2011)
9. O'Donnell, L.J., Westin, C.-F.: Automatic tractography segmentation using a high-dimensional white matter atlas. IEEE Trans. Med. Imaging **26**(11), 1562–1575 (2007)
10. Otake, Y., et al.: Patient-specific skeletal muscle fiber modeling from structure tensor field of clinical CT images. In: Descoteaux, M., et al. (eds.) MICCAI 2017, Part I. LNCS, vol. 10433, pp. 656–663. Springer, Cham (2017). https://doi.org/10.1007/978-3-319-66182-7_75
11. Popuri, K., Cobzas, D., Esfandiari, N., Baracos, V., Jägersand, M.: Body composition assessment in axial CT images using fem-based automatic segmentation of skeletal muscle. IEEE Trans. Med. Imaging **35**(2), 512–520 (2016)
12. Rajagopal, A., et al.: Full-body musculoskeletal model for muscle-driven simulation of human gait. IEEE Trans. Biomed. Eng. **63**(10), 2068–2079 (2016)
13. Rueckert, D., Sonoda, L.I., Hayes, C., Hill, D.L., Leach, M.O., Hawkes, D.J.: Non-rigid registration using free-form deformations: application to breast mr images. IEEE Trans. Med. Imaging **18**(8), 712–21 (1999)
14. Webb, J.D.: 3D finite element models of shoulder muscles for computing lines of actions and moment arms. Comput. Methods Biomech. Biomed. Eng. **17**(8), 829–37 (2014)
15. Zhou, Y.: Estimation of muscle fiber orientation in ultrasound images using revoting hough transform (RVHT). Ultrasound Med. Biol. **34**(9), 1474–81 (2008)

Atlas Propagation Through Template Selection

Hongzhi Wang[(✉)] and Rui Zhang

IBM Almaden Research Center, San Jose, USA
hongzhiw@us.ibm.com

Abstract. Template-based atlas propagation can reduce registration cost in multi-atlas segmentation. In this method, atlases and testing images are registered to a common template. We show that using a common template may be suboptimal for reducing atlas propagation errors. Instead, we propose to apply a custom selected template for each testing image by employing a large template library and a fast template selection technique. The proposed method significantly outperforms common template based atlas propagation. Using a template library with 50 images, our method produced comparable results to standard direct registration-based multi-atlas segmentation with a small fraction of registration cost.

1 Introduction

Multi-atlas label fusion (MALF) is a powerful technique for anatomy segmentation. This method relies on image registration to propagate anatomical labels from pre-labeled training images, i.e. atlases, to a target image and applies label fusion to reduce atlas propagation errors.

Template-based atlas propagation [8] has been applied for reducing registration cost in MALF. Using this approach, instead of directly registering each atlas to a target image, the pairwise registration is achieved through registering each image to one common template. Since registrations between atlases and the template can be calculated off-line, only one registration between the template and the target image needs to be calculated online.

One commonly applied criterion for choosing the propagation template is to reduce the overall atlas propagation error from atlases to the template [4,8]. We show that a more effective criterion should aim to reduce the propagation error from the template to the target image. Hence, instead of employing a common propagation template, a custom selected template should be used for each individual target image. We propose to employ a sizable template library. Given a target image, the template producing the least registration error to the target image is selected for optimal atlas propagation.

In an application of cardiac CT segmentation, we demonstrate that our method significantly outperforms standard common template based atlas propagation. Using a small fraction of computation cost, our method produces comparable results to standard MALF that uses pairwise deformable registrations.

© Springer Nature Switzerland AG 2018
A. F. Frangi et al. (Eds.): MICCAI 2018, LNCS 11070, pp. 711–719, 2018.
https://doi.org/10.1007/978-3-030-00928-1_80

1.1   Related Work

Faster atlas propagation can be achieved by: (1) using cheaper but less accurate registrations to replace deformable registration [5]; (2) reducing the number of online registrations. Employing less accurate registrations often substantially sacrifices accuracy. For instance, a recent work along this line [2] affinely warps images to common templates and applies learning-based refinement, which still underperforms deformable registration based multi-atlas segmentation.

Reducing online registrations can be achieved by atlas selection [1,10] and/or template-based propagation [8]. Atlas selection aims to select a subset of atlases that are likely to produce accurate label propagation for a target image. However, it has limited effects on reducing registration cost. The performance of multi-atlas segmentation usually increases as poorly registered atlases are excluded from label fusion. However, the performance may start decreasing after removing well registered atlases. Typically, a good number of atlases are still required for label fusion to prevent performance drop.

Template-based atlas propagation is indirect propagation, which is based on composing registrations along a registration path through intermediate image(s). Indirect propagation has been applied for improving atlas propagation accuracy. For example, each atlas is propagated through multiple registration paths to improve the chance that atlas information is accurately propagated at least once [9,12,14]. With manifold learning, instead of the brutal force approach, efficiency can be improved by decomposing a difficult-to-estimate large deformation between two images into a series of easier-to-estimate smaller deformations represented by intermediate propagation images/templates [6,13]. When applied for reducing registration cost, the indirect registration scheme is only applied through common template(s) based atlas propagation. Our contribution is a new strategy for optimal template-based propagation.

2   Method

2.1   Modeling Atlas Propagation Error

Let $\phi_{I \to K}$ be a transformation that aligns image I to image K. Let $f(\phi_{I \to K}, x)$ be registration error at location x in K, i.e. the *absolute spatial displacement* between true and estimated correspondences. Let $\phi_{I \to T \to K} = \phi_{I \to T} \circ \phi_{T \to K}$ be the composed transformation for propagating I through a template T. We have:

$$f(\phi_{I \to T \to K}, x) \le f(\phi_{I \to T}, x_T) + f(\phi_{T \to K}, x) \tag{1}$$

where x_T is the correspondence of x in T, as defined by $\phi_{T \to K}$. Let $F(I, K) = \sum_{x \in K} [f(\phi_{I \to K}, x)]$ and $F(I, T, K) = \sum_{x \in K} [f(\phi_{I \to T \to K}, x)]$ be the overall registration error in $\phi_{I \to K}$ and $\phi_{I \to T \to K}$, respectively. We have:

$$F(I, T, K) \le F(I, T) + F(T, K) \tag{2}$$

For indirect propagation, the overall registration error is upper bounded by the total registration errors in the two registrations on the registration path.

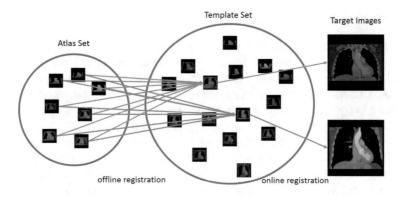

Fig. 1. Atlas propagation through a single selected template.

2.2 Biased Template Selection

Let $A = \{A_1, ..., A_n\}$ be an atlas set with n atlases. The total propagation error from an atlas set to a target image through a single template is bounded by:

$$\sum_{i=1}^{n} F(A_i, T, K) \leq \sum_{i=1}^{n} F(A_i, T) + nF(T, K) \qquad (3)$$

Our goal is to find a template T such that the total atlas propagation error is minimized, which can be achieved by choosing the template minimizing the upper bound. Based on (3), two competing schemes may minimize the upper bound: (1) **unbiased template creation/selection** that minimizes the average registration error from all atlases to a common template, i.e. minimizing $\sum_{i=1}^{n} F(A_i, T)$; (2) **biased template selection** that selects the template minimizing registration error to the target image, i.e. minimizing $nF(T, K)$.

Minimizing registration errors from all atlases to a common template is the goal for unbiased template building [4,7] and groupwise registration. However, its effect on reducing overall registration errors is limited by how tightly clustered the atlases are. The key advantage of MALF is to use diverse atlases to capture population variation for robust label propagation. Hence, it is common to have highly dissimilar images included in one atlas set, making it difficult to reduce the overall registration error from all atlases to a common template.

In contrast, the template-target registration error can be more easily minimized by choosing a template similar to the target image (see Fig. 1). Furthermore, since the template-target registration error has the highest weight in (3), the template minimizing the upper bound is also biased to reduce registration error to the target image. In fact, when $T = K$, the template-based atlas propagation becomes direct registration based propagation. Although it is intractable to consider every image as a potential template, we hypothesize that it is highly possible to find a similar template from a modestly sized and representative template library for any target image to keep the total atlas propagation error stay close to the total error produced by direct registration based atlas propagation.

2.3   Multi-template Atlas Propagation

Atlas propagation through a single template is expected to approach the performance of direct registration based atlas propagation as the template library grows. Using a finite template library, single template atlas propagation is still expected to under perform direct registration based atlas propagation. Since registrations between templates and a target image are independently calculated, the additional propagation error caused by registration composition using different templates are independent from each other, which can be effectively reduced by label fusion. Hence, employing a few templates that are similar to the target image for atlas propagation may completely remove the performance gap between template-based propagation and direct registration based propagation.

2.4   Downsampling-Based Fast Template Selection

Template selection aims to select a template from a template library that has the smallest registration error to a target image. Comparing to atlas selection [1,10], template selection has the following challenges: (1) to ensure small registration error from at least one template to any target image, a template set may contain more images than a typical atlas set; and (2) template selection needs to have low computational cost to achieve the goal of reducing overall computational cost.

To this end, each template is registered to the target image in a downsampled space. After registration, image similarity measures such as normalized mutual information (NMI) and sum squared distance (SSD) are employed for template ranking. Note that both global and region of interest based image similarity can be employed. In our experiments, both templates and target images are downsampled into a coarse resolution such that deformable registration can be finished within a few seconds, keeping the total computational cost for template selection negligible comparing to a regular registration. Registrations to the target image in the original space are only computed for selected templates.

3   Experiments

We conducted anatomy segmentation experiments using cardiac CT scans. Sixteen anatomical structures were manually traced by a clinician for 42 cases, namely, sternum, aorta (ascending/descending/arch/root), pulmonary artery (left/right/trunk), vertebrae, left/right atrium, left/right ventricle, left ventricular myocardium, superior/inferior vena cava. All images were resampled to have a $2\,\mathrm{mm}^3$ isotropic resolution. See Fig. 2(a) for one image with manual annotations.

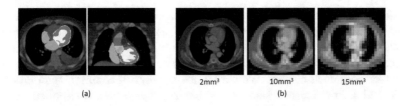

Fig. 2. (a) Axial (left) and coronal (right) views of one CT image with manual annotations. (b) One template image at 2, 10, and 15 mm^3 resolutions, respectively.

3.1   Experiment Setup

We conducted leave-one-out cross validation using the 42 labeled scans.

Image Registration. Image registration was computed using ANTS [3] by sequentially optimizing affine and deformable transform (Syn), using Mattes mutual information. Registering an image pair at 2 mm^3 resolution took ~50 min on a 2 G HZ CPU.

Performance of Direct/Indirect Registration. To compare atlas propagation accuracy produced by direct registration and indirect registration composition, we calculated pairwise deformable registrations for each pair of the 42 images with manual segmentation. The indirect registrations were produced for each image pair by taking each of the remaining images as the propagation template. The performance of direct/indirect registrations is measured by how well anatomical structures are aligned in Dice similarity coefficient (DSC).

Label Fusion. We applied joint label fusion [11] with default parameters. Note that for our method, all atlases are propagated through the selected template(s) and are used for label fusion.

Template Library. The template library was created by randomly selecting cases without manual segmentation. To investigate how the size of template library affects the performance of atlas propagation, we created four template libraries with varying sizes of 10, 20, 50, and 100, respectively.

Downsampling Space for Template Selection. To study the effect of how downsampling may affect template selection, we tested two downsampling resolutions: 10 mm^3 and 15 mm^3. Figure 2(b) shows one example template. Images in 10 mm^3 and 15 mm^3 resolutions only contain global structures, which are sufficient for a global alignment. Registration at 10 mm^3 and 15 mm^3 can be calculated within 5 s and 1 s, respectively.

Template Selection Metric. Following [8], we applied NMI and SSD for atlas/template selection. To test multi-template atlas propagation, we varied the number of selected propagation templates from 1 to 5.

Baseline Methods. MALF with direct registration atlas propagation and atlas selection was applied to set the baseline performance. We also compared with unbiased template building based atlas propagation. We iteratively applied the unbiased template building method [7] and k-means clustering to create common template(s) for the 42 testing images. For example, when k templates are created, the images are grouped into k clusters based on image similarity. One template is created from each cluster. We varied the number of common templates from 1, 2, 3, and 4. For common template(s) based propagation, we applied two label fusion schemes: (1) each training image was propagated to a target image once through its nearest neighbor template; (2) each training image was propagated through all templates and all warped atlases were applied for label fusion.

3.2   Results

Direct/Indirect Registration. Indirect registration produces more registration errors than direct registration. The average DSC scores over all anatomical structures produced by direct/indirect registrations are 0.525 and 0.456, respectively.

Baseline MALF. Figure 3(a) summarizes the performance when various number of atlases were selected for label fusion. NMI consistently outperformed SSD. Meanwhile, using fewer atlases did not produce more accurate label fusion results than using all atlases when locally weighted voting fusion was applied.

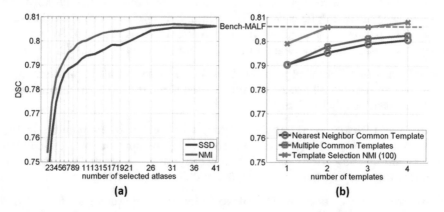

Fig. 3. (a) Segmentation performance using direct atlas propagation with atlas selection; (b) Performance using atlas propagation via common templates and templates selected from a library with 100 images. The performance of Bench-MALF, which applied 41 atlases with direct atlas-target registrations, is shown for direct comparison.

Common Template Atlas Propagation. Figure 4 shows an example when three common templates are built. The created templates capture the fact that the images may cover different body regions.

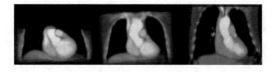

Fig. 4. Coronal views of three templates created from unbiased template building.

Figure 3(b) shows the label fusion performance when various number of common templates were created for atlas propagation. When each atlas was propagated through multiple templates, the result is slightly better than that produced by propagating each atlas only through its nearest neighbor template. As more templates were created, the registration error from each atlas to its nearest neighbor template is reduced, which results in more accurate label fusion results. Overall, common template(s) based atlas propagation underperformed standard MALF using direct atlas propagation, even when four common templates were used. The difference is significant, with $p < 0.01$ on the paired Students t-test.

Biased Template Selection Atlas Propagation. Table 1 summarizes the performance for biased template selection based atlas propagation. Again, NMI consistently outperformed SSD for template selection. Overall, using larger size template libraries produced more accurate results. The performance gain due to enlarged template library is more prominent when a single template was applied for atlas propagation. However, the performance gain diminishes as the performance approaches the accuracy level produced by standard MALF with direct registration. With NMI template selection, using a template library of size 50 or greater consistently and significantly ($p < 0.01$) outperformed common template atlas propagation (also see Fig. 3).

Table 1. Label fusion performance produced by template selection based atlas propagation. *indicates the difference from the standard MALF with direct atlas propagation is statistically significant, with $p < 0.01$ on the paired Students t-test.

Selection space		$10\,\mathrm{mm}^3$					$15\,\mathrm{mm}^3$				
	Size of template set	1	2	3	4	5	1	2	3	4	5
SSD	10	0.772*	0.792*	0.797*	0.800*	0.801*	0.773*	0.789*	0.796*	0.800*	0.802*
	20	0.776*	0.797*	0.800*	0.804	0.804	0.780*	0.797*	0.800*	0.803	0.804
	50	0.794*	0.805	0.807	0.807	0.807	0.775*	0.802*	0.805	0.807	0.807
	100	0.789*	0.802*	0.806	0.806	0.806	0.781*	0.799*	0.804	0.806	0.807
NMI	10	0.777*	0.795*	0.800*	0.802	0.804	0.781*	0.795*	0.803*	0.803	0.804
	20	0.785*	0.803	0.804	0.806	0.806	0.789*	0.800*	0.804	0.805	0.806
	50	0.796*	0.806	0.807	0.808	0.808	0.799*	0.803*	0.806	0.808	0.808
	100	0.799*	0.806	0.806	0.808	0.809*	0.796*	0.805	0.807	0.808	0.809

With a single propagation template, the best accuracy is 0.799 mean DSC produced by NMI selection in $10\,\mathrm{mm}^3$ space with a template library of 100 images. When two templates were applied for atlas propagation, the performance gap between direct-registration based MALF is completely removed with a template library of size 50. Template selection using a library of size 50 takes less than 5 minutes and 1 min in $10\,mm^3$ and $15\,mm^3$ space, respectively. Using 2 deformable registrations + template selection for atlas propagation, our method reached the performance of standard MALF, which requires 41 deformable registrations for 41 atlases. Hence, in our experiments the atlas propagation cost of our method is about 5% of standard MALF.

4   Conclusions

We provide a justification for employing a sizable template library and biased template selection to improve the performance of template-based atlas propagation. In a cardiac CT anatomy segmentation application, our method consistently outperformed common unbiased template based atlas propagation. Using 5% registration cost, our method produced comparable performance to standard direct registration based MALF.

References

1. Aljabar, P., Heckemann, R., Hammers, A., Hajnal, J., Rueckert, D.: Multi-atlas based segmentation of brain images: Atlas selection and its effect on accuracy. NeuroImage **46**, 726–739 (2009)
2. Asman, A.J., Huo, Y., Plassard, A.J., Landman, B.A.: Multi-atlas learner fusion: An efficient segmentation approach for large-scale data. MedIA **26**(1), 82–91 (2015)
3. Avants, B., Epstein, C., Grossman, M., Gee, J.: Symmetric diffeomorphic image registration with cross-correlation: Evaluating automated labeling of elderly and neurodegenerative brain. MedIA **12**(1), 26–41 (2008)
4. Avants, B.B., Yushkevich, P., Pluta, J., Minkoff, D., Korczykowski, M., Detre, J., Gee, J.C.: The optimal template effect in hippocampus studies of diseased populations. Neuroimage **49**(3), 2457–2466 (2010)
5. Coupe, P., Manjon, J., Fonov, V., Pruessner, J., Robles, N., Collins, D.: Patch-based segmentation using expert priors: Application to hippocampus and ventricle segmentation. NeuroImage **54**(2), 940–954 (2011)
6. Jia, H., Yap, P., Shen, D.: Iterative multi-atlas-based multi-image segmentation with tree-based registration. Neuroimage **59**(1), 422–430 (2012)
7. Joshi, S., Davis, B., Jomier, M., Gerig, G.: Unbiased diffeomorphism atlas construction for computational anatomy. NeuroImage 23, 151–160 (2004)
8. Lotjonen, J., Wolz, R., Koikkalainen, J., Thurfjell, L., Waldemar, G., Soininen, H., Rueckert, D.: Fast and robust multi-atlas segmentation of brain magnetic resonance images. NeuroImage **49**(3), 2352–2365 (2010)
9. Pipitone, J., Park, M., Winterburn, J., Lett, T.A., Lerch, J.P., Pruessner, J.C., Lepage, M., Voineskos, A.N., Chakravarty, M.M.: Multi-atlas segmentation of the whole hippocampus and subfields using multiple automatically generated templates. Neuroimage **101**, 494–512 (2014)
10. Rohlfing, T., Brandt, R., Menzel, R., Maurer, C.: Evaluation of atlas selection strategies for atlas-based image segmentation with application to confocal microscopy images of bee brains. NeuroImage **21**(4), 1428–1442 (2004)

11. Wang, H., Suh, J.W., Das, S., Pluta, J., Craige, C., Yushkevich, P.: Multi-atlas segmentation with joint label fusion. IEEE Trans. on PAMI **35**(3), 611–623 (2013)
12. Wang, H., Pouch, A., Takabe, M., Jackson, B., Gorman, J., Gorman, R., Yushkevich, P.A.: Multi-atlas segmentation with robust label transfer and label fusion. In: Information Processing in Medical Imaging (2013)
13. Wolz, R., Aljabar, P., Hajnal, J., Hammers, A., Rueckert, D.: Leap: Learning embeddings for atlas propagation. NeuroImage **49**(2), 1316–1325 (2010)
14. Zhuang, X., Leung, K., Rhode, K., Razavi, R., Hawkes, D., Ourselin, S.: Whole heart segmentation of cardiac mri using multiple path propagation strategy. In: MICCAI. pp. 435–443. Springer (2010)

Spatio-Temporal Atlas of Bone Mineral Density Ageing

Mohsen Farzi[1,2], Jose M. Pozo[1], Eugene McCloskey[2], Richard Eastell[2],
J. Mark Wilkinson[2], and Alejandro F. Frangi[1(✉)]

[1] Centre for Computational Imaging & Simulation Technologies in Biomedicine
(CISTIB), University of Sheffield, Sheffield, UK
a.frangi@sheffield.ac.uk
[2] Academic Unit of Bone Metabolism, University of Sheffield, Sheffield, UK

Abstract. Osteoporosis is an age-associated bone disease characterised
by low bone mass. An improved understanding of the underlying mechanism for age-related bone loss could lead to enhanced preventive and
therapeutic strategies for osteoporosis. In this work, we propose a fully
automatic pipeline for developing a spatio-temporal atlas of ageing
bone. Bone maps are collected using a dual-energy X-ray absorptiometry (DXA) scanner. Each scan is then warped into a reference template to eliminate morphological variation and establish a correspondence
between pixel coordinates. Pixel-wise bone density evolution with ageing
was modelled using smooth quantile curves. To construct the atlas, we
amalgamated a cohort of 1714 Caucasian women (20–87 years) from five
different centres in North Western Europe. As a systematic difference
exists between different DXA manufacturers, we propose a novel calibration technique to homogenise bone density measurements across the
centres. This technique utilises an alternating minimisation technique to
map the observed bone density measurements into a latent standardised
space. To the best of our knowledge, this is the first spatio-temporal atlas
of ageing bone.

1 Introduction

Ageing is associated with a gradual and progressive bone loss, which predis-
poses to osteoporosis. Osteoporosis is a bone disease characterised by low bone
mass and micro-architectural deterioration. Given the close relationship between
involutional bone loss and the underlying mechanism of osteoporosis, improving
the understanding of the bone ageing process has been of interest for the osteoporosis research community [1,2]. To facilitate this understanding, we propose a
method to develop a spatio-temporal atlas of ageing bone in the femur.

Electronic supplementary material The online version of this chapter (https://
doi.org/10.1007/978-3-030-00928-1_81) contains supplementary material, which is
available to authorized users.

A. F. Frangi et al. (Eds.): MICCAI 2018, LNCS 11070, pp. 720–728, 2018.
https://doi.org/10.1007/978-3-030-00928-1_81

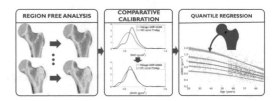

Fig. 1. Region Based Analysis. BMD values are averaged in the specified ROIs; The neck, trochanteric, and inter-trochanteric regions are shown in red, blue, and green.

Fig. 2. Bone Ageing Analysis Pipeline. BMD maps are warped into a reference template to eliminate morphological variations. Cross-calibration between different DXA manufacturers is established to homogenise BMD measurements. Smooth quantile curves are fitted to the standardised BMD values at each pixel coordinate.

Spatio-temporal atlases are useful tools for visualising and accessing a wide range of data in Medical Image Computing. For example, brain atlases demonstrated great potential for visualising age-related pathology in Alzheimer's disease [3]. However, to the best of our knowledge, no bone ageing atlas has been developed in osteoporosis research so far. Developing a comprehensive model of involutional bone loss is a challenging task. Firstly, this requires a robust and accurate quantification technique for bone mineral density (BMD) measurement and its spatial distribution. Dual-energy X-ray Absorptiometry (DXA) is the reference gold standard to measure BMD in clinical practice [4]. In conventional DXA analysis, BMD values are averaged in *a priori* specified Regions of Interest (ROIs) to compensate for shape variation between scans (Fig. 1). This data averaging, however, may reduce our insight on more focal BMD deficits. The second challenge is the ability to homogenise BMD across different technologies, as a systematic difference exists between different DXA manufacturers [5,6].

We address these challenges as follows: To maintain fidelity to high-resolution pixel BMD values, we develop a group-wise image warping technique termed region free analysis (RFA). This image warping eliminates the morphological variation between scans and establishes a correspondence between pixel coordinates. Farzi et al. presented a similar approach to analysing periprosthetic BMD change [7]. However, their method is semi-automatic and is not applicable to large-scale datasets. To amalgamate data from different scanner technologies, we propose a novel cross-calibration technique by minimising the mutual difference between the BMD probability distributions measured by each proprietary DXA scanner.

This paper describes the development of the first spatio-temporal atlas of ageing bone in the femur. To this end, we propose a fully automatic pipeline to ensure high-throughput computing applicable to large-scale datasets (Fig. 2). We also derive a set of reference quantile curves per each pixel to model the BMD evolution with ageing. The developed atlas provides new insights into the spatial pattern of bone loss, for which the conventional DXA analysis is insensitive.

2   Methods

2.1   Preprocessing

The raw data from a DXA scanner is not immediately usable for analysing BMD maps. To export BMD maps, the raw data requires processing using a computer software package specific to its vendor. We used Apex v3.2 and Encore v16 to extract pixel BMD information for Hologic Inc. (Waltham, MA) and GE-Lunar Corp. (Madison, WI) scanners, respectively.

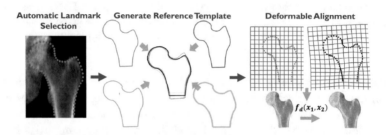

Fig. 3. Region Free Analysis. Sixty-five landmark points are automatically selected. A reference shape is learned using generalised Procrustes analysis. Each scan is warped to the template using a thin plate spline (TPS) registration.

2.2   Region Free Analysis

RFA aims to find a set of coordinate transformations such that the warped scans are aligned with each other in the template domain (Fig. 3). This warping allows pixel level inference at each coordinate in the template domain.

Automatic Landmark Extraction: Statistical shape models (SSMs) are a robust and accurate approach to automatically locate and segment the femur in radiographic imaging [8]. Here, we used a software package, called *BoneFinder*, to automatically select 65 controlling landmark points around the femur.

Template Generation: Generalised Procrustes analysis is utilised to find the reference template [9]. First, all scans are aligned to a common position, scale, and orientation. Next, the reference template is updated as the average of the aligned shapes. The algorithm iterates between these two steps until convergence.

Pairwise Registration: To eliminate morphological variation between scans, each individual scan is warped to the template domain using a thin plate spline (TPS) registration technique [10]. Since image resolution varies between different manufacturers, the space grid at the template domain was set to the finest resolution available, i.e. 0.25×0.25 mm^2.

2.3   Quantile Regression

Assume the real-valued random variable X with the cumulative distribution function (CDF) $F_X(x) = P(X \leq x)$ represents a response variable of interest, e.g. BMD at one pixel coordinate, and the real-valued random variable T represents an explanatory covariate, e.g. age. Then, the conditional quantile function $(u,t) \longmapsto Q_{X|T}(u,t)$ is defined as

$$Q_{X|T}(u,t) := \inf \left\{ x : u \leq F_{X|T=t}(x) \right\}. \tag{1}$$

For fitting the quantile curves from scattered points $\{(x_n, t_n)\}_{n=1}^{N}$, we deployed the R-package 'VGAM' using the LMS technique [11]. In this technique, a Box-Cox transformation of the response variable X with parameters λ, μ, and σ is applied to obtain normality, i.e. $Z = \psi_{\mu,\sigma,\lambda}(X)$. Given that $Q_Z(u)$ is known for a normal distribution, if smooth curves $\lambda(t)$, $\mu(t)$, and $\sigma(t)$ are estimated, then $Q_{X|T}(u,t)$ can be simply estimated using the inverse transformation, i.e. $Q_{X|T}(u,t) = \psi_{\mu(t),\sigma(t),\lambda(t)}^{-1}(Q_Z(u))$.

The smoothness of the fitted parameter curves is controlled using a vector smoothing spline. We modelled $\lambda(t)$ and $\sigma(t)$ as intercept terms and $\mu(t)$ as a smooth function with the equivalent degree of freedom 3. To assess the precision of the estimated quantile curves, we used a bootstrapping procedure. We randomly sampled subjects with replacement and re-estimated the quantile curves. We repeated this procedure 1000 times collecting a distribution of possible quantile curves. From these observations, we estimated the confidence intervals at 5% significance level [12].

2.4   Comparative Calibration

Assume the latent random variable X represents the underlying true BMD values and the random variable Y^c represents the observed BMD values measured on the machine c. Lu et al. proposed a linear model for comparative calibration between DXA scanners [6].

$$Y^c = a_c X + b_c + \epsilon_c. \tag{2}$$

$\epsilon_c \sim \mathcal{N}(0, \sigma_c^2)$ represents the measurement noise of scanner c. Lue et al. [6] proposed an expectation maximisation (EM) approach to estimate the model parameters $\{a_c, b_c, \sigma_c\}_{c=1}^{C}$ using BMD measurements based on a common group of individuals. This method cannot be used if everyone is scanned only once on each machine and no repeated measurements are available. Requiring repeated measurements of each subject across all machines is an implausible assumption in large-scale multi-centre studies. Alternatively, calibration against phantom measurements is a common pragmatic approach. However, using human measurements is preferred for calibration purposes as a significant disagreement exists between the model parameters fitted to the phantom measurements and those fitted to the human measurements [5].

Here, we propose a novel calibration technique based on human measurements where no repeated measurements are required (cf. [6]). The new technique is developed based on two assumptions. First, a unique distribution of BMD values exists independent of the manufacturers. Assuming different cohorts measured on different scanners are sampled from the same population, the estimated distributions of calibrated BMD values should match one another. Second, the signal to noise ratio is sufficiently large such that

$$Q_{Y^c}(u) \approx a_c Q_X(u) + b_c. \tag{3}$$

Note that if the noise power is zero, then the approximation would be replaced with equality in Eq. 3. With this assumption, estimation of the model parameters $\Theta = \{a_c, b_c\}$ can be decoupled from the estimation of noise variances, i.e. $\{\sigma_c^2\}$. The parameters Θ are estimated by minimizing the cost function

$$\mathcal{J} = \frac{1}{2} \sum_{c=1}^{C} \int_0^1 (Q_{Y^c}(u) - a_c Q_X(u) - b_c)^2 du, \tag{4}$$

including the latent variable X. This minimum has two degrees of freedom. More precisely, if a_c^* and b_c^* minimise the cost $\mathcal{J}$ for an X, then $a_c' = \alpha a_c^*$ and $b_c' = \beta a_c^* + b_c^*$ minimise the cost as well for a corresponding linear transformation of X by any arbitrary $\alpha \neq 0$ and β. To resolve this ambiguity, we define the true BMD as the average of expected observations given the latent variable X, i.e. $X = \frac{1}{C} \sum_c E(Y^c|X)$. This results in the two constraints

$$\sum_c b_c = 0 \quad \text{and} \quad \frac{1}{C} \sum_c a_c = 1. \tag{5}$$

Optimisation: To convert the constrained optimization problem into an unconstrained one, we can simply express the parameters a_C and b_C based on the other parameters: $a_C = C - \sum_{c \neq C} a_c$ and $b_C = -\sum_{c \neq C} b_c$

To estimate the parameters, an alternating minimisation technique is adopted: Given the model parameters, the latent variable x_n for each of the N scanned subjects can be estimated as (step 1),

$$x_n = E(X|y_n^{c_n}; a_{c_n}, b_{c_n}) \approx \frac{1}{a_{c_n}}(y_n^{c_n} - b_{c_n}), \tag{6}$$

where c_n is the corresponding machine. To update the model parameters, we set the gradients $\frac{\partial}{\partial a_c} \mathcal{J}$ and $\frac{\partial}{\partial b_c} \mathcal{J}$ to zero.

$$\frac{\partial}{\partial a_c} \mathcal{J} = (a_c + \sum_{c' \neq C} a_{c'} - C) \int_0^1 Q_X(u)^2 du + (b_c + \sum_{c' \neq C} b_{c'}) \int_0^1 Q_X(u) du$$

$$+ \int_0^1 Q_X(u)(Q_{Y^C}(u) - Q_{Y^c}(u)) du = 0, \tag{7}$$

$$\frac{\partial}{\partial b_c} \mathcal{J} = (a_c + \sum_{c' \neq C} a_{c'} - C) \int_0^1 Q_X(u)du + (b_c + \sum_{c' \neq C} b_{c'})$$

$$+ \int_0^1 (Q_{Y^c}(u) - Q_{Y^c}(u))du = 0. \tag{8}$$

Computing $Q_X(u)$ from step 1, Eqs. 7 and 8 are linear with respect to the model parameters. Hence, we have $2(C-1)$ linear equations with $2(C-1)$ parameters for which a closed-form solution exists (step 2). The algorithm iterates between these two steps until the ℓ_2-norm of the difference between estimated parameters at two consecutive iterations is less than a user-defined tolerance ϵ.

3 Results and Experiments

To construct atlas, we used $N = 1714$ femoral scans (left side) of women aged 20–87 years collected as part of the Osteoporosis and Ultrasound study (OPUS) [13]. Five centres were involved in this study: Sheffield ($N = 504$), Aberdeen ($N = 158$), Berlin ($N = 187$), Kiel ($N = 399$), and Paris ($N = 466$). Scans are collected using either a Hologic QDR 4500A (Sheffield, Paris, and Kiel) or a GE-Lunar Prodigy scanner (Aberdeen and Berlin).

3.1 DXA Cross-Calibration

We validated the proposed technique using synthetic and experimental data.

Synthetic Data: The parameters chosen to synthesise BMD measurements are as follows: $C = 3$, $N_1 = 200$, $N_2 = 300$, and $N_3 = 100$. The latent true BMD values were sampled randomly from a Gaussian distribution with $\mu_0 = 1.3$ and $\sigma_0 = 0.25$. We tested the performance at low, medium, and high noise levels; signal-to-noise ratio (SNR) were set to 28 dB, 16 dB, and 8 dB, respectively. A Monte Carlo procedure with 1000 iterations was conducted and the mean and the standard deviation of the estimated parameters are reported in Table 1.

Parameter Estimation: A prospective cohort from those scanned on each machine were selected such that they were matched for gender, age, body mass index (BMI), scan side, ethnicity, and the geographical location. Figure 4 shows the estimated calibration parameters per each pixel coordinate, i.e. the slop a_c and the intercept b_c, for the Hologic scanner.

Experimental Data: Figure 5 demonstrates the effect of calibration on fitting quantile curves. Amalgamation of Hologic and GE-Lunar scans with no calibration enforces a distinct distortion at the age of 80s onwards where the black line tilted toward the blue line (Fig. 5(a)). Following calibration, the median curves show a consistent pattern in the standardised BMD (sBMD) space (Fig. 5(b)). The fitted curves on the standardised amalgamated dataset can be mapped back to either the Hologic or the GE-Lunar space (see Fig. 5(c) and (d)).

Table 1. Cross-Calibration using synthetic dataset

	Ground Truth	Estimated [mean (standard deviation)]		
		SNR = 28 dB	SNR = 16 dB	SNR = 8 dB
a_1	0.70	0.692(0.041)	0.703(0.042)	0.740(0.045)
a_2	1.40	1.392(0.055)	1.386(0.055)	1.340(0.057)
a_3	0.90	0.916(0.060)	0.910(0.060)	0.919(0.061)
b_1	0.10	0.111(0.057)	0.097(0.056)	0.047(0.060)
b_2	−0.30	−0.291(0.074)	−0.283(0.074)	−0.222(0.076)
b_3	0.20	0.180(0.079)	0.186(0.080)	0.175(0.081)

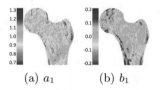

(a) a_1 (b) b_1

Fig. 4. Calibration parameters for the Hologic.

3.2 The Standardised Spatio-Temporal Ageing Atlas

We tested the RFA precision using a set of 25 scan pairs, each pair collected from the same subject on the same day with repositioning between scans. The precision expressed as the coefficient of variation (CV) at the total hip was 1.1%. Figure 6(a) shows the constructed atlas. Cortical thinning was observed consistently with ageing around the shaft from the 60s onwards. A widespread bone loss was also observed in the trochanteric area. Figure 6(b) presents the animated atlas to visualise the gradual bone loss with ageing (see supplementary

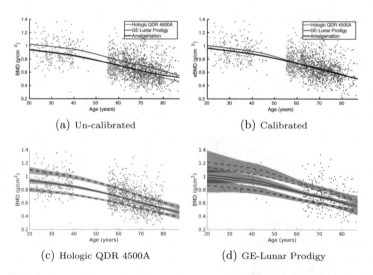

(a) Un-calibrated   (b) Calibrated

(c) Hologic QDR 4500A   (d) GE-Lunar Prodigy

Fig. 5. Fitted quantile curves for the Hologic (red), the GE-Lunar (blue), or the amalgamated (black) dataset. The solid lines represent the median and the dashed lines represent the 50% quantile range. The shaded area shows the 95% confidence interval.

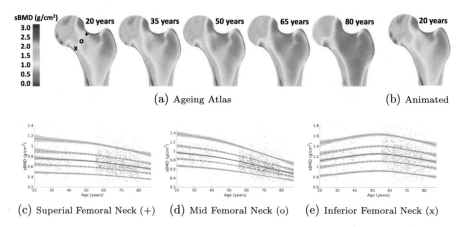

(a) Ageing Atlas

(b) Animated

(c) Superial Femoral Neck (+)   (d) Mid Femoral Neck (o)   (e) Inferior Femoral Neck (x)

Fig. 6. Bone ageing atlas. (a) The median BMD maps as a function of age. (b) Animated atlas (see supplementary material). (c,d,e) The solid, dashed, and dotted lines show the median, the 50% and the 90% quantile ranges, respectively. The green shadow shows the 95% confidence interval.

material). Figure 4(b–d) show quantile curves at the superior, mid, and inferior femoral neck. These curves demonstrated different rates of bone loss. Bone loss was observed consistently in the mid-femoral neck, whilst bone mass was preserved the most in the inferior femoral neck cortex.

4   Conclusion

This work presented the first spatio-temporal atlas of ageing bone in the femur using a large-scale multi-centre dataset (N = 1,714). We presented a region free analysis technique for DXA enabling statistical inference at the pixel level. We presented a novel cross-calibration technique to integrate data from different DXA manufacturers into an amalgamated large-scale dataset, enabling better representativeness of the estimated maps. The developed atlas provides detailed insights on spatially-complex bone loss patterns.

Acknowledgement. M Farzi was funded through a PhD Fellowship from Medical Research Council-Arthritis Research UK Centre for Integrated research into Musculoskeletal Ageing (CIMA). We are grateful for the permission from the OPUS Steering Committee to use the DXA scans.

References

1. Khosla, S., Riggs, B.L.: Pathophysiology of age-related bone loss and osteoporosis. Endocrinol. Metab. Clin. **34**(4), 1015–1030 (2005)
2. Demontiero, O., Vidal, C., Duque, G.: Ageing and bone loss: new insights for the clinician. Ther. Adv. Musculoskelet. Dis. **4**(2), 61–76 (2012)

3. Huizinga, W., Poot, D., Vernooij, M., et al.: A spatio-temporal reference model of the ageing brain. NeuroImage **169**, 11–22 (2017)
4. Adams, J.E.: Advances in bone imaging for osteoporosis. Nature Rev. Endocrinol. **9**(1), 28–42 (2013)
5. Genant, H.K., Grampp, S., Gluer, C.C., et al.: Universal standardization for dual x-ray absorptiometry: patient and phantom cross-calibration results. J. Bone Miner. Res. **9**(10), 1503–1514 (1994)
6. Lu, Y., Ye, K., Mathur, A.K., et al.: Comparative calibration without a gold standard. Stat. Med. **16**(16), 1889–1905 (1997)
7. Farzi, M., Morris, R.M., Penny, J.: Quantitating the effect of prosthesis design on femoral remodeling using high-resolution region-free densitometric analysis (DXA-RFA). J. Orthop. Res. **35**(10), 2203–2210 (2017)
8. Lindner, C., Thiagarajah, S., Wilkinson, J.M., et al.: Fully automatic segmentation of the proximal femur using random forest regression voting. IEEE Trans. Med. Imag. **32**(8), 1462–1472 (2013)
9. Goodall, C.: Procrustes methods in the statistical analysis of shape. J. Roy. Stat. Soc. **53**(2), 285–339 (1991)
10. Bookstein, F.: Principal warps: Thin-plate splines and the decomposition of deformations. IEEE Trans. Pattern Anal. Mach. Intell. **11**(6), 567–585 (1989)
11. Yee, T.W.: Quantile regression via vector generalized additive models. Stat. Med. **23**(14), 2295–2315 (2004)
12. Carpenter, J., Bithell, J.: Bootstrap confidence intervals: when, which, what? A practical guide for medical statisticians. Stat. Med. **19**(9), 1141–1164 (2000)
13. Glüer, C.C., Eastell, R., Reid, D.M., et al.: Association of five quantitative ultrasound devices and bone densitometry with osteoporotic vertebral fractures in a population-based sample: the OPUS Study. J. Bone Miner. Res. **19**(5), 782–93 (2004)

Unsupervised Learning for Fast Probabilistic Diffeomorphic Registration

Adrian V. Dalca[1,2,3]($\boxtimes$), Guha Balakrishnan[1], John Guttag[1], and Mert R. Sabuncu[3]

[1] Computer Science and Artificial Intelligence Lab, MIT, Cambridge, USA
adalca@mit.edu
[2] Martinos Center for Biomedical Imaging,
Massachusetts General Hospital, HMS, Charlestown, USA
[3] School of Electrical and Computer Engineering, Cornell University, Ithaca, USA

Abstract. Traditional deformable registration techniques achieve impressive results and offer a rigorous theoretical treatment, but are computationally intensive since they solve an optimization problem for each image pair. Recently, learning-based methods have facilitated fast registration by learning spatial deformation functions. However, these approaches use restricted deformation models, require supervised labels, or do not guarantee a diffeomorphic (topology-preserving) registration. Furthermore, learning-based registration tools have not been derived from a probabilistic framework that can offer uncertainty estimates. In this paper, we present a probabilistic generative model and derive an unsupervised learning-based inference algorithm that makes use of recent developments in convolutional neural networks (CNNs). We demonstrate our method on a 3D brain registration task, and provide an empirical analysis of the algorithm. Our approach results in state of the art accuracy and very fast runtimes, while providing diffeomorphic guarantees and uncertainty estimates. Our implementation is available online at http://voxelmorph.csail.mit.edu.

1 Introduction

Deformable registration computes a dense correspondence between two images, and is fundamental to many medical image analysis tasks. Traditional methods solve an optimization over the space of deformations, such as elastic-type models [4], B splines [25], dense vector fields [27], or discrete methods [8,12]. Constraining the allowable transformations to diffeomorphisms ensures certain desirable properties, such as preservation of topology. Diffeomorphic transforms have seen extensive methodological development, yielding state-of-the-art tools, such as LDDMM [6,29], DARTEL [2], and SyN [3]. However, these tools often demand substantial time and computational resources for a given image pair.

Recent methods have proposed to train neural networks that map a pair of input images to an output deformation. These approaches usually require ground truth registration fields, often derived via more conventional registration tools,

© Springer Nature Switzerland AG 2018
A. F. Frangi et al. (Eds.): MICCAI 2018, LNCS 11070, pp. 729–738, 2018.
https://doi.org/10.1007/978-3-030-00928-1_82

which can introduce a bias and necessitate significant preprocessing [23, 26, 28]. Some preliminary papers [9, 18] explore unsupervised strategies that build on the spatial transformer network [15], but are only demonstrated with constrained deformation models such as affine or small displacement fields. Furthermore, they have only been validated on limited volumes, such as 3D patches or 2D slices. A recent paper avoids these pitfalls, but still does not provide topology-preserving guarantees or probabilistic uncertainty estimates, which yield meaningful information for downstream image analysis [5].

In this paper we present a formulation for registration as conducting variational inference on a probabilistic generative model. This framework naturally results in a learning algorithm that uses a convolutional neural network with an intuitive cost function. We introduce novel *diffeomorphic integration* layers combined with a transform layer to enable unsupervised end-to-end learning for diffeomorphic registration. We present extensive experiments, demonstrating that our algorithm achieves state of the art registration accuracy while providing diffeomorphic deformations, fast runtime and estimates of registration uncertainty.

1.1 Diffeomorphic Registration

Although the method presented in this paper applies to a multitude of deformable representations, we choose to work with diffeomorphisms, and in particular with a stationary velocity field representation [2]. Diffeomorphic deformations are differentiable and invertible, and thus preserve topology. Let $\phi : R^3 \rightarrow R^3$ represent the deformation that maps the coordinates from one image to coordinates in another image. In our implementation, the deformation field is defined through the following ordinary differential equation (ODE):

$$\frac{\partial \phi^{(t)}}{\partial t} = v(\phi^{(t)}) \tag{1}$$

where $\phi^{(0)} = Id$ is the identity transformation and t is time. We integrate the stationary velocity field v over $t = [0, 1]$ to obtain the final registration field $\phi^{(1)}$.

We compute the integration numerically using *scaling and squaring* [1], which we briefly review here. The integration of a stationary ODE represents a one-parameter subgroup of diffeomorphisms. In group theory, v is a member of the Lie algebra and is exponentiated to produce $\phi^{(1)}$, which is a member of the Lie group: $\phi^{(1)} = \exp(v)$. From the properties of one-parameter subgroups, for any scalars t and t', $\exp((t+t')v) = \exp(tv) \circ \exp(t'v)$, where $\circ$ is a composition map associated with the Lie group. Starting from $\phi^{(1/2^T)} = p + v(p)/2^T$ where p is a map of spatial locations, we use the recurrence $\phi^{(1/2^{t-1})} = \phi^{(1/2^t)} \circ \phi^{(1/2^t)}$ to obtain $\phi^{(1)} = \phi^{(1/2)} \circ \phi^{(1/2)}$. T is chosen so that $v/2^T \approx 0$.

2   Methods

Let x and y be 3D images, such as MRI volumes, and let z be a latent variable that parametrizes a transformation function $\phi_z : R^3 \rightarrow R^3$. We use a generative model to describe the formation of x by warping y into $y \circ \phi_z$. We propose a variational inference method that uses a neural network of convolutions, diffeomorphic integration, and spatial transform layers. We learn the network parameters in an unsupervised fashion, i.e., without access to ground truth registrations. We describe how the network yields fast diffeomorphic registration of a new image pair x and y, while providing uncertainty estimates.

2.1 Generative Model

We model the prior probability of z as:

$$p(z) = \mathcal{N}(z; 0, \Sigma_z), \tag{2}$$

where $\mathcal{N}(\cdot; \mu, \Sigma)$ is the multivariate normal distribution with mean μ and covariance Σ. Our work applies to a wide range of representations z. For example, z could be a low-dimensional embedding of a dense displacement field, or even the displacement field itself. In this paper, we let z be a stationary velocity field that specifies a diffeomorphism through the ODE (1). We let $L = D - A$ be the Laplacian of a neighborhood graph defined on a voxel grid, where D is the graph degree matrix, and A is a voxel neighbourhood adjacency matrix. We encourage spatial smoothness of z by letting $\Sigma_z^{-1} = \Lambda_z = \lambda L$, where Λ_z is a precision matrix and λ denotes a parameter controlling the scale of the velocity field z.

We let x be a noisy observation of warped image y:

$$p(x|z; y) = \mathcal{N}(x; y \circ \phi_z, \sigma^2 \mathbb{I}), \tag{3}$$

where σ^2 reflects the variance of additive image noise.

We aim to estimate the posterior registration probability $p(z|x; y)$. Using this, we can obtain the most likely registration field ϕ_z for a new image pair (x, y) via MAP estimation, along with an estimate of uncertainty for this registration.

2.2 Learning

With our assumptions, computing the posterior probability $p(z|x; y)$ is intractable. We use a variational approach, and introduce an approximate posterior probability $q_\psi(z|x; y)$ parametrized by ψ. We minimize the KL divergence

$$
\begin{aligned}
\min_{\psi} &\, \mathrm{KL}\left[q_\psi(z|x; y) \| p(z|x; y)\right] \\
&= \min_{\psi} \mathrm{E}_q\left[\log q_\psi(z|x; y) - \log p(z|x; y)\right] \\
&= \min_{\psi} \mathrm{E}_q\left[\log q_\psi(z|x; y) - \log p(z, x, y)\right] + \log p(x; y) \\
&= \min_{\psi} \mathrm{KL}\left[q_\psi(z|x; y) \| p(z)\right] - \mathrm{E}_q\left[\log p(x|z; y)\right],
\end{aligned}
\tag{4}
$$

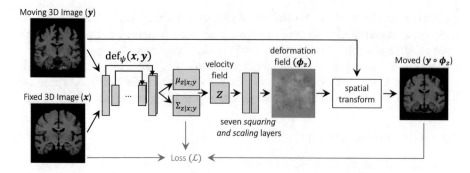

Fig. 1. Overview of end-to-end unsupervised architecture. The first part of the network, $\text{def}_\psi(\boldsymbol{x}, \boldsymbol{y})$ takes the input images and outputs the approximate posterior probability parameters representing the velocity field mean, $\boldsymbol{\mu}_{z|x;y}$, and variance, $\boldsymbol{\Sigma}_{z|x;y}$. A velocity field $\boldsymbol{z}$ is sampled and transformed to a diffeomorphic deformation field $\boldsymbol{\phi}_z$ using novel differentiable *squaring and scaling* layers. Finally, a spatial transform warps $\boldsymbol{y}$ to obtain $\boldsymbol{y} \circ \boldsymbol{\phi}_z$.

which is the negative of the *variational lower bound* of the model evidence [16]. We model the approximate posterior $q_\psi(\boldsymbol{z}|\boldsymbol{x}; \boldsymbol{y})$ as a multivariate normal:

$$q_\psi(\boldsymbol{z}|\boldsymbol{x}; \boldsymbol{y}) = \mathcal{N}(\boldsymbol{z}; \boldsymbol{\mu}_{z|x,y}, \boldsymbol{\Sigma}_{z|x,y}), \tag{5}$$

where $\boldsymbol{\Sigma}_{z|x,y}$ is diagonal.

We estimate $\boldsymbol{\mu}_{z|x,y}$, and $\boldsymbol{\Sigma}_{z|x,y}$ using a convolutional neural network $\text{def}_\psi(\boldsymbol{x}, \boldsymbol{y})$ parameterized by ψ, as described below. We can therefore learn the parameters ψ by optimizing the variational lower bound (4) using stochastic gradient methods. Specifically, for each image pair $\{\boldsymbol{x}, \boldsymbol{y}\}$ and samples $\boldsymbol{z}_k \sim q_\psi(\boldsymbol{z}|\boldsymbol{x}; \boldsymbol{y})$, we can compute $\boldsymbol{y} \circ \boldsymbol{\phi}_{z_k}$, with the resulting loss:

$$\mathcal{L}(\psi; \boldsymbol{x}, \boldsymbol{y}) = -\mathbb{E}_q\left[\log p(\boldsymbol{x}|\boldsymbol{z}; \boldsymbol{y})\right] + \text{KL}\left[q_\psi(\boldsymbol{z}|\boldsymbol{x}; \boldsymbol{y}) \| p(\boldsymbol{z})\right] \tag{6}$$

$$= \frac{1}{2\sigma^2 K}\sum_k \|\boldsymbol{x} - \boldsymbol{y} \circ \boldsymbol{\phi}_{z_k}\|^2 + \frac{1}{2}\left[\text{tr}(\lambda \boldsymbol{D}\, \boldsymbol{\Sigma}_{z|x;y} - \log|\boldsymbol{\Sigma}_{z|x;y}|) + \boldsymbol{\mu}_{z|x,y}^T \boldsymbol{\Lambda}_z \boldsymbol{\mu}_{z|x,y}\right] + \text{const},$$

where K is the number of samples used. In our experiments, we use $K = 1$. The first term encourages the warped image $\boldsymbol{y} \circ \boldsymbol{\phi}_{z_k}$ to be similar to $\boldsymbol{x}$. The second term encourages the posterior to be close to the prior $p(\boldsymbol{z})$. Although the variational covariance $\boldsymbol{\Sigma}_{z|x,y}$ is diagonal, the last term spatially smoothes the mean: $\boldsymbol{\mu}_{z|x,y}^T \boldsymbol{\Lambda}_z \boldsymbol{\mu}_{z|x,y} = \frac{\lambda}{2}\sum\sum_{j\in N(I)}(\boldsymbol{\mu}[i] - \boldsymbol{\mu}[j])^2$, where $N(i)$ are the neighbors of voxel i. We treat σ^2 and λ as fixed hyper-parameters.

2.3   Neural Network Framework

We design the network $\text{def}_\psi(\boldsymbol{x}, \boldsymbol{y})$ that takes as input $\boldsymbol{x}$ and $\boldsymbol{y}$ and outputs $\boldsymbol{\mu}_{z|x,y}$ and $\boldsymbol{\Sigma}_{z|x,y}$, based on a 3D UNet-style architecture [24]. The network includes a convolutional layer with 16 filters, four downsampling layers with 32 convolutional filters and a stride of two, and finally three upsampling convolutional layers with 32 filters. All convolutional layers use LeakyReLu activations and a 3×3 kernel.

To enable unsupervised learning of parameters ψ using (6), we must form $y \circ \phi_z$ to compute the data term. We first implement a layer that samples a new $z_k \sim \mathcal{N}(\mu_{z|x,y}, \Sigma_{z|x,y})$ using the "re-parameterization trick" [16].

We propose novel *scaling and squaring* network layers to compute $\phi_{z_k} = \exp(z_k)$. Specifically, these involve compositions within the neural network architecture using a differentiable spatial transformation operation. Given two 3D vector fields a and b, for each voxel p this layer computes $(a \circ b)(p) = a(b(p))$, a non-integer voxel location $b(p)$ in a, using linear interpolation. Starting with $\phi^{(1/2^T)} = p + z_k/2^T$, we compute $\phi^{(1/2^{t+1})} = \phi^{(1/2^t)} \circ \phi^{(1/2^t)}$ recursively using these layers, leading to $\phi^{(1)} \triangleq \phi_{z_k} = \exp(z_k)$. In our experiments, we use $T = 7$.

Finally, we use a spatial transform layer to warp volume y according to the computed diffeomorphic field ϕ_{z_k}. This network results in three outputs, $\mu_{z|x,y}, \Sigma_{z|x,y}$ and $y \circ \phi_{z_k}$, which are used in the model loss (6).

In summary, the neural network takes as input x and y, computes $\mu_{z|x,y}$ and $\Sigma_{z|x,y}$, samples a new $z_k \sim \mathcal{N}(\mu_k, \Sigma_k)$, computes a diffeomorphic ϕ_{z_k} and applies it to y. Since all the steps are designed to be differentiable, we learn the network parameters using stochastic gradient descent based methods on the loss (6). The framework is summarized in Fig. 1. We implement our method as part of the VoxelMorph package using Keras with a Tensorflow backend.

2.4   Registration and Uncertainty

Given learned parameters, we approximate registration of a new scan pair (x, y) using $\phi_{\hat{z}_k}$. We first obtain $\hat{z}_k$ using

$$\hat{z}_k = \arg \max_{z_k} p(z_k | x; y) = \mu_{z|x;y}, \tag{7}$$

by evaluating the neural network $\mathrm{def}_\psi(x, y)$ on the two input images. We then compute $\phi_{\hat{z}_k}$ using the *scaling and squaring* network layers. We also obtain $\Sigma_{z|x,y}$, enabling an estimation of the uncertainty of the velocity field z at each voxel j:

$$H(z[j]) \approx \mathbf{E}\left[-\log q_\psi(z|x,y)\right] = \frac{1}{2}\log 2\pi \Sigma_{z|x;y}[j,j]. \tag{8}$$

We also estimate uncertainty in the deformation field ϕ_z empirically. We sample several representations $z_{k'} \sim q_\psi(z|x;y)$, propagate them through the diffeomorphic layers to compute $\phi_{z'_k}$, and compute the empirical diagonal covariance $\hat{\Sigma}_{\phi_z}[j,j]$ across samples. The uncertainty is then $H(\phi[j]) \approx \frac{1}{2}\log 2\pi \hat{\Sigma}_{\phi_z}[j,j]$.

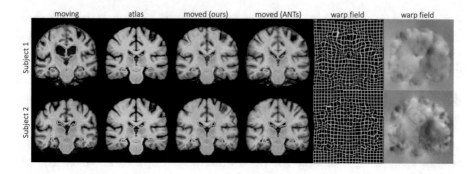

Fig. 2. Example MR slices of input moving image, atlas, and resulting warped image for our method and ANTs, with overlaid boundaries of ventricles, thalami and hippocampi. Our resulting registration field is shown as a warped grid and RGB image, with each channel representing dimension. Due to space constraints, we omit Voxel-Morph examples, which are *visually* similar to our results and ANTs.

3   Experiments

We focus on 3D atlas-based registration, a common task in population analysis. Specifically, we register each scan to an atlas computed using external data [11].

Data and Preprocessing. We use a large-scale, multi-site dataset of 7829 T1-weighted brain MRI scans from eight publicly available datasets: ADNI [22], OASIS [19], ABIDE [10], ADHD200 [21], MCIC [13], PPMI [20], HABS [7], and Harvard GSP [14]. Acquisition details, subject age ranges and health conditions are different for each dataset. We performed standard pre-processing steps on all scans, including resampling to 1mm isotropic voxels, affine spatial normalization and brain extraction for each scan using FreeSurfer [11]. We crop the final images to $160 \times 192 \times 224$. Segmentation maps including 29 anatomical structures, obtained using FreeSurfer for each scan, are used in evaluating registration results. We split the dataset into 7329, 250, and 250 volumes for train, validation, and test sets respectively, although we underscore that the training is unsupervised.

Evaluation Metric. To evaluate a registration algorithm, we register each subject to an atlas, propagate the segmentation map using the resulting warp, and measure volume overlap using the Dice metric. We also evaluate the diffeomorphic property, a focus of our model. Specifically, the Jacobian matrix $J_\phi(p) = \nabla\phi(p) \in \mathcal{R}^{3\times3}$ captures the local properties of ϕ around voxel p. The local deformation is diffeomorphic, both invertible and orientation-preserving, only at locations for which $|J_\phi(p)| > 0$ [2]. We count all other voxels, where $|J_\phi(p)| \leq 0$.

Baseline Methods. We compare our approach with the popular ANTs software package using Symmetric Normalization (SyN) [3], a top-performing algorithm [17]. We found that the default ANTs settings were sub-optimal for our task, so we performed a wide parameter and similarity metric search across a

Table 1. Summary of results: mean Dice scores over all anatomical structures and subjects (higher is better), mean runtime; and mean number of locations with a non-positive Jacobian of each registration field (lower is better). All methods have comparable Dice scores, while our method and the original VoxelMorph are orders of magnitude faster than ANTs. Only our method achieves both high accuracy and fast runtime while also having nearly zero non-negative Jacobian locations and providing uncertainty prediction.

Method	Avg. Dice	GPU sec	CPU sec	$|J_\Phi| \leq 0$	Uncertainty
Affine only	0.567 (0.157)	0	0	0	No
ANTs (SyN)	0.750 (0.135)	-	9059 (2023)	6505 (3024)	No
VoxelMorph	0.750 (0.137)	0.554 (0.017)	144 (1)	18096 (4230)	No
Ours	**0.753** (0.137)	**0.451** (0.011)	**51** (0.2)	**0.7** (2.0)	**Yes**

multitude of datasets. We identified top performing parameter values on the Dice metric and used cross-correlation as the ANTs similarity measure. We also test our recent CNN-based method, VoxelMorph, which aims to produce fast registration but does not yield diffeomorphic results or uncertainty estimates [5]. We sweep the regularization parameter using our validation set, and use the optimal parameters in our results.

Results on Test Set: Figure 2 shows representative results. Figure 3 illustrates Dice results on several anatomical structures, and Table 1 gives a summary of the results. Not only does our algorithm achieve state of the art Dice results and the fastest runtimes, but it also produces diffeomorphic registration fields (having nearly no non-negative Jacobian voxels per scan) and uncertainty estimates.

Specifically, all methods achieve comparable Dice results on each structure and overall. Our method and VoxelMorph require a fraction of the ANTs runtime to register two images: less than a second on a GPU, and less than a minute on a

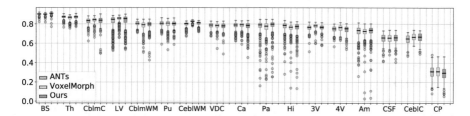

Fig. 3. Boxplots indicating Dice scores for anatomical structures for ANTs, Voxel-Morph, and our algorithm. Left and right hemisphere structures are merged for visualization, and ordered by average ANTs Dice score. We include the brain stem (BS), thalamus (Th), cerebellum cortex (CblmC), lateral ventricle (LV), cerebellum white matter (CblmWM), putamen (Pu), cerebral white matter (CeblWM), ventral DC (VDC), caudate (Ca), pallidum (Pa), hippocampus (Hi), 3rd ventricle (3V), 4th ventricle (4V), amygdala (Am), CSF (CSF), cerebral cortex (CeblC), and choroid plexus (CP).

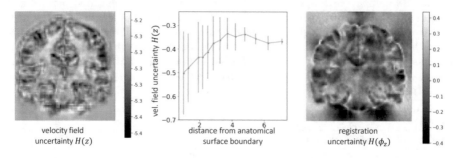

Fig. 4. Example velocity field uncertainty $H(z)$ (left) indicates low uncertainty near structure boundaries, as seen in the line graph (middle). This correlation is less obvious in the final registration field uncertainty $H(\phi_z)$ (right).

CPU (for our method). To the best of our knowledge, ANTs does not have a GPU implementation. Algorithm runtimes were computed for an NVIDIA TitanX GPU and a Intel Xeon (E5-2680) CPU, and exclude preprocessing common to all methods. Importantly, while our method achieves positive Jacobians at nearly all voxels, the flow fields resulting from the baseline methods contain a few thousand locations of non-positive Jacobians. This can be alleviated with increased spatial regularization, but this in turn leads to a drop in performance on the Dice metric.

Uncertainty. Figure 4 shows representative uncertainty maps, unique to our model. The velocity field is more certain near anatomical structure edges, and less confident in homogenous regions, such as the white matter or ventricle interior.

Parameter Analysis. We perform a grid search for the two fixed hyper-parameters λ and σ^2. We train a model for each parameter pair and evaluate Dice on the validation set. We search 30 values within two orders of magnitude around meaningful initial values for both parameters: $\sigma^2 \sim (0.07)^2$, the variance of the intensity difference between an *affinely* aligned image and the atlas, and $\lambda = 10000$, equivalent to a diagonal standard deviation of 1 voxel for ϕ_z. We found $\sigma^2 \sim (0.035)^2$ and $\lambda \in (20000, 100000)$ to perform well, and set $\lambda = 70,000$.

4   Conclusion

We propose a probabilistic model for diffeomorphic image registration and derive a learning algorithm that makes use of a convolutional neural network and an intuitive resulting loss function. To achieve unsupervised, end-to-end learning for diffeomorphic registrations, we introduce novel *scaling and squaring* differentiable layers. Our derivation is generalizable. For example, z can be a low dimensional embedding representation of a deformation field, or the displacement field itself. Our algorithm can infer the registration of new image pairs in under a second. Compared to traditional methods, our method is significantly faster, and compared to recent learning based methods, our method offers diffeomorphic guarantees, and provides natural uncertainty estimates for resulting registrations.

Acknowledgments. This research was funded by NIH grants R01LM012719, R01AG053949, and 1R21AG050122, and NSF NeuroNex Grant grant 1707312.

References

1. Arsigny, V., Commowick, O., Pennec, X., Ayache, N.: A log-euclidean framework for statistics on diffeomorphisms. In: Larsen, R., Nielsen, M., Sporring, J. (eds.) MICCAI 2006. LNCS, vol. 4190, pp. 924–931. Springer, Heidelberg (2006). https://doi.org/10.1007/11866565_113
2. Ashburner, J., et al.: A fast diffeomorphic image registration algorithm. Neuroimage **38**(1), 95–113 (2007)
3. Avants, B.B., et al.: Symmetric diffeomorphic image registration with cross-correlation: evaluating automated labeling of elderly and neurodegenerative brain. Med. Image Anal. **12**(1), 26–41 (2008)
4. Bajcsy, R., Kovacic, S.: Multiresolution elastic matching. Comput. Vis. Graph. Image Process. **46**, 1–21 (1989)
5. Balakrishnan, G., et al.: An unsupervised learning model for deformable medical image registration. arXiv:1802.02604 (2018)
6. Beg, M.F., et al.: Computing large deformation metric mappings via geodesic flows of diffeomorphisms. Int. J. Comput. Vis. **61**, 139–157 (2005)
7. Dagley, A., et al.: Harvard aging brain study: dataset and accessibility. NeuroImage **144**, 255–258 (2015)
8. Dalca, A.V., Bobu, A., Rost, N.S., Golland, P.: Patch-based discrete registration of clinical brain images. In: Wu, G., et al. (eds.) Patch-MI 2016. LNCS, vol. 9993, pp. 60–67. Springer, Cham (2016). https://doi.org/10.1007/978-3-319-47118-1_8
9. de Vos, B.D., et al.: End-to-end unsupervised deformable image registration with a convolutional neural network. In: DLMIA, pp. 204–212 (2017)
10. Di Martino, A., et al.: The autism brain imaging data exchange: towards a large-scale evaluation of the intrinsic brain architecture in autism. Mol. Psychiatry **19**(6), 659–667 (2014)
11. Fischl, B.: Freesurfer. Neuroimage **62**(2), 774–781 (2012)
12. Glocker, B., et al.: Dense image registration through MRFs and efficient linear programming. Med. Image Anal. **12**(6), 731–741 (2008)
13. Gollub, R.L., et al.: The mcic collection: a shared repository of multi-modal, multi-site brain image data from a clinical investigation of schizophrenia. Neuroinformatics **11**(3), 367–388 (2013)
14. Holmes, A.J., et al.: Brain genomics superstruct project initial data release with structural, functional, and behavioral measures. Sci. Data 2 (2015)
15. Jaderberg, M., et al.: Spatial transformer networks. In: NIPS, pp. 2017–2025 (2015)
16. Kingma, D.P., Welling, M.: Auto-encoding variational bayes. In: ICLR (2014)
17. Klein, A., et al.: Evaluation of 14 nonlinear deformation algorithms applied to human brain MRI registration. Neuroimage **46**(3), 786–802 (2009)
18. Li, H., Fan, H.: Non-rigid image registration using fully convolutional networks with deep self-supervision. arXiv preprint arXiv:1709.00799 (2017)

19. Marcus, D.S., et al.: Open access series of imaging studies (oasis): cross-sectional mri data in young, middle aged, nondemented, and demented older adults. J. Cogn. Neurosci. **19**(9), 1498–1507 (2007)
20. Marek, K., et al.: The parkinson progression marker initiative (PPMI). Prog. Neurobiol. **95**(4), 629–635 (2011)
21. Milham, M.P., et al.: The adhd-200 consortium: a model to advance the translational potential of neuroimaging in clinical neuroscience. Front. Sys. Neurosci. **6**, 62 (2012)
22. Mueller, S.G., et al.: Ways toward an early diagnosis in Alzheimer's disease: the Alzheimer's Disease Neuroimaging Initiative (ADNI). Alzheimer's Dement. **1**(1), 55–66 (2005)
23. Rohé, M.-M., Datar, M., Heimann, T., Sermesant, M., Pennec, X.: SVF-Net: learning deformable image registration using shape matching. In: Descoteaux, M., et al. (eds.) MICCAI 2017. LNCS, vol. 10433, pp. 266–274. Springer, Cham (2017). https://doi.org/10.1007/978-3-319-66182-7_31
24. Ronneberger, O., Fischer, P., Brox, T.: U-Net: convolutional networks for biomedical image segmentation. In: Navab, N., Hornegger, J., Wells, W.M., Frangi, A.F. (eds.) MICCAI 2015. LNCS, vol. 9351, pp. 234–241. Springer, Cham (2015). https://doi.org/10.1007/978-3-319-24574-4_28
25. Rueckert, D., et al.: Nonrigid registration using free-form deformation: application to breast MR images. IEEE Trans. Med. Imaging **18**(8), 712–721 (1999)
26. Sokooti, H., et al.: Nonrigid image registration using multi-scale 3D convolutional neural networks. In: Descoteaux, M., et al. (eds.) MICCAI 2017. LNCS, vol. 10433, pp. 232–239. Springer, Cham (2017). https://doi.org/10.1007/978-3-319-66182-7_27
27. Thirion, J.P.: Image matching as a diffusion process: an analogy with maxwell's demons. Med. Image Anal. **2**(3), 243–260 (1998)
28. Yang, X., et al.: Quicksilver: Fast predictive image registration-a deep learning approach. NeuroImage **158**, 378–396 (2017)
29. Zhang, M., et al.: Frequency diffeomorphisms for efficient image registration. In: Niethammer, M., et al. (eds.) IPMI 2017. LNCS, vol. 10265, pp. 559–570. Springer, Cham (2017). https://doi.org/10.1007/978-3-319-59050-9_44

Adversarial Similarity Network for Evaluating Image Alignment in Deep Learning Based Registration

Jingfan Fan[1], Xiaohuan Cao[1,2], Zhong Xue[3], Pew-Thian Yap[1],
and Dinggang Shen[1(✉)]

[1] Department of Radiology and BRIC, University of North Carolina
at Chapel Hill, Chapel Hill, NC, USA
dgshen@med.unc.edu
[2] School of Automation, Northwestern Polytechnical University, Xi'an, China
[3] Shanghai United Imaging Intelligence Co., Ltd., Shanghai, China

Abstract. This paper introduces an unsupervised adversarial similarity network for image registration. Unlike existing deep learning registration frameworks, our approach does not require ground-truth deformations and specific similarity metrics. We connect a registration network and a discrimination network with a deformable transformation layer. The registration network is trained with feedback from the discrimination network, which is designed to judge whether a pair of registered images are sufficiently similar. Using adversarial training, the registration network is trained to predict deformations that are accurate enough to fool the discrimination network. Experiments on four brain MRI datasets indicate that our method yields registration performance that is promising in both accuracy and efficiency compared with state-of-the-art registration methods, including those based on deep learning.

1 Introduction

Deformable registration establishes anatomical correspondences between a pair of images. Traditional registration methods seek to estimate smooth deformation fields based on intensity-based similarity metrics. However, these methods often involve computationally expensive high-dimensional optimization and task-dependent parameter tuning. Deep learning methods, such as convolutional neural networks (CNN), have been shown recently to be capable of addressing the limitations of conventional registration methods.

In *supervised learning* methods, the registration network is trained with ground-truth deformations. Sokooti et al. [1] proposed RegNet to estimate the displacement vector field for a pair of chest CT images. Yang et al. [2] predicted the momenta in LDDMM. Rohe et al. [3] built reference deformations for training by registering manually delineated regions of interests (ROIs). While effective, these methods are however limited by the availability of ground-truth deformations.

In *unsupervised learning* methods [4, 5], the deformable transformations are learned without ground-truth deformations by maximizing the similarity between a pair

© Springer Nature Switzerland AG 2018
A. F. Frangi et al. (Eds.): MICCAI 2018, LNCS 11070, pp. 739–746, 2018.
https://doi.org/10.1007/978-3-030-00928-1_83

of images, such as the sum of squared difference (SSD) and cross-correlation (CC). However, these similarity metrics are closely related to the nature of the images and might not be suitable when dealing with diverse datasets.

In this paper, we propose an *adversarial similarity network* to automatically learn the similarity metric for training a deformable registration network. The network is unsupervised and is inspired by generative adversarial network (GAN) [6]. More specifically, the generator is a *registration network* that predicts the deformations. The discriminator is a *discrimination network* that judges whether images are well aligned and feeds misalignment information to the registration network during training. The registration and discrimination networks are learned via *adversarial training,* learning a metric for accurate registration. The main contributions of this work are summarized as follows:

- Compared with the traditional registration methods, a robust and fast end-to-end registration network is developed for predicting the deformation in one-pass, without the need for parameter tuning.
- Compared with supervised learning registration methods, the proposed network does not need ground-truth deformations. The network is trained in an adversarial and unsupervised manner.
- The proposed *adversarial similarity network* learns a meaningful metric for effective training of the registration network.

2   Method

Image registration aims to determine a deformation field ϕ that warps a subject image $S \in \mathbb{R}^3$ to a template image $T \in \mathbb{R}^3$, so that the warped image $S \circ \phi$ is similar to T. Deformation ϕ is typically determined by minimizing energy functional

$$\phi = \underset{\phi}{argmin} \, M(S \circ \phi, T) + Reg(\phi), \tag{1}$$

where $M(S \circ \phi, T)$ quantifies the dissimilarity between the template image T and the warped subject image $S \circ \phi$. $Reg(\phi)$ is the regularization to preserve the smoothness of the deformation field ϕ.

In this paper, we design a *registration network* R, to learn the deformation field ϕ for subject and template images (S, T). The mapping can be written as $R : (S, T) \Rightarrow \phi$. **First**, the *registration network* R is trained under the guidance of image similarity, therefore no ground-truth deformation field is needed. Instead of specifying a similarity metric, the similarity guidance is derived from the *discrimination network* D, which can automatically judge whether the two images are well aligned with probability $p \in [0, 1]$. The *registration network* R is trained to register the images as accurate as possible to convince the *discrimination network* D. **Second**, in order to preserve the smoothness of the predicted deformation field ϕ, a regularization is incorporated in the training of the *registration network* R.

As shown in Fig. 1, a deformable transformation layer connects the output of the *registration network R* (i.e., the deformation field ϕ) and input of the *discrimination network D* (i.e., a pair of registered images). The input of R is $64 \times 64 \times 64$ image patches and the output is the corresponding deformation field of size $24 \times 24 \times 24$. Here, the output size is smaller than the input, in order to adapt to the displacement range in the deformable deformation. In testing stage, the deformation field is predicted by the trained R.

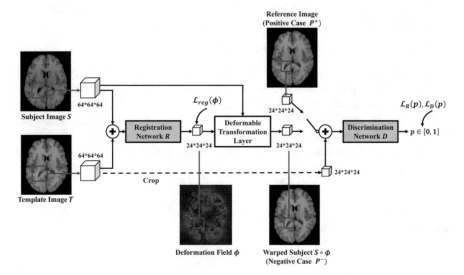

Fig. 1. The proposed adversarial similarity network for deformable image registration. The input image pair is already linearly aligned.

2.1 Adversarial Training

The adversarial training strategy, described below, is used to train *registration network R* and the *discrimination network D* is inspired by GAN [6].

(1) Training the *discrimination network D*.

The discrimination network D aims to determine whether the input image pair is similar (i.e., well registered). Two cases are fed into the network alternatively: (1) the *positive* case (P^+) where the images are well registered, and (2) the *negative* case (P^-) where the images are not well registered. The loss function of D can be defined as

$$\mathcal{L}_D(p) = \begin{cases} \log(1-p), & p \in P^+ \\ \log(p), & p \in P^- \end{cases}. \tag{2}$$

where, p is the output of the *discrimination network D* that indicates the similarity probability. During training, the *positive* case is derived from the predefined aligned images and the output of D is expected to be 1, indicating the image pair is similar. The *negative* case is derived from the registration network R, which means the image pairs are under registration and currently not well registered. Thus the output of D is expected to yield 0, indicating the image pair is dissimilar. The discrimination network can be optimized by minimizing the loss function in Eq. (2).

The ideal *positive* case is when the two images are exactly same. However, this cannot happen in real-world registration tasks. We therefore add some disturbance in the positive image pair. Specifically, for each image pair, the template image T is fixed. The perturbed subject image is created from the original subject image S as $\alpha \cdot S + (1 - \alpha) \cdot T$ with $0 < \alpha < 1$. We set $\alpha = 0.2$ in the initial training stage to weaken the similarity requirement and $\alpha = 0.1$ in later stage for greater accuracy.

(2) **Training the registration network R.**

The registration network R is supervised by the image similarity based on the discrimination network D. As mentioned, the image pair that registered by the registration network R is regarded as the negative case (P^-.) for the discrimination network D. However, the registration network aims to make the registered images as similar as possible, i.e., the output similarity probability p of discrimination network D should approximate to 1. Therefore, the loss function of registration network R can be defined as

$$\mathcal{L}_R(p) = \log(1 - p), p \in P^-. \tag{3}$$

In addition to the similarity guidance, the smoothness of the predicted deformation field ϕ is also enforced with loss

$$\mathcal{L}_{reg}(\phi) = \sum_{v \in \mathbb{R}^3} \nabla \phi(v)^2, \tag{4}$$

where v represents the voxel location. By jointly considering Eqs. (3) and (4), the total loss function for the registration network R is:

$$\mathcal{L} = \mathcal{L}_R(p) + \lambda \mathcal{L}_{reg}(\phi), \tag{5}$$

where λ is the weight of the smoothness term, which we set it to 1.

The overall network is trained by alternating between optimizing the registration network R and the discrimination network D. Convergence occurs when the discrimination network cannot distinguish the *positive* cases and the *negative* cases.

2.2 Network Details

Registration Network R. The registration network follows the same architecture in [7], which is a hierarchical U-Net regression model [8]. The network takes 3D patches from the subject and template images as input and produces the deformation fields associated with the patches as output.

Discrimination Network D. The network architecture of D is shown in Fig. 2. Basically, the input is the image pair and the output is the similarity probability $p \in [0, 1]$, with 1 indicating similarity and 0 indicating dissimilarity. Each convolution layer is followed by ReLU activations, and 0-padding is applied in each convolution layer. The fully connected (FC) layer is used to gather information from the entire image into one value.

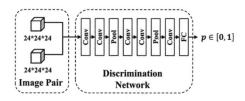

Fig. 2. The discrimination network.

Deformable Transformation Layer. A deformable transformation layer is used to warp the subject image using the deformation field ϕ. Each voxel in the warped subject image is calculated by interpolating in the corresponding location, as given by the displacement vector, in the subject image. The gradient is back propagated from the discrimination network D to train the registration network R.

Implementation Details. The network is implemented using 3D Caffe using Adam optimization. The learning rate is initially set to 1e–3, with 0.5 weight decay after every 50 K iterations. During testing, the registration network is used without the discrimination network to predict the deformation field.

3   Experiments and Results

In this section, we compare the proposed method with different training strategies and several state-of-the-art deformable registration algorithms. Four public datasets [9], including LPBA40, IBSR18, CUMC12, and MGH10, are used to validate the proposed method. After affine registration, all the images are resampled to the same size $(220 \times 220 \times 184)$ and resolution $(1 \times 1 \times 1 \text{ mm}^3)$. Two state-of-the-art registration methods, i.e., diffeomorphic demons (D. Demons) [10] and SyN [11], are used as the comparison methods. We also compare our method with other deep learning registration strategies, including (1) supervised training (i.e., ground-truth deformations obtained by SyN), (2) unsupervised training with similarity metrics SSD [4] and CC [5].

The training images are derived from LPBA40. Among the 40 subjects, 30 images are selected as the training data, in which 30×29 image pairs can be drawn. The remaining 10 images are used as the testing data. Specifically, 300 patch pairs are extracted from each training image pair, giving a total of 26,000 training samples.

3.1   Evaluation on LPBA40

For the 10 testing subjects in the LPBA40 dataset, we perform deformable registration on each image pair. The Dice Similarity Coefficient (DSC) of 54 brain ROIs (names

defined in [9]) is shown in Fig. 3. The proposed algorithm achieves the best performance for 42 out of the 54 ROIs, while the performance of the remaining 12 ROIs are
comparable, compared with other deep learning registration algorithms. The average
DSC value in Table 1 also shows the best accuracy of the proposed method, which
indicates that, the proposed adversarial similarity guidance is effective to train an
accurate registration network in an unsupervised manner.

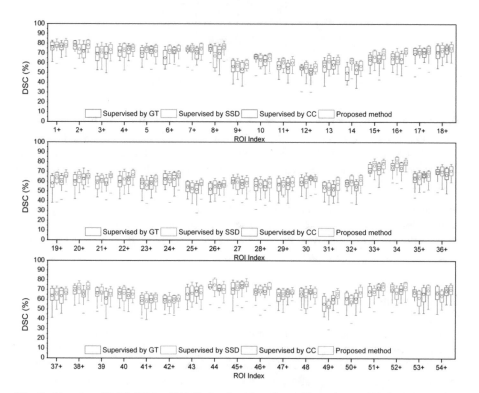

Fig. 3. Boxplot of DSC (%) in 54 ROIs for the 10 testing subjects from LPBA40 dataset, after
performing registration under different training strategies: (1) supervised learning, (2) similarity
metrics SSD and CC, and (3) the proposed adversarial similarity network. " + " marks
improvements given by the proposed method over the three other methods.

3.2   Evaluation on IBSR18, CUMC12, MGH10

To further evaluate generalizability of the proposed method, we apply the network
trained on LPBA40 dataset on a total of 40 brain images from three different datasets
(i.e., IBSR18, CUMC12, and MGH10). We register each image pair in the same
dataset. Figure 4 shows a typical set of results from MGH10. The results for Diffeomorphic Demons and SyN are obtained via careful parameter tuning.

Table 1 provides the DSC for all methods. The average DSC is calculated based on
all the ROIs for each individual dataset. The results indicate that, when applied directly

Table 1. Mean DSC (%) on LPBA40, IBSR18, CUMC12, and MGH10 datasets.

Dataset	D.Demons	SyN	Supervised by GT	Supervised by SSD	Supervised by CC	Proposed method
LPBA40	68.7 ± 2.4	71.3 ± 1.8	70.7 ± 2.3	70.4 ± 2.2	71.2 ± 2.8	$\mathbf{71.8 \pm 2.3}$
IBSR18	54.6 ± 2.2	57.4 ± 2.4	52.4 ± 3.1	53.1 ± 1.8	54.2 ± 3.4	$\mathbf{57.8 \pm 2.7}$
CUMC12	53.1 ± 3.4	54.1 ± 2.8	52.7 ± 3.1	51.6 ± 2.3	51.8 ± 4.1	$\mathbf{54.4 \pm 2.9}$
MGH10	60.4 ± 2.5	$\mathbf{62.4 \pm 2.4}$	59.7 ± 2.5	58.2 ± 1.6	59.6 ± 2.9	61.7 ± 2.1

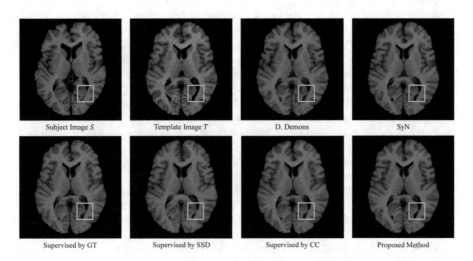

Fig. 4. Typical registration results from MGH10. The boxes mark significant improvements.

to unseen datasets, other learning strategies do not work well. Our method gives the best overall performance. Compared with the fine-tuned Diffeomorphic Demons and SyN, the proposed method exhibit better performance.

The proposed algorithm is implemented based on a single Nvidia TitanX (Pascal) GPU. The average computation time for registering a pair of 3D brain images ($220 \times 220 \times 184$) is 18.3 s, which is considered efficient for deformable registration.

4 Conclusions

In this paper, an adversarial training strategy is designed for unsupervised registration. Our network does not need ground-truth deformations or predefined similarity metrics. Instead, the similarity metric is learned automatically based on the discrimination network. The experimental results indicate that the proposed method exhibits higher registration accuracy compared with state-of-the-art registration methods.

Acknowledgment. This work was supported in part by NIH grants (EB006733, EB008374, MH100217, AG041721, AG053867).

References

1. Sokooti, H., de Vos, B., Berendsen, F., Lelieveldt, B.P.F., Išgum, I., Staring, M.: Nonrigid image registration using multi-scale 3D convolutional neural networks. In: Descoteaux, M., Maier-Hein, L., Franz, A., Jannin, P., Collins, D.L., Duchesne, S. (eds.) MICCAI 2017. LNCS, vol. 10433, pp. 232–239. Springer, Cham (2017). https://doi.org/10.1007/978-3-319-66182-7_27

2. Yang, X., et al.: Quicksilver fast predictive image registration–a deep learning approach. NeuroImage **158**, 378–396 (2017)

3. Rohé, M.-M., Datar, M., Heimann, T., Sermesant, M., Pennec, X.: SVF-Net: learning deformable image registration using shape matching. In: Descoteaux, M., Maier-Hein, L., Franz, A., Jannin, P., Collins, D.L., Duchesne, S. (eds.) MICCAI 2017. LNCS, vol. 10433, pp. 266–274. Springer, Cham (2017). https://doi.org/10.1007/978-3-319-66182-7_31

4. Li, H., Fan, Y.: Non-Rigid Image Registration Using Self-Supervised Fully Convolutional Networks without Training Data. arXiv preprint arXiv:1801.04012 (2018)

5. Balakrishnan, G., et al.: An Unsupervised Learning Model for Deformable Medical Image Registration. arXiv preprint arXiv:1802.02604 (2018)

6. Goodfellow, I., et al.: Generative adversarial nets. In: Advances in Neural Information Processing Systems (2014)

7. Fan, J., et al.: BIRNet: Brain Image Registration Using Dual-Supervised Fully Convolutional Networks. arXiv preprint arXiv:1802.04692 (2018)

8. Ronneberger, O., Fischer, P., Brox, T.: U-Net: convolutional networks for biomedical image segmentation. In: Navab, N., Hornegger, J., Wells, W.M., Frangi, A.F. (eds.) MICCAI 2015. LNCS, vol. 9351, pp. 234–241. Springer, Cham (2015). https://doi.org/10.1007/978-3-319-24574-4_28

9. Klein, A., et al.: Evaluation of 14 nonlinear deformation algorithms applied to human brain MRI registration. Neuroimage **46**(3), 786–802 (2009)

10. Vercauteren, T., et al.: Diffeomorphic demons: efficient non-parametric image registration. NeuroImage **45**(1), S61–S72 (2009)

11. Avants, B.B., et al.: Symmetric diffeomorphic image registration with cross-correlation. Med. Image Anal. **12**(1), 26–41 (2008)

Improving Surgical Training Phantoms by Hyperrealism: Deep Unpaired Image-to-Image Translation from Real Surgeries

Sandy Engelhardt[1,3]($\boxtimes$) (iD), Raffaele De Simone[2], Peter M. Full[2], Matthias Karck[2], and Ivo Wolf[3]

[1] Department of Simulation and Graphics & Research Campus STIMULATE, Magdeburg University, Magdeburg, Germany
s.engelhardt@hs-mannheim.de
[2] Department of Cardiac Surgery, Heidelberg University Hospital, Heidelberg, Germany
[3] Faculty of Computer Science, Mannheim University of Applied Sciences, Mannheim, Germany

Abstract. Current 'dry lab' surgical phantom simulators are a valuable tool for surgeons which allows them to improve their dexterity and skill with surgical instruments. These phantoms mimic the haptic and shape of organs of interest, but lack a realistic visual appearance. In this work, we present an innovative application in which representations learned from real intraoperative endoscopic sequences are transferred to a surgical phantom scenario. The term *hyperrealism* is introduced in this field, which we regard as a novel subform of surgical augmented reality for approaches that involve real-time object transfigurations. For related tasks in the computer vision community, unpaired cycle-consistent Generative Adversarial Networks (GANs) have shown excellent results on still RGB images. Though, application of this approach to continuous video frames can result in flickering, which turned out to be especially prominent for this application. Therefore, we propose an extension of cycle-consistent GANs, named *tempCycleGAN*, to improve temporal consistency. The novel method is evaluated on captures of a silicone phantom for training endoscopic reconstructive mitral valve procedures. Synthesized videos show highly realistic results with regard to (1) replacement of the silicone appearance of the phantom valve by intraoperative tissue texture, while (2) explicitly keeping crucial features in the scene, such as instruments, sutures and prostheses. Compared to the original Cycle-GAN approach, *tempCycleGAN* efficiently removes flickering between frames. The overall approach is expected to change the future design of surgical training simulators since the generated sequences clearly demonstrate the feasibility to enable a considerably more realistic training experience for minimally-invasive procedures.

© Springer Nature Switzerland AG 2018
A. F. Frangi et al. (Eds.): MICCAI 2018, LNCS 11070, pp. 747–755, 2018.
https://doi.org/10.1007/978-3-030-00928-1_84

Keywords: Generative Adversarial Networks
Minimally-invasive surgical training · Augmented reality
Mitral valve simulator · Surgical skill

1   Introduction

Surgery is a discipline that requires years of training to gain the necessary experience, skill and dexterity. With increasingly minimally invasive procedures, in which the surgeon's vision often solely relies on endoscopy, this is even more challenging. Due to the lack of appropriately realistic and elaborate endoscopic training methods, surgeons are forced to develop most of their skills in patients, which is truly undesirable. Current training methods rely on practising suturing techniques on *ex-vivo* organs ('wet labs'), virtual simulators or physical phantoms under laboratory conditions ('dry labs'). Training on authentic tissue is associated with organizational efforts and costs and is usually not accessible to the majority of the trainees. Virtual simulators overcome these requirements, but are often less realistic due to the lack of blood, smoke, lens contamination and patient-specificity. Physical phantoms, e.g. made from silicone, suffer also from these drawbacks, but they provide excellent haptic feedback and tissue properties for stitching with authentic instruments and suture material [1,2]. However, their uniform appearance does not reflect the complex environment of a surgical scene. We tackle this issue by proposing a system that is able to map patterns learned from intraoperative video sequences onto the video stream captured during training with silicone models to mimic the intraoperative domain. Our vision for a novel training simulator is to display real-time synthesized images to the trainee surgeon while he/she is operating on a phantom under restricted direct vision, such as illustrated in Fig. 1a.

Generative Adversarial Networks (GANs) demonstrate tremendous progress in the field of image-to-image translation with regard to both perceptual realism and diversity. Recently, methods have been proposed using Convolutional Neural Networks (CNNs) for deep image synthesis with paired [3] and even unpaired natural images, namely DualGAN [4] and CycleGAN [5]. These networks translate an image from one domain X to another target domain Y. The key to the success of GANs is the idea of an adversarial loss that forces the generated images to be, in principle, indistinguishable from real images, which is particularly powerful for image generation tasks. However, current solutions do not take time consistency of a video stream into account. While each frame of a generated video looks quite realistic on its own, the whole sequence lacks consistency.

In order to increase realism for endoscopic surgical training on physical phantoms, we propose the concept of *hyperrealism*.[1] We define hyperrealism as a new paradigm on the Reality-Virtuality continuum [6] as a concept closer to 'full reality' in comparison to other applications where artificial overlays are super-

---

[1] The term is related to the homonymous art form, where an excessive use of details is used to create an exaggeration of reality which cannot be seen by the human eye.

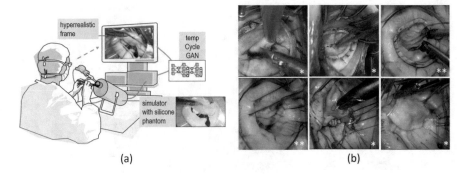

(a)   (b)

Fig. 1. (a) Vision: Augmentation of the minimally invasive training process with real-time generated *hyperrealistic* frames. (b) Visual comparison of real intraoperative frames from mitral valve surgery (*) and generated fake images (**).

imposed on a video frame. In a hyperrealistic environment, those parts of the physical phantom that look unnatural are replaced by realistic appearances.

The extended CycleGAN network, named *tempCycleGAN*, learns to translate an image stream from the source domain of *phantom data* to a target domain *intraoperative surgeries* and vice versa in the absence of paired endoscopic examples. The network's main task is to capture specific characteristics of one image set and to figure out how these characteristics could be translated into the other image domain. We evaluate the approach for the specific application of training mitral valve repair, where the network has to learn (1) how to enhance the silicon's surface appearance, at the same time not altering its shape, (2) not to replace other important features in the scene, such as surgical instruments, sutures, needles and prostheses.

2   Methods

We build upon the CycleGAN model proposed by Zhu et al. [5]. The goal of CycleGANs is to obtain mapping functions between two domains X and Y given unpaired training samples, $\{x_i | i = 1..N\} \in X$ and $\{y_j | j = 1..M\} \in Y$. Mappings in both directions are learned by two generator networks, $G : X \rightarrow Y$ and $F : Y \rightarrow X$. The generators are trained to produce output that cannot be distinguished from real images of the target domain by adversarially trained discriminators D_Y and D_X.

2.1   Temporal Cycle GAN

Temporal consistency requires to include preceding time steps into the learning process. The proposed advancement tempCycleGAN processes the current time step x_t and its two predecessors x_{t-1} and x_{t-2}, as shown in Fig. 2. In general,

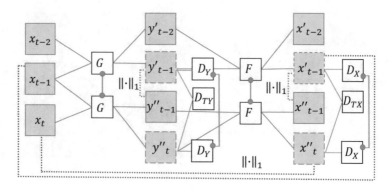

Fig. 2. Training setup of the $X \to Y \to X$ cycle of the proposed tempCycleGAN network (reverse cycle accordingly) using temporal pairs: the generators G, F and the temporal discriminators $D_{T\{X,Y\}}$ take the current frame and a single preceding frame. Each run of G (and F) synthesizes outputs for both frames. In the application of the generator, the frame of interest is the second output (y'_{t-1} and y''_t, respectively). The temporal discriminators are trained on these frames of interest, thus, the generator G needs to run twice to generate the two frames of interest (y'_{t-1} and y''_t) for D_{TY} (for F and D_{TX} accordingly). L1-distances (dotted lines) between matching time frames are used in the loss function to further enforce time consistency. $D_{\{X,Y\}}$: discriminators with 1 input; blue connections: shared weights.

it is possible to use more preceding frames and to adjust the network architecture accordingly. In the following, the general concepts of tempCycleGAN are explained and a detailed description of the setup is provided subsequently.

Temporal discriminators D_{TX} and D_{TY} (one for each domain) are introduced that take consecutive frames and try, as usual, to distinguish real from generated data. The idea is that flickering would allow the discriminators to easily identify generated data. Thus, the generators are forced to avoid flickering to successfully cheat their adversarial temporal discriminators. The generators need at least one preceding frame as additional input to be able to create a temporal consistent output for the current frame. In the current setup two frames are used as input for both the generators and the temporal discriminators.

To define a cycle consistency loss that is symmetric in G and F, we let the generators G and F create as many output frames as they get input frames. For example, $G(x_{t-1}, x_t)$ creates outputs y''_{t-1} and y''_t. Only the output for the latest frame (y''_t in the example) is the frame of interest used in the actual output video. Consecutive frames of interest (shown as dashed boxes in Fig. 2) are evaluated by the temporal discriminators. Thus, the temporal discriminators are provided with inputs of multiple runs of the generator. For example, D_{TY} takes y'_{t-1} and y''_t as input, where y'_{t-1} is the frame of interest of $G(x_{t-2}, x_{t-1})$ and y''_t is the frame of interest of $G(x_{t-1}, x_t)$. To enforce consistency between frames of matching time and domain, L1 distances to the respective frames are used as additional terms in the loss function.

2.2   Network Architectures

The network architectures of the generators and discriminators are largely the same as in the original CycleGAN approach [5]. A TensorFlow implementation provided on GitHub[2] was used as the basis and extended with the new temp-CycleGAN blocks. All discriminators take the complete input images, which is different from the 70×70 PatchGAN approach by Zhu et al. [5]. The temporal discriminators have 6 ($2\times$RGB) instead of 3 input channels. For the generators, 8 instead of 9 residual blocks are used, because experiments on our data showed better results for this configuration.

3   Experiments

The commercial minimally invasive mitral valve simulator (MICS MVR surgical simulator, Fehling Instruments GmbH & Co. KG, Karlstein, Germany) was extended with patient-specific silicone valves. Details on 3D-printed mold and valve production are elaborated on in a previous work [2]. An expert segmented mitral valves with different pathologies, such as posterior prolaps and ischemic valves on the end-systolic time step from echocardiographic data. From these virtual models, 3D printable molds and suitable annuloplasty rings were automatically generated with stitching holes using 3 different low to medium cost 3D-printers, varying material (polylactide, acrylonitrile butadiene styrene) in various colors (e.g. white, beige, red, orange). From these molds, 10 silicone valves were cast that could be anchored in the simulator on a printed valve holder. We asked an expert and a trainee to apply mitral valve repair techniques (annuloplasty, triangular leaflet resection, neo-chordae implantation) on these valves and captured the training process endoscopically.

3.1   Data and Training of Network

In total, approx. 330,000 video frames from the training procedures in full HD resolution were captured. Valves shown in videos for training were not used for testing. For training, three continuous frames after each 120th frame from a subset of approx. 160,000 frames was sampled retrospectively, such that the set comprised 1300 small sequences. Furthermore, training material for the target domain from 3 endoscopic mitral valve repair surgeries was captured. In total, approx. 320,000 frames were acquired during real surgery. For training, three continuous frames after each 240th frame were sampled retrospectively and 1294 small sequences were used for training. All streams were captured with 30fps. The scenes are highly diverse, as the valve's appearance drastically changes over time (e.g. due to cutting of tissue, implanting sutures and prostheses, fluids such as blood and saline solution), see Fig. 1b. All frames were square-cropped and re-scaled to 286×286. Data augmentation was performed by random cropping of a 256×256 region and random horizontal flipping. For all the experiments,

---

[2] https://github.com/LynnHo/CycleGAN-Tensorflow-PyTorch-Simple.

the consistency loss was weighted with $\lambda = 10$ [5]. The Adam solver with a batch size of 1 and a learning rate of 0.0001 without linear decay to zero was used. Similar to Zhu et al. [5], the objective was divided by 2 while optimizing D, which slows down the rate at which D learns relative to G. Discriminators are updated using a history of 50 generated images rather than the ones produced by the latest generative networks [5]. The tempCycleGAN network was trained for 40, 60, 80, 100 epochs to find the visually most attractive results. In analogy, the original CycleGAN networks was trained either with 1 input frame or 3 continuous frames.

3.2   Evaluation

The most important factors for the proposed application are related to perception i.e. how real the generated intraoperative videos appear to an expert with years of experience in mitral valve surgery. Furthermore, reliability plays a crucial role, as the appearance of the scene should be transferred into the target domain, while neither the shape of objects should be altered, nor additional parts should be added or taken away.

Realness: An expert was asked to score the visual quality of eleven 10s mini videos synthesized from the test set phantom frames. For assessment, the "realness score" was used, as proposed by Yi et al. [4], ranging from 0 (totally missing), 1 (bad), 2 (acceptable), 3 (good), to 4 (compelling). We decided against the conduction of a Visual Turing Test, as some shape-related features in the scene (a personalized ring shape instead of a standard commercial ring was used in the experiments) would have been easily identified by an expert surgeon.

Reliability: The result of tempCycleGAN was comprehensively compared in terms of faithfulness to the input phantom images using 39 randomly selected synthesized frames from the test set (16 showing an annuloplasty and 23 showing a triangular leaflet resection). Predefined criteria relevant for surgery were assessed, e.g. whether the instruments or all green and white sutures are completely visible or whether artifacts disturb the surgical region of interest. 12 of 39 input frames show two instruments and three frames only a single instrument. Stitching needles held by the instrument are used in six frames and a prosthetic ring is visible in 29 frames. On average, 4.9 white and 4.9 green sutures are observable in the phantom frames.

4   Results

The result of tempCycleGAN was visually most attractive after 60 epochs. Examples are provided in Fig. 3. Model training of the tempCycleGAN took 18 h for 60 epochs on a single NVIDIA GeForce Titan Xp GPU. Compared to the original CycleGAN [5] trained with a single frame or three consecutive frames, tempCycleGAN produces results with no flickering, contains fewer artifacts, and

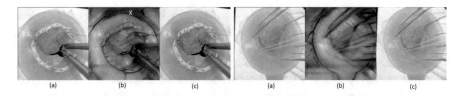

Fig. 3. tempCycleGAN results for two examples shown left and right, where (a) shows the real phantom x_t, (b) shows corresponding synthesized intraoperative images y_t'' and (c) shows the re-synthesized phantom image x_t''. X marks a synthesized atrial retractor.

better preserves content structures in the inputs and capture features (e.g., texture and/or color) of the target domain (see supplemental material videos). The tempCycleGAN approach was even capable of learning where semantically to insert blood (between the leaflets) or an atrial retractor in the scene (Fig. 3). However, it produced slightly blurred instruments and sutures.

The average "realness score" of the 11 mini-videos assessed by the expert surgeon was 3.3 (5 × category "compelling", 4 × "good", 2 ×"acceptable"). Longer versions of a compelling scene (first scene) and an acceptable scene (second scene) are provided in the supplemental video showing a ring annuloplasty[3]. The valve's texture was assessed as very realistic in general by the surgeon. Some instruments and rings appeared blurry and had minor artifacts (e.g. the projection of the sewing cuff of the original ring onto the printed ring appeared incomplete), which led to a lower realness score. However, for most of the scenes this was not crucial because relevant image regions were not effected.

The quantitative assessment of reliability (i.e. comparison of source and target frame) yielded different results for instruments, needles, sutures and silicone surface: Neither instruments, needles nor annuloplasty rings were erroneously added. One generated instrument was classified as 'not preserved', since it was partially coalesced with the valve and two (out of six) needles could not be seen in the generated images. Green sutures were better preserved (4.0 of 4.9 sutures per frame) compared to white sutures (2.2 of 4.9 sutures per frame). In 14 frames all green sutures were consistent in both source and target domain, whereas there is no such frame for white sutures. The appearance of the generated frames was evaluated to be 'overall realistic' in 82.1%. The quality of the generated valves (shape and tissue texture) was compared to the silicone valve. The visual inspection yielded 'valve differs completely' in 2.6%, 'good alignment but details differ' in 10.3% and 'good agreement' in 87.2%.

5 Discussion

According to the widely accepted definition from Azuma [7], Augmented Reality (AR) "*allows the user to see the real world, with virtual objects superimposed*

---

[3] https://youtu.be/qugAYpK-Z4M.

upon or composited with the real world. Therefore, AR supplements reality, rather than completely replacing it. Ideally, it would appear to the user that the virtual and real objects coexisted in the same space". We consider *hyperrealism* as a subform of AR where real, but artificially looking objects (in our case the silicone valves) are transfigured to appear realistically (as in a real surgery). Nothing is added to the scene of the real world, it is just altered to appear more realistic, thus the term hyperrealistic. Objects that already appear realistic ideally stay the same (in our case the instruments, sutures, needles).

The idea to use a transformer network to translate a real endoscopic image into a synthetic-like virtual image has been assessed before with the overall aim of obtaining a reconstructed topography [8,9]. We focus on the opposite transformation, synthesizing intraoperative images from real training procedures on patient-specific silicone models. Our scenes are more complex, since they contain e.g. blood and lens contamination in the target domain and moving instruments, sutures and needles in both source and target domains.

Our methodological advancement tempCycleGAN shows a substantially stabilized composition of the synthesized frames in comparison to the original CycleGAN approach. The architecture's extension by two temporal discriminators, temporal paired input frames fed into multiple runs of generators and further L1 distances in the loss function to penetrate inconsistency yields such significantly more stable results. Beyond that, tempCycleGAN reduced the number of artifacts in the reported outcomes, while slightly sacrificing image sharpness. To the best of our knowledge, our approach is the first method for unpaired image-to-image translation addressing the problem of temporal inconsistencies in moving sequences.

Acknowledgements. The authors thank Bernhard Preim for his valuable hints and Benjamin Hatscher for making the illustration in Fig. 1a. The work was supported by DFG grant DE 2131/2-1, EN 1197/2-1. The GPU was donated by NVidia small scale grant.

References

1. Kenngott, H.G., Wünscher, J.J., Wagner, M., et al.: OpenHELP (Heidelberg Laparoscopy Phantom): development of an open-source surgical evaluation and training tool. Surg. Endosc. **29**(11), 3338–3347 (2015)
2. Engelhardt, S., et al.: Elastic mitral valve silicone replica made from 3d-printable molds offer advanced surgical training. Bildverarbeitung für die Medizin 2018. I, pp. 74–79. Springer, Heidelberg (2018). https://doi.org/10.1007/978-3-662-56537-7_33
3. Isola, P., Zhu, J., Zhou, T., Efros, A.A.: Image-to-image translation with conditional adversarial networks. In: IEEE International Conference on Computer Vision (ICCV), pp. 1125–1134, October 2017
4. Yi, Z., Zhang, H., Tan, P., Gong, M.: DualGAN: unsupervised dual learning for image-to-image translation. In: IEEE International Conference on Computer Vision (ICCV), pp. 2868–2876, October 2017
5. Zhu, J.Y., Park, T., Isola, P., Efros, A.A.: Unpaired image-to-image translation using cycle-consistent adversarial networks. In: IEEE International Conference on Computer Vision (ICCV) 2017, pp. 2242–2251 (2017)

6. Milgram, P., Kishino, F.: A taxonomy of mixed reality visual displays. IEICE Trans. Inf. Syst. **77**(12), 1321–1329 (1994)
7. Azuma, R.T.: A survey of augmented reality. Presence Teleoper Virtual Environ. **6**(4), 355–385 (1997)
8. Visentini-Scarzanella, M., Sugiura, T., Kaneko, T., Koto, S.: Deep monocular 3D reconstruction for assisted navigation in bronchoscopy. Int. J. Comput. Assist. Radiol. Surg. **12**(7), 1089–1099 (2017)
9. Mahmood, F., Durr, N.: Deep learning and conditional random fields-based depth estimation and topographical reconstruction from conventional endoscopy, arXiv preprint: arXiv:1710.11216 (2017)

Computing CNN Loss and Gradients for Pose Estimation with Riemannian Geometry

Benjamin Hou[1]([⊠]), Nina Miolane[2], Bishesh Khanal[1,3], Matthew C. H. Lee[1,4], Amir Alansary[1], Steven McDonagh[1], Jo V. Hajnal[3], Daniel Rueckert[1], Ben Glocker[1], and Bernhard Kainz[1]

[1] Imperial College London, London, UK
benjamin.hou11@imperial.ac.uk
[2] INRIA and Stanford, Stanford, USA
[3] King's College London, London, UK
[4] HeartFlow, Redwood City, USA

Abstract. Pose estimation, *i.e.* predicting a 3D rigid transformation with respect to a fixed co-ordinate frame in, $SE(3)$, is an omnipresent problem in medical image analysis. Deep learning methods often parameterise poses with a representation that separates rotation and translation. As commonly available frameworks do not provide means to calculate loss on a manifold, regression is usually performed using the L2-norm independently on the rotation's and the translation's parameterisations. This is a metric for linear spaces that does not take into account the Lie group structure of $SE(3)$.

In this paper, we propose a general Riemannian formulation of the pose estimation problem, and train CNNs directly on $SE(3)$ equipped with a left-invariant Riemannian metric. The loss between the ground truth and predicted pose (elements of the manifold) is calculated as the Riemannian geodesic distance, which couples together the translation and rotation components. Network weights are updated by backpropagating the gradient with respect to the predicted pose on the tangent space of the manifold $SE(3)$. We thoroughly evaluate the effectiveness of our loss function by comparing its performance with popular and most commonly used existing methods, on tasks such as image-based localisation and intensity-based 2D/3D registration. We also show that hyper-parameters, used in our loss function to weight the contribution between rotations and translations, can be intrinsically calculated from the dataset to achieve greater performance margins.

1 Introduction

Intensity-based registration and landmark matching are the de-facto standards to align data from multiple image sources into a common co-ordinate system. Applications that require intensity-based registration include *e.g.*, atlas-based segmentation [1], motion-compensation [15], tracking [10], or clinical analysis of

© Springer Nature Switzerland AG 2018
A. F. Frangi et al. (Eds.): MICCAI 2018, LNCS 11070, pp. 756–764, 2018.
https://doi.org/10.1007/978-3-030-00928-1_85

the data visualised in a standard co-ordinate system. These often require manual initialisation of the alignment since general optimisation methods often cannot find a global minimum from any given starting position on the cost function. An initial rigid registration can be achieved by selecting common landmarks [2] through an iterative agent, which impedes hard real-time constraints or less robustly through local image descriptors [19].

Convolutional Neural Networks (CNNs) have shown promising results for intra and inter modal alignment [4,10]. These approaches show that information about a learn-able canonical co-ordinate system is encoded directly in the features of an image. Early work in this domain showed that image's pose (i.e. position and orientation) can be regressed relatively to a canonical alignment from a large set of training images sampling the canonical space [7]. Follow-up formulations for medical applications showed similar success for motion compensation and device localisation [4,10]. However, these approaches rely on heuristic approximations and manual fine-tuning of the CNN loss used to characterise the poses' prediction error. This fosters domain shift problems and limits options for interchangeable application of various deep learning pose estimation models.

Contribution: We introduce a new loss function that calculates the geodesic distance of two poses on the $SE(3)$ manifold, from a data-adaptive Riemannian metric. We derive appropriate gradients that are required for CNN back propagation. Our method couples the translation and rotation parameters, and regresses them simultaneously as one parameter on the Lie algebra $\mathfrak{se}(3)$. We show that our loss function is agnostic to the architecture by training different CNNs and can effectively predict poses that are comparable to state-of-the-art methods. In addition, we demonstrate that hyper-parameters tuning for our loss function can be directly calculated from the dataset, thus avoiding long and expensive optimisation searches to boost performance. Finally, we validate quantitatively by benchmarking the performance of our loss function with current state-of-the-art methods, and validate their statistical significance with Student's t-test.

Background: A pose, i.e. a rigid transformation in 3D, is an element of the Lie group $SE(3)$, the Special Euclidean group in 3D. A pose has two components; a rotation component of group $SO(3)$ and a translation component of $\mathbb{R}^3$. $SE(3)$ has the following matrix representation (homogeneous representation):

$$SE(3) = \left\{ X \quad \mid \quad X = \left[\begin{array}{c|c} R & t \\ \hline 0 & 1 \end{array} \right], t \in \mathbb{R}^3, R \in SO(3) \right\} \tag{1}$$

In usual implementations of $SE(3)$, the rotation ($SO(3)$) can be parameterised in any form as long as the group structure is implicitly imposed. R can be stored as Euler angles, quaternions, axis-angle or $SO(3)$ rotation matrix. The numerical properties of each parameterisation need to be considered carefully, especially when designing deep learning applications, as it can impact efficacy.

Hyunh et al. [5] have shown that Euler parameterisation is not unique, this is undesirable as two different mappings can represent the same rotation. A rotation matrix, carrying 9 parameters, is over parameterised and has a strict ordinance on orthonormality. Non-orthogonal rotation matrix can result in skewed or sheared transformations, making it undesirable also. Quaternion parameter-isation are often favoured as it can be mapped to valid transformations after normalisation. However, the parameterisation chosen for the rotation is almost never coupled with the parameterisation of the translation, thus denying the intrinsic structure of $SE(3) = SO(3) \ltimes \mathbb{R}^3$. Here, we choose to represent the rotation and the translation together as an element of the Lie algebra of $SE(3)$, i.e. its tangent space at the identity element of the group, denoted $\mathfrak{se}(3)$. It repre-sents the best linear approximation of $SE(3)$ around its identity element. Since the Lie group $SE(3)$ is 6-dimensional, an element of $\mathfrak{se}(3)$ is a 6D vector.

One can define a collection of distances on $SE(3)$, which can be used as loss functions in deep learning applications. A popular choice for the loss is the Euclidean distance associated to the L2-norm. However, the L2-norm is not desirable on $SE(3)$ since it does not respect the manifold's non-linearity and can lead to unpredictable behaviours. It is also undesirable to use two separates L2-norms on $SO(3)$ and $\mathbb{R}^3$ since $SE(3)$ is not a direct product, and $SO(3)$ itself is non-linear: this can be observed visually with quaternions, e.g., the Euclidean distance of two quaternions can be small, despite the rotation being large. This disparity causes network weight updates to be sub optimal. Hence it is desirable to have a loss function that respects the structure of $SE(3)$.

Related Work: Popular deep learning frameworks, such as Caffe, TensorFlow, Theano, PyTorch, do not provide the means to regress on $SE(3)$, as the common losses used are cross-entropy for probabilities or a p-norms for distances.

Kendall et al. [7] uses the L2-norm to regress parameters on the Lie algebra $\mathfrak{se}(3)$ directly, with a β parameter to weight the contribution between rota-tion and translation. This was similarly performed by authors in [9,10,13,17], who use the predicted parameters for registration tasks. Alternatively, [8,16] re-parameterised the pose parameters as projected co-ordinates on a 2D view plane. This was similarly performed by [3,4] with Anchor Points, where three arbitrary selected reference points on a 2D plane define the plane's location in 3D space. Using the L2-norm to calculate the Euclidean distance between a predicted pro-jection co-ordinate and the ground truth projection co-ordinate is appropriate, as the L2-norm is the appropriate metric. To the best of our knowledge, there is currently no loss function that respects the full Lie group structure of $SE(3)$, for example invariant Riemannian metrics on $SE(3)$ have not been used.

2   Method

The core of our method is to implement a new loss layer that is agnostic to the network architecture used: we define the loss as the geodesic distance on $SE(3)$ equipped with a left-invariant Riemannian metric, shown in Fig. 1.

Left-invariant Riemannian Metric On $SE(3)$: A Riemannian metric on $SE(3)$ is a smooth collection of positive definite inner products on each tangent space of $SE(3)$. Then, $SE(3)$ becomes a Riemannian manifold. With a left-invariant metric, it is enough to define an inner product on the tangent space

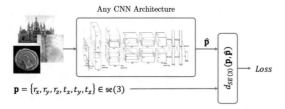

Fig. 1. CNN architecture using a Riemannian geodesic distance on $SE(3)$ as the loss.

at the identity of $SE(3)$, and then "propagate" it: the metric is s.t. $\forall u, v \in T_{p_1}SE(3)$ and $\forall p_1, p_2 \in SE(3)$: $< DL_{p_1}(p_2)u, DL_{p_1}(p_2)v >|_{L_{p_1}p_2} =< u, v >|_{p_2}$ where L_{p_1} is the left translation by p_1: $L_{p_1}(p_2) = p_1 \circ p_2$, and $DL_{p_1}(p_2)$ its differential at p_2. We define an inner product Z at p_2 = identity so that we get a metric Z_{p_1} at the tangent space of any pose p_1 of $SE(3)$ [12], and thus to compute inner products and norms of tangent vectors at p_1.

Loss and Gradient: We use the loss function: $\text{loss}(\mathbf{p}, \hat{\mathbf{p}}) = \text{dist}^Z_{SE(3)}(\mathbf{p}, \hat{\mathbf{p}})^2 = \left\| \text{Log}^Z_{\hat{\mathbf{p}}}(\mathbf{p}) \right\|^2_{Z_{\hat{\mathbf{p}}}}$ where $\text{dist}^Z_{SE(3)}$ is the geodesic distance and Log is the Riemannian logarithm at $\hat{\mathbf{p}}$ i.e. a tangent vector at $\hat{\mathbf{p}}$. We use a left-invariant Riemannian metric, thus: $\text{loss}(\mathbf{p}, \hat{\mathbf{p}}) = \| DL_{\hat{\mathbf{p}}^{-1}}.\text{Log}^Z_{\hat{\mathbf{p}}}(\mathbf{p}) \|^2_Z$, where we now have a tangent vector at the identity and we can use the inner product Z. If we take Z being the canonical inner product at identity, this is the L2-norm but on the tangent vector transported from $\hat{\mathbf{p}}$ to identity using the differential $DL_{\hat{\mathbf{p}}^{-1}}$. The backward gradient corresponding to the loss seen as a function of $\hat{\mathbf{p}}$ is $\nabla_{\hat{\mathbf{p}}}\text{loss}(\mathbf{p}, \hat{\mathbf{p}}) = -2 \cdot \text{Log}^Z_{\hat{\mathbf{p}}}(\mathbf{p})$ [14] which is a tangent vector at $\hat{\mathbf{p}}$.

Implementation: The inputs to the loss layer are the poses $\mathbf{p}$ and $\hat{\mathbf{p}}$ for ground truth and prediction respectively. We represent a pose with `geomstats` implementation [11] i.e. as the Riemannian Logarithm of canonical left-invariant metric on $SE(3)$ s.t. $p = \{r, t\} = \{r_x, r_y, r_z, t_x, t_y, t_z\} \in \mathbb{R}^6$. With this parameterisation, the rotation r is in axis-angle parameterisation, the inner product Z is a 6×6 positive definite matrix and the differential $DL_{\hat{p}}$ of the left translation is the 6×6 jacobian matrix: $J_{\hat{p}} = \begin{pmatrix} \frac{\partial L_{\hat{p}}{}^r}{\partial r} & \frac{\partial L_{\hat{p}}{}^r}{\partial t} \\ \frac{\partial L_{\hat{p}}{}^t}{\partial r} & \frac{\partial L_{\hat{p}}{}^t}{\partial t} \end{pmatrix}$. We denote $v_t = \text{Log}^Z_{\hat{\mathbf{p}}}(\mathbf{p})$ which is a tangent vector at $\hat{\mathbf{p}}$ in this parameterisation. The loss is calculated by $\text{loss}(\mathbf{p}, \hat{\mathbf{p}}) = v_t^T * J_{\hat{p}^{-1}}^T * Z * J_{\hat{p}^{-1}} * v_t$ where $*$ is the matrix multiplication and the Riemannian logarithm v_t is given by `geomstats`. The gradient is calculated by: $\nabla_{\hat{\mathbf{p}}}\text{loss}(\mathbf{p}, \hat{\mathbf{p}}) = -2 * J_{\hat{p}^{-1}}^T * Z * J_{\hat{p}^{-1}} * v_t$.

3 Experiments and Results

We evaluate our novel loss function on three datasets: **(Exp1)** the publicly available PoseNet dataset [7], which allows a direct comparison to state-of-the-art in Computer Vision and further evaluates optimisation strategies for these experiments. **(Exp2)**, C-Arm X-Ray to Computed Tomography (CT) alignment problem with data from [4]. **(Exp3)**, the pose estimation dataset for motion compensation in fetal Magnetic Resonance Imaging (MRI) from [3].

In each experiment, we benchmark existing $SE(3)$ parameterisation strategies with the respective loss function used. PoseNet: direct regression of parameters on the Lie algebra $\mathfrak{se}(3)$, where a combination of quaternion and translation parameters are regressed using L2-norms with a static β parameter to weight the respective contribution. Anchor Points formulation: a re-parameterisation of $SE(3)$ in Euclidean space, where three statically defined points in 3D space defines a plane. Each Anchor Point is regressed independently using the L2-norm. Finally, our $SE(3)$ loss, i.e., the geodesic distance on the Riemannian manifold.

All experiments are conducted using the Caffe framework, on a computer equipped with an Intel i7 6700K CPU and Nvidia Titan X Pascal GPU.

Exp.1: Metric Localisation on Natural Images: In this experiment, we replicated PoseNet's original experiment [7] on the King's College dataset as a baseline benchmark. [7] extracted images from a series of videos, and fed them into a structure from motion pipeline to create a 3D model in order to extract plane locations with respect to a world co-ordinate reference frame. The parameterisations of this dataset are quaternions with translation offsets. We mirrored the dataset using axis-angle representation instead of quaternions, and used our $SE(3)$ loss function as regressor. Both networks were trained with a GoogLeNet [18] base architecture with no parameter weighting.

Table 1. Mean error of loss functions on natural images

	R_x	R_y	R_z	t_x	t_y	t_z	G.D.
PoseNet	**4.141**	7.774	**4.597**	1.341	**1.139**	**0.154**	23.629
$SE(3)$	4.306	**6.675**	11.580	**1.307**	1.149	0.155	**14.973**
A: Without parameter weighting							
	R_x	R_y	R_z	t_x	t_y	t_z	G.D.
PoseNet	**1.790**	**2.612**	**2.371**	**1.161**	1.306	**0.154**	**13.516**
$SE(3)$	1.870	3.143	3.662	1.759	**1.240**	0.156	16.370
B: With parameter weighting							

We convert the predicted and ground truth poses to Euler angles in degrees and translation in meters, along with the geodesic distance (G.D.) on the manifold. Table 1-A shows the average errors of each parameter. It can be seen that the error is similar in each Euler and translation parameters, which is confirmed by Student's t-test to be insignificant. However, the geodesic distance error of SE(3) is much lower compared to PoseNet. Despite this, Student's t-test still shows no significant difference, which is caused by the large variance of PoseNet.

To tune the weight parameter β, Kendall et al. [7] performed grid search and found that $\beta = [120, 750]$ works best for indoor scenes and $\beta = [250, 2000]$ for outdoor scenes. Grid search is computationally very expensive, and it can be difficult to find an optimal value if the search interval is coarse. We show here that we can compute a data-adaptive Riemannian metric on $SE(3)$ to weight the contribution of each parameter in the loss.

We first train the network with no weightings, followed by an inference pass through the entire validation dataset. We compute the prediction error as the rigid transformation: $(y_{true})^{-1} \circ y_{pred}$ and consider the dataset of their Riemannian logarithms at the identity $\{X_i\}_i$. The parameter weightings are then calculated by $\text{diag}(\text{cov}(X_i)^{-1})$. The diagonal of the covariance matrix shows the variance of each parameter, whereas the inverse shows how tightly coupled it is to the mean. Thus, the higher the diagonal element, the tighter the variable is clustered. Elements, that are more sparsely coupled, are weighted less as they are likely to induce errors. The optimal weightings for the King's College dataset from [7] are: $\text{diag}(\text{cov}(X_i)^{-1}) = \{0.147, 0.954, 0.261, 0.001, 0.003, 0.002\}$.

Table 1-B shows the performance of the networks retrained with suggested weightings. Student's T-test still shows no significant difference between errors induced by PoseNet and $SE(3)$. We note that having different weightings on the rotation part induces a distance that is not a Riemannian geodesic distance anymore. The properties of this distance will be investigated in future work.

Exp.2: Plane Detection on C-ARM Imaging: [4] demonstrated the versatility of CNNs for performing 2D/3D registration of C-Arm X-ray images to CT volumes using Anchor Points. In this experiment, we replicate the 2D/3D registration task using CaffeNet and evaluate the performance with the newly proposed $SE(3)$ parameterisation and loss regressor. For comparison, a network was also trained with PoseNet's parameterisation. All weight parameters are set to a default of 1. Table 2 shows the performance of each parameterisation.

Table 2. Mean error of loss functions on DRR (Digitally reconstructed radiographs)

	R_x	R_y	R_z	t_x	t_y	t_z	G.D.
PoseNet	7.960	3.136	7.547	62.650	57.315	45.852	15201.845
Anchor points	**7.274**	**2.511**	**7.059**	59.292	**54.889**	**40.576**	15115.858
$SE(3)$	8.243	3.697	7.924	**58.647**	55.477	44.189	**14170.722***
A: Healthy patient dataset							
	R_x	R_y	R_z	t_x	t_y	t_z	G.D.
PoseNet	10.653	5.788	10.760	69.107	72.238	57.726	23495.708
Anchor points	**8.540**	**4.060**	**8.553**	65.521	**68.543**	54.133	21725.921
$SE(3)$	10.511	6.789	11.913	**62.588**	68.747	**54.110**	**19624.246***
B: Pathological patient dataset							

Here, we convert the predicted and ground truth poses to Euler angles in degrees, and translation to millimetres. Similar to Exp1, the average error for rotation and translation (for both healthy and pathological patients) are similar, and insignificant as confirmed by Student's t-test. However, there is a noticeable trend in average geodesic distance errors. Student's t-test showed significant difference (marked by *) between $SE(3)$ loss compared to PoseNet and Anchor Points for both datasets. This shows that the geodesic metric is able to quantify properties that the metric expressed in Euler-translation parameters cannot.

Exp.3: 2D/3D Registration on Fetal Brain MRI: We replicate the results evaluation method from [3], and evaluate our loss regressor for 2D/3D registration used during motion compensation of fetal MRI data in canonical organ space. [3] uses aligned, reconstructed 3D brain volumes to learn a canonical orientation space and utilises an approach based on GoogLeNet to reorient unseen 2D brain slices into their correct anatomical location in this space. To sample the canonical training space we use the same Euler iteration method (*i.e.*, 18° steps in R_x R_y R_z between −90° and +90°, and 2 mm offsets in T_z constrained between −40 and 40) to generate 1.12M images for the training set. The evaluation method is performed similarly as [3], with the performance summarised in Table 3. The validation dataset is composed of brain slices sampled with random Euler angles between −90° and +90°, and random offsets between −40 and +40.

Table 3. Mean error of loss functions on fetal brain images

	CC	MSE	PSNR	SSIM	G.D.
PoseNet	0.8199	1046.4	18.6509	0.5448	18.1708
Anchor points	0.8378	935.0	19.3564	0.5845	15.7504
$SE(3)$	**0.8732***	**724.9713***	**20.7484***	**0.6470***	**10.0836***

Our $SE(3)$ loss function shows drastic improvement in all image similarity metrics (Cross Correlation, Mean Squared Error, Peak Signal-to-Noise Ratio and Structural SIMilarity). This is confirmed by Student's t-test which shows significant difference. This is crucial for Slice-to-Volume Registration (SVR) applications as the metric for slice alignment is derived from the metrics above [6].

Discussion: A pose is a combination of rotation and translation, therefore it seems reasonable that a CNN predicting a pose should use a metric that accounts for both simultaneously. Metrics are perceptually a method of measurement with its own set of rules, *e.g.*, imperial vs. metric system for quantifying distances. Choosing a metric for a target application is not always straight forward and often a question of required precision, *e.g.*, one would not measure the diameter of a pinhead with a meter rule, nor measure distance between cities with a calliper. We have shown that our loss function, using a Riemannian geodesic distance on $SE(3)$ is better suited for medical registration tasks as shown in Exp2 and Exp3. Exp2 shows each test case yielding no significant difference on Euler and translation parameters, with significant difference on geodesic parameters. This suggests that Euler-translation parameters separately are not able to fully quantify the properties of $SE(3)$. In Exp3, our loss function was able to significantly improve the image similarity metrics, as used by SVR algorithms.

4   Conclusion

In this work, we have presented a novel loss function to regress poses on the Lie group $SE(3)$, and derived the necessary gradients required for CNN training. We showed that our method alleviates the need of re-parameterising regression parameters, which addresses the domain shift problem of deep learning applications. Our approach achieves similar results to manually fine-tuned approximations out-of-the-box, e.g., for data from a new scanner. This is demonstrated on the current state-of-the-art for pose estimation, PoseNet, where we show that our method achieves similar performance as the carefully tuned approximation used in [7]. We also show significant improvements for medical image pose estimation and outperform the state-of-the-art in this domain [3,4].

References

1. Aljabar, P.: Multi-atlas based segmentation of brain images: atlas selection and its effect on accuracy. NeuroImage **46**(3), 726–738 (2009)
2. Ghesu, F.C., Georgescu, B., Mansi, T., Neumann, D., Hornegger, J., Comaniciu, D.: An artificial agent for anatomical landmark detection in medical images. In: Ourselin, S., Joskowicz, L., Sabuncu, M.R., Unal, G., Wells, W. (eds.) MICCAI 2016. LNCS, vol. 9902, pp. 229–237. Springer, Cham (2016). https://doi.org/10. 1007/978-3-319-46726-9_27
3. Hou, B., et al.: 3D reconstruction in canonical co-ordinate space from arbitrarily oriented 2D images. IEEE Trans. Med. Imaging **PP**(99), 1 (2018)
4. Hou, B., et al.: Predicting slice-to-volume transformation in presence of arbitrary subject motion. In: Descoteaux, M., Maier-Hein, L., Franz, A., Jannin, P., Collins, D.L., Duchesne, S. (eds.) MICCAI 2017. LNCS, vol. 10434, pp. 296–304. Springer, Cham (2017). https://doi.org/10.1007/978-3-319-66185-8_34
5. Huynh, D.Q.: Metrics for 3D rotations: comparison and analysis. J. Math. Imaging Vis. **35**(2), 155–164 (2009)
6. Kainz, B.: Fast volume reconstruction from motion corrupted stacks of 2D slices. IEEE Trans. Med. Imaging **34**(9), 1901–13 (2015)
7. Kendall, A., et al.: Posenet: a convolutional network for real-time 6-DOF camera relocalization. In: ICCV, pp. 2938–2946 (2015)
8. Kendall, A., Cipolla, R.: Geometric loss functions for camera pose regression with deep learning. In: Proceedings of the IEEE CVPR (2017)
9. Liao, R., et al.: An artificial agent for robust image registration. In: AAAI, pp. 4168–4175 (2017)
10. Miao, S.: A CNN regression approach for real-time 2D/3D registration. IEEE Trans. Med. Imaging **35**(5), 1352–1363 (2016)
11. Miolane, N., Mathe, J., Donnat, C., Jorda, M., Pennec, X.: Geomstats: a python package for riemannian geometry in machine learning (2018). https://github.com/ ninamiolane/geomstats, https://arxiv.org/abs/1805.08308
12. Miolane, N., Pennec, X.: Computing bi-invariant pseudo-metrics on lie groups for consistent statistics. Entropy **17**(4), 1850–1881 (2015)

13. Pei, Y., et al.: Non-rigid craniofacial 2D-3D registration using CNN-based regression. In: Cardoso, M.J., et al. (eds.) DLMIA/ML-CDS -2017. LNCS, vol. 10553, pp. 117–125. Springer, Cham (2017). https://doi.org/10.1007/978-3-319-67558-9_14
14. Pennec, X.: Probabilities and statistics on riemannian manifolds: basic tools for geometric measurements. In: NSIP, pp. 194–198. Citeseer (1999)
15. Rousseau, F.: Registration-based approach for reconstruction of high-resolution in utero fetal MR brain images. Acad. Radiol. 13(9), 1072–1081 (2006)
16. Sarkis, M., Diepold, K.: Camera-pose estimation via projective newton optimization on the manifold. IEEE Trans. Image Process. 21(4), 1729–1741 (2012)
17. Sloan, J., et al.: Learning rigid image registration - utilizing cnns for medical image registration (2018). http://eprints.gla.ac.uk/156798/
18. Szegedy, C., et al.: Going deeper with convolutions. In: IEEE CVPR 2015 (2015)
19. Zitová, B., Flusser, J.: Image registration methods: a survey. Image Vis. Comput. 21(11), 977–1000 (2003)

GDL-FIRE^{4D}: Deep Learning-Based Fast 4D CT Image Registration

Thilo Sentker$^{1,2(\boxtimes)}$, Frederic Madesta^{1,2}, and René Werner^1

^{1} Department of Computational Neuroscience, University Medical Center
Hamburg-Eppendorf, Martinistr. 52, 20246 Hamburg, Germany
^{2} Department of Radiotherapy and Radiation Oncology, University Medical Center
Hamburg-Eppendorf, Martinistr. 52, 20246 Hamburg, Germany
{t.sentker,f.madesta,r.werner}@uke.de

Abstract. Deformable image registration (DIR) in thoracic 4D CT image data is integral for, e.g., radiotherapy treatment planning, but time consuming. Deep learning (DL)-based DIR promises speed-up, but present solutions are limited to small image sizes. In this paper, we propose a General Deep Learning-based Fast Image Registration framework suitable for application to clinical 4D CT data (GDL-FIRE^{4D}). Open source DIR frameworks are selected to build GDL-FIRE^{4D} variants. In-house-acquired 4D CT images serve as training and open 4D CT data repositories as external evaluation cohorts. Taking up current attempts to DIR uncertainty estimation, dropout-based uncertainty maps for GDL-FIRE^{4D} variants are analyzed. We show that (1) registration accuracy of GDL-FIRE^{4D} and standard DIR are in the same order; (2) computation time is reduced to a few seconds (here: 60-fold speed-up); and (3) dropout-based uncertainty maps do not correlate to across-DIR vector field differences, raising doubts about applicability in the given context.

Keywords: Non-linear image registration · Registration uncertainty
4D CT · Deep learning

1 Introduction

Acquisition of 4D image data (3D+t images, respiration-correlated data) is an integral part of current radiation therapy (RT) workflows for RT planning and treatment of thoracic and abdominal tumors. Especially 4D CT imaging is meanwhile widespread and currently estimated to be routinely applied in approximately 70% of the RT facilities in the United States [1]. Typical clinical use cases of 4D CT data are (semi-)automated target volume and organ at risk contour propagation; assessment of motion effects on dose distributions (4D RT quality assurance, dose warping) [2]; and 4D CT-based lung ventilation estimation and its incorporation into RT treatment planning [1].

T. Sentker and F. Madesta—Equal contribution.

© Springer Nature Switzerland AG 2018
A. F. Frangi et al. (Eds.): MICCAI 2018, LNCS 11070, pp. 765–773, 2018.
https://doi.org/10.1007/978-3-030-00928-1_86

At this, a key step is the application of deformable image registration (DIR) to the phase images of the 4D CT data. Traditional DIR approaches tackle the underlying task of finding an optimal transformation mapping two phase images by minimization of a dissimilarity measure that controls local correspondences of voxel intensities [3]. Yet, the algorithms are time consuming and there exists the risk of getting stuck in local minima during optimization.

Motivated by the exceptional success of deep learning (DL) and especially convolutional neural networks (CNNs) for image segmentation and classification tasks, meanwhile a number of approaches has been proposed to also solve image registration tasks by CNNs – first in the context of optical flow estimation in computer vision [4], and later similarly for medical image registration [3,5–7]. Yang *et al.* further extended a CNN-based DIR architecture to a probabilistic framework using dropouts [5], resulting in DIR uncertainty maps that could be of great value for RT treatment planning [8].

However, Uzunova *et al.* noted that "dense 3D registration with CNNs is currently computationally infeasible" [6], and focused on 2D (brain and cardiac) DIR only. To overcome this issue, patch-based approaches have been proposed for, e.g., 3D brain DIR [5], with the side effect that global information about the transformation to learn might be missing [3]. In turn, Rohé *et al.* indeed proposed using a fully convolutional architecture; with a size of $64 \times 64 \times 16$ voxel, their cardiac MR images were, however, not even close to typical sizes of 4D CT images (in the order of $512 \times 512 \times 150$ voxel per phase image).

This paper is therefore dedicated to CNN-based registration suitable for application to fast DIR in clinical thoracic 4D CT data. Taking up the afore-mentioned challenges and trends in current DL-based DIR,

C1 we propose a general and efficient CNN-based framework for deep learning of dense motion fields in clinical thoracic 4D CT, called GDL-FIRE^{4D},

C2 build variants of GDL-FIRE^{4D} using common open source DIR frameworks,

C3 perform a first comprehensive evaluation thereof using publicly available 4D CT data repositories (thereby presenting first respective benchmark baseline results for DL-based DIR in 4D CT data), and

C4 compare and discuss dropout-generated registration uncertainty maps for the different GDL-FIRE^{4D} variants.

To the best of our knowledge, all aspects C1-C4 are novel contributions in the given application context.

The remainder of the paper is structured as follows: In Sect. 2, the problem formulation and the concept of GDL-FIRE^{4D} are detailed. Applied data sets and performed experiments are described in Sect. 3 and respective results given and discussed in Sect. 4. The paper closes with concluding remarks in Sect. 5.

2   Methods: DL-Based Deformable Image Registration

A 4D CT image is a series $(I_i)_{i \in \{1,\dots,n_{\mathrm{ph}}\}}$ of 3D CT images $I_i : \Omega \to \mathbb{R}$, $\Omega \subset \mathbb{R}^3$, representing the patient geometry at different breathing phases i with n_{ph} as number of available images and breathing phases, respectively. The phases i sample the patient's breathing cycle in time and are usually denoted by cycle fractions, i.e. $\{1, \ldots, n_{\mathrm{ph}}\} \equiv \{0\%, \ldots, 50\%, \ldots\}$ with 0% as end inspiration and 50% as end expiration phase. Deformable registration in 4D CT data then aims to estimate a corresponding series of transformations $(\varphi_i)_{i \in \{1, \ldots, n_{\mathrm{ph}}\}}$ between the I_i and a reference image I_{ref}, with $\varphi_i : \Omega \to \Omega$. For the applications outlined in Sect. 1, I_{ref} usually represents one of the phase images I_i and the transformation φ_i and vector fields $u_i : \Omega \to \mathbb{R}^3$, $u_i = \varphi_i - \mathrm{id}$ (id: identity map) the respiration-induced motion of the image structures between phase i and the reference phase.

2.1 Traditional Deformable Image Registration (DIR) Formulation

In a traditional 4D CT DIR setting, the reference image is considered the fixed image, $I_{\mathrm{ref}} \equiv I_{\mathrm{F}}$, and the phase images as moving images, $I_i \equiv I_{\mathrm{M}}$, which are sequentially registered to I_{F} by $\varphi_i = \arg\min_{\varphi_i^* \in \mathcal{C}^2[\Omega]} \mathcal{J}[I_{\mathrm{F}}, I_{\mathrm{M}}; \varphi_i^*]$ to compute the sought transformations $(\varphi_i)_{i \in \{1, \ldots, n_{\mathrm{ph}}\}}$. The exact functional $\mathcal{J}$, i.e. dissimilarity measure, applied regularization approach and considered transformation model, and the optimization strategy vary in the community; see [9] for details.

2.2 Convolutional Neural Networks (CNNs) for DIR

Different to traditional DIR, we now assume a database of n_{pat} training tuples $(I_i^p, I_j^p, \varphi_{ij}^p)$, $i, j \in \{1, \ldots, n_{\mathrm{ph}}\}$, $p \in \{1, \ldots, n_{\mathrm{pat}}\}$ to be given; $\varphi_{ij}^p = \mathrm{id} + u_{ij}^p$ represents a DIR result of the phase images $I_i \equiv I_{\mathrm{F}}$ and I_j of patient p. The goal is to learn the relationship between the input data (I_i^p, I_j^p) and u_{ij}^p by a convolutional neural network.

As noted by Uzunova *et al.* [6], it is currently computationally not feasible to directly feed the entire images and vector fields into a CNN or GPU memory. Instead, we propose a slab-based approach: Let $I|_{\hat{x}} := I|_{\Omega_{\hat{x}}}$ be the restriction of image I to $\Omega_{\hat{x}} = \{(x, y, z) \in \Omega \mid x = \hat{x}\}$, i.e. the sagittal slice of I at x-position $\hat{x}$. Similarly, let $I|_{[\hat{x}_1, \hat{x}_2]}$ be the restriction of I to $\Omega_{[\hat{x}_1, \hat{x}_2]} = \{(x, y, z) \in \Omega \mid \hat{x}_1 \leq x \leq \hat{x}_2\}$, i.e. an image slab comprising the sagittal slices $\hat{x}_1, \ldots, \hat{x}_2$ of I. Using this notation, the aforementioned training tuples were converted to slab-based training samples $(I_i^p|_{[x-2, x+2]}, I_j^p|_{[x-2, x+2]}, u_{ij}^p|_x)$ with $x \in \{x_{\min}, \ldots, x_{\max}\}$ covering all sagittal slices of I. The rationale was to represent maximum information along main motion directions *inferior-superior* and *anterior-posterior* for each training sample, but also to provide some anatomical context in lateral direction.

Furthermore, the image dynamics were rescaled to $[0, 1]$, the slabs resampled to isotropic resolution of $2\,\mathrm{mm}$ and cropped/zero-padded to identical size, and the non-patient background intensity set to zero. Similar pre-processing was applied to the displacement fields (resampling and -sizing of sagittal slices, background set to zero). In addition, x-, y- and z-displacement components were z-transformed on a voxel-level to avoid unintended suppression of small displacements during CNN training. Thus, the CNN aimed to learn normalized 3D-vectors for the individual voxels of sagittal slices, which are back-transformed

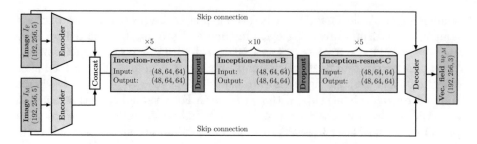

Fig. 1. CNN architecture implemented for DL-based DIR.

to actual motion fields during final reconstruction of the fields. The pre-processed slab-based samples $(\tilde{I}_i^p|_{[x-2,x+2]}, \tilde{I}_j^p|_{[x-2,x+2]}, \tilde{u}_{ij}^p|_x)$ with $x \in \{x_{\min}, \ldots, x_{\max}\}$ of the n_{pat} patients were finally shuffled and used for CNN training.

We tested different CNN architectures, including the classical U-Net [10]. Due to an observed increased robustness for DL-based DIR compared to the U-Net, we finally used an iterative CNN architecture with an Inception-ResNet-v2 [11] embedded in the encoder part of a pre-trained CT autoencoder, see Fig. 1, with MSE (mean squared error) loss function and NADAM optimizer (implemented in Tensorflow). *Iterative* means that we cascaded copies of the trained networks for improved coverage of large motion patterns.

2.3   Probabilistic CNN-Based DIR

As detailed by Yang *et al.* [5] and references therein, deterministic CNN architectures can be extended to probabilistic using dropouts [12]. Briefly speaking, the dropout layers incorporated into the CNN architecture to prevent overfitting during model training remain enabled during motion prediction. Repeated motion prediction with respectively sampled connections to be dropped eventually enable computing the sought motion field as the mean of the sampled predicted fields; further, corresponding voxel-wise variances can be interpreted as local registration uncertainty estimates [5].

3   Materials and Study Design

All experiments were run on a desktop computer with Intel Xeon CPU E5-1620 and Nvidia Titan Xp GPU. Models and scripts required can be found at https:// github.com/IPMI-ICNS-UKE/gdl-fire-4d.

3.1   Training and Testing 4D CT Data Cohorts

For CNN training and model optimization, a cohort of 69 in-house acquired RT treatment planning ten-phase 4D CT data sets of patients with small lung and liver tumors was used (image size: $512 \times 512 \times 159$ voxel) and a 85%/15% split

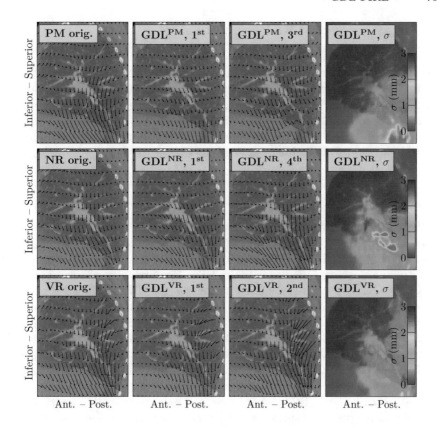

Fig. 2. Motion fields estimated by the original DIR algorithms (left column); GDL-FIRE^{4D} with only a single iteration (2nd column); GDL-FIRE^{4D} n iterations (3rd column); and GDL-FIRE^{4D} variant-specific registration uncertainty maps (right column). Data set: DIRLAB case 08, DIR of 0% and 50% phase images.

into training and testing data performed. The 4D CT images of the open data repositories DIRLAB [13] and CREATIS [14] (see also www.creatis.insa-lyon.fr/rio/popi-model) served as *external* evaluation cohort of the trained CNNs (i.e. no model optimization performed by means of the external 4D CT cohorts).

3.2 Applied DIR Frameworks and Algorithms

To provide motion field training data, the in-house 4D CT data were registered using three common open source DIR frameworks: PlastiMatch [15], NiftyReg [16], and VarReg [17]. All approaches have been proven suitable for 4D CT registration [9]; the applied parameters were similar to respective EMPIRE10 parameters [9]. However, the algorithms are applied in a plug-and-play manner (no data pre-processing or pre-registration, no masks used). For each DIR algorithm, motion fields were provided between the 20% phase image (served as I_{F}) and all other phase images.

3.3   Experiments and Evaluation Measures

For each DIR algorithm, a respective probabilistic GDL-FIRE^{4D} variant was
built (up to 4 cascaded CNNs, 20% dropouts). DIR accuracy was evaluated by
the target registration error (TRE), computed by means of the landmarks publicly available for the DIRLAB and CREATIS data. In addition, the smoothness
of transformations of the different DIR approaches and GDL-FIRE^{4D} variants
was analyzed in terms of the standard deviation of transformation Jacobian
determinant values of the lung voxels of the evaluation data.

4   Results and Discussion

Motion fields estimated by the original DIR algorithms and respective GDL-
FIRE^{4D} variants as well as corresponding registration uncertainty maps are
shown in Fig. 2 for DIRLAB case 08 (DIRLAB case with maximum motion
amplitude) and phase 50% to phase 0% DIR. The similarity of the original and
the GDL-FIRE^{4D} predicted fields is striking, i.e. the CNN obviously learned the
DIR-specific transformation properties. This includes that the NiftyReg GDL-
FIRE^{4D} variant has (similar to the original DIR) problems to directly cover
larger motion amplitudes – and thereby motivates cascading several trained
models for *iterative* CNN-based DIR. The success can be seen in Table 1, where
the NiftyReg GDL-FIRE^{4D} outperforms the original NiftyReg DIR in terms of
accuracy especially for cases with larger motion.

Still, GDL-FIRE^{4D} DIR accuracy as well as transformation properties for
the other DIR approaches also resemble respective values of the traditional registration algorithm – but GDL-FIRE^{4D} offers a reduction of the runtime from
approx. 15 min to a few seconds (speedup of approx. 60-fold).

Finally, it can be seen that the computed DIR uncertainty maps differ greatly
between the GDL-FIRE^{4D} variants. In Fig. 3, a dataset of our internal testing cohort is shown that exhibits an artifact in the liver. This artifact led to

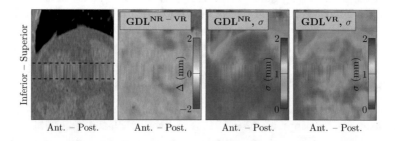

Fig. 3. From left to right: CT image serving as reference image with artifact in liver; difference of motion amplitudes estimated by the NiftyReg and the VarReg GDL-FIRE^{4D}
variants, illustrating large across-DIR approach differences; NiftyReg and VarReg GDL-
FIRE^{4D} uncertainty maps, showing negligible uncertainties for both variants.

Table 1. TRE values (in mm) and transformation smoothness (measured by standard deviation of lung voxel Jacobian determinant values), listed for the DIRLAB and CREATIS data, the individual DIR algorithms, and respective GDL-FIRE^{4D} variants (PM: PlastiMatch; NR: NiftyReg; VR: VarReg). Landmark distance before registration: (8.46 ± 6.58) mm for the DIRLAB and (8.11 ± 4.76) mm for the CREATIS data.

		Original DIR algorithms			GDL-FIRE^{4D}		
		PM [16]	NR [15]	VR [17]	PM	NR	VR
DIRLAB 4DCT	01	1.54 ± 0.98	1.46 ± 0.92	1.13 ± 0.54	1.69 ± 0.92	1.58 ± 0.80	1.20 ± 0.60
	02	1.74 ± 1.76	1.55 ± 1.06	1.17 ± 0.83	1.58 ± 1.07	1.65 ± 1.15	1.19 ± 0.63
	03	2.78 ± 2.20	2.53 ± 2.41	1.33 ± 0.69	2.39 ± 1.76	2.68 ± 1.78	1.67 ± 0.90
	04	2.70 ± 2.27	3.01 ± 2.45	3.08 ± 3.83	2.72 ± 1.97	2.48 ± 1.68	2.53 ± 2.01
	05	3.30 ± 3.06	3.21 ± 2.77	1.57 ± 1.33	2.83 ± 2.21	2.48 ± 2.50	2.06 ± 1.56
	06	3.80 ± 3.03	5.40 ± 3.94	5.23 ± 4.67	3.01 ± 1.97	2.73 ± 1.63	2.90 ± 1.70
	07	5.62 ± 5.32	8.36 ± 6.59	4.64 ± 3.91	4.48 ± 4.83	4.12 ± 4.21	3.60 ± 2.99
	08	7.65 ± 7.45	11.45 ± 9.08	4.58 ± 5.95	7.44 ± 6.87	8.26 ± 6.47	5.29 ± 5.52
	09	3.74 ± 2.60	5.66 ± 3.24	2.66 ± 2.46	3.56 ± 2.35	3.26 ± 1.90	2.38 ± 1.46
	10	3.15 ± 2.99	4.39 ± 4.21	2.14 ± 2.42	2.48 ± 1.99	2.55 ± 2.01	2.13 ± 1.88
∅ TRE		3.60 ± 1.83	4.70 ± 3.17	2.75 ± 1.57	3.22 ± 1.71	3.24 ± 1.81	2.50 ± 1.16
∅ $\sigma_{|\nabla\varphi|}$		0.10 ± 0.02	0.11 ± 0.03	0.39 ± 0.08	0.30 ± 0.13	0.24 ± 0.09	0.39 ± 0.14
CREATIS	01	1.13 ± 0.78	1.79 ± 1.26	0.90 ± 0.39	1.49 ± 0.83	1.73 ± 0.97	1.34 ± 0.74
	02	3.29 ± 3.10	4.29 ± 4.33	1.95 ± 2.87	3.59 ± 2.92	4.25 ± 3.47	2.98 ± 2.38
	03	1.95 ± 2.14	2.39 ± 2.60	1.14 ± 1.37	1.83 ± 1.42	2.05 ± 1.26	1.57 ± 1.01
	04	2.32 ± 2.95	2.51 ± 2.87	1.28 ± 2.13	1.79 ± 1.79	1.92 ± 1.73	1.64 ± 1.62
	05	1.88 ± 1.84	2.51 ± 2.73	1.17 ± 1.17	2.10 ± 1.78	2.18 ± 1.67	1.62 ± 1.09
	06	1.13 ± 0.78	1.52 ± 1.38	0.97 ± 0.72	1.60 ± 1.07	1.63 ± 1.11	1.26 ± 0.73
∅ TRE		2.01 ± 0.68	2.50 ± 0.88	1.24 ± 0.34	2.07 ± 0.78	2.29 ± 0.89	1.74 ± 0.57
∅ $\sigma_{|\nabla\varphi|}$		0.09 ± 0.02	0.11 ± 0.05	0.28 ± 0.05	0.31 ± 0.12	0.26 ± 0.08	0.30 ± 0.10

very different motion patterns estimated by the NiftyReg and the VarReg GDL-FIRE^{4D} variant, but almost no measurable uncertainty for both DIR approaches. Being a direct consequence of the concept of probabilistic CNN-based DIR, this does, however, not match our understanding of DIR uncertainty and raises doubts regarding its applicability for RT planning and estimation of uncertainties therein.

5 Conclusions

The presented GDL-FIRE^{4D} framework illustrates feasibility and potential of deep learning of dense vector fields for motion estimation in clinical thoracic 4D CT image data (TRE values of CNN-based DIR were in the same order than for the underlying DIR algorithms, accompanied by a speed-up factor of approximately 60), and thereby motivates continuing optimization of the framework.

Acknowledgments. We thank NVIDIA Corporation donating for the applied Titan Xp GPU.

References

1. Yamamoto, T., et al.: The first patient treatment of computed tomography ventilation functional image-guided radiotherapy for lung cancer. Radiother Oncol. **118**, 227–31 (2016)
2. Rosu, M., Hugo, G.D.: Advances in 4D radiation therapy for managing respiration: part II - 4D treatment planning. Z Med. Phys. **22**, 272–80 (2012)
3. Rohé, M.-M., Datar, M., Heimann, T., Sermesant, M., Pennec, X.: SVF-Net: learning deformable image registration using shape matching. In: Descoteaux, M., Descoteaux, M., et al. (eds.) MICCAI 2017. LNCS, vol. 10433, pp. 266–274. Springer, Cham (2017). https://doi.org/10.1007/978-3-319-66182-7_31
4. Dosovitskiy, A., et al.: FlowNet: learning optical flow with convolutional networks. In: 2015 IEEE International Conference on Computer Vision (ICCV), vol. 2015 Inter., pp. 2758–2766. IEEE (2015)
5. Yang, X., Kwitt, R., Styner, M., Niethammer, M.: Quicksilver: fast predictive image registration - a deep learning approach. Neuroimage **158**, 378–396 (2017)
6. Uzunova, H., Wilms, M., Handels, H., Ehrhardt, J.: Training CNNs for image registration from few samples with model-based data augmentation. In: Descoteaux, M., et al. (eds.) MICCAI 2017. LNCS, vol. 10433, pp. 223–231. Springer, Cham (2017). https://doi.org/10.1007/978-3-319-66182-7_26
7. Krebs, J., et al.: Robust non-rigid registration through agent-based action learning. In: Descoteaux, M., et al. (eds.) MICCAI 2017. LNCS, vol. 10433, pp. 344–352. Springer, Cham (2017). https://doi.org/10.1007/978-3-319-66182-7_40
8. Amir-Khalili, A., Hamarneh, G., Zakariaee, R., Spadinger, I., Abugharbieh, R.: Propagation of registration uncertainty during multi-fraction cervical cancer brachytherapy. Phys. Med. Biol. **62**, 8116–8135 (2017)
9. Murphy, K., van Ginneken, B., Reinhardt, J.M.: Evaluation of registration methods on thoracic CT: the EMPIRE10 challenge. IEEE Trans. Med. Imaging **30**, 1901–20 (2011)
10. Ronneberger, O., Fischer, P., Brox, T.: U-Net: convolutional networks for biomedical image segmentation. In: Navab, N., Hornegger, J., Wells, W.M., Frangi, A.F. (eds.) MICCAI 2015. LNCS, vol. 9351, pp. 234–241. Springer, Cham (2015). https://doi.org/10.1007/978-3-319-24574-4_28
11. Szegedy, C., Ioffe, S., Vanhoucke, V., Alemi, A.A.: Inception-v4, Inception-Resnet and the impact of residual connections on learning. In: Proceedings of the Thirty-First AAAI Conference on Artificial Intelligence (AAAI-17), pp. 4278–4284 (2017)
12. Srivastava, N., Hinton, G., Krizhevsky, A., Sutskever, I., Salakhutdinov, R.: Dropout: a simple way to prevent neural networks from overfitting. J. Mach. Learn. Res. **15**, 1929–58 (2014)
13. Castillo, R., Castillo, E., Guerra, R.: A framework for evaluation of deformable image registration spatial accuracy using large landmark point sets. Phys. Med. Biol. **54**, 1849–70 (2009)
14. Vandemeulebroucke, J., Rit, S., Kybic, J., Clarysse, P., Sarrut, D.: Spatiotemporal motion estimation for respiratory-correlated imaging of the lungs. Med. Phys. **38**, 166–78 (2011)
15. Modat, M., et al.: Fast free-form deformation using graphics processing units. Comput. Methods Programs Biomed. **98**, 278–84 (2010)

16. Shackleford, J.A., Kandasamy, N., Sharp, G.C.: On developing B-spline registration algorithms for multi-core processors. Phys. Med. Biol. **55**, 6329–51 (2010)
17. Werner, R., Schmidt-Richberg, A., Handels, H., et al.: Estimation of lung motion fields in 4D CT data by variational non-linear intensity-based registration: a comparison and evaluation study. Phys. Med. Biol. **59**, 4247–4260 (2014)

Adversarial Deformation Regularization for Training Image Registration Neural Networks

Yipeng Hu[1,2](✉), Eli Gibson[1], Nooshin Ghavami[1], Ester Bonmati[1],
Caroline M. Moore[3], Mark Emberton[3], Tom Vercauteren[1],
J. Alison Noble[2], and Dean C. Barratt[1]

[1] Centre for Medical Image Computing,
University College London, London, UK
yipeng.hu@ucl.ac.uk
[2] Institute of Biomedical Engineering, University of Oxford, Oxford, UK
[3] Division of Surgery and Interventional Science,
University College London, London, UK

Abstract. We describe an adversarial learning approach to constrain convolutional neural network training for image registration, replacing heuristic smoothness measures of displacement fields often used in these tasks. Using minimally-invasive prostate cancer intervention as an example application, we demonstrate the feasibility of utilizing biomechanical simulations to regularize a weakly-supervised anatomical-label-driven *registration network* for aligning pre-procedural magnetic resonance (MR) and 3D intra-procedural transrectal ultrasound (TRUS) images. A *discriminator network* is optimized to distinguish the registration-predicted displacement fields from the motion data simulated by finite element analysis. During training, the registration network simultaneously aims to maximize similarity between anatomical labels that drives image alignment and to minimize an adversarial *generator loss* that measures divergence between the predicted- and simulated deformation. The end-to-end trained network enables efficient and fully-automated registration that only requires an MR and TRUS image pair as input, without anatomical labels or simulated data during inference. 108 pairs of labelled MR and TRUS images from 76 prostate cancer patients and 71,500 nonlinear finite-element simulations from 143 different patients were used for this study. We show that, with *only* gland segmentation as training labels, the proposed method can help predict physically plausible deformation without any other smoothness penalty. Based on cross-validation experiments using 834 pairs of independent validation landmarks, the proposed adversarial-regularized registration achieved a target registration error of 6.3 mm that is significantly lower than those from several other regularization methods.

1 Introduction

The most recent image registration methods based on convolutional neural networks employ regularization strategies that incorporate non-application-specific prior knowledge of deformation between images to register. Unsupervised learning methods

© Springer Nature Switzerland AG 2018
A. F. Frangi et al. (Eds.): MICCAI 2018, LNCS 11070, pp. 774–782, 2018.
https://doi.org/10.1007/978-3-030-00928-1_87

that maximize similarity measures between two images, e.g. [1, 2], rely on transformation parameterization via rigid or spline-based models, and/or smoothness penalty terms, such as the norm of displacement gradients, to predict physically plausible deformation. For supervised learning approaches, e.g. [3], deformation regularization is embedded in surrogate ground-truth displacements, such as those obtained from classical registration methods, to predict detailed voxel-level displacements.

For instance, anatomical labels have been proposed to drive a so-called weakly-supervised learning method to infer dense displacements for interventional multimodal image fusion applications [4], which commonly lack a robust intensity-based similarity measure and ground-truth deformation. For training their network, more than 4,000 anatomical structures were manually delineated from prostate cancer patient images. Obtaining sufficient anatomical landmarks is constrained not only by the substantial expert effort in labelling volumetric data, but also by inherent limitations on the number of available corresponding anatomical features from different imaging modalities (in this case MR and TRUS). In the same clinical application, using fewer anatomical labels for training leads to significantly larger target registration errors (TREs), whilst we show in this paper that deformation regularization is important to avoid overfitting to limited labels.

We further argue that application-specific biologically-plausible prior on organ motion may lessen the quantity and/or quality of anatomical labels required for training data-driven registration methods. Biomechanical finite-element (FE) simulations of intraoperative prostate motion, modelling nonlinear, anisotropic and inhomogeneous properties of soft tissue, have been applied to constrain pair-wise multimodal non-rigid image fusion [5–7]. In particular, population-based motion models from previous patient data that can be instantiated to provide patient-specific constraints for unseen data, e.g. [7], have advantages in the prostate modelling: FE simulations can be generated using MR images from patients whose TRUS images are not available and the registration network can be fine-tuned for imaging-protocol-specific data without repeating large numbers of simulations. However, fully-unsupervised generative modelling of complex biomechanical simulations over the entire deformation domain (as opposed to modelling only shapes or surfaces) is non-trivial and has not been applied to neural-network-based registration methods.

We demonstrate, to our knowledge for the first time, that it is feasible to optimize an end-to-end registration network using an adversarial strategy that penalizes the divergence between the registration-predicted deformation and the FE-simulated training data. The resulting automatic registration is useful to support a wide range of interventional real-time applications, such as focal therapy and targeted biopsy [8].

2   Method

2.1   Adversarial Deformation Regularization

During the training of a registration network, the network parameters $\theta^{(reg)}$ are optimized to predict a dense displacement field (DDF) that warps the moving image to spatially align with the fixed image, by minimizing a *registration loss* $\mathcal{L}^{(reg)}$.

We propose a second neural network, the discriminator D with parameters $\theta^{(dis)}$, which is simultaneously optimized to classify the registration-network-predicted DDF and the FE-simulated DDF by minimizing a *discriminator loss* $\mathcal{L}^{(dis)}$. Considering the registration network as a DDF generator in adversarial learning [9], the registration loss can be regularized by an additive *generator loss* $\mathcal{L}^{(gen)}$, weighted by a scalar hyperparameter λ_{adv}. During every gradient-descent iteration, each of the two parameter sets $\theta^{(dis)}$ and $\theta^{(reg)}$ is updated once to minimize $\mathcal{L}^{(dis)}$ and $\left(\mathcal{L}^{(reg)} + \lambda_{adv} . \mathcal{L}^{(gen)} \right)$, respectively, while the other set is kept fixed. In Sect. 2.2, we describe a registration loss for a weakly-supervised learning method (illustrated in Fig. 1 as the lighter shaded components) for registering prostate MR- and TRUS images. In Sect. 2.3, we introduce the discriminator- and generator losses for this application, which we show lead to stable and effective training of the proposed adversarial regularization. Details of the network architectures and their training are provided in Sect. 2.4.

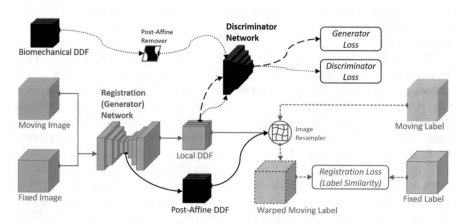

Fig. 1. The lighter shaded components connected by straight lines illustrate the weakly-supervised network training for multimodal image fusion [4]. The darker shaded components connected by curved lines depict the added elements that enable the proposed adversarial deformation regularization. Data flows required during inference, i.e. registration, are connected by solid lines, while other data connected by dotted- or dashed lines are only required for training.

2.2   Registration Loss for Weakly Supervised Multimodal Image Fusion

Assume N pairs of moving- and fixed images for training, $\{\mathbf{x}_n^A\}$ and $\{\mathbf{x}_n^B\}$, respectively, $n = 1, \ldots, N$. Further, assume M_n pairs of moving- and fixed labels, $\{\mathbf{y}_{mn}^A\}$ and $\{\mathbf{y}_{mn}^B\}$, representing corresponding anatomical structures identified in the nth image pair, $m = 1, \ldots, M_n$. The training of a registration network aims to predict inverse DDF $\boldsymbol{u}^{reg}$ that minimizes a negative *expected label similarity* over N training image pairs:

$$\mathcal{L}^{(reg)} = -\frac{1}{N}\sum\nolimits_{n=1}^{N}\frac{1}{M_n}\sum\nolimits_{m=1}^{M_n} J_{mn}\left(\mathcal{T}\left(\mathbf{y}_{mn}^{A}, \mathbf{u}_{n}^{reg}\right), \mathbf{y}_{mn}^{B}\right) \tag{1}$$

where the inner summation represents the image-level label similarity, averaging a label-level similarity measure J_{mn} over M_n labels associated with the nth image pair. Given a network-predicted displacement field $\mathbf{u}_{n}^{reg}\left(\mathbf{x}_{n}^{A}, \mathbf{x}_{n}^{B}; \boldsymbol{\theta}^{reg}\right)$, the label-level similarity is computed between the fixed label $\mathbf{y}_{mn}^{B}$ and the spatially warped moving label $\mathcal{T}\left(\mathbf{y}_{mn}^{A}, \mathbf{u}_{n}^{reg}\right)$. We adopt a differentiable, efficient and imaging-modality-independent multiscale-Dice $J_{mn} = \frac{1}{Z}\sum_{\sigma}\mathcal{S}_{Dice}\left(f_{\sigma}\left(\mathcal{T}\left(\mathbf{y}_{mn}^{A}, \mathbf{u}_{n}^{reg}\right)\right), f_{\sigma}\left(\mathbf{y}_{mn}^{B}\right)\right)$, where f_{σ} is a 3D Gaussian filter with an isotropic standard deviation σ (here, $\sigma \in \{0, 1, 2, 4, 8, 16, 32\}$ in mm and the number of scales $Z = 7$). $f_{\sigma=0}$ denotes unfiltered binary labels at the original scale included in averaging the soft probabilistic Dice values $\mathcal{S}_{Dice}$. The moving- and fixed images are the only network inputs. Therefore, the subsequent inference, i.e. registration, does not require anatomical labels, as illustrated in Fig. 1.

Displacement fields predicted by the multimodal registration network comprise of two combined geometric transformations: the biophysical deformation (deformation of anatomical structures) which should be regularized by the biomechanical simulations and the imaging-coordinate-system changes which should not. The imaging-coordinate-system changes reflect case-specific intra-procedural state (ultrasound imaging parameters such as probe position, field-of-view relative to anatomy, 3D voxel calibration and reconstruction) that is needed for intra-procedural registration and is not present in the biomechanical simulations. Therefore, to decouple these, the proposed network generates two transformations: a local DDF $\mathbf{u}_{n}^{local}$ intended to model only the biophysical deformation and an affine DDF $\mathbf{u}_{n}^{global}$ intended to model coordinate-system changes, as illustrated in Fig. 1. In minimizing the registration loss $\mathcal{L}^{(reg)}$, these are composed and optimised jointly, i.e. $\mathcal{T}\left(\mathbf{y}_{mn}^{A}, \mathbf{u}_{n}^{reg}\right) = \mathcal{T}\left(\mathcal{T}\left(\mathbf{y}_{mn}^{A}, \mathbf{u}_{n}^{local}\right), \mathbf{u}_{n}^{global}\right)$. To regularize the biophysical deformation alone, the network is trained such that the predicted local DDFs $\mathbf{u}_{n}^{local}$ match a regularizing data distribution (the FE-simulated data distribution described in Sect. 2.3) that has been normalized to exclude affine variation.

2.3 Adversarial Losses Based on Biomechanical Simulations

From a separate patient data set, assume a total of S FE simulations calculating the deformed nodal positions of the prostate glands and surrounding anatomical regions, defined on patient-specific tetrahedral meshes fitted to segmentations of the zonal structures, bladder, rectum and pelvic bones [5, 6]. For each simulation, the nonlinear neo-Hookean material properties of different regions and the boundary conditions, including initial position and movement of a virtual TRUS probe with variable-sized acoustic coupling balloon, are randomly sampled to cover the variance in intra-procedural scenarios. Inverting simulated deformation fields $\mathbf{v}_{s}^{sim}$ maps the deformed FE nodes $\mathbf{y}_{s}^{1}$ back to the undeformed $\mathbf{y}_{s}^{0}$, such that $\mathbf{y}_{s}^{0} = \mathcal{T}^{-1}\left(\mathbf{y}_{s}^{1}, \mathbf{v}_{s}^{sim}\right)$, $s = 1, \ldots, S$.

To normalize the data distribution in deformation space, each $\mathbf{v}_s^{sim}$ is decomposed into a global affine transformation $\mathbf{v}_s^{global}$ and an affine-removed local inverse displacement field $\mathbf{v}_s^{local}$, such that $\mathbf{y}_s^0 = \mathcal{T}^{-1}\left(\mathcal{T}^{-1}\left(\mathbf{y}_s^1, \mathbf{v}_s^{global}\right), \mathbf{v}_s^{local}\right)$. Using a linear least-squares method, $\mathbf{v}_s^{global}$ are computed to minimize $\left\|\mathcal{T}^{-1}\left(\mathbf{y}_s^1, \mathbf{v}_s^{global}\right) - \mathbf{y}_s^0\right\|^2$ before training. While the predicted- and simulated global transformations may have different distributions (as discussed in Sect. 2.2), the local transformations should have the same distribution. Specifically, the distribution of registration-predicted local DDFs P_{reg}, represented by random vector $\boldsymbol{u}^{local} \sim P_{reg}$ with samples $\left\{\mathbf{u}_n^{local}\right\}$, can be regularized by comparing to the FE-simulated data distribution P_{sim}, represented by random vector $\boldsymbol{v}^{local} \sim P_{sim}$ with samples $\left\{\mathbf{v}_s^{local}\right\}$. In this work, we adopt a stable discriminator loss $\mathcal{L}^{(dis)}$ and a non-saturating generator loss $\mathcal{L}^{(gen)}$ based on Jensen-Shannon divergence [10],

$$\mathcal{L}^{(dis)} = -\frac{1}{2}\mathbb{E}_{\boldsymbol{v}^{local}} \log D\left(\boldsymbol{v}^{local}\right) - \frac{1}{2}\mathbb{E}_{\boldsymbol{u}^{local}} \log \left(1 - D\left(\boldsymbol{u}^{local}\right)\right) + \frac{\gamma}{2}\Omega\left(\boldsymbol{u}^{local}, \boldsymbol{v}^{local}\right) \quad (2)$$

and

$$\mathcal{L}^{(gen)} = -\frac{1}{2}\mathbb{E}_{\boldsymbol{u}^{local}} \log D\left(\boldsymbol{u}^{local}\right) \quad (3)$$

respectively, where $\mathbb{E}$ denotes statistical expectation. A distribution smoothing term $\Omega\left(\boldsymbol{u}^{local}, \boldsymbol{v}^{local}\right)$ is added to stabilize adversarial training [10], weighted by an annealing scalar γ (here, exponentially decaying from 0.2 to 0.05 for the normalized data described in Sect. 3). Importantly, this annealing regularization also has a favorable effect on the registration network that encourages the affine branch to learn global transformation, so that the trained local DDF contains minimum affine component. It may be because that the smoothed distribution back-propagates stronger gradients from the generator loss to the local-DDF branch, relatively dominating its registration loss, especially during initial training stage when γ is large.

Without loss of generality, displacement samples from MR-, TRUS- and FE- coordinates have differently truncated finite sampling domains. As TRUS images have the most restricted fields-of-view, MR and TRUS are considered as moving- and fixed images, respectively, when computing registration loss. To avoid sampling larger-domain (MR and FE in this case) displacements from smaller-domain (TRUS) when computing adversarial losses, each FE-simulated DDF $\mathbf{v}_s^{local}$ is resampled from an estimated TRUS field-of-view before removing the affine component. The resampling coordinates are determined by matching the bounding boxes of the *deformed* prostate glands in FE- and TRUS coordinates, the latter of which is randomly sampled from the training TRUS data, i.e. the fixed labels. This estimate is also aided by data augmentation described in Sect. 2.4 to represent the variation in sampling domain.

2.4   Network Architectures and Training

As shown in Fig. 2, the registration network adapts a 3D encoder-decoder architecture taking a concatenated image pair as input, down-sampled and up-sampled by convolution (conv) and transpose-convolution (deconv), respectively, both with strides of two. The encoder consists of four residual network (resnet) blocks using $3 \times 3 \times 3$ conv kernels, with increasing numbers of feature channels n_{0-4} and decreasing feature map sizes s_{0-4}, both by a factor of two. The decoder has four *reverse* resnet blocks with, additionally, four trilinear additive up-sampling layers added over the deconv layers. Four summation skip layers shortcut the network resolution levels. Five trilinear-up-sampled displacement summands δ_{0-4} across levels s_{0-4} are summed to predict the output local DDF. 12 output affine parameters were predicted by an additional resnet block, branched out from the deepest encoder layer s_4. The discriminator shares a similar architecture with the registration network encoder, with first layer batch normalization (BN) removed and rectified linear units (relu) replaced by leaky relu (lrelu) [11]. It accepts input DDF x-, y- and z-channels and predicts binary classification logits after a fully-connected projection. Both networks start with $n_0 = 32$ initial channels.

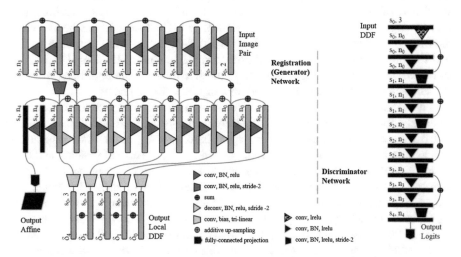

Fig. 2. The proposed registration- and discriminator networks (see details in Sect. 2.4).

The networks were implemented in TensorFlow™ with open-source code from NiftyNet [12]. For data augmentation, each image-label pair was warped by a random affine transformation and each simulated DDF was composed with a random affine for varying the sampling domain (as discussed in Sect. 2.3), before being fed into training. Using the Adam optimizer starting at a learning rate of 10^{-6} for both registration- and discriminator networks, each model was trained for 36 h with a minibatch size of 4 on a 24 GB NVIDIA® Quadro™ P6000 GPU card. The adversarial weight λ_{adv} was set to 0.01 for the reported results.

3 Experiments and Results

For computing the registration loss, a total of 108 pairs of T2-weighted MR- and TRUS images from 76 patients were acquired in multiple biopsy or therapy (ClinicalTrials.-gov Identifiers: NCT02290561, NCT02341677) clinical trials. Using a clinical ultrasound machine with a transperineal probe, 57-112 sagittal TRUS frames were acquired for each patient by rotating a digital brachytherapy stepper to reconstruct 3D volumes in Cartesian coordinates. Both MR- and TRUS volumes were normalized to zero-mean with unit-variance intensities after being resampled to $0.8 \times 0.8 \times 0.8$ mm^3 voxels. For assessing the regularization efficacy, gland segmentations were used as the only type of training landmarks, i.e. $M_n = 1$ in Eq. (1), which are arguably the most easy-to-annotate landmarks for both imaging modalities with many automated algorithms [13]. Gland segmentations on MR were acquired as per the trial protocols and those on TRUS were contoured on original slices. Both gland masks were then resampled to the voxel sizes of the associated MR or TRUS. For the adversarial training, MR images for FE meshing were acquired from an independent group of 143 patients who underwent the same procedures, without using their TRUS data in this study. For each patient, 500 FE simulations required 3–4 GPU-hours using a nonlinear FE solver [14]. Both the simulated- and predicted DDFs, as inputs of the discriminator, are normalized such that the simulated data have zero-mean and unit-variance displacements.

For quantitative validation, a total of 834 pairs of corresponding anatomical landmarks from the 108 paired images were manually labelled and further verified/edited by second observers, including apex, base, urethra, gland zonal separations, visible lesions, junctions between gland, vas deference and seminal vesicles, and other *ad hoc* landmarks such as calcifications and cysts. The annotation process took more than two hundred man-hours. Based on these independent validation landmarks, the proposed adversarial regularization was compared with two widely used smoothness regularizers, by adding a weighted L^2-norm of displacement gradients or bending energy to the registration loss in Eq. (1). For the reported results, both weights were set to 0.5, which produced the lowest median TREs from eight cross-validation experiments with four different weighting values, 0.01, 0.1, 0.5 and 1. In each fold of the 12-fold patient-level cross-validation experiments, 6–7 test patients were held out while the data from the remainder patients were used in training with all 71,500 FE simulations. The TRE was defined as root-mean-square centroid distance between the warped- and fixed validation labels. Dice similarity coefficient (DSC) was computed between the binary gland masks. These two test data results reflect quantitative clinical requirements in localizing target anatomy such as MR-visible tumors and avoiding heathy surroundings.

Approximately four 3D automatic registrations per second can be performed on the same GPU, which is adequate for many interventional applications. Figure 3 contains example registered images using the proposed network. The adversarial regularization appears more likely to preserve local details and, most interestingly, generates motion patterns unseen in those with other regularization, e.g. near-rigid motion around the rectum area where the virtual ultrasound probe is placed in FE simulations. As summarized in Table 1, the adversarial regularized registrations produced a significantly lower median TRE than the networks trained with L^2-norm or bending energy did (both *p-values* <*0.001*, paired Wilcoxon signed-rank tests at $\alpha = 0.05$), consistent with the visual inspection. The higher DSCs with L^2-norm, bending energy or without regularization may therefore indicate overfitting to the training gland labels. The obtained TRE results were based on 108 image pairs, compared to 8–19 patients validated in several previous work [5–7]. These still seem to be higher than that of 4.2 mm reported in [4], in which 4,000 training labels were required. Further comparisons, such as a comprehensive sampling of hyper-parameter values, may conclusively quantify the adversarial regularization, such as the trade-off of accuracy when using more training landmarks.

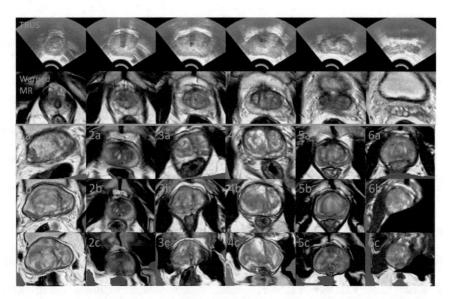

Fig. 3. The first two rows show example slices from a TRUS volume and the MR volume registered using the proposed network. The example warped MR slices (at the same slice locations in each patient, 1–6) are also compared between the proposed adversarial regularization (a), the bending energy (b) and registration without smoothness penalty (c).

Table 1. Medians [1st quatiles, 3rd quatiles] of TRE and DSC results from cross-validation

	Adversarial	Bending energy	L^2-norm	No regularization
TRE	6.3 [3.4, 8.7]	9.5 [4.6, 13.0]	10.2 [5.1, 14.7]	16.3 [14.1, 23.8]
DSC	0.82 [0.76, 0.87]	0.90 [0.83, 0.92]	0.91 [0.84, 0.92]	0.93 [0.88, 0.95]

4   Conclusion

In this work, we have proposed a novel adversarial deformation regularization, a potentially versatile strategy incorporating model-based constraints to assist data-driven image registration algorithms. We report promising results based on validation on a substantial interventional imaging data set from prostate cancer patients. Potential for further improving registration performance by, for instance, leveraging between the requirements of anatomical labels, universal smoothness measures and the proposed adversarial priors may be of interest in future research and clinical adoption.

Acknowledgement. This work received support from CRUK, the EPSRC and the Wellcome Trust (C28070/A19985, EP/M020533/1, NS/A000050/1, EP/N026993/1).

References

1. de Vos, B.D., Berendsen, F.F., Viergever, M.A., Staring, M., Išgum, I.: End-to-end unsupervised deformable image registration with a convolutional neural network. In: Cardoso, M.J., et al. (eds.) DLMIA/ML-CDS 2017. LNCS, vol. 10553, pp. 204–212. Springer, Cham (2017). https://doi.org/10.1007/978-3-319-67558-9_24
2. Cao, X., et al.: Deformable image registration based on similarity-steered CNN regression. In: Descoteaux, M., et al. (eds.) MICCAI 2017, Part I. LNCS, vol. 10433, pp. 300–308. Springer, Cham (2017). https://doi.org/10.1007/978-3-319-66182-7_35
3. Rohé, M.M., Datar, M., Heimann, T., Sermesant, M., Pennec, X.: SVF-Net: learning deformable image registration using shape matching. In: Descoteaux, M., et al. (eds.) MICCAI 2017, Part I. LNCS, vol. 10433, pp. 266–274. Springer, Cham (2017). https://doi.org/10.1007/978-3-319-66182-7_31
4. Hu, Y., et al.: Label-driven weakly-supervised learning for multimodal deformable image registration. In: 2018 IEEE 15th International Symposium on Biomedical Imaging (ISBI) (2018). arXiv:1711.01666
5. Wang, Y., et al.: Towards personalized statistical deformable model and hybrid point matching for robust MR-TRUS registration. IEEE-TMI **35**(2), 589–604 (2016)
6. Hu, Y., et al.: MR to ultrasound registration for image-guided prostate interventions. Med. Image Anal. **16**(3), 687–703 (2012)
7. Khallaghi, S., et al.: Statistical biomechanical surface registration: application to MR-TRUS fusion for prostate interventions. IEEE-TMI **34**(12), 2535–2549 (2015)
8. Valerio, M., et al.: Detection of clinically significant prostate cancer using magnetic resonance imaging-ultrasound fusion targeted biopsy. Eur. Urol. **68**(1), 8–19 (2015)
9. Goodfellow, I., et al.: Generative adversarial nets. In: NIPS 2014, pp. 2672–2680 (2014)
10. Roth, K., et al.: Stabilizing training of generative adversarial networks through regularization. In: NIPS 2017, pp. 2015–2025 (2017)
11. Radford, A., et al.: Unsupervised representation learning with deep convolutional generative adversarial networks (2015). arXiv preprint: arXiv:1511.06434
12. Gibson, E., et al.: NiftyNet: a deep-learning platform for medical imaging. Comput. Methods Programs Biomed. **158**, 113–122 (2018)
13. Litjens, G., et al.: Evaluation of prostate segmentation algorithms for MRI: the PROMISE12 challenge. Med. Image Anal. **18**(2), 359–373 (2014)
14. Johnsen, S.F., et al.: NiftySim: a GPU-based nonlinear finite element package for simulation of soft tissue biomechanics. IJCARS **10**(7), 1077–1095 (2015)

Fast Registration by Boundary Sampling and Linear Programming

Jan Kybic$^{(\boxtimes)}$ (ID) and Jiří Borovec

Faculty of Electrical Engineering, Czech Technical University in Prague,
Prague, Czech Republic
kybic@fel.cvut.cz, jiri.borovec@fel.cvut.cz

Abstract. We address the problem of image registration when speed is more important than accuracy. We present a series of simplification and approximations applicable to almost any pixel-based image similarity criterion. We first sample the image at a set of sparse keypoints in a direction normal to image edges and then create a piecewise linear convex approximation of the individual contributions. We obtain a linear program for which a global optimum can be found very quickly by standard algorithms. The linear program formulation also allows for an easy addition of regularization and trust-region bounds. We have tested the approach for affine and B-spline transformation representation but any linear model can be used. Larger deformations can be handled by multiresolution. We show that our method is much faster than pixel-based registration, with only a small loss of accuracy. In comparison to standard keypoint based registration, our method is applicable even if individual keypoints cannot be reliably identified and matched.

Keywords: Image registration · Linear programming

1 Introduction

Image registration [1] is one of the key image analysis tasks, especially in medical imaging. There are many scenarios, when image registration needs to be fast — consider matching preoperative and intraoperative images during surgery, interactive change detection of CT or MRI data for a busy radiologist, deformation compensation or 3D alignment of large histological slices for a busy pathologist, or processing large amounts of images from today's high-throughput imaging methods. On the other hand, sub-pixel or even pixel-level accuracy is not always required, which gives us the possibility to trade accuracy for speed. In this work, we shall present such a method.

Feature-based methods (e.g. [2]) are not always suitable for biomedical images, since there are few reliable and distinguishable features (e.g. corners) and weak constraints on the deformation field. The other class of registration

---

This work was supported by the Czech Science Foundation project 17-15361S.

A. F. Frangi et al. (Eds.): MICCAI 2018, LNCS 11070, pp. 783–791, 2018.
https://doi.org/10.1007/978-3-030-00928-1_88

methods, based on minimizing a pixel-based image similarity criterion, are often slow. Luckily, it turns out that criterion evaluation can be simplified, without compromising registration accuracy too much. Only a subset of the pixels can be used to evaluate the criterion [3] or its gradient [4], possibly with more weights given to pixels with a high gradient [5]. In the extreme, only edge pixels would be sampled, which leads to the idea of registering images by their segmentations, which can be done e.g. by descriptor matching [6], or region boundary matching [7].

We assume that a correspondences can be found reliably between regions but not between points in their interior. We represent the criterion as a sum of contributions from a set of sampling points placed sparsely on the region boundaries, as in [8]. Our main new insight is that if the region boundary moves in the normal direction, the criterion change is piecewise linear. This allows to formulate the optimization as a linear program (LP), which can be solved very efficiently. We present two variants of our registration method: LPSEG based on a segmentation, and LPNOSEG based on points of high gradient.

1.1   Other Related Work

Taylor and Bhusnurmath [9] create a global piecewise linear approximation of the similarity criterion, considering all pixels and all possible displacements, which is a lower bound of the true criterion. This is robust but slow. Ben-Ezra et al. [10] start by selecting a small set of keypoints using optical flow and a motion model is fitted using linear programming. This method is capable of running at several images per second but requires the motion to be small and the motion model to be simple. Linear programming can also be used for keypoint matching [11].

2   Method

2.1   Similarity Criterion

A pixel dissimilarity measure ϱ induces an image dissimilarity criterion

$$J_c(f, g) = \int\limits_{\mathbf{x} \in \Omega} \varrho\big(f(\mathbf{x}), g(\mathbf{x})\big)\, \mathrm{d}\mathbf{x} \tag{1}$$

where $\Omega \subseteq \mathbb{R}^d$ is the image domain and f, g can be intensities, but also texture features, or segmentation labels. This formulation includes directly criteria such as SSD or SAD, while other popular dissimilarity measures such as mutual information can be represented approximately, with ϱ depending on the images and updated occasionally. During registration, we calculate the criterion $J_c(f, g')$ between a reference image f and a transformed version $g'(\mathbf{x}) = (g \circ T)(\mathbf{x}) = g\big(T(\mathbf{x})\big)$ of the moving image g. Following [8], we assume to be given a set of M points $\mathbf{p}_i$ on the boundaries between regions in the image f, with normals $\mathbf{n}_i$. We are also given an a priori estimate T_0 of T, which is

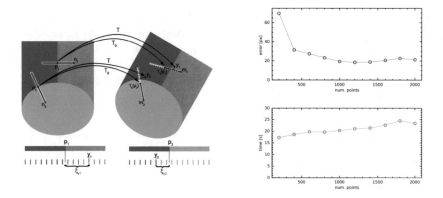

Fig. 1. *Left:* Illustration of the sampling points $\mathbf{p}_i$, their normals $\mathbf{n}_i$, and transformations T_0 and T. *Right:* The dependency of the registration error *(top graph)* and time *(bottom graph)* on the number of sampling points for LPNOSEG.

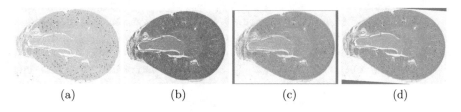

(a)   (b)   (c)   (d)

Fig. 2. Rat-kidney. Reference image (H&E) *(a)*, moving image (Podocin) *(b)*, overlay before *(c)* and after *(d)* — look e.g. at the top edge for differences.

locally close to linear. If $T_0 \approx T$, then in g there is also a boundary close to a point $\mathbf{v}_i = T_0(\mathbf{p}_i)$ with a scaled normal $\mathbf{m}_i = \big(\nabla T_0(\mathbf{p}_i)\big)\mathbf{n}_i$. The displacement along the boundary can be neglected, since both f and g are supposed to change only in the normal direction. Hence, the transformation T can be approximated by its normal projection ξ_i at points $\mathbf{p}_i$ (see Fig. 1, left)

$$T(\mathbf{p}_i) \approx \mathbf{v}_i + \mathbf{m}_i \xi_i \tag{2}$$

$$\text{where} \quad \xi_i = \big\langle T(\mathbf{p}_i) - \mathbf{v}_i, \tilde{\mathbf{m}}_i \big\rangle \quad \text{with} \quad \tilde{\mathbf{m}}_i = \mathbf{m}_i \big/ \|\mathbf{m}_i\|^2 \tag{3}$$

and the criterion J_c can be approximated as a sum of contributions at $\mathbf{p}_i$,

$$J_c(f, g') \approx J(T) + \text{const}, \qquad \text{where} \quad J(T) = \sum_{i=1}^{M} D_i(\xi_i) \tag{4}$$

The individual contributions are calculated by integration along the normals

$$D_i(\xi) = \sigma_i \int_{-h_{\max}}^{h_{\max}} \varrho\big(f(\mathbf{x}), g'(\mathbf{x})\big)\mathrm{d}h \quad \text{with} \quad \mathbf{x} = \mathbf{p}_i + \mathbf{n}_i h \tag{5}$$

with σ_i being the area corresponding to $\mathbf{p}_i$ and $h_{\max}$ the region width.

In the NLSEG method, a simple greedy strategy can provide sampling points $\mathbf{p}_i$ on the class boundaries and their normals [8], given a pixel- or superpixel-based segmentations. The NLNOSEG method differs in choosing points of high gradient, pruned with non-maxima suppression, and with $\mathbf{n}_i$ being the gradient direction. See Fig. 3ab for examples.

2.2 Piecewise Linear Approximation

Using the formula $T(\mathbf{p}_i + \mathbf{n}h) \approx \mathbf{v}_i + \mathbf{m}_i(\xi_i + h)$, the integral (5) can be approximated by a sum over h, sampling at 1 pixel intervals:

$$D_i(\xi) = \sigma_i \sum_{h=-h_{\max}}^{h_{\max}} \varrho\left(f(\mathbf{p}_i + \mathbf{n}_i h), g(\mathbf{v}_i + \mathbf{m}_i(\xi_i + h))\right) \tag{6}$$

If $\mathbf{p}_i$ is at a boundary of a segmentation f, then $f(\mathbf{p}_i + \mathbf{n}_i h)$ is going to be equal to some f^- for $h < 0$ and otherwise to f^+. Similarly, we assume that $g(\mathbf{v}_i + \mathbf{m}_i h)$ is equal to some g^- for $h < \zeta_i$ and otherwise to g^+, where ζ_i is the unknown normal shift at $\mathbf{p}_i$ due to the difference between T_0 and the true transformation.

The (continuous) contribution $D_i(\xi_t)$ is a convolution of these step functions:

$$D_i(\xi_i) = \begin{cases} u_i^0 + h_{\max} u_i^+ & \text{if } h_{\max} \leq t \\ u_i^0 + t u_i^+ & \text{if } 0 \leq t \leq h_{\max} \\ u_i^0 + t u_i^- & \text{if } -h_{\max} \leq t \leq 0 \\ u_i^0 - h_{\max} u_i^- & \text{if } t \leq -h_{\max} \end{cases} \tag{7}$$

$$\text{with} \quad t = \zeta_i - \xi_h, \qquad u_i^0 = h_{\max}\left(\varrho(f^-, g^-) + \varrho(f^+, g^+)\right)$$
$$u_i^+ = \varrho(f^+, g^-) - \varrho(f^+, g^+), \qquad u_i^- = \varrho(f^-, g^-) - \varrho(f^-, g^+)$$

For $|t| > h_{\max}$, the contribution $D_i(\xi_i)$ is constant and does not bring any information. This is avoided by choosing a suitable $\xi_{\max}$, ensuring that $D_i(\xi_i)$ is only evaluated for $|\xi_i| \leq \xi_{\max}$, assuming that the true shift also satisfies $|\zeta_i| \leq \xi_{\max}$ and choosing $h_{\max} \geq 2\xi_{\max}$.

Since the parameters in (7) are in general not known, we shall estimate them as follows: Evaluate $D_i(\xi)$ for all shifts $\xi = -\xi_{\max} \ldots \xi_{\max}$ using (6). Keeping the minimum and find the slope by least-squares fitting:

$$\hat{\zeta}_i = \arg\min_{\xi} D_i(\xi), \qquad \hat{u}_0 = D_i(\hat{\zeta}_i) \tag{8}$$

$$\hat{u}_i^+ = \arg\min_{u_i^+} \sum_{\xi=\zeta_i+1}^{\xi_{\max}} \left(D_i(\xi) - \hat{D}_i(\xi)\right)^2 = \frac{\sum_{\xi}\left(D_i(\xi) - \hat{u}_0\right)(\xi - \hat{\zeta}_i)}{\sum_{\xi}(\xi - \hat{\zeta}_i)^2}$$

and similarly for $\hat{u}_i^-$. This is both faster and more robust than fitting all four parameters. Note that the value of u_i^0 is not needed and can be dropped.

2.3   Geometric Model and Regularization

A geometrical transformation $T : \mathbb{R}^d \to \mathbb{R}^d$ is represented as a linear combination

$$T(\mathbf{x}) = \varphi_0(\mathbf{x}) + \sum_{j=1}^{N} c_j \varphi_j(\mathbf{x}) \qquad (9)$$

with some basis functions φ_j and N scalar coefficients c_j. This includes many practically used transformation functions, such as an affine transformation, radial basis functions etc. For nonlinear (elastic) transformations, we shall use uniformly spaced B-splines [12], The image registration problem is then:

$$\mathbf{c}^* = \arg\min E(\mathbf{c}) \qquad (10)$$
$$E(\mathbf{c}) = J(\mathbf{c}) + R(\mathbf{c}) \qquad (11)$$

with the data criterion $J(\mathbf{c}) = J\big(T(\mathbf{c})\big)$ defined by (4) and (9). A regularization R is needed because the image is usually not completely covered by the sampling points $\mathbf{u}_i$ and some coefficients c_j might therefore not be completely determined. We have chosen to penalize the ℓ_1 norms of the coefficients and their first-order finite differences along coordinate axes [13]:

$$R(\mathbf{c}) = \gamma \, |\Delta \mathbf{c}|_{\ell_1} + \lambda \, |\mathbf{c}|_{\ell_1} \qquad (12)$$

2.4   Linear Program

We can now proceed to formulate the linear program, which will help us recover the optimal transformation parameters c_j, given the contribution approximation parameters $\hat{u}_i^+$, $\hat{u}_i^-$, $\hat{\zeta}_i$ (8). The criterion (11) is written as

$$\min \left[\sum_{i=1}^{M} D_i + \gamma \sum_{(j,k)\in\mathcal{N}} r_{jk} + \lambda \sum_{j=1}^{N} s_j \right] \qquad (13)$$

where the absolute values from (12) were replaced using inequalities

$$c_j - c_k \le r_{jk}, \quad c_j - c_k \le r_{jk}, \qquad c_j \le s_j, \quad -c_j \le s_j \qquad (14)$$

where (j,k) are pairs of indices of neighboring B-spline coefficients c. Similarly, we replace the piecewise linear model (7) by

$$D_i \ge (\xi_i - \xi_i^0) u_i^+ \qquad\qquad \xi_i \le \xi_{\max} \qquad (15)$$
$$D_i \ge (\xi_i - \xi_i^0) u_i^- \qquad\qquad -\xi_i \le \xi_{\max} \qquad (16)$$

It remains to eliminate ξ_i from the above equations, using the linear relationship between the shifts ξ_i and transformation coefficients c_j from (3) and (9)

$$\xi_i = \big\langle \varphi_0(\mathbf{x}_i) - \mathbf{v}_i, \tilde{\mathbf{m}}_i \big\rangle + \sum_{j=1}^{N} c_j \big\langle \varphi_j(\mathbf{x}_i), \tilde{\mathbf{m}}_i \big\rangle \qquad (17)$$

The resulting LP with approximately $(2+d)N + M$ variables (neglecting the edge cases), namely D_i, c_j, r_{jk} and s_j, is solved using the simplex or interior point methods.

Table 1. *Left:* Average runtime in seconds and geometric error in pixels. *Right:* Time for solving one LP instance with 1200 sampling points and 128 B-spline coefficients for different LP solvers.

Method	Time	Error
bUnwarpJ [14]	676	129
elastix (B-splines) [15]	1286	125
FRSEG [8]	105	18
RVSS [14]	91	151
RNiftyReg (GPU)	22	67
DROP [13]	403	27
LPSEG (new)	36	50
LPNOSEG (new)	20	19

LP method	time
Gurobi simplex	54 ms
Gurobi interior point	79 ms
GLPK simplex	145 ms
GLPK interior point	failed

2.5   Iteration and Multiresolution

Iteration: When the LP is solved, the resulting sampling point positions $T(\mathbf{p}_i)$ are compared with the sampled positions used in (6). If more than a given percentage (e.g. 10 %) of the points are considered unacceptable, the procedure is repeated with the initial transformation T_0 replaced by T. A point $T(\mathbf{p}_i)$ is unacceptable if its associated shift ξ_i is close to the assumed maximum amplitude $\xi_{\max}$ (usually 5–10 pixels) or if the angular difference with $T_0(\mathbf{p}_i)$ is larger than a given threshold (e.g. 60°).

Multiresolution: At each level, the image size is reduced by a factor of two and the resulting transformation is used as the initial transformation T_0 at the next finer level. The number of sampling points is also reduced at each level by taking every second point, unless a desired minimum number of points is achieved. The final multiresolution aspect is that we usually start by an affine transformation and progressively shift to B-spline models with more and more parameters. This is controlled by the desired knot spacing.

3   Experiments

The first example in Fig. 2 shows histological slices and their alignment by the LPSEG algorithm. For these images of $\approx 800 \times 1100$ pixels, the complete registration process takes about 2 s. However, most of the time is taken by the segmentation; once sampling points are extracted, the registration itself takes only 0.2 s.

Images in Fig. 3 are already much larger ($\approx 5000 \times 3000$ pixels) and the running time of the LPSEG method has grown to 36 s, with 33 s taken by the segmentation and only 3 s by the registration itself. The segmentation-less LPNOSEG is faster, requiring around 20 s, with 15 s to identify the sampling points and 5 s for the registration itself. In this case, the registration by LPNOSEG is better (see the bottom edge of Fig. 3hi).

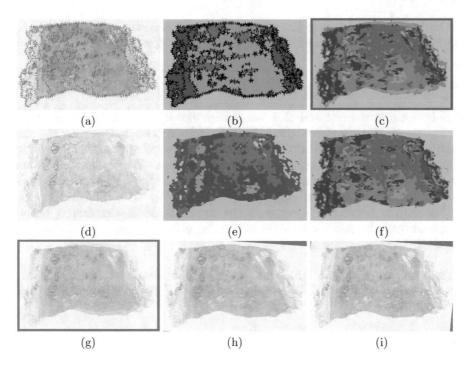

Fig. 3. Reference image with sampling points *(a)* and its segmentation *(b)* with independently extracted sampling points, segmentation overlay before registration *(c)*. Moving image *(d)*, its segmentation *(e)*, and segmentation overlay after registration *(f)*. Image overlay before registration *(g)*, image overlay after LPSEG registration using segmentation *(h)* and using LPNOSEG without segmentation *(i)*.

The graphs in the right part of Fig. 1 show the dependency of the running time and the mean registration error (measured using manually identified landmarks [8]) on the number of sampling points for the LPNOSEG algorithm. Note that the error decreases with an increasing number of sampling points and then it stagnates, as further points are probably not sufficiently reliable or accurate. The running time increases with the number of points but only slowly, the dominant part seems to be the preprocessing.

Table 1 (right) compares the GLPK[1] and Gurobi[2] LP solvers. Finally, the left part of Table 1 compares the speed and accuracy of our two proposed methods (LPSEG, LPNOSEG) with the alternatives mentioned in [8] on a subset of the same dataset with images of size around 5000×3000 (as in Fig. 3). FRSEG [8] (fast registration of segmented images) is similar to LPSEG but does not use the LP formulation. We see that LPSEG is fast and LPNOSEG even faster. The only other method with comparable speed is the GPU-accelerated version

---

[1] https://www.gnu.org/software/glpk/.

[2] http://www.gurobi.com.

of RNiftyReg. At the same time, our methods are accurate, outperformed only by the slower FRSEG, which is based on the same ideas.

4 Conclusions

We have presented two very fast image registration methods based on simplifying images using segmentations (LPSEG method) and representing the similarity criterion using contributions at a set of sampling points. The novelty here is representing the problem as a linear program, allowing an efficient and robust optimization. We have also shown that segmentation can be sometimes advantageously replaced by edge-finding (LPNOSEG), with a further increase in speed. The bottleneck is currently the segmentation or edge-finding but we hope it should be possible to avoid it by using a faster segmentation algorithm or a GPU implementation.

Acknowledgments. The authors acknowledge the support of the Czech Science Foundation project 17-15361S and the OP VVV project CZ.02.1.01/0.0/0.0/16_019/0000765.

References

1. Zitová, B., Flusser, J.: Image registration methods: a survey. Image Vis. Comput. **21**, 977–1000 (2003)
2. Lowe, D.: Distinctive image features from scale-invariant keypoints. Int. J. Comput. Vis. **60**(2), 91–110 (2004)
3. Thévenaz, P.: Halton sampling for image registration based on mutual information. Sampl. Theory Signal and Image Process. **7**(2), 141–171 (2008)
4. Klein, S., Staring, M., Pluim, J.P.W.: Evaluation of optimization methods for nonrigid medical image registration using mutual information and B-splines. IEEE Trans. Image Proc. **16**(12), 2879–2890 (2007)
5. Sabuncu, M., Ramadge, P.: Gradient based nonuniform subsampling for information-theoretic alignment methods. In: Conference of the IEEE Engineering in Medicine and Biology Society, pp. 1683–1686 (2004)
6. Domokos, C., et al.: Nonlinear shape registration without correspondences. IEEE Trans. Pattern Anal. Mach. Intell. **34**(5), 943–958 (2012)
7. Droske, M., Ring, W.: A Mumford-Shah level-set approach for geometric image registration. SIAM Appl. Math. **66**(6), 2127–2148 (2005)
8. Kybic. J., et al.: Fast registration of segmented images by normal sampling. In: CVPRW: BioImage Computing Workshop, pp. 11–19, June 2015
9. Taylor, C.J., Bhusnurmath, A.: Solving image registration problems using interior point methods. In: Forsyth, D., Torr, P., Zisserman, A. (eds.) ECCV 2008. LNCS, vol. 5305, pp. 638–651. Springer, Heidelberg (2008). https://doi.org/10.1007/978-3-540-88693-8_47
10. Ben-Ezra, M.: Real-time motion analysis with linear programming. Comput. Vis. Image Underst. **78**(1), 32–52 (2000)
11. Jiang, H., et al.: Matching by linear programming and successive convexification. IEEE Trans. Pattern Anal. Mach. Intell. **29**(6), 959–975 (2007)

12. Unser, M.: Splines: a perfect fit for signal and image processing. IEEE Signal Processing Magazine **16**(6), 22–38 (1999)
13. Glocker, B.: Dense image registration through MRFs and efficient linear programming. Med. Image Anal. **12**(6), 731–741 (2008)
14. Arganda-Carreras, I., Sorzano, C.O.S., Marabini, R., Carazo, J.M., Ortiz-de-Solorzano, C., Kybic, J.: Consistent and elastic registration of histological sections using vector-spline regularization. In: Beichel, R.R., Sonka, M. (eds.) CVAMIA 2006. LNCS, vol. 4241, pp. 85–95. Springer, Heidelberg (2006). https://doi.org/10.1007/11889762_8
15. Klein, S., Staring, M., Murphy, K.: Elastix: a toolbox for intensity-based medical image registration. IEEE Trans. Med. Imaging **29**(1), 196–205 (2010)

Learning an Infant Body Model from RGB-D Data for Accurate Full Body Motion Analysis

Nikolas Hesse[1(✉)], Sergi Pujades[2], Javier Romero[3], Michael J. Black[2], Christoph Bodensteiner[1], Michael Arens[1], Ulrich G. Hofmann[4], Uta Tacke[5], Mijna Hadders-Algra[6], Raphael Weinberger[7], Wolfgang Müller-Felber[7], and A. Sebastian Schroeder[7]

[1] Fraunhofer Institute of Optronics, System Technologies and Image Exploitation, Ettlingen, Germany
nikolas.hesse@iosb.fraunhofer.de
[2] Max Planck Institute for Intelligent Systems, Tübingen, Germany
[3] Amazon, Barcelona, Spain
[4] University Medical Center Freiburg, Faculty of Medicine, University of Freiburg, Freiburg im Breisgau, Germany
[5] University Children's Hospital Basel, Basel, Switzerland
[6] University Medical Center Groningen, University of Groningen, Groningen, Netherlands
[7] Hauner Children's Hospital, Ludwig Maximilian University, Munich, Germany

Abstract. Infant motion analysis enables early detection of neurodevelopmental disorders like cerebral palsy (CP). Diagnosis, however, is challenging, requiring expert human judgement. An automated solution would be beneficial but requires the accurate capture of 3D full-body movements. To that end, we develop a non-intrusive, low-cost, lightweight acquisition system that captures the shape and motion of infants. Going beyond work on modeling adult body shape, we learn a 3D Skinned Multi-Infant Linear body model (SMIL) from noisy, low-quality, and incomplete RGB-D data. SMIL is publicly available for research purposes at http://s.fhg.de/smil. We demonstrate the capture of shape and motion with 37 infants in a clinical environment. Quantitative experiments show that SMIL faithfully represents the data and properly factorizes the shape and pose of the infants. With a case study based on general movement assessment (GMA), we demonstrate that SMIL captures enough information to allow medical assessment. SMIL provides a new tool and a step towards a fully automatic system for GMA.

Keywords: Body models · Data-driven · Cerebral palsy
Motion analysis · Pose tracking · General movement assessment

1 Introduction

One of the most common neurodevelopmental disorders in children is *cerebral palsy* (CP), which is caused by abnormal development of, or damage to the brain.

© Springer Nature Switzerland AG 2018
A. F. Frangi et al. (Eds.): MICCAI 2018, LNCS 11070, pp. 792–800, 2018.
https://doi.org/10.1007/978-3-030-00928-1_89

Symptoms vary, but often include spasticity, abnormal muscle tone or impaired motor skills. Early intervention seems to have a positive effect on cognitive and motor outcome [18], yet requires early diagnosis. Neurological examinations or technical assessment of brain functions show a large variation in predicting developmental outcome [5], and reliable diagnoses are generally obtained between the age of one and two years [19]. Prechtl discovered that the quality of spontaneous movements, in particular of the *general movements* (GMs), at the corrected age of 2–4 months accurately reflects the state of the infant's nervous system [15]. As of today, the *general movement assessment* (GMA) method achieves the highest reliability for the diagnosis and prediction of CP at such an early age [11]. Trained experts, usually physicians, analyze video recordings of infants and rate the GM quality, ranging from *normal optimal* to *definitely abnormal* in a modified version of Prechtl's GMA [5]. Infants with abnormal movement quality have very high risk of developing CP or minor neurological dysfunction [5]. Despite being the most accurate clinical tool for early diagnosis, GMA requires a trained expert and suffers from human variability. These experts need regular practice and re-calibration to assure adequate ratings. This motivates the need for automated analysis. To allow GMA automation, a practical system must first demonstrate that is capable of capturing the relevant information needed for GMA. Moreover, to allow its widespread use, the solution needs to be seamlessly integrated into the clinical routine. Ideally it should be low-cost, easy-to-setup, and easy-to-use, producing minimal overhead to the standard examination protocol, and not affect the behavior of the infants.

We present the first work on 3D shape and 3D pose estimation of infants, as well as the first work on learning a statistical 3D body model from low-quality, incomplete RGB-D data of freely moving humans. We contribute (i) a new statistical *Skinned Multi-Infant Linear* model (SMIL), learned from 37 RGB-D low-quality sequences of freely moving infants, and (ii) a method to register the SMIL model to the RGB-D sequences, capable of handling severe occlusions and fast movements. Quantitative experiments show how SMIL properly factorizes the pose and the shape of the infants, and allows the captured data to be accurately represented in a low-dimensional space. With a case-study involving a high-risk former preterm study population, we demonstrate that the amount of motion detail captured by SMIL is sufficient to enable accurate GMA ratings. Thus, SMIL provides a fundamental tool that can form a component in a fully automatic system for the assessment of GMs. We make SMIL available to the community for research purposes.

We review related work in the fields of *medical analysis of infant motion* and *statistical body modeling*.

An overview of existing approaches for automating and objectifying the task of GMA is presented in [11]. For automated analysis, accurately capturing the motions of freely moving infants is key and has been approached in different ways. *Intrusive* systems rely on markers captured by camera systems [12], or on sensors attached to the infant's limbs, like electro-magnetical sensors [8] or accelerometers [6]. These approaches are highly accurate, since measurement

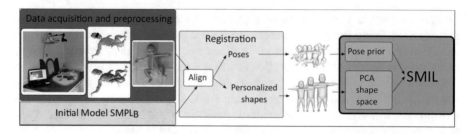

Fig. 1. Method overview. We acquire and preprocess RGB-D data. We create an initial infant model (SMPL_B) based on SMPL [9]. We register SMPL_B to the preprocessed data. We learn our new Skinned Multi-Infant Linear model (SMIL) consisting of a new shape space, and a new pose prior from the registrations.

units are directly connected to the limbs. However, the sensors/markers affect the infant's behavior. In addition, the setup and calibration of such systems can be cumbersome, the hardware is often expensive and the acquisition protocol requires time consuming human intervention. *Non-intrusive* systems rely on simple, low-cost video or depth cameras, which facilitates usage in a broad clinical environment. From raw RGB videos, different body parts are tracked using optical flow [19] or weakly supervised motion segmentation techniques [16]. RGB-D sensors allow capturing motion in all three dimensions, e.g. by estimating joint positions based on a random ferns body part classifier [7]. Most similar to our work, the authors in [13] fit a body model consisting of simplistic shapes to RGB-D data and compare their method to sparse manually annotated landmarks. Differently to [13], we (i) learn a realistic infant body model from data, (ii) resolve rotational ambiguities by capturing full body shape and pose instead of 3D joint positions, and (iii) evaluate our model with surface distances, accounting both for pose and shape accuracy.

Statistical body models aim to describe the surface of humans or animals in a low-dimensional space. These models rely on sparse [1] or dense [9] surface data captured from cooperative, easy-to-instruct subjects or 3D toy models [21]. Infants present a major challenge in terms of data acquisition as they are not cooperative and cannot be instructed. Unlike previous work on human body models, we are not aware of a repository of high quality scans of infants, and learn a 3D body model from RGB-D sequences of freely moving humans.

2   Learning the Infant Body Model

We create an initial infant model, *SMPL_B*, by adapting SMPL [9], and register it to the preprocessed data. Then, we learn our *Skinned Multi-Infant Linear* model (SMIL) from these registrations. The method overview is illustrated in Fig. 1. Manual intervention is only required in adjusting the pose priors (once for SMPL_B, once for SMIL), initial template creation (once for SMPL_B), and defining the number of clothing parts for each sequence (preprocessing).

Data Acquisition. We record freely moving infants for 3 to 5 min on the examination table without external stimulation, using a Microsoft Kinect V1 RGB-D camera. Ethics approval was obtained from Ludwig Maximilian University Munich (LMU) and all parents gave written informed consent in participating in this study.

Preprocessing. In the preprocessing step, we (i) transform depth images to 3D point clouds using the camera calibration, (ii) filter all table points not belonging to the infant by fitting a plane to the examination table, (iii) segment the infant point cloud into skin, diaper and onesie by adapting the segmentation method described in [14]. Finally, we (iv) extract landmarks from the RGB images, which provides us with 2D pose [4], hand locations [17] and facial landmarks [20], with their respective confidence estimates.

Initial Model. Learning an infant shape space is a chicken-and-egg problem: a model is needed to register the data, and registrations are needed to learn a model. We manually create our initial model $SMPL_B$, based on SMPL [9], a statistical body model learned from thousands of adult 3D scans. Simply scaling the adult model to infant size does not provide satisfactory results, as body proportions severely differ. We (i) replace the SMPL mean shape with an infant body mesh created with MakeHuman [10], (ii) leave the SMPL shape space untouched, (iii) scale the pose blendshapes to infant size, and (iv) manually adjust the pose priors. Because pose priors were learned on standing adults and not lying infants, adjusting these manually is important to prevent the model from explaining shape deformations with pose parameters.

Registration. The $SMPL_B$ registrations to the preprocessed 3D point clouds are computed by minimizing the energy

$$E(\beta, \theta) = E_{data} + E_{lm} + E_{sm} + E_{sc} + E_{table} + E_\beta + E_\theta, \tag{1}$$

where E_{data} measures the scan to registration mesh distance, E_{lm} penalizes the distance between estimated and registration landmarks projected to 2D as in [3], E_{sm} enforces temporal pose smoothness and E_{sc} penalizes model self intersections as in [3]. E_{table} integrates background information in order to keep the bottom side of the registration body close to, but not inside the table. E_β and E_θ are the shape and pose prior, that enforce the shape parameters to be close to the mean, and help to prevent unnatural poses, respectively.

Initialization. Since the optimization problem is highly non-convex, the success of the registration depends on a good initialization. Differently to adults, infants are incapable of striking poses on demand. Thus, relying on a predefined initial pose is unpractical. We overcome this by proposing a novel automatic method to select an initialization frame. We assume that a body segment is most visible if it has maximum 2D length over the sequence, since perspective projection decreases 2D body segment length. We choose the initialization frame as $f_{init} = \operatorname{argmax}_f \sum_{s \in S} \operatorname{len}(s, f) * c(s, f)$, where S is the set of segments, $\operatorname{len}(s, f)$ is the 2D length of the segment s at frame f, and $c(s, f)$ is the estimated confidence of the joints belonging to s at frame f. For f_{init} we compute the initial registration

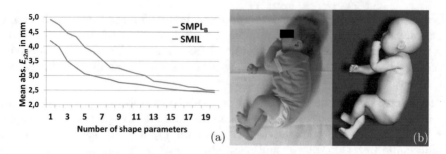

Fig. 2. (a) Average scan-to-mesh error E_{s2m} in mm w.r.t. the number of shape parameters for the two models aligned to all fusion scans. (b) Example of RGB input image and the result of SMIL registered to the data.

by optimizing a simplified version of Eq. 1. It contains a 2D body pose landmark term similar to E_{lm}, a simplified data term, a strong prior on pose, and a shape regularizer. From f_{init}, we sequentially process the neighbouring frames (forward and backward in time), using as initialization the shape and pose results of the last processed frame.

Personalized Shape. For each sequence, we "unpose" the point clouds of a randomly selected subset of 1000 frames, similarly to [2]. The process of unposing changes the pose of the model into a normalized pose, which removes the variance related to body articulation. Because large parts of the infants' backs are never visible, we add model vertices that belong to faces oriented away from the camera, and call them *virtual points*. The union of the unposed scan points and the *virtual points* is the *fusion scan*. We register the model to the fusion scan by first optimizing only shape parameters and then optimizing for the free surface to best explain the fusion scan, by coupling the free surface to the first computed shape.

SMIL. To learn our *Skinned Multi-Linear Infant model*, we compute a new infant-specific *shape space* by doing weighted PCA on all 37 personalized shapes. We use low weights for points labeled as clothing and high weights for skin points, with smooth transitions in between, to avoid including diapers and clothing wrinkles in the shape space. We retain the first 20 shape components. In order to avoid repeated poses due to the lack of motion (sequences have between 4K and 10K frames), we randomly sample 1000 poses per sequence and learn the *pose prior* from 37K poses. As the learned prior doesn't penalize illegal poses (e.g. unnatural bending of knees) we manually add penalties to avoid them. Our SMIL model is composed of the shape space, the pose prior, and a base template, which is the mean of all personalized shapes.

3   Experiments

We evaluate SMIL quantitatively with respect to $SMPL_B$ and perform a case-study on GMA ratings to demonstrate that SMIL captures enough information

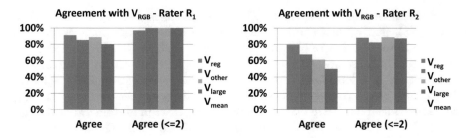

Fig. 3. Results of GMA case study. Percentage of ratings of synthetic sequences, generated using SMIL, that *agree* with the reference ratings $R_1 V_{rgb}$ (left) and $R_2 V_{rgb}$ (right), respectively. $V_{\{reg,other,large,mean\}}$ denotes different stimuli.

for medical assessment. Our dataset consists of 37 recordings of infants from a tertiary care high risk infants outpatient clinic, with an overall duration of over two hours. The infants' ages range from 9 to 18 weeks of corrected age (avg. of 14.6 weeks), their size range is 42 to 59 cm (avg. of 53.5 cm). We evaluate the SMIL model with a 9-fold cross-validation, using 33 sequences to train and 4 to test. Different clothing styles (onesie, diaper, no clothing) are distributed across all sets. We evaluate the scan distance to the model mesh (E_{s2m}) by computing the euclidean distance of each scan vertex to the mesh surface.

To evaluate the shape space, we register $SMPL_B$ and SMIL to the fusion clouds and evaluate E_{s2m} w.r.t. the number of shape parameters (Fig. 2a). SMIL is more accurate than $SMPL_B$ when using the same number of shape parameters. To evaluate how well the computed shapes and poses explain the input data we register $SMPL_B$ and SMIL to all sequences (200K frames) with the method described in Sect. 2 using 20 shape components. For $SMPL_B$, E_{s2m} is 2.67 mm (SD 0.22 mm), and for SMIL, E_{s2m} is slightly better: 2.51 mm (SD 0.21 mm). Figure 2b shows a registration sample. Manual inspection of all sequences reveals 16 unnatural leg/foot rotations, lasting altogether 41 s (= 0.54% of total duration), and 18 failure cases (in 7 sequences), lasting altogether 49 s (= 0.66% of total duration). The most common failure is "mixed up feet", i.e. feet aligned to the opposite side. Once, arm tracking is lost during side view, and one time a leg is severely twisted.

We conduct a case study on GMA to show that SMIL captures enough information to allow medical assessment. Three trained and certified GMA-experts perform GMA in different videos. We use five stimuli: (i) the original RGB videos (denoted by V_{rgb}), and (ii) the synthetic alignment videos (V_{reg}). For the next three stimuli we use the acquired poses of infants, but we animate a body with a different shape, namely (iii) a randomly selected shape of another infant (V_{other}), (iv) an extreme shape producing a very thick and large baby (V_{large}), and (v) the mean shape (V_{mean}). We exclude three of the 37 sequences, as two are too short and one has non-nutritive sucking, making it non suitable for GMA. As the number of videos to rate is high (34*5), for (iv) and (v) we only use 50% of the sequences, resulting in 136 videos. For a finer evaluation, we augment standard

GMA classes *definitely abnormal* (DA), *mildly abnormal* (MA), *normal suboptimal* (NS), and *normal optimal* (NO) [5] into a one to ten scale. Scores 1–3 correspond to DA, 4–5 to MA, 6–7 to NS, and 8–10 to NO. We consider two ratings with an absolute difference ≤ 1 to *agree*, and otherwise to *disagree*.

Rater R_1 is a long-time GMA teacher and has worked on GMA for over 25 years, R_2 has 15 years experience in GMA, and R_3 was certified one year ago, but lacks clinical routine in GMA. Average rating score (and standard deviation) for R1 is 4.7 (1.4), for R2 4.0 (1.9), and for R3 4.9 (2.3). The agreement on original RGB ratings V_{rgb} between R_3 and the more experienced raters is lower than 50%, while R_1 and R_2 agree on 65% of the ratings. This further stresses that GMA is challenging and its automation important. Due to the high rater variability we further focus on ratings of experienced raters R_1 and R_2. In Fig. 3, we present rating differences between synthetic and reference sequences. Each rater is compared to her own V_{rgb} ratings as a reference. $R_1 V_{reg}$ ratings *agree* on 91% of the reference ratings, whereas R_2 achieves an agreement rate of 79%. The agreement decreases more (R_2) or less (R_1) when the motions are presented with a different body shape. By extending the agreement threshold to ≤ 2, the percentages of all sequences become very similar. We intend to conduct further studies to elucidate the biases introduced by variation of shape.

4   Conclusions

In this paper, we contribute SMIL, a realistic, data-driven infant body model, learned from noisy, low-quality, incomplete RGB-D data, as well as a method to register SMIL to the data. Their combination allows to accurately capture the shape and the full body motion of freely moving infants. Quantitative experiments showed that SMIL's metric accuracy is ≈ 2.5 mm. We demonstrated its clinical usability with a case study on general movement assessment. Our results illustrate the challenges of human GMA ratings - raters subjectivity and raters consistency - and reinforce the need for an automated system. Two experienced raters obtained 91% and 79% agreement between GMA ratings performed on original RGB videos and on synthetic videos generated using our method, indicating that SMIL captures enough motion detail for medical assessment. The introduction of shape variations led to a degradation of rating agreement.

Future work will study which non-motion related factors (body shape, texture, lighting) most affect the GMA ratings. Furthermore, we will target the automation of GMA by learning to infer ratings from the captured data. We are also investigating the usability of the system for quantification of disease progress and the impact of early therapy in infants with spinal muscular atrophy.

References

1. Anguelov, D., Srinivasan, P., Koller, D., Thrun, S., Rodgers, J., Davis, J.: Scape: shape completion and animation of people. ACM Trans. Graph. **24**(3), 408–416 (2005)

2. Bogo, F., Black, M.J., Loper, M., Romero, J.: Detailed full-body reconstructions of moving people from monocular RGB-D sequences. In: IEEE International Conference on Computer Vision (ICCV) (2015)

3. Bogo, F., Kanazawa, A., Lassner, C., Gehler, P., Romero, J., Black, M.J.: Keep it SMPL: automatic estimation of 3D human pose and shape from a single image. In: Leibe, B., Matas, J., Sebe, N., Welling, M. (eds.) ECCV 2016, Part V. LNCS, vol. 9909, pp. 561–578. Springer, Cham (2016). https://doi.org/10.1007/978-3-319-46454-1_34

4. Cao, Z., Simon, T., Wei, S.E., Sheikh, Y.: Realtime multi-person 2D pose estimation using part affinity fields. In: IEEE Conference on Computer Vision and Pattern Recognition (CVPR) (2017)

5. Hadders-Algra, M.: General movements: a window for early identification of children at high risk for developmental disorders. J. Pediatr. **145**(2), S12–S18 (2004)

6. Heinze, F., Hesels, K., Breitbach-Faller, N., Schmitz-Rode, T., Disselhorst-Klug, C.: Movement analysis by accelerometry of newborns and infants for the early detection of movement disorders due to infantile cerebral palsy. Med. Biol. Eng. Comput. **48**(8), 765–772 (2010)

7. Hesse, N., Stachowiak, G., Breuer, T., Arens, M.: Estimating body pose of infants in depth images using random ferns. In: IEEE International Conference on Computer Vision Workshops (ICCVW) (2015)

8. Karch, D., Kim, K.S., Wochner, K., Pietz, J., Dickhaus, H., Philippi, H.: Quantification of the segmental kinematics of spontaneous infant movements. J. Biomech. **41**(13), 2860–2867 (2008)

9. Loper, M., Mahmood, N., Romero, J., Pons-Moll, G., Black, M.J.: SMPL: a skinned multi-person linear model. ACM Trans. Graph. **34**(6), 248 (2015)

10. MakeHuman: Open source tool for making 3D characters. www.makehuman.org

11. Marcroft, C., Khan, A., Embleton, N.D., Trenell, M., Plötz, T.: Movement recognition technology as a method of assessing spontaneous general movements in high risk infants. Front. Neurol. **5**, 284 (2014)

12. Meinecke, L., Breitbach-Faller, N., Bartz, C., Damen, R., Rau, G., Disselhorst-Klug, C.: Movement analysis in the early detection of newborns at risk for developing spasticity due to infantile cerebral palsy. Hum. Mov. Sci. **25**(2), 125–144 (2006)

13. Olsen, M.D., Herskind, A., Nielsen, J.B., Paulsen, R.R.: Model-based motion tracking of infants. In: Agapito, L., Bronstein, M.M., Rother, C. (eds.) ECCV 2014, Part III. LNCS, vol. 8927, pp. 673–685. Springer, Cham (2015). https://doi.org/10.1007/978-3-319-16199-0_47

14. Pons-Moll, G., Pujades, S., Hu, S., Black, M.J.: Clothcap: seamless 4D clothing capture and retargeting. ACM Trans. Graph. **36**(4), 73 (2017)

15. Prechtl, H.: Qualitative changes of spontaneous movements in fetus and preterm infant are a marker of neurological dysfunction. Early Hum. Dev. **23**(3), 151–158 (1990)

16. Rahmati, H., Dragon, R., Aamo, O.M., Adde, L., Stavdahl, Ø., Van Gool, L.: Weakly supervised motion segmentation with particle matching. Comput. Vis. Image Underst. **140**, 30–42 (2015)

17. Simon, T., Joo, H., Matthews, I., Sheikh, Y.: Hand keypoint detection in single images using multiview bootstrapping. In: IEEE Conference on Computer Vision and Pattern Recognition (CVPR) (2017)
18. Spittle, A., Orton, J., Anderson, P.J., Boyd, R., Doyle, L.W.: Early developmental intervention programmes provided post hospital discharge to prevent motor and cognitive impairment in preterm infants. The Cochrane Library (2015)
19. Stahl, A., Schellewald, C., Stavdahl, Ø., Aamo, O.M., Adde, L., Kirkerød, H.: An optical flow-based method to predict infantile cerebral palsy. IEEE Trans. Neural Syst. Rehabil. Eng. **20**(4), 605–614 (2012)
20. Wei, S.E., Ramakrishna, V., Kanade, T., Sheikh, Y.: Convolutional pose machines. In: IEEE Conference on Computer Vision and Pattern Recognition (CVPR) (2016)
21. Zuffi, S., Kanazawa, A., Jacobs, D., Black, M.J.: 3D menagerie: modeling the 3D shape and pose of animals. In: IEEE Conference on Computer Vision and Pattern Recognition (CVPR) (2017)

Consistent Correspondence of Cone-Beam CT Images Using Volume Functional Maps

Yungeng Zhang[1], Yuru Pei[1]([✉]), Yuke Guo[2], Gengyu Ma[3], Tianmin Xu[4], and Hongbin Zha[1]

[1] Key Laboratory of Machine Perception (MOE), Department of Machine Intelligence, Peking University, Beijing, China
`peiyuru@cis.pku.edu.cn`
[2] Luoyang Institute of Science and Technology, Luoyang, China
[3] uSens Inc., San Jose, USA
[4] School of Stomatology, Peking University, Beijing, China

Abstract. Dense correspondence between Cone-Beam CT (CBCT) images is desirable in clinical orthodontics for both intra-patient treatment evaluation and inter-patient statistical shape modeling and attribute transfer. Conventional 3D deformable image registration relies on time-consuming iterative optimization for correspondences. The recent forest-based correspondence methods often require large offline training costs and a separate regularization in the post-processing. In this work, we propose an efficient volume functional map for dense and consistent correspondence between CBCT images. We design a group of volume functions specifically for CBCT images and construct a reduced functional space on supervoxels. The low-dimensional map between the limited spectral bases determines the dense supervoxel-wise correspondence in an unsupervised way. Further, we perform consistent functional mapping in a collection of volume images to handle ambiguous correspondences of craniofacial structures, e.g., those due to the intercuspation. A subset of orthonormal volume functional maps is optimized on a Stiefel manifold simultaneously, which determines the cycle-consistent pairwise functional maps in the volume collection. Benefits of the proposed volume functional maps have been illustrated in label propagation and segmentation transfer with improved performance over conventional methods.

1 Introduction

Malocclusion has a high prevalence and causes aesthetic and functional problems in a large population. Cone-Beam CT (CBCT) images are widely used in clinical orthodontics to provide joint 3D geometries of the teeth, mandible, and maxilla to facilitate accurate malocclusion diagnoses and treatment evaluations. Efficient dense correspondence between CBCT images is desirable in several scenarios, including measuring shape variations due to treatments and growth [8], label propagation [5], and statistical craniofacial shape modeling [6].

© Springer Nature Switzerland AG 2018
A. F. Frangi et al. (Eds.): MICCAI 2018, LNCS 11070, pp. 801–809, 2018.
https://doi.org/10.1007/978-3-030-00928-1_90

The conventional 3D deformable registration methods, such as B-spline and Demons based registrations [11], solve the dense displacement field and correspondence under a time-consuming large-scale optimization for the craniofacial CBCT images. The importance sampling is helpful to accelerate the deformable registration by reducing the parameter space with efficient Jacobian estimation of similarity metrics [2]. However, the registration of the reduced subset also relies on the online iterative optimization. The random forest realizes efficient online dense correspondences between 3D surface meshes [10] and volume images [5,9]. Aside from the supervised classification random forest learned from a large set of labeled 3D meshes [10] or pseudo labeling obtained by supervoxel decompositions [5], the unsupervised clustering random forest realizes the self-learning of data distribution and affinity estimation without prior labeling [9]. However, the random forest built on independent data points could not guarantee the spatial consistency. A separate regularization scheme is required for smooth correspondences [9,10]. Recently the spectral methods using the Laplace Beltrami operator have gained popularity for functional mapping [7,14], co-segmentation [12], and analysis of anatomical structure [6] on surfaces and images. The functional map has a high efficiency by performing spectral mapping in a reduced functional space. However, the previous functional maps only handle 2D manifolds including images [12] and 3D surfaces [6,7].

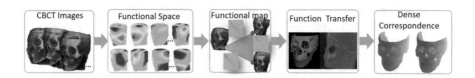

Fig. 1. Flowchart of our system.

In this paper, we propose a novel volume functional map for establishing supervoxel-wise correspondences between CBCT images (see Fig. 1). The proposed method extends the existing functional map approach from a 2D manifold, including the 2D image and 3D surface, to the 3D volume image. We design a group of volume functions, including appearances, contexts, geodesics, and label maps on supervoxel specifically for consistent correspondences between CBCT images. The spectral decomposition of the graph Laplacian produces harmonics bases of each volume image to span a linear volume functional space. The scalar-valued functions of both features and attributes over supervoxels can be reconstructed from a reduced set of functional bases. The dense supervoxel-wise correspondence is realized by finding a spectral transformation matrix between reduced functional spaces. The functional map is optimized by aligning the volume functions in an unsupervised way. Furthermore, in order to reduce correspondence ambiguities of craniofacial structures, e.g., the separation of upper and lower dentitions due to intercuspation, we exploit the cycle consistency constraints by introducing a latent functional space to a volume collection.

The pairwise orthonormal functional maps in the volume collection are optimized simultaneously on a Stiefel manifold, which meet the invertibility and transitivity requirements. The volume functional map realizes online label propagation and attribute transfer between volume images by the linear algebra with less computational complexity than conventional methods.

2   Methods

The input is a collection of clinically captured craniofacial CBCT images $\mathcal{V} = \{V_1, \ldots, V_N\}$. The goal is to build dense supervoxel-wise correspondences between volume images. Without loss of generality, we decompose each volume image into supervoxels. A volume image is represented by a graph $\mathcal{G} = (S, \mathcal{E})$ over the supervoxels $S = \{s_i | i = 1, \ldots, M\}$. $\mathcal{E}$ denotes the edges connecting adjacent supervoxels, which are weighted according to the affinity of adjacent supervoxels. In the unsupervised setting, the supervoxel-wise mapping $P_{ij} \in \mathbb{R}^{M \times M}$ between image V_i and V_j is solved based on the alignment of multi-channel features. The system also allows a user to label a small set of landmarks or region correspondences in a semi-supervised setting. With this setup, the goal is to estimate a permutation matrix P_{ij} of all supervoxels regarding CBCT images V_i and V_j.

Volume Functions. In our system, both features and attributes of supervoxels are represented by real-valued functions. Denote function $f : S \to \mathbb{R}$ to map a supervoxel s to a real value $g(s) \in \mathbb{R}$. There are four types of functions regarding the supervoxel appearance, context, geodesic distance, and label maps. The first three types are continuous real-valued functions, whereas the last one is a binary function. The appearance functions of supervoxels are composed of the normalized histograms of the original intensity and intensity gradients in x, y, and z directions. The context functions are composed of appearance differences of one supervoxel to those in a predefined contextual pattern [9]. The geodesic distance functions are defined by the sorted distance vector $\kappa(d_{i',j'} | j' = 1, \ldots, M_*)$ between supervoxel $s_{i'}$ to the rest supervoxels on the weighted graph $\mathcal{G}$, where $d_{i',j'}$ is the shortest graph distance between supervoxel $s_{i'}$ and $s_{j'}$. κ is a cubic-spline fitting and resampling operator on the sorted distance vector. In our system, we only compute geodesic vectors of M_* bony supervoxels for the computational efficiency. The label maps defined by a user are only used in the semi-supervised setting, where the indicator function $g(s) = 1$ for corresponding landmarks or regions, and $g(s) = 0$ otherwise. Let $\mathbb{G}_i$ denote all volume functions over supervoxels of image V_i. The functions $\mathbb{G}_i$ spans a linear space in $\mathbb{R}^M$.

Reduced Volume Functional Space. The Laplace-Beltrami operator on a manifold is defined as the divergence of the gradient, $\Delta g = \text{div} \nabla g$. The eigendecomposition, $\Delta \phi = \lambda \phi$, results in harmonic bases of the functional space with frequencies λ. On the discrete supervoxel decomposed volume image, the graph Laplace is used to approximate the Laplace Beltrami operator. Let W denote the weighted adjacency matrix of supervoxel graph $\mathcal{G}$, $L = D^{-1}(D - W)$, where $D_{ii} = \sum_j W_{ij}$. The eigendecomposition of L results in eigenvectors

$\Phi = (\phi_1, \ldots, \phi_M)$ as the harmonics bases and eigenvalues $(\lambda_1, \ldots, \lambda_M)$ as harmonics frequencies. The eigenvectors are sorted according to the harmonic frequencies, and the first K eigenvectors are used to represent the reduced functional space. K is set at 75 in our experiments. Eight eigenvectors related to a volume image are illustrated in Fig. 2(a). The volume function is represented as a linear combination of eigenvectors, $g = \Phi\mathfrak{g}$, where $\mathfrak{g} \in \mathbb{R}^K$. The reduced bases $\Phi^* \in \mathbb{R}^{M \times K}$.

2.1   Volume Functional Map

Given a volume image pair (V_i, V_j), and a volume function $g^{(i)} = \Phi^{(i)}\mathfrak{g}^{(i)} \in \mathbb{G}_i$, the goal of volume functional mapping is to transfer the K-dimensional vector $\mathfrak{g}^{(i)}$ to the functional space of image V_j, and reconstruct the volume function $g^{(j)} \in \mathbb{G}^{(j)}$. Given H corresponding functions $\mathbb{G}_i \in \mathbb{R}^{M \times H}$ and $\mathbb{G}_j \in \mathbb{R}^{M \times H}$ on image V_i and V_j, the corresponding supervoxels between volume images should have similar functional values. The objective function $E = \|\mathbb{G}_i - P\mathbb{G}_j\|_F^2$, where P is the unknown permutation matrix indicating the dense supervoxel correspondence between V_i and V_j. Instead of the supervoxel-wise correspondence, we handle the low-dimensional functional map C_{ij} between the reduced functional spaces. The functional map $C_{ij} = \Phi^{(i)-1}P_{ij}\Phi^{(j)}$ [6,7]. The transferred function $g^{(j)} = \Phi^{(j)}C_{ij}\mathfrak{g}^{(i)}$. The functional map is viewed as a spectral transformation of the reduced functional space $\Phi^{(i)}$ and $\Phi^{(j)}$, in which the transformation matrix accounts for the sign fliping and interchanging of eigenvectors between volume images. It is straightforward that the functional map between image V_i and V_j should transform the feature function $g^{(i)} \in \mathbb{G}_i$ to the feature function $g^{(j)} \in \mathbb{G}_j$. The functional map is optimized by minimizing feature alignment errors.

$$E(C_{ij}) = \|C_{ij}\overline{\mathfrak{g}^{(i)}} - \overline{\mathfrak{g}^{(j)}}\|_F^2 + \gamma\|\Theta_j C_{ij} - C_{ij}\Theta_i\|_F^2, \tag{1}$$

where $\|\cdot\|_F$ is the Frobenius norm. $\overline{\mathfrak{g}} \in \mathbb{R}^{K \times H}$ denotes the harmonic weight matrix in the reduced functional space. The feature space of image V_i is aligned to that of image V_j by minimizing the first term. The second term is the operator commutativity constraints. Θ is a low rank approximation of the Graph Lapidarian matrix. The constant γ is used to balance the feature alignment and the commutativity constraint, and set at 1 in our experiments. We use the linear least square to solve C_{ij}. Given functional map C_{ij}, the dense correspondence matrix $P_{ij}^* = \Phi^{(i)}C_{ij}\Phi^{(j)-1}$. Note that the matrix P_{ij}^* is not a hard permutation between image V_i and V_j, since the entries record the probability of supervoxel pair (s_i, s_j) being a counterpart to each other. The permutation matrix P_{ij} is derived from P_{ij}^* by using the column normalization and the NN scheme [7].

Consistency Regularization. When given additional images, cycle-consistent functional maps in an image collection are helpful to improve the mapping accuracies over the pairwise functional maps [12,14]. In our system, we utilize the consistency regularization to reduce the mapping ambiguity especially for the segmentation transfer of the mandible and maxilla. We follow the map decomposition [12], where the functional maps, $C_{i,j} = c_j' c_i$, are determined by a reduced mapping set $\{c_1, \ldots, c_M\}$. c_i can be viewed as the functional map from reduced functional space of V_i to a latent functional space. The decomposition of C_{ij} enforces the 3-cycle consistency of the functional maps in a volume collection. We further require the functional map $c_i, 1 \leq i \leq M$, be an orthonormal matrix in the Stiefel manifold. Thus, all the functional maps are orthonormal, and $C_{ij}' = C_{ij}^{-1}$. The functional maps satisfies the invertibility and transitivity constraints, where $C_{ij} = C_{ji}^{-1}$ and $C_{jk} C_{ij} = C_{ik}$. The objective function is rewritten as

$$E(\mathsf{c}) = \sum_{V_i, V_j \in \mathcal{V}, C_{i,j} = c_j' c_i} \|C_{ij} \overline{\mathfrak{g}^{(i)}} - \overline{\mathfrak{g}^{(j)}}\|_F^2 + \gamma \|\Theta_j C_{ij} - C_{ij} \Theta_i\|_F^2. \quad (2)$$

We implement the optimization of the functional map c on the Stiefel manifold using the trust region solver of the Manopt toolbox [3]. The functional maps c are initialized as an identity matrix and refined using the manifold optimization. In the online testing, the corresponding volume functions are extracted from the novel CBCT image. The pairwise volume functions map is computed by minimizing Eq. 1. When given additional volume images, the consistent volume functional maps are obtained by minimizing Eq. 2.

3 Experiments

Dataset. The proposed volume functional map is evaluated on a collection consisting of 10 clinically captured CBCT images of orthodontic patients, which has 90 pairwise maps. The volume image is of a resolution of $250 \times 250 \times 238$ with a voxel size of $0.8 \, \text{mm} \times 0.8 \, \text{mm} \times 0.8 \, \text{mm}$. We use the SLIC method [1] to decompose each CBCT image into $20k$ supervoxels. For each CBCT image, there are 680 functions, including 80 appearances, 500 contexts, 100 geodesics-related functions.

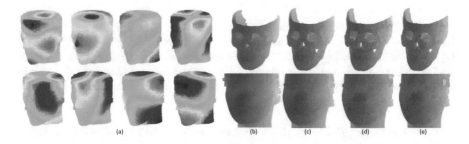

Fig. 2. (a) Eight functional bases. Supervoxel-wise correspondence between (b) the reference image and the target image by (c) the deformable B-spline registration, and the proposed (d) VFM and (e) C-VFM methods.

Qualitative Assessment. We qualitatively evaluate the supervoxel-wise label propagation of the mandible and maxilla using two metrics: the Dice similarity coefficient (DSC) and the average Hausdorff distance (AHD). We compare the proposed pairwise volume functional map (VFM) and the consistent volume functional map (C-VFM) with the conventional label propagation methods, including the patch fusion (PF) [4], the convex optimization (CO) [13], the volumetric deformable B-spline registration [11]. We also compare with the random forest-based methods, including the classification forest (Cla) [5] and the mixed metric forest (MMRF) [9] as shown in Figs. 2(b–e) and 3(a). The label propagation accuracies of the proposed method have DSCs of 0.94 ± 0.02 and 0.93 ± 0.02 when using 75 spectral bases for the mandible and the maxilla respectively, which are close to the conventional deformable B-spline registration. Moreover, the proposed volume functional map gains great efficiency and consumes approx. 20 s (1.35 s for map optimization (Eq. 1) as shown in Fig. 3(d)) when using a 75×75 functional map vs. 11 min by the B-spline registration with a $28 \times 28 \times 27$ control grid for the segmentation transfer. The running time is measured on a PC with an i7 CPU of 3.3 GHz and RAM of 32GB. The reason for the online efficiency is that the functional map exploits a low dimensional spectral transformation in the reduced function spaces. The volume functional map with a DSC of 0.94 for the mandible label propagation improves over the supervised Cla of 0.88 and the unsupervised MMRF of 0.92. The functional map and the forest-based method both realize efficient online supervoxel-based correspondences, whereas the latter requires a separate regularization and a large offline forest training cost. One sampled functional map is shown in Fig. 3(e).

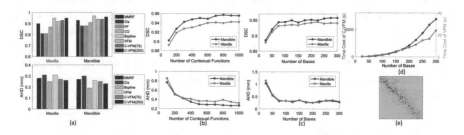

Fig. 3. (a) DSCs and AHDs of the label propagation of the mandible and maxilla by the proposed VFM and C-VFM using 75 and 250 bases compared with PF [4], CO [13], B-spline [11], Cla [5], and MMRF [9] based methods. (b) DSCs and AHDs of the label propagation with increasing number of (b) contextual functions and (c) bases. (d) Time costs of map optimizations of VFM and C-VFM. (e) Functional map of C-VFM.

Since the upper and lower dentitions are assigned to the mandible and maxilla respectively, the intercuspation causes correspondence ambiguities in segmentation transfer as shown in Fig. 4. The consistency regularization (Sect. 2.1) exploits additional volumes for consistent correspondences. In our experiments, we solve the correspondences between three volumes simultaneously.

The additional volume is helpful to avoid correspondence ambiguities (Fig. 4(f)). Furthermore, the proposed methods can work in a semi-supervised setting, where a user interactively labeled five corresponding landmarks as shown in Fig. 4(c). Corresponding landmarks are represented by pairs of volume functions as described in Sect. 2, and improve the matching even when using a small set of bases.

The functional maps are solved based on the predefined volume functions including the context and geodesic functions. Figure 3(b) illustrates that the label propagation accuracies are positively associated with the number of contextual functions. The geodesic functions facilitate the detection of connected structures. For instance, the geodesic distance between two supervoxels of the same structure is smaller than that of distinct structures. We observe that the functional maps with the geodesic functions are superior to those without the geodesic functions as constraints with mean DSC improvements of 0.53% and 0.56% for the mandible and maxilla respectively.

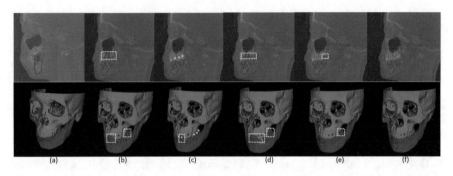

Fig. 4. Segmentation transfer from (a) the reference to the target image using VFM with (b) 25 spectral bases, (c) 25 spectral bases and 5 pairs of landmarks (yellow points), (d) 100 contextual functions, and (e) 75 bases and 500 contextual functions without consistency constraints and (f) with consistency constraints.

In our system, the reduced harmonic bases represent the original functional space compactly. Figure 3(c) shows DSCs of the label propagation with increasing number of harmonic bases. Note that, the more bases used, the more accurate label propagation. For instance, the DSC of the mandible label propagation increases from 0.94 using 75 bases to 0.96 using 250 bases. However, the additional spectral bases increase the computational costs as shown in Fig. 3(d), in which the functional map consumes from 37 s to 6850 s when using from 25 to 300 spectral bases regarding the C-VFM method.

4   Discussion and Conclusion

In this paper, we extend the conventional functional map on a 2D manifold of surfaces or images to 3D volumes. We propose a novel volume functional map for supervoxel-wise correspondences between CBCT images for label propagation. The low-dimensional functional map between reduced functional spaces realizes a spectral transformation, and uniquely determines the dense supervoxel correspondence between CBCT images. The proposed consistent volume map is promising to reduce correspondence ambiguities of craniofacial structures, such as those due to the intercuspation. The proposed method has been applied to clinically captured CBCT images for segmentation transfer of the mandible and maxilla with mean DSCs of 0.94 and 0.93 respectively when using 75 spectral bases. However, we observe that volume functional maps are limited to estimate correspondence between volumes with non-isometric deformations, e.g., the volumes of an adult and a child, due to the scale-sensitive context and geodesic functions. In the future work, we would investigate the volume functional map for more general deformations.

Acknowledgments. This work was supported by NSFC 61272342, 61632003, 81371192, ISTCPC 2014DFA31800, and NKTRDPC 2017YFB1002601.

References

1. Achanta, R., Shaji, A., Smith, K., Lucchi, A., Fua, P., Süsstrunk, S.: Slic superpixels compared to state-of-the-art superpixel methods. IEEE Trans. PAMI **34**(11), 2274–2282 (2012)
2. Bhagalia, R., Fessler, J.A., Kim, B.: Accelerated nonrigid intensity-based image registration using importance sampling. IEEE Trans. MI **28**(8), 1208–1216 (2009)
3. Boumal, N., Mishra, B., Absil, P.A., Sepulchre, R.: Manopt, a matlab toolbox for optimization on manifolds. J. Mach. Learn. Res. **15**(1), 1455–1459 (2014)
4. Coupé, P., Manjón, J.V., Fonov, V., Pruessner, J., Robles, M., Collins, D.L.: Patch-based segmentation using expert priors: application to hippocampus and ventricle segmentation. NeuroImage **54**(2), 940–954 (2011)
5. Kanavati, F., Tong, T., Misawa, K., Fujiwara, M., Mori, K., Rueckert, D., Glocker, B.: Supervoxel classification forests for estimating pairwise image correspondences. Pattern Recogn. **63**, 561–569 (2017)
6. Lombaert, H., Arcaro, M., Ayache, N.: Brain transfer: spectral analysis of cortical surfaces and functional maps. In: Ourselin, S., Alexander, D.C., Westin, C.-F., Cardoso, M.J. (eds.) IPMI 2015. LNCS, vol. 9123, pp. 474–487. Springer, Cham (2015). https://doi.org/10.1007/978-3-319-19992-4_37
7. Ovsjanikov, M., Ben-Chen, M., Solomon, J., Butscher, A., Guibas, L.: Functional maps: a flexible representation of maps between shapes. ACM Trans. Graph. **31**(4), 30 (2012)
8. Pei, Y., Ma, G., Chen, G., Zhang, X., Xu, T., Zha, H.: Superimposition of cone-beam computed tomography images by joint embedding. IEEE Trans. BME **64**(6), 1218–1227 (2017)
9. Pei, Y., et al.: Mixed metric random forest for dense correspondence of cone-beam computed tomography images. In: Descoteaux, M., Maier-Hein, L., Franz, A., Jannin, P., Collins, D.L., Duchesne, S. (eds.) MICCAI 2017. LNCS, vol. 10433, pp. 283–290. Springer, Cham (2017). https://doi.org/10.1007/978-3-319-66182-7_33
10. Rodolà, E., Rota Bulo, S., Windheuser, T., Vestner, M., Cremers, D.: Dense non-rigid shape correspondence using random forests. In: CVPR, pp. 4177–4184 (2014)

11. Sotiras, A., Davatzikos, C., Paragios, N.: Deformable medical image registration: a survey. IEEE Trans. MI **32**(7), 1153–1190 (2013)
12. Wang, F., Huang, Q., Guibas, L.J.: Image co-segmentation via consistent functional maps. In: ICCV, pp. 849–856 (2013)
13. Wang, L., et al.: Automated segmentation of CBCT image using spiral CT atlases and convex optimization. In: MICCAI 2013, pp. 251–258 (2013)
14. Zhang, C., Smith, W.A., Dessein, A., Pears, N., Dai, H.: Functional faces: groupwise dense correspondence using functional maps. In: CVPR, pp. 5033–5041 (2016)

Elastic Registration of Geodesic Vascular Graphs

Stefano Moriconi[1]([✉]), Maria A. Zuluaga[2], H. Rolf Jäger[3], Parashkev Nachev[3], Sébastien Ourselin[4], and M. Jorge Cardoso[1,4]

[1] Translational Imaging Group, CMIC, University College London, London, UK
stefano.moriconi.15@ucl.ac.uk
[2] Universidad Nacional de Colombia, Bogotá, Colombia
[3] Institute of Neurology, University College London, London, UK
[4] School of Biomedical Engineering and Imaging Sciences,
King's College London, London, UK

Abstract. Vascular graphs can embed a number of high-level features, from morphological parameters, to functional biomarkers, and represent an invaluable tool for longitudinal and cross-sectional clinical inference. This, however, is only feasible when graphs are co-registered together, allowing coherent multiple comparisons. The robust registration of vascular topologies stands therefore as key enabling technology for group-wise analyses. In this work, we present an end-to-end vascular graph registration approach, that aligns networks with non-linear geometries and topological deformations, by introducing a novel over-connected geodesic vascular graph formulation, and without enforcing any anatomical prior constraint. The 3D elastic graph registration is then performed with state-of-the-art graph matching methods used in computer vision. Promising results of vascular matching are found using graphs from synthetic and real angiographies. Observations and future designs are discussed towards potential clinical applications.

1 Introduction

Vascular graphs can be obtained from angiographies using connectivity paradigms and network extraction algorithms by embedding high-level features, such as spatial location, direction, scale, and bifurcations. However, the correct extraction of subject-specific vascular topologies, in complex (cerebro)vascular networks, can be challenging when rather tortuous and tangled structures are present. In other cases, anatomical cycles and their variants (i.e. the circle of Willis, anastomoses and fenestrations) [7], the presence of pathology (e.g. tangled arterio-venous malformations, neoplastic and embryologic plexiforms), and image-related limitations (e.g. unresolved kissing vessels) dramatically increase the network complexity, and sometimes impede the extraction of the vascular topology as a tree. A viable approach is to consider a data-driven vectorial prior from an early group-wise vascular graph registration. Defining a group-wise vectorial prior first embeds the likelihood of connectivity patterns from a

© Springer Nature Switzerland AG 2018
A. F. Frangi et al. (Eds.): MICCAI 2018, LNCS 11070, pp. 810–818, 2018.
https://doi.org/10.1007/978-3-030-00928-1_91

population, and subsequently injects a probabilistic prior towards the inference of the most meaningful subject-specific vascular topology. The same vectorial prior could also embed morphometric parameters, functional and hemodynamic descriptors and surrogate biomarkers, constituting thus a labelled multi-spectral vascular atlas. By registering the obtained vectorial atlas over a set of similar vascular graphs, a number of group-level clinical analyses would be allowed, from inter-subject comparisons of the underlying vascular morphology, to longitudinal studies of vascular pathologies, on which clinical prediction and therapeutic inference ultimately depend. The robust alignment of multiple topologies is of critical relevance and represents a methodological bottleneck for population-level analyses. The alignment of networks and vectorial graphs raised increasing interest among the scientific community in the last decade. Motivated by registering acyclically connected structures from biomedical imaging, (e.g. vascular and respiratory trees), [1,4,13–16] introduced different registration techniques, which mostly rely on pairwise matching distances between junction nodes and connecting edges. Following an initial alignment, these methods usually minimise a similarity cost function or maximise a probabilistic likelihood between pairs of nodes/edges or sub-trees and graph kernels, and hierarchically evaluate the correspondences at different levels of tree-depth. Whilst only few formulations would register generic spatial graphs [14], in all cases the considered topologies were either hierarchically pre-defined as trees, or determined beforehand on a specific anatomical compartment. Also, since these methods exploit node locations, branches geometry, arborescence depth, or the parent-child relation of a rooted tree, they require the explicit tree topology to accurately capture the underlying vasculature, where each bifurcation is correctly annotated as its connectivity pattern. The registration of noisy topologies, (i.e. mis-connections, missing branches and short-cuts), and non-linearly deformed geometries remains a challenging and open problem. In this preliminary work, we address vascular graph matching (GM) by relaxing assumptions on the acyclic (un)directed graph structure and the anatomical hierarchical prior from any vascular compartment. The idea is to consider and register the vasculature as an over-connected graph: a redundant topology encoding the likelihood of connections between neighbouring nodes with minimal paths. This enhanced connectivity pattern would compensate for topological inaccuracies, for non-linear deformations of branches, and would enrich the registration space-search with distinctive features. The pairwise graph registration problem can be subsequently solved using generic GM algorithms. In the following sections, the proposed approach is first described, then, an experimental set-up is presented, comprising graphs from synthetic and real angiographies. The accuracy of different GM algorithms is evaluated on correct nodes correspondences. Observations and conclusions are discussed, focusing on future developments and potential applications.

2   Methods

Aiming at the pairwise alignment of vascular topologies within a deformable and anatomical prior-free framework, we first introduce a novel over-connected

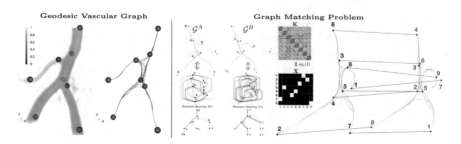

Fig. 1. Geodesic Vascular Graph and GM problem of non-linearly deformed topologies. Extraction of a fully-connected topology from an initial set of nodes (left). Associated graph representations and minimum spanning trees for two topologically different instances ($\mathcal{G}^A$ and $\mathcal{G}^B$) of the same underlying vascular anatomy (center). Graphs alignment and nodes matching for the generalised GM problem (right).

geodesic vascular graph (GVG), then the generic GM problem is presented together with the proposed affinity metrics based on vessels geometry and their redundant geodesic connectivity. The two-steps registration pipeline is described also listing the considered GM algorithms.

Geodesic Vascular Graph. We define the undirected geodesic vascular graph $\mathcal{G} = (N, E)$ in $\mathbb{R}^3$, as the set of nodes $\mathbf{n}_i \in N$, and the associated set of connecting geodesic edges $\mathbf{e}_v \in E$, encoding the graph adjacency list. Each geodesic edge $\mathbf{e}_v$ is defined as the 3D shortest path joining a generic pair of nodes, by solving the Eikonal equation [8] over a vascular smoothly connected manifold as in [12]. However, an exhaustive search is here performed by connecting all pairs of nodes independently, or up to a pre-defined spatial neighborhood ν. This determines an over-connected vascular graph of minimal paths, which fully captures the underlying vasculature with enhanced geodesic redundancy (Fig. 1). Together with the formulation of the over-connected $\mathcal{G}$, we also introduce a set of edge- and node-attributes. The edge-attributes $\mathbf{e}_v = \{\mathbf{p}_v, l_v, u_v\}$ comprise the dense sampling $\mathbf{p}_v$ of each shortest path in 3D (i.e. the point coordinates sequence as in Figs. 2 and 3), its associated euclidean length l_v and the geodesic integral energy u_v integrated along the path, as in [12]. The node-attributes $\mathbf{n}_i = \{\mathbf{c}_i, d_i\}$ include the spatial location $\mathbf{c}_i$ as coordinates in $\mathbb{R}^3$, and the geodesic node degree $d_i = \frac{1}{|\tilde{\mathbf{e}}_v|} \sum_{\tilde{\mathbf{e}}_v} u_v$, with $\tilde{\mathbf{e}}_v$ the set of incident edges of cardinality $|\tilde{\mathbf{e}}_v|$.

Graph Matching Problem and Affinity Metrics. As presented in [19], the problem of matching a pair of graphs $\mathcal{G}^A$ and $\mathcal{G}^B$ requires the definition of an affinity matrix $\mathbf{K}$ to measure the similarity between each pair of nodes and edges. Given the node cardinality $i = |\mathbf{n}_i^A|$, and $j = |\mathbf{n}_j^B|$, the symmetric affinity matrix $\mathbf{K} \in \mathbb{R}^{ij \times ij}$ encodes the similarity between nodes along its diagonal elements, whereas the edges similarity is encoded in the off-diagonal ones. Given $\mathbf{K}$, the problem of graph matching consists in finding the optimal correspondence

X between all the nodes (Fig. 1), so that a compatibility functional $J(\mathbf{X})$ is maximised with a quadratic assignment problem (QAP) [11],

$$\max \; J(\mathbf{X}) = \text{vec}(\mathbf{X})^t \; \mathbf{K} \; \text{vec}(\mathbf{X}), \tag{1}$$

where **X** is constrained to be a one-to-one mapping between the sets of nodes $\mathbf{n}_i^A$ and $\mathbf{n}_i^B$, and vec(**X**) denotes the vectorisation of the correspondence matrix. We formulate both node- and edge-similarity metrics for the definition of the affinity matrix **K**, by adopting the matrix factorisation as in [19], i.e. $\mathbf{K_{n}}_{AB}$ and $\mathbf{K_{e}}_{AB}$ respectively. In detail, we define

$$\mathbf{K_{n}}_{AB} = e^{-\left(\alpha_1 \frac{\mathbf{C}^{AB}}{\sigma_{\mathbf{C}}} + \alpha_2 \frac{\mathbf{D}^{AB}}{\sigma_{\mathbf{D}}}\right)} \quad \text{with} \; \alpha_1 + \alpha_2 = 1, \quad \text{and} \tag{2}$$

$$\mathbf{K_{e}}_{AB} = e^{-\left(\beta_1 \frac{\mathbf{P}^{AB}}{\sigma_{\mathbf{P}}} + \beta_2 \frac{\mathbf{L}^{AB}}{\sigma_{\mathbf{L}}} + \beta_3 \frac{\mathbf{U}^{AB}}{\sigma_{\mathbf{U}}}\right)} \quad \text{with} \; \beta_1 + \beta_2 + \beta_3 = 1, \tag{3}$$

where $\mathbf{C}^{AB}$ and $\mathbf{D}^{AB}$ are the pairwise ℓ^2-norm matrices between the two sets of node coordinates $\{\mathbf{c}_i^A, \mathbf{c}_j^B\}$, and geodesic degrees $\{d_i^A, d_j^B\}$, as well as $\mathbf{P}^{AB}$, $\mathbf{L}^{AB}$ and $\mathbf{U}^{AB}$ are the pairwise average symmetric distance matrices of the connecting minimal paths $\{\mathbf{p}_v^A, \mathbf{p}_w^B\}$, and the pairwise ℓ^2-norm matrices between the sets of the euclidean lengths $\{l_v^A, l_w^B\}$ and geodesic integral energies $\{u_v^A, u_w^B\}$, respectively. The normalisation factors $\sigma_{\mathbf{C,D,P,L,U}}$ are the standard deviations estimated from the off-diagonal elements of the associated distance matrices over the considered population of graphs. Lastly, α_1, β_1 and β_2 weight the geometrical similarities among nodes and edges, whereas α_2 and β_3 represent the respective geodesic trade-off. We refer to [19] for the composition of **K** from the factorised components $\mathbf{K_{n}}_{AB}$ and $\mathbf{K_{e}}_{AB}$, and for the QAP solver implementation.

Graph Registration. Although some GM algorithms do not require any spatial initialisation of the graphs, we present a two-steps approach (Figs. 2 and 3) by combining an early coarse alignment strategy to facilitate the further registration by reducing biases due to pure rigid mis-alignment.

Rigid Alignment. The globally-optimal iterative closest point (Go-ICP) [17] is run on $\mathcal{G}^A$ and $\mathcal{G}^B$ as coarse geometrical initialisation. Here, the dense cloud of samples, i.e. the nodes coordinates $\{\mathbf{c}_i^A, \mathbf{c}_j^B\}$ and the sequences of edge points $\{\mathbf{p}_v^A, \mathbf{p}_w^B\}$, is retrieved for the spatial rigid pre-alignment. Go-ICP searches the entire 3D motion space, and, under the minimisation of an L_2 error metric based on a branch-and-bound scheme, guarantees the global optimality of the rigid mapping, even in presence of noisy data, outliers, and partial samples overlap.

Fine Graph Matching. Classic GM algorithms employed in computer vision, are considered for the fine registration. We account for Graduated Assignment (GA) [5], Spectral Matching (SM) [9], Spectral Matching with Affine Constraints (SMAC) [3], Probabilistic Matching (PM) [18], Integer Projected Fixed Point (IPFP-U/SM) [10], Re-weighted Random Walk Matching (RRWM) [2], and the current state-of-the-art, the non-rigid Factorized Graph Matching

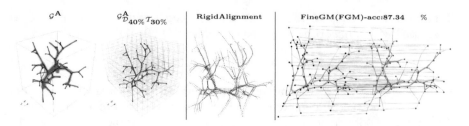

Fig. 2. Example of sGVG, simulated deformations, rigid alignment and resulting GM.

(FGM) [19]. The deformable graph matching problem, detailed in [19], formulates the unknown graph correspondence being constrained with a geometric transformation T. A composition of transformations (i.e. similar, affine, and non-rigid) are incorporated into the compatibility function (Eq. 1), and subsequently estimated by optimising jointly the correspondence matrix $\mathbf{X}$ and the composite transformation T itself. We employed the undirected-graph versions of the listed algorithms. Implementations and configurations are available from authors' websites.

3   Experiments and Results

Dataset. A set of 10 synthetic over-connected geodesic vascular graphs (sGVG) and associated minimum spanning trees (sGVT) are obtained from 3D vascular tree images [6] (isotropic $100\times100\times100$ voxels), as in Sect. 2. Each graph comprises 80 nodes, i.e. the vascular junction and end-points, over-connected within a neighbourhood of radius $\nu = 35$ (Fig. 2). A total of 10 fully over-connected geodesic vascular graphs (aGVG) as well as the respective minimum spanning trees (aGVT) of the basilar artery are derived as in Sect. 2 from Time-of-Flight MRI angiographies ($0.35 \times 0.35 \times 0.5$ mm), where anatomical vascular junctions and endpoints were manually labelled (Fig. 3) following [7].

Synthetic Graphs. We randomly deform the synthetic datasets sGVG and sGVT with a non-linear geometrical displacement field (i.e. max magnitude $\mathcal{D}_{30\%}$, $\mathcal{D}_{40\%}$, $\mathcal{D}_{50\%}$ of the graph spatial embedding), a topological pruning (i.e. reducing by $\mathcal{T}_{30\%}$, $\mathcal{T}_{40\%}$, $\mathcal{T}_{50\%}$ the original connectivity), and a combination of both, for a representative set of alterations (Fig. 2). The deformed graphs were then registered with the respective unaltered topologies. The accuracy of the GM is given by the percentage of correct correspondences, and differences of registration performances between sGVG and sGVT are evaluated with a paired Wilcoxon signed rank test.

Angiographic Graphs. Both aGVG and aGVT are pairwise aligned, covering all possible inter-subject combinations within the same dataset. The matching accuracy is given by the percentage of correct correspondence among the labelled nodes. Differences between aGVG and aGVT are evaluated with a paired Wilcoxon signed rank test.

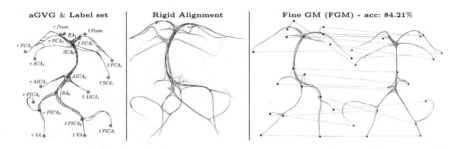

Fig. 3. aGVG label set [7] and pairwise registration of anatomical topologies.

Synthetic Graph Matching. In Fig. 4 (charts), the GM accuracy is reported for the synthetic datasets, for each algorithm and for the simulated levels of deformation. The affinity metrics trade-offs are arbitrarily defined as $\alpha = [0.5, 0.5]$, and $\beta = [0.25, 0.25, 0.5]$ in all cases, to balance the similarity features. Similar trends of performances are observed for the considered GM algorithms across different levels of increasing deformation. Overall, FGM reported the best matching accuracy together with RRWM in both sGVG and sGVT, whereas the other algorithms showed globally varying performances. Purely geometrical displacements did not affect the registration, whereas more severe topological pruning showed a visible drop of accuracy in both sGVG and sGVT, as well as the combination of joint deformations at different degrees. Overall, better matching is found for sGVG compared to sGVT at the same level of alteration. A significant accuracy drop ($p < 0.05$) is found for the registration of tree-like structures, proportional to the combined deformation. This suggests that the proposed registration pipeline would benefit from both geometrical and geodesic information arising from a more dense and redundant over-connected pattern, rather than an explicit vascular tree hierarchy, in presence of non-linear deformations.

Angiographic Graph Matching. The accuracy of the pairwise registration for both aGVG and aGVT datasets is reported in Fig. 4 (table). The affinity metrics trade-offs adopted here are the same as those for the synthetic experiments. Overall, discrete matching is obtained for the state-of-the-art FGM ($61.26 \pm 21.91\%$), as well as for GA ($65.16 \pm 20.39\%$) and SM ($62.83 \pm 22.96\%$). The considered angiographic dataset presented large deformations and anatomically different variants (Fig. 3). In line with results of Sect. 3, the registration of over-connected topologies (aGVG) showed significantly higher accuracy ($p < 0.05$), compared to the respective hierarchical minimum spanning trees (aGVT). Globally, nodes mismatch occurred in correspondence of nodes with lower degree and centrality, where higher confusion is found for spatially close vascular end-points and neighbouring branches. Conversely, the correspondence of superior/inferior and left/right branches was correctly preserved in the majority of cases.

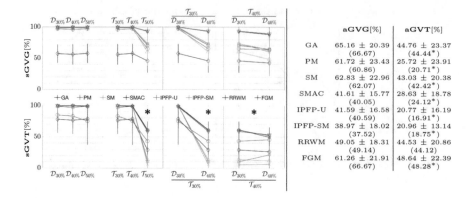

Fig. 4. Accuracy of GM: synthetic datasets sGVG vs. sGVT (charts), and angiographic datasets aGVG vs. aGVT (table). Values are mean ± SD, (median), $* = p < 0.05$.

4   Discussion and Conclusions

We presented a vascular graph matching approach to pairwise and elastically register similar topologies, in presence of non-linear deformations. A novel formulation of the vascular network is first introduced using an over-connected geodesic vascular graph. Then, the non-rigid nodes correspondence assignment is solved with a two-steps alignment comprising an optimal rigid registration of the network geometrical embedding, and a set of graph matching algorithms employed in computer vision. For the first time, a general registration of vascular graphs, accounting for noisy over-connected topologies with possible cycles, could be performed by relaxing the explicit hierarchical vessel-tree structure or connectivity patterns specific of a vascular compartment. The use of multiple GM strategies, on the one hand, is motivated by the unconstrained formulation of the GVG, on the other hand, it is justified by the different connectivity lattice of the introduced GVG. The latter can dramatically differ from the connectivity patterns found in computer vision applications (i.e. 3D polygonal subdivision and/or triangulations in 2D), therefore, established GM algorithms may show rather different performances. Early results show, however, good matching from synthetic vascular graphs even in presence of mild-to-moderate non-linear deformations. With the same registration pipeline, we aligned over-connected and redundant topologies, as well as hierarchical undirected tree-structures. Despite these share the same similarity features, the graph matching reported significantly different accuracies, where better nodes correspondences are found for the over-connected topologies. This suggests that the overhead information from the redundant connectivity may enrich the registration space-search with more distinctive cues. Similarly, the registration of geodesic vascular graphs from angiographic datasets reported appreciable matching, even in cases of large spatial deformations and anatomically different topologies, whereas the registration of the associated tree-like structures showed significantly lower accuracies, in line with the synthetic experiments. On the basis of this early evidence, we assume the problem of vascular tree- and graph-registration could be generalised with a multi-spectral network alignment, where further developments towards a more robust design for vascular applications may better incorporate both geometrical and geodesic vascular features. Although most of the GM algorithms considered in this work are used for 2D applications in computer vision, their general formulation allows the alignment of any generic network, regardless the dimensional embedding, and offer a rich ground for ad-hoc methodological developments. From a clinical perspective, the successful vascular graph alignment would lead to the definition of a co-registered group-wise prior to improve the inference of patient specific anatomical topologies. In last instance, the co-registration of a vascular vectorial prior would pave the way for group-wise analyses with potential applications in neurovascular cross-sectional and longitudinal studies.

Acknowledgements. The study is co-funded from the Wellcome Trust, the EPSRC grant EP/H046410/1, and the National Institute for Health Research, University College London Hospitals, Biomedical Research Centre.

References

1. Charnoz, A., Agnus, V., Malandain, G., Nicolau, S., Tajine, M., Soler, L.: Design of robust vascular tree matching: validation on liver. In: Christensen, G.E., Sonka, M. (eds.) IPMI 2005. LNCS, vol. 3565, pp. 443–455. Springer, Heidelberg (2005). https://doi.org/10.1007/11505730_37

2. Cho, M., Lee, J., Lee, K.M.: Reweighted random walks for graph matching. In: Daniilidis, K., Maragos, P., Paragios, N. (eds.) ECCV 2010. LNCS, vol. 6315, pp. 492–505. Springer, Heidelberg (2010). https://doi.org/10.1007/978-3-642-15555-0_36

3. Cour, T., Srinivasan, P., Shi, J.: Balanced graph matching. In: NIPS (2007)

4. Feragen, A., et al.: A hierarchical scheme for geodesic anatomical labeling of airway trees. In: Ayache, N., Delingette, H., Golland, P., Mori, K. (eds.) MICCAI 2012. LNCS, vol. 7512, pp. 147–155. Springer, Heidelberg (2012). https://doi.org/10.1007/978-3-642-33454-2_19

5. Gold, S., Rangarajan, A.: A graduated assignment algorithm for graph matching. IEEE Trans. Pattern Anal. Mach. Intell. **18**, 377–388 (1996)

6. Hamarneh, G., Jassi, P.: VascuSynth: simulating vascular trees for generating volumetric image data with ground-truth segmentation and tree analysis. Comput. Med. Imaging Graph. **34**, 605–616 (2010)

7. Jinkins, J.R.: Atlas of Neuroradiologic Embryology, Anatomy, and Variants. Lippincott Williams & Wilkins, Philadelphia (2000)

8. Kimmel, R., Sethian, J.A.: Computing geodesic paths on manifolds. Proc. Nat. Acad. Sci. **95**, 8431–8435 (1998)

9. Leordeanu, M., Hebert, M.: A spectral technique for correspondence problems using pairwise constraints. In: IEEE ICCV (2005)

10. Leordeanu, M., Hebert, M., Sukthankar, R.: An integer projected fixed point method for graph matching and map inference. In: NIPS (2009)

11. Loiola, E.M., de Abreu, N.M.M., Boaventura-Netto, P.O., Hahn, P., Querido, T.: A survey for the quadratic assignment problem. Eur. J. Oper. Res. **176**(2), 657–690 (2007)

12. Moriconi, S., Zuluaga, M.A., Jäger, H.R., Nachev, P., Ourselin, S., Cardoso, M.J.: VTrails: inferring vessels with geodesic connectivity trees. In: Niethammer, M., et al. (eds.) IPMI 2017. LNCS, vol. 10265, pp. 672–684. Springer, Cham (2017). https://doi.org/10.1007/978-3-319-59050-9_53

13. Petersen, J., Modat, M., Cardoso, M.J., Dirksen, A., Ourselin, S., de Bruijne, M.: Quantitative airway analysis in longitudinal studies using groupwise registration and 4D optimal surfaces. In: Mori, K., Sakuma, I., Sato, Y., Barillot, C., Navab, N. (eds.) MICCAI 2013. LNCS, vol. 8150, pp. 287–294. Springer, Heidelberg (2013). https://doi.org/10.1007/978-3-642-40763-5_36

14. Serradell, E., Pinheiro, M.A., Sznitman, R., Kybic, J., Moreno-Noguer, F., Fua, P.: Non-rigid graph registration using active testing search. IEEE Trans. Pattern Anal. Mach. Intell. **37**(3), 625–638 (2015)

15. Wang, X.: Automatic labeling of vascular structures with topological constraints via HMM. In: Descoteaux, M., Maier-Hein, L., Franz, A., Jannin, P., Collins, D.L., Duchesne, S. (eds.) MICCAI 2017. LNCS, vol. 10434, pp. 208–215. Springer, Cham (2017). https://doi.org/10.1007/978-3-319-66185-8_24

16. Xue, H., Malamateniou, C., Allsop, J., Srinivasan, L., Hajnal, J.V., Rueckert, D.: Automatic extraction and matching of neonatal cerebral vasculature. In: IEEE International Symposium on Biomedical Imaging Nano to Macro (2006)

17. Yang, J., Li, H., Campbell, D., Jia, Y.: Go-ICP: a Globally optimal solution to 3D ICP point-set registration. IEEE Trans. Pattern Anal. Mach. Intell. (2016)

18. Zass, R., Shashua, A.: Probabilistic graph and hypergraph matching. In: IEEE CVPR (2008)

19. Zhou, F., De la Torre, F.: Factorized graph matching. IEEE Trans. Pattern Anal. Mach. Intell. **38**(9), 1774–1789 (2016)

Efficient Groupwise Registration of MR Brain Images via Hierarchical Graph Set Shrinkage

Pei Dong[1,2], Xiaohuan Cao[1,2,3], Pew-Thian Yap[2],
and Dinggang Shen[2(✉)]

[1] Shanghai United Imaging Intelligence Co., Ltd., Shanghai 201807, China
[2] Department of Radiology and BRIC,
University of North Carolina at Chapel Hill, Chapel Hill, NC, USA
dgshen@med.unc.edu
[3] School of Automation, Northwestern Polytechnical University, Xi'an, China

Abstract. Accurate and efficient groupwise registration is important for population analysis. Current groupwise registration methods suffer from high computational cost, which hinders their application to large image datasets. To alleviate the computational burden while delivering accurate groupwise registration result, we propose to use a hierarchical graph set to model the complex image distribution with possibly large anatomical variations, and then turn the groupwise registration problem as a series of simple-to-solve graph shrinkage problems. Specifically, first, we divide the input images into a set of image clusters hierarchically, where images within each image cluster have similar anatomical appearances whereas images falling into different image clusters have varying anatomical appearances. After clustering, two types of graphs, i.e., intra-graph and inter-graph, are employed to hierarchically model the image distribution both within and across the image clusters. The constructed hierarchical graph set divides the registration problem of the whole image set into a series of simple-to-solve registration problems, where the entire registration process can be solved accurately and efficiently. The final deformation pathway of each image to the estimated population center can be obtained by composing each part of the deformation pathway along the hierarchical graph set. To evaluate our proposed method, we performed registration of a hundred of brain images with large anatomical variations. The results indicate that our method yields significant improvement in registration performance over state-of-the-art groupwise registration methods.

1 Introduction

Groupwise registration is key to population analysis of medical images. Unbiased groupwise registration is important for population analysis for discovering imaging biomarkers of neurological disorders, such as Alzheimer's disease (AD) [1]. Unlike conventional pairwise registration, which aligns one image to another, groupwise registration aims to simultaneously align a set of images to their common space, i.e., the population center, thus facilitating the subsequent data analysis.

For over a decade, many groupwise registration methods have been proposed. The most straightforward way is to register each image to a selected template. To reduce the

© Springer Nature Switzerland AG 2018
A. F. Frangi et al. (Eds.): MICCAI 2018, LNCS 11070, pp. 819–826, 2018.
https://doi.org/10.1007/978-3-030-00928-1_92

bias, Park *et al.* [2] chose the template image as the geometrical mean of the image set. Hamm *et al.* [3] built a spanning tree on a learned intrinsic geodesic image manifold, where the template image was selected as the median of the manifold. One major drawback of these methods is that the selected template image will inevitably introduce bias to the subsequent image analysis result, since the brain anatomies vary across individuals [4].

To avoid the bias introduced by selecting a specific subject as the template, unbiased groupwise registration methods were proposed [5–7], where the population center is estimated in a data-driven manner. Joshi *et al.* [5] proposed to calculate the initial tentative group mean by averaging the images after affine registration. Then, all images were aligned to this initial mean image by using diffeomorphic Demons [8]. These two steps were alternatively repeated until convergence, i.e., computing the group mean image from the warped images and aligning the warped images to the newly computed group mean image. However, one major drawback of this method is that the final registration accuracy could be limited by an initial blurry group mean image, especially for registering a group of images with large anatomical variations. To alleviate this limitation, data distribution was taken into consideration. Jia *et al.* [6] proposed a method called ABSORB to progressively move each image towards the group center by using the average deformation field calculated from its neighbor images in the image manifold. In a later study, Ying *et al.* [7] proposed a method called HUGS, which harnessed the image distribution in the image manifold using a graph. Then, the groupwise registration task was formulated as a dynamic graph shrinkage problem. Although these proposed groupwise registration methods can produce accurate group mean images, the computational cost is very expensive, which makes them less effective in real clinical application, especially when dealing with the large-scale dataset.

In this paper, we propose an efficient groupwise registration method for aligning MR brain images, which may potentially have large anatomical variations by using hierarchical graph set shrinkage. To handle images with large anatomical variation, we propose to use a hierarchical graph set to model the heterogeneous image distribution. The main idea is to divide the complex registration problem into multiple easy-to-solve registration problems. Thus, the whole registration process can be conducted accurately and efficiently. The main contributions can be summarized as follows.

(1) We hierarchically divide the whole image set into multiple clusters. Then, we employ two types of graph shrinkage to register the heterogeneous distributed image set: (1) using *intra-graph shrinkage* to register the images within each cluster, and (2) using *inter-graph shrinkage* to register the cluster exemplar images from different clusters. Thus, the whole registration framework considers image distribution both locally and globally.

(2) The registration can be performed efficiently by using the hierarchical graph set, where the deformation field of each image to the population center can be calculated by composing multiple small deformation fields of the neighboring images throughout the graph set.

We evaluated our method in registering 100 images with large anatomical variations from ADNI dataset and also compared it with two state-of-the-art groupwise registration methods, i.e., ABSORB [6] and HUGS [7].

2 Method

Our goal is to accurately register a set of brain images to their group center in an efficient manner. To achieve this goal, *first*, we divide the whole image set into multiple clusters hierarchically by using affinity propagation (AP) [9]. Then, we use two types of graphs, i.e., intra-graph and inter-graph, to hierarchically model the image distribution both *within* each cluster and *across* different clusters. Next, we formulate the groupwise registration into a series of simple graph shrinkage problems, where the entire image set can be registered to its population center both accurately and efficiently.

2.1 Hierarchical Image Clustering

Given a set of linearly aligned images $I = \{I_i | i = 1, \ldots N\}$, we aim to hierarchically divide the image set into multiple clusters, where images within each cluster have similar image appearance, while images falling into different image clusters exhibit anatomical variability. Specifically, we employ the affinity propagation (AP) to perform the image clustering. Compared to other clustering methods, the advantage of using AP clustering method is that no pre-defined number of clusters is required. The method clusters the image set by using an image similarity matrix S. The non-diagonal elements of the similarity matrix $s(i,j)(i,j \in [1,N], i \neq j)$ are calculated as the negative sum of squared distance (SSD) of the two images I_i and I_j, i.e., $s(i,j) = -d_{i,j} = -\left\| I_i - I_j \right\|^2$. The diagonal element of matrix S is set to the preference value p. Since no prior knowledge is available for the input image set, all the diagonal elements of S are set to the same value, i.e., equal to the median of the input similarities, to generate a moderate number of clusters. Because the AP clustering method has no regulation on the number of images within each cluster, after the first round of AP clustering, some clusters may still contain a large number of images, as shown in Fig. 1. Thus, for the clusters with a large number of images, we iteratively perform the AP clustering method for these clusters until the number of images within each cluster is below a pre-defined number. Finally, we can divide the whole image set into hierarchical clusters.

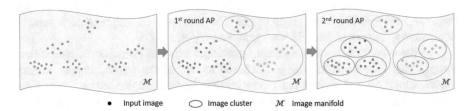

Fig. 1. Illustration of a simple 2-round AP clustering on the image manifold.

2.2   Construction of Hierarchical Graph Set

Upon obtaining the hierarchical image clusters, we build a series of graphs to model both the local and global image distribution using two types of graphs, i.e., intra-graph and inter-graph, as illustrated in Fig. 2. The intra-graph models the image distribution within each cluster, and the inter-graph models the image distribution across different clusters.

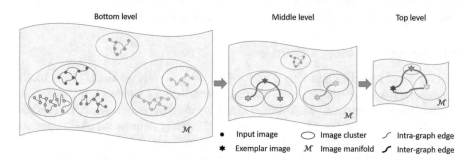

Fig. 2. Illustration of construction of hierarchical graph set.

For the construction of intra-graph, we follow the graph construction method used in [7]. Specifically, by using a line-search based method, all images within the cluster are linked to a single graph, and the number of edges within the graph is minimized. The vertices of the graph represent all images within the same cluster, and the edge of the graph suggests that two connected images are similar. The topology of each constructed intra-graph is kept throughout the registration process to maintain the image distribution locally on the manifold within the image cluster. To move each image unbiasedly towards their group center within the cluster, each vertex of the graph is associated with a vertex label, which is defined by the degree of the graph vertex, i.e., the number of edges connected to the vertex. It will influence the speed of the image moving along the image manifold. Clearly, the larger the value of the vertex label, the more similar the current image is compared with other images, and the slower the image will move towards the group center. The advantage of assigning each vertex a label value is important for achieving unbiased registration.

For the construction of inter-graph, each vertex is the exemplar image of each cluster, where the exemplar image is chosen as one of the warped images in each cluster, which has the highest label vertex value. Each exemplar image is also associated with a vertex label value, which equals to the value of total vertex degree of the represented image cluster. As shown in Fig. 2, by constructing both intra-graph and inter-graph, the graph set can be constructed hierarchically from the clusters at the bottom level to the clusters at the top level.

2.3   Groupwise Image Registration via Hierarchical Graph Shrinkage

With the constructed hierarchical graph set, the groupwise registration for the entire dataset can be achieved by solving a series of dynamic simple graph shrinkage problems through the hierarchical graph set from the image clusters at the bottom level towards the image clusters at the top level. Specifically, for a certain image I_i located in an image cluster at the bottom level, we first obtain the deformation field φ_i^1 using the *intra-graph shrinkage*, which warps the image I_i to the group center at the bottom level. Then, by using the *inter-graph shrinkage* at the next level, we can obtain the deformation field that warps the exemplar image to the group center at the next level. In this way, by performing the graph shrinkage hierarchically from the bottom level to the top level along the hierarchical graph set, a set of deformation fields $\varphi_i = \{\varphi_i^p | p = 1, \ldots, P(i)\}$ can be obtained, where $P(i)$ denotes the total number of deformation fields for image I_i warped from the bottom level to the whole-image-set group center I_{GC}. Finally, the whole deformation pathway ψ_i, which warps the image I_i to I_{GC}, can be obtained by composing each part of the deformation fields in φ_i:

$$\psi_i = \varphi_i^1 \circ \varphi_i^2 \circ \cdots \circ \varphi_i^{P(i)}. \tag{1}$$

In this way, the final deformation field set $\Psi = \{\psi_i | i = 1, \ldots, N\}$ can be obtained, which can be used to warp every respective image to the group center I_{GC}.

There are two reasons that why the whole groupwise registration process can be efficiently performed. *First*, for *intra-graph shrinkage*, the registration process can be converged with only a few iterations, since all image appearances within the image cluster are similar. *Second*, for *inter-graph shrinkage*, the total number of the graph vertices (exemplar image) is small, since only one exemplar image is used for each cluster. Thus, the computational cost is not expensive. Therefore, our method can significantly reduce the computational time.

3   Experiments and Results

To verify the effectiveness of our method, we evaluated the method for registering one hundred brain images, which were randomly selected from ADNI dataset. For the selected images, we randomly selected 50 subjects from the normal control (NC) group and the other 50 images from the AD group. Before performing groupwise registration, all images were pre-processed by the following steps. *First*, all images were resampled and cropped to an image size of $196 \times 164 \times 176$ with a voxel size of $1 \times 1 \times 1$ mm^3. Then, we used N3 algorithm [10] to correct the intensity inhomogeneity. After that, we employed Brain Extraction Tool (BET) [11] for skull stripping. Then, we selected one image sitting in the median of the geodesic image manifold as the template image, and all the remaining images were linearly aligned to this template by using FLIRT [12]. Next, we segmented each image into three brain tissues of gray matter (GM), white matter (WM) and cerebrospinal fluid (CSF) by using FAST [13]. These tissue segmentations were then manually corrected by visual inspection and were used as the ground truth for evaluating the registration performance. Figure 3 illustrates

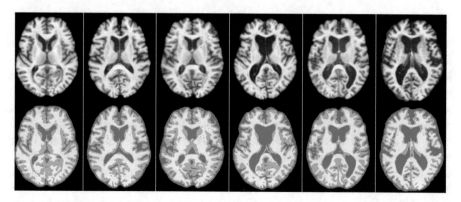

Fig. 3. Typical MR brain images and the corresponding tissue labels from ADNI dataset. The darker yellow, light yellow and blue represent brain tissue types of GM, WM, and CSF, respectively.

typical intensity images and their corresponding segmented images from the NC group (left three columns) and the AD group (right three columns).

To quantitatively evaluate our method, we employed Dice ratio to measure the tissue overlap after groupwise registration. The Dice ratio is defined as $DR = 2 \times |A \cap B|/(|A| + |B|)$, where A and B are the two corresponding tissue regions in the two aligned brain images. Since no label image was available in the common space of the group center, we used a majority voting method on all registered images to compute a label image in the common space. The Dice ratio of different brain tissue type for each image can be then calculated *with respect to* the created label image in the common space.

To illustrate the registration performance of our method compared with the state-of-the-art groupwise registration methods, Fig. 4(a) shows the progression curve of the overall Dice ratio at each iteration when performing groupwise registration. It can be observed that our method achieved the best registration accuracy with only a few iterations, compared with the other methods. By regarding the maximum performance as the one with the slope of progression curve smaller than 0.001, the ABSORB method reached its maximum performance at 11th iteration with Dice ratio of 83.6%. HUGS attained its maximum performance at 15th iteration with Dice ratio of 89.3%. Our proposed method (HML) obtained its maximum Dice ratio at 6th iteration with overall Dice ratio of 90.3%. By using a *t*-test, our method significantly outperformed state-of-the-art registration methods. In addition, our method can also significantly reduce the computational time compared with the best counterpart method (HUGS). Figure 4(b) illustrates the computational time of each method for reaching their maximum performance. It shows that our method saves about six times the computational cost compared with the HUGS method. Figure 5 shows the group mean images of all registered 100 brain images by the three groupwise registration methods in achieving their maximum registration performance. As can be seen, the group mean image of our method has more anatomical details compared to the other two methods.

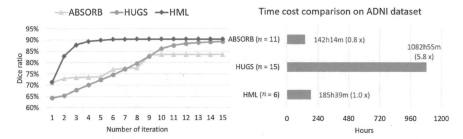

Fig. 4. (a) Progression curve of the overall Dice ratio of the three brain tissue types, i.e., GM, WM, and CSF, during the groupwise registration by the three methods on the ADNI dataset. (b) Time cost comparison between our method and the other two methods in registering 100 images from ADNI dataset for achieving the maximum registration performance at the n-th iteration.

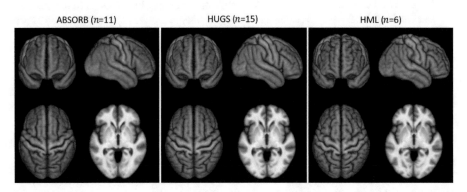

Fig. 5. Group mean images of the three groupwise registration methods (left: ABSORB; middle: HUGS; right: HML) at their maximum performance.

4   Conclusion

In this paper, we proposed an accurate and efficient groupwise registration method for registering MR brain images that may pose large anatomical variations. After hierarchically dividing the whole image set into multiple image clusters, we employed two types of graphs, i.e., intra-graph and inter-graph, to model the local and the global image distributions hierarchically. Then, the whole image registration can be achieved by solving a series of simple graph shrinkage problems, where each simple graph shrinkage can be calculated both accurately and efficiently. Our method was successfully applied to registering 100 brain images with large anatomical variations. Experimental results showed that our method could an provide more accurate registration result while significantly reducing the computational cost, compared to state-of-the-art groupwise registration methods.

References

1. Viergever, M.A., Maintz, J.B.A., Klein, S., Murphy, K., Staring, M., Pluim, J.P.W.: A survey of medical image registration – under review. Med. Image Anal. **33**, 140–144 (2016)
2. Park, H., Bland, P.H., Hero, A.O., Meyer, C.R.: Least biased target selection in probabilistic atlas construction. In: Duncan, J.S., Gerig, G. (eds.) MICCAI 2005, Part II. LNCS, vol. 3750, pp. 419–426. Springer, Heidelberg (2005). https://doi.org/10.1007/11566489_52
3. Hamm, J., Davatzikos, C., Verma, R.: Efficient large deformation registration via geodesics on a learned manifold of images. In: Yang, G.-Z., Hawkes, D., Rueckert, D., Noble, A., Taylor, C. (eds.) MICCAI 2009, Part I. LNCS, vol. 5761, pp. 680–687. Springer, Heidelberg (2009). https://doi.org/10.1007/978-3-642-04268-3_84
4. Toga, A.W., Thompson, P.M.: The role of image registration in brain mapping. Image Vis. Comput. **19**, 3–24 (2001)
5. Joshi, S., Davis, B., Jomier, M., Gerig, G.: Unbiased diffeomorphic atlas construction for computational anatomy. NeuroImage **23**, S151–S160 (2004)
6. Jia, H., Wu, G., Wang, Q., Shen, D.: ABSORB: atlas building by self-organized registration and bundling. In: 2010 IEEE Computer Society Conference on Computer Vision and Pattern Recognition, pp. 2785–2790 (2010)
7. Ying, S., Wu, G., Wang, Q., Shen, D.: Hierarchical unbiased graph shrinkage (HUGS): a novel groupwise registration for large data set. NeuroImage **84**, 626–638 (2014)
8. Vercauteren, T., Pennec, X., Perchant, A., Ayache, N.: Non-parametric diffeomorphic image registration with the demons algorithm. In: Ayache, N., Ourselin, S., Maeder, A. (eds.) MICCAI 2007, Part II. LNCS, vol. 4792, pp. 319–326. Springer, Heidelberg (2007). https://doi.org/10.1007/978-3-540-75759-7_39
9. Frey, B.J., Dueck, D.: Clustering by passing messages between data points. Science **315**, 972–976 (2007)
10. Sled, J.G., Zijdenbos, A.P., Evans, A.C.: A nonparametric method for automatic correction of intensity nonuniformity in MRI data. IEEE Trans. Med. Imaging **17**, 87–97 (1998)
11. Smith, S.M.: Fast robust automated brain extraction. Hum. Brain Mapp. **17**, 143–155 (2002)
12. Jenkinson, M., Smith, S.: A global optimisation method for robust affine registration of brain images. Med. Image Anal. **5**, 143–156 (2001)
13. Zhang, Y., Brady, M., Smith, S.: Segmentation of brain MR images through a hidden Markov random field model and the expectation-maximization algorithm. IEEE Trans. Med. Imag. **20**(1), 45–57 2001

Initialize Globally Before Acting Locally: Enabling Landmark-Free 3D US to MRI Registration

Julia Rackerseder[1(✉)], Maximilian Baust[2], Rüdiger Göbl[1], Nassir Navab[1,3], and Christoph Hennersperger[1,4]

[1] Technische Universität München, Munich, Germany
`julia.rackerseder@tum.de`
[2] Konica Minolta Laboratory Europe, Munich, Germany
[3] Johns Hopkins University, Baltimore, USA
[4] Trinity College Dublin, Dublin, Ireland

Abstract. Registration of partial-view 3D US volumes with MRI data is influenced by initialization. The standard of practice is using extrinsic or intrinsic landmarks, which can be very tedious to obtain. To overcome the limitations of registration initialization, we present a novel approach that is based on Euclidean distance maps derived from easily obtainable coarse segmentations. We evaluate our approach on a publicly available brain tumor dataset (RESECT) and show that it is robust regarding minimal to no overlap of target area and varying initial position. We demonstrate that our method provides initializations that greatly increase the capture range of state-of-the-art nonlinear registration algorithms.

1 Introduction

Image registration, i.e. the process of establishing a common reference frame for two or more image data sets, is an important step for a number of medical image computing tasks and computer aided medical procedures. As noted by Viergever *et al.* [1] in their recent review article on medical image registration, intensity-based approaches are now forming the basis for the vast majority of registration methods, and research in this field focuses almost exclusively on nonlinear image registration. However, initialization plays a crucial role in convergence of such intensity-based and nonlinear methods. In case of mono- or multi-modal tomographic registration tasks, such a initialization might be obtained based on the information stored in the header of the respective datasets. The situation is entirely different for registering 3D ultrasound (US) data, as it lacks a canonical orientation. Thus, the registration task is particularly challenging when a common reference frame for 3D US data and Magnetic Resonance Imaging (MRI)

This project has received funding from the European Union's Horizon 2020 research and innovation program EDEN2020 under grant agreement No 688279 as well as the GPU grant program from NVIDIA Corporation.

© Springer Nature Switzerland AG 2018
A. F. Frangi et al. (Eds.): MICCAI 2018, LNCS 11070, pp. 827–835, 2018.
https://doi.org/10.1007/978-3-030-00928-1_93

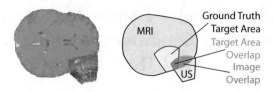

Fig. 1. Limited overlap in registration. To initialize registration, a sufficient overlap of images is required. In case of limited overlap landmark selection is challenging. Target Area Overlap is defined as pixels where Target Area and US volume are superimposed (blue), Image Overlap is the part where MRI and US are superimposed before initialization (green + blue).

data has to be established, because US scans usually depict only a substantially reduced portion of the anatomy. This is in strong contrast to the capture range of state-of-the-art registration methods, requiring an initial error not greater than 15 mm, as reported recently [2].

Thus, the application of such nonlinear or *local registration* methods requires a sufficiently close *global initialization*. If external fiducials are not available or feasible, such an initialization is obtained via the selection of 3D landmarks in common clinical practice. In view of the aforementioned observations by Viergever *et al.* [1], we argue that the problem of global initialization has received too little attention so far – particularly for the targeted application of 3D US to MRI registration with limited overlap (see Fig. 1). Although the process of defining a single landmark requires little user interaction (1 click), it depends on profound geometrical understanding of the targeted anatomy as well as the modality-specific appearance. Particularly in case of 3D US, this process puts a high mental load on the observer, as visual inspection of three dimensional images is difficult due to the lack of predefined orientations as well as the limited volumetric coverage of the anatomy. While a high precision can be achieved in theory [3], it is tedious and time consuming. In practice, this often results in impaired accuracies and high inter-observer variability due to the limited time in daily routine. Moreover, many works show that the learning curve can be steep when evaluating 3D US, even if the rater had previous training in 2D US [4]. Contrary to identifying landmarks in 3D, we argue that obtaining coarse segmentations and using them for global initialization is a much more convenient alternative. The reason is that they can be obtained either with state-of-the-art automatic segmentation techniques, or sophisticated slice-wise and semi-automatic methods. Furthermore, experts are not required to perform a mental mapping of multiple 3D data sets with partially limited field of view to precisely identify specific and corresponding anatomical landmarks in the data.

We thus propose a novel initialization procedure based on segmentation-derived distance maps. We validate this approach on the publicly available REtroSpective Evaluation of Cerebral Tumors (RESECT) dataset [3] and compare it to the global initialization based on landmarks.

2   Discussion of Related Work

For the nonlinear, deformable registration of 3D US and MRI data, several state-of-the-art methods are available. They all have in common that initial conditions are stringent in terms of target registration error: for instance, about 15 mm are reported by Fürst *et al.* [2] and below 10 mm are reported by Coupé *et al.* [5]. In order to obtain an initialization of sufficient quality, three possible methods exist: Usage of external tracking data, landmarks identified in the image data and registration of geometrical entities, e.g. rigid registration of segmentations. If external tracking is not available, such as for retrospective studies, only the latter two strategies are available. From a clinical point of view, landmark-based initialization appears to be the more widely-used approach, but it requires a sufficient geometrical understanding of the target anatomy and employed imaging modalities as mentioned before. Reports of inter-observer variation of landmark selection range from 0.33 ± 0.08 mm [3] up to 1.6 mm [6] even in case of clearly discernible landmarks. As we focus on situations where tracking data is not available, we regard landmark-based initialization as the baseline approach for evaluation, where the aforementioned studies have been used to define a realistic experiment setup, c.f. Sect. 4.

Segmentation-based registration initialization has been studied in context of prostate fusion biopsy [7], where trans-rectal US has to be registered to MRI data. Both this example and the situation studied in this work (see Fig. 1) are challenging in terms of limited view of the US volume and the target organ being highly symmetrical, where the global registration of even perfect segmentations would suffer from many ambiguities.

As a consequence, the initialization problem requires further regularization, for which we employ distance transforms which have been shown to be very useful for correspondence estimation [7–9]. Together with an adaptive gradient-based optimization strategy, c.f. Sect. 3, we thus are able to satisfy initialization conditions for state-of-the-art deformable registration methods, even in case of very limited views of the US data and coarse semi-automatic US segmentations.

3   Methods

In this section, we derive a novel initialization procedure that only requires low-resolution coarse segmentations to initialize multi-modal deformable 3D US to MRI registration methods. These segmentations can be easily obtained via coarse annotations or any segmentation method. From these label maps, multi-class distance maps are computed, which are registered simultaneously by optimizing our proposed similarity measure via a gradient-based optimization strategy.

3.1   Coarse Segmentation

Let $V_f : \Omega_f \to \mathbb{R}$ denote the fixed and $V_m : \Omega_m \to \mathbb{R}$ the moving volumes defined on their respective domains $\Omega_f, \Omega_m \subset \mathbb{R}^3$. The first step of our method comprises the creation of N coarse segmentations for both V_f and V_m, i.e. we assume two, not necessarily disjoint and complete, partitions of Ω_f and Ω_m:

$$\bigcup_{\ell=1}^{N} \Omega_{f,\ell} \subset \Omega_f \quad \text{and} \quad \bigcup_{\ell=1}^{N} \Omega_{m,\ell} \subset \Omega_m. \tag{1}$$

The choice of the segmentation algorithm itself depends on targeted anatomy and specific application, but can be automated in most cases. In Sect. 4 we evaluate our approach for the application of intra-operative brain imaging, where the US volume takes the role of V_f and the MRI volume takes the role of V_m.

3.2 Initialization Procedure

Registering the two sets of label masks obtained via segmentation could be formulated as a (pseudo-)mono-modal registration problem for which plenty of classical intensity-based registration techniques are available. However, this approach would suffer from the following issues: Firstly, computing the similarity of label maps containing all labels encoded by numerical values would bare the possibility of trading label errors in an unfavorable way: two erroneously registered voxels with a label distance of one would yield the same error as one erroneously registered voxel with label distance two. Secondly, registering label maps with bad initialization would suffer from low capture range as homogeneous label regions (particularly in case of the background label) would not yield meaningful information for optimization. In order to overcome these two problems, we propose a similarity measure which computes label-specific distances (taking into account the first problem) and employs distance maps to increase the capture range (solving the latter issue). We chose distance maps due to their suitability for correspondence estimation, see [8,9] for an example. Therefore, a Euclidean distance transform ϕ is applied to each of the N classes individually and the resulting distance maps are denoted by

$$\phi_{f,\ell} = \phi(\chi(\Omega_{f,\ell})) \quad \text{and} \quad \phi_{m,\ell} = \phi(\chi(\Omega_{m,\ell})), \tag{2}$$

where χ denotes the characteristic function applied to the respective set. This allows us to formulate the initialization task as a minimization problem

$$\min_{T \in SE(3)} \sum_{\ell=1}^{N} \int_{\Omega_f} |(\phi_{m,\ell} \circ T)(x) - \phi_{f,\ell}(x)|^p \, dx, \tag{3}$$

where $p = 1, 2$ and $T \in SE(3)$ denotes the rigid transformation. As Eq. (3) is differentiable, gradient-based optimization techniques can be applied[1]. In order to avoid parameter updates from becoming too large and yielding unstable behavior, we employ the following modified gradient descent scheme:

$$p_{i+1} = p_i - \tau \text{sign}(\delta_i) \min\{|\delta_i|, p_{\max}\}, \tag{4}$$

---

[1] In case of $p = 1$ a differentiable relaxation can be found.

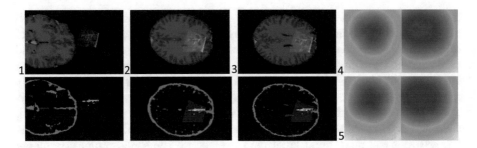

Fig. 2. Volumes and label map with (1) −80 mm offset in x direction, −0.1 rad rotation around α and β for the MRI (2) after initialization with our method and (3) ground truth provided by RESECT (4) distance map for surface (5) and foreground label.

where p_i denotes the optimized rotation angle or translation parameter and δ_i the partial derivative of Eq. (3) w.r.t. p at iteration step i. Furthermore, $\tau > 0$ is a positive step size parameter and $p_{\max} > 0$ regulates the maximum parameter update per iteration. This way, unstable behavior can be avoided by restricting the maximum parameter update to $\tau p_{\max}$ (measured in radians or mm, respectively). For $|\delta_i| < p_{\max}$, however, the update scheme corresponds to a regular gradient descent optimization.

The distance maps not only ensure a large capture range, but also cause the cost function in Eq. (3) to enjoy favorable properties, as they a more regular than the piecewise constant label maps. Moreover, from an implementation point of view, it is advisable to employ a foreground mask Ω_F to restrict the computation of Eq. (3) to the target domain $\Omega_F \cap \Omega_f$.

4   Experiments and Results

We evaluate our proposed initialization method on the example of the publicly available RESECT dataset [3]. It is comprised of imaging data for 23 patients with low-grade gliomas, containing co-registered 3T Gadolinium-enhanced T1w and T2-FLAIR MRI, as well as B-mode ultrasound sweeps from before, during and after tumor resection, reconstructed into 3D volumes. Retrospectively, up to 17 high accuracy anatomical landmarks were annotated across all three registered US sweeps and between US and MRI volumes for 22 patients. Only these patients are included in our evaluation. For easier and faster computation, we downsample all US volumes to match the MRI isotropic resolution of 1 mm in 3D Slicer [10].[2] [10]. We mask the foreground in ultrasound and MRI volumes.

With regard to the coarse registration, the idea is to provide clearly distinguishable and salient labels in both MRI and US, focusing on unique features which are partly visible from any angle the US transducer could be positioned at

---

[2] https://www.slicer.org/.

(see Fig. 2). For brain imaging, included classes are for example (lateral) ventricles, longitudinal fissure and sulci, such as the prominent central and precentral sulcus. In other applications, features such as vessel trees, bones, or fasciae could be considered for coarse segmentations. Due to the penetration depth of the ultrasound in the RESECT dataset, we employ superficial structures, namely sulci, cerebellar tentorium and longitudinal fissure. Skull stripping and gray-white matter segmentations are automatically performed in FreeSurfer[3] [11], yielding labels in all MRI datasets that satisfy the characteristics defined above. For creating the ultrasound label map, we choose the semi-automatic random walk approach [12], where only few pre-labeled pixels are needed. From the extracted labels, a multi-channel distance map (here, 2 channels: 1 = foreground, 2 = surface) is created for both modalities respectively. The proposed metric (see Eq. 3) is estimated and minimized with gradient descent for the distance maps to find the optimal transformation matrix T. We set the step size τ to 0.5, p_{max} to 0.004 rad, and 0.5 mm, keeping updates per step minimal.

4.1   Evaluation

In view of providing a global initialization for following local multi-modal registration, we evaluate the robustness of the proposed initialization, and compare it to manual landmark-annotation as the de-facto standard in practice.

As a standard error metric for any registration method, the quality of the initialization is evaluated by means of the mean target registration error [13] (TRE_{mean}), computed on all landmarks L provided by the RESECT dataset.

We consider initialization to be a success if the position is within the capture range of state-of-the-art (deformable) registration methods, otherwise we score it as a failure. With respect to application in neurosurgery, automatic US–MRI registration using the LC^2 metric has a capture range of 15 mm [2]. Thus we define the following quality criteria: If $TRE_{mean} \leq 15$ mm the initialization is considered acceptable, 10–15 mm good and ≤ 5 mm very good.

Robustness. In order to test the robustness with regard to target area overlap and image overlap (see Fig. 1) we conduct convergence tests for increasing translation in x,y,z direction of up to ±200 mm, as well as rotation around Euler angles α, β, γ of up to ±0.3 rad. In total, this results in 2244 conducted initializations, of which 24.96% are very good, 32.62% good, 26.75% acceptable and 15.64% fail. All of the failed cases have below 10% overlap with the target area. Furthermore, all cases with image overlap over 30% converge with $TRE_{mean} \leq 15$ mm, showing the robustness of the initialization. Of these, 25.48% are considered very good, 40.61% good and 33.91% acceptable results. Even 24.94% of cases with no initial overlap of MRI and US converge with very good results, 19.82% with good, 15.83% with acceptable.

Comparison to Standard in Practice. As discussed in Sect. 2, the widely used practice is to initialize volumes with non-overlapping positions by manual

---

[3] http://surfer.nmr.mgh.harvard.edu/fswiki/.

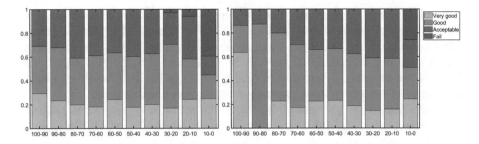

Fig. 3. Robustness test for decreasing overlap percentage. These barplots show the fraction of experiments that fall into each quality measure category $(y - axis)$ considering the percentage of overlap $(x - axis)$ for image overlap (left) and target area overlap right image (right).

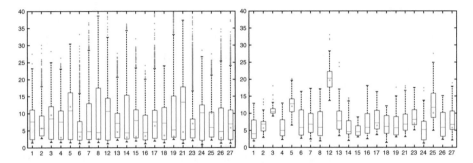

Fig. 4. Comparison to manual landmark selection. Shown are errors for all patient TREs for initialization with four random landmarks selected from all available landmark pairs disturbed with Gaussian ($\sigma = 1.5$ mm) noise (left) in comparison to errors for our initialization (right). Circles mark the TRE given by RESECT

selection of landmarks. We simulate this behaviour by randomly choosing 4 landmarks given by the dataset and disturbing them with Gaussian noise with $\sigma = 1.5$ mm, since this is a commonly reported inter-observer variation (see Sect. 2). For each patient this is repeated 10,000 times and the TRE_{mean} is calculated on all ground truth landmarks. Results are visualized in Fig. 4 on the left side. For comparison, on the right side, we show the distribution of TRE_{mean} for our conducted initialization test.

5   Discussion and Conclusion

Despite the fact that our results partially show outliers in terms of initialization accuracy, especially the comparison to manual landmark registration, reflects the potentially high inter-operator variability in initialization performance. In particular for challenging anatomies, landmark-based registration is demanding for non-experts, because even finding a sufficient number of landmark pairs is often difficult. In view of applications in practice, it should be noted that many experts are not trained in ultrasound imaging, and thus finding appropriate features can be unclear, also due to quality of US in 3D data. Even for placing landmarks in MRI high inter-observer variation has been reported [14].

Furthermore, the presented initialization is robust with respect to both the target area overlap, as well as the specific image overlap, cf. Fig. 3. This can be accounted to the specific choice of distance maps in combination with coarse features, providing anatomical context as well as coverage even when the actual volumes do not overlap. We hope that the proposed method can lead to a simplified clinical routine and more robust results in 3D image registration.

References

1. Viergever, M.A., Maintz, J.A., Klein, S., Murphy, K., Staring, M., Pluim, J.P.: A survey of medical image registration–under review. Med. Image Anal. **33**, 140–144 (2016)
2. Fuerst, B., Wein, W., Müller, M., Navab, N.: Automatic ultrasound-MRI registration for neurosurgery using the 2D and 3D LC2 metric. Med. Image Anal. **18**(8), 1312–1319 (2014)
3. Xiao, Y., Fortin, M., Unsgård, G., Rivaz, H., Reinertsen, I.: Retrospective evaluation of cerebral tumors (RESECT): a clinical database of pre-operative MRI and intra-operative ultrasound in low-grade glioma surgeries. Med. Phys. **44**, 3875–3882 (2017)
4. Rodriguez, A., Guillén, J.J., López, M.J., Vassena, R., Coll, O., Vernaeve, V.: Learning curves in 3-dimensional sonographic follicle monitoring during controlled ovarian stimulation. J. Ultrasound Med. **33**(4), 649–655 (2014)
5. Coupé, P., Hellier, P., Morandi, X., Barillot, C.: 3D rigid registration of intraoperative ultrasound and preoperative MR brain images based on hyperechogenic structures. J. Biomed. Imaging **2012**, 1 (2012)
6. Mabee, M., Dulai, S., Thompson, R.B., Jaremko, J.L.: Reproducibility of acetabular landmarks and a standardized coordinate system obtained from 3D hip ultrasound. Ultrason. Imaging **37**(4), 267–276 (2015)
7. Fedorov, A., et al.: Open-source image registration for MRI–TRUS fusion-guided prostate interventions. Int. J. Comput. Assist. Radiol. Surg. **10**(6), 925–934 (2015)
8. Itti, L., Chang, L., Mangin, J.F., Darcourt, J., Ernst, T.: Robust multimodality registration for brain mapping. Hum. Brain Mapp. **5**(1), 3–17 (1997)
9. Slavcheva, M., Kehl, W., Navab, N., Ilic, S.: SDF-2-SDF: highly accurate 3D object reconstruction. In: Leibe, B., Matas, J., Sebe, N., Welling, M. (eds.) ECCV 2016. LNCS, vol. 9905, pp. 680–696. Springer, Cham (2016). https://doi.org/10.1007/978-3-319-46448-0_41
10. Fedorov, A., et al.: 3D slicer as an image computing platform for the quantitative imaging network. Magn. Reson. Imaging **30**(9), 1323–1341 (2012)
11. Fischl, B., et al.: Whole brain segmentation: automated labeling of neuroanatomical structures in the human brain. Neuron **33**(3), 341–355 (2002)

12. Grady, L.: Random walks for image segmentation. IEEE Trans. Pattern Anal. Mach. Intell. **28**(11), 1768–1783 (2006)
13. Fitzpatrick, J.M., West, J.B., Maurer, C.R.: Predicting error in rigid-body point-based registration. IEEE Trans. Med. Imaging **17**(5), 694–702 (1998)
14. Park, A., Nam, D., Friedman, M.V., Duncan, S.T., Hillen, T.J., Barrack, R.L.: Inter-observer precision and physiologic variability of MRI landmarks used to determine rotational alignment in conventional and patient-specific TKA. J. Arthroplast. **30**(2), 290–295 (2015)

Solving the Cross-Subject Parcel Matching Problem Using Optimal Transport

Guillermo Gallardo[1]([⊠]), Nathalie T. H. Gayraud[1], Rachid Deriche[1],
Maureen Clerc[1], Samuel Deslauriers-Gauthier[1], and Demian Wassermann[1,2]

[1] Inria Sophia Antipolis, Université Côte d'Azur, Nice, France
`guillermo.gallardo-diez@inria.fr`
[2] Inria, CEA, Université Paris-Saclay, Paris, France

Abstract. Matching structural parcels across different subjects is an open problem in neuroscience. Even when produced by the same technique, parcellations tend to differ in the number, shape, and spatial localization of parcels across subjects. In this work, we propose a parcel matching method based on Optimal Transport. We test its performance by matching parcels of the Desikan atlas, parcels based on a functional criteria and structural parcels. We compare our technique against three other ways to match parcels which are based on the Euclidean distance, the cosine similarity, and the Kullback-Leibler divergence. Our results show that our method achieves the highest number of correct matches.

1 Introduction

Brain organization displays high variability across individuals and species. Studying brain connectivity therefore faces the challenge of locating homogeneous regions while accounting for this variability. Different techniques have been proposed to parcellate the brain based on its structural connectivity. However, matching the resulting parcels across different subjects is still an open problem in neuroscience. Even when produced by the same technique, parcellations tend to differ in the number, shape, and spatial localization of parcels across subjects [8]. Current theories hold that long-range structural connectivity, namely, extrinsic connectivity, is strongly related to brain function [14]. Therefore, being able to match parcels with similar connectivity across subjects can help to understand brain function while also enabling the comparisons of cortical areas across different species [9].

Most of the current methods to match parcels across subjects are strongly linked to the technique used to create them. For example, Moreno-Dominguez et al. [11] seek correspondences between dendrograms created by means of Hierarchical Clustering. Parisot et al. [13] impose the consistence of parcels across subjects while creating the parcellation. In recent works Mars et al. propose to

---

G. Gallardo and N. T. H. Gayraud contributed equally in this work.

A. F. Frangi et al. (Eds.): MICCAI 2018, LNCS 11070, pp. 836–843, 2018.
https://doi.org/10.1007/978-3-030-00928-1_94

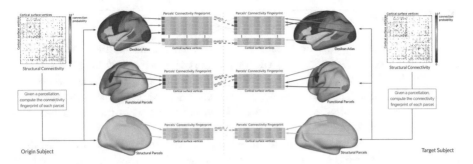

Fig. 1. From the cortico-cortical structural connectivity matrix of a subject, we can estimate the connectivity fingerprints of each parcel in three different types of parcellations. For each parcellation we compute the amount of correct matches (green lines) that each matching technique produces.

use the Manhattan distance, cosine similarity [10] or the Kullback–Leibler (KL) divergence [9] to compare and match connectivity fingerprints, successfully identifying common areas across humans and primates.

In this work, we propose to match parcels based on their extrinsic connectivity fingerprint using Optimal Transportation theory. Optimal Transport (OT) is a technique that seeks the optimal way to transport mass between probability distributions. While KL divergence computes the difference between two distributions, OT computes a matching between them. In particular, our method adopts a discrete regularized version of Optimal Transport (OT), which has been presented in Gayraud et al. [6] and Courty et al. [2] as a solution to the domain adaptation problem.

We validate our method with four different experiments. In the first experiment, we test the feasibility of our method by generating parcels with synthetic connectivity fingerprints and matching them. In the second one, we show that our technique is able to match parcels of the same atlas across subjects. We use the anatomical atlas of Desikan [4] as its parcels have high spatial coherence and consistent connectivity profiles across subjects [16]. Finally, we show the capacity of our method to match parcels generated with the same criteria but have some spatial cross-subject variability. We assess this for two different situations. In the first one, we derive the parcels from functional activations [1]. We use responses to motor and visual stimuli since they have been shown to be strongly related to structural connectivity [12,15]. In the second one, we divide the Lateral Occipital Gyrus in 3 parcels using a structurally-based parcellation technique [5]. We use the Lateral Occipital Gyrus since it has been shown to have a consistent parcellation across subjects [5,17]. The outline of the last three experiments can be seen in Fig. 1.

In each experiment, we compare our technique against three other ways to match parcels based on the Euclidean distance; the cosine similarity; and the Kullback-Leibler divergence. Our results on real data show that our method based on OT always achieves the highest number of correct matches.

2 Methods

Given two subjects with their respective parcellations, we compute their parcel matching by considering one as the origin and the other one as target. More formally, let $X^a = \{x_i^a\}_{i=1}^{N_a}$, $x_i^a \in \Omega^a \subset \mathbb{R}^n$ be an origin dataset where N_a denotes the number of parcels; x_i^a is the extrinsic connectivity fingerprint of parcel i; and n denotes its dimension. We wish to recover a matching between X^a and a target dataset $X^b = \{x_i^b\}_{i=1}^{N_b}$, $x_i^b \in \Omega^b \subset \mathbb{R}^n$.

In this section, we start by formulating our regularized discrete OT-based method and proceed by presenting three ways of computing this matching that are based on the Euclidean distance; the cosine similarity; and the KL-divergence.

2.1 Discrete Regularized Optimal Transport

Optimal Transport (OT) theory boils down to finding the optimal way to transport or redistribute mass from one probability distribution to another with respect to some cost function. In this work, since the datasets X^a and X^b are discrete datasets, we use their empirical probability distributions and apply the discrete formulation of OT [2,6] to solve the parcel matching problem. A simplified example of how our method proceeds is presented in Fig. 2.

Assume that X^a and X^b follow probability distributions $p_a(x^a)$ and $p_b(x^b)$, respectively. We suppose that X^a has undergone a transformation $\mathbf{T} : \Omega^a \to \Omega^b$, such that $p_b(\mathbf{T}(x^a)) = p_b(x^b)$. We wish to recover $\mathbf{T}$ and use it to match the parcels of X^a and X^b. Using discrete regularized OT we compute a transport plan γ_0 between these two probability distributions. This transport plan is a doubly stochastic matrix which minimizes a certain transportation cost C over the vectors of X^a and X^b. In other words, it defines the optimal exchange of mass between the two probability distributions. We use γ_0 to compute an estimation $\hat{\mathbf{T}}$ by selecting the pairs of vectors, i.e., parcels that exchange the most mass.

Since $p_a(x^a)$ and $p_b(x^b)$ are not known, we use the corresponding empirical distributions $\mu_a = \sum_{i=1}^{N^a} p_i^a \delta_{x_i^a}$ and $\mu_b = \sum_{j=1}^{N^b} p_j^b \delta_{x_j^b}$ instead, where p_i^a and p_j^b are the probability masses associated to each sample. However, given that the dimension of our data depends on the number of vertices in the cortical mesh, the curse of dimensionality makes the estimation of μ_a and μ_b intrinsically difficult. We therefore simply assume a uniform probability distribution over all vectors, $p_i^a = \frac{1}{N^a}$ and $p_j^b = \frac{1}{N^b}$. We compute the transport plan γ_0 such that, if

$$\mathcal{B} = \left\{\gamma \in (\mathbb{R}^+)^{N_a \times N_b} \mid \gamma \mathbf{1}_{N_b} = \frac{1}{N^a}\mathbf{1}_{N_a}, \gamma^{\mathbf{T}}\mathbf{1}_{N_a} = \frac{1}{N^b}\mathbf{1}_{N_b}\right\} \tag{1}$$

denotes the set of all doubly stochastic matrices whose marginals are the probability measures μ_a and μ_b, where $\mathbf{1}_N$ is an N-dimensional vector of ones, then $\gamma_0 \in \mathcal{B}$ is the output of the following minimization problem.

$$\gamma_0 = \arg\min_{\gamma \in \mathcal{B}} \langle \gamma, C \rangle_F + \lambda \sum_{i,j} \gamma(i,j) \log \gamma(i,j) \tag{2}$$

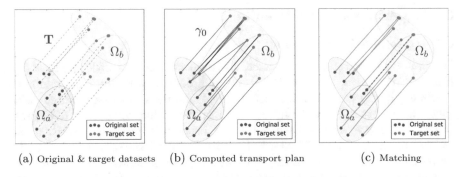

(a) Original & target datasets   (b) Computed transport plan   (c) Matching

Fig. 2. A 2-d example of using OT to compute the matching between two different datasets. On the left we show the original and target datasets. The real matchings are displayed as green dashed edges. In the middle, the edge densities represent the values of the computed coupling γ_0, which denote the amount of mass that is exchanged between vectors x_i^a and x_j^b. On the right, we see the recovered matching. The blue edges represent the correct matchings, while the red dotted edges represent the incorrect ones.

The matrix C, where $C(i, j) = \|x_i^a - x_j^b\|_2^2$, represents the cost of moving probability mass from location x_j^a to location x_i^b, in terms of their squared Euclidean distance. The rightmost term is a regularization term based on the negative entropy of γ allows us to solve this optimization problem using the Sinkhorn-Knopp algorithm [3] which improves the computation time.

Matrix γ_0 contains information about the exchange of probability mass between the vectors of X^a and X^b. By construction, this exchange depends on the selected cost function. The choice of the squared euclidean distance is motivated both by the fact that it renders the optimization problem convex and because it will allow the parcels to be matched according to the vicinity of their feature vectors. Hence, the origin feature vectors will distribute their corresponding probability mass to the target feature vectors that are closest to them. Consequently, we define $\hat{\mathbf{T}} : \Omega^a \to \Omega^b$ as $\hat{\mathbf{T}}(x_i^a) = x_{\hat{j}}^b$ where $\hat{j} = \arg\max_j \gamma_0(i, j)$. Therefore, i will be matched to the parcel $\hat{j}$ that it sent the most mass to.

2.2 Matching Parcels Based on Dissimilarity Between Features

Let $d(x_i^a, x_j^b)$ be some dissimilarity measure between the elements of X^a and X^b. Then, we say that parcel i matches parcel j if $\arg\min_k d(x_i^a, x_k^b) = j$. We compare three dissimilarity measures against our method. First, we use the Euclidean distance, which can be interpreted as matching the parcel i to the parcel j whose feature vector x_j^b is the closest to x_i^a. Then, we use the cosine similarity, which is minimized when two feature vectors are colinear. Lastly, we use the Kullback-Leibler divergence, which measures the difference between two probability distributions in terms of their relative entropy. Note that we need to convert our vectors into probability vectors in order to evaluate d_{KL}.

3   Experiments and Results

3.1   Data and Preprocessing

For this work we randomly selected 20 subjects from the S500 group of the Human Connectome Project (HCP), all preprocessed with the HCP minimum pipeline [7]. Fiber orientation distributions functions where computed using spherical constrained deconvolution with a spherical harmonic order of 8. Probabilistic tractography was then performed using 1000 seeds per vertex of the cortical mesh provided with the HCP data. For each subject, we computed a connectivity matrix by counting the number of streamlines that connect each pair of vertices of the cortical mesh. Each row in the matrix is a vertex connectivity vector, representing the probability that a connection exists between a surface vertex and the rest of the surface's vertices.

Given a whole brain cortical parcellation, we compute the connectivity fingerprint of each parcel by averaging the connectivity fingerprint of its vertices. Because the mesh's vertices are coregistered across subjects [7], we are able to compare the connectivity fingerprints across subjects. The criterion to compute the parcel matching between two subjects is the similarity between connectivity fingerprints. That is, we match two parcels if they are connected to the rest of the brain in a similar manner. Due to the distance bias that occurs in tractography, a parcel tends to be highly connected to the vertices that compose it. To prevent the matching to be influenced by this bias, we disconnect each parcel from its own vertices.

3.2   Matching Parcels

In this section we evaluate the performance of our method by comparing it to the methods presented in Sect. 2.2. For each experiment we compute parcel matchings between all possible pairs of connectivity matrices. To quantify the result of each technique, we compute the accuracy in terms of percentage of correctly matched parcels per pairwise matching.

Matching Parcels with Synthetic Fingerprints. In this first experiment, we test the feasibility of our method by generating parcels with synthetic connectivity fingerprints and matching them. We start by generating a connectivity matrix M using probabilistic Constrained Spherical Deconvolution based tractography to use as ground truth. Our ground truth matrix is a square matrix that represents the connectivity between the 64 parcels of the Desikan atlas in one subject of the HCP dataset. Each coefficient $M(i,j) = \theta_{ij}$ is the parameter of a random variable that follows a Bernoulli distribution $X_{ij} B(\theta_{ij})$. This variable X_{ij} represents the probability of a connection existing between the parcels i and j. Using M, we generate 20 synthetic matrices in such a way that the coefficients of each synthetic connectivity matrix are random variables that follow a binomial distribution $X(i,j) \sim B(p = M(i,j), n)$. By doing this we simulate doing tractography for various values of the number n of particles. Figure 3a shows the performance of each method as a function of n.

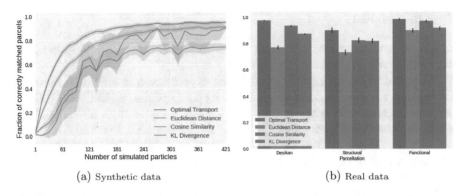

(a) Synthetic data   (b) Real data

Fig. 3. Proportion of parcels correctly matched by each method (see Sect. 2.2) when matching: (a) synthetic connectivity fingerprints and (b) connectivity fingerprints of a cortical parcellation, for three different parcellations (as described in Sect. 3.2). OT always performs significantly better.

Matching Parcels of the Desikan Atlas. For each subject, we compute the connectivity fingerprint of each parcel in their Desikan atlas as explained in Sect. 3.1. When matching parcels across subjects, Fig. 3b shows that on average OT achieves an accuracy of $98\% \pm 2\%$, followed by cosine similarity ($94\% \pm 3\%$), KL divergence ($87\% \pm 4\%$), and finally Euclidean distance ($77\% \pm 11\%$).

Matching Parcels Created Using Functional criteria. Each subject in the HCP dataset possesses z-score maps representing responses to different stimuli obtained with functional MRI (fMRI) [1]. We derive parcels for each subject from the responses to motor (hand, foot and tongue movement) and visual stimuli (faces vs shape recognition). We do so by keeping only the vertices whose z-score is in the top 35%. Figure 3b shows that OT performs best with an average of $98\% \pm 6\%$. The cosine similarity, KL divergence, and Euclidean distance achieve average accuracies of $97\% \pm 6\%$, $92\% \pm 10\%$, and $90\% \pm 13\%$ respectively.

Matching Parcels Created Using Structural criteria. For each subject, we first mask their Lateral Occipital Gyrus using the Desikan atlas. Then, we divide it into 3 parcels using the structural based parcellation technique of Gallardo et al. [5]. Once more, we can see on Fig. 3b that optimal transport has the highest average accuracy, equal to $92\% \pm 16\%$. It is followed by the cosine similarity, the KL divergence, and the Euclidean distance, whose average accuracies equal $85\% \pm 17\%$, $84\% \pm 17\%$, and $75\% \pm 17\%$

4   Discussion

In this work we proposed a method to match parcels across subjects based on the connectivity fingerprint of a parcel.

We tested our method with four different experiments. In the first experiment our technique correctly matched connectivity fingerprints created in a synthetic way. Specifically, each entry in a fingerprint was sampled from a Binomial distribution, whose parameter was chosen as the corresponding value of a ground truth connectivity matrix. This can be thought as a simulation of the process of tracking in tractography with different number of streamlines.

Our second experiment shows that we can correctly match parcels of the Desikan atlas across subjects with a 98% of correct matches. The parcels of the Desikan atlas are known to have high spatial coherence and consistent connectivity profiles across subjects [16]. We therefore use this experiment as a reference point to benchmark our technique. The last two experiments show that our technique can match parcels generated with a same criteria, even when they have some spatial variability across-subjects. The first experiment uses parcels created from the functional response to specific motor and visual stimuli, known to be strongly linked to functional connectivity [12, 15]. The second one, parcels created from the structural parcellation of the Lateral Occipital Gyrus, a structure documented to have a consistent structural division [5, 17].

It's important to notice that our technique achieved more than a 90% of correct matches in every experiment with real data. Given that we used 20 subjects, this represents a total of $20 \times 19 = 380$ cross-subject matches. In the case of the Desikan atlas, which possesses 64 parcels, this translates into a total of 24320 matches, from which 98% where correctly matched. Furthermore, when tested with a paired t-test to compare the number of correct matches, our method always performs significantly better than the other three ($p < 10^{-256}$).

5   Conclusion

Matching structural parcels across different subjects is an open problem in neuroscience. In this work, we proposed a novel parcel matching method based on Optimal Transport. We tested its performance with four different experiments, always obtaining the highest number of correctly matched parcels, which is an improvement over the results of the currently used techniques. Our technique could have major implications in the study of brain connectivity and its relationship with brain function, allowing for the location of parcels with similar connectivity but not high spatial coherence. Also, it could help to understand the link between different brain atlases, and improve the comparisons of cortical areas between higher primates.

Acknowledgements. This work has received funding from the European Research Council (ERC) under the Horizon 2020 research and innovation program (ERC Advanced Grant agreement No 694665: CoBCoM), and from the ANR NeuroRef.

References

1. Barch, D.M., Burgess, G.C., Harms, M.P., et al.: Function in the human connectome: Task-fMRI and individual differences in behavior. Neuroimage **80**, 169–189 (2013)
2. Courty, N., Flamary, R., Tuia, D., Rakotomamonjy, A.: Optimal transport for domain adaptation. IEEE Trans. Pattern Anal. Mach. Intell. **39**(9), 1853–1865 (2017)
3. Cuturi, M.: Sinkhorn distances: lightspeed computation of optimal transport. In: Advances in Neural Information Processing Systems, pp. 2292–2300 (2013)
4. Desikan, R.S., Ségonne, F., Fischl, B., et al.: An automated labeling system for subdividing the human cerebral cortex on MRI scans into gyral based regions of interest. Neuroimage **31**(3), 968–980 (2006)
5. Gallardo, G., Wells, W., Deriche, R., Wassermann, D.: Groupwise structural parcellation of the whole cortex: a logistic random effects model based approach. Neuroimage **170**, 307–320 (2018)
6. Gayraud, N.T., Rakotomamonjy, A., Clerc, M.: Optimal transport applied to transfer learning for P300 detection. In: 7th Graz Brain-Computer Interface Conference 2017 (2017)
7. Glasser, M.F., et al.: The minimal preprocessing pipelines for the Human Connectome Project. Neuroimage **80**, 105–124 (2013)
8. Jbabdi, S., Behrens, T.E.: Long-range connectomics. Ann. N. Y. Acad. Sci. **1305**(1), 83–93 (2013)
9. Mars, R.B., Sotiropoulos, S.N., Passingham, R.E.: Whole brain comparative anatomy using connectivity blueprints. bioRxiv (2018). https://doi.org/10.1101/245209
10. Mars, R.B., Verhagen, L., Gladwin, T.E., Neubert, F.X., Sallet, J., Rushworth, M.F.S.: Comparing brains by matching connectivity profiles. Neurosci. Biobehav. Rev. **60**, 90–97 (2016)
11. Moreno-Dominguez, D., Anwander, A., Knösche, T.R.: A hierarchical method for whole-brain connectivity-based parcellation. Hum. Brain Mapp. **35**(10), 5000–5025 (2014)
12. Osher, D.E., Saxe, R.R., Koldewyn, K., Gabrieli, J.D.E., Kanwisher, N., Saygin, Z.M.: Structural connectivity fingerprints predict cortical selectivity for multiple visual categories across cortex. Cereb. Cortex **26**(4), 1668–1683 (2016)
13. Parisot, S., Arslan, S., Passerat-Palmbach, J., Wells, W.M., Rueckert, D.: Tractography-driven groupwise multi-scale parcellation of the cortex. Inf. Process. Med. Imaging **24**, 600–12 (2015)
14. Passingham, R.E., Stephan, K.E., Kötter, R.: The anatomical basis of functional localization in the cortex. Nat. Rev. Neurosci. **3**(8), 606–616 (2002)
15. Penfield, W., Jasper, H.: Epilepsy and the Functional Anatomy of the Human Brain, Boston (1954)
16. de Reus, M.A., van den Heuvel, M.P.: The parcellation-based connectome: limitations and extensions. Neuroimage **80**, 397–404 (2013)
17. Rostro-caudal architecture of the frontal lobes in humans: Thiebaut de Schotten, M., et al. Cereb. Cortex **27**, 1–15 (2016). https://academic.oup.com/cercor/article/27/8/4033/3056313

GlymphVIS: Visualizing Glymphatic Transport Pathways Using Regularized Optimal Transport

Rena Elkin[1]([envelope]), Saad Nadeem[2], Eldad Haber[3], Klara Steklova[3], Hedok Lee[4],
Helene Benveniste[4], and Allen Tannenbaum[1,5]

[1] Department of Applied Mathematics and Statistics,
Stony Brook University, Stony Brook, NY, USA
rena.elkin@stonybrook.edu
[2] Department of Medical Physics, Memorial Sloan Kettering Cancer Center,
New York City, NY, USA
[3] Department of Mathematics, University British Columbia, Vancouver, Canada
[4] Department of Anesthesiology, Yale School of Medicine, New Haven, CT, USA
[5] Department of Computer Science, Stony Brook University, Stony Brook, NY, USA

Abstract. The glymphatic system (GS) is a transit passage that facilitates brain metabolic waste removal and its dysfunction has been associated with neurodegenerative diseases such as Alzheimer's disease. The GS has been studied by acquiring temporal contrast enhanced magnetic resonance imaging (MRI) sequences of a rodent brain, and tracking the cerebrospinal fluid injected contrast agent as it flows through the GS. We present here a novel visualization framework, GlymphVIS, which uses regularized optimal transport (OT) to study the flow behavior between time points at which the images are taken. Using this regularized OT approach, we can incorporate diffusion, handle noise, and accurately capture and visualize the time varying dynamics in GS transport. Moreover, we are able to reduce the registration mean-squared and infinity-norm error across time points by up to a factor of 5 as compared to the current state-of-the-art method. Our visualization pipeline yields flow patterns that align well with experts' current findings of the glymphatic system.

1 Introduction

The glymphatic system (GS) is the structural entity whereby waste products are transported from the brain and into lymphatic vessels located outside, in the meninges and along the neck vasculature [8]. Importantly, the GS also flushes out of the brain soluble amyloid beta (Aβ) and tau proteins, the main culprits of Alzheimer's disease (AD) in humans and animals [5]. Despite the potential implications of the GS for AD and other neurodegenerative conditions, there are significant gaps in our understanding of the waste clearance mechanisms and the physical forces controlling transport.

Glymphatic transport behavior can be observed with a temporal series of contrast enhanced MR images of the rodent brain. Briefly, the small molecular

© Springer Nature Switzerland AG 2018
A. F. Frangi et al. (Eds.): MICCAI 2018, LNCS 11070, pp. 844–852, 2018.
https://doi.org/10.1007/978-3-030-00928-1_95

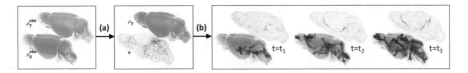

Fig. 1. GlymphVIS Pipeline: **(a)** The generalized regularized OT procedure (GR-OT) takes initial and final 'observed' density images as input and returns the 'clean' or 'believed true' final density image along with the corresponding velocity vector field describing the deformation. **(b)** The output density images and velocity are then subsequently passed to the flow pattern analysis procedure (FPA) which returns pathway and streamline clustering visualization for the whole time domain.

weight gadolinium (Gd) contrast agent (tracer) is infused into the cerebrospinal fluid (CSF) reservoir of the cisterna magna and its spatial distribution into the brain is captured by the successive acquisition of 3D T1-weighted images (234 μm resolution) every $\sim$4 minutes, for a total of $\sim$3 hours [6]. However, these MRIs do not provide directional information on the tracer movement between time points. Therefore, there is an urgent need for a mathematical framework that can capture and help visualize the dynamic tracer behavior in a manner aligning well with the biological understanding.

In this work, we present a novel visualization framework, GlymphVIS, for studying glymphatic transport pathways using regularized optimal transport (OT). The theory of OT seeks the most feasible way to redistribute mass from one given distribution to another while minimizing the associated cost of transportation ([9],[12]). OT has been used for registration and connectivity analysis of brain white matter [7], image morphing [4], and has recently been extended to the case of measures of different total mass [2].

Ratner *et al.* [10] modeled the glymphatic flow using the traditional OT formulation. This approach yielded promising results, but at the expense of some unrealistic assumptions: (1) the movement of the contrast agent is not affected by diffusion, (2) the total mass of the tracer remains constant over time, and (3) the given MRIs represent the true density distribution at that time. From the implementation perspective, the mass conservation constraint requires normalizing the density distribution which can be drastically altered by the presence of noise in the data and additional noise interference is caused by taking the given images as fixed endpoints. Finally, the authors of [10] do not explicitly model time which means the resulting deformation field cannot reflect time-varying dynamics. In this work, we introduce a new and more physiologically relevant model inspired by the work of Benamou and Brenier [1] that relaxes the above-mentioned unrealistic constraints. Specifically, the contributions of this paper are enumerated as follows:

1. We replace the continuity equation with the advection-diffusion equation to more accurately model the flow behavior and smoothen the deformation field;
2. We no longer enforce total mass conservation, so normalization of the density distributions is not needed;

3. We treat the final time condition as a free endpoint which prevents overfitting to noise;
4. We explicitly model the time domain, which allows for a direct temporal analysis of the dynamic flow behavior.

This project was supported by AFOSR grant FA9550-17-1-0435), ARO grant (W911NF-17-1-049), grants from National Institutes of Health (1U24CA1809240 1A1, R01-AG048769), MSK Cancer Center Support Grant/Core Grant (P30 CA008748), and a grant from Breast Cancer Research Foundation (grant BCRF-17-193).

2   GlymphVIS

Benamou and Brenier [1] recast the OT problem in the context of fluid mechanics that explicitly yields a time-interpolant between the two densities. This naturally motivates an ideal framework for studying the glymphatic pathways because it allows for more direct control and variation in modeling its dynamic flow behavior. Here, we introduce the following two terms to the original Benamou and Brenier OT formulation: (1) a regularization term to alleviate the effect of noise and (2) a diffusion term in the standard continuity equation to better model both advection and diffusion in the glymphatic system. We then clusters the streamlines from the resulting velocity field in order to elucidate and visualize the conduits of glymphatic flow and efflux; see Fig. 1.

2.1   Regularized OT

In order to motivate our model formulation, we begin with our assumptions about the data:

Assumption 1. *Image intensity is proportional to tracer mass,* (and we therefore refer to the intensity as mass).

Assumption 2. *Tracer is transported via glymphatic pathway,* as supported by experimental findings [5].

Assumption 3. *Apparent motion of glymphatic transport is governed by the advection-diffusion equation (ADE),*

$$\frac{\partial \rho}{\partial t} + \nabla \cdot (\rho v) = \nabla \cdot \sigma^2 \boldsymbol{\nabla} \rho, \tag{1}$$

where $0 \leq \rho : [0,T] \times \mathcal{D} \to \mathbb{R}$ is a density with compact support, $\mathcal{D} \subset \mathbb{R}^d$, $v : [0,T] \times \mathcal{D} \to \mathbb{R}^d$ is velocity and $0 \leq \sigma \in \mathbb{R}$ is diffusivity.

Assumption 4. *The MR images we are given are noisy observations of the tracer's conditions at time $t = T_i$,*

$$\rho(T_i, x) + \epsilon = \rho_{T_1}^{\mathrm{obs}}(x), \quad i = 0, ..., N, \tag{2}$$

where ϵ is a random Gaussian iid with covariance Σ.

Given initial and final observations of tracer density ρ_0^{obs} and ρ_T^{obs} at times $t = 0$ and $t = T$ respectively, our goal is to find the velocity field v and the 'believed true' or 'clean' image ρ_T such that the constraint (1) is satisfied. To this end, we propose to minimize the objective function

$$\mathcal{J}[\rho, v] = \int_0^T \int_{\mathcal{D}} \frac{1}{2} \rho \|v\|^2 \, dx dt + \alpha \|\rho(T, x) - \rho_T^{\mathrm{obs}}(x)\|_\Sigma^2, \qquad (3)$$

subject to the ADE constraint (1) with the initial condition $\rho(0, x) = \rho_0^{\mathrm{obs}}(x)$. Here, we have added the second term to the Benamou and Brenier energy functional [1] so that noise, which is inherent in all sensor-derived data, is explicitly taken into account. The parameter α weighs the balance between fitting the data and minimizing the energy associated with transporting the mass. We refer to (3) as the **generalized regularized OT** problem (GR-OT) and note that supplemental regularization can easily be implemented by adding intermediate densities to help guide the optimization procedure toward more accurate results.

Remark:
In the original Benamou-Brenier formulation of OT, $\sigma = 0$ and endpoint distribution is specified in Eq. (1), and $\alpha = 0$ in Eq. (3).

Proposed Minimization Method. While it is possible to solve the optimization problem (3) as a constrained one, it is straightforward to eliminate the ADE (1) and solve the problem for v alone. Accordingly, consider solving the PDE for a given v, obtaining the smooth, differentiable map

$$F(v) = \rho(t, x), \quad t \in [0, 1]. \qquad (4)$$

Discretization. Suppose the given images are $(n_1 \times \ldots \times n_d)$ in size, let $s = n_1 * \ldots * n_d$ denote the total number of voxels, and let m denote the number of time steps such that $m * \delta t = T$. We will use bold font to denote linearized variables.

We use mimetic methods, designed to keep their properties when considering inner products, for the discretization of the problem. First, we use operator splitting to discretize the ADE (1) as an advection step and diffusion step, independently. In the first step, we consider the advection equation and solve the problem

$$\frac{\partial \rho}{\partial t} + \nabla \cdot (\rho v) = 0 \quad \rho(t_n, x) = \rho_n.$$

Using a particle in cell (PIC) method, we obtain the discrete equivalent $\boldsymbol{\rho}_{n+1}^* = \mathbf{S}(\mathbf{v}_n)\boldsymbol{\rho}_n$ where $\mathbf{S}$ is a linear interpolation matrix. The method is conservative which means that no mass is lost during this step. For the second step, we consider the diffusion equation and solve the problem

$$\frac{\partial \rho}{\partial t} = \nabla \cdot \sigma^2 \boldsymbol{\nabla} \rho \quad \rho(t_n, x) = \rho_{n+1}^*.$$

Using the backward Euler method, we obtain the discrete equivalent

$$(\mathbf{I} - \delta t \mathbf{A})\boldsymbol{\rho}_{n+1} = \boldsymbol{\rho}_{n+1}^* \tag{5}$$

where $\mathbf{I}$ is the identity matrix and $\mathbf{A}$ is a discretization of the diffusion operator $\nabla \cdot \sigma^2 \nabla$ on a cell centered grid. Combining these two steps, we obtain the corresponding discrete forward problem $(\mathbf{I} - \delta t \mathbf{A})\boldsymbol{\rho}_{n+1} = \mathbf{S}(\mathbf{v}_n)\boldsymbol{\rho}_n, n = 0, \ldots, m$. Clearly, the density at any time step depends only on the initial density $\boldsymbol{\rho}_0$ and the velocity $\mathbf{v}$, allowing us to define the discrete map $F(\mathbf{v})$ (4) that maps the velocity to the density at all times. Next, defining $\boldsymbol{\rho} = [\boldsymbol{\rho}_1^\top, \ldots, \boldsymbol{\rho}_{m+1}^\top]^\top$ and $\mathbf{v} = [\mathbf{v}_0^\top, \ldots, \mathbf{v}_m^\top]^\top$, a straightforward discretization of the energy yields

$$\int_0^T \int_{\mathcal{D}} \rho\|v\|^2 dx\, dt \approx h^d \delta t \boldsymbol{\rho}^\top (\mathbf{I}_m \otimes \mathbf{A}_v)(\mathbf{v} \odot \mathbf{v}), \tag{6}$$

where h^d is the volume of each cell, $\mathbf{I}_k$ is the $k \times k$ identity matrix, $\mathbf{A}_v$ is a $1 \times d$ block matrix of $\mathbf{I}_s$, $\otimes$ denotes the Kronecker product and $\odot$ denotes the Hadamard product. We then solve the discrete optimization problem which now reads

$$\min \; \phi(\mathbf{v}) = \frac{1}{2}h^d\, \delta t \boldsymbol{\rho}^\top (\mathbf{I}_m \otimes \mathbf{A}_v)(\mathbf{v} \odot \mathbf{v}) + \alpha\|\boldsymbol{\rho}_n - \boldsymbol{\rho}_n^{\mathrm{obs}}\|^2 \tag{7}$$

$$\text{subject to} \; \begin{cases} (\mathbf{I} - \delta t \mathbf{A})\boldsymbol{\rho}_{n+1} - \mathbf{S}(\mathbf{v}_n)\boldsymbol{\rho}_n = 0 \\ \boldsymbol{\rho}_0 = \boldsymbol{\rho}_0^{\mathrm{obs}}. \end{cases}$$

Note that the objective function is quadratic with respect to $\mathbf{v}$ and the interpolation matrix $\mathbf{S}$ is linear with respect to $\mathbf{v}$ as it contains the weights on the linear interpolation. Following [11], one can use a Gauss-Newton like method to solve the problem.

2.2   Flow Pattern Analysis

The time-interpolant of density images and corresponding time-varying velocity vector field $\mathbf{v}(t, x)$ directly output by the GR-OT procedure is then fed into our flow pattern analysis procedure (FPA). For each time step, we construct streamlines by integrating the velocity field $\mathbf{v}$. By looking at the streamline density through each voxel, we get a global visualization of the GS 'pathways'. In order to supplement this with local information, we cluster the streamlines using the QuickBundles algorithm [3]. Significant clusters provide more information regarding different flow trajectories within different pathways and fluid reservoirs. Both the pathways and clusters are converted to NIfTI files where they are analyzed by overlaying anatomical masks using Amira software specifically designed for visualization of data in 3D and 4D. We discuss these results in the following section.

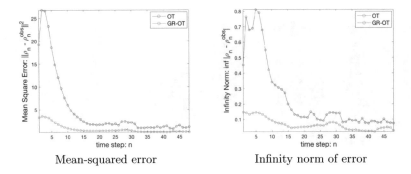

Mean-squared error   Infinity norm of error

Fig. 2. Registration error between model returned final density and target image density for the traditional OT model [10] (shown in blue) and our GR-OT model (shown in red).

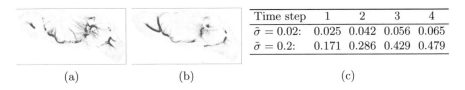

Time step	1	2	3	4
$\tilde{\sigma} = 0.02$:	0.025	0.042	0.056	0.065
$\tilde{\sigma} = 0.2$:	0.171	0.286	0.429	0.479

(a)   (b)   (c)

Fig. 3. Robustness of diffusion parameter. (a) Pathways obtained with $\sigma = 0.002$ and (b) pathways obtained with $\sigma = 0.2$. (c) Root mean square error between 'clean' densities obtained with $\sigma = 0.002$ and $\sigma = \tilde{\sigma}$. Top row: $\tilde{\sigma} = 0.02$. Bottom row: $\tilde{\sigma} = 0.2$.

3   Results

In order to quantitatively assess the performance of our model, we look at the registration error between the model returned 'clean' density and the target image density. Taking the mean square of the error and the infinity norm of the error, our model (with no diffusion, i.e. $\sigma = 0$) yields up to 5 times smaller errors than the traditional OT model proposed in [10] (Fig. 2). This large improvement was possible due to the aforementioned adjustments made to account for noise in the data. We then introduce a little diffusion ($\sigma = 0.002$) and look at the root mean square error between the returned 'clean' densities with the 'clean' densities obtained by increasing the diffusion parameter by factors of 10 ($\sigma = 0.02, 0.2$). The robustness of the diffusion parameter is shown by these errors, given in Fig. 3c, as well as by the consistent pathways found with multiple values of σ, see Figs. 3a and b.

The utility of GlymphVIS is further validated by its success in reproducing known aspects of glymphatic transport. This is illustrated by the pathways and clusters derived from the MRIs at 1.2hr after contrast infusion into the CSF, shown respectively in Figs. 4 and 5. In particular, Fig. 4 demonstrates that pathways found by our methodology have accurately captured glymphatic periarterial transport along the MCA and in other areas such as the CSF reservoirs.

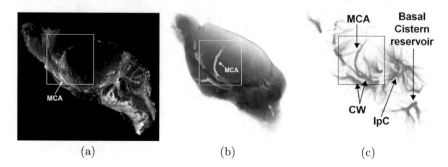

Fig. 4. GlymphVIS pathways. (a) Original contrast enhanced MRI highlighting the MCA area. (b) 3D volume rendering of the GlymphVIS pathways in relation to the whole rat brain (grey scale, volume rendered) demonstrating that GlymphVIS pathways track CSF transport along the MCA from the level of the Circle of Willis (CW) to where it crosses the olfactory tract (not shown) and proceeds dorsally onto the surface of the brain. (c) GlymphVIS pathways without the whole brain. Details of the pathways in other areas are now visible including pathway reservoirs associated with the basal cistern, the interpenduncular cistern (IpC) and cleft between the hippocampus and other brain nuclei.

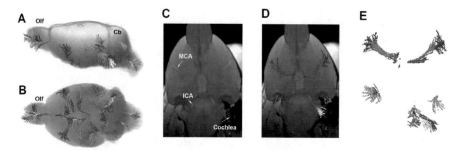

Fig. 5. GlymphVIS clusters. (A,B) Clusters shown in different colors (Olf=olfactory bulb and Cb=cerebellum). (C) Anatomical MRI from the ventral surface, where the MCA and internal carotid artery (ICA) can be visualized as single, vascular structures running along the surface of the brain. In addition, the acoustic nerve and inner ear complex (cochlea) is included. (D) Selected streamline clusters related to the MCA and the cochlea overlaid on anatomical template. (E) Selected streamline clusters related to the MCA and the cochlea.

Even more promising, are the trajectories shown by the streamline clusters in Fig. 5. This is the first time that specific contrast relevant streamlines have been captured moving towards the inner ear, and illustrates the promise of GlymphVIS and the new GR-OT flow analysis pipeline.

4   Conclusions and Future Work

In this paper, we considered a modification of the Benamou-Brenier formulation of OT in which both the continuity and energy cost functionals were modified. This was done to take into account noise as well as possible diffusion in the glymphatic flows for "normal" rat brains. In the future, we also intend to consider cases in which there may be some pathologies, in particular, rat brain models in which there is evidence of AD and vascular dementias. The concept and hypothesis to be tested would be to see if using these mathematical techniques, one could quantitatively differentiate between normal and aberrant CSF flow inside as well as outside the brain, which specifically relate to evolving neuropathology. Finally, one can consider the technique we have proposed as one of deformable registration. In contrast to other deformable methods such as LDDMM, we are not constrained by only considering diffeomorphic transformations. Moreover, in our setting, we have explicitly taken into account the advection-diffusion nature of the flow, and thus the underlying physics.

References

1. Benamou, J.D., Brenier, Y.: A computational fluid mechanics solution to the Monge-Kantorovich mass transfer problem. Numerische Mathematik **84**(3), 375–393 (2000)
2. Feydy, J., Charlier, B., Vialard, F.-X., Peyré, G.: Optimal transport for diffeomorphic registration. In: Descoteaux, M., Maier-Hein, L., Franz, A., Jannin, P., Collins, D.L., Duchesne, S. (eds.) MICCAI 2017. LNCS, vol. 10433, pp. 291–299. Springer, Cham (2017). https://doi.org/10.1007/978-3-319-66182-7_34
3. Garyfallidis, E., Brett, M., Correia, M.M., Williams, G.B., Nimmo-Smith, I.: Quickbundles, a method for tractography simplification. Front. Neurosci. **6**, 175 (2012)
4. Haker, S., Tannenbaum, A., Kikinis, R.: Mass preserving mappings and image registration. In: Niessen, W.J., Viergever, M.A. (eds.) MICCAI 2001. LNCS, vol. 2208, pp. 120–127. Springer, Heidelberg (2001). https://doi.org/10.1007/3-540-45468-3_15
5. Iliff, J.J., Wang, M., Liao, Y., Plogg, B.A., et al.: A paravascular pathway facilitates CSF flow through the brain parenchyma and the clearance of interstitial solutes, including amyloid β. Sci. Transl. Med. **4**(147), 147ra111–147ra111 (2012)
6. Lee, H., Mortensen, K., Sanggaard, S., Koch, P.: Quantitative gd-dota uptake from cerebrospinal fluid into rat brain using 3D vfa-spgr at 9.4 t. Magn. Reson. Med. **79**(3), 1568–1578 (2018)
7. Marigonda, A., Orlandi, G.: Optimal mass transportation-based models for neuronal fibers. In: Lirkov, I., Margenov, S., Waśniewski, J. (eds.) LSSC 2011. LNCS, vol. 7116, pp. 131–138. Springer, Heidelberg (2012). https://doi.org/10.1007/978-3-642-29843-1_14
8. Nedergaard, M.: Garbage truck of the brain. Science **340**(6140), 1529–1530 (2013)
9. Rachev, S.T., Rüschendorf, L.: Mass Transportation Problems, Vol. I and II. Springer, New York (1998)
10. Ratner, V., Gao, Y., Lee, H., Elkin, R., et al.: Cerebrospinal and interstitial fluid transport via the glymphatic pathway modeled by optimal mass transport. NeuroImage **152**, 530–537 (2017)

11. Steklova, K., Haber, E.: Joint hydrogeophysical inversion: state estimation for sea-water intrusion models in 3D. Comput. Geosci. **21**(1), 75–94 (2017)
12. Villani, C.: Topics in Optimal Transportation. American Mathematical Society, Providence (2003)

Hierarchical Spherical Deformation for Shape Correspondence

Ilwoo Lyu[1]([✉]), Martin A. Styner[2], and Bennett A. Landman[1]

[1] Electrical Engineering and Computer Science,
Vanderbilt University, Nashville, TN, USA
ilwoo.lyu@vanderbilt.edu
[2] Psychiatry, The University of North Carolina at Chapel Hill,
Chapel Hill, NC, USA

Abstract. We present novel spherical deformation for a landmark-free shape correspondence in a group-wise manner. In this work, we aim at both addressing template selection bias and minimizing registration distortion in a single framework. The proposed spherical deformation yields a non-rigid deformation field without referring to any particular spherical coordinate system. Specifically, we extend a rigid rotation represented by well-known Euler angles to general non-rigid local deformation via spatial-varying Euler angles. The proposed method employs spherical harmonics interpolation of the local displacements to simultaneously solve rigid and non-rigid local deformation during the optimization. This consequently leads to a continuous, smooth, and hierarchical representation of the deformation field that minimizes registration distortion. In addition, the proposed method is group-wise registration that requires no specific template to establish a shape correspondence. In the experiments, we show an improved shape correspondence with high accuracy in cortical surface parcellation as well as significantly low registration distortion in surface area and edge length compared to the existing registration methods while achieving fast registration in 3 m per subject.

Keywords: Shape correspondence
Spherical harmonics interpolation · Spherical mapping
Surface registration

1 Introduction

Understanding of morphology in medical imaging is a fundamental step for statistical analyses of cortical structures such as anatomy, pathology, and physiology. This typically requires well establishment of a shape correspondence, which might otherwise result in an unacceptable analysis. For example, studies of brain degeneration such as Alzheimer's disease rely on a proper shape correspondence of cortical structures for a valid comparison of local cortical measurements. However, most cortical structures are highly variable in general; therefore, it is quite challenging to define a formal consensus in the existence of such variability.

© Springer Nature Switzerland AG 2018
A. F. Frangi et al. (Eds.): MICCAI 2018, LNCS 11070, pp. 853–861, 2018.
https://doi.org/10.1007/978-3-030-00928-1_96

Spherical deformation has been widely used for surface registration [3,4,6, 7]. Several template-based methods have been proposed without referring to a specific spherical coordinate system [3,6,7]. In [7], spherical displacements are represented as local geodesics in the local tangent space but only capture local deformation after applying an initial rigid rotation. [6] discretized the local spherical deformation using fixed sampling points. The degree of freedom of deformation is limited to the number of the points. Alternatively [4] proposed a template-free method via spherical harmonics interpolation of local angular displacements. However, the quality of their deformation depends on a spherical coordinate system due to linear interpolation of non-linear polar angles. This yields an inconsistent deformation field having instability around the poles.

A desirable property to surface registration is to reduce registration distortion while maximizing similarity metrics. Even with high registration accuracy, registration distortion could still exist due to template bias or missing anatomy, which potentially affects secondary statistical shape analyses. For instance, [6] showed that a shape correspondence with reduced registration distortion improves statistical sensitivity in secondary analyses. Such registration distortion can be reduced with deformation regularization [3,6,7] or without employing a template in an unbiased fashion [4]. In addition to the smoothness of deformation fields, an optimal rigid alignment can minimally allow non-rigid local deformation. However, most surface registration methods typically use either a specific template or an initial rigid alignment once before non-rigid deformation.

In this paper, we propose novel spherical deformation that minimizes registration distortion. The proposed method harmonizes rigid and non-rigid deformation in a single framework. Specifically, it achieves global rigid alignment during the optimization while simultaneously allowing spatial-varying local deformation as a function of each spherical location. Moreover, the proposed method is group-wise registration without referring to a specific template. Our method is inspired by spherical harmonics interpolation of deformation fields [4]. In contrast to their spherical deformation relying heavily on initial optimal pole selection, however, the proposed method does not refer to any particular spherical coordinate system. This thus yields a well-established shape correspondence with lower registration distortion in 3 m per subject than the existing methods [3,7].

2   Methods

2.1   Problem Definition

We consider a set of N cortical surfaces with their initial spherical mappings. For the ith subject, the goal is to estimate a continuous spherical deformation field $M^i : \mathbb{S}^2 \to \mathbb{S}^2$ such that

$$M^1(\mathbf{x}^1) = M^2(\mathbf{x}^2) = \cdots = M^N(\mathbf{x}^N) \,, \tag{1}$$

where $\mathbf{x}^i \in \mathbb{S}^2$ is the corresponding location of the ith subject. In principle, M provides displacements carrying any spherical locations to their corresponding ones. A desirable deformation field is smooth and continuous. Here, a key component is thus to represent spherical displacements of the corresponding locations appropriately that meet such a demand. In the following sections, we first describe the proposed displacement encoding scheme represented by a rigid rotation and then extend the idea to non-rigid deformation.

2.2 Displacement Encoding

We consider a displacement on the unit sphere. We seek a consistent displacement encoding scheme free from a non-linear spherical polar coordinate system. Here, an Euler rotation can efficiently encode such a displacement by the composition of two independent rotations: rotation of an Euler axis followed by rotation about the Euler axis. Figure 1 shows a schematic illustration of the proposed encoding.

Euler Axis. Any reference Euler axis can sufficiently implement a target rigid rotation. Euler's rotation theorem implies that intermediate rotations (of and about an Euler axis) vary depending on a reference Euler axis but their composite rotation is equivalent to any target rotation independent of a reference Euler axis. Therefore we choose an arbitrary Euler axis (e.g., north pole) denoted by $\mathbf{z} \in \mathbb{S}^2$.

Rotation of Euler Axis. We consider $\mathbf{z}$ is rotated to be at $\hat{\mathbf{z}} \in \mathbb{S}^2$. The location of $\hat{\mathbf{z}}$ is given as a function of two polar angles $(\alpha, \beta) \in [0, \pi] \times [-\pi, \pi]$.

$$\hat{\mathbf{z}}(\alpha, \beta) = [\sin(\alpha_{\mathbf{z}} + \alpha)\cos(\beta_{\mathbf{z}} + \beta), \sin(\alpha_{\mathbf{z}} + \alpha)\sin(\beta_{\mathbf{z}} + \beta), \cos(\alpha_{\mathbf{z}} + \alpha)]^T , \quad (2)$$

where $\alpha_{\mathbf{z}}$ and $\beta_{\mathbf{z}}$ are inclination and azimuth of $\mathbf{z}$, respectively. To rotate $\mathbf{z}$ to $\hat{\mathbf{z}}$, we define an additional rotation axis $\mathbf{z}^\perp$ and its rotation angle τ as follows:

$$\mathbf{z}^\perp(\alpha, \beta) = \frac{\mathbf{z} \times \hat{\mathbf{z}}(\alpha, \beta)}{\|\mathbf{z} \times \hat{\mathbf{z}}(\alpha, \beta)\|_2} \text{ and } \tau = \arccos(\mathbf{z}^T \cdot \hat{\mathbf{z}}(\alpha, \beta)) . \quad (3)$$

Unfortunately, α and β are non-linear and vary with respect to a spherical coordinate system. To overcome this issue, we instead compute α and β as functions of unit-speed geodesics on the local tangent plane at $\mathbf{z}$ via the exponential map $\varphi_{\mathbf{z}} : T_{\mathbf{z}}\mathbb{S}^2 \to \mathbb{S}^2$. In this way, we can thus find a unique location $\mathbf{z}_T \in T_{\mathbf{z}}\mathbb{S}^2$ that corresponds to $\hat{\mathbf{z}}$. For two arbitrary orthonormal bases $\mathbf{u}_1, \mathbf{u}_2 \in T_{\mathbf{z}}\mathbb{S}^2$, α and β are determined by a linear combination of the two bases as follows:

$$[\alpha, \beta]^T = \varphi_{\mathbf{z}}(\mathbf{z}_T) = \varphi_{\mathbf{z}}(c_{\mathbf{u}_1}\mathbf{u}_1 + c_{\mathbf{u}_2}\mathbf{u}_2) , \quad (4)$$

where $c_{\mathbf{u}_1}$ and $c_{\mathbf{u}_2}$ are coefficients associated with $\mathbf{u}_1$ and $\mathbf{u}_2$, respectively. Note that $\mathbf{u}_1$ and $\mathbf{u}_2$ define a reference frame on the tangent space, which has no influence on geodesics themselves on $T_{\mathbf{z}}\mathbb{S}^2$.

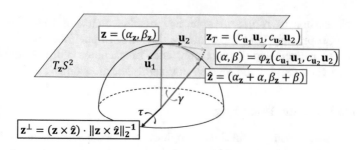

Fig. 1. A schematic illustration of the proposed rotation by Euler angles α, β, and γ. For the rotation of a given location, the rotation axis $\mathbf{z}$ (*red*) is rotated to $\hat{\mathbf{z}}$ (*blue*) by α and β (i.e., τ about $\mathbf{z}^\perp$), followed by a rotation about $\hat{\mathbf{z}}$ by γ (*green*). Since α and β are inconsistent subject to the poles of a spherical coordinate system, the exponential map φ (*violet*) at $\mathbf{z}$ is employed to encode local geodesics (*orange*). Overall, the rotation axis $\hat{\mathbf{z}}$ and its associated rotation angle γ smoothly vary on the unit sphere as functions of spherical locations. A half sphere is used for better visualization.

Rotation About Euler Axis. Given a rotation angle $\gamma \in [-\pi, \pi]$ about $\hat{\mathbf{z}}$, we compute the rigid rotation using the following Rodrigues rotation formula:

$$\mathbf{R}(\alpha, \beta, \gamma) = (\mathbf{I} + (\sin \gamma)[\hat{\mathbf{z}}]_\times + (1 - \cos \gamma)[\hat{\mathbf{z}}]_\times^2) \cdot (\mathbf{I} + (\sin \tau)[\mathbf{z}^\perp]_\times + (1 - \cos \tau)[\mathbf{z}^\perp]_\times^2) , \quad (5)$$

where $[\hat{\mathbf{z}}]_\times$ and $[\mathbf{z}^\perp]_\times$ are the 3×3 skew symmetric matrices of $\hat{\mathbf{z}}$ and $\mathbf{z}^\perp$, which represent cross products, respectively. For $\forall \mathbf{x} \in \mathbb{S}^2$, this encodes a new location:

$$M(\mathbf{x}) = \hat{\mathbf{x}}(\alpha, \beta, \gamma) = \mathbf{R}(\alpha, \beta, \gamma) \cdot \mathbf{x}. \quad (6)$$

The resulting deformation M yields an identical rigid rotation at every location and globally drives the corresponding locations to the closest location by finding an optimal set of α, β, and γ, which needs an extension to non-rigid deformation.

2.3   Extension to Hierarchical Spherical Deformation

In general, all the corresponding locations are not completely aligned after the rigid rotation. This leads to an extension of the rigid rotation to non-rigid deformation. Here, we propose smoothly spatially-varying rotation angles (α, β, γ) as functions of spherical locations rather than constants. For this purpose, we use a spherical harmonics interpolation technique that allows smooth interpolation of signals defined on the unit sphere. At a spherical location (θ, ϕ), the spherical harmonics basis function of degree l and order m $(-l \leq m \leq l)$ is given by

$$Y_l^m(\theta, \phi) = \sqrt{\frac{2l + 1}{4\pi} \frac{(l - m)!}{(l + m)!}} P_l^m(\cos \theta) e^{im\phi} , \quad (7)$$

$$Y_l^{-m}(\theta, \phi) = (-1)^m Y_l^{m*}(\theta, \phi) \,, \tag{8}$$

where Y_l^{m*} denotes the complex conjugate of Y_l^m, and P_l^m is the associated Legendre polynomial

$$P_l^m(x) = \frac{(-1)^m}{2^l l!} (1 - x^2)^{\frac{m}{2}} \frac{d^{(l+m)}}{dx^{(l+m)}} (x^2 - 1)^l \,. \tag{9}$$

In particular, α and β are obtained by plugging a set of spherical harmonics coefficients $\mathbf{c}_{\mathbf{u}_1} = \{c_{l,\mathbf{u}_1}^m\}$ and $\mathbf{c}_{\mathbf{u}_2} = \{c_{l,\mathbf{u}_2}^m\}$ into Eq. (4):

$$[\alpha(\theta, \phi), \beta(\theta, \phi)]^T = \varphi_{\mathbf{z}} \left(\sum_{l=0}^{\infty} \sum_{m=-l}^{l} \left(c_{l,\mathbf{u}_1}^m \mathbf{u}_1 + c_{l,\mathbf{u}_2}^m \mathbf{u}_2 \right) \cdot Y_l^m(\theta, \phi) \right) \,. \tag{10}$$

This locally defines $\hat{\mathbf{z}}$. Similarly, γ is obtained by the spherical harmonics interpolation as a function of spherical harmonics coefficients $\mathbf{c}_\gamma = \{c_{l,\gamma}^m\}$.

$$\gamma(\theta, \phi) = \sum_{l=0}^{\infty} \sum_{m=-l}^{l} c_{l,\gamma}^m \cdot Y_l^m(\theta, \phi) \,. \tag{11}$$

This locally defines a rotation about $\hat{\mathbf{z}}$ at each spherical location (θ, ϕ), which implies that the rotation smoothly changes across spherical locations. The proposed deformation is hierarchically represented since the spherical harmonics basis functions are linearly independent; the lower spherical harmonics degree, the smoother, more global deformation. Thus, the smoothness is easily controllable. Note that the deformation is equivalent to a rigid (global) rotation if $l = 0$.

2.4 Optimization

We use scalar maps (e.g., mean curvature) defined on the cortical surfaces for the registration metric. We evaluate the agreement of the deformed scalar maps on the unit sphere to find the optimal Euler angles. Since an explicit correspondence of scalar maps is unavailable, we instead put S icosahedral sampling points on each subject's sphere and evaluate the agreement of the deformed scalar maps at the corresponding sampling locations. Given estimates of $\mathbf{c}_{\mathbf{u}_1}^i, \mathbf{c}_{\mathbf{u}_2}^i, \mathbf{c}_\gamma^i$ of the ith subject, we consider its scalar map m^i and the corresponding location $\mathbf{x}_j^i$ to the jth sampling location $\mathbf{x}_j$ such that $\mathbf{x}_j = \mathbf{R}(\mathbf{c}_{\mathbf{u}_1}^i, \mathbf{c}_{\mathbf{u}_2}^i, \mathbf{c}_\gamma^i) \cdot \mathbf{x}_j^i$ (see Eq. (6)). By letting $\bar{m}_j$ be the mean across scalar maps at $\mathbf{x}_j$, the energy function is given by

$$E(\mathbf{c}_{\mathbf{u}_1}, \mathbf{c}_{\mathbf{u}_2}, \mathbf{c}_\gamma) = \frac{1}{2SN} \sum_{j=1}^{S} \sum_{i=1}^{N} \frac{1}{\sigma_{\mathbf{x}_j}^2} \cdot \left(m^i(\mathbf{x}_j^i; \mathbf{c}_{\mathbf{u}_1}^i, \mathbf{c}_{\mathbf{u}_2}^i, \mathbf{c}_\gamma^i) - \bar{m}_j \right)^2 \,, \tag{12}$$

where $\sigma_{\mathbf{x}_j}^2$ is feature variance at $\mathbf{x}_j$. By assuming that $\bar{m}$ and $\sigma_{\mathbf{x}}^2$ are constant, we have the following gradients by some algebra:

$$-\frac{\partial E}{\partial c_{l,\mathbf{u}}^m} = \frac{1}{SN} \sum_{j=1}^{S} \sum_{i=1}^{N} \frac{1}{\sigma_{\mathbf{x}_j}^2} \cdot Y_l^m(\theta_{\mathbf{x}_j^i}, \phi_{\mathbf{x}_j^i}) \cdot ([\mathbf{z} \times \mathbf{u}]_\times \cdot \mathbf{x}_j)^T \cdot \nabla_{\mathbf{x}_j} m^i \cdot (\bar{m}_j - m^i(\mathbf{x}_j^i)) \,, \tag{13}$$

$$-\frac{\partial E}{\partial c_{l,\gamma}^{m}} = \frac{1}{SN} \sum_{j=1}^{S} \sum_{i=1}^{N} \frac{1}{\sigma_{\mathbf{x}_j}^2} \cdot Y_l^m(\theta_{\mathbf{x}_j^i}, \phi_{\mathbf{x}_j^i}) \cdot ([\hat{\mathbf{z}}]_\times \cdot \mathbf{x}_j)^T \cdot \nabla_{\mathbf{x}_j} m^i \cdot (\bar{m}_j - m^i(\mathbf{x}_j^i)),$$

(14)

where $\nabla_{\mathbf{x}} m$ is a spatial gradient that can be efficiently computed as proposed in [7]. The optimal coefficients are then obtained by a standard gradient descent technique. Due to the nonlinearity of the energy function, the optimization is first preformed incrementally on each individual degree from $l = 0$ for the initial guess [4]. We also estimate $\bar{m}$ and $\sigma_{\mathbf{x}}^2$ from initial scalar maps and then update them during the initial guess to employ improved population statistics. Finally, the spherical harmonics coefficients are tuned simultaneously, which drives all the deformation fields with rigid and non-rigid deformation at the same time.

3   Results

We randomly chose 14 subjects out of the OASIS dataset [5]. Each hemisphere was manually labeled by an expert via the brainCOLOR protocol (49 ROIs)[1]. The evaluation was based on the surface parcellation and registration distortion. The cortical surfaces were reconstructed via a standard FreeSurfer pipeline [2], and the left hemispheres were used. We compared the proposed method with two existing methods with their default parameter settings: FreeSurfer (fixed template) [3] and Spherical Demons (fixed population average) [7]. In our method, we empirically set $l = 10$. All experiments were conducted with a single thread (Intel Xeon E5-2630 2.20 GHz). For each subject, the proposed method and Spherical Demons took less than 3 m, whereas FreeSurfer took more than an hour.

3.1   Registration Metrics

First, we computed the registration results using convexity (*sulc*) and rough/fine curvature (*curv*) features of the FreeSurfer's outputs that are optimized for FreeSurfer and Spherical Demons. In these methods, the registration was achieved in a multi-scale manner by aligning *sulc* and rough *curv* maps followed by fine *curv* maps. Similarly, we varied the number of the sampling points at four different levels of icosahedral subdivision from 4 ($S = 2,562$) to 7 ($S = 163,842$). Unlike [7], we performed only a single round of co-registration, which yields much faster registration. Second, we evaluated the three methods for their flexibility of deformation with only a fine *curv* feature having many local homogeneous regions. Here, we used $S = 163,842$. Figure 2 shows the average fine *curv* features. Overall, similar patterns were observed in the three methods with all features since rough features provided well initial alignments in the low scales. On the other hand, the use of a fine *curv* feature yielded a less alignment in FreeSurfer and Spherical Demons, whereas the proposed method offered a comparable alignment to that with all features. Our method also produced less biased average population patterns than FreeSurfer that refers to a specific template.

---

[1] Neuromorphometrics, Inc. http://www.neuromorphometrics.com/.

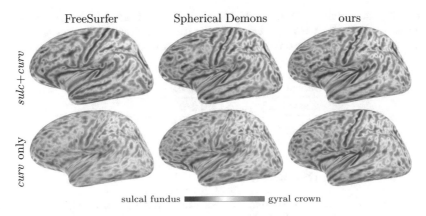

Fig. 2. The average fine *curv* feature maps. The three methods achieve similar *curv* patterns with *sulc+curv*. On the other hand, FreeSurfer and Spherical Demons show less aligned *curv* maps with only a fine *curv* feature due to the local homogeneity, whereas the proposed method provides a comparable result to that with *sulc+curv*.

3.2 Cortical Surface Parcellation

Since no ground-truth parcellation was available, we computed the mode parcellation map across the subjects. Then, we computed a Dice coefficient for each region with the mode map. We performed one-sided t-tests to reveal regions with statistically significant improvement on Dice coefficients. In addition, we corrected p-values via multi-comparisons using a standard false discovery rate [1] at $q = 0.05$. Tables 1 and 2 summarize the Dice coefficients and the revealed regions, respectively. One improved region was found with all features compared to FreeSurfer, while showing comparable results to Spherical Demons. The proposed method achieved a high Dice coefficient even with only a fine *curv* feature; a large number of regions were revealed with significant improvement because the ambiguity in the local homogeneity of the highly localized feature maps was reduced by harmonizing rigid and non-rigid deformation.

Table 1. Overall Dice coefficient in cortical surface parcellation. Compared to FreeSurfer and Spherical Demons, the proposed method achieves comparable Dice coefficients with *sulc+curv* and better overlaps with *curv* ($^*p \ll 0.001$). See Table 2 for more details about individual regions with significantly improved Dice coefficients.

Metric	FreeSurfer	Spherical Demons	Ours
sulc+curv	0.782 ± 0.132	0.784 ± 0.133	0.785 ± 0.129
curv only	0.692 ± 0.164	0.728 ± 0.155	$0.774 \pm 0.130^*$

Table 2. The number of regions with statistical significance (# of increases/# of decreases). One-sided t-tests reveal regions with statistical significance after multi-comparison correction ($q = 0.05$). No region is found with a decreased Dice coefficient.

Metric	FreeSurfer	Spherical Demons
sulc+curv	1/0	0/0
curv only	40/0	23/0

3.3   Registration Distortion

Again, measuring registration distortion is important to evaluate bias introduced by deformation fields, which could affect secondary statistical shape analyses. We measured area and length distortion for each triangle and edge as the absolute log ratio between before and after registration [6]. Table 3 summarizes registration distortion in the three methods. Our method provided significantly reduced registration distortion compared to FreeSurfer and Spherical Demons regardless of registration metrics. We emphasize that such reduced distortion is achieved while keeping comparable registration accuracy to the existing methods.

Table 3. Registration distortion: absolute log ratio (mean $\pm$ std (max)) in surface area and edge length. For both *sulc+curv* and *curv* features, the proposed method yields significantly less registration distortion than FreeSurfer and Spherical Demons by showing statistical significance ($^*p \ll 0.001$).

	Metric	FreeSurfer	Spherical Demons	Ours
Area	*sulc+curv*	0.268 ± 0.217 (8.045)	0.194 ± 0.166 (2.986)	0.164 ± 0.130 (1.050)*
	curv only	0.243 ± 0.214 (10.722)	0.113 ± 0.101 (3.007)	0.090 ± 0.075 (0.662)*
Len	*sulc+curv*	0.178 ± 0.150 (4.330)	0.129 ± 0.108 (1.980)	0.102 ± 0.083 (0.747)*
	curv only	0.156 ± 0.138 (5.398)	0.072 ± 0.066 (1.316)	0.055 ± 0.046 (0.438)*

4   Conclusion

We presented novel spherical deformation for a shape correspondence. The proposed method extends the rigid rotation represented by Euler angles to general non-rigid deformation. Both rigid rotation and non-rigid deformation are updated simultaneously in a single framework. Moreover, the proposed method is group-wise registration that does not require a specific template. Consequently, the resulting deformation field is smooth, continuous, and independent of a particular spherical coordinate system. In the experiments, the proposed method showed high accuracy in cortical surface parcellation as well as low registration distortion compared to the existing methods.

Acknowledgments. This work was supported in part by the National Institutes of Health (NIH) under Grant R01EB017230, Grant R01MH102266, Grant R01MH091645, Grant R01MH098098, Grant P30HD003110, and Grant U54HD079124, and in part by the VISE/VICTR under Grant VR3029.

References

1. Benjamini, Y., Hochberg, Y.: Controlling the false discovery rate: a practical and powerful approach to multiple testing. J. Roy. Stat. Soc. Ser. B (Methodol.) **57**, 289–300 (1995)
2. Dale, A.M., Fischl, B., Sereno, M.I.: Cortical surface-based analysis: I. Segmentation and surface reconstruction. Neuroimage **9**(2), 179–194 (1999)
3. Fischl, B., Sereno, M., Tootell, R., Dale, A.: High-resolution intersubject averaging and a coordinate system for the cortical surface. Hum. Brain Mapp. **8**(4), 272–284 (1999)
4. Lyu, I., et al.: Robust estimation of group-wise cortical correspondence with an application to macaque and human neuroimaging studies. Front. Neurosci. **9**, 210 (2015)
5. Marcus, D.S., Wang, T.H., Parker, J., Csernansky, J.G., Morris, J.C., Buckner, R.L.: Open access series of imaging studies (OASIS): cross-sectional MRI data in young, middle aged, nondemented, and demented older adults. J. Cogn. Neurosci. **19**(9), 1498–1507 (2007)
6. Robinson, E.C., et al.: Multimodal surface matching with higher-order smoothness constraints. Neuroimage **167**, 453–465 (2018)
7. Yeo, B., Sabuncu, M., Vercauteren, T., Ayache, N., Fischl, B., Golland, P.: Spherical demons: fast diffeomorphic landmark-free surface registration. IEEE Trans. Med. Imaging **29**(3), 650–668 (2010)

Diffeomorphic Brain Shape Modelling Using Gauss-Newton Optimisation

Yaël Balbastre$^{(\boxtimes)}$, Mikael Brudfors, Kevin Bronik, and John Ashburner

Wellcome Centre for Human Neuroimaging, University College London, London, UK
y.balbastre@ucl.ac.uk

Abstract. Shape modelling describes methods aimed at capturing the natural variability of shapes and commonly relies on probabilistic interpretations of dimensionality reduction techniques such as principal component analysis. Due to their computational complexity when dealing with dense deformation models such as diffeomorphisms, previous attempts have focused on explicitly reducing their dimension, diminishing *de facto* their flexibility and ability to model complex shapes such as brains. In this paper, we present a generative model of shape that allows the covariance structure of deformations to be captured without squashing their domain, resulting in better normalisation. An efficient inference scheme based on Gauss-Newton optimisation is used, which enables processing of 3D neuroimaging data. We trained this algorithm on segmented brains from the OASIS database, generating physiologically meaningful deformation trajectories. To prove the model's robustness, we applied it to unseen data, which resulted in equivalent fitting scores.

1 Introduction

In neuroimaging studies, or more generally in shape analysis, normalising a set of subjects consists in deforming them towards a common space that allows one-to-one correspondence. Finding this common space usually reduces to finding an optimal shape in terms of distance to all subjects in the space of deformations. However, the covariance structure of these deformations is not known *a priori* and the deformation metric generally involves penalising roughness. Yet, in a Bayesian setting, a prior that is informative of population variance would make the registration process, which relies on *a posteriori* estimates, more robust. Shape models aim to learn this covariance structure from the data. As deformations are parameterised in a very high-dimensional space, learning their covariance is computationally intractable. Dimensionality reduction techniques are therefore commonly used, even though some have tackled this problem by parameterising deformations using location-adaptive control points [8].

For a long time, due to their computational complexity, shape modelling approaches had only been applied to simple models of deformations [7] or simple data sets [6,9]. Recently, Zhang and Fletcher applied a probabilistic shape model, named principal geodesic analysis, to densely sampled diffeomorphisms

© Springer Nature Switzerland AG 2018
A. F. Frangi et al. (Eds.): MICCAI 2018, LNCS 11070, pp. 862–870, 2018.
https://doi.org/10.1007/978-3-030-00928-1_97

and 3D MR images of the brain [14]. Diffeomorphisms correspond to a particular family of deformations that are ensured to be invertible, allowing for very large deformations. Geodesic shooting of diffeomorphisms involves specifying a Riemannian metric on their tangent space and allows a diffeomorphism to be entirely parameterised by its initial velocity [3, 11]. However, because Zhang and Fletcher's optimisation scheme relies either on Gradient descent or on Monte Carlo sampling of the posterior, they have focused on effectively reducing the dimensionality of velocity fields. It results in an effective approach for studying the principle modes of variations, but may give less accurate alignment than with classical approaches. In particular, they do not explicitly model "anatomical noise", $i.e.$, deformations that are not captured by the principal modes.

Here, we propose a generative shape model, whose posterior is inferred using variational inference and Laplace approximations. A residual velocity field capturing anatomical noise is explicitly defined and its magnitude is inferred from the data. An efficient Gauss-Newton optimisation is used to obtain the maximum a $posteriori$ latent subspace as well as individual coordinates, minimising the chances of falling into local minima, and making the registration more robust.

2 Methods

2.1 Generative Shape Model

First, let us define a generative model of brain shape. Here, the observed variables are supposed to be categorical images ($i.e.$, segmentations) comprising K classes—e.g. grey matter, white matter, background—stemming from a categorical distribution. This kind of data term has proved very effective for driving registration [2] and is compatible with unified models of registration and segmentation. If needed, it is straightforward to replace this term with a stationary Gaussian noise model. The template μ encodes prior probabilities of finding each of the K classes in a given location, and is deformed towards the n-th subject according to the spatial transform ϕ_n. In practice, its log-representation a is encoded by trilinear basis functions, and the deformed template is recovered by softmax interpolation [2]:

$$\mu_n^{(k)}(x) = [\text{softmax}(a \circ \phi_n(x))]_k = \frac{\exp(a^{(k)} \circ \phi_n(x))}{\sum_{l=1}^{K} \exp(a^{(l)} \circ \phi_n(x))}. \tag{1}$$

Note that the discrete operation $a \circ \phi_n$ can be equivalently written as the matrix multiplication, $\Phi_n a$, where Φ_n is a large and sparse matrix that depends on ϕ_n and performs the combined "sample and interpolate" operation. We will name this operation $pulling$, while the multiplication by its transpose, Φ_n^T, will be named $pushing$.

Let $\{f_n \in \mathbb{R}^{I \times K}; 1 \leqslant n \leqslant N\}$ be the set of observed images[1]. For each subject, let $\phi_n \in \mathbb{R}^{I \times 3}$ be the diffeomorphic transformation, and let

---

[1] We assume that they all have the same lattice, but this condition can be waived by composing each diffeomorphic transform with a fixed "change of lattice" transform, which can even embed a rigid-body alignment.

$\boldsymbol{\mu}_n = \text{softmax}\,(\boldsymbol{a} \circ \boldsymbol{\phi}_n)$ be the deformed template. The likelihood of observed voxel values at locations $\{\boldsymbol{x}_i \; ; \; 1 \leqslant i \leqslant I\}$ is:

$$p(\boldsymbol{f}_n(\boldsymbol{x}_i) \mid \boldsymbol{\mu}_n(\boldsymbol{x}_i)) = \text{Cat}(\boldsymbol{f}_n(\boldsymbol{x}_i) \mid \boldsymbol{\mu}_n(\boldsymbol{x}_i)) = \prod_{k=1}^{K} \mu_n^{(k)}(\boldsymbol{x}_i)^{f_n^{(k)}(\boldsymbol{x}_i)}. \tag{2}$$

In this work, diffeomorphisms are defined as geodesics, according to a Riemannian metric[2] defined by a positive definite operator named L, and are thus entirely parameterised by their initial velocity [11]. A complete transformation $\boldsymbol{\phi}$ is recovered by integrating the velocity in time, knowing that the momentum $\boldsymbol{u}_t = L\boldsymbol{v}_t$, is conserved at any t:

$$\boldsymbol{u}_t(\boldsymbol{x}) = \left| D\boldsymbol{\phi}_t^{-1}(\boldsymbol{x}) \right| \left(D\boldsymbol{\phi}_t^{-1}(\boldsymbol{x}) \right)^T \left(\boldsymbol{u}_0 \circ \boldsymbol{\phi}_t^{-1}(\boldsymbol{x}) \right). \tag{3}$$

The velocity field can be retrieved from the momentum field by performing the inverse operation $\boldsymbol{v}_t = K\boldsymbol{u}_t$, where K is L's Green's function Because we want to model inter-individual variability, we need them to be all defined in the same (template) space, which is achieved by using the initial velocity of their inverse[3], that we name $\{\boldsymbol{v}_n \in \mathbb{R}^{I \times 3} \; ; \; 1 \leqslant n \leqslant N\}$. Following [13], we use the probabilistic principal component analysis (PPCA) framework to regularise initial velocity fields, which leads to writing them as a linear combination of principal modes plus a residual field. Let us assume that we want to model them with $M \ll 3I$ principal components. Then, let $\boldsymbol{W}$ be a $3I \times M$ matrix (called the *principal subspace*), each column being one principal component, let $\boldsymbol{z}_n$ be the latent representation of a given velocity field in the principal subspace and let $\boldsymbol{r}_n$ be the corresponding residual field. This yields $\boldsymbol{v}_n = \boldsymbol{W}\boldsymbol{z}_n + \boldsymbol{r}_n$. In [13], latent coordinates $\boldsymbol{z}_n$ stem from a standard Gaussian and $\boldsymbol{r}_n$ is i.i.d. Gaussian noise, and a maximum-likelihood estimate of the principal subspace is retrieved. A Bayesian version can be designed by placing a Gaussian prior on each principal component [5]. Smooth velocities can be enforced with a smooth prior over each principal component and over the residual field, and a Gaussian prior over the latent coordinates, yielding:

$$p(\boldsymbol{W}) = \prod_{m=1}^{M} \mathcal{N}\left(\boldsymbol{w}_m \mid \boldsymbol{0}, \boldsymbol{L}^{-1}\right), \tag{4}$$

$$p(\boldsymbol{z}_n \mid \boldsymbol{A}) = \mathcal{N}\left(\boldsymbol{z}_n \mid \boldsymbol{0}, \boldsymbol{A}^{-1}\right), \tag{5}$$

$$p(\boldsymbol{r}_n \mid \lambda) = \mathcal{N}\left(\boldsymbol{r}_n \mid \boldsymbol{0}, (\lambda \boldsymbol{L})^{-1}\right), \tag{6}$$

where $\boldsymbol{L}$ is the discretisation of L and λ is the anatomical noise precision. However, this approach is often not regularised enough. Zhang and Fletcher [14] proposed a different prior, which can be seen as being set over the reconstructed velocities. In practice, it takes the form of a joint distribution over all latent coordinates, residual fields and the principal subspace:

$$p(\boldsymbol{z}_{1...N}, \boldsymbol{r}_{1...N}, \boldsymbol{W}) \propto \prod_{n=1}^{N} \mathcal{N}\left(\boldsymbol{W}\boldsymbol{z}_n + \boldsymbol{r}_n \mid \boldsymbol{0}, \boldsymbol{L}^{-1}\right). \tag{7}$$

---

[2] In this work, it is a combination of membrane, bending and linear-elastic energies.
[3] The initial velocity of $\boldsymbol{\phi}$ is the opposite of the final velocity of $\boldsymbol{\phi}^{-1}$, and *vice versa*.

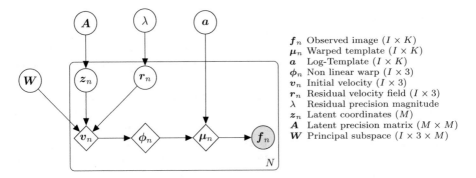

$\boldsymbol{f}_n$	Observed image $(I \times K)$
$\boldsymbol{\mu}_n$	Warped template $(I \times K)$
$\boldsymbol{a}$	Log-Template $(I \times K)$
$\boldsymbol{\phi}_n$	Non linear warp $(I \times 3)$
$\boldsymbol{v}_n$	Initial velocity $(I \times 3)$
$\boldsymbol{r}_n$	Residual velocity field $(I \times 3)$
λ	Residual precision magnitude
$\boldsymbol{z}_n$	Latent coordinates (M)
$\boldsymbol{A}$	Latent precision matrix $(M \times M)$
$\boldsymbol{W}$	Principal subspace $(I \times 3 \times M)$

Fig. 1. Generative shape model, in the form of a graphical model. Circles indicate random variables while diamonds indicate deterministic variables. Shaded variables are observed. Plates indicate replication.

The advantage of the first formulation (4–6) is that it explicates the covariance matrix of the latent coordinates and the noise precision, which can then be inferred from the data. Additionally, it could be extended to multimodal latent distributions such as Gaussian mixtures. However, the second formulation (7) is better at effectively regularising the principal subspace and, in general, the reconstructed velocities. In practice, we use a weighted combination of these two formulations, and call the weights γ_1 and γ_2.

The noise precision, λ, can be inferred in a Bayesian fashion by introducing a conjugate Gamma prior[4] with $\alpha = \frac{\nu_0 \times 3I}{2}$ and $\beta = \frac{\nu_0 \times 3I}{2\lambda_0}$ as shown in [12]. Similarly, the latent covariance matrix is given a conjugate Wishart prior, which is made as non-informative as possible by setting its degrees of freedom to M, and whose expected value is the identity matrix, *i.e.*, $p(\boldsymbol{A}) = \mathcal{W}\left(\boldsymbol{A} \mid \frac{1}{M}\boldsymbol{I}, M\right)$. This prior has the opposite effect of an automatic relevance determination prior, since it prevents principal components from collapsing during the first iterations by promoting non-null variances.

Finally, we look for a maximum *a posteriori* estimate of the template, $\boldsymbol{a}$, with a very uninformative log-Dirichlet prior that prevents null probabilities (a smooth prior could also be used following [2]). The complete model is depicted in the form of a graphical model in Fig. 1.

2.2 Inference[5]

A basic inference scheme would be to search for a mode of the model likelihood, by optimising in turn each parameter of the model. It is however more consistent to tackle this problem as one of missing data, which is dealt with by computing the posterior distribution over all latent variables. Unfortunately, the

---

[4] The Gamma prior is a parameterised such that $\mathbb{E}[\lambda] = \lambda_0$.

[5] $\boldsymbol{q}$ is used for approximate posteriors and $\mathbb{E}_q$ for posterior expected values. Superscript stars denote optimal approximations. $\overset{c}{=}$ means "equal up to an additive constant".

posterior does not possess a tractable form. A solution is to use variational inference to describe an approximate posterior q that can be more easily computed, by restricting the search space to distributions that factorise over a subset of variables [4]. This method allows the uncertainty about parameters estimates to be accounted for when inferring other parameters. Here, for computational reasons, we do not perform a fully Bayesian treatment of the problem and look for mode estimates of the principal subspace and template. We still marginalise over all subject-specific parameters (latent coordinates and residual field), as recommended by [1]. We state that the set of marginalised latent variables is $\boldsymbol{\Upsilon} = \{z_{1...N}, \boldsymbol{r}_{1...N}, \boldsymbol{A}, \lambda\}$ and make the (mean field) approximation that the posterior factorises over $(z_{1...N})$, $(\boldsymbol{r}_{1...N})$, $(\boldsymbol{A})$ and (λ).

Since we used conjugate priors for the latent precision matrix and the anatomical noise precision, their posterior have the same form as their prior and update equations are equivalent to computing a weighted average between their prior expected value and their maximum likelihood estimator. In contrast, posterior distributions of z_n and $\boldsymbol{r}_n$ have no simple form. We thus make a Laplace approximation and estimate their mean $(z_n^\star, \boldsymbol{r}_n^\star)$ and covariance $(\boldsymbol{S}_{z,n}^\star, \boldsymbol{S}_{r,n}^\star)$ with their mode and second derivatives about this mode. They are obtained by Gauss-Newton optimisation and the corresponding derivations are provided in Sect. 2.3. Because of the non-linearity induced by geodesic shooting and template interpolation, we first make the approximation that:

$$\mathbb{E}_q\Big[p\left(\boldsymbol{f}_n \mid z_n, \boldsymbol{r}_n, \boldsymbol{W}, a\right)\Big] \approx p\left(\boldsymbol{f}_n \mid z_n^\star, \boldsymbol{r}_n^\star, \boldsymbol{W}, a\right) = p\left(\boldsymbol{f}_n \mid \boldsymbol{\mu}_n^\star\right), \qquad (8)$$

where $\mathbb{E}_q$ means the posterior expected value and $\boldsymbol{\mu}_n^\star$ is the template deformed according to the above parameter estimates. Consequently, we find:

$$\ln q^\star(z_n) \stackrel{c}{=} \ln p\left(\boldsymbol{f}_n \mid \boldsymbol{\mu}_n^\star\right) - \frac{1}{2} z_n^T \left(\gamma_1 \boldsymbol{A} + \gamma_2 \boldsymbol{W}^T \boldsymbol{L} \boldsymbol{W}\right) z_n - \gamma_2 z_n^T \boldsymbol{W}^T \boldsymbol{L} \boldsymbol{r}_n^\star \qquad (9)$$

$$\ln q^\star(r_n) \stackrel{c}{=} \ln p\left(\boldsymbol{f}_n \mid \boldsymbol{\mu}_n^\star\right) - \frac{\gamma_1 \lambda^\star + \gamma_2}{2} \boldsymbol{r}_n^T \boldsymbol{L} \boldsymbol{r}_n - \gamma_2 \boldsymbol{r}_n^T \boldsymbol{L} \boldsymbol{W} z_n^\star. \qquad (10)$$

2.3   Gauss-Newton Optimisation

Gauss-Newton (GN) optimisation of an objective function $\mathcal{E}$ with respect to a vector of parameters $\boldsymbol{x}$ consists of iteratively improving the objective function by making, locally, a second-order approximation. The gradient, $\boldsymbol{g}$, and Hessian matrix, $\boldsymbol{H}$, are computed about the current best estimate of the optimal parameters, $\boldsymbol{x}_i$, and the new optimum is found according to $\boldsymbol{x}_{i+1} = \boldsymbol{x}_i - \boldsymbol{H}^{-1}\boldsymbol{g}$. In practice, this update scheme sometimes overshoots it is therefore common to perform a backtracking line search along the direction $-\boldsymbol{H}^{-1}\boldsymbol{g}$.

Differentiating the Data Term: Let us write $\mathcal{E}$ the (negative) data term for an arbitrary subject:

$$\mathcal{E} = -\ln p\left(\boldsymbol{f} \mid \boldsymbol{\mu}\right) = -\sum_{i=1}^{I} \ln \operatorname{Cat}\left(\boldsymbol{f}(\boldsymbol{x}_i) \mid \operatorname{softmax}\left(\boldsymbol{\Phi}\boldsymbol{a}(\boldsymbol{x}_i)\right)\right) = \mathcal{C}_f\left(\boldsymbol{\Phi}\boldsymbol{a}\right). \quad (11)$$

Following [3], differentiating $\mathcal{E}$ with respect to $\boldsymbol{v}$ can be approximated by differentiating with respect to $\boldsymbol{\Phi}$ and applying the chain rule, which yields:

$$\tfrac{\partial \mathcal{E}}{\partial v} = \left(\boldsymbol{\Phi}^T \boldsymbol{\nabla}\mathcal{C}_f\left(\boldsymbol{\Phi}\boldsymbol{a}\right)\right)\boldsymbol{\nabla}\boldsymbol{a}, \quad (12)$$

where $\boldsymbol{\nabla}\mathcal{C}_f$ is the gradient of the log-Categorical distribution and takes the form of an $I \times K$ vector field, and $\boldsymbol{\nabla}\boldsymbol{a}$ contains spatial gradients of the log-template and takes the form of an $I \times 3$ vector field. Second derivatives can be approximated by:

$$\tfrac{\partial^2 \mathcal{E}}{\partial v^2} = \boldsymbol{\nabla}\boldsymbol{a}^T \left(\boldsymbol{\Phi}^T \boldsymbol{\nabla}^2\mathcal{C}_f\left(\boldsymbol{\Phi}\boldsymbol{a}\right)\right)\boldsymbol{\nabla}\boldsymbol{a}, \quad (13)$$

where $\boldsymbol{\nabla}^2\mathcal{C}_f$ is the Hessian of the log-Categorical distribution and takes the form of an $I \times K \times K$ symmetric tensor field. The gradient and Hessian of $\mathcal{C}_f$ were derived in [2] and can be computed in each voxel according to:

$$\tfrac{\partial \mathcal{C}_f(a)}{\partial a_k} = \mu_k\left(\sum_{l=1}^{K} f_l\right) - f_k, \quad \tfrac{\partial^2 \mathcal{C}_f(a)}{\partial a_k \partial a_m} = \mu_k(\delta_k^m - \mu_m)\sum_{l=1}^{K} f_l. \quad (14)$$

Since $\boldsymbol{v} = \boldsymbol{W}\boldsymbol{z} + \boldsymbol{r}$, derivatives with respect to $\boldsymbol{r}$, $\boldsymbol{z}$ and $\boldsymbol{W}$ are obtained by applying the chain rule.

Orthogonalisation: The PPCA formulation is invariant to rotations inside the latent space [13]. Consequently, it allows finding an optimal subspace but does not enforce the individual bases $\boldsymbol{w}_{1...M}$ to be the eigenmodes of the complete covariance matrix. It makes sense, however, to transform the subspace so that it corresponds to the first eigenmodes as it eases the interpretation. Also, in order to enforce a sparse Hessian matrix over $\boldsymbol{W}$, we require $\boldsymbol{Z}\boldsymbol{Z}^T$ to be diagonal, where the columns of $\boldsymbol{Z}$ are the individual $\boldsymbol{z}_n$. This leads us to look for an $M \times M$ transformation matrix $\boldsymbol{T}$ that keeps the actual diffeomorphisms untouched ($\boldsymbol{W}\boldsymbol{z} = \boldsymbol{W}\boldsymbol{T}^{-1}\boldsymbol{T}\boldsymbol{z}$), while diagonalising both $\boldsymbol{Z}\boldsymbol{Z}^T$ and $\boldsymbol{W}^T\boldsymbol{L}\boldsymbol{W}$. This is done by a series of singular value decompositions that insure that $\boldsymbol{T}\boldsymbol{Z}\boldsymbol{Z}^T\boldsymbol{T}^T$ is diagonal and $\boldsymbol{T}^{-T}\boldsymbol{W}^T\boldsymbol{L}\boldsymbol{W}\boldsymbol{T}^{-1}$ is the identity. However, the distribution of diagonal weights between $\boldsymbol{W}^T\boldsymbol{L}\boldsymbol{W}$ and $\boldsymbol{Z}\boldsymbol{Z}^T$ is not optimal and we optimise an additional diagonal scaling matrix $\boldsymbol{Q}$ by alternating between updating $\boldsymbol{A}$ from the rotated $\mathbb{E}\left[\boldsymbol{Z}\boldsymbol{Z}^T\right]$, and updating the scaling weights by Gauss-Newton optimisation of the remaining terms of the lower bound that depend on them:

$$\mathcal{E}_Q = -\tfrac{1}{2}\left(\operatorname{Tr}\left(\boldsymbol{Q}\boldsymbol{T}\boldsymbol{Z}\boldsymbol{Z}^T\boldsymbol{T}^T\boldsymbol{Q}\boldsymbol{A}\right) + \operatorname{Tr}\left(\boldsymbol{Q}^{-1}\boldsymbol{T}^{-T}\boldsymbol{W}^T\boldsymbol{L}\boldsymbol{W}\boldsymbol{T}^{-1}\boldsymbol{Q}^{-1}\right)\right). \quad (15)$$

3   Experiments and Results

We ran the algorithm on a training set consisting of the first 38 subjects of the OASIS cross-sectional database [10]. We used the provided FSL segmentations, which we transformed into tissue probability maps by extracting the grey and

| 0 | 2 | 8 | 16 | 32 | 32+R |

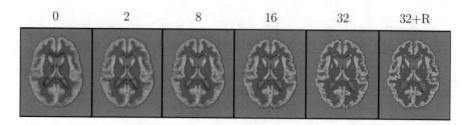

Fig. 2. Template reconstructed using an increasing number of principal modes, and with the addition of the residual field.

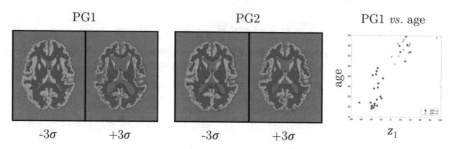

PG1   PG2   PG1 *vs.* age

-3σ $+3\sigma$ -3σ $+3\sigma$ z_1

Fig. 3. Left: deformed template along the first two principal modes. Right: latent coordinates *vs.* subject ages. Probable AD subjects are marked with a red cross.

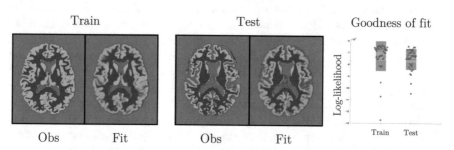

Train   Test   Goodness of fit

Obs   Fit   Obs   Fit   Train   Test

Fig. 4. Left: two random examples of fit from the train and test sets. Right: distribution of categorical log-likelihood values for the train and test sets.

white matter classes and smoothing them with a 1-voxel FWHM Gaussian kernel. We set the number of principal components to 32, the parameters of the membrane, bending and linear-elastic energies were respectively set to 0.001, 0.02 and $(0.0025, 0.005)$, and we used $\gamma_1 = \gamma_2 = 1$. We set the prior parameters of the residual precision magnitude based on tests conducted on 2D axial slices ($\lambda_0 = 17$, $\nu_0 = 10$). Templates reconstructed with a varying number of principal modes, and with or without the residual field, are presented in Fig. 2, while Fig. 3 shows the template deformed along the first two principal modes, the first one being typical of brain ageing. This pattern is validated by plotting coordinates along the first dimension against actual ages. Finally, the learnt model was tested by registering the template towards 38 unseen images from the OASIS database. The distribution of categorical log-likelihood values for the training and testing sets are depicted in Fig. 4, along with two example fits that were randomly selected. Both sets have similar distributions (mean $\pm$ std $\times 10^5$. Train: -7.23 ± 1.26 ; Test: -7.55 ± 0.88), showing the model's robustness.

4 Conclusion

We presented a generative model of brain shape that does not limit the space of diffeomorphisms, allowing learning regularisation while preserving enough flexibility for accurate normalisation. We showed how principal modes of variation correlate with known factors of brain shape variability, hinting towards the fact that this low-dimensional representation might allow to discriminate between physiological states. Future research will focus on applying this framework to very large databases, and on combining it with segmentation models in order to work directly with raw data. The latent distribution may be improved by using multimodal priors such as Gaussian mixtures. Our main limitation is the small number of principal basis that can be learned due to their large size. This could be overcome by explicitly modelling sparse and local covariance patterns.

References

1. Allassonnière, S., Amit, Y., Trouvé, A.: Towards a coherent statistical framework for dense deformable template estimation. J. R. Stat. Soc. Ser. B Stat. Methodol. **69**(1), 3–29 (2007)
2. Ashburner, J., Friston, K.J.: Computing average shaped tissue probability templates. NeuroImage **45**(2), 333–341 (2009)
3. Ashburner, J., Friston, K.J.: Diffeomorphic registration using geodesic shooting and Gauss-Newton optimisation. NeuroImage **55**(3), 954–967 (2011)
4. Bishop, C.: Pattern Recognition and Machine Learning. Information Science and Statistics. Springer, New York (2006)
5. Bishop, C.M.: Bayesian PCA. In: Kearns, M.J., Solla, S.A., Cohn, D.A. (eds.) NIPS, vol. 11, pp. 382–388. MIT Press (1999)
6. Cootes, T.F., Twining, C.J., Babalola, K.O., Taylor, C.J.: Diffeomorphic statistical shape models. Image Vis. Comput. **26**(3), 326–332 (2008)
7. Cootes, T., Hill, A., Taylor, C., Haslam, J.: Use of active shape models for locating structures in medical images. Image Vis. Comput. **12**(6), 355–365 (1994)
8. Durrleman, S., Allassonnière, S., Joshi, S.: Sparse adaptive parameterization of variability in image ensembles. Int. J. Comput. Vis. **101**(1), 161–183 (2013)
9. Fletcher, P.T., Lu, C., Pizer, S.M., Joshi, S.: Principal geodesic analysis for the study of nonlinear statistics of shape. IEEE Trans. Med. Imaging **23**(8), 995–1005 (2004)
10. Marcus, D.S., Wang, T.H., Parker, J., Csernansky, J.G., Morris, J.C., Buckner, R.L.: Open access series of imaging studies (OASIS): cross-sectional MRI data in young, middle aged, nondemented, and demented older adults. J. Cognit. Neurosci. **19**(9), 1498–1507 (2007)

11. Miller, M.I., Trouvé, A., Younes, L.: Geodesic shooting for computational anatomy. J. Math. Imaging Vis. **24**(2), 209–228 (2006)
12. Simpson, I.J.A., Schnabel, J.A., Groves, A.R., Andersson, J.L.R., Woolrich, M.W.: Probabilistic inference of regularisation in non-rigid registration. NeuroImage **59**(3), 2438–2451 (2012)
13. Tipping, M.E., Bishop, C.M.: Probabilistic principal component analysis. J. R. Stat. Soc. Ser. B Stat. Methodol. **61**(3), 611–622 (1999)
14. Zhang, M., Fletcher, P.T.: Bayesian principal geodesic analysis for estimating intrinsic diffeomorphic image variability. Med. Image Anal. **25**(1), 37–44 (2015)

Multi-task SonoEyeNet: Detection of Fetal Standardized Planes Assisted by Generated Sonographer Attention Maps

Yifan Cai[✉], Harshita Sharma, Pierre Chatelain, and J. Alison Noble

Institute of Biomedical Engineering, University of Oxford,
Old Road Campus Research Building, Oxford OX3 7DQ, UK
yifan.cai@eng.ox.ac.uk

Abstract. We present a novel multi-task convolutional neural network called Multi-task SonoEyeNet (*M-SEN*) that learns to generate clinically relevant visual attention maps using sonographer gaze tracking data on input ultrasound (US) video frames so as to assist standardized abdominal circumference (AC) plane detection. Our architecture consists of a generator and a discriminator, which are trained in an adversarial scheme. The generator learns sonographer attention on a given US video frame to predict the frame label (standardized AC plane/background). The discriminator further fine-tunes the predicted attention map by encouraging it to mimick the ground-truth sonographer attention map. The novel model expands the potential clinical usefulness of a previous model by eliminating the requirement of input gaze tracking data during inference without compromising its plane detection performance (Precision: 96.8, Recall: 96.2, F-1 score: 96.5).

Keywords: Multi-task learning · Generative Adversarial Network
Gaze tracking · Fetal ultrasound · Saliency prediction
Standardized plane detection

1 Introduction

The detection of fetal Intra-Uterine Growth Restriction using ultrasound-based diagnostic methods relies on the detection of standardized 2D ultrasound (US) planes for several biometric measurements, such as the abdominal circumference (AC), the head circumference (HC), the bi-parietal diameter (BPD), and the femur length (FL) [1]. Increasing demand for sonographers [2] has encouraged attempts to automate standardized plane detection using Random Forests [3] and, more recently, convolutional neural networks (CNNs) [4]. However, the large amount of labeled data required to train traditional classification CNNs is normally not available in medical image analysis, which requires more efficient

© Springer Nature Switzerland AG 2018
A. F. Frangi et al. (Eds.): MICCAI 2018, LNCS 11070, pp. 871–879, 2018.
https://doi.org/10.1007/978-3-030-00928-1_98

use of the limited time of clinical experts available for labeling data. In the clinical domain of interest here, sonographer eye movements are a strong prior for human interpretation of US video frames. Recently, the SonoEyeNet [5] architecture was proposed that used sonographer gaze tracking data in tandem with US video frames as two inputs to detect standard AC planes. However, SonoEyeNet requires sonographer gaze tracking data for inference, which significantly limits its usefulness in a clinical setting. In this paper, we address this limitation by proposing a novel framework that learns sonographer gaze tracking data to predict visual attention maps which assist in standardized plane detection without the requirement of gaze tracking data for inference.

Contributions. This paper proposes an end-to-end multi-task CNN called Multi-task SonoEyeNet (*M-SEN*) with a primary task to classify abdominal fetal ultrasound video frames into standard AC planes or background, and an auxiliary task to predict sonographer visual attention on those frames to assist the primary task. This novel architecture (I) substantially expands the potential usefulness of SonoEyeNet [5] in a clinical setting as a biometry assistance tool by removing the requirement of input gaze tracking data for inference without compromising frame classification performance; (II) adopts a novel adversarial regulariser to improve the quality of the generated attention map, which subsequently improves frame classification results; (III) demonstrates that the novel gaze tracking data collected during clinical experts' labeling time can also be learnt to improve model performance on a moderately-sized dataset, which makes the approach attractive for modeling other medical imaging problems.

Related Work. Two themes related to this work are saliency prediction and US image classification. Many attempts have been made to model human visual attention: from models built purely from hand-crafted features [6] to the state-of-the-art that learns image features using deep neural networks [7]. Generative Adversarial Networks (GAN) were recently used to model human attention on natural images [8]. For US image classification using images alone, Yaqub *et al.* [3] automated standardized plane detection using Random Forests; Baumgartner *et al.* used transfer learning and a FCN to detect 12 standard planes [4]. The first attempt to use sonographer gaze tracking data to assist standard AC plane detection was [9], which mimicked sonographer's visual behavior using a pictorial structures model inspired by observing human eye movement patterns. Recently, SonoEyeNet [5] was the first to implement gaze tracking data assisted standardized plane detection within a deep learning framework.

2   Methods

M-SEN **Architecture.** The *M-SEN* architecture consists of two CNN modules: the generator (G) and the discriminator (D). It is summarized in Fig. 1. **Generator Architecture.** G is a multi-task module that can be trained independently without D to generate both a predicted visual attention map $\hat{A}$ and a classification score vector of the input frame $\hat{y}$: $(\hat{A}, \hat{y}) = G(I; \theta_G)$, where I represents the US video frame and θ_G represents weights of the generator network. First, image features are extracted using the first three convolutional blocks of a pre-trained SonoNet [4]. All layers use 3×3 convolutional kernels and the number of kernels used can be seen in Fig. 1. Feature maps are down-sampled by a factor of 2 after each block using max pooling. The network separates into two branches after the third convolutional block: one branch for the auxiliary task of saliency prediction so as to mimic sonographer visual attention on US video frames; the other for frame classification. Feature maps ϕ_{c3} are first spatially down-sampled by 4 and then passed through 3 convolutional layers with 3×3 kernels in each branch. This produces ϕ_{c4S} and ϕ_{c4C} for saliency prediction and classification respectively. Convolution with 1×1 kernels is performed on ϕ_{c4S} to generate $\hat{A}$. The attention map $\hat{A}$ is then fused with ϕ_{c4C} through element-wise multiplication. The resultant feature maps are passed through another convolutional block, and then through two adaptation layers [4] which used 256 and two 1×1 kernels respectively. Global average pooling on the two resultant feature maps is performed before softmax so as to predict class scores for the standard AC plane and background. Classification loss L_C is defined between the predicted class scores and actual label, and saliency loss L_S between the predicted and the actual sonographer visual attention maps.

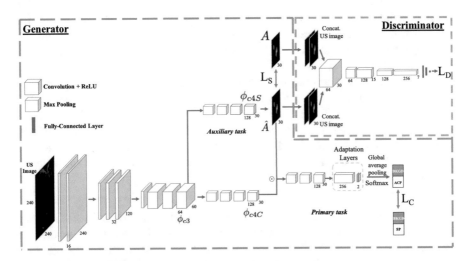

Fig. 1. Architecture of the multi-task SonoEyeNet (*M-SEN*). It has two modules: the generator (in Green-dashed polygon) and the discriminator (Orange-dashed box). The generator has two tasks: a primary task to classify frames (bottom) and an auxiliary task to predict visual attention map ($\hat{A}$). The discriminator differentiates between real (A) and predicted ($\hat{A}$) attention maps. The dotted circle $\odot$ indicates element-wise multiplication. L_S, L_C and L_D represent the losses of saliency prediction, frame classification, and the discriminator respectively.

Discriminator Architecture. The discriminator module is a CNN with three convolutional layers with 64, 128 and 256 3 × 3 kernels respectively, each with max pooling and leaky rectified linear unit (leaky ReLU) activation, followed by three fully-connected (FC) layers. Hyperbolic tangent (tanh) activation was used for the first two FC layers and sigmoid activation for the last FC layer. As sonographer attention is conditional on the US video frame, I is concatenated to A or $\hat{A}$ as inputs into D.

Loss Functions. The discriminator loss L_D and the generator loss L_G for each mini-batch with m samples are defined [10] as:

$$L_D = -\frac{1}{m} \sum_{i=1}^{m} \log(D(I_i, A_i; \theta_D)) + \log(1 - D(I_i, \hat{A}_i; \theta_D)) \tag{1}$$

$$L_G = \lambda_1 L_S + \lambda_2 L_C - \frac{\lambda_3}{m} \sum_{i=1}^{m} \log(D(I_i, \hat{A}_i; \theta_D)) \tag{2}$$

where $D(I, A; \theta_D)$ is the probability that the discriminator successfully recognizes the real attention map, while $D(I, \hat{A}; \theta_D)$ is the probability that the discriminator is fooled. θ_D represents the weights of D. The generator loss is designed to include both classification and saliency losses L_C and L_S as well as an adversarial regulariser by using the discriminator loss on $\hat{A}$; this regulariser was not used during generator pre-training. Hyper-parameters λ_1, λ_2, and λ_3 determine the relative contributions of the three losses. The saliency loss L_S is defined as the pixel-level content loss between $\hat{A}$ and A, which is used to train the generator of the attention maps. Two loss functions were experimented with in the models shown in Table 1: *M-SEN MSE* uses the mean squared error (MSE) loss, a base-line loss as it has been used in many visual saliency prediction works [11]; *M-SEN BCE* uses binary cross-entropy (BCE) loss, which is mathematically equivalent to Kullback-Leibler divergence, arguably the best metric to measure saliency prediction performance [12]. For the classification task, cross-entropy loss was used as L_C, the same as in [5].

Training Details. The generator was independently pre-trained for 30 epochs before adding the discriminator as the adversarial regulariser. The network was initialized using the first three convolutional blocks of SonoNet [4]; all other layers were initialized using a zero-mean Gaussian distribution with standard deviation 0.01. Batch normalization and dropout (rate = 0.2) were used for each convolutional layer before the adaptation layers. The weight λ_1 was dynamically changed from 2 to 1 over epochs so as to allow the generator to focus on learning attention maps first and then frame classification. The weight λ_2 was set to 1, as classification was the primary task of the network. After 30 epochs, the network was further fine-tuned for 2000 steps using an adversarial training scheme by training the discriminator and the generator once per step in an alternating manner. When training the discriminator, one-sided label smoothing [13] was used; when training the generator, the weights of discriminator were not updated. The network was trained using adaptive moment estimation (Adam) with an initial learning rate 2×10^{-4}. Batch size was set to 64. Five-fold cross-validation was used.

US Dataset and Preprocessing. The dataset was acquired following a free-hand US sweep protocol by moving the probe from the bottom to the top of pregnant women's abdomens. The dataset consists of 1616 frames from 33 fetal abdominal US video clips, each belonging to a unique patient. Each frame was assigned a class either the standard AC plane (ACP) or background (BG). Data augmentation by horizontal flipping and rotation was performed; equal number of ACP and BG frames were sampled for each batch during training. All frames were cropped at the positions of the abdominal wall and resized to 240×240 pixels. The dataset was separated video-wise into training and testing sets: frames from 25 videos clip (80% of all clips) were used for training, and those from remaining clips for testing.

Eye Movement Acquisition and Filtering. Gaze tracking data (x-y coordinates and time stamps) were acquired and filtered following the protocol in [5]. An eye tracker (The EyeTribe) recorded sonographer gaze tracking data at 30 Hz when they identified standard ACPs in each US video clips. A temporal moving average filter of window size 3 (100 ms) was applied to remove high frequency noise caused by eye tremor. Angular velocity threshold of $30°/s$ [14] was applied to separate fixations from saccades. Fixations $0.5°$ visual angle apart were merged, and those shorter than 80 ms in durations were discarded. A binary map of fixation points (1) and saccades or background (0) of 240×240 pixels was thus created. Since the human field of view typically extends to $1.5°$ visual angle [15] around a fixation point, the binary map was convolved with a 2-D Gaussian kernel with $\sigma = 30$ pixels, given an observer-to-screen distance of 0.5 m and screen dimensions of 20.7 cm $\times$ 33.2 cm. Attention maps corresponding to each frame, as detailed in the next section, were processed the same way by cropping, rotation and flipping.

3 Results and Discussion

Frame Classification Performance. Classification results of all models are presented in Table 1. Two observations can be made. First, all *M-SEN* models that use learned saliency maps to assist frame detection outperform the *SonoNet* models [4], which are supervised only by image-level labels. The classification precision of 79.3% for the *SonoNet-32* model was increased to 96.8% ($p < 0.05$) in *M-SEN BCE + GAN*, which uses BCE as saliency loss and is further fine-tuned using adversarial regulariser. Recall increased from 82.1% to 96.2% ($p < 0.05$). Second, models that adopted adversarial regularizers achieve better results: performances of both BCE and MSE models are improved by training with an adversarial discriminator. For example, introducing adversarial regularizer to *M-SEN MSE* increased its precision from 92.4% to 94.8% ($p < 0.05$), recall from 75.6% to 91.9% ($p < 0.05$), and F-1 score from 83.2% to 93.3% ($p < 0.05$). The best performing *M-SEN BCE + GAN* model achieves performance competitive to that of *SonoEyeNet-Late FT* [5] ($p = 0.692$), which uses both the US frame and sonographer visual attention map for inference. *SS-cls Net* that attempts to classify US video frames solely on sonographer visual attention map achieved a performance similar to that of *SonoEyeNet-Late FT*.

Saliency Prediction Performance. Examples of predicted visual attention maps generated by variations of *M-SEN* models on the test set US video frames can be seen in Fig. 2. All independently trained *M-SEN* models generate visually good quality attention maps that capture the salient regions fixated by sonographers, e.g. edges of the stomach bubble. Interestingly, *M-SEN BCE* extends

Table 1. Comparative evaluation of classification performance. In column "Inputs", "I" and "A" refer to US images and attention maps, respectively. "SS-cls Net" refers to single-stream network trained only on attention maps to classify US video frames.

Models	Inputs	Precision	Recall	F1-score
M-SEN BCE + GAN	I	96.8	96.2	96.5
M-SEN BCE	I	96.7	90.5	93.5
M-SEN MSE + GAN	I	94.8	91.9	93.3
M-SEN MSE	I	92.4	75.6	83.2
SonoNet-32 [4]	I	79.3	82.1	80.7
SonoNet-16 [4]	I	73.6	74.1	73.8
SS-cls Net	A	71.5	76.4	73.9
SonoEyeNet-Late FT [5]	I and A	96.5	99.0	97.8

Table 2. Quantitative metrics of saliency prediction on the test set. "SS-att" indicates those single-stream models for saliency prediction without a classification branch. Saliency metrics include information gain (IG), pearson's cross-correlation (CC), normalized saliency scan path (NSS), similarity (SIM), and area under curve (AUC) [16].

Models	IG	CC	NSS	SIM	AUC
M-SEN BCE + GAN	**0.543**	0.693	**2.525**	0.512	0.775
M-SEN BCE	0.429	0.615	2.144	0.469	0.726
M-SEN MSE + GAN	0.307	0.634	2.327	0.309	0.616
M-SEN MSE	0.288	0.556	2.253	0.310	0.603
SS-att BCE	0.192	**0.708**	1.480	**0.570**	**0.801**
SS-att MSE	0.152	0.546	1.329	0.532	0.788

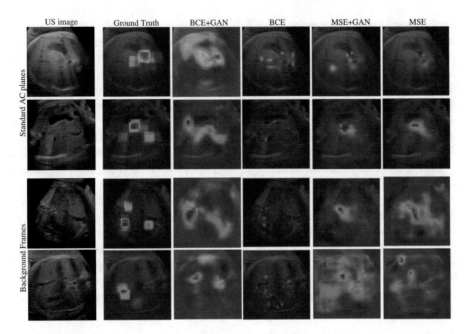

Fig. 2. Attention maps generated by different variations of the Generator. From left to right: US image, Gound-truth (Sonographer's actual attention map), *M-SEN BCE + GAN, M-SEN BCE, M-SEN MSE + GAN, M-SEN MSE.*

beyond the constraint of the ground-truth salient regions and explores other key anatomical structures, e.g. the umbilical veins, that the sonographers had not necessarily looked at during examination. In addition, we observe a similar trend previously observed in Table 1 that adding an adversarial regulariser improves model performance. *M-SEN BCE + GAN* is able to learn a more realistic visual attention map while retaining the ability to assign confidence to other key anatomical structures. Adding an adversarial discriminator regularises the predicted saliency map by reducing confidence in its false-positive points, as can be observed in Fig. 2; this can also be observed in Table 2, where saliency scores measured by all five metrics increase.

Discussion. The best performing *M-SEN BCE + GAN* model outperforms baseline models (*SS-att BCE* and *SS-att MSE*) in IG and NSS, but not in CC, SIM and AUC. It shows that tasks in the multi-task network influence each other, which strikes a balance between mimicking a ground truth attention map as close as possible and generating an attention map that includes clinically useful information on the US video frame.

In general, MSE models generate attention maps with more false-negatives (predicted as non-salient while fixated by sonographer), while BCE models generate more false-positives (predicted as salient but not fixated by sonographer). A change of loss function from *M-SEN MSE* to *M-SEN BCE* improves saliency performance measured by four out of five metrics. The performance improvement is consistent with the way gaze tracking data was collected. Our experiments allow sonographers to inspect each frame as long as they want, so each pixel can be modelled as an independent binary variable (fixated or not), which is best modelled using BCE loss; MSE, on the other hand, does not assume pixel independence and models the probability distribution of fixation on a frame in a brief glimpse. As confirmed by other literature [8], BCE loss performs better than MSE loss. The only exception is in NSS, where *M-SEN MSE* outperforms *M-SEN BCE*. This can be attributed to the fact that NSS is extremely sensitive to false positives, which *M-SEN BCE* exploits to cover non-fixated anatomical structures to benefit classification task.

Since sonographers view each frame for as long as they want, fixations on background frames, where there's no relevant anatomical structure, are non-specific; frames closer to the standardized planes exhibit a more consistent gaze pattern. Thus, attention maps provide a coarse distinction between backgrounds and frames that contain relevant anatomical structures. On the other hand, for frames close to the standardized plane, attention maps can look similar, and this is where image features (i.e. intensity values) become more important for our task.

4   Conclusion

This paper presents a novel and effective algorithm that models sonographer visual attention on US video frames to assist frame classification in an end-to-end deep learning framework. The multi-task network surpasses a previously reported model in classification performance [4]; it has great potential to be used in a clinical setting as it doesn't require gaze tracking data during inference. Our result suggests that it is better to model saliency prediction as a binary classification problem (using BCE loss), rather than a simple regression (using MSE loss). Adopting an adversarial regulariser proves to be effective in fine-tuning the generated attention maps, which further assists the classification task. The presented approach is general; the pipeline of gaze-tracking data collection, multi-task network design and adversarial regulation could be generalized to a wide range of other medical imaging challenges.

Acknowledgments. We acknowledge the ERC (ERC-ADG-2015 694581 for project PULSE) and the EPSRC (EP/GO36861/1, and EP/MO13774/1).

References

1. Hack, M., et al.: Outcomes of extremely low birth weight infants. Pediatrics **98**(5), 931–937 (1996)
2. Sarris, I., et al.: Intra- and inter-observer variability in fetal ultrasound measurements. Ultrasound Obstet. Gynecol. **39**(3), 266–273 (2012)

3. Yaqub, M., Kelly, B., Papageorghiou, A.T., Noble, J.A.: Guided random forests for identification of key fetal anatomy and image categorization in ultrasound scans. In: Navab, N., Hornegger, J., Wells, W.M., Frangi, A.F. (eds.) MICCAI 2015. LNCS, vol. 9351, pp. 687–694. Springer, Cham (2015). https://doi.org/10.1007/978-3-319-24574-4_82

4. Baumgartner, C.F., et al.: SonoNet: real-time detection and localisation of fetal standard scan planes in freehand ultrasound. IEEE Trans. Med. Imaging **36**(11), 2204–2215 (2017)

5. Cai, Y., et al.: SonoEyeNet: standardized fetal ultrasound plane detection informed by eye tracking. In: IEEE ISBI, pp. 1475–1478 (2018)

6. Koch, C., Ullman, S.: Shifts in selective visual attention: towards the underlying neural circuitry. In: Vaina, L.M. (ed.) Matters of Intelligence. Synthese Library (Studies in Epistemology, Logic, Methodology, and Philosophy of Science), vol. 188, pp. 115–141. Springer, Dordrecht (1987). https://doi.org/10.1007/978-94-009-3833-5_5

7. Kümmerer, M., et al.: DeepGaze II: Reading fixations from deep features trained on object recognition. arXiv preprint arXiv:1610.01563 (2016)

8. Pan, J., et al.: SalGAN: Visual Saliency Prediction with Generative Adversarial Networks. In: arXiv:1701.0181v2 [cs.CV] (2017)

9. Ahmed, M., et al.: An eye-tracking inspired method for standardised plane extraction from fetal abdominal ultrasound volumes. In: ISBI, pp. 1084–1087. IEEE (2016)

10. Goodfellow, I., et al.: Generative adversarial nets. In: NIPS, pp. 2672–2680 (2014)

11. Kruthiventi, S.S., et al.: Deepfix: a fully convolutional neural network for predicting human eye fixations. IEEE Trans. Image Process. **26**(9), 4446–4456 (2017)

12. Huang, X., et al.: SALICON: Reducing the semantic gap in saliency prediction by adapting deep neural networks. In: ICCV, pp. 262–270 (2015)

13. Radford, A., et al.: Unsupervised representation learning with deep convolutional generative adversarial networks. arXiv preprint arXiv:1511.06434 (2015)

14. Fuchs, A.F.: The saccadic system. In: The Control of Eye Movements, pp. 343–362 (1971)

15. Mathe, S., Sminchisescu, C.: Dynamic eye movement datasets and learnt saliency models for visual action recognition. In: Fitzgibbon, A., Lazebnik, S., Perona, P., Sato, Y., Schmid, C. (eds.) ECCV 2012. LNCS, pp. 842–856. Springer, Heidelberg (2012). https://doi.org/10.1007/978-3-642-33709-3_60

16. Bylinskii, Z., et al.: What do different evaluation metrics tell us about saliency models? arXiv preprint arXiv:1604.03605 (2016)

Efficient Laplace Approximation for Bayesian Registration Uncertainty Quantification

Jian Wang[1]([✉]), William M. Wells III[2,3], Polina Golland[2], and Miaomiao Zhang[1]

[1] Computer Science and Engineering Department,
Lehigh University, Bethlehem, PA, USA
`jiw917@lehigh.edu`
[2] Computer Science and Artificial Intelligence Laboratory, MIT,
Cambridge, MA, USA
[3] Brigham and Women's Hospital, Harvard Medical School, Boston, MA, USA

Abstract. This paper presents a novel approach to modeling the posterior distribution in image registration that is computationally efficient for large deformation diffeomorphic metric mapping (LDDMM). We develop a Laplace approximation of Bayesian registration models entirely in a bandlimited space that fully describes the properties of diffeomorphic transformations. In contrast to current methods, we compute the inverse Hessian at the mode of the posterior distribution of diffeomorphisms directly in the low dimensional frequency domain. This dramatically reduces the computational complexity of approximating posterior marginals in the high dimensional imaging space. Experimental results show that our method is significantly faster than the state-of-the-art diffeomorphic image registration uncertainty quantification algorithms, while producing comparable results. The efficiency of our method strengthens the feasibility in prospective clinical applications, e.g., real-time image-guided navigation for brain surgery.

1 Introduction

Diffeomorphic image registration has been widely studied in the fields of computational anatomy [3,8], atlas-based image segmentation [2], and anatomical shape analysis [9,16], as it provides smooth and invertible smooth spatial correspondences between images. The problem of 'inexact' registration is an ill-posed problem since the image data are usually contaminated by unknown noise. Providing efficient measures to quantify the registration uncertainty or error is critical to fair assessment on estimated transformations and subsequent improvement on the accuracy of predictive models. This also forms the basis for model-assisted decision making, for example, image-guided neurosurgery system, where surgeons need a better understanding of registration uncertainty to identify residual tumors [10].

© Springer Nature Switzerland AG 2018
A. F. Frangi et al. (Eds.): MICCAI 2018, LNCS 11070, pp. 880–888, 2018.
https://doi.org/10.1007/978-3-030-00928-1_99

Motivated by probabilistic modeling, several works have proposed to quantify registration uncertainty by having a probability distribution over the space of transformation parameters [4,11,13,14]. These approaches formulate Bayesian image registration as an image matching likelihood term regularized by a prior that encourages smooth deformations. The spread of the posterior of unknown registration parameters is then considered as a measure of the registration uncertainty. Existing methods including stochastic [13] and sampling [4,5,10] methods have been investigated to estimate the uncertainty, due to the fact that the posterior does not have a closed form and is computationally problematic to solve. A large computational effort is required to sample over high dimensional parameter spaces. To alleviate the excessive computational demands of sampling methods, a multivariate Gaussian approximation to the mode over the posterior was presented in [14]. In spite of the advantages of constructing Bayesian models, the extremely high computational cost and large memory footprint of the algorithms mentioned above have limited their usage in important applications that require computational efficiency.

In this paper, we are the first to introduce an efficient Bayesian image registration uncertainty quantification model that employs a low dimensional Fourier representation of the tangent space of diffeomorphisms [17]. We develop a novel Laplace approximation of the log posterior distribution that characterizes the deformation uncertainty at the optimal solution in a bandlimited space. More specifically, we assume a complex Gaussian distribution at the mode of the posterior, and approximate its covariance matrix to quantify the registration uncertainty. Our method dramatically reduces the computational complexity of approximating posterior marginals, which makes the uncertainty analysis for diffeomorphic image registration tractable in time. Another major benefit of our algorithm is that the covariance matrix can be easily computed and stored through the inverse Hessian of the log posterior defined by the low dimensional representations of transformation fields. We demonstrate the effectiveness of our model in both synthetic and real brain MRI data. A promising clinical application of our method is to provide key information on brain shifts; hence helping neurosurgeons to identify residual tumor tissue in real time, while lowering the risk of collateral tissue damage.

2   Background: LDDMM with Geodesic Shooting

Consider a source image S and a target image T as square-integrable functions defined on a torus domain $\Omega = \mathbb{R}^d / \mathbb{Z}^d$ ($S(x), T(x) : \Omega \to \mathbb{R}$). The problem of diffeomorphic image registration is to find the shortest path of diffeomorphic transformations $\psi_t \in \mathrm{Diff}(\Omega) : \Omega \to \Omega, t \in [0,1]$, such that the deformed image $S \circ \psi_1$ at time point $t = 1$ is similar to T. An explicit energy function of LDDMM with geodesic shooting [12,15] is formulated as an image matching term plus a regularization term that guarantees the smoothness of the transformation fields

$$E(v_0) = \frac{\lambda}{2} \mathrm{Dist}(S \circ \psi_1, T) + \frac{1}{2}(\mathcal{L}v_0, v_0), \quad s.t. \ \ geodesic \ constraint, \quad (1)$$

where λ is a positive weight parameter and $\text{Dist}(\cdot, \cdot)$ is a distance function that measures the similarity between images. The deformation ψ is defined as an integral flow of the time-varying Eulerian velocity field v_t that lies in the tangent space of diffeomorphisms $V = T\text{Diff}(\Omega)$. Here $\mathcal{L} : V \to V^*$ is a symmetric, positive-definite differential operator that maps a tangent vector $v \in V$ into the dual space $m \in V^*$, with its inverse $\mathcal{K} : V^* \to V$. The $(\cdot, \cdot)$ denotes a paring of a momentum vector $m \in V^*$ with a tangent vector $v \in V$.

The geodesic at the minimum of (1) is uniquely determined by integrating the geodesic constraint, a.k.a. Euler-Poincaré differential equation (EPDiff) [1, 7], which is computationally expensive in high dimensional image spaces. A recent work demonstrated that the entire optimization of LDDMM with geodesic shooting can be efficiently carried in a low dimensional bandlimited space with dramatic speed improvement [17,18]. We briefly review the basic concepts below.

Let $\widetilde{\text{Diff}}(\Omega)$ and $\tilde{V}$ denote the space of Fourier representations of diffeomorphisms and velocity fields respectively. Given time-dependent velocity field $\tilde{v}_t \in \tilde{V}$, the diffeomorphism $\tilde{\psi}_t \in \widetilde{\text{Diff}}(\Omega)$ in the finite-dimensional Fourier domain can be computed as

$$\tilde{\psi}_t = \tilde{e} + \tilde{u}_t, \quad \frac{d\tilde{u}_t}{dt} = -\tilde{v}_t - \tilde{\mathcal{D}}\tilde{u}_t * \tilde{v}_t, \qquad (2)$$

where $\tilde{e}$ is the frequency of an identity element, $\tilde{\mathcal{D}}\tilde{u}_t$ is a tensor product $\tilde{\mathcal{D}} \otimes \tilde{u}_t$, representing the Fourier frequencies of a Jacobian matrix $\tilde{\mathcal{D}}$ with central difference approximation, and $*$ is a circular convolution with zero padding to avoid aliasing[1].

The Fourier representation of the geodesic constraint (EPDiff) is defined as

$$\frac{\partial \tilde{v}_t}{\partial t} = \text{ad}_{\tilde{v}_t}^\dagger \tilde{v}_t = -\tilde{\mathcal{K}} \left[(\tilde{\mathcal{D}}\tilde{v}_t)^T \star \tilde{m}_t + \tilde{\nabla} \cdot (\tilde{m}_t \otimes \tilde{v}_t) \right], \qquad (3)$$

where $\star$ is the truncated matrix-vector field auto-correlation and $\text{ad}^\dagger$ is an adjoint operator to the negative Lie bracket of vector fields, $\text{ad}_{\tilde{v}}\tilde{w} = -[\tilde{v}, \tilde{w}] = \tilde{\mathcal{D}}\tilde{v} * \tilde{w} - \tilde{\mathcal{D}}\tilde{w} * \tilde{v}$. The operator $\tilde{\nabla} \cdot$ is the discrete divergence of a vector field. Here $\tilde{\mathcal{K}}$ is a smoothing operator with its inverse $\tilde{\mathcal{L}}$, which is the Fourier transform of a commonly used Laplacian operator $(-\alpha\Delta + I)^c$, with a positive weight parameter α and a smoothness parameter c. The Fourier coefficients of $\tilde{\mathcal{L}}$ is, i.e., $\tilde{\mathcal{L}}(\xi_1, \ldots, \xi_d) = \left(-2\alpha \sum_{j=1}^d (\cos(2\pi\xi_j) - 1) + 1 \right)^c$, where $(\xi_1, \ldots, \xi_d)$ is a d-dimensional frequency vector.

3   Low-Dimensional Bayesian Registration Uncertainty

We introduce a Bayesian model of diffeomorphic image registration represented in the bandlimited velocity space $\tilde{V}$, with registration uncertainty explicitly encoded as latent variables of the model.

---

[1] To prevent the domain from growing infinity, we truncate the output of the convolution in each dimension to a suitable finite set.

Assuming i.i.d. Gaussian noise on image intensities, we obtain the likelihood

$$p(T \mid S, \sigma^2) = \frac{1}{(\sqrt{2\pi\sigma^2})^M} \exp\left(-\frac{1}{2\sigma^2}\|S \circ \psi_1 - T\|_2^2\right), \qquad (4)$$

where σ^2 is the noise variance and M is the number of image voxels. The deformation ψ_1 corresponds to $\tilde{\psi}_1$ in Fourier space via the Fourier transform $\mathcal{F}(\psi_1) = \tilde{\psi}_1$, or its inverse $\psi_1 = \mathcal{F}^{-1}(\tilde{\psi}_1)$.

We define a prior on the initial velocity field $\tilde{v}_0$ to be a complex multivariate Gaussian distribution that ensures the smoothness of the geodesic path, i.e.,

$$p(\tilde{v}_0) = \frac{1}{(2\pi)^{\frac{Md}{2}}|\tilde{\mathcal{L}}^{-1}|^{\frac{1}{2}}} \exp\left(-\frac{1}{2}(\tilde{\mathcal{L}}\tilde{v}_0, \tilde{v}_0)\right), \qquad (5)$$

where $|\cdot|$ is matrix determinant.

Combining the likelihood (4) and prior (5) together, we obtain the negative log posterior distribution on the deformation parameter parameterized by $\tilde{v}_0$ as

$$-\ln p(\tilde{v}_0 \mid S, T, \sigma^2) = \frac{1}{2}(\tilde{\mathcal{L}}\tilde{v}_0, \tilde{v}_0) + \frac{\|S \circ \psi_1 - T\|_2^2}{2\sigma^2} + M \ln \sigma + \text{const.} \qquad (6)$$

In most probabilistic formulations of image-based registration, the likelihood function (4), as a function of the transformation parameters, is highly non-Gaussian because of the complex spatial structure of the images. This brings difficulties in the inference of such a non-Gaussian posterior.

3.1 Laplace Approximation

In this section, we introduce Laplace's method to approximate the covariance matrix at the mode of the posterior in a low dimensional bandlimited space. We first minimize the negative log posterior in (6) to the optimum, denoted as $\tilde{v}_0^{opt}$ (details are introduced in the following Sect. 4). We then assume a local complex Gaussian distribution at the optimal solution.

To simplify the notation, we use $f(\tilde{v}_0) \triangleq -\ln p(\tilde{v}_0 \mid S, T, \sigma^2)$. The function $f(\tilde{v}_0)$ is approximated to quadratic order by using second order Taylor series expansion at the optimal solution $\tilde{v}_0$ as

$$f(\tilde{v}_0) \approx f(\tilde{v}_0^{opt}) + \nabla f^T(\tilde{v}_0^{opt})(\tilde{v}_0 - \tilde{v}_0^{opt}) + \frac{1}{2}(\tilde{v}_0 - \tilde{v}_0^{opt})^T \mathcal{H} f(\tilde{v}_0^{opt})(\tilde{v}_0 - \tilde{v}_0^{opt}),$$

where ∇ denotes the first derivative and $\mathcal{H}$ is a second order Hessian. Since the first derivative of f vanishes at the optimal solution $\tilde{v}_0^{opt}$, we have

$$f(\tilde{v}_0) \approx f(\tilde{v}_0^{opt}) + \frac{1}{2}(\tilde{v}_0 - \tilde{v}_0^{opt})^T \mathcal{H} f(\tilde{v}_0^{opt})(\tilde{v}_0 - \tilde{v}_0^{opt}). \qquad (7)$$

The posterior is approximately a Gaussian $\mathcal{N}(\tilde{v}_0^{opt}, \mathcal{H}^{-1} f(\tilde{v}_0^{opt}))$. The inverse Hessian corresponds to the covariance matrix of the registration parameters.

4   Inference

Following optimal control theory [12], we first develop a gradient decent algorithm to minimize the negative log posterior distribution (6) w.r.t. the initial velocity $\tilde{v}_0$ and the image noise variance σ^2. Analogous to [14], we then derive the second variation of (6) to compute the Hessian-vector product via a linearized forward-backward sweep.

Parameter Estimation. We add Lagrange multipliers to constrain the diffeomorphism $\tilde{\psi}_t$ to be a geodesic path in the frequency domain. This is done by introducing time-dependent adjoint variables, $\hat{v}_t$ and $\hat{u}_t$, and writing the augmented energy[2],

$$E(\tilde{v}_0) = -\ln p(\tilde{v}_0 \mid S, T, \sigma^2) + \int_0^1 \langle \hat{v}_t, \dot{\tilde{v}}_t + \mathrm{ad}^\dagger_{\tilde{v}_t} \tilde{v}_t \rangle + \langle \hat{u}_t, \dot{u}_t + \tilde{v}_t + \tilde{\mathcal{D}}\tilde{u}_t * \tilde{v}_t \rangle \, dt, \quad (8)$$

where the last two terms correspond to Lagrange multipliers enforcing the geodesic constraint (3) and deformation transport Eq. (2) that is proved mathematically equivalent to the evolution equation [12].

The optimality conditions for the adjoints $\hat{v}_t, \hat{u}_t$ are given by the following time-dependent system of ordinary differential equations, termed the adjoint equations (equivalent to error-back propagation):

$$-\dot{\hat{v}}_t + \mathrm{ad}_{\tilde{v}_t}\hat{v}_t - \mathrm{ad}^\dagger_{\hat{v}_t}\tilde{v}_t + \hat{u}_t + (\tilde{\mathcal{D}}\tilde{u}_t)^T \star \hat{u}_t = 0, \quad -\dot{\hat{u}}_t - \mathrm{div}(\hat{u}_t \otimes \tilde{v}_t) = 0, \quad (9)$$

subject to initial conditions $\hat{v}_1 = 0$ and $\hat{u}_1 = -\frac{1}{\sigma^2}\mathcal{F}[\langle \nabla S(1), S(1) - T \rangle]$, where $S(1) = S \circ \psi_1$.

After integrating the geodesic equations (state equations) (3) forward in time to $t = 1$ and then backward integrating the adjoint Eqs. (9) in time to $t = 0$, the gradient of E w.r.t. $\tilde{v}_0$ is $\nabla_{\tilde{v}_0} E = \tilde{v}_0 - \hat{v}_0$.

Setting the gradient w.r.t. σ^2 to zero, we have a closed form update $\sigma^2 = \frac{1}{M}\|S(1) - T\|_2^2$.

Covariance Estimation. To estimate the full covariance matrix as an inverse Hessian, we develop a similar forward-backward approach to compute the Hessian-vector products that involves the second variation of the augmented energy function (8). In particular, after deriving the second variation in the direction $\delta\tilde{v}_0$ as $\frac{\partial^2}{\partial\epsilon^2}E(\tilde{v}_0 + \epsilon \cdot \delta\tilde{v}_0)|_{\epsilon=0} = \langle \delta\tilde{v}_0, \mathcal{H}E\,\delta\tilde{v}_0 \rangle$, we read off the Hessian-vector product $\mathcal{H}E\,\delta\tilde{v}_0$. Given an initial condition $\delta\tilde{v}_0$, we can compute the Hessian-vector product as $\mathcal{H}E\,\delta\tilde{v}_0 = \delta\tilde{v}_0 - \delta\hat{v}_0$, where $\delta\hat{v}_0$ is the adjoint variable of $\delta\tilde{v}_0$.

The second variation can be accomplished by forward-sweeping the linearized geodesic constraint around the optimal solution, followed by a backward sweep of the linearized adjoint system. Introducing time-dependent adjoint variables $\delta\hat{v}_t$ and $\delta\hat{u}_0$, the forward linearized geodesic equations are

$$\delta\dot{\tilde{v}}_t = -\mathrm{ad}^\dagger_{\delta\tilde{v}_t}\tilde{v}_t - \mathrm{ad}^\dagger_{\tilde{v}_t}\delta\tilde{v}_t, \qquad \delta\dot{\tilde{u}}_t = -\tilde{\mathcal{D}}_{\delta\tilde{u}_t} * \tilde{v}_t - \tilde{\mathcal{D}}_{\tilde{u}_t} * \delta\tilde{v}_t - \delta\tilde{v}_t.$$

---

[2] For notation simplification, we define the time derivative $\dot{\tilde{v}}_t \triangleq d\tilde{v}_t/dt$.

The linearized adjoint system for the backward integration is

$$\delta \dot{\hat{v}}_t = \text{sym}_{\tilde{v}_t}^\dagger \delta \hat{v}_t - \text{sym}_{\delta \hat{v}_t}^\dagger \hat{v}_t + \delta \hat{u}_t + (\tilde{\mathcal{D}} \tilde{u}_t)^T \star \delta \hat{u}_t + (\tilde{\mathcal{D}} \delta \tilde{u}_t)^T \star \hat{u}_t,$$

$$\delta \dot{\hat{u}}_t = -\text{div}(\delta \hat{u}_t \otimes \tilde{v}_t + \hat{u}_t \otimes \delta \tilde{v}_t),$$

subject to initial conditions $\delta \hat{u}_1 = -\frac{2}{\sigma^2} \mathcal{F}[\nabla S(1) \cdot \nabla S(1) + (S(1) - T) \cdot \nabla^2 S(1)]$ and $\delta \hat{v}_1 = 0$, with $\text{sym}_{\tilde{v}_t}^\dagger \delta \hat{v}_t = \text{ad}_{\delta \tilde{v}_t} \hat{v}_t - \text{ad}_{\hat{v}_t}^\dagger \delta \tilde{v}_t$.

5 Results

To evaluate our model, we first estimate the covariance matrix by using $\alpha = 3, c = 6$ for the operator $\tilde{L}$. We set each dimension of the initial velocity field $\tilde{v}_0$ as 16, which is similar to the settings used in the pairwise diffeomorphic image registration [17]. The number of time steps for Euler integration in geodesic shooting is set to 10. We then compare our results with an uncertainty quantification method computed in a full dimensional image space [14] on the same dataset. For a fair comparison, we keep all the parameters including regularization and time steps for numerical integration fixed across both algorithms.

Data. We test the proposed approach both on 2D synthetic data and 3D brain MRI scans from the OASIS dataset [6]. We generate a collection of binary image with resolution 100^2. The MRIs are of dimension 128^3, 1.25 mm^3 isotropic voxels, and underwent skull-stripping, downsampling, intensity normalization, bias field correction, and co-registration with affine transformations.

Experimental Results. Figure 1 visualizes the uncertainty information estimated from both our method and the baseline algorithm performed in high dimensional space on 2D data. We extract the local covariance matrix of each voxel and visualize it as an ellipse on the source image, with the color representing the matrix determinant. The smaller determinants are closer to the non-isotropic area (e.g., circle boundaries), which indicate more confident registration results.

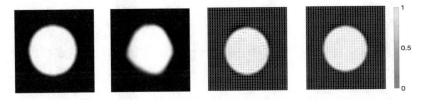

Fig. 1. Left to right: source image, target image, covariance matrix determinant estimated by baseline algorithm and our method.

Figure 2 visualizes an example of 3D brain registration uncertainty. Note that due to the difficulty of computing a full covariance matrix by inverse Hessian In a high dimensional image space, we need to use an approximated low-rank Hessian with a number of dominant eigenmodes [14]. We choose the first 3000 eigenmodes with non-zero values to represent the most effective uncertainty results estimated from the baseline method (see the left panel of Fig. 3). Both methods show that the high uncertainty (with less confidence) appears in isotropic areas (e.g., inside the ventricle), while the low uncertainty (with high confidence) appears around non-isotropic areas (e.g. ventricle boundaries). The subtle differences hardly affect the uncertainty visualization between these two methods. Figure 3 reports the comparison of time and memory consumption. Our algorithm offers significant improvements in computational efficiency.

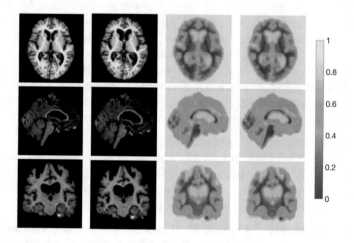

Fig. 2. Left to right: source image, target image, and uncertainty (visualized as the trace of covariacne) estimated by baseline algorithm and our method.

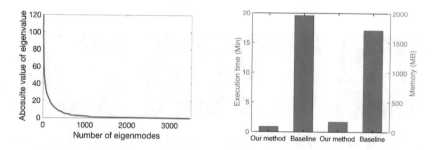

Fig. 3. Left: eigenvalues of the Hessian matrix estimated by baseline algorithm; Right: comparison of runtime and memory consumption.

6   Conclusion

We presented a low dimensional Bayesian model for registration uncertainty quantification in the space of diffeomorphic transformations. Our method dramatically reduces the computational cost of the registration posterior approximation effectively in a bandlimited velocity space. This work is the first step toward efficient probabilistic models of registration uncertainty quantification based on high dimensional diffeomorphisms. The next future work will be investigating sampling based methods to assess our developed model uncertainty. While in this paper we focus on the context of LDDMM, our method can be generalized to other transformation parameterizations such as stationary velocity fields.

Acknowledgments. This work is sponsored by NIH grants P41EB015898 and P41EB015902.

References

1. Arnol'd, V.I.: Sur la géométrie différentielle des groupes de Lie de dimension infinie et ses applications à l'hydrodynamique des fluides parfaits. Ann. Inst. Fourier **16**, 319–361 (1966)
2. Ashburner, J., Friston, K.J.: Unified segmentation. Neuroimage **26**(3), 839–851 (2005)
3. Joshi, S., Davis, B., Jomier, M., Gerig, G.: Unbiased diffeomorphic atlas construction for computational anatomy. NeuroImage **23**, S151–S160 (2004)
4. Kybic, J.: Bootstrap resampling for image registration uncertainty estimation without ground truth. IEEE Trans. Image Process. **19**(1), 64–73 (2010)
5. Le Folgoc, L., Delingette, H., Criminisi, A., Ayache, N.: Quantifying registration uncertainty with sparse bayesian modelling. IEEE Trans. Med. Imaging **36**(2), 607–617 (2017)
6. Marcus, D.S., et al.: Cross-sectional MRI data in young, middle aged, nondemented and demented older adults. Cogn. Neurosci. **19**, 1489–1507 (2007)
7. Miller, M.I., Trouvé, A., Younes, L.: Geodesic shooting for computational anatomy. J. Math. Imaging Vis. **24**(2), 209–228 (2006)
8. Miller, M.I.: Computational anatomy: shape, growth, and atrophy comparison via diffeomorphisms. NeuroImage **23**, S19–S33 (2004)
9. Qiu, A., Younes, L., Miller, M.I.: Principal component based diffeomorphic surface mapping. IEEE Trans. Med. Imaging **31**(2), 302–311 (2012)
10. Risholm, P., Pieper, S., Samset, E., Wells, W.M.: Summarizing and visualizing uncertainty in non-rigid registration. In: Jiang, T., Navab, N., Pluim, J.P.W., Viergever, M.A. (eds.) MICCAI 2010. LNCS, vol. 6362, pp. 554–561. Springer, Heidelberg (2010). https://doi.org/10.1007/978-3-642-15745-5_68
11. Risholm, P., Samset, E., Wells, W.: Bayesian estimation of deformation and elastic parameters in non-rigid registration. In: Fischer, B., Dawant, B.M., Lorenz, C. (eds.) WBIR 2010. LNCS, vol. 6204, pp. 104–115. Springer, Heidelberg (2010). https://doi.org/10.1007/978-3-642-14366-3_10
12. Vialard, F.X., Risser, L., Rueckert, D., Cotter, C.J.: Diffeomorphic 3d image registration via geodesic shooting using an efficient adjoint calculation. Int. J. Comput. Vis. **97**(2), 229–241 (2012)

13. Wassermann, D., Toews, M., Niethammer, M., Wells, W.: Probabilistic diffeo-morphic registration: representing uncertainty. In: Ourselin, S., Modat, M. (eds.) WBIR 2014. LNCS, vol. 8545, pp. 72–82. Springer, Cham (2014). https://doi.org/10.1007/978-3-319-08554-8_8

14. Yang, X., Niethammer, M.: Uncertainty quantification for LDDMM using a low-rank hessian approximation. In: Navab, N., Hornegger, J., Wells, W.M., Frangi, A.F. (eds.) MICCAI 2015. LNCS, vol. 9350, pp. 289–296. Springer, Cham (2015). https://doi.org/10.1007/978-3-319-24571-3_35

15. Younes, L., Arrate, F., Miller, M.I.: Evolutions equations in computational anatomy. NeuroImage **45**(1), S40–S50 (2009)

16. Zhang, M., Fletcher, P.T.: Bayesian principal geodesic analysis in diffeomorphic image registration. In: Golland, P., Hata, N., Barillot, C., Hornegger, J., Howe, R. (eds.) MICCAI 2014. LNCS, vol. 8675, pp. 121–128. Springer, Cham (2014). https://doi.org/10.1007/978-3-319-10443-0_16

17. Zhang, M., Fletcher, P.T.: Finite-dimensional lie algebras for fast diffeomorphic image registration. In: Ourselin, S., Alexander, D.C., Westin, C.-F., Cardoso, M.J. (eds.) IPMI 2015. LNCS, vol. 9123, pp. 249–260. Springer, Cham (2015). https://doi.org/10.1007/978-3-319-19992-4_19

18. Zhang, M., et al.: Frequency diffeomorphisms for efficient image registration. In: Niethammer, M., et al. (eds.) IPMI 2017. LNCS, vol. 10265, pp. 559–570. Springer, Cham (2017). https://doi.org/10.1007/978-3-319-59050-9_44

Correction to: Medical Image Computing and Computer Assisted Intervention – MICCAI 2018

Alejandro F. Frangi(ID), Julia A. Schnabel, Christos Davatzikos(ID),
Carlos Alberola-López(ID), and Gabor Fichtinger

Correction to:
A. F. Frangi et al. (Eds.): *Medical Image Computing*
and Computer Assisted Intervention – MICCAI 2018,
LNCS 11070, https://doi.org/10.1007/978-3-030-00928-1

In the originally published version of chapter 47, the Acknowledgements section was missing a grant number. This has been corrected.

In the originally published version of chapters 25 and 38, the Acknowledgements section was missing. This has been corrected and an Acknowledgements section has been added.

The updated version of these chapters can be found at
https://doi.org/10.1007/978-3-030-00928-1_25
https://doi.org/10.1007/978-3-030-00928-1_38
https://doi.org/10.1007/978-3-030-00928-1_47

© Springer Nature Switzerland AG 2020
A. F. Frangi et al. (Eds.): MICCAI 2018, LNCS 11070, p. C1, 2020.
https://doi.org/10.1007/978-3-030-00928-1_100

Author Index

Adam, Dan   126
Aertsen, Michael   313
Al Arif, S. M. Masudur Rahman   430
Alansary, Amir   277, 392, 563, 756
Alexander, Andrew L.   629
Alexander, Daniel C.   118
Ames, David   65
Antani, Sameer   457
Anton, Gisela   137
Araújo, Teresa   82
Arbel, Tal   655
Arens, Michael   792
Armitage, Paul A.   39
Arnold, Douglas L.   655
Ashburner, John   862
Aughwane, Rosalind   313
Awate, Suyash P.   338, 673
Ayton, Scott   65
Azuma, Takashi   73

Bagheri, Mohammadhadi   511
Bai, Wenjia   259, 268, 277
Balakrishnan, Guha   729
Balbastre, Yaël   862
Barratt, Dean C.   774
Batmanghelich, Kayhan N.   502
Baumgartner, Christian   476
Baust, Maximilian   827
Bekkers, Erik J.   440
Benveniste, Helene   844
Berger, Martin   137
Bieri, Oliver   198
Biffi, Carlo   383
Bisdas, Sotirios   691
Black, Michael J.   792
Blatti-Moreno, Marcela   682
Blondheim, David   126
Blumberg, Stefano B.   118
Bodensteiner, Christoph   792
Bonmati, Ester   774
Bopp, Johannes   137
Borovec, Jiří   783
Bourgeat, Pierrick   65

Boyle, Alec   347
Bradley, Andrew P.   546
Bragman, Felix   691
Brand, Lodewijk   555
Breininger, Katharina   145
Bria, Alessandro   82
Bronik, Kevin   862
Bronstein, Alex   126
Brudfors, Mikael   862
Brun, Emilie   401
Bush, Ashley I.   65
Bustin, Aurelien   250

Cai, Ruojin   620
Cai, Yifan   871
Calabresi, Peter A.   100
Campilho, Aurélio   82
Cao, Xiaohuan   739, 819
Carass, Aaron   100
Cardoso, M. Jorge   48, 691, 810
Carneiro, Gustavo   546
Castro, Daniel C.   206, 259
Cattin, Philippe C.   198
Cerrolaza, Juan J.   383, 392, 563
Chaitanya, Krishna   476
Chang, Weitang   215
Chatelain, Pierre   871
Chen, Jialei   537
Chen, Terrence   171
Chen, Yong   215
Chen, Yuhua   91
Chen, Zhaolin   338
Chen, Zhixiang   620
Cheng, Jie-Zhi   410
Chevalier, Jérôme-Alexis   638
Chevillard, Sylvie   401
Christlein, Vincent   232
Christodoulou, Anthony G.   91
Chung, Moo K.   629
Clerc, Maureen   836
Cohen, Joseph Paul   529
Conjeti, Sailesh   493, 664
Cook, Stuart   268

Cooper, Anthony   365
Costa, Pedro   82
Cruz, Gastao   250

Dalca, Adrian V.   729
David, Anna L.   313
Davidson, Richard J.   629
Davies, Mike E.   39
Dawant, Benoit M.   3
De Luca, Alberto   304
de Marvao, Antonio   268
De Simone, Raffaele   747
Deprest, Jan   313
Deriche, Rachid   836
Deslauriers-Gauthier, Samuel   836
Dewey, Blake E.   100
Diouf, Ibrahima   65
Doecke, James   65
Doel, Tom   313
Dong, Pei   819
Duan, Jinming   259
Duits, Remco   440

Eastell, Richard   720
Eaton-Rosen, Zach   21, 691
Ebner, Michael   313
El Basha, Mohammad D.   12
Elkin, Rena   844
Emberton, Mark   774
Engelhardt, Sandy   747
Eo, Taejoon   241
Eppenhof, Koen A. J.   440
Ermis, Ekin   682

Fan, Jingfan   739
Fang, Ruogu   12
Farzi, Mohsen   720
Fazlollahi, Amir   65
Felsner, Lina   137
Feng, Jianjiang   620
Ferreira, Pedro   295
Firmin, David   232, 295
Folgoc, Loic Le   277
Fotouhi, Javad   356
Frangi, Alejandro F.   720
Fripp, Jurgen   65
Fukuda, Norio   703
Full, Peter M.   747

Galdran, Adrian   82
Gallardo, Guillermo   836
Gao, Zhifan   374
Garbi, Rafeef   365
Garg, Saurabh   673
Gayraud, Nathalie T. H.   836
Ghavami, Nooshin   774
Gibson, Eli   774
Giger, Alina   198
Glocker, Ben   206, 277, 756
Göbl, Rüdiger   827
Golland, Polina   880
Gomez, Alberto   383
Gong, Mingming   502
Gorodezky, Margarita   295
Grall, Romain   401
Guerrero, Ricardo   277
Guo, Jun   590
Guo, Yimo   286
Guo, Yufan   449
Guo, Yuke   801
Gupta, Chandni   392, 563
Gur, Yaniv   449
Guttag, John   729

Haber, Eldad   844
Hadders-Algra, Mijna   792
Hajnal, Jo V.   259, 756
Hamarneh, Ghassan   57
Hatami, Nima   467
Hennersperger, Christoph   827
Hermosillo, Gerardo   286
Herrmann, Evelyn   682
Hervella, Álvaro S.   321
Hesse, Nikolas   792
Hill Goldsmith, H.   629
Hodgson, Antony J.   365
Hofmann, Ulrich G.   792
Honari, Sina   529
Hong, Sungmin   286
Hou, Benjamin   277, 392, 756
Hu, Lingjing   611
Hu, Yipeng   774
Huang, Heng   555
Huang, Jiashuang   647
Huang, Junzhou   590
Huang, Ruobing   572
Huang, Xiaolei   457

Huang, Yixing   145
Huo, Zhimin   154
Hutton, Brian F.   48
Hwang, Dosik   241

Izadi, Saeed   57
Jäger, H. Rolf   810
Jiang, Rui   485
Jiao, Jieqing   48
Jud, Christoph   198
Jun, Yohan   241
Jungo, Alain   682

Kaczmarz, Stephan   30
Kaeppler, Sebastian   137
Kainz, Bernhard   277, 383, 392, 563, 756
Kamnitsas, Konstantinos   277
Karani, Neerav   476
Karck, Matthias   747
Kaur, Prabhjot   109
Keegan, Jennifer   232, 295
Khalique, Zohya   295
Khanal, Bishesh   392, 563, 756
Kim, Dongchan   189
Kim, Hyo-Eun   520
Kim, Seungwook   520
Kim, Taeseong   241
King, Andrew P.   250
Kläser, Kerstin   48
Knapp, Karen   430
Knight, Caroline   392, 563
Knight, Caronline   383
Kokkinos, Iasonas   118
Konukoglu, Ender   476
Krauss, Andreas   171
Kuang, Tao   224
Kwon, Kinam   189
Kybic, Jan   783

Lafarge, Maxime W.   440
Lahoti, Geet   537
Lalush, David S.   329
Landman, Bennett A.   853
Lauritsch, Günter   145
Lee, Hedok   844
Lee, Jaehwan   520
Lee, Matthew C. H.   756
Leemans, Alexander   304
Lemaire, Hermine   401

Leow, Alex D.   629
Li, Debiao   91
Li, Hongying   163
Li, Shuo   374
Li, Wenqi   313
Li, Yangjunyi   12
Li, Yu   180
Li, Yuanwei   277, 383, 392, 563
Liao, Haofu   154
Liao, Peng   590
Liao, Shu   286
Limousin, Olivier   401
Lin, Hongxiang   73
Lin, Weili   215, 329
Linguraru, Marius George   347
Lisowska, Anna   599
Liu, Jiulong   224
Liu, Ling   145
Liu, Mingxia   647
Liu, Peng   12
Liu, Tianming   286
Liu, Zhi   374
Lu, Jiwen   620
Luck, Margaux   529
Ludwig, Veronika   137
Luo, Jianwen   374
Luo, Jiebo   154
Luo, Zhan   629
Lyu, Ilwoo   853

Ma, Gengyu   801
Ma, Kai   171
Madani, Ali   449
Madesta, Frederic   765
Maicas, Gabriel   546
Maier, Andreas   137, 145, 232, 356
Maier, Daniel   401
Makin, Stephen D.   39
Manhart, Michael   356
Markiewicz, Pawel J.   48
Marlow, Neil   21
Masters, Colin L.   65
Matthew, Jacqueline   383, 392, 563
McCloskey, Eugene   720
McDonagh, Steven   277, 756
McGill, Laura-Ann   295
Meier, Raphael   682
Melbourne, Andrew   21, 48, 313
Mendonça, Ana Maria   82
Menze, Bjoern H.   30, 39

Michailovich, Oleg   126
Michel, Thilo   137
Miolane, Nina   756
Mohiaddin, Raad   232
Moore, Caroline M.   774
Moradi, Mehdi   449
Moriarty, Kathleen P.   57
Moriconi, Stefano   810
Müller-Felber, Wolfgang   792
Mulpuri, Kishore   365

Nachev, Parashkev   810
Nadeem, Saad   844
Nair, Tanya   655
Namburete, Ana I. L.   572
Nascimento, Jacinto C.   546
Navab, Nassir   356, 421, 493, 664, 827
Navarro, Fernando   493
Nguyen, Damien   198
Noble, J. Alison   572, 774, 871
Noble, Jack H.   3
Novo, Jorge   321

O'Regan, Declan   268
Oh, Jiwon   100
Oksuz, Ilkay   250
Oktay, Ozan   232, 259, 268, 277
Ortega, Marcos   321
Otake, Yoshito   703
Ourselin, Sébastien   21, 48, 313, 691, 810
Owen, David   21

Pacheco, Carolina   581
Park, HyunWook   189
Paschali, Magdalini   493
Paserin, Olivia   365
Passerat-Palmbach, Jonathan   277
Patel, Premal A.   313
Pei, Yuru   801
Pelzer, Georg   137
Pennell, Dudley   295
Pham, Dzung L.   100
Pluim, Josien P. W.   440
Poczos, Barnabas   502
Porras, Antonio R.   347
Pozo, Jose M.   720
Precup, Doina   655
Preibisch, Christine   30

Preuhs, Alexander   356
Prieto, Claudia   250
Prince, Jerry L.   100
Pujades, Sergi   792
Puyol-Antón, Esther   250

Qian, Zhen   537
Qin, Chen   259

Rackerseder, Julia   827
Raeper, Rory   599
Raniga, Parnesh   65
Ratiney, Hélène   467
Ravanbakhsh, Siamak   502
Reich, Daniel S.   100
Reid, Ian   546
Rekik, Islem   599
Renaud, Diana   401
Reyes, Mauricio   682
Riess, Christian   137
Risacher, Shannon   555
Robini, Marc   163
Rodney Long, L.   457
Roehl, Malte   295
Rohrer, Jonathan   21
Romero, Javier   792
Rouco, José   321
Rowe, Christopher C.   65
Roy, Abhijit Guha   421, 664
Rueckert, Daniel   232, 250, 259, 268, 277,
            295, 383, 392, 563, 756
Ruijsink, Bram   250

Sabuncu, Mert R.   729
Salmon, Joseph   638
Salvado, Olivier   65
Sandkühler, Robin   198
Sao, Anil Kumar   109
Sati, Pascal   100
Sato, Yoshinobu   703
Saykin, Andrew   555
Schlemper, Jo   232, 259, 295
Schnabel, Julia A.   250
Schott, Jonathan M.   48
Schuh, Andreas   268
Sciurba, Frank   502
Scott, Andrew   295

Scott, Catherine J.   48
Sdika, Michaël   467
Sebastian Schroeder, A.   792
Sehnert, William J.   154
Seitzer, Maximilian   232
Senouf, Ortal   126
Sentker, Thilo   765
Sharma, Harshita   871
Shen, Dinggang   215, 329, 410, 647, 739,
    819
Shen, Li   555
Shi, Feng   91
Shin, Hyungseob   241
Sicard, Cécile   401
Sinclair, Matthew   268, 383, 392, 563
Singh, Vivek   171
Singla, Sumedha   502
Slabaugh, Greg   430
Steklova, Klara   844
St-Jean, Samuel   304
Stolidi, Adrien   401
Styner, Martin A.   853
Sudarshan, Viswanath P.   338
Sugano, Nobuhiko   703
Summers, Ronald M.   511
Sun, Xinwei   611
Suzuki, Hideaki   268
Syeda-Mahmood, Tanveer   449

Tacke, Uta   792
Takagi, Shu   73, 703
Takao, Masaki   703
Tamersoy, Birgi   171
Tang, Wei   163
Tannenbaum, Allen   844
Tanno, Ryutaro   118
Tarroni, Giacomo   268
Teixeira, Brian   171
Tetteh, Giles   30, 39
Thirion, Bertrand   638
Thoma, George R.   457
Thomas, David L.   21
Thrippleton, Michael J.   39
Tu, Liyun   347

Ulas, Cagdas   30, 39
Unberath, Mathias   356
Unlu, Mehmet Burcin   73

Vaillant, Ghislain   277
Vannan, Mani A.   537
Vedula, Sanketh   126
Vercauteren, Tom   313, 774
Veta, Mitko   440
Vidal, René   581
Vienne, Caroline   401
Viergever, Max A.   304
Villemagne, Victor L.   65

Wachinger, Christian   421, 664
Wang, Ben   537
Wang, Fusheng   180
Wang, Guotai   313
Wang, Hongzhi   711
Wang, Hua   555
Wang, Jian   880
Wang, Jianing   3
Wang, Kaiwen   485
Wang, Kan   537
Wang, Lei   329
Wang, Mingliang   647
Wang, Qian   215
Wang, Yan   329
Wang, Yizhou   611
Wang, Zih Huei   537
Wardlaw, Joanna M.   39
Wassermann, Demian   836
Weber, Thomas   137
Weinberger, Raphael   792
Wells, William M.   880
Werner, René   765
Wiest, Roland   682
Wilkinson, J. Mark   720
Wolf, Ivo   747
Wong, Tom   232
Woo, Jonghye   100
Wu, Sitong   374
Wu, Xi   329
Wu, Yifan   171
Würfl, Tobias   145, 232

Xiang, Lei   215, 410
Xie, Yibin   91
Xie, Yujia   537
Xu, Min   485
Xu, Tao   457
Xu, Tianmin   801
Xu, Wei   180
Xu, Zheng   590

Xue, Yuan   457
Xue, Zhiyun   457
Xue, Zhong   739

Yamamura, Naoto   703
Yan, Ke   511
Yan, Zhennan   286
Yang, Guang   232, 295
Yang, Liu   590
Yao, Yuan   611
Yap, Pew-Thian   410, 739, 819
Yu, Biting   329

Zha, Hongbin   801
Zhan, Yiqiang   215, 286
Zhang, Chuck   537
Zhang, Daoqiang   647
Zhang, Fandong   611
Zhang, Heye   374
Zhang, Miaomiao   880
Zhang, Pengyue   180
Zhang, Rui   711

Zhang, Xiaoqun   224
Zhang, Yongqin   410
Zhang, Yungeng   801
Zhao, Can   100
Zhao, Guannan   485
Zhao, Liang   286
Zhao, Yiyuan   3
Zhao, Yu   286
Zhou, Bo   485
Zhou, Jie   620
Zhou, Jiliu   329
Zhou, Luping   329
Zhou, Shaohua Kevin   154
Zhou, Xiang Sean   286
Zhou, Zhengwei   91
Zhou, Zhongwei   163
Zhu, Feiyun   590
Zhu, Yuemin   163
Zibulevsky, Michael   126
Zu, Chen   329
Zuluaga, Maria A.   810
Zurakhov, Grigoriy   126